BERGEY'S MANUAL® OF

Systematic Bacteriology

Volume 3

BERGEY'S MANUAL® OF
Systematic Bacteriology
Volume 3

JAMES T. STALEY
EDITOR, VOLUME 3

MARVIN P. BRYANT
ASSOCIATE EDITOR, VOLUME 3

NORBERT PFENNIG
ASSOCIATE EDITOR, VOLUME 3

JOHN G. HOLT
EDITOR-IN-CHIEF

WITH CONTRIBUTIONS FROM
90 COLLEAGUES

WILLIAMS & WILKINS
Baltimore • Hong Kong • London • Sydney

Editor: William R. Hensyl
Associate Editor: Harriet Felscher
Copy Editors: Bill Cady and Klementyna L. Bryte
Design: Norman W. Och
Illustration Planning: Lorraine Wrzosek
Production: Raymond E. Reter

Printed in the United States of America

Library of Congress Cataloging-in-Publication Data
(Revised for vol. 3)

Bergey's manual of systematic bacteriology.

Based on: Bergey's manual of determinative bacteriology.
Vol. 2: Peter H. A. Sneath, editor; v. 3, James T. Staley, editor.
Includes bibliographies and indexes.
1. Bacteriology—Classification—Collected works. I. Bergey, D. H. (David Hendricks), 1860-1937. II. Krieg, Noel R. III. Holt, John G. IV. Title: Bergey's manual of determinative bacteriology. [DNLM: 1. Bacteriology—Terminology. 2. Bacteria—Classification. QW 4 B832m]
QR81.B46 1984   589.9′0012   82-21760
ISBN 0-683-04108-8 (v. 1)
ISBN 0-683-07893-3 (v. 2)
ISBN 0-683-07908-5 (v. 3)

89 90 91 92 93
10 9 8 7 6 5 4 3 2 1

Contributors

H.-D. Babenzien
Akademie der Wissenschaften der DDR, Zentralinstitut für Mikrobiologie und Experimentelle Therapie, Abteilung Limnologie, DDR-1431 Neuglobsow, German Democratic Republic

D. A. Bazylinski
Graduate Department of Biochemistry, Brandeis University, Waltham, Massachusetts 02254 U.S.A.

N. A. Blakemore
Department of Microbiology, Spaulding Hall, University of New Hampshire, Durham, New Hampshire 03824 U.S.A.

R. P. Blakemore
Department of Microbiology, Spaulding Hall, University of New Hampshire, Durham, New Hampshire 03824 U.S.A.

Eberhard Bock
Mikrobiologische Abteilung, Institut für Allgemeine Botanik, Universität Hamburg, Jungiusstr. 6-8, D-2000 Hamburg 36, Federal Republic of Germany

David R. Boone
Environmental Science and Engineering, Oregon Graduate Center, 19600 von Neumann Drive, Beaverton, Oregon 97006-1999 U.S.A.

Thomas D. Brock
Department of Bacteriology, University of Wisconsin, Madison, Wisconsin 53706 U.S.A.

Ellis R. Brockman
Department of Biology, Central Michigan University, Mount Pleasant, Michigan 48859 U.S.A.

Marvin P. Bryant
Department of Dairy Science, University of Illinois, Urbana, Illinois 61801 U.S.A.

T. Burger-Wiersma
University of Amsterdam, 1018 WS Amsterdam, The Netherlands

Douglas E. Caldwell
Department of Applied Microbiology and Food Science, University of Saskatchewan, Saskatoon, Saskatchewan S7N 0W0, Canada

L. Earl Casida, Jr.
Pennsylvania State University, S101 Frear Building, University Park, Pennsylvania 16802 U.S.A.

Richard W. Castenholz
Department of Biology, University of Oregon, Eugene, Oregon 97403 U.S.A.

Penelope Christensen
No. 11 Quesnell Road, Edmonton, Alberta T5R 5N1, Canada

N. V. Doronina
Institute of Biochemistry and Physiology of Microorganisms, U.S.S.R. Academy of Sciences, Pushchino on the Oka, Moscow Region, U.S.S.R.

G. A. Dubinina
Institute of Microbiology, Academy of Sciences of the U.S.S.R., Profsojuznaya 7, Moscow B-133, U.S.S.R.

K. B. Easterbrook
Department of Microbiology, Dalhousie University, Halifax, Nova Scotia B3H 4H7, Canada

Jeffrey L. Favinger
Jordan Hall 436, Department of Biology, Indiana University, Bloomington, Indiana 47405 U.S.A.

James G. Ferry
Anaerobe Laboratory, Virginia Polytechnic Institute and State University, Blacksburg, Virginia 24060 U.S.A.

G. Fiala
Universität Regensburg, Institut für Biochemie, Universitätsstr. 31, 8400 Regensburg, Federal Republic of Germany

Peter D. Franzmann
Department of Agricultural Science, University of Tasmania, Hobart, Tasmania, 7001, Australia

John A. Fuerst
Department of Microbiology, University of Queensland, St. Lucia, 4067, Brisbane, Australia

Ranier Gebers
Institut für Allgemeine Mikrobiologie der Universität Kiel, D-2300 Kiel, Federal Republic of Germany

Howard Gest
Jordan Hall 436, Department of Biology, Indiana University, Bloomington, Indiana 47405 U.S.A.

Norman E. Gibbons (Deceased)
Ottawa, Ontario, Canada

Jane Gibson
Biochemistry Division of Biology, Wing Hall, Cornell University, Ithaca, New York 14853 U.S.A.

Steven J. Giovannoni
Department of Biology, University of Oregon, Eugene, Oregon 97403 U.S.A.

Vladimir M. Gorlenko
Institute of Microbiology, Academy of Sciences of the U.S.S.R., Profsojuznaya 7, Moscow B-133, U.S.S.R.

Jennifer Gossling
Apartment 2D, 7553 Buckingham Drive, Clayton, Missouri 63105 U.S.A.

William D. Grant
Department of Microbiology, The Medical School, University of Leicester, Leicester LE1 7RH, England

D. J. Griffiths
Department of Botany, James Cook University of North Queensland, Townsville, 4811, Queensland, Australia

Hans H. Hanert
Institut für Mikrobiologie der Technische Universität, Mendelssohnstrasse 4, 3300 Braunschweig, Federal Republic of Germany

Heinz Harms
Mikrobiologische Abteilung, Institut für Allgemeine Botanik, Universität Hamburg, Jungiusstr. 6-8, D-2000 Hamburg 36, Federal Republic of Germany

Arthur P. Harrison, Jr.
Division of Biological Sciences, Tucker Hall, University of Missouri, Columbia, Missouri 65201 U.S.A.

Peter Hirsch
Institut für Allgemeine Mikrobiologie der Universität Kiel, 23 Kiel, Federal Republic of Germany

John G. Holt
Department of Microbiology, 205 Sciences I, Iowa State University, Ames, Iowa 50011 U.S.A.

Stanley C. Holt
Department of Periodontics, Dental School, The University of Texas, San Antonio, Texas 78284 U.S.A.

Alan B. Hooper
Department of Genetics and Cell Biology, University of Minnesota, St. Paul, Minnesota 55108 U.S.A.

Johannes F. Imhoff
Institut für Mikrobiologie, Rheinische Friedrich-Wilhelms Universität, 5300 Bonn 1, Federal Republic of Germany

John L. Johnson
Department of Anaerobic Microbiology, Virginia Polytechnic Institute and State University, Blacksburg, Virginia 24061 U.S.A.

Dorothy Jones
Department of Microbiology, The Medical School, University of Leicester, Leicester LE1 7RH, England

T. Kawasumi
National Food Research Institute, Ministry of Agriculture, Forestry and Fisheries, 2-1-2 Kannondai, Yatabe-Mache, Tsukuba-Gun, Ibaraki-Ken 305, Japan

D. P. Kelly
Department of Environmental Sciences, University of Warwick, Coventry CV4 7AL, England

S. A. Kinder
Department of Periodontics, Dental School, The University of Texas, San Antonio, Texas 78284 U.S.A.

Helmut König
Abteilung für Angewandte Mikrobiologie und Mykologie, Universität Ulm, Oberer Eselsberg M23, 8400 Regensburg, Federal Republic of Germany

Hans-Peter Koops
Mikrobiologische Abteilung, Institut für Allgemeine Botanik, Universität Hamburg, Jungiusstr. 6-8, D-2000 Hamburg 36, Federal Republic of Germany

Noel R. Krieg
Department of Biology, Virginia Polytechnic Institute and State University, Blacksburg, Virginia 24061 U.S.A.

J. Gijs Kuenen
Laboratory of Microbiology, Delft University of Technology, Julianalaan 67a, Delft 8, The Netherlands

Thomas A. Langworthy
Department of Microbiology, School of Medicine, University of South Dakota, Vermillion, South Dakota 57069 U.S.A.

Jan W. M. la Riviére
International Institute for Hydraulic and Environmental Engineering, Oude Delft 95, Delft, The Netherlands

John M. Larkin
Department of Microbiology, Louisiana State University, Baton Rouge, Louisiana 70803 U.S.A.

Helge Larsen
Department of Biochemistry, University of Trondheim, 7034 Trondheim – NTH, Norway

Edward R. Leadbetter
Department of Molecular and Cell Biology, The University of Connecticut, U-131, 354 Mansfield Road, Room 321, Storrs, Connecticut 06268 U.S.A.

Ralph A. Lewin
Scripps Institution of Oceanography, University of California San Diego, La Jolla, California 92093 U.S.A.

Robert A. Mah
Division of Environmental and Nutritional Science, School of Public Health, University of California, Los Angeles, California 90024 U.S.A.

Siegfried Maier
Department of Zoology and Microbiology, Ohio University, Athens, Ohio 45701 U.S.A.

Howard D. McCurdy
4758 Wyandotte Street East, Windsor, Ontario N8Y 1H7, Canada

Terry L. Miller
Wadsworth Center for Laboratories and Research, New York State Department of Health, Box 509, Albany, New York 12201-0509 U.S.A.

Thomas T. Moench
Boeing Computer Services, P.O. Box 24346, Seattle, Washington 98124 U.S.A.

Richard L. Moore
Department of Microbiology, Faculty of Medicine, University of Calgary, Calgary, Alberta T2N 4N1, Canada

E. G. Mulder
Professor Emeritus, Department of Microbiology, Agricultural University, Hesselink van Suchtelenweg 4, Wageningen, The Netherlands

Luuc R. Mur
University of Amsterdam, 1018 WS Amsterdam, The Netherlands

R. G. E. Murray
Department of Bacteriology and Immunology, University of Western Ontario, London, Ontario N6A 5C1, Canada

Malcomb J. B. Paynter
Department of Microbiology, Clemson University, Long Hall, Clemson, South Carolina 29631 U.S.A.

Norbert Pfennig
Fakultät für Biologie, Universität Konstanz, Postfach 5560, D-7750 Konstanz 1, Konstanz, Federal Republic of Germany

Beverly K. Pierson
Biology Department, University of Puget Sound, Tacoma, Washington 98416 U.S.A.

Jeanne S. Poindexter
Science Division, Long Island University, University Plaza, Brooklyn, New York 11201-5372 U.S.A.

Hans Reichenbach
Ges. Biotechn. Forsch., Mascheroder Weg 1, D-3300 Braunschweig, Federal Republic of Germany

Rosmarie Rippka
Institut Pasteur, 75724 Paris Cedex 15, France

L. A. Robertson
Laboratory of Microbiology, Delft University of Technology, Julianalaan 67A, Delft 8, The Netherlands

James A. Romesser
Central Research-Development Department, Experimental Station, E. I. DuPont, Wilmington, Delaware 19898 U.S.A.

Jean M. Schmidt
Department of Botany and Microbiology, Arizona State University, Tempe, Arizona 85281 U.S.A.

Karin Schmidt
Institut für Mikrobiologie, Universität Göttingen, Göttingen, Federal Republic of Germany

A. Segerer
Universität Regensburg, Institut für Biochemie, Universitätsstr. 31, 8400 Regensburg, Federal Republic of Germany

V. B. D. Skerman
Department of Microbiology, University of Queensland, St. Lucia, 4067, Brisbane, Australia

Paul F. Smith
Department of Microbiology, School of Medicine, University of South Dakota, Vermillion, South Dakota 57069 U.S.A.

Peter H. A. Sneath
Department of Microbiology, The Medical School, University of Leicester, Leicester LE1 7RH, England

Kevin R. Sowers
Department of Microbiology, Life Sciences 5304, University of California Los Angeles, 405 Hilgard Avenue, Los Angeles, California 90024 U.S.A.

James T. Staley
Department of Microbiology, University of Washington, Seattle, Washington 98195 U.S.A.

Mortimer P. Starr
Department of Microbiology, University of California, Davis, California 95616 U.S.A. Permanent mailing address: 751 Elmwood Drive, Davis, California 95616 U.S.A.

Karl O. Stetter
Universität Regensburg, Institut für Biochemie, Universitätsstr. 31, 8400 Regensburg, Federal Republic of Germany

William R. Strohl
Department of Microbiology, The Ohio State University, 484 West 12th Avenue, Columbus, Ohio 43210 U.S.A.

Luong-Van Thinh
Department of Botany, James Cook University of North Queensland, Townsville, 4811, Queensland, Australia

Yuri A. Trotsenko
Institute of Biochemistry and Physiology of Microorganisms, U.S.S.R. Academy of Sciences, Pushchino on the Oka, Moscow Region, U.S.S.R.

Hans G. Trüper
Institut für Mikrobiologie, Rheinische Friedrich-Wilhelms Universität, 5300 Bonn 1, Federal Republic of Germany

Olli H. Tuovinen
Department of Microbiology, The Ohio State University, Columbus, Ohio 43210 U.S.A.

L. V. Vasilyeva
Institute of Microbiology, Academy of Sciences of the U.S.S.R., Profsojuznaya 7, Moscow B-133, U.S.S.R.

John B. Waterbury
Woods Hole Oceanographic Institute, Woods Hole, Massachusetts 02543 U.S.A.

Stanley W. Watson
Woods Hole Oceanographic Institute, Woods Hole, Massachusetts 02543 U.S.A.

R. M. Weiner
Department of Microbiology, University of Maryland, College Park, Maryland 20742 U.S.A.

David White
Department of Biology, Indiana University, Bloomington, Indiana 47401 U.S.A.

William B. Whitman
Department of Microbiology, University of Georgia, Athens, Georgia 30602 U.S.A.

Brian Whitton
Department of Botany, University of Durham, Durham, DH1 3LE, England

Friedrich Widdel
Mikrobiologie, FB Biologie, Philipps Universität, Lahnberge, D-3550 Marburg/Lahn, Federal Republic of Germany

G. A. Zavarzin
Institute of Microbiology, Academy of Sciences of the U.S.S.R., Profsojuznaya 7, Moscow B-133, U.S.S.R.

Alexander J. B. Zehnder
Department of Microbiology, Agricultural University, Hesselink von Suchletenweg 4, Wageningen, The Netherlands

Wolfram Zillig
Max Planck Institut für Biochemie, D-8033 Martinsried bei München, Federal Republic of Germany

Advisory Committee Members

The Board of Trustees is grateful to all who served on the Advisory Committees and assisted materially in the preparation of this edition of the *Manual*. Chairs of the committees are indicated by an asterisk.

Section 18. *Anoxygenic Phototrophic Bacteria:* E. N. Kondratieva, N. Pfennig,*
H. G. Trüper

Section 19. *Oxygenic Photosynthetic Bacteria:* R. W. Castenholz,* G. L. Gherna,
R. Lewin, R. Rippka, J. B. Waterbury, B. A. Whitton

Section 20. *Aerobic Chemolithotrophic Bacteria and Associated Organisms:* D. P. Kelly,
S. Watson, G. A. Zavarzin*

Section 21. *Budding and/or Appendaged Bacteria:* P. Hirsch, J. Schmidt,
J. S. Poindexter, J. T. Staley,* G. A. Zavarzin

Section 22. *Sheathed Bacteria:* J. G. Holt,* P. Hirsch, E. G. Mulder

Section 23. *Nonphotosynthetic, Nonfruiting Gliding Bacteria:* D. Kuhn, J. Larkin,*
H. Reichenbach

Section 24. *Fruiting Gliding Bacteria: The Myxobacteria:* E. R. Brockman, H. McCurdy*

Section 25. *Archaeobacteria:* M. P. Bryant,* D. Boone, H. Larsen, R. A. Mah,
K. O. Stetter, R. S. Wolfe

Preface to First Edition of *Bergey's Manual® of Systematic Bacteriology*, Volume 3

Many microbiologists advised the Trust that a new edition of the *Manual* was urgently needed. Of great concern to us was the steadily increasing time interval between editions; this interval reached a maximum of 17 years between the seventh and eighth editions. To be useful the *Manual* must reflect relatively recent information; a new edition is soon dated or obsolete in parts because of the nearly exponential rate at which new information accumulates. A new approach to publication was needed, and from this conviction came our plan to publish the *Manual* as a sequence of four subvolumes concerned with systematic bacteriology as it applies to taxonomy. The four subvolumes are divided roughly as follows: (a) the Gram-negatives of general, medical or industrial importance; (b) the Gram-positives other than actinomycetes; (c) the archaeobacteria, cyanobacteria and remaining Gram-negatives; and (d) the actinomycetes. The Trust believed that more attention and care could be given to preparation of the various descriptions within each subvolume, and also that each subvolume could be prepared, published, and revised as the area demanded, more rapidly than could be the case if the *Manual* were to remain as a single, comprehensive volume as in the past. Moreover, microbiologists would have the option of purchasing only that particular subvolume containing the organisms in which they were interested.

The Trust also believed that the scope of the *Manual* needed to be expanded to include more information of importance for systematic bacteriology and bring together information dealing with ecology, enrichment and isolation, descriptions of species and their determinative characters, maintenance and preservation, all focused on the illumination of bacterial taxonomy. To reflect this change in scope, the title of the *Manual* was changed and the primary publication becomes *Bergey's Manual® of Systematic Bacteriology*. This contains not only determinative material, such as diagnostic keys and tables useful for identification, but also all of the detailed descriptive information and taxonomic comments. Upon completion of each subvolume, the purely determinative information will be assembled for eventual incorporation into a much smaller publication which will continue the original name of the *Manual, Bergey's Manual® of Determinative Bacte-*

riology, which will be a similar but improved version of the present *Shorter Bergey's Manual®*. So, in the end there will be two publications, one systematic and one determinative in character.

An important task of the Trust was to decide which genera should be covered in the first and subsequent subvolumes. We were assisted in this decision by the recommendations of our Advisory Committees, composed of prominent taxonomic authorities to whom we are most grateful. Authors were chosen on the basis of constant surveillance of the literature of bacterial systematics and by recommendations from our Advisory Committees.

The activation of the 1976 Code had introduced some novel problems. We decided to include not only those genera that had been published in the Approved Lists of Bacterial Names in January 1980 or that had been subsequently validly published, but also certain genera whose names had no current standing in nomenclature. We also decided to include descriptions of certain organisms which had no formal taxonomic nomenclature, such as the endosymbionts of insects. Our goal was to omit no important group of cultivated bacteria and also to stimulate taxonomic research on "neglected" groups and on some groups of undoubted bacteria that have not yet been cultivated and subjected to conventional studies.

Some readers will note the consistent use of the stem -var instead of -type in words such as biovar, serovar and pathovar. This is in keeping with the recommendations of the Bacteriological Code and was done against the wishes of some of the authors.

We have deleted much of the synonymy of scientific names which was contained in past editions. The adoption of the new starting date of January 1, 1980 and publication of the Approved Lists of Bacterial Names has made mention of past synonymy obsolete. We have included synonyms of a name only if they have been published since the new starting date, or if they were also on the Approved Lists and, in rare cases, if the mention of an old name would help readers associate the organism with a clinical problem. If the reader is interested in tracing the history of a name we suggest he or she consult past editions of the *Manual* or the *Index Bergeyana* and its *Supplement*. In citations of names we have used the abbreviation *AL* to denote the inclusion of the name on the Approved Lists of Bacterial Names and *VP* to show the name has been validly published.

In the matter of citation of the *Manual* in the scientific literature, we again stress the fact that the *Manual* is a collection of authored chapters and the citation should refer to the author, the chapter title and its inclusive pages, not the Editors.

To all contributors, the sincere thanks of the Trust is due; the Editors are especially grateful for the good grace with which the authors accepted comments, criticisms and editing of their manuscripts. It is only because of the voluntary and dedicated efforts of these authors that the *Manual* can continue to serve the science of bacteriology on an international basis.

A number of institutions and individuals deserve special acknowledgment from the Trust for their help in bringing about the publication of this volume. We are grateful to the Department of Microbiology of the University of Washington for providing space, facilities and, above all, tolerance for the diverted time taken by the Edi-

tor during the preparation of the book. The Department of Microbiology at Iowa State University of Science and Technology continues to provide a welcome home for the main editorial offices and archives of the Trust, and we acknowledge their continued support.

A number of individuals deserve special mention and thanks for their help. Professor Emeritus Thomas O. MacAdoo of the Department of Foreign Languages and Literature at the Virginia Polytechnic Institute and State University has given invaluable advice on the etymology and correctness of scientific names. Those assisting the Editors in the Seattle office were Nancy B. Pellerin, John A. Fuerst, and Russell P. Herwig. Their excellent help is sincerely appreciated. In the Ames office, we were ably assisted by Cynthia Pease, who had the major responsibility for keying and sorting the list of references and index.

Comments on this edition of the *Manual* will be welcomed and should be addressed to the Bergey's Manual® Trust, c/o Williams & Wilkins, 428 E. Preston St., Baltimore, Maryland 21202 U.S.A.

Preface to First Edition of *Bergey's Manual®* *of Determinative Bacteriology*

The elaborate system of classification of the bacteria into families, tribes and genera by a Committee on Characterization and Classification of the Society of American Bacteriologists (1917, 1920) has made it very desirable to be able to place in the hands of students a more detailed key for the identification of species than any that is available at present. The valuable book on "Determinative Bacteriology" by Professor F. D. Chester, published in 1901, is now of very little assistance to the students, and all previous classifications are of still less value, especially as earlier systems of classification were based entirely on morphologic characters.

It is hoped that this manual will serve to stimulate efforts to perfect the classification of bacteria, especially by emphasizing the valuable features as well as the weaker points in the new system which the Committee of the Society of American Bacteriologists has promulgated. The Committee does not regard the classification of species offered here as in any sense final, but merely a progress report leading to more satisfactory classification in the future.

The Committee desires to express its appreciation and thanks to those members of the society who gave valuable aid in the compilation of material and the classification of certain species . . .

The assistance of all bacteriologists is earnestly solicited in the correction of possible errors in the text; in the collection of descriptions of all bacteria that may have been omitted from the text; in supplying more detailed descriptions of such organisms as are described incompletely; and in furnishing complete descriptions of new organisms that may be discovered, or in directing the attention of the Committee to publications of such newly described bacteria.

DAVID H. BERGEY, *Chairman*
FRANCIS C. HARRISON
ROBERT S. BREED
BERNARD W. HAMMER
FRANK M. HUNTOON
Committee on Manual

August, 1923.

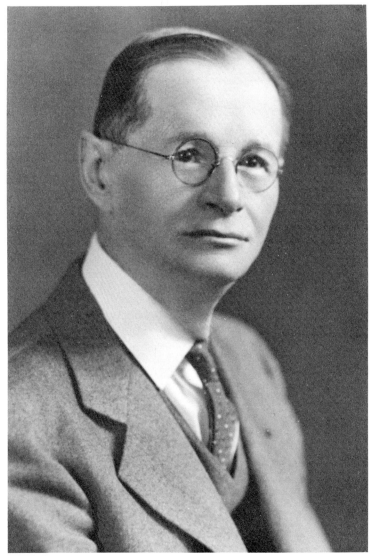

Archives of the ASM

DAVID HENDRICKS BERGEY
1860–1937
Bergey set up the Trust on January 2, 1936

History of the *Manual*

The first edition of *Bergey's Manual® of Determinative Bacteriology* was initiated by action of the Society of American Bacteriologists (now called the American Society for Microbiology) by appointment of an Editorial Board consisting of David H. Bergey, Chairman, Francis C. Harrison, Robert S. Breed, Bernard W. Hammer, and Frank M. Huntoon. This Board, under auspices of the Society of American Bacteriologists who, then as now, published the *Journal of Bacteriology* as a service to science, brought the first edition of the *Manual* into print in 1923. The Board, with some changes in membership and Dr. David Bergey as Chairman, published a second edition of the *Manual* in 1925 and a third edition in 1930.

In 1934, during preparation of the fourth edition, Dr. Bergey requested that the Society of American Bacteriologists make available the royalties paid to the Treasurer of the Society from the sale of the earlier editions to defray the expense of preparing the fourth edition for publication. The Society made such provision, but the use of the Society's fiscal machinery proved cumbersome, to both the Society and the Editorial Board. Subsequently, it was agreed by the Society and Dr. Bergey that the Society would transfer to Dr. Bergey all of its rights, title, and interest in the *Manual* and that Dr. Bergey would, in turn, create an educational trust to which all rights would be transferred.

Dr. Bergey was then the nominal owner of the *Manual*, and he executed a Trust Indenture on January 2, 1936, designating David H. Bergey, Robert S. Breed, and E. G. D. Murray as the initial trustees, and transferring to the Trustees and their successors the ownership of the *Manual*, its copyrights, and the right to receive the income arising from its publication. The Trust is a nonprofit organization, and its income is used solely for the purpose of preparing, editing, and publishing revisions and successive editions of the *Manual* and any supplementary publications, as well as providing for any research that may be necessary or desirable in such activities.

Since the creation of the Trust, the Trustees have published, successively, the fourth, fifth, sixth, seventh, and eighth editions of the *Manual* (dated 1934, 1939, 1948, 1957, and 1974, respectively). In 1977 the Trust published an abbreviated version of the eighth edition, called *The Shorter Bergey's Manual® of Determinative Bacteriology;* this contained the outline classification of the bacteria, the descriptions of all genera and higher taxa, all of the keys and tables for the diagnosis of species, all of the illustrations, and two of the introductory chapters; however, it did not contain the detailed species descriptions, most of the taxonomic comments, the etymology of names, and references to authors.

Other ventures in producing books to assist those engaged in bacteriology and bacterial taxonomy in particular include the *Index Bergeyana* (1966), a *Supplement to Index Bergeyana* (1981), and a planned future volume bringing the lists of published names up to date. The Trust is presently publishing the first edition of *Bergey's Manual® of Systematic Bacteriology,* which has a much broader scope than the previous publications and is intended to act as the amplified source for revision of the determinative *Manual.*

Through the years the *Manual* has become a widely used international reference work for bacterial taxonomy. Similarly, the Bergey's Manual® Trust has become international in its composition, in the location of its meetings and in the breadth of its consultations. In addition to its publication activities, the Trust attempts to foster and support various aspects of taxonomic research. One of the ways in which it does this is by recognizing those individuals who have made outstanding contributions to bacterial taxonomy, through its periodic presentation of the Bergey Award, an effort jointly supported by funds from the Trust and Williams & Wilkins who have been involved in the production of the *Manual* from its beginning.

The following individuals have served as members of the Editorial Board and Board of Trustees.

On Using the *Manual**

James T. Staley

ARRANGEMENT OF THE *MANUAL*

One important goal of the *Manual* is to assist in the identification of bacteria, but another, equally important goal is to indicate the relationships that exist between the various kinds of bacteria. The methods of molecular biology have now made it possible to envision the eventual development of a comprehensive classification of bacteria based on their phylogenetic relatedness to one another. Such a general classification scheme would lead, hopefully, to more unifying concepts of bacterial taxa, to greater stability and predictability, to the development of more reliable identification schemes, and to an understanding of how bacteria have evolved.

Such a general scheme, however, cannot yet be perceived fully. The relatedness within and between some bacterial groups has been intensively studied, but for other groups very little work has been done. Moreover, the relatedness studies that have been done often have involved the use of one or another method without confirmation by other methods. Studies have been done at differing levels of resolution, and the interpretation of the data may not yet be entirely clear. Still another major difficulty is the conflict between "practical" classification vs. strange groupings that may be indicated by molecular biology methods. This is because some of the phenotypic characteristics traditionally used in bacterial classification (cell shape, flagellar arrangement, fermentative vs. respiratory types of metabolism, etc.) do not always correlate well with groups established on the basis of relatedness. This conflict will, one hopes, eventually be relieved by the finding of nontraditional, easily determined, phenotypic characteristics that *do* correlate well with relatedness groups, but much work needs to be done in this regard.

Such considerations have forced the present edition of the *Manual* to adhere largely to traditional characteristics in arranging bacterial taxa. It should be understood, however, that reassessments of these groupings will soon need to be made on a broad, comprehensive scale. The present classification, although of considerable practical value, must be regarded as only an interim arrangement.

THE SECTIONS

Volume 3 contains a very diverse collection of procaryotes, undoubtedly the most diverse collection of all of the volumes of this first edition of the *Manual.* Included here are sections with vernacular titles for the various groups treated, including the oxygenic and anoxygenic photosynthetic bacteria, the chemolithotrophs, the budding and appendaged bacteria, the fruiting bacteria, the nonfruiting gliding bacteria, the sheathed bacteria and the archaeobacteria.

The cyanobacteria and their oxygenic photosynthetic associates have not been previously included in *Bergey's Manual® of Determinative Bacteriology* or other publications of the Trust. The decision to include them here was the result of discussions with bacteriologists, phycologists and botanists. From a holistic standpoint it seems appropriate that all procaryotes should be included within a single classification, and it is in this spirit that the cyanobacteria are now classified in *Bergey's Manual®.* However, for the foreseeable future these organisms will continue to be treated by a dual system of nomenclature, i.e. within the framework of the Botanical Code and the Bacteriological Code, as well as by a dual system of classification.

Readers will note the provisional nature of classification in this volume at the higher taxonomic levels. Few groups have a rigorous classification at the level of families and orders. A single notable exception is the *Archaeobacteria.* The phylogenetic relatedness among the *Archaeobacteria* has been determined by analyses of ribosomal RNA (rRNA). This has resulted in the first complete phylogenetic classification of a bacterial group based on a strong scientific foundation. This group is also phenotypically distinct from the so-called "eubacteria," in that the *Archaeobacteria* lack peptidoglycan in their cell walls, a fact that supports the ribosomal analyses. The classification of *Archaeobacteria* provides a model that is being used in the reexamination of the classification of all other procaryotes.

As a result of the introduction of molecular phylogenetic approaches, many previous elaborate and inclusive classifications of families and orders are now in question. For example, it is clear that the formal familial and ordinal taxa of the anoxygenic phototrophic (photosynthetic) bacteria presented in the eighth edition of *Bergey's Manual® of Determinative Bacteriology* are not correct phylogenetically, at least when rRNA analyses are considered. Therefore, the former hierarchical classification of *Rhodospirillales* has given way to a transitional but functional vernacular classification.

In contrast, the classification of some groups has changed little since the eighth edition of *Bergey's Manual® of Determinative Bacteriology.* For example, the fruiting bacteria (*Myxococcales*) remain largely as they were classified then. This is not necessarily an indication that this classification is accurate, but, rather, it is an indication that this group has received very little taxonomic attention, particularly with respect to modern molecular analyses.

---

*The material in this article is based largely on that prepared by Noel Krieg for Volume 1.

Another result of molecular phylogeny is the recognition that the bacteria placed within some phenotypic groups are not as closely related to one another as they are to taxa in other groups. An example of this is the nonfruiting gliding bacteria. For instance, the genus *Cytophaga* is apparently related to *Bacteroides* and *Flavobacterium*. However, both *Bacteroides* and *Flavobacterium* were treated in previous volumes of the series before this information was appreciated. To address this situation, the issues of relatedness are discussed within the text when the appropriate groups are described.

Rapid changes are occurring in systematics. New taxa such as the order *Planctomycetales*, a group of organisms recognized recently to be peptidoglycanless eubacteria, are clearly justified both phenotypically and on the basis of their 16S rRNA analyses, but their proposal came too late to permit them to be treated as a new order. Thus, they are included as a vernacular group within the budding and/or appendaged bacteria.

It will be apparent from using this volume that the field of bacterial classification is still very exciting and rapidly evolving. There is yet much work to be done with determination of the relatedness of well-known taxa as well as in the discovery of new taxa. Our conception of bacterial diversity is determined perhaps not so much by the techniques we use for the isolation and growth of new organisms as by our limited perceptions and imaginations in understanding the niche of the undiscovered bug. Clearly, the entire field of bacterial systematics, from microbe hunting to nucleic acid sequencing, will remain a fertile area for future generations of microbiologists.

Some specific noteworthy comments regarding the taxa treated in Volume 3 follow.

Section 18: Anoxygenic Phototrophic Bacteria

The genus *Erythrobacter* is a nonphotosynthetic bacterium that is included in Section 18 because it contains bacteriochlorophyll *a*. The relationship between this genus and certain facultatively methylotrophic bacteria (genus "*Protaminobacter ruber*" and the "*Pseudomonas*" species) that also contain bacteriochlorophyll *a* is presently unclear.

Section 19: Oxygenic Photosynthetic Bacteria

Section 19 includes the cyanobacteria as well as the *Prochlorales* group, neither of which has been treated in previous classifications of the bacteria in *Bergey's Manual®*.

Section 20: Aerobic Chemolithotrophic Bacteria and Associated Organisms

Not all of the bacteria in Section 20 are chemolithotrophs. Those that are not are included because they either grow in association with chemolithotrophs or are involved in the specific processes of metal oxidation and/or deposition.

Although they are not expected to be a phylogenetically cohesive group, the magnetotactic bacteria have been included in Section 20 as a means of encouraging their further study.

Section 21: Budding and/or Appendaged Bacteria

Section 21 includes the spinate bacteria that produce large fimbriae termed spinae. Although these organisms do not appear to be related to one another or to the other bacteria in this section, they have been included to encourage their further study.

Section 22: Sheathed Bacteria

The grouping of bacteria in Section 22 is based upon the occurrence of a single morphologically distinctive feature. This section has been retained in this edition for deterministic purposes without phylogenetic implications.

Section 23: Nonphotosynthetic, Nonfruiting Gliding Bacteria

Considerable interest has been aroused in the phylogenetic relatedness between certain *Cytophaga* species and members of the genera *Bacteroides* and *Flavobacterium*. *Cytophaga* is treated here, whereas *Bacteroides* and *Flavobacterium* were treated previously in Volume 1.

Section 25: Archaeobacteria

A new order is proposed for the extreme halophilic bacteria, *Halobacteriales*. Although the extreme halophiles were treated in Volume 1, they have been included here because they comprise a group of the *Archaeobacteria*. Several new genera have been added to the group since its treatment in Volume 1.

The taxonomy of the other *Archaeobacteria* is also changing rapidly with the discovery of new orders such as "*Archaeoglobales*" and the recognition of others such as *Sulfolobales*. Every attempt has been made to provide the most recent information at the time of press.

SECTIONS VS. TAXONOMIC NAMES

Each section bears a vernacular name, but it sometimes also bears the name of a taxon. For example, Section 24 ("Fruiting Gliding Bacteria: The Myxobacteria") is the order *Myxococcales*. As indicated previously, no attempt has been made to provide a complete formal hierarchy of higher taxa throughout the *Manual*, and the vernacular names of the sections form the primary basis for the organization of the *Manual*; however, a suggested hierarchy for higher taxa has been proposed in one of the introductory articles (see "The Higher Taxa, or, a Place for Everything. . . ?").

ARTICLES

Each article dealing with a bacterial genus is presented wherever possible in a definite sequence as follows.

(a) *Name of the Genus.* Accepted names are in **boldface,** followed by the authority for the name, the year of the original description, and the page on which the taxon was named and described. The superscript *AL* indicates that the name was included on the Approved Lists of Bacterial Names, published in January 1980. The superscript *VP* indicates that the name, although not on the Approved Lists of Bacterial Names, has subsequently been validly published in the *International Journal of Systematic Bacteriology*. Names given within quotation marks have no standing in nomenclature; as of the date of preparation of the *Manual* they had not been validly published in the *International Journal of Systematic Bacteriology*, although they had been "effectively published" elsewhere. Names followed by the term "gen. nov." are newly proposed but will not be validly published until they appear in the *International Journal of Systematic Bacteriology*; their proposal in the *Manual* constitutes only "effective publication," not valid publication.

(b) *Name of Author(s).* The person or persons who prepared the article are indicated. The address of each author can be found in the list of contributors at the beginning of the *Manual*.

(c) *Synonyms.* In some instances a list is given of synonyms which have been used in the past for the same genus. The synonymy may not always be complete, and usually is not given at all, as the Editorial Board believes that the earlier synonyms have been covered adequately in the *Index Bergeyana* or in the *Supplement to the Index Bergeyana*.

(d) *Etymology of the Genus Name.* Etymologies are provided as in previous editions, and many (but undoubtedly not all) errors have been corrected. It is often difficult, however, to determine why a particular name was chosen, or the nuance intended, if the details were not provided in the original publication. Those authors who propose new names are urged to consult a Greek and Latin authority before publishing, in order to ensure grammatical correctness and also to ensure that the name means what it is intended to mean. An excellent authority to communicate with in this regard is Dr. Thomas O. MacAdoo, Department of Foreign Languages, Virginia Polytechnic Institute and State University, Blacksburg, Virginia 24061 U.S.A.

(e) *Capsule Description.* This is a brief resume of the salient features of the genus. The most important characteristics are given in **boldface.** The name of the type species of the genus is also indicated.

(f) *Further Descriptive Information.* This portion elaborates on the various features of the genus, particularly those features having significance for systematic bacteriology. The treatment serves to acquaint the reader with the overall biology of the organisms but is not meant to be a comprehensive review. The information is represented in sequence, as follows:

> Morphological characteristics
> Colonial morphology and pigmentation
> Growth conditions and nutrition
> Physiology and metabolism
> Genetics, plasmids and bacteriophages
> Antigenic structure
> Pathogenicity
> Ecology

(g) *Enrichment and Isolation Procedures.* A few methods are presented, together with the pertinent media formulations.

(h) *Maintenance Procedures.* Methods used for maintenance of stock cultures and preservation of strains are given.

(i) *Procedures for Testing Special Characters.* This portion provides methodology for testing for unusual characteristics or performing tests of special importance.

(j) *Differentiation of the Genus from Other Genera.* Those characteristics that are especially useful for distinguishing the genus from

similar or treated organisms are indicated here, usually in a tabular form.

(k) *Taxonomic Comment.* This summarizes the available information about the taxonomic placement of the genus and indicates the justification for considering genus to be a distinct taxon. Particular emphasis is given to the methods of molecular biology for estimating the relatedness to other taxa, where such information is available. Taxonomic information regarding the arrangement and status of the various species within the genus follows. Where taxonomic controversy exists, the problems are delineated and the various alternative viewpoints are discussed.

(l) *Further Reading.* A list of selected references, usually of a general nature, is given to enable the reader to gain access to additional sources of information about the genus.

(m) *Differentiation of the Species of the Genus.* Those characteristics that are important for distinguishing from one another the various species within the genus are presented, usually with reference to a table summarizing the information.

(n) *List of Species of the Genus.* The citation of each species is given, followed in some instances by a brief list of objective synonyms. The etymology of the specific epithet is indicated. Descriptive information for the species is usually presented in tabular form, but special information may be given in the text. Because of the emphasis on tabular data the species descriptions are usually brief. The type strain of each species is indicated, together with the collection in which it can be found. (Addresses of the various culture collections are given in the chapter "List of Culture Collections.")

(o) *Species Incertae Sedis.* The "List of Species of the Genus" may be followed in some instances by a listing of additional species, under the heading "Species Incertae Sedis." The taxonomic placement or status of such species is questionable, and the reasons for the uncertainty are presented.

(p) *Literature Cited.* All references given in the article are listed alphabetically at the end of the volume rather than at the end of each article.

TABLES

In each article dealing with a genus, there are generally three kinds of tables: (a) those that differentiate the genus from similar or related genera, (b) those that differentiate the species within the genus, and (c) those that provide additional information about the species, with such information not being particularly useful for differentiation. Unless otherwise indicated, the meanings of symbols are as follows:

+, 90% or more of the strains are positive.

d, 11–89% of the strains are positive.

−, 90% or more of the strains are negative.

D, different reactions occur in different taxa (species of a genus or genera of a family).

v, strain instability (NOT equivalent to "d").

Exceptions to use of these symbols, as well as the meaning of additional symbols, are clearly indicated in footnotes to the tables.

USE OF THE *MANUAL* FOR DETERMINATIVE PURPOSES

Entry into the *Manual* is best achieved by studying the titles of the various sections, as listed in the "Contents." These titles provide an elementary, but by no means perfect, key to the various kinds of bacteria. Each section has keys or tables for differentiation of the various taxa contained therein. Suggestions on identification may be found in the article "Identification of Bacteria." For identification of species, it is important to read both the generic and species descriptions because characteristics listed in the generic descriptions are not usually repeated in the species descriptions.

The "Index" is useful in locating the names of unfamiliar taxa or in discovering what has been done with a particular taxon. Every bacterial name mentioned in the *Manual* is listed in the "Index."

ERRORS, COMMENTS, SUGGESTIONS

As indicated in the "Preface to First Edition of *Bergey's Manual® of Determinative Bacteriology,*" the assistance of bacteriologists is earnestly solicited in the correction of possible errors in the text. Comments on the presentation will also be welcomed, as well as suggestions for future editions. Correspondence should be addressed to the Bergey's Manual® Trust, c/o Williams & Wilkins, 428 E. Preston St., Baltimore, Maryland 21202 U.S.A.

Contents

SECTION 20
Aerobic Chemolithotrophic Bacteria and Associated Organisms 1807

SECTION 21
Budding and/or Appendaged Bacteria 1890

Classification of Procaryotic Organisms: An Overview

James T. Staley and Noel R. Krieg

CLASSIFICATION, NOMENCLATURE AND IDENTIFICATION

Classification, nomenclature and identification are the three separate, but interrelated, areas of taxonomy. **Classification** is the arranging of organisms into taxonomic groups (taxa) on the basis of similarities or relationships. **Nomenclature** is the assignment of names to the taxonomic groups according to international rules. **Identification** is the process of determining that a new isolate belongs to one of the established, named taxa.

There are numerous procaryotic organisms and great diversity in their types. In any endeavor aimed at an understanding of large numbers of entities it is convenient to arrange, or classify, the objects into groups based upon their similarities. Thus, classification has been used to organize the bewildering and seemingly chaotic array of individual bacteria into an orderly framework.

Classification of organisms requires knowledge of their characteristics. For procaryotes, this knowledge is obtained by experimental as well as observational techniques, because biochemical, physiological and genetic characteristics are often necessary, in addition to morphological features, for an adequate description of a taxon.

The process of classification may be applied to existing, named taxa or to newly described organisms. If the taxa have already been described, named, and classified, either new characteristics about the organisms or a reinterpretation of existing knowledge of characteristics is used to formulate a new classification. However, if the organisms are new, i.e. cannot be identified as existing taxa, they are named according to the rules of nomenclature and placed in an appropriate position in an existing classification.

Taxonomic Ranks

Several levels or ranks are used in bacterial classification. All procaryotic organisms are placed in the kingdom *Procaryotae*. Divisions, classes, orders, families, genera and species are successively smaller, nonoverlapping subsets of the kingdom, and the names of these subsets are given formal recognition (have "standing in nomenclature"). An example is given in Table I.1.

In addition to these formal, hierarchical taxonomic categories, informal or vernacular groups that are defined by common descriptive names are often used; the names of such groups have no official standing in nomenclature. Examples of such groups are: the procaryotes, the spirochetes, dissimilatory sulfate- and sulfur-reducing bacteria, the methane-oxidizing bacteria, etc.

Species

The basic taxonomic group in bacterial systematics is the species. The concept of a bacterial species is less definitive than for higher organisms. This difference should not seem surprising, because bacteria, being procaryotic organisms, differ markedly from higher organisms. Sexuality, for example, is not used in bacterial species definitions because relatively few bacteria undergo conjugation. Likewise, morphological features alone are usually of little classificatory significance; this is because most procaryotic organisms are too simple morphologically to provide much useful taxonomic information. Consequently, morphological features are relegated to a less important role in bacterial taxonomy in comparison with the taxonomy of higher organisms.

A bacterial species may be regarded as a collection of strains that share many features in common and differ considerably from other strains. (A strain is made up of the descendants of a single isolation in pure culture, and usually is made up of a succession of cultures ultimately derived from an initial single colony.) One strain of a species is designated as the **type strain**; this strain serves as the name-bearer strain of the species and is the permanent example of the species, i.e. the *reference specimen for the name.* (See the chapter on "Bacterial Nomenclature" for more detailed information about nomenclatural types.) The type strain has great importance for classification at the species level, because *a species consists of the type strain and all other strains that are considered to be sufficiently similar to it as to warrant inclusion with it in the species.* This concept of a species obviously involves making subjective judgments, and it is not surprising that some bacterial species have greater phenotypic

Table I.1.

Taxonomic ranks

Formal rank	Example
Kingdom	*Procaryotae*
Division	*Gracilicutes*
Class	*Scotobacteria*
Order	*Spirochaetales*
Family	*Leptospiraceae*
Genus	*Leptospira*
Species	*Leptospira interrogans*

and genetic diversity than others. A more uniform and rigorous species definition would be desirable. For example, the level of DNA homology exhibited among a group of strains might be used as a basis for defining a species, i.e. definition on the basis of a particular degree of genetic relatedness. The advantage of adopting this or a similarly restrictive species definition must be weighed against its potential impact on well established and accepted bacterial groups. For practical reasons, classifications and nomenclature should remain stable because changes create confusion, particularly at the genus and species levels, and result in costly modifications of identification schemes and texts. However, classifications have *never* remained static and probably never will, because new information bearing on the taxonomy of bacteria is continually being generated by researchers.

Though classification schemes based on genetic relatedness are rather recent, they promise to be quite reliable and stable. This view may have to be reassessed, however, when we more fully understand the impact that transposable elements might have upon the stability of the procaryotic genome. Genetic studies have already resolved many instances of confusion concerning which strains belong to a given species, and DNA homology is increasingly being used for establishing new species and for resolving taxonomic problems at the species level.

Subspecies

A species may be divided into two or more subspecies based on minor but consistent phenotypic variations within the species or on genetically determined clusters of strains within the species. It is the lowest taxonomic rank that has official standing in nomenclature.

Infrasubspecific Ranks

Ranks below subspecies, such as biovars, serovars, and phagovars, are often used to indicate groups of strains that can be distinguished by some special character, such as antigenic makeup, reactions to bacteriophage, or the like. Such ranks have no official standing in nomenclature but often have great practical usefulness. A list of some common infrasubspecific categories is given in Table I.2.

Table I.2.
Infrasubspecific ranks

Preferred name	Synonym	Applied to strains having:
Biovar	Biotype	Special biochemical or physiological properties
Serovar	Serotype	Distinctive antigenic properties
Pathovar	Pathotype	Pathogenic properties for certain hosts
Phagovar	Phagotype	Ability to be lysed by certain bacteriophages
Morphovar	Morphotype	Special morphological features

Genus

All species are assigned to a genus (although not always with a high degree of certainty as to which genus is the best choice). In this regard, bacteriologists conform to the binomial system of nomenclature of Linnaeus in which the organism is designated by its combined genus and species name. The bacterial genus is usually a well-defined group that is clearly separated from other genera, and the thorough descriptions of genera in this edition of *Bergey's Manual*® exemplify the depth to which this taxonomic group is usually known. However, there is so far no general agreement on the *definition* of a genus in bacterial taxonomy, and considerable subjectivity is involved at the genus level. Indeed, what is perceived to be a genus by one person may be perceived as being merely a species by another systematist. The use of genetic relatedness (e.g. ribosomal RNA (rRNA) homology or rRNA oligonucleotide cataloging) offers hope for greater objectivity and has already been useful in several instances.

Higher Taxa

Classificatory relationships at the familial and ordinal levels are even less certain than those at the genus and species levels. Frequently there is little basis for ascription of taxa at these higher levels, except in a few cases (e.g. the family *Enterobacteriaceae*) where there is evidence for genetic relatedness. Thus, rather than formalize families and orders upon uncertain relationships, many systematists frequently adopt a provisional, ad hoc ranking in which purely descriptive and vernacular names for groups are applied (e.g. in this edition of *Bergey's Manual*® see Section 7 on "Dissimilatory Sulfate- or Sulfur-reducing Bacteria"). As more is learned about the similarities among these bacteria, familial and ordinal placements will likely ensue. A recent example that illustrates the effect that increased knowledge has on the taxonomy of groups concerns the methane-producing bacteria. In the eighth edition of the *Manual*, the methanogens were treated as a single family of bacteria, with three genera. Authorities for this group now propose that three *orders* are required for the circumscription of these organisms (Balch et al., 1979).

In this edition of the *Manual* the procaryotes have been classified into four divisions, these being subdivided into classes (see the chapter by Murray on "The Higher Taxa"). There is no general agreement about this or any other arrangement of divisions and classes, however, and even at the kingdom level of classification controversy exists. Recent information based on rRNA oligonucleotide catalogs and biochemical features has led some authorities to propose that not all bacteria are procaryotes and that some represent a kingdom of life distinct from both procaryotes and eucaryotes (i.e. the so-called "*Archaebacteria*")(see Fox et al., 1980, and Woese, 1981, for summaries). That this group possesses a number of unique features is beyond question, and there is strong evidence that it has taken an evolutionary path distinct from that of other bacteria, but so far there is no general agreement as to what level of classification is applicable to the group.

MAJOR DEVELOPMENTS IN BACTERIAL CLASSIFICATION

A century elapsed between Antonie van Leeuwenhoek's discovery of bacteria and Müller's initial acknowledgment of bacteria in a classification scheme (Müller, 1773). Another century passed before techniques and procedures had advanced sufficiently to permit a fairly inclusive and meaningful classification of these organisms. For a comprehensive review of the early development of bacterial classification, readers should consult the introductory sections of the first, second, and third editions of *Bergey's Manual*®. A less detailed treatment of early classifications can be found in the sixth edition of the *Manual* in which post-1923 developments were emphasized.

Two primary difficulties beset early bacterial classification systems. First, they relied heavily upon morphological criteria. For example, cell shape was often considered to be an extremely important feature. Thus,

the cocci were often classified together in one group (family or order). In contrast, contemporary schemes rely much more strongly on physiological characteristics. For example, the fermentative cocci are now separated from the photosynthetic cocci, which are separated from the methanogenic cocci, which are in turn separated from the nitrifying cocci, and so forth. Second, the pure culture technique which revolutionized microbiology was not developed until the latter half of the 19th century. In addition to dispelling the concept of "polymorphism," this technical development of Robert Koch's laboratory had great impact on the development of modern procedures in bacterial systematics. Pure cultures are analogous to herbarium specimens in botany. However, pure cultures are much more useful because they can be (a) maintained in a viable state, (b) subcultured, (c) subjected indefinitely to experimental tests, and (d) shipped from one laboratory to another. A natural outgrowth of the pure culture technique was the establishment of *type strains* of species which are deposited in repositories referred to as "culture collections" (a more suitable term would be "strain collections"). These type strains can be obtained from culture collections and used as reference strains for direct comparison with new isolates.

Before the development of computer-assisted numerical taxonomy and subsequent taxonomic methods based on molecular biology, the traditional method of classifying bacteria was to characterize them as thoroughly as possible and then to arrange them according to the intuitive judgment of the systematist. Although the subjective aspects of this method resulted in classifications that were often drastically revised by other systematists who were likely to make different intuitive judgments, many of the arrangements have survived to the present day, even under scrutiny by modern methods. One explanation for this is that the systematists usually *knew their organisms thoroughly,* and their intuitive judgments were based on a wealth of information. Their data, while not computer processed, were at least processed by an active mind to give fairly accurate impressions of the relationships existing between organisms. Moreover, some of the characteristics that were given great weight in classification were, in fact, highly correlated with many other characteristics. This principle of *correlation of characteristics* appears to have started with the Winslows (1908), who noted that parasitic cocci tended to grow poorly on ordinary nutrient media, were strongly Gram-positive, and formed acid from sugars, in contrast to saprophytic cocci which grew abundantly on ordinary media, were generally only weakly Gram-positive, and formed no acid. This division of the cocci that were studied by the Winslows (equivalent to the present genus *Micrococcus* (the saprophytes) and the genera *Staphylococcus* and *Streptococcus* (the parasites)) has held up reasonably well even to the present day.

Other classifications have not been so fortunate. A classic example of one which was not is that of the genus "*Paracolobactrum.*" This genus was proposed in 1944 and is described in the seventh edition of *Bergey's Manual®* published in 1957. It was created to contain certain lactose-negative members of the family *Enterobacteriaceae.* Because of the importance of a lactose-negative reaction in *identification* of enteric pathogens (i.e. *Salmonella* and *Shigella*), the reaction was mistakenly given great taxonomic weight in *classification* as well. However, for the organisms placed in "*Paracolobactrum,*" the lactose reaction was not highly correlated with other characteristics. In fact, the organisms were merely lactose-negative variants of other lactose-positive species; for example, "*Paracolobactrum coliforme*" resembled *Escherichia coli* in every way except in being lactose-negative. Absurd arrangements such as this eventually led to the development of more objective methods of classification, i.e. numerical taxonomy, in order to avoid giving great weight to any single characteristic.

Phylogenetic Classifications

Classification systems for many higher organisms are based to a large extent upon evolutionary evidence obtained from the fossil record and appropriate sedimentary dating procedures. Such classifications are termed "natural" or "phylogenetic" and are distinguished from "practical" or "artificial" classifications, which are based entirely on phenotypic characteristics. Until about 20 years ago, however, there was no convincing evidence of fossil microorganisms. Now, micropaleontological evidence indicates that microorganisms existed during the Precambrian period. Indeed, many scientists believe that bacteria existed at least 3.5 billion years ago on an earth that is 4.5 billion years old. Of course, the discovery of fossil microorganisms in early sedimentary rocks tells very little about the phylogeny of procaryotic groups. Micropaleontologists are far from reconstructing an evolutionary scheme based upon the presently available fossil record.

Despite the absence of a complete fossil record, proposals have been made since the early part of this century regarding the evolution of bacteria. Until recently, these proposals have been entirely speculative in nature. Orla-Jensen (1909) proposed that autotrophic bacteria were the most primitive group, and he devised an extensive phylogenetic scheme

based on this premise. Today, most microbiologists would agree that the premise is probably incorrect, but Orla-Jensen's classification did provide a coherent framework for thinking about the relationships among bacteria. Another notable phylogenetic scheme was that devised by Kluyver and van Niel (1936); in contrast to Orla-Jensen's scheme, which had been based almost entirely on physiological characteristics, Kluyver and van Niel's scheme was based on morphology. The basic premise was that the simplest morphological form, the coccus, was also the most primitive, and from this form developed more complex forms such as spirilla, rods, and branching filaments.

As recently as the seventh edition of *Bergey's Manual®* (i.e. 1957), before convincing evidence of Precambrian microbes had been discovered, the view was expressed that bacteria were a primitive group of organisms, and the classification scheme presented in that edition of the *Manual* claimed to be a natural scheme in which the photosynthetic bacteria were treated first, because they were regarded as the most primitive bacterial group. However, because of the lack of objective evidence for this (or any other) phylogenetic scheme, the eighth edition of the *Manual* abandoned all attempts at a phylogenetic approach to bacterial classification and concentrated instead on providing groupings of organisms under vernacular headings for purposes of recognition and identification; i.e. it was a purely practical and admittedly artificial classification.

Phylogenetic information has increased since the eighth edition, however, largely through the increasing use of methods for measuring genetic relatedness (i.e. DNA/DNA hybridization, DNA/rRNA hybridization, rRNA oligonucleotide cataloging, and protein sequencing). A record of bacterial evolution appears to exist in the amino acid sequences of bacterial proteins and in the nucleotide sequences of bacterial DNA and RNA. Unfortunately, the phylogenetic information is still in a fragmentary form, and it seems probable that the interpretation of the data is still not entirely clear. Not all of the bacterial groups have been surveyed, and it is likely that surprises and strange associations will continue to come from further work. Available phylogenetic information is presented throughout this *Manual* in the "Taxonomic Comments" sections of the various chapters, and some preliminary rearrangements of taxa have already been made based upon phylogenetic information.

Official Classifications

Some microbiologists seem to have the impression that the classification presented in *Bergey's Manual®* is the "official classification" to be used in microbiology. It seems important to correct that impression. **There is no "official" classification of bacteria.** (This is in contrast to bacterial *nomenclature,* where each taxon has one and only one valid name, according to internationally agreed-upon rules, and judicial decisions are rendered in instances of controversy about the validity of a name.) The closest approximation to an "official" classification of bacteria would be one that is widely accepted by the community of microbiologists. A classification that is of little use to microbiologists, no matter how fine a scheme or who devised it, will soon be ignored or significantly modified.

It also seems worthwhile to emphasize something that has often been said before, viz. **bacterial classifications are devised for microbiologists, not for the entities being classified.** Bacteria show little interest in the matter of their classification. For the systematist, this is sometimes a very sobering thought!

Further Reading

Cowan, S.T. 1971. Sense and nonsense in bacterial taxonomy. J. Gen. Microbiol. *67*: 1–8.
An incisive, personal view of bacterial taxonomy, with some "heretical" suggestions.
Cowan, S.T. 1974. Cowan and Steel's Manual for the Identification of Medical Bacteria. Cambridge University Press, Cambridge, England.
Chapters 1 and 9 of this work provide a concise statement of many principles of bacterial taxonomy.
Gerhardt, P., R.G.E. Murray, R.N. Costilow, E.W. Nester, W.A. Wood, N.R. Krieg and G.B. Phillips (Editors). 1981. Manual of Methods for General Bacteriology. American Society for Microbiology, Washington, D.C.

Section V of this book gives a brief introduction to phenotypic characterization, numerical taxonomy, genetic characterization, and classification of bacteria.

Johnson, J.L. 1973. Use of nucleic acid homologies in the taxonomy of anaerobic bacteria. Int. J. Syst. Bacteriol. *23:* 308–315.

This paper proposes a unifying concept of a bacterial species and stresses the importance of correlating nucleic acid homology with phenotypic tests to allow differentiation among species.

Margulis, L. 1968. Evolutionary criteria in thallophytes: a radical alternative. Science (Washington) *161:* 1020–1022.

This paper presents the hypothesis that eucaryotic organisms evolved from procaryotic organisms through endosymbioses.

Schopf, J.W. 1978. The evolution of the earliest cells. Sci. Am. *239:* 110–138.

A micropaleontologist's view of microbial evolution.

Schwartz, R.M. and M.O. Dayhoff. 1978. Origins of procaryotes, eucaryotes, mitochondria, and chloroplasts. Science (Washington) *199:* 395–403.

A discussion of results obtained from the analysis of protein and nucleic acid sequence data as they pertain to the phylogeny of organisms.

Sneath, P.H.A. 1978. Classification of microorganisms. *In* Norris and Richmond (Editors), Essays in Microbiology. John Wiley, Chichester, England, pp. 9/1–9/31.

An excellent general introduction to bacterial classification.

Trüper, H.G. and J. Krämer. 1981. Principles of characterization and identification of prokaryotes. *In* Starr, Stolp, Trüper, Balows and Schlegel (Editors), The Prokaryotes. A Handbook on Habitats, Isolation, and Identification of Bacteria. Springer-Verlag, Berlin, pp. 176–193.

A brief overview of systematic bacteriology, including developments and trends in taxonomy.

Woese, C.R. and G.E. Fox. 1977. Phylogenetic structure of the procaryotic domain: the primary kingdoms. Proc. Natl. Acad. Sci. U.S.A. *74:* 5088–5090.

The authors recognize three distinct groups: the eubacteria, the archaebacteria, and the urcaryotes (cytoplasmic components of eucaryotes).

BACTERIAL CLASSIFICATION II

Numerical Taxonomy

Peter H. A. Sneath

Numerical taxonomy (sometimes called **taxometrics**) developed in the late 1950s as part of multivariate analyses and in parallel with the development of computers. Its aim was to devise a consistent set of methods for classification of organisms. Much of the impetus in bacteriology came from the problem of handling the tables of data that result from examination of their physiological, biochemical and other properties. Such tables of results are not readily analyzed by eye, in contrast to the elaborate morphological detail that is usually available from examination of higher plants and animals. There was thus a need for an objective method of taxonomic analyses, whose first aim was to sort individual strains of bacteria into homogeneous groups (conventionally species) and which would also assist in the arrangement of species into genera and higher groupings. Such numerical methods also promised to improve the exactitude in measuring taxonomic, phylogenetic, serological, and other forms of relationship, together with other benefits that can accrue from quantitation (such as improved methods for bacterial identification; see the discussion by Sneath on "Numerical Identification" on p. 1626 of this *Manual*).

Numerical taxonomy has been broadly successful in most of these aims, particularly in defining homogeneous **clusters** of strains and in integrating data of different kinds (morphological, physiological, antigenic). There are still problems in constructing satisfactory groups at high taxonomic levels, e.g. families and orders, although this may be due to inadequacies in the available data rather than any fundamental weakness in the numerical methods themselves.

The application of the concepts of numerical taxonomy was made possible only through the use of computers, because of the heavy load of routine calculations. However, the principles can easily be illustrated in hand-worked examples. In addition, two problems had to be solved: the first was to decide how to weight different variables or characters; the second was to analyze similarities so as to reveal the **taxonomic structure** of groups, species, or clusters. A full description of numerical taxonomic methods may be found in Sneath (1972) and Sneath and Sokal (1973). Briefer descriptions and illustrations in bacteriology are given by Skerman (1967), Lockhart and Liston (1970), and Sneath (1978a). A thorough review of applications to bacteria is that of Colwell (1973).

It is important to bear in mind certain definitions. Relationships between organisms can be of several kinds. Two broad classes are as follows.

Similarity on Observed Properties, Similarity, or resemblance, refers to the attributes that an organism possesses today, without reference to how those attributes arose. It is expressed as proportions of similarities and differences, for example, in existing attributes and is called **phenetic relationship.** This includes similarities both in phenotype (e.g. motility) and in genotype (e.g. DNA pairing).

Relationship by Ancestry, or Evolutionary Relationship. This refers to the **phylogeny** of organisms and not necessarily to their present attributes. It is expressed as the time to a common ancestor, or the amount of change that has occurred in an evolutionary lineage. It is not expressed as a proportion of similar attributes or as the amount of DNA pairing and the like, although evolutionary relationship may sometimes by *deduced* from phenetics *on the assumption* that evolution has indeed proceeded in some orderly and defined way. As an analogy, individuals from different nations may occasionally look more similar than brothers or sisters of one family: their phenetic resemblance (in the properties observed) may be high, though their evolutionary relationship is distant.

Numerical taxonomy is concerned primarily with phenetic relationships. It has, in recent years, been extended to phylogenetic work by using rather different techniques: these seek to build up on the assumed regularities of evolution so as to give, from *phenetic data,* the *most probable phylogenetic reconstructions.* Relatively little has been done so far in bacteriology, but a review of the area is given by Sneath (1974).

The basic taxonomic category is the species. In the chapter on "Bacterial Nomenclature" it is noted that it is useful to distinguish a **taxospecies** (a cluster of strains of high mutual phenetic similarity) from a **genospecies** (a group of strains capable of gene exchange) and both of these from a **nomenspecies** (a group bearing a binominal name, whatever its status in other respects). Numerical taxonomy attempts to define taxospecies. Whether these are justified as genospecies or nomenspecies turns on other criteria. It should be emphasized that groups with high genomic similarity are not necessarily genospecies: genomic resemblance is included in phenetic resemblance; genospecies are defined by gene exchange.

Groups can be of two important types. In the first, the possession of certain invariant properties defines the group without permitting any exception. All triangles, for example, have three sides, not four. Such groupings are termed **monothetic.** Taxonomic groups are, however, not of this kind. Exceptions to the most invariant characters are always possible. Instead, taxa are **polythetic;** i.e. they consist of assemblages whose members share a high proportion of common attributes but not necessarily any invariable set. Numerical taxonomy produces polythetic groups and thus permits the occasional exception on any character.

LOGICAL STEPS IN CLASSIFICATION

The steps in the process of classification are as follows:

1. Collection of data. The **bacterial strains** that are to be classified have to be chosen, and they must be examined for a number of relevant properties (**taxonomic characters**).
2. The data must be coded and scaled in an appropriate fashion.
3. The **similarity** or **resemblance** between the strains is calculated. This yields a table of similarities (**similarity matrix**) based on the chosen set of characters.
4. The similarities are analyzed for **taxonomic structure**, to yield the groups or clusters that are present, and the strains are arranged into **phenons** (phenetic groups), which are broadly equated with taxonomic groups (**taxa**).
5. The properties of the phenons can be tabulated for publication or further study, and the most appropriate characters (**diagnostic characters**) can be chosen on which to set up **identification systems** that will allow the best identification of additional strains.

It may be noted that those steps must be carried out in the above order. One cannot, for example, find diagnostic characters before finding the groups of which they are diagnostic. Furthermore, it is important to obtain complete data, determined under well-standardized conditions.

Data for numerical taxonomy

The data needed for numerical taxonomy must be adequate in quantity and quality. It is a common experience that data from the literature are inadequate on both counts: most often it is necessary to examine bacterial strains afresh by an appropriate set of tests.

Organisms

Most taxonomic work with bacteria consists of examining individual strains of bacteria. However, the entities that can be classified may be of various forms—strains, species, genera—for which no common term is available. These entities, t in number, are therefore called **operational taxonomic units (OTUs)**. In most studies, OTUs will be strains. A numerical taxonomic study, therefore, should contain a good selection of strains of the groups under study, together with type strains of the taxa and of related taxa. Where possible, recently isolated strains, and strains from different parts of the world, should be included.

Characters

A **character** is defined as any property that can vary between OTUs. The values it can assume are **character states.** Thus, "length of spore" is a character, and "1.5 μm" is one of its states. It is obviously important to compare the same character in different organisms, and the recognition that characters are the same is called the **determination of homology.** This may sometimes pose problems, but in bacteriology these are seldom serious. A single character treated as independent of others is called a **unit character.** Sets of characters that are related in some way are called **character complexes.**

There are many kinds of characters that can be used in taxonomy. The descriptions in the *Manual* give many examples. For numerical taxonomy, the characters should cover a broad range of properties: morphological, physiological, biochemical. It should be noted that certain data are not characters in the above sense. Thus the degree of serological cross-reaction or the percent pairing of DNA is analogous, not to character states, but to similarity measures.

Numbers of Characters

Although it is well to include a number of strains of each known species, numerical taxonomies are not greatly affected by having only a few strains of a species. This is not so, however, for characters. The similarity values should be thought of as estimates of values that would be obtained if one could include a very large number of phenotypic features. The accuracy of such estimates depends critically on having a reasonably large number of characters. The number, n, should be 50 or more. Several hundred are desirable, though the taxonomic gain falls off with very large numbers.

Quality of Data

The quality of the characters is also important. Microbiological data are prone to more experimental error than is commonly realized. The average difference in replicate tests on the same strain is commonly about 5%. Efforts should be made to keep this figure low, particularly by rigorous standardization of test methods. It is very difficult to obtain reasonably reproducible results with some tests, and they should be excluded from the analysis. As a check on the quality of the data, it is useful to reduplicate a few of the strains and carry them through as separate OTUs: the average test error is about half the percentage discrepancy in similarity of such replicates (e.g. 90% similarity implies about 5% experimental variation).

Coding of Results

The test reactions and character states now need coding for numerical analysis. There are several satisfactory ways of doing this, but for the present purposes of illustration only one common scheme will be described. This is the familiar process of coding the reactions or states into positive and negative form. The resulting table, therefore, contains entries + and − (or 1 and 0, which are more convenient for computation) for t OTUs scored for n characters. Naturally, there should be as few gaps as possible.

The question arises as to what weight should be given to each character relative to the rest. The usual practice in numerical taxonomy is to give each character equal weight. More specifically, it may be argued that unit characters should have unit weight, and if character complexes are broken into a number of unit characters (each carrying one unit of taxonomic information), it is logical to accord unit weight to each unit character. The difficulties of deciding what weight should be given *before* making a classification (and hence in a fashion that does not prejudge the taxonomy) are considerable. This philosophy derives from the opinions of the 18th century botanist Adanson, and therefore numerical taxonomies are sometimes referred to as Adansonian.

Similarity

The $n \times t$ table can then be analyzed to yield similarities between OTUs. The simplest way is to count, for any pair of OTUs, the number of characters in which they are identical (i.e. both are positive or both are negative). These **matches** can be expressed as a percentage or a proportion, symbolized as S_{SM} (for simple matching coefficient). This is the commonest coefficient in bacteriology. Other coefficients are sometimes used because of particular advantages. Thus the Gower coefficient, S_G, accommodates both presence-absence characters and quantitative ones; the Jacquard coefficient, S_J, discounts matches between two negative results; and the Pattern coefficient, S_P, corrects for apparent differences that are caused solely by differences between strains in growth rate and hence metabolic vigor. These coefficients emphasize different aspects of the phenotype (as is quite legitimate in taxonomy), so one cannot regard one or the other as necessarily the correct coefficient, but fortunately this makes little practical difference in most studies.

The similarity values between all pairs of OTUs yield a checkerboard of entries, a square table of similarities known as a **similarity matrix** or **S matrix.** The entries are percentages, with 100% indicating identity and 0% indicating complete dissimilarity between OTUs. Such a table is symmetrical (the similarity of a to b is the same as that of b to a), so that usually only one half, the left lower triangle, is filled in.

These similarities can also be expressed in a complementary form as *dissimilarities*. Dissimilarities can be treated as analogs of distances, when "taxonomic maps" of the OTUs are prepared, and it is a convenient property that the quantity $d = \sqrt{(1 - S_{SM})}$ is equivalent geometrically to a *distance* between points representing the OTUs in a space of many dimensions (a **phenetic hyperspace**).

Taxonomic structure

A table of similarities does not of itself make evident the **taxonomic structure** of the OTUs. The strains will be in an arbitrary order which will not reflect the species or other groups. These similarities therefore require further manipulation. It will be seen that a table of serological cross-reactions, if complete and expressed in quantitative terms, is analogous to a table of percentage similarities, and the same is true of a table of DNA pairing values. Such tables can be analyzed by the methods described below, though in serological and nucleic studies there are some particular difficulties on which further work is needed.

There are two main types of analyses to reveal the taxonomic structure, **cluster analysis** and **ordination.** The result of the former is a treelike diagram or **dendrogram** (more precisely a **phenogram,** because it expresses phenetic relationships), in which the tightest bunches of twigs represent clusters of very similar OTUs. The result of the latter is an **ordination diagram** or **taxonomic map,** in which closely similar OTUs are placed close together. The mathematical methods can be elaborate, so only a nontechnical account is given here.

In cluster analysis, the principle is to search the table of similarities for high values that indicate the most similar pairs of OTUs. These form the nuclei of the clusters and the computer searches for the next highest similarity values and adds the corresponding OTUs onto these cluster nuclei. Ultimately all OTUs fuse into one group, represented by the basal stem of the dendrogram. Lines drawn across the dendrogram at descending similarity levels define, in turn, phenons that correspond to a reasonable approximation to species, genera, etc. The commonest cluster methods are the **unweighted pair group method with averages (UPGMA)** and **single linkage.**

In ordination, the similarities (or their mathematical equivalents) are analyzed, so that the phenetic hyperspace is summarized in a space of only a few dimensions. In two dimensions this is a scattergram of the positions of OTUs from which one can recognize clusters by eye. Three-dimensional perspective drawings can also be made. The commonest ordination methods are **principal components analysis** and **principal coordinates analysis.**

A number of other representations are also used. One example is a similarity matrix in which the OTUs have first been rearranged into the order given by a clustering method and then the cells of the matrix have been shaded, with the highest similarities shown in the darkest tone. In these "shaded S matrices," clusters are shown by dark triangles. Another representation is a table of the mean similarities between OTUs of the same cluster and of different clusters (**intergroup** and **intragroup** similarity table): if based on S_{SM} with UPGMA clustering, this table expresses the positions and radii of clusters (Sneath, 1979a) and, consequently, the distance between them and their probable overlap— properties of importance in numerical identification as discussed later.

For general purposes a dendrogram is the most useful representation, but the others can be very instructive, since each method emphasizes somewhat different aspects of the taxonomy.

The analysis for taxonomic structure should lead logically to the establishment or revision of taxonomic groups. We lack, at present, objective criteria for different taxonomic ranks; i.e. one cannot automatically equate a phenon with a taxon. It is, however, commonly found that phenetic groups formed at about 80% S are equivalent to bacterial species. Similarly, we lack good tests for the statistical significance of clusters and for determining how much they overlap, though some progress is being made here (Sneath, 1977, 1979b). The fidelity with which the dendrogram summarizes the S matrix can be assessed by the **cophenetic correlation coefficient**, and similar statistics can be used to compare the **congruence** between two taxonomies if they are in quantitative form (e.g. phenetic and serological taxonomies). Good scientific judgment in the light of other knowledge is indispensable for interpreting the results of numerical taxonomy.

Descriptions of the groups can now be made by referring back to the original table of strain data. The better diagnostic characters can be chosen—those whose states are very constant within groups but vary between groups. It is better to give percentages or proportions than to use symbols such as +, (+), v, d, or − for varying percentages, because significant loss of statistical information can occur with these simplified schemes. It would, however, be superfluous to list percentages based on very few strains. As systematic bacteriology advances, it will be increasingly important to publish the actual data on an individual strain or deposit it in archives; such data will show its full value when test methods become very highly standardized.

It is evident that numerical taxonomy *and* numerical identification (see the chapter on "Identification of Bacteria" in this *Manual*) place considerable demands on laboratory expertise. New test methods are continually being devised. New information is continually being accumulated. It is important that progress should be made toward agreed data bases (Krichevsky and Norton, 1974), as well as toward improvements in standardization of test methods in determinative bacteriology, if the full potential of numerical methods is to be achieved.

Nucleic Acids in Bacterial Classification

John L. Johnson

Historically, classification of bacteria has been based on similarities in phenotypic characteristics. Although this method has been quite successful, it has not been precise enough for distinguishing superficially similar organisms or for determining phylogenetic relationships among the bacterial groups. Nucleic acid studies were first applied to such problems in bacterial classification more than 20 years ago and have since become of major importance. There are several advantages to be gained by basing classification on genomic relatedness:

1. A more unifying concept of a bacterial species is possible.
2. Classifications based on genomic relatedness tend not to be subject to frequent or radical changes.

3. Reliable identification schemes can be prepared after organisms have been classified on the basis of genomic relatedness.
4. Information can be obtained that is useful for understanding how the various bacterial groups have evolved and how they can be arranged according to their ancestral relationships.

The purpose of this chapter is to provide an overview of the principles involved in nucleic acid methodology, to give a brief description of the procedures being used, to compare the results obtained by one procedure with those obtained by another, and to indicate how the results are being used in bacterial classification.

PROPERTIES OF NUCLEIC ACIDS

DNA Base Composition

The first unique feature of DNA that was recognized as having taxonomic importance was its mole percent guanine plus cytosine content (mol% G + C). Among the bacteria, the mol% G + C values range from ∼25 to 75, and the value is constant for a given organism. Closely related bacteria have similar mol% G + C values. However, it is important to recognize that two organisms that have similar mol% G + C values are not necessarily closely related; this is because the mol% G + C values *do not take into account the linear arrangement of the nucleotides in the DNA.*

Mol% G + C values were initially determined by acid-hydrolyzing the DNA, separating the nucleotide bases by paper chromatography, and then eluting and quantifying the individual bases. Other methods have since become more popular.

Thermal Denaturation Method. During the controlled heating of a preparation of double-stranded DNA in a ultraviolet spectrophotometer, the absorbance increases by ∼40%. This is due to the disruption of the hydrogen bonds between the base pairs that link the two DNA strands. *The temperature at the midpoint of the curve obtained by plotting temperature vs. absorbance is called the "melting temperature" or T_m.* The T_m is correlated in a linear manner with the mol% G + C content of the DNA (Marmur and Doty, 1962). The higher the T_m, the higher the mol% G + C of the DNA (see Johnson, J.L. (1981) for further details).

Buoyant Density Method. When DNA is subjected to centrifugation in a cesium chloride density gradient (isopycnic centrifugation), it will become located in the form of a band at a position where its density exactly matches that of the cesium chloride solution. The higher the density of cesium chloride where the DNA forms a band, the higher the mol% G + C value of the DNA (Schildkraut et al. (1962); also see Mandel et al. (1968) for further details).

Although these methods are widely used for estimating DNA base composition, technical problems occasionally do arise because of contamination of the DNA preparation by polysaccharides or pigments or because of excessive fragmentation of the DNA during its purification. Recent developments in high pressure liquid chromatography have resulted in methods that will accurately and rapidly quantify the free bases, nucleosides, or nucleotides of DNA (see, for example, Ko et al., 1977).

DNA Denaturation and Renaturation

A unique physical property of double-stranded (native) DNA is that under certain conditions (high temperature of high pH) the complementary strands will dissociate (denature). When the resulting single-stranded DNA is then subjected to a somewhat lower temperature and a rather high salt concentration, the complementary strands will reassociate (renature) to form double-stranded DNA/DNA structures (duplexes) that are very similar if not identical to the native DNA (Marmur and Doty, 1961). The renaturation rate is inversely proportional to the genome size (see the following references for further details: Wetmur and Davidson, 1968; Wetmur, 1976).

RNA/DNA Hybrids

Since only one strand of DNA is used by a cell as a template for RNA synthesis, RNA is complementary only to that strand. Since RNA is single-stranded, RNA molecules do not associate with other RNA molecules; however, when mixed with denatured DNA, they can pair with a complementary DNA strand (hybridization) (see Galau et al., 1977, for further details).

Heterologous DNA Duplexes or RNA Hybrids

If denatured DNA from one organism is mixed with denatured DNA from a second organism, heterologous duplexes may form (i.e. duplexes consisting of one strand from the first DNA hybridized with one strand from the second DNA). Similarly, heterologous RNA duplexes may be formed when RNA from one organism is mixed with denatured DNA from a second organism. However, in order for heterologous DNA duplexes or RNA hybrids to occur, the two strands must be complementary in their nucleotide base sequence. A perfect match is not required, and estimates of the amount of base pair mismatch that is tolerated range from ~8 to 10% (Ullman and McCarthy, 1973). The thermal stability is usually determined by measuring strand separation during stepwise increases in temperature, and the results mimic the optical melting profile previously discussed under "DNA Base Composition." The thermal stability is usually represented by the term "$T_{m(e)}$," which is the midpoint of the thermal stability profile (i.e. analogous to T_m of native DNA). The difference between the $T_{m(e)}$ of a heterologous duplex and that of a homologous duplex is referred to as the $\Delta T_{m(e)}$ and is used as a measure of the degree of base pair mismatching in the heterologous duplex. The $\Delta T_{m(e)}$ values for heterologous duplexes range from 0 (no mismatching) to 18°C (considerable mismatching). In general, as the fractions of the genomes which can form heterologous duplexes decrease, the thermal stabilities of the duplexes that do form also decrease.

DNA AND RNA HOMOLOGY EXPERIMENTS

Such experiments attempt to answer one question: does DNA or RNA from organism A have a base sequence that is sufficiently similar to that from organism B to allow the formation of DNA heteroduplexes or heterologous RNA hybrids?

DNA Homology Values

These are average measurements of similarity in which the *entire genome of one organism is compared with that of another.*

RNA Homology Values

These values are specific for each type of RNA:

Messenger RNA (mRNA) Homology Values. These are similar to those obtained by DNA homology (at least for bacteria), because a large portion of the genome is used for transcribing the mRNA molecules. For this reason, and because mRNA is difficult to label, mRNA homology has not been widely used in bacterial taxonomy.

Ribosomal RNA (rRNA) and Transfer RNA (tRNA) Homology Values. In contrast to mRNA, rRNA and tRNA are coded for by *only a small fraction of the bacterial genome;* therefore, in homology experiments using either of these two types of RNA, only those fractions of the genome are being compared, not the entire genome. In all groups of bacteria so far studied, the arrangement of nucleotides in the rRNA and tRNA cistrons of the DNA appears to have evolved less rapidly than the bulk of the cistrons in the DNA. This is probably due to their role in determining the structural and functional aspects of the ribosome (Woese et al., 1975).

Therefore, DNA homology experiments are used to detect similarities between *closely related* organisms, whereas RNA homology experiments are used to detect similarities between *more distantly related* organisms.

METHODS FOR HOMOLOGY EXPERIMENTS

Many procedures have been developed for detecting heterologous DNA duplexes or RNA hybrids. A brief description of some of these follows.

Heavy Isotopes

The earliest efforts to quantify the formation of heteroduplexes were made by incorporating a heavy base (5-bromouracil) or a heavy isotope (^{15}N) into one of the DNA preparations. After the labeled and unlabeled DNA preparations were mixed and allowed to reassociate, the mixture was subjected to ultracentrifugation with cesium chloride. This allowed the separation of heteroduplexes (which had an intermediate buoyant density) from the homologous duplexes (which had either a light or a heavy density). These experiments were time-consuming and worked best only for small genomes such as those of viruses.

Agarose Gels

In 1963, McCarthy and Bolton immobilized high molecular weight denatured DNA in an agarose gel. The gel was then cut into small particles by forcing the agar through a small mesh screen. The agar particles were then incubated with radioactive-labeled RNA or fragmented DNA. The smaller RNA molecules or DNA fragments could diffuse through the agar and form hybrids or duplexes with complementary immobilized DNA. The immobilization of the high molecular weight DNA prevented it from reassociating with other high molecular weight DNA and also provided a means for washing unreacted labeled nucleic acid fragments away from those that had formed hybrids or duplexes with the immobilized DNA. The results from such experiments were quantitative and could readily be applied to broad taxonomic studies (Hoyer et al., 1964).

Binding to Nitrocellulose

In 1963, Nygaard and Hall found that native DNA, denatured DNA, and RNA/DNA hybrids would bind to nitrocellulose, whereas RNA would not. This provided another means for immobilizing denatured DNA for use in RNA/DNA hybridization experiments and also for separating RNA/DNA hybrids from free RNA. The parameters for these experiments were worked out in detail by Gillespie and Spiegelman (1965).

In 1966, Denhardt described a procedure for covering the DNA binding sites on nitrocellulose membranes. This made it possible first to immobilize a given amount of denatured DNA on the membrane and then to treat the membrane with a mixture that prevented additional DNA from binding to the membrane (unless it was complementary to the immobilized DNA on the membrane). Thus the membrane procedure became readily applicable to DNA homology experiments and has completely replaced the agarose gel method.

By the use of nitrocellulose membranes, DNA or RNA homology values can be determined by either *direct binding* or *competition* experiments.

Direct Binding Method. In the direct binding method, a given amount of denatured labeled DNA or RNA is incubated under standardized conditions with various single-stranded DNA preparations that have been immobilized on nitrocellulose membranes. After incubation the unbound labeled nucleic acid is washed away, and the radioactivity remaining on the membrane (due to duplex or hybrid formation) is measured. The *percent homology* is expressed as the *amount of heterologous binding divided by the amount of homologous binding $\times$ 100*. The results are somewhat variable because it is difficult to consistently get the same amounts of DNA on the membranes. This problem is circumvented with the competition method.

Competition Method. In the competition method, unlabeled denatured reference DNA is fixed onto nitrocellulose membranes. A direct binding reaction, used for a reference point, is performed between the homologous denatured labeled DNA in solution and membrane-bound reference DNA. The competitive reactions have the same components as the direct binding reaction but additionally contain high concentrations of unlabeled denatured DNA fragments in solution. If the competitor DNA is homologous to the labeled DNA in solution and to the unlabeled DNA bound to the membrane, the competitor DNA will form duplexes with both the labeled DNA and the immobilized DNA; consequently, the amount of labeled DNA that forms duplexes with the immobilized DNA will be much lower than that occurring in the direct binding reaction. The homologous competition will be ~90% effective. On the other hand, if the competitor DNA is not related, it will not form duplexes with the labeled DNA and immobilized DNA, and there will be no competition. The percent homology is the ratio of the heterologous competition to the homologous competition $\times$ 100. Such competition experiments give very reproducible results but do require relatively large quantities of DNA (Johnson, J.L., 1981).

Free Solution Reassociation

In this method, all of the component nucleic acids are in solution rather than being immobilized in some manner. Reassociation of DNA may be monitored optically by ultraviolet spectrophotometry or by means of a labeled probe.

Optical Procedure. In the optical procedure, the rates of reassociation are determined. Since DNA reassociation is a second-order reaction, the rate will be proportional to the square of the concentration. The general procedure for comparing the DNAs from two organisms is to measure the reassociation rates of equivalent concentrations from each of the organisms separately and compare those rates with that of an equal mixture of the two DNA preparations. If the two organisms are identical, the reassociation rates in the three cuvettes will be the same. If the two organisms are unrelated, then each kind of DNA in the mixture will reassociate independently of the other, and since they are each at half the concentration as that used in the cuvettes with a single DNA component, the overall rate will be one-half. De Ley et al. (1970) have studied the parameters of the method in detail and have derived equations for calculating the homology values.

Labeled DNA Probe. The most popular procedure for free solution reassociation involves the use of a labeled DNA probe. As discussed above, the rate of DNA reassociation is a function of DNA concentration, and because the labeled probe DNA is used at a very low concentra-

tion, very little of it will reassociate. The unlabeled test DNA with which the probe DNA is incubated is at a much higher concentration, and most of it will reassociate. Therefore, if the probe DNA is identical with the unlabeled test DNA, it will reassociate with the unlabeled DNA at the rate at which the unlabeled DNA is reassociating. On the other hand, if the two DNAs are unrelated, the unlabeled DNA will reassociate, but most of the probe DNA will remain single-stranded. To determine the amount of probe DNA that has duplexed with the unlabeled DNA, either *hydroxylapatite* or *S1 nuclease* is usually used.

Hydroxylapatite is used to separate single-stranded (denatured) DNA from double-stranded DNA. At a phosphate concentration of 0.14 M, only double-stranded DNA will adsorb to hydroxylapatite, and single-stranded DNA can be washed away. The double-stranded DNA can then be desorbed by increasing the phosphate concentration. Although originally used as a column chromatography procedure (Bernardi, 1969a, b; Miyazawa and Thomas, 1965), the batch procedure described by Brenner et al. (1969) has been widely used.

Under suitable conditions, S1 nuclease will have little effect on double-stranded DNA but will hydrolyze single-stranded DNA. Consequently, the extent of the duplex formation by the probe DNA can be determined by the amount of S1 nuclease-resistant (i.e. acid-precipitable) radioactivity (Crosa et al., 1973).

Comparison of Various Homology Methods

In spite of the diversity of the DNA homology methods, they are all used to measure the same phenomenon, and so it is comforting to find that, for the most part, they all give similar results. The major experimental parameters that affect homology results are the sodium ion concentration and the reassociation temperatures. The most commonly used sodium ion concentration is about 0.4 M, although concentrations up to 1 M do not alter the results significantly. The reassociation temperature can have a profound effect on the homology values, and therefore a standardized temperature of about 25°C below the T_m ($T_m - 25$°C) is most commonly used (Marmur and Doty, 1961). The reassociation temperature effect is approximately linear for the membrane competition and the hydroxylapatite procedures: for organisms having less that 50% homology, the homology values will increase by about 20% at 10°C below the $T_m - 25$°C temperature and decrease by about 20% at 10°C above the $T_m - 25$°C temperature. Reassociation temperature differences do not have as great an effect on the optical (De Ley et al., 1970) or the S1 nuclease methods (Grimont et al., 1980).

Under similar conditions of reassociation, the hydroxylapatite, membrane competition and spectrophotometric methods give very similar results (Kurtzman et al., 1980). The S1 nuclease procedure results in somewhat lower (15–20%) homology values, particularly between organisms having less than 50% homology.

The rRNA cistrons have been found to be very conserved in all groups of organisms that have been investigated. The nitrocellulose membrane procedures, such as competition, direct binding and thermal stability of hybrids, have been used for most of the rRNA homology studies. Results from these experiments appear to reflect nucleotide sequence differences that are similar to those found in the DNA homology experiments discussed above.

rRNA OLIGONUCLEOTIDE CATALOGS

Besides the use of RNA/DNA homology experiments for comparison of the rRNA cistrons from various bacteria, rRNA molecules have been compared directly by determining the nucleotide sequences in oligonucleotides. The rRNA preparation is first digested with T1 ribonuclease which cleaves between the 3′-guanylic acid and the 5′-hydroxyl group of the adjacent nucleotide. This results in an guanine residue at the 3′ end of each oligonucleotide. The oligonucleotides are then separated by two-

dimensional electrophoresis (Sanger et al., 1965; Uchida et al., 1974). The first dimension is on cellulose acetate at pH 3.5. The oligonucleotides are then transferred from the cellulose acetate strip onto DEAE cellulose and electrophoresed in the second dimension in 6.5% formic acid. The oligonucleotide spots form three-to-four series of wedge-shaped patterns (Sanger et al., 1965). Within each pattern the oligonucleotides contain a constant number of uracil residues, and the locations of the spots within a pattern indicate the number of adenine and cytosine residues. Therefore, by inspecting the pattern one can predict the nucleotide sequence of the shorter oligonucleotides and the base compositions for the longer ones. The spots containing the longer nucleotides are then cut out for secondary analysis. After digestion with other ribonucleases, they are again electrophoresed on DEAE cellulose. If the nucleotide sequence still is not clear, a tertiary analysis is required. The unique oligonucleotides (usually only one per rRNA molecule) of each organism are entered (cataloged) into computer storage. The oligonucleotide catalog from one organism can then be compared with that of another. The similarity values between two organisms is the number of unique oligonucleotides (in each of their rRNA molecules) that they share, divided by the average total number of unique oligonucleotides. This procedure compares the sequence for a rather large portion of the rRNA molecules.

Most recently, procedures have been developed for rapidly sequencing long segments of DNA and RNA (Maxam and Gilbert, 1977; Peattie, 1979; Sanger et al., 1977). DNA from several viruses has been sequenced. Sequencing all of the DNA of a bacterium would generate a rather formidable amount of data; however, specific cistrons have been compared by sequence analysis, such as the genes of the tryptophan operon of *Escherichia coli* and *Salmonella typhimurium* (Crawford et al., 1980).

CONTRIBUTIONS OF NUCLEIC ACID STUDIES TO BACTERIAL TAXONOMY

Concept of a Bacterial Species

A major contribution of DNA homology studies has been to provide a more unifying concept of a bacterial species. Although the exact level of DNA homology above which one considers organisms as belonging to the same species is arbitrary, similar homology clusters have been found in all bacterial groups that have been investigated. I have previously suggested what seemed to be reasonable cut-off points for delineating subspecies, species, and closely related species (Johnson, 1973). These are illustrated in Figure III.1. DNA heterogeneity in the species range (*A*) has been found for many bacterial groups that are phenotypically very similar. In some instances the homology values will tend to cluster in the 80–90% homology range (*B*). Examples of this are the clustering of *Propionibacterium acnes* (Johnson and Cummins, 1972) and *Bacteroides uniformis* (Johnson, 1978). In other instances there may also be clustering at the lower end of the species range (*C*). *Bacteroides fragilis*, for example, clusters into two groups where the intergroup homology values are in the range of 60–70% and the intragroup homology values are in the 80–90% range (Johnson, 1978). It is important to note that the thermal stabilities of heteroduplexes between organisms in the 80–90% DNA homology range will be very similar to those of homoduplexes ($\Delta T_{m(e)}$ values of 0–3°C), whereas with heteroduplexes between 60 and 70% homology they will be substantially lower ($\Delta T_{m(e)}$ values of 6–9°C). Therefore, it appears that 60–70% homology is a transitional point between genetic events that may be largely cistron-rearranging in nature and genetic events where there are also many changes in the base sequences (Johnson, 1973). In other instances, e.g. *Bacteroides ovatus* (Johnson, 1978), multiple groups within the 60–70% homology range make subgrouping at this level rather complicated so that, unless there are other important considerations, such as pathogenicity (Krych et al., 1980), it may not be justified.

The DNA homology groups in the lower homology range (*D* in Fig. III.1) often are quite distinct phenotypically from the species with which they are being compared, although in some instances they may differ only in a few characters (Johnson and Ault, 1978; Johnson, 1981; Mays et al., 1982).

It is important to remember that few bacteria have read Figure III.1; therefore, the exact limits chosen for a given group of organisms will have to remain at the discretion of the individual investigator.

Identification Schemes

A major practical use of DNA homology data is for correlation with individual phenotypic tests. It is common to find variability for a trait among strains within a DNA homology group as well as distinct DNA homology groups that differ from each other by only a few traits (Johnson and Ault, 1978; Johnson, 1980; Mays et al., 1982; Holdeman et al., 1982). Correlating phenotypic test results with DNA homology groups enables investigators to select phenotypic tests that are required for the accurate identification of organisms belonging to these groups.

Concept of a Bacterial Genus and Higher Taxa

Comparisons of rRNA cistrons by rRNA homology experiments and by 16S oligonucleotide catalog similarities are providing data from which a more unifying phylogenetic concept for higher bacterial taxa is possible. De Ley and his associates (De Ley et al., 1978; De Smedt et al., 1980) have proposed the establishment of several genera on the basis of rRNA homology results. On the basis of 16S rRNA oligonucleotide similarity, Woese (in Fox et al., 1980) has proposed the reestablishing of the higher bacterial taxa which were dropped from the eighth edition of *Bergey's Manual*® because it was thought that the higher taxa listed in the seventh edition did not represent phylogenetic relationships. As examples, the 16S rRNA oligonucleotide similarity values have contributed greatly to the present taxonomic scheme of the methanogenic bacteria (Balch et al., 1979) and to the establishment of division IV *Mendosicutes* in the kingdom *Procaryotae* (see the chapter on "The Higher Taxa" by Murray in this *Manual*).

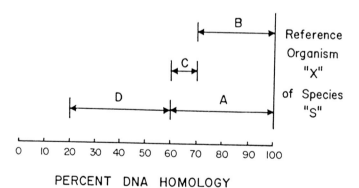

PERCENT DNA HOMOLOGY

Figure III.1. Proposed taxonomic groupings based upon DNA homology data. *A*, organisms belong to species "S"; *B*, varieties within subspecies to which "X" belongs; *C*, other subspecies that belong to "S"; *D*, species that are closely related to species "S."

Genetic Methods

Dorothy Jones

The use of genetic characteristics in bacterial classification is comparatively recent. It dates from the mid-1950s when bacterial gene transfer was discovered and Watson and Crick demonstrated the molecular basis of genetic information in the sequence of bases on the deoxyribonucleic acid (DNA) molecule. Since that time the development of physicochemical techniques for the analysis of the genetic material, together with the exploitation of bacteria as genetic tools, had resulted in the accumulation of material which has proved significant for bacterial systematics.

In the past 2 decades it has become clear that the genetic complement of a bacterial cell lies not only in the main chromosome but, in many cases, also in extrachromosomal elements such as plasmids, transposons and lysogenic or temperate phages. All these elements carry genetic material capable of phenotypic expression. What contribution such extrachromosomal entities make to a particular bacterial phenotype, by either direct expression or interaction with the chromosomal DNA of the cell, is only just beginning to be understood (see Broda, 1979; Harwood, 1980; Hardy, 1981).

For the bacterial taxonomist the genetic approach to systematics has great appeal both for its potential to reveal biologically significant, stable groupings (taxa) and for the elucidation of bacterial evolutionary relationships (phylogeny). Consequently, several of the newer taxonomic methods have been and are being directed towards the characterization of the genetic complement of bacteria.

Physicochemical methods for the analysis of bacterial genomes have been discussed in the previous chapter. The present chapter is concerned with genetic methods used in bacterial classification, i.e. methods based on the transfer of genes between bacteria.

CHROMOSOMAL GENE EXCHANGE

The three main classes of chromosomal gene exchange are: (a) those in which genes are transferred as soluble DNA molecules, i.e. **transformation**; (b) those involving transfer by bacteriophage, i.e. **transduction**; and (c) those involving cell contact followed by transfer of whole or part of the bacterial chromosome, i.e. **conjugation.** Of these classes, transformation studies have so far proved the most useful for determining relationships between bacteria.

Transformation

Transformation has been demonstrated usually between different taxospecies and only rarely between taxa presently recognized as different genera. Interspecific transformation has revealed three distinct homology groups among neisseriae and moraxellae. Transformation studies have indicated a close relationship between *Rhizobium leguminosarum* and *Agrobacterium tumefaciens*. Studies with the micrococci have shown a close relationship between *Micrococcus luteus* and *M. lylae* that, in this case, was confirmed by DNA reassociation studies in vitro. Similar studies have shown a low rate of transformation between *Pasteurella multocida, P. haemolytica, P. ureae* and *P. pneumotropica*, taxa which are also closely related on phenetic and DNA reassociation criteria. A great deal of transformation work has been done on the genus *Haemophilus. Haemophilus influenzae, H. aegyptius* and *H. parainfluenzae* appear to be closely related.

Transformation of chromosomal DNA has been demonstrated also among other taxa, and there is no doubt that it is a good indication of the degree of relatedness between different taxospecies and can highlight areas of taxonomic homogeneity and heterogeneity (Jones and Sneath, 1970; Bøvre, 1980).

Transduction

In transduction, host chromosomal material is incorporated into a bacteriophage by several mechanisms and transmitted from one bacteriophage host to another by phage-mediated transduction. Only a small range of bacterial groups are presently known to be susceptible to transduction, e.g. the *Enterobacteriaceae*, the genus *Bacillus*, pseudomonads and some streptococci. Not much is known about how readily strains of the same species can be transduced, but the host range pattern of the transducing bacteriophages is probably a major limiting factor. It has been suggested also that the greater difficulties associated with transduction are due to the larger sizes of the DNA fragments involved in transduction compared with those involved in transformation, with the larger fragments being less easily integrated into the recipient chromosome. Again this mechanism of genetic transfer appears to have significance for bacterial classification only at the taxospecies level, and its usefulness is further restricted by the host range of bacteriophages (see Jones and Sneath, 1970).

It is appropriate here to mention the other roles of bacteriophages in bacterial classification. As noted earlier, a temperate bacteriophage can lysogenize in a host bacterium and express its genetic information as phenotypic characters different from those typical of the bacterium devoid of phage. The consequences of this for bacterial classification will be dealt with later (see "Extrachromosomal Elements"). Additionally, and this is perhaps their best known feature, virulent bacteriophages infect and lyse bacteria. The process is referred to as **phage lysis.**

The inclusion of phage lysis in a section dealing with genetic methods may cause the reader some surprise. Phage lysis of the bacterial cell (as distinct from the much less specific phage adsorption, or killing of the cell followed by lysis from without) involves phage infection with phage multiplication but without lysogenization. In bacteriophage infection, the genes of the virulent phage are transferred and expressed, even though they are not integrated into the host chromosome or, of course, in the lineage of the recipient. Specific phage receptors are necessary for the adsorption of virulent phage on to the recipient bacterial cell; once in the cell the phage may be repressed if the bacterium is carrying a homologous prophage, or it may be restricted enzymically. The ability of two bacterial strains to support the growth of a given virulent phage may reflect similarity in only one or two host genes. Therefore, the technique has little value for *bacterial classification.* However, the value of phage lysis cross-reactions for *bacterial identification* is high. The reported host range of bacteriophages extends from those specific for very few strains of one taxospecies, to those that can lyse bacteria which are currently placed in different bacterial genera, families and even orders. However, most reports in the literature show that most phages lyse a significant proportion of strains belonging to the same taxospecies as the propagating strain. Phage-typing schemes are playing increasingly important epidemiological and identification roles among a number of bacterial groups, e.g. some pyogenic streptococci, staphylococci and enterobacteria.

Conjugation

This method of gene exchange refers to the transfer of the whole or a portion of the bacterial chromosome following cell-to-cell contact. The conjugation system is best understood among the coliforms (Curtiss, 1969). Similar systems have been noted among other genera, such as *Pseudomonas, Vibrio, Pasteurella* and *Rhizobium,* and are known to occur among other groups, but the mechanism is less well understood. In the streptococci there is evidence that in some cases the bacteria make use of sex pheromones to generate cell-to-cell contact (Clewell, 1981). Transfer of bacterial chromosomal material by conjugation has not been reported so frequently as has transfer by transformation or transduction. However, evidence suggests that it takes place only between closely related taxa.

Bacterial taxonomy has not, to date, benefited greatly from studies involving genetic exchange of chromosomal material and the concept of a bacterial genospecies is far from being realized. However, bacteriologists no longer believe that gene transfer is so rare among bacteria that it is of no consequence for natural bacterial populations. In the past 2 decades it has been recognized that gene transfer, particularly involving phages, plasmids and transposons, their interaction with each other, and the bacterial chromosome together with the gene transfer mediated by insertion sequences, can be a significant factor in bacterial variation. This variation has obvious consequences for bacterial systematics.

EXTRACHROMOSOMAL ELEMENTS

Plasmids, transposons and phages are collectively referred to as extrachromosomal elements (Novick, 1969; Broda, 1979; Hardy, 1981). Their transfer between bacteria is essentially by the same mechanisms as those described under "Chromosomal Gene Exchange." Phages play a role in the transduction of all genetic material between bacteria, and it is now recognized that the F' factor is a plasmid. It is therefore probably artificial to make too clear a distinction between the transfer of chromosomal DNA and that of extrachromosomal elements between bacteria. Transformation by chromosomal DNA may or may not be accompanied by plasmid DNA. In transduction, phages can carry a portion of the chromosomal or plasmid DNA, and in conjugation, plasmid and chromosomal DNA can be transferred at the same time. The situation is far more complex than was previously realized (Novick, 1969; Hardy, 1981; Clewell, 1981).

A range of methods now exists for the isolation of extrachromosomal genetic elements from bacteria and for their analyses by physicochemical methods. A good account is given by Hardy (1981).

The two aspects of extrachromosomal elements which are of prime interest to the bacterial taxonomist are their ability to code for phenotypic traits in a range of bacteria and their significance in evolution.

Phenotypic Traits

Plasmids have been observed in virtually every bacterial genus examined. Many plasmids detected by physical screening methods are not known to code for any phenotypic trait in the host bacterium. They are called **cryptic plasmids.** The fact that their presence has not been correlated with a phenotypic characteristic does not mean that they do not code for such a trait. It may be that their particular phenotypic traits have not been identified.

Phenotypic traits known to be coded for by plasmids include resistance to a variety of antibiotics, heavy metal ions and ultraviolet light; production of enterotoxin, exfoliate toxin, the surface antigens K88 and K89, hemolysins, proteases, bacteriocins, urease and H_2S; metabolism of lactose, sucrose, raffinose and citrate; degradation of a variety of organic compounds such as camphor, octanol and toluene (at least part of the remarkable diversity shown by pseudomonads in the degradation of organic compounds is due to the presence of degradative plasmids); and nitrogen fixation. Preliminary evidence suggests that the production of gas vacuoles in *Halobacterium* is controlled by a plasmid. There is also evidence that pigment, coagulase, and fibrolysin production in staphylococci are plasmid determined. It also seems highly probable that among the streptococci the production of serum opacity factor, M protein production, nisin production and the ability to ferment galactose and xylose are plasmid-coded.

Transposons found on the plasmids of Gram-negative bacteria have been shown to code for resistance to a number of antibiotics, lactose fermentation (in *Yersinia enterocolitica*), heat stable toxin (in *Escherichia coli*), and doubtless others coding for other phenotypic traits will be found. Full accounts of the phenotypic traits conferred on bacteria by plasmids and transposons are given by Harwood (1980), Clewell (1981) and Hardy (1981).

The classic example of a phage-encoded phenotypic trait is the diphtheria toxin which was shown by Freeman in 1950 to be produced only when *Corynebacterium diphtheriae* is lysogenized by a particular phage. The structural gene for the protein toxin is on the phage chromosome. This phage can lysogenize and synthesize toxin in a number of closely related corynebacteria, viz. *C. diphtheriae, C. ulcerans* and *C. ovis* (Barksdale, 1970).

Effect of Extrachromosomal Elements on Classification and Identification

Since these elements confer extra phenotypic traits on their hosts, they could have a marked effect on bacterial classification if those characters were ones on which the classification was based. Two examples of the presence of plasmids which relate to species nomenclature are the plasmid-coded hemolysin of *Streptococcus faecalis,* which resulted in the naming of such plasmid-bearing strains as *Streptococcus faecalis* var. *zymogenes,* and the plasmid-determining citrate utilization in *Streptococcus lactis,* which appears to be responsible for the name *Streptococcus lactis* subsp. *diacetylactis.* However, the effect of an extrachromosomal coded trait on a classification based on a large number of characters would normally be expected to be small, and this has proved to be the case in the few preliminary studies so far conducted.

Such characters can, however, affect the identification of bacteria when the identification is based on a small number of characters and considerable weight is placed on individual features, e.g. lactose fermentation in the identification of enterobacteria. It is best therefore if identification schemes are based on stable features chosen as a result of a taxonomic study where a large number of characters have been employed, e.g. computer-assisted classifications (numerical taxonomy). Ideally, computer-based identification matrices derived from such studies should be employed. The risk of a misidentification due to the loss or gain of one or two phenotypic characters is thereby reduced to a minimum.

It has been suggested that strains known to carry extrachromosomal elements should be excluded from taxonomic studies. Such a policy is not practical because present methods do not always detect such strains; further, it is believed that many bacterial populations depend on the presence of these elements for their survival. It has also been suggested that known or suspected extrachromosomal coded characters should be excluded when classifications are constructed. Again, present methods do not allow all such characters to be determined; besides, such characters may have taxonomic relevance.

Bacteriologists should accept that extrachromosomal elements do contribute to bacterial variation. This variation should therefore be recognized, and due allowance made, when bacterial taxa are described and when identification schemes are constructed.

Extrachromosomal Elements and Evolution

At the present time the relative contributions of mutation and recombination to bacterial evolution are difficult to assess. Mutation results in changes in the protein structure of the organism. Recombination leads to the rearrangement of existing genes. Until recently, little attention was paid to the possible involvement of gene rearrangement in evolution. The recognition that gene transfer involving extrachromosomal elements can be a significant factor in bacterial variation has led to a view that these elements have played an important role in bacterial evolution. Whether or not the role which these elements play in contemporary bacterial variation and adaptation is one of the major ways in which bacteria have evolved from the earliest times is still not resolved (Cullum and Saedler, 1981; Hardy, 1981; Koch, 1981; Reanney, 1976).

BACTERIAL CLASSIFICATION V

Serology and Chemotaxonomy

Dorothy Jones and Noel R. Krieg

Serology and chemotaxonomy are both methods for investigating the molecular architecture of the bacterial cell, although the methodologies used in the two techniques are quite different.

SEROLOGY

Serological techniques depend on the ability of the chemical constituents of bacterial cells to behave as antigens, i.e. to elicit the production of antibodies in vertebrate animals. The antibodies used in serological studies are the humoral antibodies found in the blood serum and referred to as antiserum. Monoclonal antibodies, highly specific serological agents directed against specific antigenic determinants (epitopes), are now being used increasingly in serological studies (Macario and Conway de Macario, 1985).

Serological techniques used include agglutination, precipitation (including many refinements, e.g. use of gels and electrophoretic techniques), complement fixation and immunofluorescence. Details of the techniques may be found in a number of immunological or microbiological textbooks.

Serological studies of value in bacterial taxonomy can be divided into two broad classes: (a) those concerned with detecting differences or similarities between bacteria **on the basis of their cell surface and associated antigenic complement** (e.g. flagella, pili, cell walls, cytoplasmic membranes, capsules and slime layers) and (b) the use of antisera raised against purified enzymes to assess **structural similarities between homologous proteins from different bacteria.**

Cell Surface and Associated Antigens

On the basis of the antigenic complexity of their surface antigens (cell wall lipopolysaccharide, flagella and capsule constituents), the genera of the family *Enterobacteriaceae* can be divided into many serovars; e.g. more than 1000 serovars have been detected within the genus *Salmonella* (Kauffmann, 1966). Contrary to the view of Kauffmann (1966) these serovars do not represent separate taxospecies. The information derived from serological studies of a group such as the enterobacteria is now so large, and so many cross-reactions occur, that in the absence of any methods (e.g. computer programs) for analyzing the plethora of data in an objective fashion, it is generally accepted that these techniques are of little value in classification but are valuable in epidemiological studies.

Serological studies of the streptococci based on the use of acid-extracted polysaccharide antigens (Lancefield, 1933, 1934) have resulted in the division of the genus *Streptococcus* into a number (now approaching 30) of serological groups labeled A, B, C, etc. Until fairly recently, very great emphasis was placed on the serological grouping of streptococci for purposes of both classification and identification.

Although some serological groups correspond to distinct taxospecies (e.g. serological group A (*S. pyogenes*) and serological group B (*S. agalactiae*)), other serological groups comprise more than one taxospecies (e.g. serological groups C, D and N), while serological groups G, H and K do not serve to define any good taxa (see Jones, 1978).

Other serological studies of this kind have been based on the use of different classes of antigenic material, e.g. cell walls, spore suspensions. A review of the serochemical specificity and location of antigens in the bacterial cell, together with observations on the significance of such serological studies for bacterial classification, has been provided by Cummins (1962). A comprehensive review on the use of monoclonal antibodies as molecular probes for complex structures such as the bacterial cell surface, cell membrane and spores is that of Macario and Conway de Macario (1985).

Use of Antisera Raised against Purified Proteins

The basis of this approach is that one antiserum raised against a purified enzyme can be used to detect the serological cross-reactions of homologous proteins in crude extracts of other bacteria if the bacteria possess the same enzyme. The use of microcomplement fixation techniques makes this approach a very sensitive one. Comparative studies on purified proteins of known primary structure have indicated that there is a very high correlation between the amino acid sequence of the proteins and the degree of serological similarity (see later section on "Amino Acid Sequences"). Examples of this approach include studies of the muconate-lactonizing enzymes of the *Pseudomonadaceae* (Stanier et al., 1970), the fructose diphosphate aldolases of the lactic acid bacteria (London and Kline, 1973), and the catalases of staphylococci and micrococci. In the instance of the staphylococci, a very high correlation has been shown to exist between the serological relationships of their catalases and genetic relatedness based on DNA/DNA homology data (see Kandler and Schleifer, 1980).

Similar studies on the transaldolases of several species of bifidobacteria (Sgorbati and Scardovi, 1979; Sgorbati, 1979) indicate that the genus *Bifidobacterium* contains several distinct clusters based on the index of dissimilarity of their respective aldolases. In some instances there was good correlation between the clusters so obtained and clusters formed on the basis of other criteria, but in others the correlation was not so high.

Baumann et al. (1980) and Bang et al. (1981) found the immunological relationships among glutamine synthetases and superoxide dismutases of *Vibrio* and *Photobacterium* species were in good agreement with relationships based on rRNA/DNA homology experiments. The amino acid sequence of the glutamine synthetases was conserved to a greater extent than was that of the superoxide dismutases, and this supports the idea that the study of proteins having different evolutionary rates can permit the resolution of close, intermediate and distant relationships among organisms.

It should be noted that serological homology studies of proteins, like many other techniques, have their limitations. There is evidence that the approach is useful only for the study of proteins with relatively high (70% or greater) sequence homologies. Further, serological techniques measure similarities only at the surface of proteins, and it is at the protein surface that the greatest number of amino acid changes occur. The results can be influenced also by the number of antigenic sites per protein molecule. Nevertheless, serological techniques of this kind provide a rapid and convenient method for assessing structural similarities between homologous proteins and are useful in the classification of bacteria and can also cast some light on possible phylogenetic relationships. The use of monoclonal antibodies to detect particular cell constituents, enzymes and toxins in vitro and in vivo is reviewed by Macario and Conway de Macario (1985).

CHEMOTAXONOMY

During the past 20 years or so, the application of chemical and physical techniques to elucidate the chemical composition of whole bacterial cells or parts of cells has produced information of great value in the classification and identification of bacteria. Indeed, so useful have some of the data generated proved to be that the word "chemotaxonomy," used to describe the classification of bacteria on the basis of their chemical composition, is now firmly entrenched in the literature (see Schleifer and Stackebrandt, 1983; Goodfellow and Minnikin, 1985).

In addition, techniques such as gas chromatography have allowed the more precise analysis of the products of fermentation, and there is a growing awareness of the taxonomic significance of enzyme systems and their regulation as opposed to the detection of individual enzymes.

Cell Wall Composition

The characteristic cell wall polymer of many procaryotes, present in Gram-negative and Gram-positive bacteria and in the cyanobacteria, is peptidoglycan (murein). Peptidoglycan is not found in the mycoplasmas, and conventional peptidoglycan (containing muramic acid) is not present in the *Archaeobacteria*. The chemical structure of the peptidoglycan of Gram-negative bacteria is, with few exceptions, reasonably uniform. However, the variation in qualitative amino acid and/or sugar composition, especially the variation in the primary structure of the peptidoglycans of various Gram-positive bacteria, has provided information of enormous taxonomic value.

The cell wall composition of Gram-positive bacteria was one of the earliest useful chemotaxonomic characters. On the basis of the analysis of the purified cell walls of Gram-positive bacteria, Cummins and Harris (1956) suggested that the cell wall amino acid composition might prove to be an important taxonomic criterion at the generic level and that the sugar composition might help to distinguish between species. Subsequent studies have indicated this to be the case. The amino acids present in the cell wall are now an accepted important part of the generic description. Information from cell wall analysis of the type done by Cummins and Harris (1956) has proved of especial value among the coryneform group of bacteria (see Keddie and Bousfield, 1980, for a comprehensive review).

Information of even greater taxonomic value has resulted from the methods devised by Schleifer and Kandler (1967) and used by them and their associates to determine the peptidoglycan types of a wide range of Gram-positive bacteria (see Schleifer and Kandler, 1972; Kandler and Schleifer, 1980; Schleifer and Seidl, 1985). This approach has revealed differences between bacteria which could not possibly have been detected by qualitative cell wall analysis. The methods for determining differences in peptidoglycan types are, however, quite specialized and cannot be used routinely to screen large numbers of bacteria.

More recently, a number of "rapid" methods have been developed for the routine screening of bacteria to determine those cell wall components which have been shown to be of the greatest discriminatory value in bacterial classification and identification. The reviews of Keddie and Bousfield (1980), Kandler and Schleifer (1980), Bousfield et al. (1985) and Schleifer and Seidl (1985) contain references to the pertinent literature.

A novel peptidoglycan, the so-called pseudomurein, characterized by the replacement of muramic acid by talosaminouronic acid, has been found to be the typical cell wall constituent of the genus *Methanobacterium,* which taxon is now recognized as a member of the *Archaeobacteria* (see Kandler and Schleifer, 1980). The same cell wall polymer has been detected in the archaeobacterial genus *Methanobrevibacter.* Other of the *Archaeobacteria* possess a thick cell wall composed of heteropolysaccharides or a cell envelope consisting of glycoproteins or proteins. *Thermoplasma* lacks a cell wall but contains a glycoprotein in the cell membrane (see Schleifer and Stackebrandt (1983).

Lipid Composition

Among the procaryotes there are two quite distinct lipid categories. The *Archaeobacteria* contain isopranyl-branched ether-linked lipids but not aliphatic ester-linked lipids which are present in other bacteria. The presence of isopranyl-branched ether-linked lipids serves to distinguish the *Archaeobacteria.* Further details of archaeobacterial lipids are given by Kates (1978), Langworthy (1982) and Schleifer and Stackebrandt (1983).

Lipids occur in the cytoplasmic membranes of all eubacteria and in the cell wall complex of Gram-negative bacteria and certain Gram-positive bacteria such as the genera *Corynebacterium* and *Mycobacterium.* The eubacterial lipids comprise a number of different classes, and in the past decade, it has become increasingly clear that at least some of these lipids have chemotaxonomic potential (see Lechevalier, 1977; Schleifer and Stackebrandt, 1983; Goodfellow and Minnikin, 1985).

The fatty acid composition of the bacterial cell has proved useful in the classification of certain bacteria, and in some cases the fatty acid pattern may be characteristic for a particular taxon (see Lechevalier, 1977). However, it should be noted that the fatty acid patterns obtained may be influenced by a number of factors: composition of growth medium, temperature of incubation, age of culture, and techniques employed to analyze the sample.

A special category of fatty acids free from the aforementioned limitations are the mycolic acids. These long-chain 3-hydroxy 2-branched acids have been found, so far, only in the taxa *Bacterionema, Corynebacterium, Micropolyspora, Mycobacterium, Nocardia* and *Rhodococcus.* Differences in the structure of their component mycolic acids have proved to be a valuable criterion in the classification and identification of members of these taxa (see Minnikin and Goodfellow, 1980; Collins et al., 1982; Goodfellow and Minnikin, 1985).

Another class of lipids of recognized chemotaxonomic potential are the polar lipids which occur in all bacteria. The most common polar lipid types are the phospholipids and the glycolipids. Phospholipids occur in many bacteria, but certain actinomycetes and coryneform bacteria contain very characteristic phospholipids, the phosphatidylinositol mannosides. Other highly characteristic phospholipids include phosphosphingolipids found in certain Gram-negative taxa, e.g. *Bacteroides* (see Lechevalier, 1977). Glycolipids (glycosyldiacylglycerols) are widely distributed among Gram-positive bacteria and can also be used as chemotaxonomic markers (see Shaw, 1975; Schleifer and Stackebrandt, 1983).

Other lipids with chemotaxonomic potential include hopanoids, hydrocarbons and carotenoids.

Isoprenoid Quinones

Isoprenoid quinones are a class of terpenoid lipids located in the cytoplasmic membranes of many bacteria. They play important roles in electron transport, oxidative phosphorylation and, possibly, active transport. Their potential as an aid to the classification of bacteria was recognized by Jeffries et al. (1969), Yamada et al. (1976) and others (see Collins and Jones, 1981). Representatives of one, or more than one, of the three main types, ubiquinones, menaquinones and demethylmenaquinones, are present in the majority of procaryotes so far examined. The cyanobacteria contain neither ubiquinones nor menaquinones. However, they do contain phylloquinones and plastoquinones which are indigenous to the plant kingdom but not normally found in bacteria. All the mycoplasmas so far examined contain menaquinones only. Among the *Achaeobacteria* no isoprenoid quinones have been detected in the fastidious anaerobic species *Methanobacterium thermoautotrophicum*, a situation in keeping with that most commonly, but not invariably, found among the strictly anaerobic eubacteria. An unusual terpenoid, caldariellaquinone, has been detected in the extreme acidophile "*Caldariella acidophila*." The other *Archaeobacteria* examined possess menaquinones.

The majority of the strictly aerobic, Gram-negative bacteria produce only ubiquinones, with the exception of cytophagas and myxobacters which produce only menaquinones. Facultatively anaerobic, Gram-negative bacteria contain ubiquinones, menaquinones or demethylmenaquinones or a combination of the three. Strictly anaerobic, Gram-negative bacteria (e.g. the genus *Bacteroides*) produce only menaquinones.

The majority of the aerobic and facultatively anaerobic Gram-positive bacteria produce only menaquinones. Most streptococci do not contain any isoprenoid quinones, but demethylmenaquinones are present in *Streptococcus faecalis*, and menaquinones have been detected in "*S. faecium* subsp. *casseliflavus*" and *S. lactis*. Similarly, members of the genus *Lactobacillus* generally lack isoprenoid quinones, but recently, low levels of an uncharacterized menaquinone have been detected in one strain of *L. brevis*. Uncharacterized menaquinones have also been reported in some strains of the strictly anaerobic genus *Clostridium*, although, in general, this genus lacks quinones.

The current data on isoprenoid quinone structural types in bacteria and their implications for taxonomy are reviewed by Collins and Jones (1981). From the available data on procaryotes in general, it appears that menaquinones have far greater discriminatory value that ubiquinones. Menaquinones possess not only a greater range of isoprenologs, but additional modifications such as ring demethylation and partial hydrogenation of the polyprenyl side chain occur. The available data strongly suggest that these compounds will be of considerable value in the classification of micrococci, staphylococci, coryneform bacteria and certain actinomycetes (see Collins and Jones, 1981).

Cytochrome Composition

Cytochromes are specialized forms of hemoproteins which are involved in a variety of redox processes in the procaryote cell. They can be assigned to four main classes, *a*, *b*, *c*, and *d*, according to the structures of their heme prosthetic groups. Cytochrome *o* is an autoxidizable *b* type cytochrome.

Two basic methods are available which use cytochromes as an aid to classification and identification of bacteria; the "pattern" and the "structure" approach. The former compares the cytochrome patterns of different bacterial species as compared by conventional difference spectrophotometry (see Meyer and Jones, 1973); the latter compares primary structures and, where possible, the tertiary structures of easily purified cytochrome *c* as determined by amino acid sequence and x-ray diffraction (see Ambler, 1976, and the later section on "Amino Acid Sequences").

Cytochrome patterns show greater variation among the procaryotes than among eucaryotes and can therefore be a useful aid in bacterial classification. Qualitative analyses of the cytochrome composition of over 200 species of bacteria have now been done. The results indicate that the heterotrophic Gram-positive bacteria comprise a rather homogeneous grouping, with cytochromes $bcaa_3o$ forming the predominant pattern. There are some variations, however, and cytochrome *c* is often absent from facultatively anaerobic Gram-positive bacteria. Some lactic acid bacteria, when grown on a heme-containing medium, contain only cytochrome *b*. Propionibacteria exhibit a cytochrome bda_1 pattern. The genus *Clostridium* lacks cytochromes. It is of interest that the cytochrome $bcaa_3o$ pattern of logarithmic growth-phase cells of the aerobe *Arthrobacter globiformis* changes to $bcaa_3od$ when the cells become oxygen-limited and lose their ability to retain the crystal violet-iodine complex in the Gram stain. Cytochrome *d* is characteristic of many Gram-negative bacteria.

In contrast, the Gram-negative heterotrophic bacteria form a much less homogeneous group on the basis of cytochrome composition. The majority have the basic pattern $bcdoa_1$ from which *c* may often be absent. Cytochrome c_{co} appears to be characteristic of methylotrophs; however, it is also present in the nonmethylotrophic genus *Chromobacterium*. The phototrophic bacteria contain cytochromes *b* and *c* when grown photosynthetically, but when grown aerobically in the absence of light, there are differences between the taxa. The obligately aerobic chemolithotrophs exhibit the cytochrome pattern $bcaa_3oq$, with some occasional omissions. Neither the phototrophs nor the chemolithotrophs have been shown to produce cytochrome *d*.

There is now sufficient evidence available to indicate that cytochrome patterns, in conjunction with other evidence, are useful guides in bacterial classification. There is, however, little evidence that cytochrome patterns will be useful for purposes of identification, mainly because bacteria contain relatively few types of spectrally distinct cytochromes. A comprehensive review of the use of cytochrome patterns in bacterial classification is that of Jones (1980).

It should be stressed that when cytochrome patterns are used for taxonomic purposes, the influence of the growth environment should be taken into account. Growth conditions can influence the quantitative and, to a lesser extent, the qualitative cytochrome content of bacteria.

Amino Acid Sequences of Various Proteins

Comparison of the amino acid sequence of specific kinds of proteins or of properties, such as antigenic reactivity, which reflect the amino acid sequence of these proteins has been used as a measure of phylogenetic relationships among organisms. The fundamental concept involved is that most extant proteins are likely to have evolved from a very small number of archetypal proteins by the processes of genetic duplication and modification. In comparing the proteins of any particular group (such as cytochrome *c*, superoxide dismutase, ferredoxin or other enzymes), the greater the difference in amino acid sequence between the protein of one organism and the corresponding protein of another organism, the greater is believed to be the evolutionary divergence between the two organisms. Conversely, if the amino acid sequence of corresponding proteins from two organisms is very similar, the two organisms are believed to be closely related phylogenetically. Even distant relationships between organisms can be deduced by this approach, and various phylogenetic schemes have been constructed to reflect the perceived evolutionary development of a great variety of organisms, both procaryotic and eucaryotic (see the review by Schwartz and Dayhoff, 1978). Among the proteins that have been used for such studies are ferredoxins, flavodoxins, azurins, plastocyanins, and cytochrome *c*. For example, a remarkable similarity in the structure of cytochrome *c* exists between certain nonsulfur purple photosynthetic bacteria (i.e. *Rhodopseudomonas capsulatus* and *R. sphaeroides*), the nonphotosynthetic respiring bacterium *Paracoccus denitrificans,* and the mitochondria of eucaryotic organisms; this and other kinds of congruent data have led to the view that *P. denitrificans* descended from nonsulfur purple bacteria by loss of photosynthetic properties and that this species is the procaryote that most closely resembles the putative procaryotic ancestor of mitochondria (see the exposition by Dickerson (1980) as well as a critical review of the various theories for the endosymbiont origin of mitochondria and chloroplasts by Gray and Doolittle (1982)). Reservations about many of the conclusions based on cytochrome *c* sequences have been expressed by Ambler et al. (1979a, b), and an analysis of some of the limitations involved in comparing amino acid sequences of proteins has been given by Doolittle (1981).

Protein Profiles

The basic premise here is that closely related organisms should have similar or identical kinds of cellular proteins. Two-dimensional electrophoretic and isoelectric focusing procedures (O'Farrell, 1975) have made it possible to resolve several hundred proteins from a cell extract. The protein "fingerprint" so obtained for one bacterial strain is a reflection of the genetic background of that strain and can be compared with the "fingerprints" from other strains as a measure of relatedness. For examples of the application of this method, see the comparison of *Rhizobium* strains made by Roberts et al. (1980) and the comparison of *Spiroplasma* strains made by Mouches et al. (1979). The method requires a considerable degree of standardization in order to yield optimum results.

One-dimensional polyacrylamide gel electrophoresis (PAGE) of cellular proteins can yield patterns of up to ~30 bands, and although it is not comparable in resolving power to the two-dimensional separation method, it can distinguish related organisms from unrelated organisms. In general, whole cells or cellular membrane fractions are used, and the proteins are solubilized by means of a detergent such as sodium dodecyl sulfate (SDS); however, many studies have employed merely the water-soluble proteins ("soluble" fraction) from disintegrated cells. A few examples of the application of PAGE are: identification of mycoplasmas (Razin and Rottem, 1967), taxonomy of *Haemophilus* strains (Nicolet et al., 1980), comparison of isolates from gingival crevice floras (Moore et al., 1980), and differentiation of isolates of indigenous *Rhizobium* populations (Noel and Brill, 1980). By use of rigorously standardized conditions, extremely reproducible protein patterns can be obtained which are amenable to rapid, computerized, numerical analysis (Kersters and De Ley, 1975).

In an analysis of the patterns of soluble cellular proteins from strains of 70 *Clostridium* species, Cato et al. (1982) found that strains having >80% DNA/DNA homology usually produced identical patterns, strains related by ~70% homology showed overall similarity of the total patterns but also showed minor differences, and strains unrelated by DNA homology showed major differences. In many instances, the patterns obtained within 24 h of isolating an organism were sufficiently distinctive so that the identity of the organism could be strongly suspected.

Enzyme Characterization

It is now recognized that the functional and structural patterns displayed by certain bacterial enzymes provide data of use in classification.

Good examples are the diverse regulatory and molecular size patterns exhibited by bacterial citrate synthases and succinate thiokinases. Both of these are enzymes of the citric acid (Krebs) cycle, and the near universal occurrence of this cycle in living cells makes it a very suitable pathway for comparative studies between different organisms (see Weitzman, 1980).

In general, the citrate synthases of Gram-negative bacteria are inhibited by reduced nicotinamide adenine dinucleotide (NADH), while those of Gram-positive bacteria are not. The citrate synthases of Gram-negative bacteria can be further divided into two classes on the basis of whether their NADH sensitivity is overcome by adenosine monophosphate (AMP). Citrate synthases from the majority of strictly aerobic Gram-negative bacteria are reactivated by AMP, while those of the facultatively anaerobic Gram-negative bacteria are not. Citrate synthases of the Gram-negative facultative anaerobes are also inhibited by α-oxoglutarate, but the enzymes from the aerobic Gram-negative bacteria and from Gram-positive bacteria are not. Citrate synthases of the cyanobacteria are not inhibited by NADH, but they are inhibited by α-oxoglutarate and by succinylcoenzyme A.

Bacterial citrate synthases fall into two groups, "large" and "small," on the basis of molecular size. The majority of Gram-negative bacteria possess large citrate synthases (mol. wt. ~250,000), while the majority of Gram-positive bacteria produce citrate synthases of the small type (mol. wt. ~100,000).

Exceptions to the broad general pattern occur. The citrate synthases of the Gram-negative genus *Acetobacter* do not appear to be inhibited by NADH, although the enzyme is of the large type. On the other hand, the citrate synthase of *Thermus aquaticus* is both insensitive to NADH and of the small type. In both respects it resembles the citrate synthases of the archaeobacterial genus *Halobacterium* and the majority of the citrate synthases of Gram-positive bacteria.

Similar molecular size patterns occur among bacterial succinate thiokinases. All succinate thiokinases from the Gram-positive bacteria so far studied are of the small type (mol. wt. 70,000–75,000), whereas those of Gram-negative bacteria, cyanobacteria and *Halobacterium* species are of the large type (mol. wt. 140,000–150,000). Bacterial succinate thiokinases can be further subdivided on the basis of their specificity for nucleotide substrates (guanosine diphosphate or inosine diphosphate), and preliminary results point to interesting patterns of enzyme diversity of possible potential in bacterial classification.

Rapid methods are now available for the routine laboratory screening of bacterial citrate synthases, and as further such methods are developed, it is likely that the regulatory and molecular properties of these and other enzymes will prove useful in the classification of bacteria (see Weitzman, 1980).

Fermentation Product Profiles

The use of gas-liquid chromatographic methods to analyze the fatty acids formed as end products of protein or carbohydrate metabolism is particularly useful in the classification and identification of the anaerobic genera *Clostridium, Bacteroides, Eubacterium*, etc. (see Holdeman et al., 1977).

Bacterial Nomenclature

Peter H. A. Sneath

SCOPE OF NOMENCLATURE

Nomenclature has been called the handmaid of taxonomy. The need for a stable set of names for living organisms, and rules to regulate them, has been recognized for over a century. The rules are embodied in international codes of nomenclature. There are separate codes for animals, noncultivated plants, cultivated plants, bacteria and viruses. But partly because the rules are framed in legalistic language (so as to avoid imprecision), they are often difficult to understand. Useful commentaries are found in Ainsworth and Sneath (1962), Cowan (1978) and Jeffrey (1977).

The nomenclature of the different kinds of living creatures falls into two parts: (a) informal or vernacular names, or very specialized and restricted names, and (b) scientific names of taxonomic groups (taxon, plural taxa).

Examples of the first are vernacular names from a disease, strain numbers, the symbols for antigenic variants, and the symbols for genetic variants. Thus one can have a vernacular name such as the tubercle bacillus, a strain with the designation K12, a serological form with the antigenic formula Ia, and a genetic mutant requiring valine for growth labeled *val*. These names are usually not controlled by the codes of nomenclature, although the codes may recommend good practice for them.

Examples of scientific names are the names of species, genera and higher ranks. Thus *Mycobacterium tuberculosis* is the scientific name of the tubercle bacillus, a species of bacterium.

These scientific names are regulated by the codes (with few exceptions) and have two things in common: (a) they are all Latinized in form so as to be easily recognized as scientific names, and (b) they possess definite positions in the taxonomic hierarchy. These names are international: thus microbiologists of all nations know what is meant by *Bacillus anthracis,* but few would know it under vernacular names such as Milzbrandbacillus or Bactéridie de charbon.

The scientific names of bacteria are regulated by the International Code of Nomenclature of Bacteria, which is also known as the Revised Code and was most recently published in 1975 (Lapage et al.). This edition authorized a new starting date for names of bacteria on January 1, 1980, and the starting document is the Approved Lists of Bacterial Names (Skerman et al., 1980), which contains all the scientific names of bacteria that retain their nomenclatural validity from the past. The operation of these Lists will be referred to later. The Code and the Lists are under the aegis of the International Committee on Systematic Bacteriology, which is a constituent part of the International Union of Microbiological Societies. The Committee is assisted by a number of Taxonomic Subcommittees on different groups of bacteria and by the Judicial Commission which considers amendments to the Code and any exceptions that may be needed to specific Rules.

LATINIZATION

Since scientific names are in Latinized form, they obey the grammar of classic or medieval Latin. Fortunately the necessary grammar is not very difficult, and the commonest point to watch is that adjectives agree in gender with the substantives they qualify. Some examples are given later. The names of genera and species are normally printed in italics (or underlined in manuscripts to indicate italic font). For higher categories, conventions vary: in Britain they are often in ordinary roman type, but in the United States they are usually in italics, which is preferable because this reminds the reader they are Latinized scientific names.

TAXONOMIC HIERARCHY

The taxonomic hierarchy is a conventional arrangement. Each level above the basic level of species is increasingly inclusive. The names belong to successive **categories**, each of which possesses a position in the hierarchy called its **rank.** The lowest category ordinarily employed is that of species, though sometimes these are subdivided into subspecies.

The main categories in decreasing rank, with their vernacular and Latin forms and examples, are shown in Table VI.1.

Additional categories may sometimes be intercalated (e.g. subclass below class, and tribe below family.)

Table VI.1.
Ranking of taxonomic categories

Category	Example[a]
Kingdom (*Regnum*)	*Procaryotae*
Phylum (*Phylum*) in zoology or Division (*Divisio*) in botany and bacteriology	*Gracilicutes*
Class (*Classis*)	*Scotobacteria*
Order (*Ordo*)	*Rickettsiales*
Family (*Familia*)	*Rickettsiaceae*
Genus (*Genus*)	*Coxiella*
Species (*Species*)	*Coxiella burnetii*

[a]Based on the classification given by Murray in the chapter on "The Higher Taxa" in this *Manual.*

FORM OF NAMES

The form of Latinized names differs with the category. The species name consists of two parts. The first is the **genus name.** This is spelled with an initial capital letter and is a Latinized substantive. The second is the **specific epithet** and is spelled with a lower case initial letter. The epithet is a Latinized adjective in agreement with the gender of the genus name, or a Latin word in the genitive case, or occasionally a noun in apposition. Thus in *Mycobacterium tuberculosis,* the epithet *tuberculosis* means "of tubercle," so the species name means the mycobacterium of tuberculosis. The species name is called a **binominal name, or binomen,** because it has two parts. When subspecies names are used, a trinominal name results, with the addition of an extra **subspecific epithet.** An example is the subspecies of *Lactobacillus casei* that is called *Lactobacillus casei* subsp. *rhamnosus.* In this name, *casei* is the specific epithet and *rhamnosus* is the subspecific epithet. The existence of a subspecies such as *rhamnosus* implies the existence of another subspecies, in which the subspecific and specific epithets are identical, i.e. *Lactobacillus casei* subsp. *casei.*

One problem that frequently arises is the scientific status of a species. It may be difficult to know whether an entity differs from its neighbors in certain specified ways. A useful terminology was introduced by Ravin

(1963). It may be believed, for example, that the entity can undergo genetic exchange with a nearby species, in which event they could be considered to belong to the same **genospecies.** It may be believed that the entity is not phenotypically distinct from its neighbors, in which event they could be considered to belong to the same **taxospecies.** Yet the conditions for genetic exchange may vary greatly with experimental conditions, and the criteria of distinctness may depend on what properties are considered, so that it may not be possible to make clear-cut decisions on these matters. Nevertheless, it may be convenient to give the entity a species name and to treat it in nomenclature as a separate species, a **nomenspecies.** It follows that all species in nomenclature should strictly be regarded as nomenspecies.

Genus names, as mentioned above, are Latinized nouns, and so are subgenus names (now rarely used) which are conventionally written in parentheses after the genus name; e.g. *Bacillus (Aerobacillus)* indicates the subgenus *Aerobacillus* of the genus *Bacillus.* As in the case of subspecies, this implies the existence of a subgenus *Bacillus (Bacillus).*

Above the genus level most names are plural adjectives in the feminine gender, agreeing with the word *Procaryotae,* so that *Brucellaceae* means *Procaryotae Brucellaceae,* for example.

PURPOSES OF THE CODES OF NOMENCLATURE

The codes have three main aims:

1. Names should be stable.
2. Names should be unambiguous.
3. Names should be necessary.

These three aims are sometimes contradictory, and the rules of nomenclature have to make provision for exceptions where they clash. The principles are implemented by three main devices: (a) priority of publication to assist stability, (b) establishment of nomenclatural types to ensure the names are not ambiguous, and (c) publication of descriptions to indicate that different names do refer to different entities. These are supported by subsidiary devices, such as the Latinized forms of names, and the avoidance of synonyms for the same taxon.

PRIORITY OF PUBLICATION

In order to achieve stability, the first name given to a taxon (provided the other rules are obeyed) is taken as the correct name. This is the **principle of priority.** But to be safeguarded in this way a name obviously has to be made known to the scientific community: one cannot use a name that has been kept secret. Therefore, names have to be published in the scientific literature, together with sufficient indication of what they refer to. This is called **valid publication.** If a name is merely published in the scientific literature it is called **effective publication**: to be valid it also has to satisfy additional requirements, which are summarized later.

The earliest names that must be considered are those published after an official starting date. For many groups of organisms this is Linnaeus' *Species Plantarum* of 1753, but the difficulties of knowing to what the early descriptions refer, and of searching of voluminous and growing literature, have made the principle of priority increasingly hard to obey.

The code of nomenclature for bacteria, therefore, has established a new starting date of 1980, with a new starting document, the Approved Lists of Bacterial Names (Skerman et al., 1980). This list contains names of bacterial taxa that are recognizable and in current use. Names not on the Lists lost standing in nomenclature on January 1, 1980, although there are provisions for reviving them if the taxa are subsequently rediscovered or need to be reestablished. In order to prevent the need to search the voluminous scientific literature, the new provisions for bacterial nomenclature require that for valid publication new names (including new names in patents) must be published in certain official publications. Alternatively, if the new names were effectively published in other scientific publications they must be announced in the official publications to become validly published. Priority dates from the official publication concerned. At present, the only official publication is the *International Journal of Systematic Bacteriology.*

NOMENCLATURAL TYPES

In order to make clear what names refer to, the taxa must be recognizable by other workers. In the past it was thought sufficient to publish a description of a taxon. This has been found over the years to be inadequate. Advances in techniques and in knowledge of the many undescribed species in nature have shown that old descriptions are usually insufficient. Therefore, an additional principle is employed, that of **nomenclatural types.** These are actual specimens (or names of subordinate taxa that ultimately relate to actual specimens). These type specimens are deposited in museums and other institutions. For bacteria (like some other microorganisms that are classified according to their properties in artificial culture), instead of type specimens, **type strains** are employed. The type specimens or strains are intended to be typical specimens or strains which can be compared with other material when classification or identification is undertaken, hence the word "type." However, a moment's thought will show that if a type specimen has to be designated when a taxon is *first* described and named, this will be done at a time when little has yet been found out about the new group. Therefore, it is impossible to be sure that it is indeed a typical specimen. By the time a completely typical specimen can be chosen, the taxon may be so well known that a type specimen is unnecessary: no one would now bother to designate a type specimen of a bird so well known as the common house sparrow.

The word "type" thus does *not* mean that it is typical but simply that it is a **reference specimen for the name.** This use of the word, type, is a very understandable cause for confusion that may well repay attention by the taxonomists of the future.

In recent years other type concepts have been suggested. Numerical taxonomists have proposed the hypothetical median organism (Liston et al., 1963), or the centroid: these are mathematical abstractions, not actual organisms. The most typical strain in a collection is commonly taken to be the **centrotype** (Silvestri et al., 1962), which is broadly equivalent to the strain closest to the center (centroid) of a species cluster. Some workers have suggested that several type strains should be designated. Gordon (1967) refers to this as the "population concept." One strain, however, must be the official nomenclatural type in case the species must later be divided. Gibbons (1974) proposed that the official type strain should be supplemented by reference strains that indicated the range of variation in the species, and that these strains could be termed the "type constellation." It may be noted that some of these concepts are intended to define not merely the center but, in some fashion, the limits of a species. Since these limits may well vary in different ways for different characters, or classes of characters, it will be appreciated that there may be difficulties in extending the type concept in this way. The centrotype, being a very typical strain, has often been chosen as the type strain, but otherwise these new ideas have not had much application to bacterial nomenclature.

Type strains are of the greatest importance for work on both classification and identification. These strains are preserved (by methods to minimize change to their properties) in culture collections from which they are available for study. They are obviously required for new classificatory work, so that the worker can determine whether he has new species among his material. They are also needed in diagnostic microbiology, because one of the most important principles in attempting to identify a microorganism that presents difficulties is to compare it with authentic strains of known species. The drawback that the type strain may not be entirely typical is outweighed by the fact that the type strain is, by definition, authentic.

Not all microorganisms can be cultured, and for some the function of a type can be served by a preserved specimen, a photograph, or some other device. In such instances, these are the nomenclatural types, though it is commonly considered wise to replace them by type strains when this becomes possible.

Sometimes types become lost, and new ones (**neotypes**) have to be set up to replace them: the procedure for this is described in the Code. In the past it was necessary to define certain special classes of types, but most of these are now not needed.

Types of species and subspecies are type specimens or type strains. For categories above the species the function of the type—to serve as a point of reference—is assumed by a *name*, e.g. that of a species or subspecies. The species or subspecies is, of course, tied to its type specimen or type strain.

Types of genera are **type species** (one of the included species) and types of higher names are usually **type genera** (one of the included genera). This principle applies up to and including the category, order. This can be illustrated by the types of an example of a taxonomic hierarchy shown in Table VI.2.

Just as the type specimen, or type strain, must be considered a member of the species whatever other specimens or strains are excluded, so the **type species of a genus must be retained in the genus even if all other species are removed from it.** A type, therefore, is sometimes called a **nominifer** or **name bearer**: it is the reference point for the name in question.

Table VI.2.

Example of taxonomic types

Category	Taxon	Type
Family	*Pseudomonadaceae*	*Pseudomonas*
Genus	*Pseudomonas*	*Pseudomonas aeruginosa*
Species	*Pseudomonas aeruginosa*	American Type Culture Collection strain number 10145

DESCRIPTIONS

The publication of a name, with a designated type, does in a technical sense create a new taxon—insofar as it indicates that the author believes he has observations to support the recognition of a new taxonomic group. But this does not afford evidence that can be readily assessed from the bald facts of a name and designation of a type. From the earliest days of systematic biology it was thought important to describe the new taxon for two reasons: (a) to show the evidence in support of a new taxon and (b) to permit others to identify their own material with it—indeed this antedated the type concept (which was introduced later to resolve difficulties with descriptions alone).

It is, therefore, a requirement for valid publication that a description of a new taxon is needed. However, just how full the description should be and what properties must be listed are difficult to prescribe.

The codes of nomenclature recognize that the most important aspect of a description is to provide a list of properties that distinguish the new taxon from others that are very similar to it, and that consequently fulfill the two purposes of adducing evidence for a new group and allowing another worker to recognize it. Such a brief differential description is called a **diagnosis,** by analogy with the characteristics of diseases that are associated with the same word. Although it is difficult to legislate for adequate diagnoses, it is usually easy to provide an acceptable one: inability to do so is often because insufficient evidence has been obtained to support the establishment of the new taxon.

The Code provides guidance on descriptions, in the form of recommendations. Failure to follow the recommendations does not of itself invalidate a name, though it may well lead later workers to dismiss the taxon as unrecognizable or trivial. The Code recommends that as soon as minimum standards of description are prepared for various groups, workers should thereafter provide that minimum information; this is intended as a guide to good practice and should do much to raise the quality of systematic bacteriology. For an example of minimum standards, see the report of the International Committee on Systematic Bacteriology Subcommittee on the Taxonomy of *Mollicules* (1979).

CLASSIFICATION DETERMINES NOMENCLATURE

The student often asks how an organism can have two different names. The reason lies in the fact that a name implies acceptance of some taxonomy, and on occasion no taxonomy is generally agreed. Scientists are entitled to their own opinions on taxonomies: there are no rules to force the acceptance of a single classification.

Thus opinions may be divided on whether the bacterial genus *Pectobacterium* is sufficiently separate from the genus *Erwinia*. The soft-rot bacterium was originally called *Bacterium carotovorum* in the days when most bacteria were placed in a few large genera such as *Bacillus* and *Bacterium*. As it became clear that these unwieldy genera had to be divided into a number of smaller genera, which were more homogeneous and convenient, this bacterium was placed in the genus *Erwinia* (established for the bacterium of fireblight, *Erwinia amylovora*) as *Erwinia carotovora*. When further knowledge accumulated, it was considered by some workers that the soft-rot bacterium was sufficiently distinct to merit a new genus, *Pectobacterium*. The same organism, therefore, is also known as *Pectobacterium carotovorum*. Both names are correct in their respective positions. If one believes that two separate genera are justified, then the correct name for the soft-rot bacterium is *Pectobacterium carotovorum*. If one considers that *Pectobacterium* is not justified as a separate genus, the correct name is *Erwinia carotovora*.

Classification, therefore, determines nomenclature, not nomenclature classification. Although unprofitable or frivolous changes of name should be avoided, the freezing of classification in the form it had centuries ago is too high a price to pay for stability of names. Progress in classification must reflect progress in knowledge (e.g. no one now wants to classify all rod-shaped bacteria in *Bacillus*, as was popular a century ago). Changes in name must reflect progress in classification: some changes in name are thus inevitable.

CHANGES OF NAME

Most changes in name are due to moving species from one genus to another or dividing up older genera. Another cause, however, is the rejection of a commonly used name because it is incorrect under one or more of the Rules. A much-used name, for example, may not be the earliest, because the earliest name was published in some obscure journal and had been overlooked. Or there may already be another identical name for a different microorganism in the literature. Changes can be very inconvenient if a well-established name is found to be **illegitimate** (contrary to a Rule) because of a technicality. The codes of nomenclature therefore make provision to allow the organizations that are responsible for the codes to make exceptions if this seems necessary. A name thus retained by international agreement is called a **conserved name**, and when a name is conserved, the type may be changed to a more suitable one.

When a species is moved from one genus into another, the specific epithet is retained (unless there is, by chance, an earlier name which forms the same combination, when some other epithet must be chosen), and this is done in the interests of stability. The new name is called a **new combination**. An example has been given above. When the original *Bacterium carotovorum* was moved to *Erwinia*, the species name became *Erwinia carotovora*. The gender of the species epithet becomes the same as that of the genus *Erwinia*, which is feminine, so the feminine ending, *-a*, is substituted for the neuter ending, *-um*.

NAMES SHOULD BE NECESSARY

The codes require that names should be necessary; i.e. **there is only one correct name for a taxon** in a given or implied taxonomy. This is sometimes expressed by the statement that an organism with a given position, rank and circumscription can have only one correct name.

NAMES ARE LABELS, NOT DESCRIPTIONS

In the early days of biology there was no regular system of names, and organisms were referred to by long Latin phrases which described them briefly, such as *Tulipa minor lutea italica folio latiore*, "the little yellow Italian tulip with broader leaves." The Swedish naturalist Linnaeus tried to reduce these to just two words for species, and in doing so he founded the present *binominal system* for species. This tulip might then become *Tulipa lutea*, just "the yellow tulip." Very soon it would be noted that a white variant sometimes occurred. Should it then still be named "the yellow tulip?" Why not change it to "the Italian tulip?" Then someone would find it in Greece and point out that the record from Italy was a mistake anyway. Twenty years later an orange form would be found in Italy after all. Soon the nomenclature would be confused again.

After a time it was realized that the original name had to be kept, even if it was not descriptive, just as a man keeps his name of Fairchild Goldsmith as he grows older, and even if he becomes a farmer. The scientific names or organisms are today only **labels**, to provide a means of referring to taxa, just like personal names.

A change of name is therefore only rarely justified, even if it sometimes seems inappropriate. Provisions exist for replacement when the name causes great confusion.

CITATION OF NAMES

A scientific name is sometimes amplified by a *citation,* i.e. by adding after it the author who proposed it. Thus the bacterium that causes crown galls is *Agrobacterium tumefaciens* (Smith and Townsend) Conn. This indicates that the name refers to the organism first named by Smith and Townsend (as *Bacterium tumefaciens,* in fact, though this is not evident in the citation) and later moved to the genus *Agrobacterium* by Conn, who therefore created a **new combination**. Sometimes the citation is expanded to include the date (e.g. *Rhizobium* Frank 1889) and, more rarely, to include also the publication, e.g. *Proteus morganii* Rauss 1936 *Journal of Pathology and Bacteriology* Vol. 42, p. 183.

It will be noted that citation is only necessary to provide a suitable reference to the literature or to distinguish between inadvertent duplication of names by different authors. A citation is *not* a means of giving credit to the author who described a taxon: the main functions of citation would be served by the bibliographic reference without mentioning the author's name. Citation of a name is to provide a **means of referring** to a name, just as a name is a means of referring to a taxon.

SYNONYMS AND HOMONYMS

A homonym is a name identical in spelling with another name but based on a different type, so they refer to different taxa under the same name. They are obviously a source of confusion, and the one that was published later is suppressed. The first published name is known as the **senior homonym,** and later published names are known as **junior homonyms.** Names of higher animals and plants that are the same as bacterial names are not treated as homonyms of names of bacteria, but to reduce confusion among microorganisms, bacterial names are suppressed if they are junior homonyms of names of fungi, algae, protozoa or viruses.

A synonym is a name that refers to the same taxon under another scientific name. Synonyms thus come in pairs or even swarms. They are of two kinds:

1. **Objective synonyms** are names with the same nomenclatural type, so that there is no doubt that they refer to the same taxon. These are often called nomenclatural synonyms. An example is

Erwinia carotovora and *Pectobacterium carotovorum:* they have the same type strain, American Type Culture Collection strain 15713.

2. **Subjective synonyms** are names that are believed to refer to the same taxon but which do not have the same type. They are matters of taxonomic opinion. Thus *Pseudomonas geniculata* is a subjective synonym of *P. fluorescens* for a worker who believes that these taxa are sufficiently similar to be included in one species, *P. fluorescens.* They have different types, however (American Type Culture Collection strains 19374 and 13525, respectively), and another worker is entitled to treat them as separate species if he so wishes.

There are senior and junior synonyms, as for homonyms. The synonym that was first published is known as the **senior synonym,** and those published later are known **junior synonyms.** Junior synonyms are normally suppressed.

PROPOSAL OF NEW NAMES

The valid publication of a new taxon requires that it be named. The Code insists that an author should make up his mind about the new taxon: if he feels certain enough to propose a new taxon with a new name, then he should say he does so propose; if he is not sure enough to make a definite proposal, then his name will not be afforded the protection of the Code. He cannot expect to suggest provisional names—or possible names, or names that one day might be justified—and then expect others to treat them as definite proposals at some unspecified future date: how can a reader possibly know when such vague conditions have been fulfilled?

If a taxon is too uncertain to receive a new name, it should remain with a vernacular designation (e.g. the marine form, group 12A). If it is already named, but its affinities are too uncertain to move it to another genus or family, it should be left where it is. There is one exception, and that is that a new species should be put into some genus even if it is not very certain which is the most appropriate, or if necessary, a new genus should be created for it. Otherwise, it will not be validly published, it will be in limbo, and it will be generally overlooked, because no one else will

know how to index it or whether they should consider it seriously. If it is misplaced, it can later be moved to a better genus.

The basic needs for publication of a new taxon are four: (a) the publication should contain a new name in proper form that is not a homonym of an earlier name of bacteria, fungi, algae, protozoa or viruses; (b) the taxon should not be a synonym of an earlier taxon; (c) a description or at least a diagnosis should be given; (d) the type should be designated. A new species is indicated by adding the Latin abbreviation *sp. nov.;* a new genus, by adding *gen. nov.;* and a new combination, by adding *comb. nov.* The most troublesome part is the search of the literature to cover the first two points. This is now greatly simplified for bacteria, because the new starting date means that one need only search the Approved Lists of Bacterial Names and the issues of the *International Journal of Systematic Bacteriology* from January 1980 onwards for all validly published names that have to be considered. However, the new name has to be published in that journal, with its description and designation of type, or if published elsewhere, the name must be announced in that journal to render it validly published.

Identification of Bacteria

Noel R. Krieg

NATURE OF IDENTIFICATION SCHEMES

Identification schemes are not classification schemes, although there may be a superficial similarity. An identification scheme for a group of organisms can be devised only **after** that group has first been classified (i.e. recognized as being different from other organisms); it is based on one or more characters, or on a pattern of characters, which all the members of the group have and which other groups do not have. The characters used are often not those that were involved in classification of the group; e.g. classification might be based on a DNA/DNA hybridization study, whereas identification might be based on a phenotypic character that is found to correlate well with the genetic information. In general, the characters chosen for an identification scheme should be **easily determinable**, whereas those used for classification may be quite difficult to determine (such as DNA homology values). The characters should also be **few in number**, whereas classification may involve large numbers of characters, such as in a numerical taxonomy study. These ideal features of an identification scheme may not always be possible, particularly with genera or species that are not susceptible to being characterized by traditional biochemical or physiological tests. In such cases, one may need to resort to relatively difficult procedures in order to achieve an accurate identification—procedures such as polyacrylamide gel electrophoresis (PAGE) of cellular proteins, cellular lipid patterns, genetic transformation, or even nucleic acid hybridization.

Serological reactions, which generally have only limited value for classification, often have enormous value for identification. Slide agglutination tests, fluorescent antibody techniques, and other serological methods can be performed simply and rapidly and are usually highly specific; therefore, they offer a means for achieving quick, presumptive identification of bacteria. Their specificity is frequently not absolute, however, and confirmation of the identification by additional physiological or biochemical tests is usually required.

With many genera and species, identification may not be based on only a few tests, but rather on the pattern given by applying a whole battery of tests. The members of the family *Enterobacteriaceae* represent one example of this. To alleviate the need for inoculating large numbers of tubed media, a variety of convenient and rapid multitest systems have been devised and are commercially available for use in identifying various taxa, particularly those of medical importance. A summary of some of these systems has been given by Smibert and Krieg (1981), but new systems are being developed continually. Each manufacturer provides charts, tables, coding systems, and characterization profiles for use with the particular multitest system being offered.

NEED FOR STANDARDIZED TEST METHODS

One difficulty of devising identification schemes is that the results of characterization tests may vary depending on the size of the inoculum, incubation temperature, length of the incubation period, composition of the medium, the surface-to-volume ratio of the medium, and the criteria used to define a "positive" or "negative" reaction. Therefore, the results of characterization tests obtained by one laboratory often do not match exactly those obtained by another laboratory, although the results within each laboratory may be quite consistent. The blind acceptance of an identification scheme without reference to the particular conditions employed by those who devised the scheme can lead to error (and, unfortunately, such conditions are not always specified). Ideally, it would be desirable to standardize the conditions used for testing various characteristics, but this is easier said than done, especially on an international basis. The use of commercial multitest systems offers some hope of increasing the standardization among various laboratories because of the high degree of quality control exercised over the media and reagents, but no one system has yet been agreed on for universal use for any given taxon. **It is therefore always advisable to include strains whose identity has been firmly established** (type or reference strains, available from national culture collections) **for comparative purposes when making use of an identification scheme**, to make sure that the scheme is valid for the conditions employed in one's own laboratory.

NEED FOR DEFINITIONS OF "POSITIVE" AND "NEGATIVE" REACTIONS

Some tests may be found to be based on plasmid- or phage-mediated characteristics; such characteristics may be highly mutable and therefore unreliable for identification purposes. Even with immutable characteristics, certain tests may not be well suited for use in identification schemes because they may not give highly reproducible results (e.g. the catalase test, oxidase test, Voges-Proskauer test and gelatin liquefaction test are notorious in this regard). Ideally, a test should give reproducible results that are clearly either positive or negative, without equivocal reactions. In fact, no such test may exist. The Gram reaction of an organism may be "Gram-variable," the presence of endospores in a strain that makes only a few may be very difficult to determine by staining or by heat resistance tests, acid production from sugars may be difficult to distinguish from no aid production if only small amounts of acid are produced, and a weak growth response may not be clearly distinguishable from "no growth." A precise (although arbitrary) definition of what constitutes a "positive" and a "negative" reaction is often important in order for a test to be useful for an identification scheme.

PURE CULTURES

Although a few bacteria are so morphologically remarkable as to make them identifiable without isolation, pure cultures are nearly always a necessity before one can attempt identification of an organism. **It is important to realize that the single selection of a colony from a plate does not assure purity.** This is especially true if selective media are used; live but nongrowing contaminants may often be present in or near a colony and can be subcultured along with the chosen organism. It is for this reason that **nonselective media are preferred for final isolation**, because they allow such contaminants to develop into visible colonies. Even with nonselective media, apparently well-isolated colonies should not be isolated too soon; some contaminants may be slow-growing and may appear on the plate only after a longer incubation. Another difficulty occurs with bacteria that form extracellular slime or that grow as a network of chains or filaments; contaminants often become firmly embedded or entrapped and are difficult to penetrate. In the instance of cyanobacteria, contaminants frequently penetrate and live in the gelatinous sheaths that surround the cells, making pure cultures difficult to obtain.

In general, colonies from a pure culture that has been streaked on a solid medium are similar to one another, providing evidence of purity. Although this is generally true, there are exceptions, as in the case of S → R variation, capsular variants, pigmented or nonpigmented variants, etc., which may be selected by certain media, temperatures or other growth conditions. Another criterion of purity is morphology: organisms from a pure culture generally exhibit a high degree of morphological similarity in stains or wet mounts. Again, there are exceptions, depending on the age of the culture, the medium used and other growth conditions: coccoid body formation, cyst formation, spore formation, pleomorphism, etc. For example, examination of a broth culture of a marine spirillum after 2 or 3 days may lead one to believe the culture is highly contaminated with cocci unless one is previously aware that such spirilla generally develop into thin-walled coccoid forms following active growth.

APPROACHES TO IDENTIFICATION OF AN ISOLATE

The vernacular headings of the various sections of *Bergey's Manual®* indicate major categories of the procaryotes and are a good starting point for identification. The categories are concerned with such phenotypic characteristics as the Gram-staining reactions, morphology, and general type of metabolism. It is therefore important to establish whether the new isolate is a chemolithotrophic autotroph, a photosynthetic organism or a chemoheterotrophic organism. Living cells should be examined by phase-contrast microscopy, and Gram-stained cells, by light microscopy; other stains can be applied if this seems appropriate. If some outstanding morphological property, such as endospore production, sheaths, holdfasts, acidfastness, cysts, stalks, fruiting bodies, budding division, or true branching, is obvious, then further efforts in identification can be confined to those groups having such a property. Whether or not the organisms are motile, and the type of motility (swimming, gliding), may be very helpful in restricting the range of possibilities. Gross growth characteristics, such as pigmentation, mucoid colonies, swarming, or a minute size, may also provide valuable clues to identification. For example, a motile, Gram-negative rod that produces a water-soluble fluorescent pigment is likely to be a *Pseudomonas* species, whereas one that forms bioluminescent colonies is likely to belong to the *Vibrionaceae.*

The source of the isolate can also help to narrow the field of possibilities. For example, a spirillum isolated from coastal seawater is likely to be an *Oceanospirillum*, whereas Gram-positive cocci occurring in grapelike clusters and isolated from the human nasopharynx are likely to belong to the genus *Staphylococcus.*

The relation of the isolate to oxygen (i.e. whether it is aerobic, anaerobic, facultatively anaerobic, or microaerophilic) is often of fundamental importance in identification. For example, a small, microaerophilic vibrio isolated from a case of diarrhea is likely to be a *Campylobacter,* whereas an anaerobic, Gram-negative rod isolated from a wound infection is probably a member of the *Bacteroidaceae*. Similarly, it is important to test the isolate for its ability to dissimilate glucose (or other simple sugar) to determine whether the type of metabolism is oxidative or fermentative or whether sugars are catabolized at all.

Above all, at each stage where the possibilities are narrowed, common sense should be used in deciding what additional tests should be performed. There should be a reason for the selection of each test, in contrast to a "shotgun" type of approach where many tests are used but most provide little pertinent information for the particular isolate under investigation. As the category to which the isolate belongs becomes increasingly delineated, one should follow the specific tests indicated in the particular diagnostic tables or keys that apply to that category.

The following summary is taken from "The Mechanism of Identification" by S. T. Cowan and J. Liston in the eighth edition of the *Manual*, with some modifications:

1. Make sure that you have a pure culture.
2. Work from broad categories down to a smaller, specific category of organism.
3. Use all the information available to you in order to narrow the range of possibilities.
4. Apply common sense at each step.
5. Use the minimum number of tests to make the identification.
6. Compare your isolate to type or reference strains of the pertinent taxon to make sure the identification scheme being used actually is valid for the conditions in your particular laboratory.

If, as may well happen, you cannot identify your isolate from the information contained in the *Manual*, neither despair nor immediately assume that you have isolated a new genus or species; many of the problems of microbial classification are the result of people jumping to this conclusion prematurely. When you fail to identify your isolate, check: (a) its **purity,** (b) that you have carried out the **appropriate tests**, (c) that your **methods are reliable**, and (d) that you have used correctly the various keys and tables of the *Manual.* It has been said that the most frequent cause of mistaken identity of bacteria is error in the determination of shape, Gram-staining reaction, and motility. In most cases, you should have little difficulty in placing your isolate into a genus; allocation to a species or subspecies may need the help of a specialized reference laboratory.

On the other hand, it is always possible that you have actually isolated a new genus or species. A comparison of the present edition of the *Manual* with the previous edition indicates that a number of new genera and species have been added. Some prime examples can be found in the family *Legionellaceae*, "Other Genera" of the family *Enterobacteriaceae*, the genus *Azospirillum*, "Dissimilatory Sulfate- or Sulfur-reducing Bacteria," the genus *Meniscus*, etc. Undoubtedly, there exist in nature a great number of bacteria that have not yet been classified and, therefore, cannot yet be identified by existing schemes. Yet, before describing and naming a new taxon, one must be **very sure that it is really a new taxon** and not merely the result of an inadequate identification.

Further Reading

Goodfellow, M. and R.G. Board (Editors). 1980. Microbiological Classification and Identification, Society for Applied Bacteriology Symposium Series No. 8. Academic Press, London.

Hedén, C. and T. Illéni (Editors). 1975. New Approaches to the Identification of Microorganisms. John Wiley & Sons, New York.

Holding, J.A. and J.G. Colee. 1971. Routine biochemical tests. Methods Microbiol. *6A:* 1–32.

Mitruka, B.J. 1976. Methods of Detection and Identification of Bacteria. CRC Press, Cleveland, Ohio.

Skerman, V.B.D. 1967. A Guide to the Identification of the Genera of Bacteria, 2nd Ed. Williams & Wilkins, Baltimore.

Skerman, V.B.D. 1969. Abstracts of Microbiological Methods. Wiley-Interscience, New York.

Skerman, V.B.D. 1974. A key for the determination of the generic position of organisms listed in the *Manual*. *In* Buchanan and Gibbons (Editors), Bergey's Manual® of Determinative Bacteriology, 8th Ed. Williams & Wilkins, Baltimore, pp. 1098–1146.

Skinner, F.A. and D.W. Lovelock. 1979. Identification Methods for Microbiologist. Society for Applied Bacteriology Technical Series No. 14. Academic Press, New York.

Smibert, R.M. and N.R. Krieg. 1981. General characterization. *In* Gerhardt, Murray, Costilow, Nester, Wood, Krieg and Phillips (Editors), Manual of Methods for General Bacteriology. American Society for Microbiology, Washington, D.C., pp. 409–443.

NUMERICAL IDENTIFICATION

Peter H. A. Sneath

The success of numerical taxonomy has in recent years led to the development of a new diagnostic method based upon it, called **numerical identification**. The rapidly growing field is well reviewed by Lapage et al. (1973) and Willcox et al. (1980). The essential principles can be illustrated geometrically (Sneath, 1978) by considering the columns of percent positive test reactions in a new table, a table of q taxa for m diagnostic characters. If an object is scored for two variables, its position can be represented by a point on a scatter diagram. Use of three variables determines a position in a three-dimensional model. Objects that are very similar on the variables will be represented by clusters of points in the diagram or the model, and a circle or sphere can be drawn round each cluster so as to define its position and radius. The same principles can be extended to many variables or tests, which then represent a multidimensional space or "hyperspace." A column representing a species defines, in effect, a region in hyperspace, and it is useful to think of a species as being represented by a hypersphere in that space, whose position and radius are specified by the numerical values of these percentages. The tables form a reference library, or data base, of properties of the taxa.

The operation of numerical identification is to compare an unknown strain with each column of the table in turn and to calculate a distance (or its analog) to the center of each taxon hypersphere. If the unknown lies well within a hypersphere, this will identify it with that taxon. Furthermore, such systems have important advantages over most other diagnostic systems. The numerical process allows a likelihood to be attached to an identification, so that one can know to some order of magnitude the certainty that the identity is correct. The results are not greatly affected by an occasional aberrant property of the unknown or by an occasional experimental mistake in performing the tests. Furthermore, the system is robust toward missing information, and quite good identifications can be obtained if only a moderate proportion of the tests have been performed.

Numerous applications of numerical identification are now being made. Most commercial testing kits or automatic instruments for microbial identification are based on these concepts, and they require the comparison of results on an unknown strain with a data base, using computer software, or with printed material prepared by such means. Research sponsored by the *Bergey's Manual®* Trust (Feltham et al., 1984) shows that these concepts can be extended to a very wide range of genera.

Further Reading

Feltham, R.K.A., P.A. Wood and P.H.A. Sneath. 1984. A general-purpose system for characterizing medically important bacteria to genus level. J. Appl. Bacteriol. *57:* 279–290.

Lapage, S.P., S. Bascomb, W.R. Willcox and M.A. Curtis. 1973. Identification of bacteria by computer. I. General aspects and perspectives. J. Gen. Microbiol. *77:* 273–290.

Sneath, P.H.A. 1978. Identification of microorganisms. *In* Norris and Richmond (Editors), Essays in Microbiology. John Wiley, Chichester, England, pp. 10/1–10/32.

Willcox, W.R., S.P. Lapage and B. Holmes. 1980. A review of numerical methods in bacterial identification. Antonie van Leeuwenhoek J. Microbiol. Serol. *46:* 233–299.

Reference Collections of Bacteria—
The Need and Requirements
for Type Strains

The Late Norman E. Gibbons
Revised by Peter H. A. Sneath and Stephen P. Lapage

As it became possible to grow bacteria in liquid and solid media, microbiologists began to exchange cultures with their colleagues for information and comparison. Each investigator kept his own isolates, added those received from others, and in this way built up his own reference and working collection.

About the turn of the century, Professor František Král of Prague realized the value of a central collection and began to collect cultures which he made available for a fee to other workers. After Král's death in 1911, the collection was acquired by Professor Ernst Pribram and transferred to the University of Vienna in 1915. Pribram brought part of the collection to Loyola University in Chicago some years before the Second World War. He was killed in a car accident in 1940, but the fate of his collection is not known. The cultures left in Vienna were destroyed during World War II.

The next oldest collection—Centraalbureau voor Schimmelcultures—was founded in 1906 by the Association internationale des Botanistes. Although the founding association did not survive the First World War, the collection is still in existence at Baarn under the auspices of The Royal Netherlands Academy of Sciences. This collection provides a holding and distribution center for fungi and an identification service.

Since then, many other collections have developed—some general, some specialized, and some oriented to service. A full account of the history of culture collections is given by Porter (1976). Some salient developments may be mentioned briefly. About 1946, Professor P. Hauduroy established a centralized information facility at Lausanne, the "Centre de Collections de Types Microbiens" which provided information on which collections held cultures of various bacterial species. In 1947, the Lausanne Centre became associated with the International Association of Microbiological Societies (IAMS, now the International Union of Microbiological Societies, IUMS), and in cooperation with it, an International Federation of Type Culture Collections was formed. This Federation had ambitious plans which were never realized, and the Federation went out of existence within a few years.

In 1962, therefore, a Conference on Culture Collections (Martin, 1963), held after the Seventh International Congress for Microbiology, asked IAMS to form a Section on Culture Collections. The Section was set up in 1963 and, on the reorganization of IAMS in 1970, became the World Federation of Culture Collections (WFCC). The WFCC is also a multidisciplinary Commission of the International Union of Biological Sciences in the Divisions of Botany and Zoology, linking it with other organizations concerned with problems of biological preservation, such as herbaria, zoological gardens, and museums. It has collected information on several hundred collections throughout the world, and the *World Directory of Collections of Cultures of Microorganisms* (Martin and Skerman, 1972) has been published. This has recently been updated (McGowan and Skerman, 1982). Pridham (1974) has also compiled a useful list of the acronyms and abbreviations for numerous culture collections. A number of national Federations of Culture Collections have also been formed which are affiliated with the WFCC. The aims of the WFCC include the collection of information on strains held by the collections and more detailed information on the strains themselves.

In the preservation of cultures, satisfactory methods of maintenance, with minimal change in the cultures, are essential, and an accepted system of taxonomy should be used. Particularly stringent standardization is required in the case of cooperative and comparative studies. In pursuit of these and similar aims, the WFCC has held training courses for curators and workers in culture collections at which other important functions of culture collections are also discussed. The WFCC also works in close cooperation with the International Committee on Systematic Bacteriology (ICSB) and its Judicial Commission and other related national or international bodies dealing with all aspects of the preservation of various groups of microorganisms. It has also sponsored a number of international conferences on culture collections. A list of these, together with a summary of other WFCC activities, is given by Lapage (1975). The WFCC supports the development of the World Data Centre at the University of Queensland, Brisbane, Australia, which is collecting cultural, physiological and other data on strains of microorganisms and is exploring methods of recording such information in a standard format.

NEED FOR CULTURE COLLECTIONS

It is essential for the orderly development of bacteriology that cultures of organisms described or mentioned in publications be available for independent study. Because microbiologists are mortal and their interests vary during their working life, collections are necessary to provide an element of stability and continuity.

Although some microbiologists spend a lifetime on one or two groups of organisms and build up large specialized collections, others move from one organism to another, abandoning old favorites. Both approaches generate problems in the preservation of organisms. The specialized collection may become so large and so specialized that it is hard to find a willing successor to the original enthusiastic curator. The worker whose interests are more fickle seldom worries about the systematic aspects, which make the preservation of cultures so desirable to the taxonomist.

Until the 1920s, the main reason for the existence of collections was their value for taxonomic and epidemiological studies. In the 1930s, the burgeoning interest in microbial physiology and biochemistry gave rise to a need for preserving organisms that produced or gave better yields of specific compounds. This greatly increased the value of culture collections.

More recently, studies on bacterial genetics have resulted in the isolation of numerous mutants which have, in turn, necessitated specialized collections. Some of these mutants are concerned with genetic loci useful in studies of nutrient and of biochemical pathways. The 1972 Stockholm Conference on the Environment recognized the importance of genetic pools and of collections of microorganisms.

Current developments in culture collections are diverse. Reviews of these can be found in Lapage (1971), the volume edited by Colwell (1976), and in Kirsop (1985). Methods of preservation are undergoing change, with increasing use of storage at very low temperatures to reduce the risk of genetic change. Loss of plasmids is a problem with some methods. Preservation methods are described in Kirsop and Snell (1984). Recent legislation on patents has led to the need for deposition of strains used in industry. A review of requirements for patents is given by Crespi (1982). Cultures are also needed for teaching of microbiology and for quality control in many fields. The growth of numerous new diagnostic aids requires that large sets of strains from numerous species shall be available for establishing the data bases that are needed (Sneath, 1977). Culture collections in the future may also expand associated activities, such as storage and supply of dried material of microbial origin, standard antisera, nucleic acid preparations, and the like.

TYPE STRAINS

A particularly important function of culture collections is to preserve type strains and make them available to microbiologists who are undertaking taxonomic revisions. The nomenclatural aspects of type strains are discussed in the article on "Bacterial Nomenclature," but some related points are briefly summarized here.

Type strains of bacterial species and subspecies are essential for the advance of taxonomy. They are required for comparison with strains that an author may believe belong to a new species or subspecies. Descriptions have never proved to be sufficient, because new techniques in systematics are continually being devised, and there is no substitute for an authentic strain when one wishes to make a critical comparison.

Type strains are of such taxonomic and nomenclatural importance that in this edition as many of them as possible are listed by their designation and catalog number in the main collections; a list of collections mentioned is given in the next article.

The new International Code of Nomenclature of Bacteria (or Revised Code) (see Lapage et al., 1975) has made several special provisions for types. It is now a requirement for valid publication of a cultivable new species or subspecies of bacteria that a type strain shall be designated (alternative provisions exist for noncultivable bacteria). The Code urges that a type strain should be deposited in one or more of the permanently established culture collections. The numerous problems caused in the past by taxa for which there were no type strains should thus be largely overcome. Type cultures should, in the future, be available for all cultivable species of bacteria.

In the past, it was frequently necessary to distinguish between different classes of type culture, in particular between types and neotypes, but the Revised Code has made most of these distinctions unnecessary. The new starting document for bacterial nomenclature, which came into force on January 1, 1980 (Approved Lists of Bacterial Names, Skerman et al., 1980) lists the type strains for the names of bacterial species that are currently recognized and given in the Lists. In the past, when many species had no type strains, it was necessary to establish **neotypes** for taxa where no type existed or the type had been lost. A neotype was thus a replacement for a type, and there should rarely be a need in the future for neotypes, except in the case of loss of the types. The procedure for establishing a neotype is given in the Revised Code; of course, the neotype should be deposited in one or, preferably, several of the main culture collections.

Although culture collections maintain type strains and neotypes as described above, they also keep typical and atypical strains, reference strains, and strains with particular properties of interest to biochemistry, genetics, serology, bacteriophage studies and the like; they also carry out many other functions, of which a general account can be found in Lapage (1971). Culture collections are therefore of great value not only to systematists but to all bacteriologists and are essential to the development of the subject.

List of Culture Collections

There are several hundred culture collections in the world, with the majority being small specialized collections, often collected by one individual. Details of most of these may be found in the *World Directory of Collections of Cultures of Microorganisms* (edited S. M. Martin and V. B. D. Skerman, 1972). This has recently been updated (McGowan and Skerman, 1982). A smaller number of collections are frequently referred to in bacteriological work, and a selection of these is given below with commonly used abbreviations.

AMRC   FAO-WHO International Reference Centre for Animal Mycoplasmas, Institute for Medical Microbiology, University of Aarhus, Aarhus, Denmark.

ATCC   American Type Culture Collection, 12301 Parklawn Drive, Rockville, Maryland 20852, U.S.A.

BKM   See VKM.

BKMW   See VKM.

CBS   Centraalbureau voor Schimmelcultures, Oosterstraat 1, Baarn, The Netherlands.

CCEB   Culture Collection of Entomophagous Bacteria, Institute of Entomology, Czechoslovak Academy of Sciences, Flemingovo N2, Prague 6, Czechoslovakia.

CCM   Czechoslovak Collection of Microorganisms, J. E. Purkyne University, Tr. Obr. Miru 10, Brno, Czechoslovakia.

CDC   Centers for Disease Control, Atlanta, Georgia 30333, U.S.A.

CIP   Collection of the Institut Pasteur, Rue du Dr. Roux, Paris 15, France.

CNC   Czechoslovak National Collection of Type Cultures, Institute of Epidemiology and Microbiology, Srobarova 48, Prague 10, Czechoslovakia.

DSM   Deutsche Sammlung von Mikroorganismen, Grisebachstrasse 8, Gottingen, Federal Republic of Germany.

IAM   Institute of Applied Microbiology, University of Tokyo, Bunkyo-ku, Tokyo, Japan.

ICPB   International Collection of Phytopathogenic Bacteria, University of California, Davis, California 95616, U.S.A.

IFO   Institute for Fermentation, 4-54 Jusonishinocho, Osaka, Japan.

IMET   Institutes für Mikrobiologie und Experimentelle Therapie, Deutsche Akademie der Wissenschaften zu Berlin, Beuthenbergstrasse 11, Jena 69, German Democratic Republic.

IMRU   Institute of Microbiology, Rutgers—The State University, New Brunswick, New Jersey 08903, U.S.A.

IMV   Institute of Microbiology and Virology, Academy of Sciences of the Ukrainian S.S.R., Kiev, U.S.S.R.

INA   Institute for New Antibiotics, Bolshaya Pirogovskaya II, Moscow, U.S.S.R.

INMI   Institute for Microbiology, U.S.S.R. Academy of Sciences, Moscow, U.S.S.R.

IPV   Istituto di Patologia Vegetale, Milan, Italy.

KCC   Kaken Chemical Company Ltd., 6-42 Jujodai-1-Chome, Tokyo 114, Japan.

LIA   Museum of Cultures, Leningrad Research Institute of Antibiotics, 23 Ogorodnikov Prospect, Leningrad L-20, U.S.S.R.

LSU   Louisiana State University, Baton Rouge, Louisiana 70803, U.S.A.

LMD   Laboratorium voor Microbiologie, Technische Hogeschool, Julianalaan 67a, 2623 BC Delft, The Netherlands.

NCDO   National Collection of Dairy Organisms, National Institute for Research in Dairying, University of Reading, Shinfield, Reading, England, U.K.

NCIB   National Collection of Industrial Bacteria, Torry Research Station, Aberdeen AB9 8DG, Scotland, U.K.

NCPPB   National Collection of Plant Pathogenic Bacteria, Plant Pathology Laboratory, Hatching Green, Harpenden, England, U.K.

NCTC   National Collection of Type Cultures, Central Public Health Laboratory, Colindale, London NW9 5HT, England, U.K.

NIAID   National Institute of Allergy and Infectious Diseases, Hamilton, Montana 59840, U.S.A.

NIHJ   National Institute of Health, Tokyo, Japan.

NRC   National Research Council, Sussex Drive, Ottawa 2, Canada.

NRL   Neisseria Reference Laboratory, U.S. Public Health Service Hospital, Seattle, Washington 98114, U.S.A.

NRRL   Northern Utilization Research and Development Division, U.S. Department of Agriculture, Peoria, Illinois 61604, U.S.A.

NTHC   North Technical Hogskolles Collection, Department of Biochemistry, Technical University of Norway, Trondheim MTH, Norway.

OEU   Tennoji Branch, Osaka University of Liberal Arts and Education, Minami-Kawabori-Cho, Tennojiku, Osaka, Japan.

PDDCC   Culture Collection of Plant Diseases Division, New Zealand Department of Scientific and Industrial Research, Auckland, New Zealand.

TC   Thaxter Collection, Farlow Herbarium, Harvard University, Cambridge, Massachusetts 02138, U.S.A.

TPH   Microbiological Culture Collection, Public Health Laboratory, Ontario Department of Health, Toronto 116, Canada.

UMH   University of Missouri Herbarium, Columbia, Missouri 65201, U.S.A.

UQM   Culture Collection, Department of Microbiology, University of Queensland, Herston, Brisbane 4006, Australia.

VKM   Department of Culture Collection, Institute of Biochemistry and Physiology of Microorganisms, U.S.S.R. Academy of Sciences, Pushchino, Moscow region, 142292, U.S.S.R.

VPI   Anaerobe Laboratory, Virginia Polytechnic Institute and State University, Blacksburg, Virginia 24061, U.S.A.

WINDSOR   Culture Collection, University of Windsor, Windsor, Ontario, Canada.

WVU   West Virginia University, Department of Microbiology, Medical Center, Morgantown, W. Virginia 26506, U.S.A.

The Higher Taxa, or,
A Place for Everything . . . ?

R. G. E. Murray

"Quot homines tot sententiae; suo quoque mos." ("So many men, so many opinions; each to his own taste.")

Terence, Phormio

When the eighth edition of *Bergey's Manual*® was in preparation, a major taxonomic concern was the provision of a clear statement of where the bacteria fitted among living things. This was set out in "A Place for Bacteria in the Living World" (Murray, 1974), which summarized the reasons for recognizing the kingdom *Procaryotae,* inclusive of the bacteria and the "blue-green algae" (cyanobacteria). This concept, based on cellular organization, is now a part of the fundamental training of all biologists, and a formal repetition is no longer a necessity. The student who wishes to relive that era should consult the major essays for details and references (Stanier, 1961; Stanier and van Niel, 1962; Murray, 1962; Allsopp, 1969; Stanier, 1970). Taxonomy is not static, however, and new horizons are being explored that give perspective and greater definition to higher taxa as well as the lower categories of genus and species.

The prefatory chapter mentioned above included a tentative proposal of appropriate higher taxa. The arguments and proposals that have arisen since then concern the levels of dissection of the kingdoms of the living world (Whittaker and Margulis, 1978; Woese and Fox, 1977a), the definition and levels of dissection of the major procaryotic groups (Gibbons and Murray, 1978; Whittaker and Margulis, 1978), and the integration of evolutionary information (Stackebrandt and Woese, 1981). There is a renewal of interest in bacterial taxonomy stimulated by the recognition of novel groups of bacteria that do not fit comfortably into current systematic schemes and by new understanding of the taxonomic utility and phylogenetic significance of molecular and genetic data. The system of "superphyla" and phyla proposed by Whittaker and Margulis (1978) is not sensitive to current interpretations of biochemical relatedness based on wall chemistry or other unique features of well-established groups of procaryotes. There is no advantage, at this stage of our understanding, in debating the relative value of recognizing "super kingdoms" (Whittaker and Margulis, 1978) or "primary kingdoms" (the "Urkingdoms" of Woese and Fox, 1977a) to accommodate views of cellular organization in protists, plants and animals as well as speculations about the nature of putative progenitors. We should be content for now to deal with the *Procaryotae* and the systematic problems that arise within that circumscription; there must be sufficient time for assimilation and consolidation of the burgeoning data. There are attractive features in the dendrograms generated by C. R. Woese and his colleagues; their time will come when the patterns of associations are less fragmentary. For now it would appear sensible to look to the Gibbons and Murray (1978) proposal as capable of modification as an interim broad classification with a few areas of taxonomic validity.

The conceptual changes deriving from genetic and molecular studies are making inroads into the cherished beliefs of taxonomists and bacteri-

ologists. We have to agree with the moderate statement taken from Stackebrandt and Woese (1981): ". . . what bacterial classification we have (say up through the eighth edition of *Bergey's Manual,* 1923-1974) is probably not in very good accord with the natural relationships that exist among organisms." This is true enough because it is only in the past decade that sequencing of biopolymers and molecular genetics has provided convincing data on relatedness and because the intent and role of *Bergey's Manual*® has always been to provide a basis for the determination of the identity of a pure culture. It is unfortunate that the expression of nomenclatural decisions, hierarchical arrangements (even if all but abandoned in the eighth edition), and the mask of authority has tended to induce undue confidence in the relationships implied in earlier editions.

Even if our perception of "natural relationships" is flawed by ignorance as well as inadequate information, the practical bacteriologist needs a simple scheme of classification as a framework for recognition. At this stage, for example, the possibility that some micrococci are more closely related to *Arthrobacter* than to other spherical Gram-positive cocci and the implication for a further splitting of the genus *Micrococcus* (Stackebrandt and Woese, 1979, 1981) would be confusing to the practical bench worker or the physician and is unhelpful. At the higher taxonomic levels some sort of serviceable scheme that can recognize and, to a degree, accommodate the possibilities will be of service, will cushion the shocks to come, and will stimulate appropriate research. This sort of practicality is almost realized in the proposal by Gibbons and Murray (1978). But any scheme will require future modification because it will take time to attain a complete reassessment of the taxonomic significance and validity of those characters that are reasonably easy to determine and apply effectively to each level of identification. The alternative possibility is that we should maintain two entirely independent schemes: a practical taxonomy and an academic (phylogenetic) taxonomy. The dichotomy of these phenotypic and genotypic approaches is with us because people of such persuasions work in semi-isolation and because, as argued by Stackebrandt and Woese (1981), ". . . the classically defined taxonomic categories, the genera and families, do not correspond to fixed (minimal) S_{AB} values." Furthermore, the genetics of today is beginning to clarify the mechanisms operating in the grand evolutionary experiment, blessed with minimal constraints of time and circumstance, conducted in nature's laboratory. It is clear that point mutations are less important than effective reassociations of determinants with their modifying segments and the mechanisms allowing the exchange, chromosomal integration and amplification of operative sets of determinants (Campbell, 1981; Cullum and Saedler, 1981). It is conceivable, now, that major complex characters of physiological and taxonomic significance (involving a considerable number of genes) could be transferred between organisms both closely and distantly related in the clonal arborizations of the phylogenetic tree. All that is required is an occasional evolutionarily successful experiment in a time frame measured in thousands, millions or billions of years (or cell divisions, for that matter).

An overall taxonomic scheme that is capable of incorporating phylogenetic data (as well as providing a primary key) would be helpful in minimizing the dichotomy of interests and understanding among bacteriologists. It is desirable to bridge the growing gap between the practical applied fields and the academic substratum with something more than the perfidy of plasmids and technological legerdemain. The perpetual quandary is how and when to incorporate into systematic bacteriology the generalizations derived by intensive and expensive study of "model" organisms or of a limited set.

The most exciting and evocative of recent explorations of the possibilities of extracting phylogenetic information from highly conserved biopolymers (the "semantides" of Zuckerkandl and Pauling, 1965) are the comparisons of 16S ribosomal RNA (rRNA) catalogs undertaken by Carl Woese and his colleagues (Woese and Fox, 1977b). This approach, together with that involving the functional structural homologies and interchangeability of whole ribosome parts and some protein components, shows promise of providing comparative data with evolutionary significance for the whole living world (Brimacombe et al., 1978; Kandler, 1981). Of most interest to us is the capability of the technique of RNA nucleotide analysis, expensive and slow though it may be, in spanning the widest range of procaryotic clones. The stability of most of this fairly large (1540 residues) molecule is the basis of the application to assessment of taxa at the level of family and higher. The fact that a few variable domains exist in the molecule allows for the partially realized possibility of contributing a degree of resolution at the level of genus. This could add to the data on relations within genus and species generated by utilizing DNA/DNA (Johnson, 1973) and RNA/DNA hybridization (De Smedt and De Ley, 1977). The figures that are generated (either the number of shared oligonucleotides or an association coefficient, the S_{AB} value) are based on a computer comparison of the catalogs of oligonucleotides (liberated from the 16S RNA by ribonuclease T_1) large enough to show individuality (larger than pentamers). This means that a considerable portion of the molecule yielding oligonucleotides smaller than hexamers is not taken into account, and therefore, the sequence data cannot directly be related to all other hybridization data. Nevertheless, the results of comparing some 200 representative bacteria, surprises and all, support the directing thesis that most of the 16S rRNA sequence has drifted only slowly with time. We surmise (q.v. Stackebrandt and Woese, 1981) that the comparison provides a measure of the "depth" of the separation between the phylogenetic units or branches of the phylogenetic tree. It is an article of faith that the degree of cleavage (a low S_{AB} value) is proportional to time and is reasonable for initial purposes, although the time scale may be different for different major taxa.

Clones giving rise to unique and now recognizable groups of bacteria must have separated at various stages of procaryotic evolution (Fox et al., 1980). Earliest among these departures from the main stem so far detected by this oligonucleotide cataloging are the *Archaeobacteria*,* which comprise the methanogens, halobacteria and thermoacidophiles; these, it is now known (Kandler, 1981), possess peculiar lipids and either no murein or a pseudomurein in their cell walls. The eight or so major groups of photosynthetic and chemosynthetic bacteria (all designated "eubacteria" in the papers cited) arose somewhat later in this imprecise evolutionary time scale. The data suggest that some genera are truly ancient (e.g. *Clostridium*, *Spirochaeta*) and older, in fact, than some very complex associations of genera (e.g. the actinomycetes).

Those involved in the comparative studies of 16S rRNA, ribosomes and ribosomal proteins have come to the enthusiastic conclusion that the procaryotes are made up of two kingdoms, the eubacteria and the *Archaeobacteria*. The molecular and biochemical bases for the separation have been summarized by Woese (1981) and Kandler (1981). There is no doubt whatever that the *Archaeobacteria* are distinguished by a

number of specialized characters from the rest of the procaryotes ("eubacteria" has had too many meanings in the past to be a useful term). They include the number of ribosomal proteins, the size and shape of the ribosomal S unit, the proportion of acidic ribosomal proteins, the constitution of transfer RNA initiator, the presence of ether-linked rather than ester-linked lipids, and the absence of muramic acid or the normal form of peptidoglycan from cell walls. These and some other intimate features make for interesting thoughts about eucaryotes, mitochondria and chloroplasts, as well as the procaryotes. But these distinctions are not suitable to kingdom status. Stackebrandt and Woese (1981) sum up the situation as follows: ". . . the general conclusion that seems to be emerging with regard to the differences among archaebacteria, true bacteria and eucaryotes is that all are identical in the basic aspects of their basic processes, yet all differ from one another in the details of these processes." An examination of any of the methanogens, strict halophiles or thermoacidophiles would place them in the kingdom *Procaryotae* as presently defined. It is not appropriate to separate kingdoms on any basis but a major, reasonably easily determined difference in organization. Therefore, it seems sensible to treat the *Archaeobacteria* as a major taxon within the *Procaryotae* and, if necessary, amend its status at some later date when more evidence is collected and digested. Perhaps we will soon recognize other equally distinctive clones that diverged very early from the stem clones of primitive microbes.

There is a comforting sequel to pondering compilations of articles regarding biochemical evolution (Wilson et al., 1977; Carlile et al., 1981). Although these studies suggest that "strange bedfellows" may be assigned to some of the more complex groups or point to unexpected separations (e.g. among the photosynthetic bacteria, Gibson et al., 1979; among the micrococci, Stackebrandt and Woese, 1979), there are concordant features. Gram-positiveness and Gram-negativeness are still unassailable characters except in what are now known to be phylogenetically and biochemically separate groups, the *Archaeobacteria* (Balch et al., 1979), the radiation-resistant cocci (Brooks et al., 1980) and, of course, the wall-less *Mollicutes*. Among the Gram-positives, it is encouraging to see that the many peptidoglycan types form consistent patterns in the branches of the dendrograms generated by comparison of the oligonucleotide catalogs (Schleifer and Kandler, 1972; Kandler and Schleifer, 1980; Kandler, 1981).

The infinitely diverse groupings of Gram-negative bacteria have yet to be surveyed to an extent that allows of any decisive taxonomic proposals, and many of those included up to now exhibit phylogenetic and phenotypic incoherence. A major surprise arising from the analysis of rRNA oligonucleotides has been that each of the three coherent phylogenetic groupings of anoxygenic photosynthesizers contain a variety of seemingly related, diverse and well-known nonphotosynthetic genera showing subordinate S_{AB} values (Gibson et al., 1979; Stackebrandt and Woese, 1981). The implication is that photosynthetic clones may spawn apochlorotic derivatives, a thesis often directed to the cyanobacteria in the past (Pringsheim, 1967) but not yet subjected to this sort of phylogenetic analysis. It would seem wise not to make phototrophism an overriding taxonomic unit until the situation clarifies. This makes for difficulties in more conventional schemes such as that of Gibbons and Murray (1978), which separated in simplistic fashion the photosynthetic (*Photobacteria*) and the nonphotosynthetic (*Scotobacteria*) included in the Gram-negative bacteria (*Gracilicutes*). But it may be too early to be either discouraged or encouraged, and there is still room for the exercise of one's prejudices.

Classifications cannot be final, and there are many ways in which bacteria can be classified (Cowan, 1968); this one has no more permanence than those that went before it. But the doubts and criticisms that come to the mind of the reader are the stimuli to further work and a deeper consideration of the taxonomic implications of the new mix of biochemical and phylogenetic data. Changes from the earlier versions (Murray, 1974;

---

* Equivalent to the term *Archaebacteria*. Because the word is formed by a combination of two Greek words (*archaios*, ancient, and *bakterion*, a small rod), the letter *o* should be used as the combining vowel, hence, *Archaeobacteria*.

Gibbons and Murray, 1978) were inevitable. The hierarchical levels needed to be raised to give greater scope for classifying the range of organisms included at each major level. For example, students of the cyanobacteria, even those most sympathetic to their incorporation into bacterial taxonomy, despair of being able to accommodate their charges within the single order assigned by Gibbons and Murray (1978). As already indicated, it would take more than ordinary taxonomic agility to make a phylogenetically sensitive classification of the phototrophic bacteria and their derivatives in our present state of understanding.

The following is proposed as an arrangement of higher taxa which can serve during this time of taxonomic transition. It involves some amendments of rank and new names.

Kingdom *Procaryotae* Murray 1968, 252.

Division I. *Gracilicutes* Gibbons and Murray 1978, 3.

Class I. *Scotobacteria* Gibbons and Murray 1978, 4.

Class II. *Anoxyphotobacteria* (Gibbons and Murray) classis nov.^{VP†} (Subclassis *Anoxyphotobacteria* Gibbons and Murray 1978, 4.)

Class III. *Oxyphotobacteria* (Gibbons and Murray) classis nov.^{VP} (Subclassis *Oxyphotobacteria* Gibbons and Murray 1978, 3.)

Division II. *Firmicutes* Gibbons and Murray 1978, 5. (*Firmacutes* (sic) Gibbons and Murray 1978, 5.)

Class I. *Firmibacteria* classis nov.^{VP}; L. adj. *firmus* strong; Gr. dim. n. *bakterion* a small rod; M.L. fem. pl. n. *Firmibacteria* strong bacteria, indicative of simple Gram-positive bacteria.

Class II. *Thallobacteria* classis nov.; Gr. n. *thallos* branch; Gr. dim. n. *bakterion* a small rod; M.L. fem. pl. n. *Thallobacteria* branching bacteria.
(These new names are proposed to express the general basis of splitting the division into the simple Gram-positive bacilli and those Gram-positive bacteria showing a branching habit, the actinomycetes and related organisms.)

Division III. *Tenericutes* div. nov.^{VP}; L. adj. *tener* soft, tender; L. fem. n. *cutis* skin; M.L. fem. n. *Tenericutes* procaryotes of pliable, soft nature, indicative of lack of a rigid cell wall.

Class I. *Mollicutes* Edward and Freundt 1967, 267.
(The *Mollicutes* are a distinctive group of wall-less procaryotes of sufficiently diverse phylogenies that separate classes may well be required in the future.)

Division IV. *Mendosicutes* Gibbons and Murray 1978, 2. (*Mendocutes* (sic) Gibbons and Murray 1978, 2.)

Class I. *Archaeobacteria* (Woese and Fox) classis nov.^{VP} (Kingdom *Archaebacteria* (sic) Woese and Fox 1977a, 5089.)
(The *Archaeobacteria* are defined in terms of being procaryotes with unusual walls, membrane lipids, ribosomes and RNA sequences (Kandler, 1981). The future may bring further classes into the *Mendosicutes* when (and if) truly primitive organisms as envisioned by Woese and Fox (1977b) are isolated and recognized as related to a "universal ancestor" or progenote.)

This arrangement of the procaryotes continues to recognize the absence or presence and nature of cell walls as determinative at the highest level. The omission of *Photobacteria* (Gibbons and Murray, 1978) as a class and the elevation of *Oxyphotobacteria* and *Anoxyphotobacteria* to class status is intended to provide more scope than is offered by Gibbons and Murray (1978) for the inevitable arrangement and rearrangement of the lower taxa within these categories as new understanding of lineage and relationships is brought to bear. For instance, the groups of phototrophic bacteria are formed of several major subgroups; separation of these from the level of class would be appropriate to the deep phylogenetic clefts that may be established in both the *Oxyphotobacteria* (the cyanobacteria and the *Prochlorales*) and the *Anoxyphotobacteria,* as pointed out by Stackebrandt and Woese (1981). Furthermore, it may not be appropriate to place all the nonphotosynthetic, Gram-negative bacteria in the *Scotobacteria* if the molecular evidence points clearly to derivation from photosynthetic ancestors; undoubtedly this would require separation at a high level within the class. The same need for broad scope is apparent in the *Firmicutes* with its two major divisions, the simple Gram-positive bacteria (*Clostridium* and relatives) and the actinomycetes.

The *Tenericutes* would have less support from the molecular phylogenetic evidence as a taxon at the highest level because of their probable origin from Gram-positive bacteria and the possibility that they may not have a single common ancestry (Woese et al., 1980). However, they form a stable and distinctive group; they are not obviously a subset of the *Firmicutes,* and their wall-less state puts them clearly in a division by themselves as long as we base our classification on the presence or absence and character of the cell wall. On the other hand, we must recognize that an organism may lose a component of a very complex wall and still merit consideration as a member of that class; e.g. the members of the genus *Chlamydia* have no muramic acid, but other characters, including some concerned with the relict wall, suggest a relationship to organisms that are definitive members of the *Gracilicutes.*

The *Archaeobacteria,* for their part, are a very diverse group in terms of cell wall attributes (all the way from a complex wall including pseudomurein to wall-less), and there are at least five groupings with S_{AB} values of < 0.3. There is sufficient scope within a division for the apparent complexity laid out by Balch et al. (1979) and any extraordinary "primitive" organisms that may be isolated. The sensible approach would seem to be maintenance of the consistency of the higher taxa by including in the class *Mendosicutes* all those procaryotes with a cell wall composition inconsistent with that defined for *Gracilicutes* and *Firmicutes* (e.g. in simplest terms, not possessing muramic acid). This view is supported by Starr and Schmidt (1981). The inclusion of wall-less thermoacidophiles among the *Archaeobacteria* will be necessary even if seemingly inconsistent. There will come a time, without doubt, when we can set up taxa that are precisely defined in terms of molecular genetics, but that time has not yet arrived.

We cannot assume that all possible procaryotic organisms have been observed and isolated for study. The possibility exists that organisms will be found that are even more "primitive" (i.e. separated from the main stem even earlier) than the *Archaeobacteria* and have a constitution revealing more of the nature of the "universal common ancestor" (Woese and Fox, 1977; Stackebrandt and Woese, 1981). A class can be formed in the future as a suitable home for any organism whose proteins and genetic translation apparatus do not fit into the line of evolution represented by the procaryotes and eucaryotes studied up to now. They may have characteristics that foreshadow the fundamental eucaryotic cell.

No place is provided in our scheme for the fossil microbes being described from specimens of Precambrian and, possibly, archean cherts (see Walter, 1977). This is because they can only be described in terms of size, shape and associations. The oldest are in stratified structures closely resembling the stromatolites and "algal mats" that can be found today, which are complex consortia of cyanobacteria, algae and bacteria with equally complex layering of metabolic and physiological characteristics. There are several attractive morphological resemblances. Size is about all that distinguishes the interpretation of forms as bacterial or

---

†*VP* denotes that this name, although not on the Approved Lists of Bacterial Names, has been validly published in the official publication, *International Journal of Systematic Bacteriology.*

algal. A further interpretation that a particular form is photosynthetic is entirely circumstantial and assumptive. Names have been assigned in binominal form (usually based on the Botanical Code) as a means of classifying the varied types being observed. This is a legitimate and stimulating activity, but it is not yet helpful in terms of procaryotic classification or evolutionary taxonomy. Because of the uncertainties of alignment, they should be classified for determinative purposes in a separate group of microbiota.

Our view of classification and the taxonomic edifice is based on a century of experience supporting the contention that there is a reasonable degree of fixity in the characters describing a species. Such variation as there is within the clusters (as we now see in computer-assisted studies) can be included in the circumscription offered in describing the species or other categories. Certainly the species is a concept, not an entity (Cowan, 1968); but phenetic studies utilizing large numbers of strains and the widest possible range of characters has, if anything, clarified our concept of taxonomic groups (Sneath, 1978). Despite a growing appreciation of the Adansonian approach to species, the attitude to the definition of higher taxa involves the selection of seemingly single but very complex characters as exemplified by this essay.

The alternative and extreme view that the bacteria are so pleomorphic that the species concept has no reality is misleading and draws the attention away from the important facts of life in clonal populations. Views of this character have been put forward by Sonea (1971) and Sonea and Panisset (1976, 1980). They believe, along with the rest of us, that the procaryotic clones are united by their lineage, but these investigators differ in their interpretations of the stability of taxonomic units. They argue that genetic exchange (and "communications" of all sorts) between diverse clones makes nonsense of the species concept. The extension of their analysis into a concept of unity for the entire world population of bacteria and their interactions with the environment (a sort of global organism as real as a horse or an elephant) is an interesting but philosophical curiosity. The approach stimulates thought, but it seems evident that modern pleomorphists will have to modify and adapt their views to practical necessities dictated by new knowledge as much as our views, expressed in this chapter, will have to bend with the winds of change. A century of bacteriological analysis and studies of cultures can convince one that there is sufficient stability to allow of the recognition of most taxonomic clusters.

No doubt, there are many and variant attitudes to the details of bacterial taxonomy. But the substratum of fact is now beginning to be revealed beneath the veneer of fancy or prejudice and to allow judgment to operate. Perhaps bacteriology is maturing after about 150 years of seeking a stable basis for classification.

"For now we see through a glass, darkly; but then face to face: now I know in part. . . ."

The First Epistle of Paul
to the Corinthians (XIII:12)

That we can now perceive, albeit dimly, aspects of classification and phylogeny in the macromolecules of the *Procaryotae* is the legacy of many more scientists than have been cited so far in the prefatory chapters. The views that we espouse today still reflect the prejudices and enthusiasms of our teachers, our teachers' teachers and the influential observers and exponents of each stage in the maturation of bacteriology. The praise and the blame cannot easily be apportioned, but undoubtedly we can recognize the pervasive influence of strong-minded people of the modern era who enjoyed trying to make order out of chaos. These included D. H. Bergey, R. S. Breed, R. E. Buchanan and N. E. Gibbons whose efforts have brought *Bergey's Manual®* into print in its various editions. But they, like others before and after them and despite their special interests, not to say prejudices, were collectors of the intellections and arrangements of "authorities." Despite the arguments concerning validity that undoubtedly surfaced at the time, their efforts could not prevent the perpetuation of numerous unstable taxa that we still struggle with today: form genera, color genera, physiological genera, etc., encompassing diverse and probably unrelated species, as genetical and biochemical criteria now force us to realize. But it is more important, perhaps, to realize that the most pervasive influences on all manner of approaches have been the writings of the "Delft school" (M. W. Beijerinck and A. J. Kluyver) and the product of that school, C. B. van Niel. The discussions accompanying "the van Niel course" (attended by an equally remarkable collection of microbiologists) started many thinking about microbes in new ways and set them and their students on productive lines of work. The comparative studies that resulted from these stimuli were of great significance in microbial biochemistry, physiology and ecology; a high proportion of the studies resulted in significant contributions being made to systematic bacteriology. Not least among those influenced by van Niel was R. Y. Stanier, whose death came just as this volume was being readied for the press. It is obvious that we owe a particular debt to this lineage of bacteriologists. Stanier's arguments in our meetings, when he was a member of the Board of Trustees, were largely responsible for major changes in attitude and format expressed in the eighth and in this edition of the *Manual;* we sharpened our judgments with the help of other well-established heretics such as S. T. Cowan (1970). And now, as strongly expressed and supported in this essay, a new breed of heretic is influencing bacterial systematics, as we had been warned would be the case by another former trustee, A. W. Ravin.

In the end, a reassessment of the diverse characters used in classifications will have as important consequences as the major generalization based on cellular organization used in defining the kingdom. We must identify characters of proven reliability and validity encompassing more of the genome than seems to be the case today. The techniques must allow the comparison of groups whatever their ecological niche or the professional proclivities of those that study them. Happily, we can echo the Rabbi ben Ezra and proclaim: "The best is yet to be."

Editorial note: A publication presenting much of the data and examining the perspectives revealed in research on the *Archaeobacteria* appeared after the completion of this essay. It includes contributions from most if not all of the laboratories engaged in this thrilling task and starts with "an overview" by C. R. Woese. This comprehensive collection of papers is in *Zentralblatt für Bakteriologie, Mikrobiologie und Hygiene*, I Abt. Orig. C.3(1/2):1–345, March/May 1982.

SECTION 18

Anoxygenic Phototrophic Bacteria

Norbert Pfennig and Hans G. Trüper

The anoxygenic phototrophic (photosynthetic) bacteria represent an assemblage of predominantly aquatic bacteria that are able to grow under anaerobic conditions by photosynthesis without oxygen production. Common to all species is the presence of bacteriochlorophylls (see Table 18.1.) and of carotenoid pigments (Table 18.2.) All species contain cytochromes, quinones and non-heme iron proteins of the ferredoxin type. The photosynthetic metabolism differs from that of the cyanobacteria, algae and green plants in that water cannot serve as electron donor substrate; photosynthetic CO_2 assimilation depends on the utilization of external electron donors, such as reduced sulfur compounds, molecular hydrogen or organic compounds. Carbon dioxide is photoassimilated through the reductive pentose phosphate cycle or the reductive citric acid cycle. Fixation of dinitrogen has been demonstrated in representatives of all groups.

The Gram-negative cells are spherical, spiral, rod- or vibrioid-shaped; unicellular or uniseriately multicellular filamentous forms also occur. The diameter of individual cells ranges from 0.3 to >6 μm. In most cases, multiplication is by binary fission; some species have a polar type of cell growth and multiply by budding. Colors of cell suspensions are from purple-violet to purple, red, orange-brown, yellowish-brown, brown and green. In the presence of sulfide and light, cells of purple sulfur bacteria form highly refractile globules of elemental sulfur.

The anoxygenic phototrophic bacteria comprise essentially two cytologically different groups that are only distantly related phylogenetically (S_{AB} value about 0.2; see Fig. 18.1):

I. **Purple bacteria** in which the photosynthetic pigments are located in intracytoplasmic membrane systems that are continuous with the cytoplasmic membrane.
II. **Green bacteria** in which the photosynthetic pigments are located in the cytoplasmic membrane and in the chlorosomes that underlie and are attached to the cytoplasmic membrane.
III. **Genera incertae sedis**, i.e., two genera of bacteriochlorophyll-containing bacteria which, at present, cannot be affiliated with the purple or green bacteria.

Table 18.1.
Nomenclature of bacteriochlorophylls

Bacteriochlorophyll	Designation by	Characteristic absorption maxima in living cells (nm)
a	Jensen et al. (1964)	375, 590, 805, 830–890
b		400, 605, 835–850, 1020–1030
c		Long wavelength abs. max. 745–755
d		Long wavelength abs. max. 710–740
e	Gloe et al. (1975)	Long wavelength abs. max. 700–710
g	Brockmann and Lipinski (1983)	370, 419, 575, 670, 788

Table 18.2.
Carotenoid groups of anoxygenic phototrophic bacteria[a]

Group	Name	Major components
1	Normal spirilloxanthin series	Lycopene, rhodopin, spirilloxanthin
2	Alternative spirilloxanthin series	Chloroxanthin, spheroidene, spheroiden-one, (spirilloxanthin)
3	Okenone series	Okenone
4	Rhodopinal series (variation of group 1)	Lycopene, lycopenal, lycopenol, rhodopin, rhodopinal, spirilloxanthin
5	Chlorobactene series	Chlorobactene, isorenieratene, β-carotene, γ-carotene

[a]Data are from Schmidt, 1978.

Figure 18.1. Dendrogram showing the relationships of most groups of the anoxygenic phototrophic bacteria and some nonphototrophic relatives, as revealed by comparative oligonucleotide cataloging of their 16S rRNA. Compiled from data published by Gibson et al. (1979) and Stackebrandt and Woese (1984).

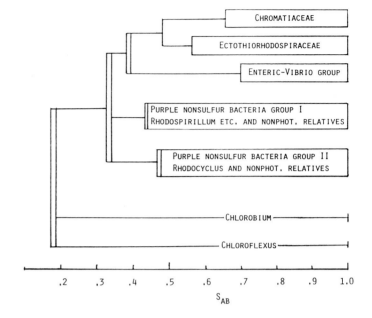

Key to the groups and families of the phototrophic **Purple** *and* **Green Bacteria** *and to the* **Genera Incertae Sedis**

Cells able to grow by a photoautotrophic and/or photoorganotrophic metabolism under anaerobic conditions.

I. Cells contain bacteriochlorophyll *a* or *b* and various carotenoids of groups 1–4 (Table 18.2.); photosynthetic pigments located in the cytoplasmic membrane and in intracytoplasmic membrane systems of different fine structure, which are continuous with the cytoplasmic membrane.
Purple Bacteria
A. Cells able to grow with sulfide and elemental sulfur as the sole photosynthetic electron donor. In the presence of both sulfide and light, globules of elemental sulfur are formed inside the cells and further oxidized to sulfate.
Family I. *Chromatiaceae*
B. Cells able to grow by photoautotrophic and/or photoorganotrophic metabolism. Sulfide and elemental sulfur are used for photoautotrophic growth. In the presence of both sulfide and light, globules of elemental sulfur are formed outside the cells and may be further oxidized to sulfate. Growth dependent on saline and alkaline growth conditions.
Family II. *Ectothiorhodospiraceae*
C. Cells preferably grow by a photoorganotrophic metabolism with simple organic substances; most species also able to grow photolithoautotrophically with molecular hydrogen as electron donor. Some species capable of using sulfide or thiosulfate as electron donor; if elemental sulfur is formed as an oxidation product, sulfur globules appear only outside the cells, never inside. Elemental sulfur rarely oxidized further to sulfate. Most species require one or more growth factors.
Purple Nonsulfur Bacteria
II. Cells contain low concentrations of bacteriochlorophylls *a* and, in most cases, *c, d* or *e* as the major bacteriochlorophyll components, as well as various carotenoids of group 5 (Table 18.2.). Light-harvesting photosynthetic pigments located in the chlorosomes which underlie and are attached to the cytoplasmic membrane.
Green Bacteria
A. Cells able to grow with sulfide or elemental sulfur as sole photosynthetic electron donor. In the presence of both sulfide and light, globules of elemental sulfur are formed outside the cells, never inside. All species are strictly anaerobic and obligately phototrophic. Simple organic substrates may be photoassimilated in the presence of both sulfide and light; therefore; cells are potentially mixotrophic.
Green Sulfur Bacteria
B. Cells uniseriately arranged in multicellular filaments that may be capable of gliding motility. Species with bacteriochlorophylls and various carotenoids.
Multicellular Filamentous Green Bacteria
III. Genera Incertae Sedis
A. Gram-negative, long, rod-shaped bacteria with gliding motility and strictly anaerobic, obligately photoorganotrophic metabolism. Cells lack intracytoplasmic membranes or chlorosomes but contain bacteriochlorophyll *g* and carotenoids. Color of cultures brownish-green.

Genus *Heliobacterium*

B. Gram-negative, rod-shaped bacteria with subpolar flagellation. Metabolism aerobic and chemoorganotrophic. Unable to grow phototrophically under any conditions. Cells contain bacteriochlorophyll *a* and carotenoids; color of cell material pale orange or red.

Genus *Erythrobacter*

Further Reading

Brockmann, H. Jr. and A. Lipinski. 1983. Bacteriochlorophyll *g*. A new bacteriochlorophyll from *Heliobacterium chlorum*. Arch. Microbiol. *136:* 17–19.

Gloe, A., N. Pfennig, H. Brockmann Jr. and W. Trowitzsch. 1975. A new bacteriochlorophyll from brown-colored *Chlorobiaceae*. Arch. Microbiol. *102:* 103–109.

Jensen, A., O. Aasmundrud and K.E. Eimhjellen. 1964. Chlorophylls of photosynthetic bacteria. Biochim. Biophys. Acta *88:* 466–479.

Schmidt, K. 1978. Biosynthesis of carotenoids. *In* Clayton and Sistrom (Editors), The Photosynthetic Bacteria. Plenum Press, New York, pp. 729–750.

Stackebrandt, E., V.J. Fowler, W. Schubert, J.F. Imhoff. 1984. Towards a phylogeny of phototrophic purple sulfur bacteria—the genus *Ectothiorhodospira*. Arch. Microbiol. *137:* 366–370.

I. PURPLE BACTERIA

FAMILY I. **CHROMATIACEAE** BAVENDAMM 1924, 125,[AL*] EMENDED DESCRIPTION IMHOFF 1984, 339

NORBERT PFENNIG AND HANS G. TRÜPER

Chro.ma.ti.a′ce.ae. M.L. neut. n. *Chromatium* type genus of the family; *-aceae* ending to denote a family; M.L. fem. pl. n. *Chromatiaceae* the *Chromatium* family.

Cells spherical, ovoid, spiral, rod- or vibrioid-shaped; multiplication by binary fission. Species with or without gas vacuoles; motile or nonmotile. Motile forms have polar flagella and are either monotrichous or multitrichous. The internal photosynthetic membrane system is continuous with the cytoplasmic membrane and of vesicular type (Fig. 18.2); only one species (*Thiocapsa pfennigii*) contains tubular membranes (Fig. 18.3) and bacteriochlorophyll *b*. All other species contain bacteriochlorophyll *a* and carotenoids of groups 1, 3 or 4. In general, cultures of strains with carotenoids of group 1 appear orange-brown to brownish-red or pink; those of group 3, purple-red; and those of group 4, purple-violet.

Under anaerobic conditions, all species are capable of photolithoautotrophic growth with sulfide or elemental sulfur as electron donor.

Elemental sulfur accumulates intermediarily as globules inside the cells. Sulfate is the ultimate oxidation product of sulfur compounds. Many species are able to use molecular hydrogen as an electron donor under reducing culture conditions. All species are potentially mixotrophic and photoassimilate a number of simple organic compounds, of which acetate and pyruvate are the most widely used. Some species are able to photoassimilate organic substances in the absence of sulfide or sulfur. Many species are strictly anaerobic and obligately phototrophic. Some species are capable of chemolithoautotrophic or chemoorganotrophic growth under microaerobic to aerobic conditions in the dark.

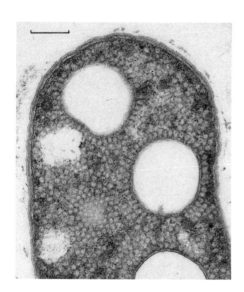

Figure 18.2. *Chromatium vinosum.* The intracytoplasmic membrane system of vesicular type extends throughout the cell. The *large white roundish areas* are former sites of sulfur globules. Electron micrograph of thin section. *Bar,* 0.3 μm.

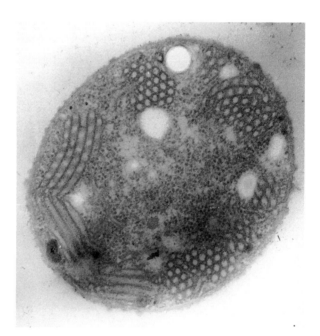

Figure 18.3. *T. pfennigii* strain DSM 228. Note the bundled tube type of the intracytoplasmic membrane system. Electron micrograph (× 60,000). (Courtesy of S. W. Watson, J. B. Waterbury and C. C. Remsen.)

*AL denotes inclusion of this name on the Approved Lists of Bacterial Names (1980).

The pathway of autotrophic CO_2 assimilation was shown to be the reductive pentose phosphate cycle in all species tested so far.

The fixation of dinitrogen has been demonstrated in several species. Storage materials are polysaccharides, poly-β-hydroxybutyrate and polyphosphate. Vitamin B_{12} is required by several species.

In nature, the *Chromatiaceae* occur in the anaerobic and sulfide-containing parts of all kinds of aquatic environments from moist and muddy soils to ditches, ponds, lakes, rivers, sulfur springs, salt lakes, estuaries and marine habitats.

Depending on the environmental conditions in nature or the culture conditions, all species are able to develop either in the form of single cells or in nonmotile cell aggregates of variable size and shape embedded in slime. The different modes of growth described by Winogradsky (1888) may be obtained experimentally by varying sulfide concentration, light intensity, pH, salinity, temperature and oxygen tension. At high sulfide concentration (2–4 mM) and high light intensity (2000–4000 lx), all flagellated species become nonmotile as the result of slime formation embedding groups of cells. For a given light intensity the various species differ from each other with respect to the sulfide concentration at which the cells develop functional flagella and become motile. For a given sulfide concentration the species differ with respect to the light intensity and mode of illumination (diurnal light and dark periods) which allow the cells to become motile. The lower the light intensity (100–200 lx), the higher the sulfide concentration at which a given strain can persist in the motile stage. These characteristics must be considered for reliable identification of pure cultures.

The mol% G + C of the DNA is 45–71 (Bd).

Type genus: *Chromatium* Perty 1852, 174.

The present arrangement of genera and species of the *Chromatiaceae* is entirely based on simple phenotypic characteristics as used in the eighth edition of the *Manual* (Pfennig and Trüper, 1974). Much systematic work is required to rearrange the existing species and genera in a taxonomic order that may reflect the phylogenetic relationships established by Fowler et al. (1984); these results are presented in the dendrogram shown in Figure 18.4.

The major differentiating characteristics of the genera of *Chromatiaceae* are presented in Table 18.3.

Further Comments

In the eighth edition of *the Manual* the *Chromatiaceae* were described to include the genus *Ectothiorhodospira*, purple sulfur bacteria that form sulfur globules outside the cells (Pfennig and Trüper, 1974). Studies of the 16S rRNA oligonucleotide catalogs of *Ectothiorhodospira* species strongly supported the intention to remove this genus from the *Chromatiaceae* (Stackebrandt et al., 1984). The new family *Ectothio-*

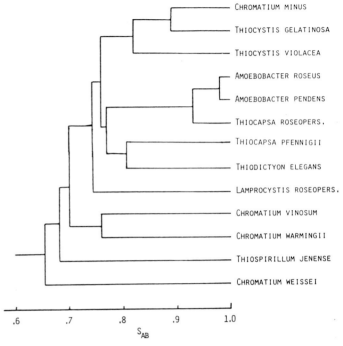

Figure 18.4. Dendrogram showing the relationships of the genera of the *Chromatiaceae* as revealed by comparative oligonucleotide cataloging of their 16S rRNA. The data are taken from Fowler et al. (1984).

rhodospiraceae was established for the *Ectothiorhodospira* species, and an emended description of the *Chromatiaceae* Bavendamm 1924 was given (Imhoff, 1984a). The *Chromatiaceae* now exclusively comprise phototrophic sulfur bacteria capable of depositing globules of elemental sulfur inside the cells. This description agrees with Molisch's (1907) definition of the "*Thiorhodaceae*," purple sulfur bacteria.

Similarity coefficients calculated on the basis of the oligonucleotide catalogs of the 16S rRNA of the type strains of most species and genera of the *Chromatiaceae* clearly demonstrated that photosynthetic sulfide oxidation with intermediate deposition of sulfur globules inside the cells is not just a feature of phenotypic similarity. All these bacteria are phylogenetically closely related to each other and form a uniform group, fairly well separated from both the *Ectothiorhodospiraceae* and the three major groups of the purple nonsulfur bacteria (Fowler et al.,

Table 18.3.
Differential characteristics of the genera of the family **Chromatiaceae**[a]

Characteristic	I. *Chromatium*	II. *Thiocystis*	III. *Thiospirillum*	IV. *Thiocapsa*	V. *Lamprobacter*	VI. *Lamprocystis*	VII. *Thiodictyon*	VIII. *Amoebobacter*	IX. *Thiopedia*
Motile by polar flagella	+	+	+	−	+	+	−	−	−
Gas vacuoles	−	−	−	−	+	+	+	+	+
Cells spherical	−	+	−	+	−	+	−	+	−
Cells spherical to ovoid, arranged in flat sheets	−	−	−	−	−	−	−	−	+
Cells ovoid to rod-shaped	+	−	−	−	+	−	+	−	−
Cells spiral or vibrioid-shaped	−	−	+	−	−	−	−	−	−
Cells aways with slime capsules	−	−	−	+	−	−	−	+	−

[a]Symbols: +, 90% or more of strains are positive; and −, 90% or more of strains are negative.

1984). Also, no other purely chemotrophic bacteria have so far been found to be more closely related to the species of both the *Ectothiorhodospiraceae* and the *Chromatiaceae* than are these bacteria related among themselves. All these facts were considered to be sufficiently significant to maintain the use of the higher taxon, the family *Chromatiaceae*. The phylogenetic position of the *Chromatiaceae* among the purple bacteria is shown in the dendrogram of relationships given in Figure 18.4.

Further Reading

Fowler, V.J., N. Pfennig, W. Schubert and E. Stackebrandt. 1984. Towards a phylogeny of phototrophic purple sulfur bacteria—16S rRNA oligonucleotide cataloguing of 11 species of *Chromatiaceae*. Arch. Microbiol. *139:* 382–387.

Imhoff, J. 1984. Reassignment of the genus *Ectothiorhodospira* Pelsh 1936 to a new family, *Ectothiorhodospiraceae* fam. nov., and emended description of the *Chromatiaceae* Bavendamm 1924. Int. J. Syst. Bacteriol. *134:* 338–339.
Molisch, H. 1907. Die Purpurbakterien nach neuen Untersuchungen. G. Fischer, Jena, pp. 1–95.
Pfennig, N. and H.G. Trüper. 1974. Family II. *Chromatiaceae. In* Buchanan and Gibbons (Editors), Bergey's Manual of Determinative Bacteriology, 8th ed. Williams & Wilkins, Baltimore, pp. 34–51.
Stackebrandt, E., V.J. Fowler, W. Schubert and J.F. Imhoff. 1984. Towards a phylogeny of phototrophic purple sulfur bacteria—the genus *Ectothiorhodospira*. Arch. Microbiol. *137:* 366–370.
Winogradsky, S. 1888. Beiträge zur Morphologie und Physiologie der Bakterien. Heft 1. Zur Morphologie und Physiologie der Schwefelbakterien. Arthur Felix, Leipzig, pp. 1–120.

Genus I. **Chromatium** *Perty 1852, 174*[AL]

Norbert Pfennig

Chro.ma′ti.um. Gr. n. *chromatium* color, paint.

Cells straight to slightly curved rod-shaped or ovoid, with rounded ends. Multiplication by binary fission, **motile by monotrichous or multitrichous polar flagella.** Cells occur singly or in pairs or may stick together and form clumps. Gram-negative. **Contain internal photosynthetic membrane systems of vesicular type** in which the photosynthetic pigments bacteriochlorophyll *a* and carotenoids of groups 1–4 are located. Do not contain gas vacuoles.

Under anaerobic conditions, **all species are capable of photolithoautotrophic growth with sulfide or elemental sulfur as electron donor**; elemental sulfur is formed as an intermediate oxidation product **and stored in the form of highly refractile globules inside the cells.** Sulfate is the ultimate oxidation product. Molecular hydrogen may be used as electron donor. All species are potentially mixotrophic and able to photoassimilate a number of simple organic compounds; acetate or pyruvate are most widely used. *Chromatium* species are mesophilic with optimal growth temperatures between 20 and 40°C. Storage materials: polysaccharides, poly-β-hydroxybutyrate, polyphosphates.

The mol% G + C of the DNA is 48.0–70.4 (Bd).

Type species: *Chromatium okenii* (Ehrenberg 1838) Perty 1852, 174.

Further Descriptive Information

Depending on the environmental or culture conditions, all species of the genus *Chromatium* can be pleomorphic. Individual cells may be irregularly swollen by the content of large globules of elemental sulfur or large granules of poly-β-hydroxybutyrate. Insufficient or excessive amounts of NaCl and $MgCl_2$ or unfavorable pH values may cause aberrant cell forms of long, extended shape and of variable diameter. The characteristic self-consistent morphology of each species is preferably obtained under optimal photoautotrophic growth conditions with sulfide as the electron donor substrate and at light intensities below saturation (1000–2000 lx). Diurnal light and dark phases may be required to sustain active flagellar motility. Particularly with the large species, optimal growth conditions are clearly recognized by the bioconvection patterns that arise as a result of the swarming activity of the cells (Pfennig, 1962).

The large *Chromatium* species, *C. okenii, C. weissei, C. warmingii* and *C. buderi,* have a polar tuft of multitrichous flagella that can be seen in the light microscope with either brightfield or phase-contrast illumination. The large species are strictly anaerobic and obligately phototrophic and require vitamin B_{12} for growth. Organic substrates can be photoassimilated by these species only in the presence of sulfide or sulfur and bicarbonate. Most of the small species are able to photoassimilate various organic substrates under reducing conditions in the absence of reduced sulfur compounds. The small species, *C. minus, C. vinosum, C. violascens* and *C. gracile,* are capable of chemolithoautotrophic or chemoorganotrophic growth under microaerobic to aerobic conditions in the dark (Kämpf and Pfennig, 1980). Under such conditions, thiosulfate is used as an electron donor substrate for autotrophic growth.

All species use ammonia as nitrogen source; nitrate is not reduced. Dinitrogen fixation was demonstrated only for two species (Yoch, 1978).

The large *Chromatium* species *C. okenii, C. weissei* and *C. warmingii* have so far been found only in sulfide-containing freshwater habitats exposed to light. *C. buderi* and all other species may occur in marine, estuarine and freshwater habitats. It remains to be established how closely related are the phenotypically similar strains isolated from marine or freshwater habitats.

Enrichment and Isolation Procedures

The large *Chromatium* species, *C. okenii, C. weissei* and *C. warmingii,* have so far been found only in sulfide-containing freshwater habitats is of primary importance for the results of enrichment experiments. In liquid enrichment cultures, strains or species that were not detected in the original sample from the natural habitat may become dominant. When certain species that were detected microscopically in reasonable numbers in a given sample are to be isolated, agar shake dilution series should be prepared directly from the sample without enrichment experiments in liquid medium. The incubation conditions for the agar cultures should closely resemble the conditions to be used for liquid enrichment cultures of the particular species. The defined medium* proved to be relatively nonspecific and may be used for the cultivation

---

* Defined medium for *Chromatiaceae*: The medium is prepared in an Erlenmeyer flask with an outlet near the bottom at one side. Connected to the outlet is a silicon rubber tube with a pinchcock and a bell for aseptic distribution of the medium into bottles or tubes. The flask is closed by a silicon rubber stopper with an inlet and an outlet for gas and a screw-capped glass tube through which additions can be made or samplings taken. The defined basal medium has the following composition (per liter of distilled water): KH_2PO_4, 0.25 g; NH_4Cl, 0.34 g; KCl, 0.34 g; $CaCl_2·2H_2O$, 0.25 g; NaCl (only for seawater medium), 20.0 g; $MgSO_4·7H_2O$, 0.5 g (for seawater medium, 3.0 g); and trace element solution (see below), 0.5 ml. After the medium has been autoclaved and cooled under an atmosphere of 90% N_2 plus 10% CO_2, the following components are added aseptically per liter of medium from sterile stock solutions while access of air is prevented by continuous flushing with the gas mixture of 90% N_2 plus 10% CO_2: 15 ml of a 10% (w/v) solution of $NaHCO_3$ (saturated with CO_2 and autoclaved under a CO_2 atmosphere); 4 ml of a 10% (w/v) solution of $Na_2S·9H_2O$) (autoclaved under an N_2 atmosphere); and 1 ml of a vitamin B_{12} solution containing 2 mg vitamin B_{12} in 100 ml of distilled water. The pH of the medium is adjusted to 7.2 with sterile 2 M H_2SO_4 or 2 M Na_2CO_3 solution while the medium is magnetically stirred. The medium is then dispensed aseptically into sterile 100-ml bottles with metal screw caps containing autoclavable rubber seals. A small air bubble is left in each bottle to meet possible pressure changes. Trace element solution (modified SL4 of Pfennig and Lippert, 1966) contains the following amounts per liter of distilled water: ethylenediaminetetraacetate-Na_2, 3.0 g; $FeSO_4·7H_2O$, 1.1 g; $CoCl_2·6H_2O$, 190 mg; $MnCl_2·4H_2O$, 100 mg; $ZnCl_2$, 70 mg; $Na_2MoO_4·2H_2O$, 18 mg; $NiCl_2·6H_2O$, 24 mg; H_3BO_3, 300 mg; and $CuCl_2·2H_2O$, 2 mg. The EDTA-Na_2 is dissolved first, followed by the other components.

of all known *Chromatiaceae*. A somewhat simpler culture medium, which is, however, less widely applicable, was described by Pfennig and Trüper (1981).

The small and fast-growing *Chromatium* species are preferentially enriched at high sulfide concentrations (3–4 mM), at high light intensities of 1000–2000 lx and at incubation temperatures of about 30°C. The large *Chromatium* species have a selective advantage when cultures with lower sulfide concentrations (1–2 mM) are incubated at about 20°C and low light intensities of 50–300 lx with diurnal light and dark phases (e.g. 16 h light, 8 h dark). The large species keep swarming in the whole bottle (Pfennig, 1962) and can be further enriched by using cell suspensions from the upper part of the enrichment culture as inoculum for subsequent enrichments.

The sulfide concentration that is initially provided in fresh culture medium does not support much growth. To achieve reasonably high population densities in enrichments or pure cultures, repeated additions of neutralized sodium sulfide solution are necessary. Additions are made when the previously added sulfide is consumed and the transiently stored elemental sulfur is nearly oxidized. The sulfide solution for feeding of cultures is prepared by neutralizing (pH to about 7.3) a stirred sodium sulfide solution (60 mM) with a certain amount of sterile 2 M sulfuric acid. The neutralized solution has to be applied immediately. Alternatively, a special device for preparation and storage of sterile neutral sulfide solution may be used (Siefert and Pfennig, 1984).

In agar shake dilution cultures, growth may be enhanced by the addition of 3 mM acetate to the defined medium.

Pure cultures are obtained by repeated application of the agar shake dilution method. Water agar is prepared with 3.3% (w/v) of agar; before the solution is prepared, the agar should be washed several times in distilled water. Depending on the salinity of the sample from nature or the enrichment culture medium, corresponding amounts of NaCl and MgCl$_2$·6H$_2$O per liter of water agar are added. The agar solution is dispensed in 3-ml amounts into test tubes, which become stoppered with cotton plugs and are autoclaved. The agar tubes are kept molten in a water bath at 55°C. Ready prepared defined culture medium is prewarmed to 40°C, and 6-ml amounts are added to the tubes of liquefied agar; exposure to air is minimized by dipping the tip of the pipette into the agar medium. Starting with a few drops of sample from

nature or an enrichment culture as inoculum and using 6–8 tubes, serial dilutions are made. All tubes are then hardened in cold water and immediately sealed with a sterile overlay consisting of 1 part paraffin wax and 3 parts paraffin oil; the overlay should be 2 cm thick. The tubes are finally flushed with 90% N$_2$ plus 10% CO$_2$ and sealed with butyl rubber stoppers. The tubes are kept in the dark for 12 h and subsequently incubated at the desired light intensity and temperature. During the first 2 days of incubation, the paraffin overlay is gently reheated to achieve a complete sealing effect. Well-separated pink, purple-red, purple-violet or orange-brown colonies that occur in the higher dilutions can be removed with sterile Pasteur pipettes and without breaking the tube. The cells are suspended in 0.5–1.0 ml of anaerobic medium and used as the inoculum for subsequent agar shake cultures. The process is repeated until a pure culture is achieved.

When pure agar cultures are obtained, individual colonies are isolated and inoculated into liquid medium. It is advisable to start with small-sized bottles or screw-capped tubes (10 or 25 ml) and then to scale up to the regularly used sizes. Purity is checked both microscopically and by use of A-C medium (Difco), adjusted to the respective salinities.

Maintenance Procedures

Pure cultures of all *Chromatium* species can be maintained in the defined mineral medium; 100-ml screw-capped bottles are preferred as culture vessels. The freshly grown cultures are supplemented with neutralized sulfide solution to a final concentration of 1.5 mM and kept in the light for about 2 h until the cells have formed intracellular sulfur globules. At this stage, the stock cultures can be stored at 4°C for 2–3 months. The cultures keep well if they are put back under dim light at room temperature and again become supplemented with neutralized sulfide solution. After formation of sulfur globules, the cultures are put back into the refrigerator.

Long term preservation of purple sulfur bacteria is successfully done by storage in liquid nitrogen. For this purpose, heavy cell suspensions of liquid cultures are supplemented with DMSO as a protective agent to a final concentration of 5%. Such suspensions are filled into 2-ml plastic ampuls, sealed, and freeze-stored. Many *Chromatium* species cannot be preserved by lyophilization.

Differentiation of the genus **Chromatium** from other genera

The genus *Chromatium* is separated from other motile genera of the purple sulfur bacteria with intracellular sulfur globules by its rod-shaped morphology and the lack of gas vacuoles. Only in the case of very short rod-shaped *Chromatium* strains may problems of delineation from the genus *Thiocystis* arise. In this case, stages of cell division should be compared. Under optimal growth conditions and also during division, cells of *Thiocystis* are consistently spherical. In contrast, cells of *Chromatium* before division appear to be short rod-shaped.

Taxonomic Comments

The differentiation of species within the genus *Chromatium* is entirely based on phenotypic similarities, e.g. the size (width) of the cells and the color of the cultures (carotenoid groups). Already the DNA base ratios of the genus (48.0–70.4 mol% G + C) indicate that genetically only distantly related species are grouped together. Studies of the

16S rRNA oligonucleotide catalogs of the type strains of four *Chromatium* species yielded similar results (Fig. 18.4). The same problem exists on the species level; the broad range of mol% G + C shows that some species may embrace a heterogenous collection of only phenotypically similar strains (e.g. *C. vinosum*, 61–66 mol% G + C). The situation will be improved if more strains of each species are isolated in pure culture and compared with respect to their phenotypic traits and genetic relationships. Further nucleic acid studies, such as rRNA oligonucleotide cataloging and DNA/DNA hybridization, will be helpful in establishing a genetically more meaningful classification.

Further Reading

Fowler, V.J., N. Pfennig, W. Schubert and E. Stackebrandt. 1984. Towards a phylogeny of phototrophic purple sulfur bacteria—16S rRNA oligonucleotide cataloguing of 11 species of *Chromatiaceae*. Arch. Microbiol. *139*: 382–387.

Differentiation of the species of the genus **Chromatium**

The few taxonomically significant phenotypic characteristics that can presently be correlated with the existing species are listed in Table 18.4.

List of species of the genus **Chromatium**

1. **Chromatium okenii** (Ehrenberg 1838) Perty 1852, 174.[AL] (*Monas okenii* Ehrenberg 1838, 15.)

o.ken'i.i. M.L. gen. n. *okenii* of Oken; named for L. Oken, a German naturalist.

Cells straight or slightly curved rod-shaped, 4.5–6.0 μm wide, 8–16 μm long, occasionally longer. Polarly situated flagellar tuft usually 1.5–2 times the cell length, visible by brightfield (Fig. 18.5) or phase-contrast microscopy. In the presence of sulfide and light, globules of

Table 18.4.
Differentiation of the species of the genus **Chromatium**[a]

Characteristic	1. *C. okenii*	2. *C. weissei*	3. *C. warmingii*	4. *C. buderi*	5. *C. minus*	6. *C. violascens*	7. *C. vinosum*	8. *C. purpuratum*	9. *C. gracile*	10. *C. minutissimum*
Cell diameter (μm)										
4.5–6.0	+	−	−	−	−	−	−	−	−	−
3.5–4.5	−	+	+	+	−	−	−	−	−	−
2.0	−	−	−	−	+	+	+	−	−	−
1.2–1.7	−	−	−	−	−	−	−	+	−	−
1.0	−	−	−	−	−	−	−	−	+	+
Color of culture, carotenoid series										
Purple-red, okenone	+	+	−	−	+	−	−	+	−	−
Purple-violet, rhodopinal	−	−	+	+	−	+	−	−	−	−
Brown-red, normal spirillo-xanthin	−	−	−	−	−	−	+	−	+	+
Vitamin B$_{12}$ requirement	+	+	+	+	−	−	−	−	−	−
NaCl requirement (%)	0	0	0	2	0	0	0	5	2	0
Mol% G + C of DNA	48–50	48–50	55–60	62–63	62	62–64	61–66	68–69	69–70	64

[a]Symbols: +, 90% or more of strains are positive; −, 90% or more of strains are negative.

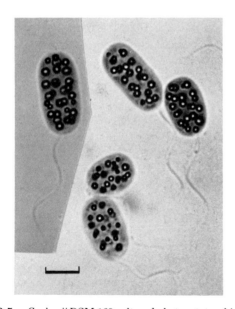

Figure 18.5. *C. okenii* DSM 169 cultured photoautotrophically with sulfide. Note the evenly distributed intracellular globules of elemental sulfur and the spiral tufts of polar flagella. Brightfield micrograph. *Bar,* 5 μm.

elemental sulfur appear evenly distributed within the cell. Color of individual cells and of cell suspensions purple-red. Photosynthetic pigments are bacteriochlorophyll *a* and carotenoid okenone.

Obligately phototrophic; strictly anaerobic. Requires sulfide-reduced media. Photosynthetic electron donors: sulfide, sulfur. In the presence of sulfide and bicarbonate, acetate and pyruvate are photoassimilated. Assimilatory sulfate reduction lacking. Not utilized: thiosulfate, molecular hydrogen, sugars, sugar alcohols, alcohols, higher fatty acids, amino acids, benzoate, formate and most intermediates of the tricarboxylic acid cycle. Nitrogen sources: ammonium salts, urea. Vitamin B$_{12}$ required. pH range: 6.5-7.3; optimum pH: 7.0. Optimum growth tempera-

ture: 25–30°C. Habitat: ditches, ponds and lakes with stagnant freshwater containing hydrogen sulfide and exposed to light.

The mol% G + C of the DNA of the neotype strain is 48 (Bd).

Type strain: DSM 169 (strain 1111, Ostrau, of Schlegel and Pfennig, 1961).

2. **Chromatium weissei** Perty 1852, 174.[AL]

weis′se.i. M.L. gen. n. *weissei* of Weisse; named for J. F. Weisse, a German zoologist.

Cells rod-shaped, 3.5–4.5 μm wide, 7–14 μm long. Other characteristics as for *C. okenii*. Nitrogenase activity present.

The mol% G + C of the DNA of the neotype strain is 48 (Bd).

Type strain: DSM 171 (strain 2111, Göttingen).

3. **Chromatium warmingii** (Cohn 1875) Migula 1900, 1048.[AL]
(*Monas warmingii* Cohn 1875, 167.)

war.min′gi.i. M.L. gen. n. *warmingii* of Warming; named for E. Warming, a Danish botanist.

Cells ovoid to rod-shaped, 3.5–4.0 μm wide, 5–11 μm long, sometimes longer. Flagellar tuft usually 1.5–2 times the cell length visible by brightfield or phase-contrast microscopy. In the presence of sulfide and light, globules of elemental sulfur are predominantly located at the two poles of the cell; dividing cells form additional sulfur globules near the central division plane (Fig. 18.6). Color of individual cells grayish to slightly pink, color of cell suspensions pinkish to purple-violet. Photosynthetic pigments are bacteriochlorophyll *a* and carotenoids of the rhodopinal series.

Obligately phototrophic; strictly anaerobic. Photosynthetic electron donors: sulfide, sulfur. In the presence of sulfide and bicarbonate, acetate and pyruvate are photoassimilated. Assimilatory sulfate reduction lacking. Not utilized: thiosulfate, sugars, alcohols, higher fatty acids, amino acids, benzoate, formate and most intermediates of the tricarboxylic acid cycle. Nitrogen sources: ammonium salts, urea, dinitrogen. Requires sulfide-reduced media. Vitamin B$_{12}$ required. pH range: 6.5–7.3; optimum pH: 7.0. Optimum growth temperature: 25–30°C. Habitat: ditches, ponds and lakes with stagnant freshwater containing hydrogen sulfide and exposed to light.

The mol% G + C of the DNA is 55.1–60.2 (Bd) (neotype strain: 55.1).

Type strain: DSM 173; ATCC 14959 (strain 6512, Melbourne).

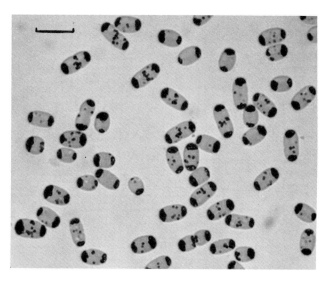

Figure 18.6. *C. warmingii* DSM 173 cultured photoautotrophically with sulfide. Note the polarly located globules of elemental sulfur. Dividing cells also deposited sulfur globules at the newly formed crosswalls. Brightfield micrograph. *Bar, 5 μm.*

4. **Chromatium buderi** Trüper and Jannasch 1968, 364.[AL]

bu'der.i. M.L. gen. n. *buderi* of Buder; named for J. Buder, a German plant physiologist.

Cells ovoid to rod-shaped, 3.5–4.5 μm wide, 4.5–9 μm long during exponential growth, about 3–4 μm in the stationary phase. Flagellar tuft, usually 1.5–2 times the cell length, may be visible in the light microscope. Globules of elemental sulfur appear evenly distributed within the cell. Color of individual cells grayish, color of cell suspensions pinkish-violet to purple-violet. Photosynthetic pigments are bacteriochlorophyll *a* and carotenoids of the rhodopinal series.

Obligately phototrophic, strictly anaerobic. Photosynthetic electron donors: sulfide, sulfur. In the presence of sulfide and bicarbonate, acetate and pyruvate are photoassimilated. Incapable of assimilatory sulfate reduction. Not utilized: thiosulfate, molecular hydrogen, sugars, alcohols, higher fatty acids, amino acids, benzoate, formate and most intermediates of the tricarboxylic acid cycle. Nitrogen sources: ammonium salts. Vitamin B_{12} required. Salinity of 1–3% (w/v) NaCl required, otherwise extremely pleomorphic. pH range: 6.5–7.6. Optimum growth temperature: 25–30°C. Habitat: estuarine salt flats and salt marshes.

The mol% G + C of the DNA is 62.2–62.8 (Bd) (type strain: 62.2).

Type strain: DSM 176; ATCC 25588 (Santa Cruz/Galapagos).

5. **Chromatium minus** Winogradsky 1888, 99.[AL]

mi'nus. L. comp. adj. *minor* (neut. *minus*) less, smaller.

Cells rod-shaped, about 2 μm wide, 2.5–6 μm long; polarly flagellated. Globules of elemental sulfur evenly distributed within the cell. Single cells appear colorless to pinkish, color of cell suspensions purple-red. Photosynthetic pigments are bacteriochlorophyll *a* and carotenoid okenone.

Phototrophic under anaerobic conditions; facultatively chemoautotrophic or mixotrophic under microaerobic to semiaerobic conditions (Kämpf and Pfennig, 1980). Photosynthetic electron donors: sulfide, sulfur, thiosulfate. In the presence of sulfide and bicarbonate, acetate, pyruvate and glucose are photoassimilated. Incapable of assimilatory sulfate reduction. Not utilized: sugar-alcohols, alcohols, higher fatty acids, amino acids, benzoate, formate and most intermediates of the tricarboxylic acid cycle (Thiele, 1968). Nitrogen sources: ammonium salts, dinitrogen. pH range: 6.5–7.6. Optimum growth temperature: 30°C. Habitat: ponds and lakes with stagnant freshwater containing hydrogen sulfide and exposed to light.

The mol% G + C of the DNA is 62.2 (Bd).

Type strain: DSM 178 (1211, Reyershausen).

6. **Chromatium violascens** Perty 1852, 174.[AL]

vi.o.las'cens. L. part. *violascens* becoming violet.

Cells rod-shaped, about 2 μm wide, 2.5–6.0 μm long, occasionally longer. Color of cell suspensions purple-violet. Photosynthetic pigments are bacteriochlorophyll *a* and carotenoids of the rhodopinal series. Other characteristics are the same as those for *C. vinosum* except that *C. violascens* does not utilize fumarate, malate and succinate (Thiele, 1968).

The mol% G + C of the DNA is 1.8–64.3 (Bd) (type strain: 62.2).

Type strain: DSM 198; ATCC 17096 (6111, Carmel River.)

7. **Chromatium vinosum** (Ehrenberg 1838) Winogradsky 1888, 99.[AL] (*Monas vinosa* Ehrenberg 1838, 11.)

vi.no'sum. L. neut. adj. *vinosum* full of wine.

Cells rod-shaped, 2 μm wide, 2.5–6 μm long, occasionally longer. Globules of elemental sulfur evenly distributed within the cell (Fig. 18.7). Single cells colorless; color of growing cultures at first yellowish to orange-brown, later reddish-brown. Photosynthetic pigments are bacteriochlorophyll *a* and carotenoids of the normal spirilloxanthin series.

Phototrophic under anaerobic conditions; facultatively chemoautotrophic or mixotrophic under microaerobic to semiaerobic conditions (Kämpf and Pfennig, 1980). Photosynthetic electron donors: sulfide, sulfur, thiosulfate, sulfite, molecular hydrogen, formate, acetate, propionate, pyruvate, fumarate, malate, succinate. Some strains utilize butyrate. Not utilized: sugars, sugar alcohols, alcohols, benzoate, citrate, amino acids. Capable of assimilatory sulfate reduction (Thiele, 1968). Nitrogen sources: ammonium salts, dinitrogen. pH range: 6.5–7.6. Optimum growth temperature: 30–35°C. Marine isolates require 1–2% NaCl. Habitat: ponds and lakes with stagnant freshwater or seawater containing hydrogen sulfide; sewage lagoons, estuaries, salt marshes; the most widespread occurring species of the genus *Chromatium*.

The mol% G + C of the DNA is 61.3–66.3 (Bd) (type strain: 64.3).

Type strain: ATCC 17899 (strain D. Roelofsen, 1934, 660).

8. **Chromatium purpuratum** Imhoff and Trüper 1980b, 601.[VP†] (Effective publication: Imhoff and Trüper 1980a, 69.)

pur.pur.a'tum. L. neut. adj. *purpuratus* dressed in purple.

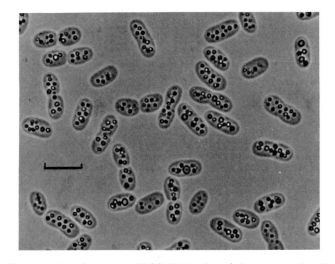

Figure 18.7. *C. vinosum* ATCC 17899 cultured photoautotrophically with sulfide. The cells contain sulfur globules. Brightfield micrograph. *Bar, 5 μm.*

---

† VP denotes that this name, although not on the Approved Lists of Bacterial Names (1980), has been validly published in the official publication, *International Journal of Systematic Bacteriology.*

Cells rod-shaped, 1.2–1.7 μm wide, 3–4 μm long if grown under autotrophic conditions. Polarly flagellated. Color of cell suspensions purple-red. Photosynthetic pigments are bacteriochlorophyll *a* and carotenoids of the okenone series.

Obligately phototrophic, strictly anaerobic. Photosynthetic electron donors: sulfide, sulfur, thiosulfate. Photoorganotrophic growth in the presence of bicarbonate with acetate, propionate, butyrate, valerate, lactate, pyruvate, fumarate, malate, succinate. Not utilized: sugars, sugar-alcohols, alcohols, higher fatty acids, benzoate, amino acids. Nitrogen sources: ammonium salts. pH range: 7.2–7.6. Salinity range: between 2 and 7% NaCl; optimum salinity: 5% NaCl. Temperature range: 25–30°C. Habitat: anoxic marine sediments and hydrogen sulfide-containing water above the sediment exposed to light; marine sponges.

The mol% G + C of the DNA of the type strain is 68.9 (T_m).

Type strain: DSM 1591 (strain BN 5500).

9. **Chromatium gracile** Strzeszewski 1913, 321.[AL]
gra′ci.le. L. neut. adj. *gracile* thin, slender.

Cells rod-shaped, 1–1.3 μm wide, 2–6 μm long. NaCl of 2–3% required for growth. Other characteristics are the same as those for *C. vinosum*; the following substrates are used in addition: lactate, propionate, butyrate (Imhoff and Trüper, 1980a).

The mol% G + C of the DNA is 68.9–70.4 (Bd) (type strain: 69.9).

Type strain: DSM 203 (strain 8611, marine, Hadley Harbor).

10. **Chromatium minutissimum** Winogradsky 1888, 100.[AL]
mi.nu.tis′si.mum. L. neut. sup. adj. *minutissimum* very small, smallest.

Cells rod-shaped, 1–1.2 μm wide, 2 μm long. Other characteristics are the same as those for *C. vinosum*.

The mol% G + C of the DNA is 63.7 (Bd).

Type strain: DSM 1376 (strain MSV, Glubokoe Lake, U.S.S.R.).

Addendum

New species recently described by M. T. Madigan (1986): *Chromatium tepidum*.

Genus II. **Thiocystis** *Winogradsky 1888, 60* [AL]

NORBERT PFENNIG

Thi.o.cys′tis. Gr. n. *thios* sulfur; Gr. n. *cystis* the bladder, a bag; M.L. fem. n. *Thiocystis* sulfur bag.

Cells spherical to slightly ovoid; before cell division, diplococcus-shaped. Multiplication by binary fission; **motile by means of a single flagellum.** Cells occur singly or in pairs or may grow in irregular aggregates surrounded by slime. Gram-negative. **Contain internal photosynthetic membrane systems of vesicular type** in which the photosynthetic pigments bacteriochlorophyll *a* and carotenoids of groups 3 or 4 are located. Do not contain gas vacuoles.

Under anaerobic conditions, cells are **capable of photolithoautotrophic growth with sulfide or sulfur as electron donor**; during sulfide oxidation, globules of elemental sulfur are transiently stored inside the cells. The final oxidation product is sulfate. **Facultatively chemoautotrophic under microaerobic to aerobic conditions.**

Storage materials: polysaccharide, poly-β-hydroxybutyrate, polyphosphate. Habitat: anoxic sulfide-containing water and mud of fresh and brackish water and marine environments.

The mol% G + C of the DNA is 61.3–67.9 (Bd).

Type species: *Thiocystis violacea* Winogradsky 1888, 65.

Further Descriptive Information

The spherical, motile, gas vacuole-free purple sulfur bacteria of the genus *Thiocystis* are frequently found in the same natural habitats as the small *Chromatium* species of the *C. vinosum* type. Physiologically the small *Chromatium* species closely resemble the *Thiocystis* species. This is true not only for the phototrophic metabolism of reduced sulfur compounds and organic substrates but also for the facultatively chemoautotrophic or chemoorganotrophic metabolism under microaerobic to aerobic conditions in the dark (Kämpf and Pfennig, 1980).

Enrichment and Isolation Procedures

The methods to be used are the same as those described for the small *Chromatium* species (see page 1640).

Maintenance Procedures

Maintenance of strains in liquid culture medium and long term preservation in liquid nitrogen are carried out as described for the genus *Chromatium*.

Differentiation of the genus **Thiocystis** *from other genera*

Characteristics useful for differentiation of the genus *Thiocystis* from other genera of the *Chromatiaceae* are listed in Table 18.3.

Taxonomic Comments

The genus *Thiocystis* is delineated from the genus *Chromatium* solely on the basis of its spherical morphology. A second genus for spherical, motile purple sulfur bacteria, *Thiothece* Winogradsky 1888, was distinguished by Winogradsky from *Thiocystis* on the basis of the location of the intracellular sulfur globules. In the monotypic genus *Thiothece* the sulfur globules are located at the inner periphery of the cells, whereas in *Thiocystis* the globules are distributed at random in

the cell. Pfennig and Trüper (1971) included *Thiothece gelatinosa* Winogradsky 1888 in the genus *Thiocystis*, since they did not consider the maintenance of *Thiothece* besides *Thiocystis* justified. The results of similarity studies on the 16S rRNA oligonucleotide catalogs of *Chromatiaceae* (Fowler et al., 1984) not only substantiated the close relationship of *Thiocystis gelatinosa* with *T. violacea* (see Fig. 18.4) but also revealed a close genetic relationship between *Thiocystis* and *Chromatium minus*. Further studies with more strains are required to uncover whether the spherical *Thiocystis* strains indeed form a group of related bacteria separate from rod-shaped *Chromatium* species.

Differentiation of the species of the genus **Thiocystis**

I. Sulfur globules appear randomly distributed within the cell; cells contain carotenoids of the rhodopinal series, and cultures are purple-violet.

1. *T. violacea*

II. Sulfur globules occur only at the inner periphery of the cell; cells contain carotenoids of the okenone series, and cultures are purple-red.

2. *T. gelatinosa*

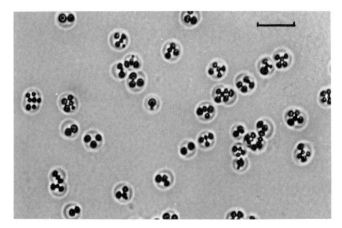

Figure 18.8. *T. violacea* DSM 207 cultured photoautotrophically with sulfide. The cells contain sulfur globules. Brightfield micrograph. *Bar,* 5 μm.

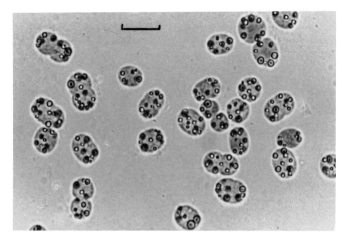

Figure 18.9. *T. gelatinosa* DSM 215 cultured photoautotrophically with sulfide. The peripheral deposition of the sulfur globules is clearly visible in some of the cells. Brightfield micrograph. *Bar,* 5 μm.

List of species of the genus **Thiocystis**

1. **Thiocystis violacea** Winogradsky 1888, 65.[AL]

vi.o.la′ce.a. L. fem. adj. *violacea* violet-colored.

Cells are spherical, about 2.5–3 μm in diameter; depending on the culture conditions, larger individual cells may occur. Under unfavorable conditions, irregular aggregates of cells surrounded by slime are formed. Sulfur globules appear randomly distributed within the cell (Fig. 18.8). Color of individual cells grayish, color of cell suspensions purple-violet. Photosynthetic pigments are bacteriochlorophyll *a* and carotenoids of the rhodopinal series (Schmidt et al., 1965).

Phototrophic under anaerobic conditions, facultatively chemoautotrophic or mixotrophic under microaerobic to aerobic conditions in the dark. Photosynthetic electron donors: sulfide, sulfur, thiosulfate, and sulfite (used by some strains). In the presence of sulfide and bicarbonate, acetate and pyruvate are photoassimilated; in addition, some strains use fumarate, succinate, oxoglutarate, fatty acids and glucose or fructose. Some strains capable of assimilatory sulfate reduction. Nitrogen sources: ammonium salts, urea, dinitrogen. pH range: 6.5–7.6; optimum pH: 7.3. Growth temperature: 25–35°C. Marine isolates require 1–2% NaCl. Habitat: ponds and lakes with stagnant freshwater and brackish water or seawater containing hydrogen sulfide; sewage lagoons, estuaries, salt marshes, sulfur springs.

The mol% G + C of the DNA is 62.8–67.9 (Bd) (type strain: 63.1).

Type strain: DSM 207 (strain 2711, Grünenplan).

2. **Thiocystis gelatinosa** (Winogradsky 1888) Pfennig and Trüper 1971, 11.[AL] (*Thiothece gelatinosa* Winogradsky 1888, 82.)

ge.la.ti.no′sa. L. part. adj. *gelatus* frozen, stiffened; M.L. n. *gelatinum* that which stiffens; M.L. fem. adj. *gelatinosa* gelatinous.

Cells are spherical, about 3 μm in diameter; under unfavorable conditions, elongated ovoid cells may occur. At high sulfide concentration (4–6 mM) and light intensity (>1000 lx), cells are nonmotile, growing in irregular aggregates surrounded by slime. Under optimal growth conditions, globules of elemental sulfur occur only in the peripheral part of the cytoplasm (Fig. 18.9). Color of individual cells is slightly pink; color of cell suspensions is purple-red. Photosynthetic pigments are bacteriochlorophyll *a* and carotenoids of the okenone series (Pfennig et al., 1968).

Phototrophic under anaerobic conditions, facultatively chemoautotrophic or mixotrophic under microaerobic to semiaerobic conditions. Photosynthetic electron donors: sulfide, sulfur. In the presence of sulfide and bicarbonate, acetate and pyruvate are photoassimilated. Nitrogen sources: ammonium salts. pH range: 6.5–7.6. Optimum growth temperature: 30°C. A salinity of at least 1% NaCl is required by the type strain. Habitat: stagnant water containing hydrogen sulfide; hypolimnion of meromictic lakes.

The mol% G + C of the DNA of the type strain is 61.3 (Bd).

Type strain: DSM 215 (strain 2611, Langvik).

Genus III. **Thiospirillum** Winogradsky 1888, 104[AL]

NORBERT PFENNIG

Thi.o.spi.ril′lum. Gr. n. *thios* sulfur; M.L. dim. neut. n. *Spirillum* a bacterial genus; M.L. neut. n. *Thiospirillum* sulfur *Spirillum.*

Cells curved rod-shaped or spiral (sigmoid), dividing by binary fission, **motile by means of (multitrichous) polar flagella.** Under certain conditions, cells may be nonmotile and grow in irregular aggregates surrounded by slime. Gram-negative. **Contain internal photosynthetic membrane systems of vesicular type** in which the photosynthetic pigments are located. Do not contain gas vacuoles.

Obligately phototrophic, strictly anaerobic. Capable of photolithoautotrophic growth with sulfide or sulfur as electron donor; elemental sulfur is transiently stored inside the cells. Sulfate is the ultimate oxidation product. Storage materials are polysaccharides, poly-β-hydroxybutyrate and polyphosphate.

The mol% G + C of the DNA is 45.5 (Bd).

Type species: *Thiospirillum jenense* (Ehrenberg) Winogradsky 1988, 104.

Further Descriptive Information

Only one species of *Thiospirillum* has so far been studied in pure culture: *T. jenense.* The cells of this species are generally sigmoid; however, curved rod- or vibrioid-shaped cells may occur under optimum growth conditions. *T. jenense* is a typical freshwater bacterium; it remains to be elucidated whether spirilloid purple sulfur bacteria of similar size occurring in marine habitats belong to the same species.

Enrichment and Isolation Procedures

The culture conditions for *T. jenense* are essentially the same as those described in detail for the large *Chromatium* species (see page 1640). Most likely because of their large size (generally 30–40 μm in length), the cells of *T. jenense* do not grow well in agar shake cultures suitable for the large *Chromatium* species. However, growth could be obtained if the concentration of thoroughly washed agar was lowered to 0.6–0.8% (w/v). In such agar cultures, colonies of *Thiospirillum* appeared irregular and wisp-shaped; the individual cells could be recognized by using a low power, binocular dissecting microscope. Cultures with not more than 4-6 mM sulfide should be incubated at low light intensity (200-500 lx). Colonies from agar shake cultures grew well in liquid medium, provided culture vessels of small volume were used first, e.g. screw-capped test tubes of 10–15-ml volume.

Maintenance Procedures

Maintenance of strains in liquid culture medium and long term preservation in liquid nitrogen are carried out as described for the genus *Chromatium* (see page 1640). *Thiospirullum* cannot be preserved by lyophilization.

Differentiation of the genus **Thiospirillum** *from other genera*

Characteristics useful for differentiation of the genus *Thiospirillum* from other genera of the *Chromatiaceae* are listed in Table 18.3.

Taxonomic Comments

In addition to *T. jenense*, two other species of *Thiospirillum* had been described from observations of water and mud samples collected in nature: "*T. sanguineum*" and "*T. rosenbergii*." The former species was described as being the same size and morphology as *T. jenense*, with which it could have been confused. More recent reports on the existence of "*T. rosenbergii*" are lacking. Further studies of strains obtained in pure culture are required in order for the species of the genus *Thiospirillum* to be recognized.

List of species of the genus **Thiospirillum**

1. **Thiospirillum jenense** (Ehrenberg 1838) Migula 1900, 1050.[AL] (*Ophidomonas jenensis* Ehrenberg 1838, 44.)

je.nen'se. M.L. neut. adj. *jenense* pertaining to Jena, Germany, the city where Ehrenberg discovered this organism.

Cells curved rod- or vibrioid-shaped, sigmoid or spiral, 2.5–4.0 μm wide; sigmoid cells usually 30–40 μm long; spiral cells up to 100 μm long. Complete turns may measure 15-40 μm and have a coil depth of 3-7 μm. Polarly situated flagellar tuft usually 10-12 μm long, visible by brightfield or phase-contrast microscopy (Fig. 18.10). Cells rarely tufted at both ends. Color of individual cells pale yellow, color of cell suspensions yellowish to orange-brown. Photosynthetic pigments are bacteriochlorophyll *a* and carotenoids lycopene and rhodopin (Schmidt et al., 1965).

Obligately phototrophic and anaerobic. Photosynthetic electron donors: sulfide, sulfur. Thiosulfate not utilized. In the presence of sulfide and bicarbonate, acetate is photoassimilated. Nitrogen sources: ammonium salts. Vitamin B_{12} is required for growth. pH range: 6.5–7.5; optimum pH: 7.0. Growth temperature: 20-25°C. Habitat: mud and stagnant water of ditches and freshwater ponds containing hydrogen sulfide.

The mol% G + C of the DNA of the type strain is 45.5

Type strain: DSM 216 (strain 1112, Ostrau).

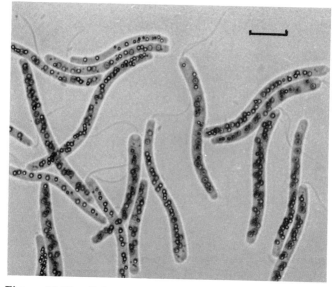

Figure 18.10. *T. jenense* DSM 216 cultured photoautotrophically with sulfide. Note the intracellular sulfur globules and the short, slightly sigmoidal tufts of polar flagella. Brightfield micrograph. *Bar,* 10 μm.

Genus IV. **Thiocapsa** *Winogradsky 1888, 84*[AL]

NORBERT PFENNIG

Thi.o.cap'sa. Gr. n. *thios* sulfur; L. n. *capsa* box; M.L. fem. n. *Thiocapsa* sulfur box.

Cells spherical to slightly ovoid, 1.2–3 μm in diameter; multiplication by binary fission; **nonmotile.** Tetrads may be formed as a result of consecutive divisions in two perpendicular planes. Under unfavorable culture conditions and in many natural habitats, cells may grow in irregular clumps surrounded by slime. Gram-negative. **Contain internal photosynthetic membrane systems of vesicular or tubular type** in which the photosynthetic pigments bacteriochlorophyll *a* or *b* and carotenoids are located. **Do not contain gas vacuoles.**

Phototrophic under anaerobic conditions; may be chemoautotrophic or mixotrophic under microaerobic to aerobic conditions in the dark. Capable of photolithoautotrophic growth with sulfide or sulfur as electron donor; elemental sulfur transiently stored inside the cells; the final oxidation product is sulfate.

The mol% G + C of the DNA is 63.3–69.9 (Bd).

Type species: *Thiocapsa roseopersicina* Winogradsky 1888, 84.

Further Descriptive Information

The phototrophic sulfur bacteria of the genus *Thiocapsa* are spherical, nonmotile and free of gas vacuoles. Under unfavorable growth conditions, the *Thiocapsa* species may form aggregates of cells embedded in slime similar to *Thiocystis* or small *Chromatium* species. The species of these genera can be distinguished and identified only when they are obtained in pure culture and studied under optimal growth conditions during which no aggregates are formed and the potentially flagellated species are motile. Depending on the culture conditions, the cell diameter of the spherical purple sulfur bacteria may vary considerably.

Enrichment and Isolation Procedures

The methods to be used are the same as those described for the small *Chromatium* species (see page 1640). *Thiocapsa reseopersicina* is one of the most common purple sulfur bacteria in nature. It is particularly abundant in ponds, pools or lagoons receiving sewage or wastewater rich in organic matter. Since this is the most nonfastidious purple sulfur bacterium known, its isolation presents no problems. The other species of *Thiocapsa*, *T. pfennigii*, is the only purple sulfur bacterium known so far that contains bacteriochlorophyll *b*. Owing to this bacteriochlorophyll, the bacterium has an in vivo absorption maximum in the infrared region of the spectrum between 1020 and 1030 nm. This specific absorption has been successfully used for the selective enrichment culture of bacteriochlorophyll *b*-containing *Thiocapsa* strains (Eimhjellen et al., 1967). In contrast to the facultatively photoorganotrophic *T. roseopersicina*, *T. pfennigii* is strictly anaerobic and dependent on sulfide or sulfur as photosynthetic electron donor. This must be taken into account for the isolation of pure cultures.

Maintenance Procedures

Maintenance of strains in liquid culture medium and long term perservation in liquid nitrogen are carried out as described for the genus *Chromatium* (see page 1640).

Differentiation of the genus **Thiocapsa** *from other genera*

Characteristics useful for differentiation of the genus *Thiocapsa* from other genera of the *Chromatiaceae* are listed in Table 18.3. *Thiocapsa* cells may form tetrads; thus this genus has repeatedly been mistaken for *Thiopedia rosea*. The cells of the latter genus are, however, readily distinguishable from *Thiocapsa* by their conspicuous gas vacuoles as well as their formation of platelets, which usually consist of 8, 16 or more regularly arranged cells.

Taxonomic Comments

The genus *Thiocapsa* is defined as the spherical, nonmotile, gas vacuole-free *Chromatiaceae*. The two species of the genus differ, however, in the structure of their intracytoplasmic membrane systems and in their photosynthetic pigments. *T. roseopersicina* contains bacteriochlorophyll *a* and a vesicular photosynthetic membrane system (Takács and Holt, 1971). *T. pfennigii* contains bacteriochlorophyll *b* and a tubular membrane system (Eimhjellen et al., 1967; Eimhjellen, 1970).

Comparison of the 16S rRNA oligonucleotide catalogs of the two species revealed an S_{AB} value of 0.77 which is higher than the S_{AB} values for all other species of the *Chromatiaceae* with the exception of *Thiodictyon elegans* (S_{AB} value of 0.81 to *Thiocapsa pfennigii*). This result indicates that the particular phenotypic traits of *T. pfennigii* are not the expression of a distant relationship to the other *Chromatiaceae*. In fact, the nearest relatives of *T. pfennigii* are *Thiodictyon elegans*, *Thiocapsa roseopersicina* and the two *Amoebobacter* species (see Fig. 18.4).

Further Reading

Eimhjellen, K.E. 1970. *Thiocapsa pfennigii* sp. nov. a new species of the phototrophic sulfur bacteria. Arch. Microbiol. *73:* 193–194.

Eimhjellen, K.E., H. Steensland and J. Traetteberg. 1967. A *Thiococcus* sp. nov. gen., its pigments and internal membrane system. Arch. Microbiol. *59:* 82–92.

Takács, B.J. and S.C. Holt. 1971. *Thiocapsa floridana*; a cytological physiological and chemical characterization. I. Cytology of whole cells and isolated chromatophore membranes. Biochim. Biophys. Acta *233:* 258–277.

Differentiation of the species of the genus **Thiocapsa**

I. Cells contain bacteriochlorophyll *a* and, as the major carotenoid, spirilloxanthin and culture definitively pink. Photosynthetic membrane system of vesicular type. All strains able to grow under microaerobic to aerobic conditions in the dark.

         1. *T. roseopersicina*

II. Cells contain bacteriochlorophyll *b* and, as the major carotenoid, tetrahydrospirilloxanthin and culture light yellow to orange-brown. Photosynthetic membrane system consists of bundles of ribbonlike branched tubes. Strictly anaerobic.

         2. *T. pfennigii*

List of species of the genus **Thiocapsa**

1. **Thiocapsa roseopersicina** Winogradsky 1888, 84.[AL]

ro.se.o.per.si.ci′na. L. adj. *roseus* rosy; Gr. n. *persicus* the peach; M.L. fem. adj. *roseopersicina* rosy peach-colored.

Cells spherical, 1.2–3.0 µm, usually 1.5 µm in diameter (Fig. 18.11). Individual cells surrounded by a strong slime capsule. Aggregates of two, four or more cells are common; irregular clumps of cells are usually surrounded by slime. Photosynthetic membrane system of vesicular type. Individual cells colorless, color of cell suspensions pink to rose-red, although orange-brown and purple-violet strains may occur. Photosynthetic pigments are bacteriochlorophyll *a* and carotenoids of the normal spirilloxanthin series (Schmidt et al., 1965).

Phototrophic under anaerobic conditions, facultatively chemoautotrophic or chemoorganotrophic under microaerobic to aerobic conditions in the dark. Photosynthetic electron donors: sulfide, sulfur, thiosulfate or molecular hydrogen. Acetate, pyruvate, fumarate malate, succinate, glycerol and fructose are photoassimilated. Not utilized: lactate, propionate, butyrate, tartrate, α-oxoglutarate, citrate, benzoate and alcohols. Most strains capable of assimilatory sulfate reduction. Nitrogen sources: ammonium salts. Nitrogenase activity present. pH range: 6.5–7.5; optimum pH: 7.3. Growth temperature: 20–35°C. Habitat: stagnant water and the mud of ponds, pools or wastewater lagoons containing degradable organic substances and hydrogen sulfide. Common also in estuaries and salt marshes.

The mol% G + C of the DNA is 63.3–66.3 (Bd) (type strain: 65.3).

Type strain: DSM 217 (strain 1711, Hardenberg).

2. **Thiocapsa pfennigii** Eimhjellen 1970, 193.[AL]

pfen.nig′i.i. M.L. gen. n. *pfennigii* of Pfennig; named after N. Pfennig, a German microbiologist.

Cells spherical, 1.2–1.5 µm in diameter; diplococcus-shaped division stages about 2.5 µm long. Stationary phase cells 0.8–1.0 µm in diameter. Internal photosynthetic membrane system consisting of bundles of ribbonlike branched tubes continuous with the cytoplasmic membrane. Individual cells colorless, color of cell suspensions yellowish to orange-brown. Photosynthetic pigments are bacteriochlorophyll *b* and carotenoid 3,4,3′,4′-tetrahydrospirilloxanthin (Eimhjellen et al., 1967).

Obligately phototrophic and strictly anaerobic. Photosynthetic electron donors: sulfide, sulfur. In the presence of sulfide and bicarbonate, acetate and propionate and photoassimilated. Not utilized: thiosulfate, butyrate. Nitrogen sources: ammonium salts, dinitrogen. pH range: 6.5–7.5; optimum pH: 7.0 Growth temperature: 20–35°C. Habitat: river freshwater mud and brackish water mud containing hydrogen sulfide and exposed to light.

The mol% G + C of the DNA is 69.4–69.9 (Bd).

Type strain: RG3, Nidelven (Department of Biochemistry, Technical University, Trondheim, Norway).

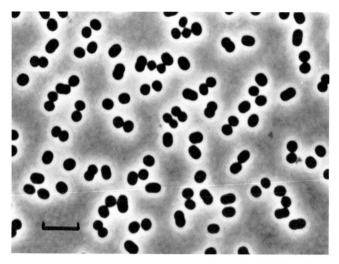

Figure 18.11. *T. roseopersicina* DSM 219 cultured photoautotrophically with sulfide. Phase-contrast micrograph *Bar*, 5 μm.

Genus V. **Lamprobacter** Gorlenko, Krasil'nikova, Kikina and Tatarinova 1988, 220[VP] (Effective publication: Gorlenko, Krasil'nikova, Kikina and Tatarinova 1979, 765)

VLADIMIR M. GORLENKO

Lam′pro.bac′ter. Gr. adj. *lamprus* bright, brilliant; M.L. masc. n. *bacter* equivalent of Gr. neut. n. *bacterion* a rod; M.L. masc. n. *Lamprobacter* brilliant rod.

Cells rod-shaped or ovoid, multiply by binary fission. Do not form typical aggregates. **Possess gas vacuoles** located in the periphery or in the entire cytoplasm. Accumulate **intracellular globules of sulfur** when growing on media with sulfide or thiosulfate. **Motile by means of flagella** during a certain stage of development. Motile cells are normally devoid of gas vacuoles. Gram-negative. **Bacteriochlorophyll *a* as well as carotenoid pigments** are localized in the intracytoplasmic membrane system of vesicular type.

Capable of photoautotrophic growth under anaerobic conditions with reduced sulfur compounds as electron donor. Facultatively microaerophilic and capable of chemoautotrophic growth in the dark.

The mol% G + C of the DNA is 64 (chem. anal.).

Type species: *Lamprobacter modestohalophilus* Gorlenko, Krasil'nikova, Kikina and Tatarinova 1988, 220.

Further Descriptive Information

L. modestohalophilus exhibits considerable polymorphism when grown under various growth conditions (Gorlenko et al., 1979). On the mineral medium of Pfennig (1965) with sulfide or thiosulfate, rod-shaped or ovoid cells of different strains may vary in size, 0.5–1.5 μm wide, 2.5–4 μm long.

These cells display dimorphism during normal development of cultures on bicarbonate-containing media with acetate, glycerol or other organic compounds. On the first day, cells are rod-shaped, motile by means of flagella, and generally devoid of gas vacuoles and contain globules of sulfur. On the third or fourth day, cells lose their motility, gas vacuoles appear, and slimy capsules are formed. Slimy capsules consolidate and cells are transformed into a cyst. Multiple passages on a mineral medium result in a temporary disability to produce motile cells. Bacteria contain gas vacuoles throughout the period of growth and are surrounded by loose or dense slimy capsules.

Involution cells are large and irregularly shaped at excessive NaCl concentrations and an acid pH of 5.9–6.6 and are thin, elongated and slightly bent at a pH of 8.0 or higher.

Cells stain Gram-negative. The cell wall is of the Gram-negative type; characteristically, the outer membrane is overlain by an external layer consisting of hexagonal subunits 20 nm long. Vegetative cells possess a loose fibrous slimy capsule. Slimy capsules of the cystlike cells are dense, with a clear margin.

Photosynthetic membrane system is of vesicular type. Vesicles are 70 nm in diameter, extend from the cytoplasmic membrane, and occupy the major part of the protoplasm in bacteria growing anaerobically in the light. Vesicles are confined by a triple membrane similar to the cytoplasmic membrane.

DNA filaments and polyribosomes were not observed, owing to the abundance of photosynthetic structures.

Storage materials are especially abundantly produced on a medium with glycerol both in the light and, aerobically, in the dark.

Cells with gas vacuoles tend to concentrate in the upper part of the bottle at room temperature. Gas vesicles, short point-ended cylinders of 60 × 80 nm to 120 × 140 nm, are grouped near the periphery of the cell; sulfur is deposited in the central vesicle-free part of the cell.

Suspension of bacteria grown anaerobically in the light appears purple-pink. In vivo absorption spectrum maxima at 370, 655, 804 and 827 nm indicate the presence of bacteriochlorophyll *a*, while a major peak at 518 nm and shoulders at 486 and 549 nm reveal the presence of carotenoids of the okenone series.

Examined strains of *L. modestohalophilus* are only capable of photoautotrophic growth on mineral medium in the presence of vitamin B$_{12}$. Bacteria lack assimilatory sulfate reduction (Krasil'nikova, 1985). Oxidize H$_2$S and Na$_2$S$_2$O$_3$ to S^0 and further to SO$_4$$^{2-}$ in the light, with the accumulation of S^0 and generation of sulfate being parallel. CO$_2$ is assimilated via the Calvin cycle.

L. modestohalophilus are moderate halophiles with optimum 1–2% NaCl; growth is possible with up to 9% NaCl. Favorable growth pH: 7.4–7.6. Optimum temperature: 25–27°C.

Lamprobacter utilizes a number of organic compounds besides CO$_2$; glycerol, acetate, pyruvate, lactate, maltose and lactose sharply increase the yield.

Glycerol metabolism involves the functioning of glycerol kinase and α-glycerophosphate dehydrogenase independent of pyridine nucleotides (Krasil'nikova et al., 1979).

Organic acids are assimilated through the incomplete tricarboxylic acid cycle. The glyoxylate cycle is absent (Krasil'nikova, 1985; Krasil'nikova and Kondrat'eva, 1979).

Sugars are utilized through the Embden-Meyerhof pathway.

Nitrogen sources: ammonium salts, urea, casein hydrolysate, glutamic acid. Capable of nitrogen fixation.

Aerobic growth: for facultative microaerophiles, the best growth occurs in the dark with 10% O_2 in the gas phase; growth is suppressed in the light with an O_2 concentration above 2%. Thiosulfate or S^0 is required as donor and as the S source for assimilatory purposes (Krasil'nikova, 1981). Optimum concentration of thiosulfate is 0.1–0.2%. At a concentration of 0.5% $Na_2S_2O_3$, growth of aerobic cultures is sharply inhibited.

In the dark, $Na_2S_2O_3$ is oxidized to S^0 and SO_4^{2-}. Molecular sulfur is deposited intracellularly as an intermediate product. These cells are capable of chemolithotrophic aerobic growth in the presence of vitamin B_{12} (Kondrat'eva et al., 1981). Best growth occurs in the dark with additional glycerol. Moreover, lactate, pyruvate and propionate stimulate growth.

Enrichment and Isolation Procedures

L. modestohalophilus widely occurs in shallow saline water bodies (0.5–10% NaCl) with high sulfide content. Found only in well-warmed water bodies in southern areas of the U.S.S.R: the Crimea, Donetsk region (Ukraine), Turkmenia. In the White Sea littoral, *Lamprobacter* could not be found.

When water and mud samples are inoculated into a medium containing 0.5–2% NaCl, 500 mg $Na_2S \cdot 9H_2O$/l, 1 g $Na_2S_2O_3$/l and 1 g sodium acetate/l, microorganisms with gas vacuoles are concentrated in the upper part of the bottle. This fraction is removed by using a sterile capillary and is transferred with dilutions into 0.8% agar medium of the same composition. Grown colonies are then purified by repeated application of agar shake dilution cultures.

Maintenance Procedures

Cultures are maintained in liquid medium that is stored in a refrigerator at low light intensity for 1–3 months.

Differentiation of the genus **Lamprobacter** from other genera

Major features of differentiation from similar genera of purple sulfur bacteria are presented in Table 18.3

The genus *Lamprobacter* occupies an intermediate position between the genera *Thiodictyon* and *Lamprocystis*, which also contain gas vacuoles. Major differences are in cell shape, motility and peculiarities in the development cycle. Cells of the genus *Lamprobacter* differ from those of genus *Chromatium* in that they contain gas vacuoles.

Taxonomic Comments

Generic differentiation from purple sulfur bacteria will have to be ascertained by future molecular genetic investigations.

List of species of the genus **Lamprobacter**

1. **Lamprobacter modestohalophilus** Gorlenko, Krasil'nikova, Kikina and Tatarinova 1988, 220.[VP] (Effective publication: Gorlenko, Krasil'nikova, Kikina and Tatarinova 1979, 765.)

mo.des'to.ha.lo.phi'lus. L. n. *modestus* moderate; Gr. n. *halos* salt; Gr. adj. *philus* loving; M.L. masc. adj. *modestohalophilus* moderate salt-loving.

Cells rod-shaped or ovoid, 2–2.5 µm wide and 4–5 µm long, and polymorphous under changing conditions of incubation (Fig. 18.12). Have a complex life cycle with two alternating morphological forms: nonmotile cells with gas vacuoles and slimy capsules, and cells motile by means of flagella and devoid of gas vacuoles. Gas vacuoles are more frequently located in the periphery, while the globules of elemental sulfur are located in the center of the cell. Contain bacteriochlorophyll *a* and carotenoid pigments of the okenone series. The photosynthetic structures are of the vesicular type. Vesicles in cells grown on mineral medium measure about 70 nm.

Cultures: capable of growth under anaerobic conditions in the light and under microaerobic conditions in the dark. Under anaerobic conditions in the light, cell suspensions appear purple-pink. Under aerobic conditions in the dark, the synthesis of pigments is reduced and cultures become colorless.

In a stab culture in 0.8% agar medium in the dark, growth occurs 1 cm below the surface. Optimum growth temperature: 23–27°C. Favorable light intensity: 3000 lx. Optimum pH: 7.4–7.6. Optimum salinity: 1–2%. Growth is absent in the absence of sodium chloride.

Electron donors in the light: sulfide, thiosulfate, elemental sulfur, hydrogen (sulfite is not utilized). Electron donors in the dark: thiosulfate, sulfur.

In the light in the the presence of sulfide (or thiosulfate) and bicarbonate, the carbon sources utilized are alcohols (glycerol, *n*-propanol, *n*-butanol, ethanol, isobutanol, isopropanol) and organic acids (lactate, pyruvate and acetate). Methanol, isoamyl alcohol, sorbitol, dulcitol, mannitol, succinate, fumarate, malate, lactose, maltose, xylose, galactose, and fructose are not utilized. Growth is inhibited by *n*-amyl alcohol, allyl alcohol, formate, propionate, benzoate, arabinose, ramnose and raffinose. Strain differences in the spectrum of organic

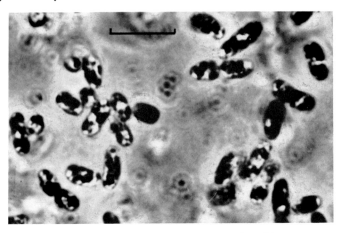

Figure 18.12. *L. modestohalophilus* strain RO-1. Phase-contrast micrograph. *Bar*, 10 µm. (Reproduced with permission from V. M. Gorlenko, E. N. Krasil'nikova, O. G. Kikina and N. Y. Tatarinova, Izvestiya Akademii Nauk S.S.S.R. Seriya Biologicheskaya (Moskva) 5: 765, 1979.)

compounds utilized are possible. Nitrogen sources: ammonium salts, urea, casein hydrolysate, glutamic acid, molecular nitrogen. Vitamin B_{12} is required as a growth factor. Lack assimilatory sulfate reduction, require reduced sulfur compounds, sulfide or thiosulfate for biosynthesis. Hydrogenase and catalase activity is present.

Storage materials: sulfur, poly-β-hydroxybutyrate, polyphosphate and polysaccharide.

Habitat: hydrogen sulfide-containing mud and water of saline water bodies. Occur at salinity of 1–4% together with the following other phototrophic bacteria: *Chromatium vinosum*, *Chromatium buderi*, *Pelodictyon phaeum*, *Pelodictyon luteolum*, *Prosthecochloris aestuarii*.

The mol% G + C of the DNA is 64 ± 0.5 (chem. anal.).

Type strain: RO-1 (Institute of Microbiology, Academy of Sciences of the U.S.S.R., Moscow, U.S.S.R.), isolated from Lake Rozovyi Por-

sugel': salinity, 4%; H_2S, 12 mg/l; pH, 8.4–8.7; temperature, 20°C; O_2, traces.

Genus VI. **Lamprocystis** Schroeter 1886, 151[AL]

NORBERT PFENNIG

Lam.pro.cys'tis. Gr. adj. *lampros* bright, brilliant; Gr. n. *cystis* the bladder, a bag; M.L. fem. n. *Lamprocystis* brilliant bag.

Cells spherical to ovoid, 2–3.5 μm in diameter, diplococcus-shaped before cell division. Multiplication by binary fission, **motile by means of a single flagellum.** At high sulfide concentration (4–6 mM) and light intensity (1000–2000 lx), **cells may grow in long and branching cell aggregates which are embedded in slime.** At more favorable growth conditions, **the cell aggregates may break up into smaller clusters and more or less spherical colonies which become motile by the flagella of the composing cells; finally, individual motile cells are liberated.** Gram-negative. Contain internal photosynthetic membrane systems of vesicular type in which the photosynthetic pigments bacteriochlorophyll *a* and carotenoids are located. **Contain gas vacuoles in the central part of the cell.**

Obligately phototrophic and strictly anaerobic. Capable of photolithoautotrophic growth with sulfide or sulfur as electron donor. During sulfide oxidation, globules of elemental sulfur are transiently stored in the gas vacuole-free peripheral part of the cell. Final oxidation product is sulfate. Habitat: mud and stagnant water of ponds and lakes containing hydrogen sulfide; most common planktonic bacterium in the sulfide-containing hypolimnion of freshwater lakes.

The mol% G + C of the DNA is 63.8 (Bd).

Type species: *Lamprocystis roseopersicina* (Kützing 1849) Schroeter 1886, 151.

Enrichment and Isolation Procedures

Lamprocystis and other gas vacuole-containing purple sulfur bacteria may be selectively enriched by making use of their buoyancy at lower temperatures (4–10°C). For enrichment cultures, an inoculum from a

natural habitat should be used in which the presence of *Lamprocystis* cells and cell aggregates was established microscopically. The culture medium and incubation conditions are the same as described for the large *Chromatium* species (see page 1639). Low sulfide concentration (1–2 mM) and low light intensity (100–300 lx) with diurnal light and dark periods (e.g. 18 h light, 6 h dark) are employed at a room temperature of about 20°C. The bottles are incubated in a lying position to avoid accumulation of cells in the nonilluminated area under the screw cap. After two or three supplementations of the enrichment culture with neutralized sulfide solution, the well-developed culture is stored in a refrigerator in an upright position. This is not done until the various types of purple sulfur bacteria have almost completely oxidized the sulfur globules inside the cells. After 1–2 weeks of storage at a temperature between 4–10°C, gas vacuole-containing purple sulfur bacteria, including *Lamprocystis*, will have accumulated at the surface of the liquid medium under the screw cap. A small amount of the floating purple-violet material is removed with an inoculation loop and inspected microscopically under brightfield illumination. For further enrichment, the floating cell mass is carefully pipetted from the surface and transferred to fresh medium. Alternatively or in addition, the enriched material is used to inoculate one or two series of agar shake cultures as described for the isolation of *Chromatium* species.

Maintenance Procedures

Maintenance of strains in liquid culture medium and long term preservation in liquid nitrogen are carried out as described for the genus *Chromatium* (see page 1640).

Differentiation of the genus **Lamprocystis** from other genera

Characteristics useful for differentiation of the genus *Lamprocystis* from other genera of the *Chromatiaceae* are listed in Table 18.3.

Taxonomic Comments

Only a few strains of *Lamprocystis roseopersicina* have thus far been studied in pure culture. From observations of this characteristic cell type in samples from nature, it is apparent that strains of fairly different cell diameter occur. Further studies with many pure culture isolates will have to show whether clusters of strains of different cell diameter may represent different species.

Determinations of the similarity coefficients of the 16S rRNA oligonucleotide catalogs of the type strains of *Lamprocystis roseopersi-*

cina, *Thiodictyon elegans* and *Amoebobacter roseus* indicate that these morphologically clearly distinguishable genera of gas-vacuolate bacteria also constitute phylogenetically well-separated lines (Fowler et al., 1984; see Fig. 18.4). The S_{AB} value for *Lamprocystis* and *Thiodictyon* is 0.74; the value for *Thiodictyon* and *Amoebobacter* is 0.77. Future studies will have to show the range of variation of these cell types on the species and genus level.

Further Reading

Pfennig, N., M.C. Markham and S. Liaaen-Jensen. 1968. Carotenoids of *Thiorhodaceae*. 8. Isolation and characterization of a *Thiothece*, *Lamprocystis* and *Thiodictyon* strain and their carotenoid pigments. Arch. Mikrobiol. *62:* 178-191.

List of species of the genus **Lamprocystis**

1. **Lamprocystis roseopersicina** (Kützing 1849) Schroeter 1886, 151.[AL] (*Protococcus roseopersicinus* Kützing 1849, 196.)

ro.se.o.per.si.ci'na. L. adj. *roseus* rosy; Gr. n. *persicus* the peach; M.L. fem. adj. *roseopersicina* rosy peach-colored.

Cells spherical to ovoid, 2.0–3.5 μm in diameter (Fig. 18.13). Color of cell suspensions pinkish-violet to purple-violet. Photosynthetic pigments are bacteriochlorophyll *a* and carotenoids of the rhodopinal

series; lycopenal is the main component (Pfennig et al., 1968).

In the presence of sulfide and bicarbonate, acetate and pyruvate are photoassimilated. Nitrogen sources: ammonium salts. pH range: 6.7–7.3. Growth temperature: 20–30°C.

The mol% G + C of the DNA of the neotype strain is 63.8 (Bd).

Neotype strain: DSM 229 (strain 3012, Bergkamen).

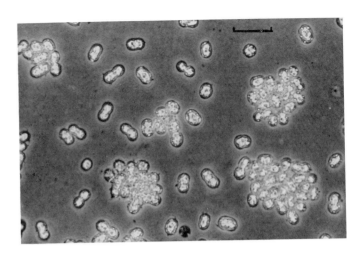

Figure 18.13. L. *roseopersicina* DSM 229 cultured photoautotrophically with sulfice. Single cells and cell colonies are motile in liquid medium. The *irregular whitish areas* within the cells are the gas vacuoles. The *small spherical bodies* in the cells are the sulfur globules. Phase-contrast micrograph. *Bar*, 10 μm.

Genus VII. **Thiodictyon** *Winogradsky 1880, 80* [AL]

NORBERT PFENNING

Thi.o.dic′ty.on. Gr. n. *thios* sulfur; Gr. n. *dictyon* a net; M.L. neut. n. *Thiodictyon* sulfur net.

Cells rod-shaped with rounded ends, sometimes appearing spindle-shaped. Multiplication by binary fission, **nonmotile under all conditions. May form aggregates in which the cells are arranged end to end in an irregular netlike structure,** the shape of which is not constant. **May also form more compact clumps or break up into individual cells.** Gram-negative. Contain internal photosynthetic membrane systems of vesicular type in which the photosynthetic pigments bacteriochlorophyll *a* and carotenoids are located. **Contain large, irregularly shaped gas vacuoles in the central part of the cell.**

Obligately phototrophic and strictly anaerobic. Capable of photolithoautotrophic growth with sulfide or sulfur as electron donor. During sulfide oxidation, globules of elemental sulfur are transiently stored in the gas vacuole-free peripheral part of the cell. Final oxidation product is sulfate. Habitat: mud and stagnant water of ponds and lakes containing hydrogen sulfide; not uncommon as planktonic bacterium in the sulfide-containing hypolimnion of freshwater lakes.

The mol% G + C of the DNA is 65.3–66.3 (Bd).

Type species: *Thiodictyon elegans* Winogradsky 1888, 82.

Enrichment and Isolation Procedures

Prerequisite for the successful enrichment and isolation of *Thiodictyon* from anoxic water or mud samples is the microscopic establishment of the bacterium in the particular sample. Since in its natural habitats *Thiodictyon* almost regularly grows in the form of the readily recognizable netlike cell aggregates, the recognition of this bacterium does not present problems.

For the isolation of pure cultures, it is advisable to prepare both liquid enrichment cultures as well as agar shake dilution cultures that are directly inoculated from the sample of the natural habitat. In liquid enrichment cultures, *Thiodictyon* may be outgrown by other gas vacuole-containing purple sulfur bacteria. The culture medium and incubation conditions are the same as those described for the large *Chromatium* species (see page 1639) and for *Lamprocystis* (see page 1649).

Maintenance Procedures

Maintenance of strains in liquid culture medium and long term preservation in liquid nitrogen are carried out as described for the genus *Chromatium* (see page 1640).

Differentiation of the genus **Thiodictyon** from other genera

Characteristics useful for differentiation of the genus *Thiodictyon* from other genera of the *Chromatiaceae* are listed in Table 18.3.

Taxonomic Comments

The genus *Thiodictyon* presently comprises two species: *T. elegans*, the type species of the genus, and *T. bacillosum*. The latter species was originally described by Winogradsky (1888) as *Amoebobacter bacillosus*.

Pfennig and Trüper (1971) transferred the species *Amoebobacter bacillosus* Winogradsky to the genus *Thiodictyon*, since the rod-shaped

cells are very similar to those of *Thiodictyon elegans* Winogradsky. In accordance with the original description of the type species of the genus *Amoebobacter* (*Amoebobacter roseus* Winogradsky 1888), this genus should comprise only spherical, nonmotile, gas-vacuolated species. Future studies on similarity coefficients of nucleic acids of these species will show whether this morphology-based classification can be substantiated.

The mol% G + C of the DNA of the two *Thiodictyon* species are very close.

Differentiation of the species of the genus **Thiodictyon**

I. Cells able to grow in form of typical netlike aggregates under certain culture conditions.
   1. *T. elegans*
II. Cells that do not form netlike aggregates, usually growing in the form of free single cells.
   2. *T. bacillosum*

List of species of the genus Thiodictyon

1. **Thiodictyon elegans** Winogradsky 1888, 82.[AL]

e'le.gans. L. adj. *elegans* choice, elegant.

Cells rod-shaped, 1.5–2.0 μm wide, 3–8 μm long. Growth in the form of irregular netlike aggregates is dependent on high sulfide concentration and light intensity (Fig. 18.14). In cultures of higher population densities, cell chains break apart and the cultures contain predominantly single cells (Fig. 18.15). Color of single cells grayish, color of cell suspensions light violet to purple-violet. Photosynthetic pigments are bacteriochlorophyll *a* and carotenoids of the rhodopinal series; rhodopinal and rhodopin are major carotenoid components (Pfennig et al., 1968). In the presence of sulfide and bicarbonate, acetate and pyruvate are photoassimilated. Nitrogen sources: ammonium salts. pH range: 6.7–7.3. Growth temperature: 20–25°C.

The mol% G + C of the DNA is 65.3–66.3 (Bd) (neotype strain: 65.4).

Neotype strain: DSM 232 (strain 3011, Bergkamen).

2. **Thiodictyon bacillosum** (Winogradsky 1888) Pfennig and Trüper 1971, 12.[AL] (*Amoebobacter bacillosus* Winogradsky 1888, 78.)

ba.cil.lo'sum. L. dim. n. *bacillus* a small rod; M.L. neut. adj. *bacillosum* full of or made up of small rods.

Cells rod-shaped, 1.5–2.0 μm wide, 3–6 μm long. Cells may grow in irregular clumps surrounded by slime; no netlike aggregates are formed. Color of cell suspensions light violet to purple-violet. Photosynthetic pigments are bacteriochlorophyll *a* and carotenoids of the rhodopinal series; a major component is rhodopinal (Schmidt et al, 1965).

In the presence of sulfide and bicarbonate, acetate and pyruvate are photoassimilated. Nitrogen sources: ammonium salts. pH range: 6.7–7.3. Growth temperature: 20–30°C.

The mol% G + C of the DNA of the neotype strain is 66.3 (Bd).

Neotype strain: DSM 234 (strain 1814, Zeulenroda).

Genus VIII. **Amoebobacter** Winogradsky 1888, 71 [AL]

NORBERT PFENNIG

A.moe.bo.bac'ter. Gr. n. *amoebe* change, transformation; M.L. n. *bacter* a rod; M.L. masc. n. *Amoebobacter* changeable rod.

Cells spherical, multiplication by binary fission, **nonmotile. Individual cells are surrounded by slime; cells may stick together, forming irregular aggregates.** Gram-negative. **Cells contain irregularly shaped gas vacuoles in the central part.** Photosynthetic pigments bacteriochlorophyll *a* and carotenoids are located in internal membrane systems of vesicular type.

Phototrophic under anaerobic conditions; may be chemoautotrophic or mixotrophic under microaerobic to aerobic conditions in the dark. Capable of photolithoautotrophic growth with sulfide or sulfur as electron donor. During sulfide oxidation, globules of elemental sulfur are transiently stored in the gas vacuole-free peripheral part of the cells. Final oxidation product is sulfate.

Habitat: mud and stagnant water of ponds and lakes containing hydrogen sulfide; may occur as dominant bloom-forming bacteria together with *Thiocapsa roseopersicina* in wastewater lagoons containing degradable organic substances.

The mol% G + C of the DNA is 64.3–65.3 (Bd).

Type species: *Amoebobacter roseus* Winogradsky 1888, 77.

Enrichment and Isolation Procedures

No particular enrichment or isolation procedures are available for *Amoebobacter*. Samples collected in nature are used directly as inoculum for agar shake dilution cultures, as is described for the *Chromatium* species (see page 1639). The color of colonies in agar is characteristically pinkish, which is similar to that for *Thiocapsa*. In contrast to the latter, colonies of *Amoebobacter* maintain a somewhat chalky appearance even if the cells are free of elemental sulfur. This appearance is due to the presence of gas vacuoles in the cells of *Amoebobacter* species. Individual colonies have to be isolated and checked for the presence of gas vacuoles in cells of spherical morphology.

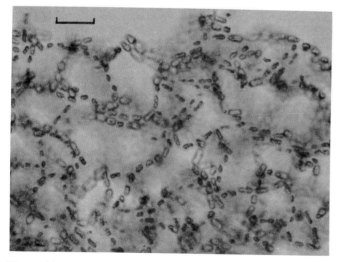

Figure 18.14. *T. elegans* DSM 232 showing the typical, somewhat irregular netlike arrangement of the cells. Brightfield micrograph. *Bar, 12* μm.

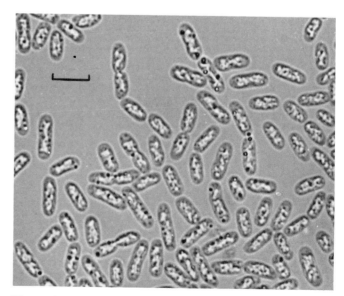

Figure 18.15. *T. elegans* DSM 232 cultured photoautotrophically with sulfide. The irregular whitish areas within the cells are the gas vacuoles. The cells also contain small, blackish-appearing globules of elemental sulfur. Brightfield micrograph. *Bar, 5* μm.

Maintenance Procedures

Maintenance of strains in liquid culture medium and long term

preservation in liquid nitrogen are carried out as described for the genus *Chromatium* (see page 1640).

Differentiation of the genus **Amoebobacter** *from other genera*

Characteristics useful for differentiation of the genus *Amoebobacter* from other genera of the *Chromatiaceae* are listed in Table 18.3. The color of *Amoebobacter* cultures is pink to rose-red, which is similar to that of *Thiocapsa* cultures.

bobacter species are closely related to each other; the S_{AB} value is 0.98. The genus *Amoebobacter* is most closely related to the genus *Thiocapsa*; the S_{AB} value is 0.93 (Fowler et al., 1984).

Taxonomic Comments

In accordance with the original description of the type species of the genus *Amoebobacter*, this genus comprises only spherical, nonmotile, gas-vacuolated species (Pfennig and Trüper, 1971). Analyses of the oligonucleotide catalogs of the 16S rRNA showed that the two *Amoe-*

Further Reading

Fowler, V.J., N. Pfennig, W. Schubert and E. Stackebrandt. 1984. Towards a phylogeny of phototrophic purple sulfur bacteria—16S rRNA oligonucleotide cataloguing of 11 species of *Chromatiaceae*. Arch. Microbiol. *139*: 382–387

Pfennig, N. and H.G. Trüper. 1971. New nomenclatural combinations in the phototrophic sulfur bacteria. Int. J. Syst. Bacteriol. *21*: 11–14.

Differentiation of the species of the genus **Amoebobacter**

I. Cells 2-3 µm in diameter.

          1. *A. roseus*

II. Cells 1.5-2 µm in diameter. Pronounced slime formation under most culture conditions causes a highly viscous culture medium.

          2. *A. pendens*

List of species of the genus **Amoebobacter**

1. **Amoebobacter roseus** Winogradsky 1888, 77.[AL]

ro′se.us. L. adj. *roseus* rosy, rose-colored, pink.

Cells spherical, 2.0–3.0 µm in diameter. Individual cells and irregular cell aggregates surrounded by slime. Individual cells appear colorless, color of cell suspensions pink to rose-red. Photosynthetic pigments are bacteriochlorophyll *a* and carotenoids of the spirilloxanthin series with spirilloxanthin as the major component.

Photoautotrophic under anaerobic conditions and facultatively chemoautotrophic or mixotrophic under microaerobic to aerobic conditions in the dark. Photosynthetic electron donors: sulfide, sulfur, thiosulfate or molecular hydrogen. Acetate, pyruvate, malate, fructose and casamino acids are photoassimilated. Not utilized: other sugars, alcohols, fatty acids, lactate, succinate, tartrate, benzoate or citrate. Nitrogen sources: ammonium salts. Sulfate not used as sole sulfur source. Vitamin B$_{12}$ required for growth. pH range: 6.7–7.5. Growth temperature: 20–35°C.

The mol% G + C of the DNA is 64.3 (Bd).

Neotype strain: DSM 235 (strain 6611, Davis).

2. **Amoebobacter pendens** (Molisch) Pfennig and Trüper 1971, 13.[AL] (*Rhodothece pendens* Molisch 1906, 230.)

pen′dens. L. part. adj. *pendens* hanging.

Cells spherical, 1.5–2.0 µm in diameter. A few cells up to 2.5 µm in diameter may occur. Individual cells surrounded by slime capsules which give rise to irregular cell aggregates of different size. Because of copious slime formation the culture medium becomes rather viscous. Individual cells appear colorless, color of cell suspensions pink to rose-red. Photosynthetic pigments are bacteriochlorophyll *a* and carotenoids of the spirilloxanthin series with spirilloxanthin as the dominant component.

Obligately phototrophic, no growth under microaerobic to aerobic conditions in the dark. Photosynthetic electron donors: sulfide, sulfur, thiosulfate, sulfite or molecular hydrogen. Acetate, pyruvate and glucose are the only organic substrates photoassimilated. Sulfate not used as sole sulfur source. Vitamin B$_{12}$ required for growth. pH range: 6.7–7.5. Growth temperature: 20–35°C.

The mol% G + C of the DNA is 65.3 (Bd).

Neotype strain: DSM 236 (strain 1314, Klein-Kalden).

Addendum

New species recently described by B. Eichler and N. Pfennig (1986): *Amoebobacter pedioformis*.

Genus IX. **Thiopedia** *Winogradsky 1888, 85* [AL]

NORBERT PFENNIG

Thi.o.pe′di.a Gr. n. *thios* sulfur; Gr. n. *pedium* a plain, a flat area; M.L. fem. n. *Thiopedia* sulfur plain.

Cells spherical to ovoid, multiplication by binary fission. **Owing to consecutive divisions in two perpendicular planes, rectangular platelets with 4, 8, 16, 32 or more regularly arranged cells** (up to 128 or 256 cells may stick together) **are formed. Nonmotile. Gram-negative. Cells contain irregularly shaped gas vacuoles in the central part.** Photosynthetic pigments bacteriochlorophyll *a* and carotenoids are located in internal membrane systems of the vesicular or the stack lamellar type.

Phototrophic under anaerobic conditions. Capable of photolithotrophic growth with sulfide or sulfur as electron donor; during sulfide oxidation, globules of elemental sulfur are transiently formed in the gas vacuole-free peripheral part of the cells. Sulfate is the final

oxidation product. Habitat: mud and stagnant water of ponds and lakes containing hydrogen sulfide; common planktonic bacterium in the sulfide-containing hypolimnion of freshwater lakes.

Type species: *Thiopedia rosea* Winogradsky 1888, 85.

Enrichment and Isolation Procedures

Prerequisite for the successful enrichment and isolation of *Thiopedia* is the use of an inoculum from anoxic water or mud samples in which the characteristic *Thiopedia* platelets were microscopically detected. For the isolation of pure cultures, it is advisable to prepare enrichment cultures in liquid media as well as agar shake dilution cultures that are directly inoculated from the sample of the natural habitat. In liquid media, *Thiopedia* may be outgrown by other gas vacuole-containing purple sulfur bacteria. The culture medium and incubation conditions are similar to those described for the large *Chromatium* species (see page 1639) and for *Lamprocystis* (see page 1649). Not more than 1.5 mM sulfide and 3 mM acetate should be used for *Thiopedia*, and the trace element solution must not contain a chelating agent (e.g. EDTA). Incubation is carried out at a temperature of 20-25°C and a light intensity of 100-200 lx. *Thiopedia* grows in the form of individual cells or platelets with between 4 and 128 cells. Colonies and cell suspensions of

Thiopedia rosea exhibit a unique bright purple-red and can, therefore, readily be differentiated from other purple sulfur bacteria.

Maintenance Procedures

Stock cultures may be maintained in liquid medium in tightly closed 100-ml screw-capped bottles at 4-8°C. Such cultures should be transferred every 2 months. For long term preservation, vials with cell suspensions in anoxic culture medium containing 5% (v/v) DMSO are stored in liquid nitrogen.

Differentiation of the genus **Thiopedia** from other genera

The differentiating characteristics between the other genera of the purple sulfur bacteria and the only species of the genus *Thiopedia* so far studied in pure culture are: (a) the arrangement of the cells in rectangular platelets, (b) possession of gas vacuoles, and (c) the purple-red of cell material, which is caused by the carotenoid okenone.

Taxonomic Comments

Purple sulfur bacteria of the morphology first described by Winogradsky for *Thiopedia rosea* are widely distributed in sulfide-containing ponds and lakes (Utermöhl, 1925). Since only one strain has so far been isolated in pure culture and studied physiologically (Pfennig, 1973), our knowledge of this genus is in its infancy. Fine structure studies of *Thiopedia*-like cell material collected from a purple bacteria bloom in a small Michigan (U.S.A.) forest pond revealed that at least two *Thiopedia* types with different internal membrane systems exist (Hirsch, 1973). One type contained a vesicular membrane system, while

the other type contained a membrane system which consisted of stacks of disk-shaped lamellae. Thin sections of the *Thiopedia* type with a vesicular membrane system were published by Remsen (1978). More work is required to reveal how many different types or species with *Thiopedia* morphology exist and whether they are genetically related.

Further Reading

Hirsch, P. 1973. Fine structure of *Thiopedia* spp. *In* Drews (Editor), Abstracts of Symposium on Prokaryotic Photosynthetic Organisms, Freiburg, pp. 184–185.

Pfennig, N. 1973. Culture and ecology of *Thiopedia* rosea. *In* Drews (Editor), Abstracts of Symposium on Prokaryotic Photosynthetic Organisms, Freiburg, pp. 75–76.

Remsen, C.C. 1978. Comparative subcellular architecture of photosynthetic bacteria. *In* Clayton and Sistrom (Editors), The Photosynthetic Bacteria. Plenum Press, New York, pp. 31–60.

Utermöhl, H. 1925. Limnologische Phytoplanktonstudien. Arch. Hydrobiol. Suppl. *5*: 251–277.

List of species of the genus **Thiopedia**

1. **Thiopedia rosea** Winogradsky 1888, 85.[AL]

ro'se.a. L. adj. *rosea* rosy, rose-colored, pink.

Cells spherical to ovoid or elongated ovoid, 1.2–1.6 μm wide, 1.5–2.0 μm long, regularly arranged in rectangular platelets with up to 64 or more cells (Fig. 18.16). Individual cells appear colorless, color of cell suspensions bright purple-red. Photosynthetic pigments are bacteriochlorophyll *a* and the carotenoid okenone as major components. Photosynthetic membrane system of vesicular type.

Obligately anaerobic and phototrophic. Capable of photolithoorganotrophic growth with sulfide or sulfur as electron donor. Only low sulfide concentrations up to 1.5 mM are tolerated. In the presence of sulfide and bicarbonate, the following substrates are photoassimilated: acetate, butyrate or valerate (not more than 0.03% (w/v) of each to be added); less well photoassimilated are succinate, fumarate, malate and fructose (0.05%). Ammonium salts serve as nitrogen source. Reduced sulfur compounds are required as sulfur source. Growth is enhanced by the use of 100 μM dithionite. Vitamin B$_{12}$ is required for growth. Optimum pH: 7.3. Growth temperature: 20°C. Only one strain studied in pure culture (strain 4211, Schmarksee; Pfennig, 1973). No neotype strain designated.

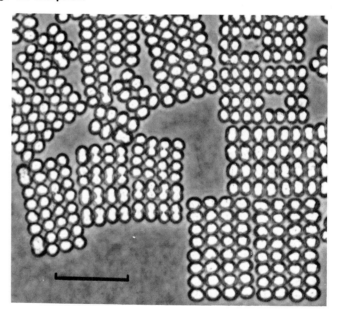

Figure 18.16. *T. rosea* strain 4211 cultured phototrophically with sulfide and acetate. The light areas inside the cells are the gas vacuoles. In some of the platelets, synchronously dividing cells can be recognized. Phase-contrast micrograph. *Bar,* 10 μm.

FAMILY II. **ECTOTHIORHODOSPIRACEAE** IMHOFF 1984, 33[VP]

JOHANNES F. IMHOFF

Ec.to.thi.o.rho.do.spi.ra′ce.ae. M.L. fem. n. *Ectothiorhodospira* type genus of the family; *-aceae* ending to denote a family; M.L. fem. pl. n. *Ectothiorhodospiraceae* the *Ectothiorhodospira* family.

Cells are spiral or vibrioid- or rod-shaped, are motile by means of polar flagella, divide by binary fission, with or without gas vacuoles, and are Gram-negative. Able to perform anoxygenic photosynthesis with bacteriochlorophylls and carotenoids as photosynthetic pigments. Growth occurs anaerobically in the light with reduced sulfur compounds as electron donors. Sulfide is oxidized to elemental sulfur, which is deposited outside the cells and may be further oxidized to sulfate. In nature, members of the *Ectothiorhodospiraceae* are found in marine to extremely saline environments containing sulfide and having neutral to extremely alkaline pH.

The mol% G + C of the DNA is 50.5–69.7 (T_m).

Type genus: *Ectothiorhodospira* Pelsh 1936, 120.

Taxonomic Comments

The position of the *Ectothiorhodospira* species among the phototrophic purple bacteria has been disputed since their discovery by Pelsh (1936). He distinguished these bacteria, which he called "Ectothiorhodaceae," from those purple bacteria with elemental sulfur inside their cells, which he called "Endothiorhodaceae" (Pelsh, 1937). Pelsh's isolates were poorly characterized and were lost soon after their isolation. Trüper (1968) reisolated *Ectothiorhodospira mobilis*, and Pfennig and Trüper (1971) included *Ectothiorhodospira* as an exceptional genus into the *Chromatiaceae*, because of its ability to perform a dissimilatory sulfur metabolism. Because the *Ectothiorhodospira* species showed significant differences to all other genera of the *Chromatiaceae* and because, meanwhile, representatives of the Purple Nonsulfur Bacteria were found performing oxidation of sulfide to extracellular elemental sulfur, Pfennig (1977) proposed to remove the genus *Ectothiorhodospira* from the *Chromatiaceae* and to place it in the Purple Nonsulfur Bacteria. Imhoff et al. (1982a) distinguished three groups of phototrophic

purple bacteria on the basis of polar lipid compositions: *Chromatiaceae,* the genus *Ectothiorhodospira,* and the Purple Nonsulfur Bacteria. Differences were also found in the fatty acid and quinone composition to the two other groups of phototrophic purple bacteria (Imhoff, 1982). The separation of *Ectothiorhodospira* as a distinct family, the *Ectothiorhodospiraceae,* has been discussed on a similar basis (Tindall, 1980) and on the basis of 16S rRNA analyses (Stackebrandt et al., 1984) (Fig. 18.17). A formal proposal for the reassignment of the genus *Ectothiorhodospira* to the new family *Ectothiorhodospiraceae* has been made by Imhoff (1984).

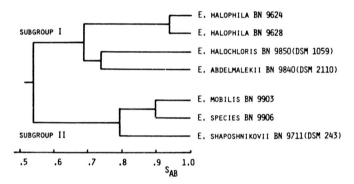

Figure 18.17. Similarity dendrogram of *Ectothiorhodospira* species, derived from 16S rRNA oligonucleotide catalogs. (Reproduced with permission from E. Stackebrandt, V. J. Fowler, W. Schubert and J. F. Imhoff, *Archives of Microbiology 137:* 369, 1984.)

Genus **Ectothiorhodospira** *Pelsh 1936, 120*[AL]

JOHANNES F. IMHOFF

Ec.to.thi.o.rho.do.spi′ra. Gr. prep. *ectos* outside; Gr. n. *thios* sulfur; Gr. n. *rhodos* the rose; Gr. n. *spira* the spiral; M.L. fem. n. *Ectothiorhodospira* rose spiral with sulfur outside.

Cells are vibrioid- or rod-shaped to spiral, 0.5–1.5 µm in diameter, and **motile by polar flagella; they multiply by binary fission** and are Gram-negative. **Internal photosynthetic membranes are present as lamellar stacks** that are continuous with the cytoplasmic membrane. Photosynthetic pigments are bacteriochlorophyll *a* or *b* and carotenoids.

Growth occurs photoautotrophically under anaerobic conditions with reduced sulfur compounds or hydrogen as electron donors or photoheterotrophically with a limited number of simple organic compounds. **Sulfide is oxidized to elemental sulfur, which is deposited outside the cells,** and may be further oxidized to sulfate. Some species are able to grow under microaerobic to aerobic conditions in the dark. **Growth is dependent on saline and alkaline conditions.** Growth factors are not required, but vitamin B_{12} enhances growth of some strains. Storage products are polysaccharides, poly-β-hydroxybutyrate and polyphosphate.

Ectothiorhodospira species can be found in marine to extremely saline environments with neutral to extremely alkaline pH and containing sulfide, such as estuaries, salt flats, salt lakes, soda lakes and others; occasionally they may be found in soil.

The mol% G + C of the DNA is 50.5–69.7 (T_m).

Type species: *Ectothiorhodospira mobilis* Pelsh 1936, 120.

Further Descriptive Information

Cell morphology of the *Ectothiorhodospira* species varies with the growth conditions, in particular with pH and salinity. *E. halophila* and *E. halochloris* are clearly spirals. *E. mobilis* and *E. abdelmalekii* are spirals under proper growth conditions, but they tend to form vibrioid-shaped cells or more or less bent rods. *E. shaposhnikovii* and *E. vacuolata* form straight or slightly bent rods at suitable growth conditions. The photosynthetic membranes of *E. halochloris* in negatively stained preparations under the electron microscope have been found to have a regularly granulated structure (Imhoff and Trüper, 1977). The photosynthetic complexes are actually arranged in a regular hexagonal array in *E. halochloris, E. abdelmalekii* and other bacteria containing bacteriochlorophyll *b* (Engelhardt et al., 1983). Bacteriochlorophyll *b* of *E. halochloris* and *E. abdelmalekii* is esterified with Δ2,10-phytadienol, not with phytol as is bacteriochlorophyll *a* of the other *Ectothiorhodospira* species (Steiner et al., 1981; and R. Steiner, personal communication). Carotenoids of the normal spirilloxanthin series are present in those species containing bacteriochlorophyll *a*. Spirilloxanthin is always the predominant component, and the content of rhodopin, which is about 10–20% in the less halophilic species, is negligible in *E. halophila* (Schmidt and Trüper, 1971). The content of carotenoids in *E. halochloris* and *E. abdelmalekii* is low; methoxyrhodopin glucoside (major), rhodopin glucoside and rhodopin have mainly been found (K. Schmidt, personal communication).

All species grow well under anaerobic conditions in the light with reduced sulfur compounds as photosynthetic electron donors and in the presence of organic carbon sources and inorganic carbonate. *E. mobilis* and *E. shaposhnikovii* also grow microaerobically in the dark if sulfide is present. During phototrophic growth with sulfide as electron donor, the oxidation of sulfide and elemental sulfur strictly follow each other, as has been shown for *E. mobilis* (see Trüper, 1978). Under the alkaline growth conditions, which are optimal for *Ectothiorhodospira* species, polysulfides are stable intermediates in sulfide oxidation. As a result, polysulfides are the first measurable oxidation products, probably formed by chemical reaction of elemental sulfur with sulfide, and the media become yellow-translucent at this stage. After sulfide depletion, elemental sulfur droplets are formed rather rapidly, and the medium becomes whitish-opaque. During further growth, cultures become pinkish and finally red, if elemental sulfur disappears. These color changes are best observed under photoautotrophic growth conditions with the red species. The knowledge of enzymes involved in the oxidation of reduced sulfur compounds by *Ectothiorhodospira* species has been summarized by Trüper and Fischer (1982).

Under autotrophic growth conditions, the fixation of carbon dioxide via the ribulosebisphosphate pathway is apparently the major route of carbon assimilation in *E. shaposhnikovii* (Firsov et al., 1974). High activities of ribulosebisphosphate carboxylase have been found in *E. shaposhnikovii* (Firsov et al., 1974), *E. mobilis* (Sahl and Trüper, 1977) and *E. halophila* (Tabita and McFadden, 1972). The assimilation of several organic carbon sources, such as acetate and propionate, depends on the presence of carbon dioxide and proceeds via several carboxylation reactions (Firsov and Ivanovskii, 1974, 1975). Under these conditions, considerable proportions of the cellular carbon are therefore derived from carbon dioxide, which is not assimilated via the ribulosebisphosphate pathway. Phosphoenolpyruvate carboxylase, ferredoxin-dependent pyruvate synthase and oxoglutarate synthase were found in *E. shaposhnikovii* (Firsov et al., 1974); phosphoenolpyruvate carboxylase, phosphoenolpyruvate carboxykinase and pyruvate carboxylase were found in *E. mobilis* (Sahl and Trüper, 1977). All enzymes of the glycolytic pathway and the tricarboxylic acid cycle with the exception of oxoglutarate dehydrogenase are present in *E. shaposhnikovii* (Krasil'nikova, 1975). Cells grown on acetate demonstrated increased activities of isocitrate lyase, which is indicative of the function of the glyoxylic acid pathway. From acetate and butyrate the major reserve material formed in the absence of carbon dioxide is poly-β-hydroxybutyric acid. From other organic carbon sources and from acetic acid and butyric acid in the presence of carbon dioxide preferably, carbohydrates are formed (Novikova, 1971).

Ammonia and glutamine are suitable nitrogen sources for all species. Dinitrogen fixation has been demonstrated for some of the species and is probably a property inherent to all of them. Glutamate dehydrogenase (NADH-dependent) and glutamine synthetase/glutamate synthase (NADH-dependent) have been found in *E. mobilis* (Bast, 1977). Nitrate can be used as a nitrogen source by *E. shaposhnikovii*, and its reduction is catalyzed by a ferredoxin-dependent nitrate reductase, which is associated or bound to the membranes and induced during growth with nitrate (Malofeeva et al., 1975).

To adapt to the high and sometimes varying concentrations of salts, *Ectothiorhodospira* species accumulate organic solutes to balance the outside osmotic pressure. In *Ectothiorhodospira halochloris*, glycine betaine has been found as the main osmotic active cytoplasmic component (Galinski and Trüper, 1982).

Enrichment and Isolation Procedures

Ectothiorhodospira species have been isolated from marine sources and salt lakes from many parts of the world. Alkaline soda lakes show a natural abundance of *Ectothiorhodospira* species, which can be taken as proof for their successful adaptation to these environments. From such sources, isolation can be achieved in agar dilution series with natural samples without prior enrichment. For the extremely halophilic species, the tolerance of and the dependence on high salinity and alkalinity are strongly selective conditions for their enrichment. Marine strains of *Ectothiorhodospira* can selectively be enriched under photoautotrophic conditions with sulfide as electron donor and in saline and alkaline media (3% NaCl and pH 8.5–9.0) even in the presence of high proportions of *Chromatium* species in the natural sample. With use of a medium (Imhoff and Trüper, 1977) based on the mineral composition of the soda lakes of the Wadi Natrun (Jannasch, 1957; Imhoff et al., 1979) or modifications thereof, many *Ectothiorhodospira* strains have been isolated from various locations. A recipe for a medium containing 20% salts is given below.* For adapting this medium to different salinities, the amounts of sodium salts (sulfates, carbonates and chloride) are changed by maintaining the proportions of the basic mineral composition.

Maintenance Procedures

Standard maintenance procedures can be used for storage in liquid nitrogen

Taxonomic Comments

After reassignment, *Ectothiorhodospira* is at present the only genus of this new family *Ectothiorhodospiraceae*. It is clear from the literature cited, however, that *Ectothiorhodospira* species form two subgroups, which are represented by the extremely halophilic species on the one hand and by the species with lower salt requirement on the other hand. The formation of two subgroups is also depicted in the similarity coefficients of the 16S rRNA (Stackebrandt et al., 1984; and Fig. 18.17). Future studies will have to show whether these differences warrant separation into genera.

Differentiation of the species of the genus Ectothiorhodospira

The main differentiating properties of the species are summarized in Tables 18.5 and 18.6.

---

*The medium contains (per liter): 0.8 g KH₂PO₄, 0.8 g NH₄Cl, 0.05 g CaCl₂·2H₂O, 0.1 g MgCl₂·6H₂O, 1 ml trace element solution SLA (ingredients are given below), 200 mM sodium carbonate buffer pH 9.0, 20 g Na₂SO₄ and 160 g NaCl. This basal medium may be sterilized by filtration. As organic carbon source, 2 g sodium acetate and, as reduced sulfur source, 0.5–1.0 g Na₂S·9H₂O are sterilized separately and added. If this medium is autoclaved, NH₄Cl and magnesium and calcium salts are also sterilized separately and added afterwards. Sodium thiosulfate, if used as electron donor, may be sterilized together with the basal medium. Sodium sulfate, which may be replaced by sodium chloride, is added to 10% of the total salt content (5 and 20 g/l for a 5% and a 20% medium, respectively). The remaining amount is added as sodium chloride.

The trace element solution SLA has the following composition: 1.8 g FeCl₂·4H₂O, 250 mg CoCl₂·6H₂O, 10 mg NiCl₂·6H₂O, 10 mg CuCl₂·5H₂O, 70 mg MnCl₂·4H₂O, 100 mg ZnCl₂, 500 mg H₃BO₃, 30 mg Na₂MoO₄·2H₂O and 10 mg Na₂SeO₃·5H₂O. These components are dissolved in 1 l of bidistilled water. The pH of the solution is adjusted with HCl to 2–3.

Table 18.5.
Differentiating characteristics of the species of the genus **Ectothiorhodospira**[a]

Characteristic	1. E. mobilis	2. E. shaposhnikovii	3. E. vacuolata	4. E. halophila	5. E. halochloris	6. E. abdelmalekii
Cell diameter (μm)	0.7–1.0	0.8–0.9	1.5	0.6–0.9	0.5–0.6	0.9–1.2
Mol% G + C of DNA (T_m)	62.2–63.7	62.0	61.4–63.6	67.5–69.7	50.5–52.9	63.3–63.8
Type of flagellation	Polar tuft	Polar tuft	Polar tuft	Bipolar	Bipolar	Bipolar
Color of cell suspensions	Red	Red	Red	Red	Green	Green
Major carotenoid	sp	sp	sp	sp	rp	rp
Bacteriochlorophyll	a_p	a_p	a_p	a_p	b_{pd}	b_{pd}
Gas vacuoles	−	−	+	−	−	−
Nitrate utilization	−	+	−	−	−	−
Optimal salinity range (%)	2–10	1–7	1–6	11–32	14–27	12–18

[a] Symbols: sp, spirilloxanthin; rp, rhodopin and derivatives thereof; a_p, bacteriochlorophyll a esterified with phytol; b_{pd}, bacteriochlorophyll b esterified with phytadienol; +, present or positive; −, absent or negative.

Table 18.6.
Photosynthetic electron donors and carbon sources used by species of the genus **Ectothiorhodospira**[a]

Donor/source	1. E. mobilis	2. E. shaposhnikovii	3. E. vacuolata	4. E. halophila	5. E. halochloris	6. E. abdelmalekii	Donor/source	1. E. mobilis	2. E. shaposhnikovii	3. E. vacuolata	4. E. halophila	5. E. halochloris	6. E. abdelmalekii
Formate	−	−	−	−	−	−	Glucose	−	+	±	−	−	−
Acetate	+	+	+	+	+	+	Fructose	(+)	+	±	−	−	−
Propionate	+	+	±	+	+	+	Glycerol	−	−	−	−	−	o
Butyrate	−	+	±	−	−	−	Methanol	−	−	−	−	−	−
Pyruvate	+	+	+	+	+	+	Ethanol	−	−	−	−	−	−
Lactate	−	+	±	±	−	−	Hydrogen	o	+	+	o	o	o
Malate	+	+	+	+	+	+	Sulfide	+	+	+	+	+	+
Succinate	+	+	+	+	+	+	Thiosulfate	+	+	+	+	−	−
Fumarate	+	+	+	+	+	+							

[a] Symbols: −, negative in most strains; +, positive in most strains; ±, positive in some strains but negative in other strains; o, not tested.

List of species of the genus **Ectothiorhodospira**

1. **Ectothiorhodospira mobilis** Pelsh 1936, 120.[AL]

mo′bi.lis. L. adj. *mobilis* mobile.

Cells are vibrioid-shaped or curved in a short spiral or, sometimes, appear as slightly bent rods, 0.7–1.0 μm wide and 2.0–2.6 μm long; the length of a full turn of a spiral is 3.6–4.8 μm (Fig. 18.18). Cells are motile by means of polar tufts of flagella and are Gram-negative. Internal photosynthetic membranes are present as lamellar stacks. Color of cell suspensions that are free of polysulfides and elemental sulfur is red. Absorption spectra of living cells show maxima at 378, 488, 516, 550, 590, 797, and 835–847 nm. Photosynthetic pigments are bacteriochlorophyll a (esterified with phytol) and carotenoids of the spirilloxanthin series with spirilloxanthin as the major component.

Cells grow preferably under anaerobic conditions in the light with reduced sulfur compounds or organic carbon sources as electron donor. Photoautotrophic growth is possible with sulfide, thiosulfate, elemental sulfur, sulfite and hydrogen. Acetate, pyruvate, malate, succinate and fumarate are used as organic carbon source and electron donor. Some strains also use fructose, glucose, lactate, butyrate and propionate. Ammonia, glutamine and some other amino acids are used as nitrogen source. Sulfate can be used as sole sulfur source. Growth of some strains is enhanced by vitamin B_{12}. Optimal development is at 25–40°C, pH 7.6–8.0, and 2–10% salts.

The mol% G + C of the DNA is 67.3–69.9 (Bd) and 62.2–63.7 (T_m). *Type strain:* DSM 237 (Trüper: 8112).

2. **Ectothiorhodospira shaposhnikovii** Cherni, Solovieva, Fedorova and Kondratieva 1969, 483.[AL]

sha.posh.ni.kov′i.i. M.L. gen. n. *shaposhnikovii* of Shaposhnikov; named for D. I. Shaposhnikov, a Russian microbiologist.

Cells are rod-shaped, usually slightly bent; with propionate as carbon source, they have a vibrioid or short spirillar shape and are 0.8–0.9 μm wide and 1.5–2.5 μm long, motile by means of a tuft of polar flagella, and Gram-negative. Internal photosynthetic membranes are present as lamellar stacks. Color of cell suspensions in the absence of polysulfides and elemental sulfur is red. Absorption spectra of living cells show maxima at 378, 488, 516, 550, 590, 798 and 854 nm. Photosynthetic pigments are bacteriochlorophyll a (esterified with phytol) and carotenoids of the spirilloxanthin series with spirilloxanthin as the major component.

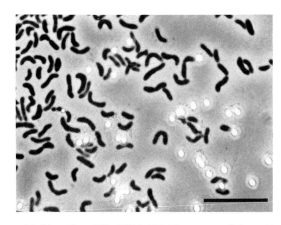

Figure 18.18. *E. mobilis* DSM 237. Note extracellular sulfur globules. Phase-contrast micrograph. *Bar,* 10 μm. (Reproduced with permission from H. G. Trüper and J. F. Imhoff. 1977. *In* Starr, Stolp, Trüper, Balows and Schlegel (Editors), The Prokaryotes. A Handbook on Habitats, Isolation, and Identification of Bacteria. Springer-Verlag, Berlin, p. 277.)

Cells preferably grow under anaerobic conditions in the light. Photoautotrophic growth is possible with reduced sulfur compounds or molecular hydrogen as electron donor. Chemoautotrophic and chemoheterotrophic growth is possible under microaerobic conditions in the dark. The photosynthetic electron donors used are sulfide, elemental sulfur, thiosulfate, sulfite, molecular hydrogen, acetate, propionate, butyrate, lactate, pyruvate, malate, succinate, fumarate and fructose. Not used are formate, methanol, ethanol, glycerol, citrate and benzoate. Ammonia, dinitrogen, nitrate and some amino acids are used as nitrogen source. Sulfate is used as sole sulfur source under photoheterotrophic conditions. Growth factors are not required. Optimal development is at 30–35°C, pH 8.0–8.5, and 1–7% salts.

The mol% G + C of the DNA is 62.3 (Bd), 64.0 (chem. anal.) and 62.0 (T_m).

Type strain: DSM 243 (Kondratieva: N1).

3. Ectothiorhodospira vacuolata Imhoff, Tindall, Grant and Trüper 1982b, 266.[VP] (Effective publication: Imhoff, Tindall, Grant and Trüper 1981, 240.)

va.cu.o.la′ta. L. adj. *vacuolatus* containing vacuoles.

Cells are rod-shaped, sometimes slightly bent, 1.5 μm wide and 2–4 μm long, and motile by means of polar tufts of flagella; divide by binary fission; and are Gram-negative. Motile forms often develop gas vacuoles and later become immotile and float to the top because of the presence of these vacuoles. At low sulfide concentrations and low light intensities, motile nonvacuolated cells predominate. Stationary phase cells generally become immotile and vacuolated. Internal photosynthetic membranes are present as lamellar stacks. Color of cell suspensions is pink to red. Absorption spectra of living cells show maxima at 376, 488, 515, 550, 590, 797 and 860 nm. Photosynthetic pigments are bacteriochlorophyll *a* (esterified with phytol) and carotenoids of the spirilloxanthin series with spirilloxanthin as the major component.

Cells grow preferably under anaerobic conditions in the light. Photoautotrophic growth with sulfide, thiosulfate or elemental sulfur is possible. The organic carbon sources and electron donors used are acetate, propionate, pyruvate, malate, succinate and fumarate. Ammonia and dinitrogen are used as nitrogen source. Cysteine, not sulfate and methionine, is used as sole sulfur source under photoheterotrophic growth conditions. Growth factors are not required. Optimal development is at 30–40°C, pH 7.5–9.5, and 1–6% salts.

The mol% G + C of the DNA is 61.4–63.6 (T_m).

Type strain: ATCC 43036, DSM 2111, BN 9512 (Imhoff: β1).

4. Ectothiorhodospira halophila Raymond and Sistrom 1969, 125.[AL]

ha.lo′phi.la. Gr. n. *halos* salt; Gr. adj. *philos* loving; M.L. fem. adj. *halophila* salt-loving.

Cells are curved in a spiral, 0.6–0.9 μm wide and 2–8 μm long, and motile by means of bipolar flagella; divide by binary fission; and are Gram-negative (Fig. 18.19). Internal photosynthetic membranes are present as lamellar stacks. Color of cell suspensions in the absence of polysulfides and elemental sulfur is red. Absorption spectra of living cells show maxima at 378, 488, 516, 550, 590, 797, 832–835 and 873–885 nm. Photosynthetic pigments are bacteriochlorophyll *a* (esterified with phytol) and carotenoids of the spirilloxanthin series with spirilloxanthin as the predominant component.

Cells grow under strictly anaerobic conditions and are obligately phototrophic. Photoautotrophic growth is possible with sulfide and thiosulfate as electron donors. In the presence of inorganic carbonate, acetate, propionate, pyruvate, malate, succinate and fumarate are used as organic carbon source. Ammonia, glutamate and glutamine serve as nitrogen source. Sulfate is not assimilated. Cysteine is used as sulfur source under photoheterotrophic growth conditions. Growth factors are not required; vitamin B_{12} enhances growth in some strains. Optimal development is at 30–40°C, pH 8.5–9.0, and 11–32% salts. Cells lyse below about 0.5 M NaCl.

The mol% G + C of the DNA is 67.5–69.7 (T_m).

Type strain: DSM 244 (Raymond: Summer Lake 1 = SL1).

5. Ectothiorhodospira halochloris Imhoff and Trüper 1977, 120.[AL]

ha.lo.chlo′ris. Gr. n. *hals* salt; Gr. adj. *chloros* green; M.L. adj. *halochloris* green-colored and salt-loving.

Cells are spiral, 0.5–0.6 μm wide and, depending on the culture conditions, 2.5–8.0 μm long, and motile by means of bipolar flagella; multiply by binary fission; and are Gram-negative (Fig. 18.20). Internal photosynthetic membranes are present as lamellar stacks. Color of cell suspensions is pale green to gooseberry-green, in dense populations with a brownish tinge. Living cells have absorption maxima at 374, 389, 598, 796, 884 and 1018 nm. Photosynthetic pigments are bacteriochlorophyll *b* (esterified with phytadienol) and small amounts of carotenoids (mainly rhodopin glucoside and its methoxy derivative).

Cells grow under strictly anaerobic conditions and are obligately phototrophic. In the presence of sulfide as photosynthetic electron donor and inorganic carbonate, acetate, propionate, pyruvate, succinate, fumarate and malate are used. Ammonia and glutamine are used as nitrogen sources. Growth factors are not required. Optimal development is at 30–44°C, pH 8.1–9.1, and 14–27% salts; there is no growth below the level of 10% salts.

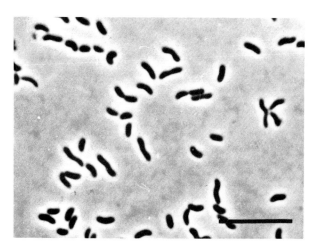

Figure 18.19. *E. halophila* BN 9621. Phase-contrast micrograph. *Bar,* 10 μm. (Reproduced with permission from H. G. Trüper and J. F. Imhoff. 1977. *In* Starr, Stolp, Trüper, Balows and Schlegel (Editors), The Prokaryotes. A Handbook on Habitats, Isolation, and Identification of Bacteria. Springer-Verlag, Berlin, p. 277.)

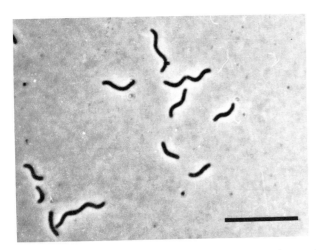

Figure 18.20. *E. halochloris* DSM 1059. Phase-contrast micrograph. *Bar*, 10 µm. (Reproduced with permission from H. G. Trüper and J. F. Imhoff. 1977. *In* Starr, Stolp, Trüper, Balows and Schlegel (Editors), The Prokaryotes. A Handbook on Habitats, Isolation, and Identification of Bacteria. Springer-Verlag, Berlin, p. 277.)

The mol% G + C of the DNA is 50.5–52.9 (T_m).

Type strain: ATCC 35916, DSM 1059, BN 9850 (Imhoff: A).

6. **Ectothiorhodospira abdelmalekii** Imhoff and Trüper 1982, 266.[VP] (Effective publication: Imhoff and Trüper 1981, 232.)

abd.el.ma.lek'i.i. M.L. gen. n. *abdelmalekii* of Abd-El-Malek; named for Y. Abd-El-Malek, an Egyptian microbiologist.

Cells are spiral and, under some conditions, appear as rods, 0.9.–1.2 µm wide and 4–6 µm long or, at some growth conditions, even longer; are motile by means of bipolar and sheathed flagella; multiply by binary fission; and are Gram-negative. Internal photosynthetic membranes are present as lamellar stacks. Color of cell suspensions is pale green, sometimes with a brownish tinge. Photosynthetic pigments are bacteriochlorophyll *b* (esterified with phytadienol) and small amounts of carotenoids.

Cells grow under strictly anaerobic conditions in the presence of sulfide, inorganic carbonate, and an organic carbon source. Acetate, propionate, pyruvate, succinate and fumarate are used as carbon source and electron donor. Growth factors are not required. Ammonia is used as nitrogen source. Optimal development is at 30–44°C, pH 8.0–9.2, and 12–18% salts.

The mol% G + C of the DNA is 63.3–63.8 (T_m).

Type strain: ATCC 35917, DSM 2110, BN 9840 (Imhoff: 51/20).

PURPLE NONSULFUR BACTERIA *(RHODOSPIRILLACEAE* PFENNIG AND TRÜPER 1971, 17[AL])

JOHANNES F. IMHOFF AND HANS G. TRÜPER

Cells are spherical or ovoid or are of short or long rods or spirals of various width; are motile by polar, subpolar or peritrichous flagella or are nonmotile; and divide by binary fission or show polar growth and budding. None of the described species contains gas vacuoles. **Gram-negative.** Internal photosynthetic membranes are continuous with the cytoplasmic membrane and consist of fingerlike intrusions, vesicles or lamellae. Color of cell suspensions is green, yellowish-green, yellowish-brown, brown, brown-red, red or purple-violet. **Photosynthetic pigments are located in the cytoplasmic membrane and the internal membrane systems and are bacteriochlorophyll *a* or *b* (esterified with phytol or geranylgeraniol) and various types of carotenoids.** In most species, the formation of pigments and of the internal membrane systems are repressed under aerobic conditions but become derepressed at oxygen tensions below a certain level.

Under anaerobic conditions in the light, all species grow as photoheterotrophs with various organic substrates or as photoautotrophs with either molecular hydrogen or, in some species, sulfide, thiosulfate or elemental sulfur as electron donor and CO_2 as sole carbon source (growth factors are required in most cases). **Under microaerobic to aerobic conditions in the dark, many representatives can grow as chemoheterotrophs, and some grow as chemoautotrophs.** Some species may metabolize anaerobically in the dark with sugars and either nitrate, DMSO or trimethylamine-*N*-oxide as electron sink or, though poorly, with metabolic intermediates as electron acceptors.

Some representatives are very sensitive to oxygen; others grow equally well under aerobic conditions in the dark at the full oxygen tension of air and under anaerobic conditions in the light. Ammonia, dinitrogen and several organic nitrogen compounds are generally used as nitrogen source; nitrate is also used by some strains. The majority of the species are able to assimilate sulfate as sole surfur source; only a few species depend on the presence of reduced sulfur compounds as sulfur source. Sulfide is inhibitory for many species already at low concentrations; some, however, exhibit a remarkable tolerance towards this compound. **One or more vitamins are generally required as growth factors**; most commonly required are biotin, thiamine, niacin and *p*-aminobenzoic acid. These compounds are rarely needed by species of the *Chromatiaceae* and *Ectothiorhodospiraceae*, which may require vitamin B_{12} as sole growth factor. Growth of most species is enhanced by small amounts of yeast extract, and some species have a complex nutrient requirement. **As storage materials, polysaccharides, poly-*β*-hydroxybutyric acid and polyphosphate have been found.**

Members of this group are widely distributed in nature and found not only in freshwater, marine and hypersaline environments but also in moist soils and paddy fields. They live preferably in aquatic habitats with significant amounts of soluble organic matter and low oxygen tension, but they rarely form colored blooms, which are characteristically formed by representatives of other families of anoxygenic phototrophic bacteria.

The mol% G + C of the DNA is 52.0–73.2 (Bd and T_m).

Further Comments

Bacteria with a pigmentation similar to the purple sulfur bacteria (*Rhodobacteriaceae* Migula 1900) were described in some detail by Molisch (1907). He considered these bacteria, which were not sulfur bacteria but depended on organic carbon sources for development, as members of a new order, *Rhodobacteria* Molisch 1907. This order comprised the Purple Nonsulfur Bacteria (*Athiorhodaceae*) and the purple sulfur bacteria (*Thiorhodaceae*). This combination was not without problems, since Molisch had to remove the purple sulfur bacteria from the *Thiobacteria* Migula 1900, where they had been combined with the colorless sulfur bacteria (*Beggiatoaceae* Migula 1900). Since that time, pigmentation and, later, the ability to perform anoxygenic photosynthesis were considered so important that these properties were taken as the first criterion for assigning a bacterium to the *Rhodobacteria*, later called *Rhodospirillales* Pfennig and Trüper 1971.

In the seventh edition of the *Manual*, van Niel (1957) consequently stated: "*Rhodomicrobium vannielii* does not conform to the criteria of the order *Pseudomonadales*. Physiologically it is a typical nonsulfur purple bacterium in that it is capable of development in strictly anaerobic media only when the cultures are illuminated and carries out a photosynthetic metabolism without oxygen evolution." In that edition of the *Manual*, *Rhodomicrobium* was, however, still included in the *Hyphomicrobiales;* in the eight edition, it was placed with the *Rhodospirillales* (Pfennig and Trüper, 1974).

The dissimilatory sulfur metabolism and the formation of sulfur globules inside the cells remained the main criteria for the distinction between the two families of the phototrophic purple bacteria, the *Athiorhodaceae* Molisch 1907 (*Rhodospirillaceae* Pfennig and Trüper 1971) and the *Thiorhodaceae* Molisch 1907 (*Chromatiaceae* Bavendamm 1924). However, difficulties in the definitions of the families arose when phototrophic purple bacteria were discovered, with sulfide used as an electron donor for photosynthesis but with elemental sulfur deposited outside rather than inside the cells (*Ectothiorhodospira mobilis* Pelsh 1937; Trüper, 1968). In their physiological properties these bacteria resembled the *Chromatiaceae*. So that these bacteria could be classified with this family, the definition was emended, and they were recognized as the genus *Ectothiorhodospira* (Pelsh, 1937; Trüper, 1968) of the *Chromatiaceae*. Further difficulties arose with the finding of bacteria, which were recognized as members of the *Rhodospirillaceae*, that were, however, able to use sulfide as a photosynthetic electron donor and oxidize it to sulfate (Hansen and van Gemerden, 1972; Hansen and Veldkamp, 1973). Other representatives of the Purple Nonsulfur Bacteria that oxidize sulfide to sulfate and intermediately deposit elemental sulfur outside the cells have now been isolated (Hansen et al., 1975; Neutzling et al., 1984a; Hansen and Imhoff, 1985). With these recent findings, all previous definitions to distinguish the purple sulfur bacteria from the Purple Nonsulfur Bacteria became unsuitable. Therefore, the *Chromatiaceae* were defined as those phototrophic bacteria that deposit globules of elemental sulfur inside their cells under the proper growth conditions (Imhoff, 1984a). In consequence, the genus *Ectothiorhodospira*, which comprises six species, was removed from the *Chromatiaceae* and is recognized as a separate family, the *Ectothiorhodospiraceae* Imhoff 1984.

The most diverse group of the phototrophic purple bacteria is, by far, the Purple Nonsulfur Bacteria. This diversity is reflected in greatly varying morphology, internal membrane structure, carotenoid composition, utilization of carbon sources and electron donors, etc. In view of the lack of significant common properties of all species of this group, which would at the same time distinguish it from the *Chromatiaceae* and *Ectothiorhodospiraceae*, a clear descriptive separation from these two families is difficult. A clear separation of the Purple Nonsulfur Bacteria from the purple sulfur bacteria, as well as their own diversity, is, however, depicted in the oligonucleotide patterns of 16S rRNA molecules, which are considered phylogenetically conservative (Stackebrandt and Woese, 1981). The similarity coefficients derived from these patterns are higher than 0.6 within the *Chromatiaceae* (Fowler et al., 1984) and higher than 0.5 within the *Ectothiorhodospiraceae* (Stackebrandt et al., 1984) but considerably lower between most of the species of the Purple Nonsulfur Bacteria. Binary similarity coefficients higher than 0.6 have been obtained only for the couples *Rhodobacter capsulatus* and *Rhodobacter sphaeroides*, *Rhodospirillum rubum* and *Rhodospirillum photometricum*, and *Rhodocyclus tenuis* and *Rhodocyclus gelatinosus* (Gibson et al., 1979; C. R. Woese, personal communication). Similarity coefficients between species of the Purple Nonsulfur Bacteria and species of the purple sulfur bacteria are between 0.3 and 0.4. Furthermore, not only are the Purple Nonsulfur Bacteria heterogeneous in themselves, but also, on the basis of similarities of the structures of some molecular cell constituents, representatives of this group are much more similar to nonphototrophic chemoheterotrophic bacteria than to each other. High similarities were revealed, for example, in 16S rRNA oligonucleotide patterns and cytochrome c_2 amino acid sequences between *Paracoccus denitrificans* and *Rhodobacter capsulatus* (Ambler et al., 1979; Gibson et al., 1979), in 16S rRNA oligonucleotide patterns, lipid A structure, and internal membrane structures

between *Nitrobacter winogradskyi* and *Rhodopseudomonas palustris* (Seewaldt et al., 1982; Mayer et al., 1983), and in 16S rRNA oligonucleotide patterns between *Sphaerotilus natans* and *Rhodocyclus gelatinosus* (Gibson et al., 1979). These similarities were taken as evidence for the development of some nonphototrophic bacteria from phototrophic ancestors, and on the basis of 16S rRNA similarities the relations within three major groups of Gram-negative bacteria, the alpha, beta, and gamma subdivisions, have been described (Woese et al., 1984a, b; 1985). Although only the species of the genus *Rhodocyclus* were found in the beta subdivision, all other Purple Nonsulfur Bacteria were in the alpha subdivision (Fig. 18.21).

For systematics, the question arises as to whether the phototrophic bacteria should be treated separately or together with their nonphototrophic relatives. In our opinion, the phototrophic bacteria should be treated separately from the nonphototrophic bacteria, since pigmentation and ability to grow phototrophically are easily recognizable determinative properties. This treatment is, however, not without problems: Bacteria such as *Erythrobacter longus* are known to contain bacteriochlorophyll and carotenoids but are unable to grow under anaerobic conditions in the light as phototrophs, as is demanded for the members of this group. At present, our knowledge of these bacteria is too poor for a clear decision to be made about their taxonomic position. A quite similar situation exists for strains of *Rhodospirillum rubrum*, which lose the ability to grow phototrophically by the simple loss of a plasmid (Kuhl et al., 1983). By definition, these strains would not belong to the phototrophic bacteria if their relations would not be known.

For all of the foregoing reasons, we decided to treat the *Rhodospirillaceae* Pfennig and Trüper 1971 as a taxonomic group of the photo-

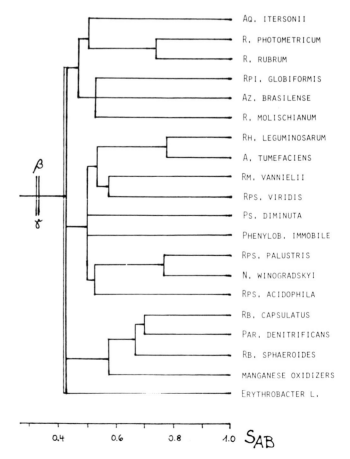

Figure 18.21. Dendrogram of the alpha subdivision of Gram-negative bacteria. (Redrawn after Woese et al., 1984a.)

trophic purple bacteria besides the "genetically well defined" *Chromatiaceae* and the *Ectothiorhodospiraceae* but to omit the use of a true family name. We proposed to classify them under the term Purple Nonsulfur Bacteria (Imhoff et al., 1984a), abbreviated PNSB.

There are problems in the classification of species and genera within the PNSB group. Seven of 23 well-recognized species are characterized on the basis of information on a single strain, and 7 species are characterized on the basis of a few strains only. Furthermore, there is, on the one hand, considerable high variability in the physiological properties (e.g. carbon nutrition, relations to oxygen, and the ability to grow under microaerobic to aerobic conditions in the dark) between different species in most of the genera, while on the other hand, some species from different genera are physiologically quite similar. The physiological similarities are not in accordance with similarities in the organization of the internal membrane systems, in 16S rRNA oligonucleotide patterns, in cytochrome c_2 amino acid sequences and in lipid

A structures. As a consequence, the assignment of new species to the genera on the basis of only physiological properties is not suitable; therefore, the morphological properties and the similarities in molecular structures of certain cell constituents must also be taken into consideration and used. A number of such properties are shown in Table 18.7 for representatives of the genera of the PNSB group. Some of the problems in the use of physiological properties for taxonomic purposes are discussed further in the article on *Rhodobacter* (under Further Descriptive Information).

Despite the fundamental background for the description of the genera and some of the species (obtained by analyses of molecular structures of various cell constituents, which were revealed in many years work in several specialized laboratories), the presently known species can be identified by rather simple methods. In general, the knowledge of cell form and size (microscopic observation), the color of the cell suspensions and their in vivo absorption spectra (spectrophotometric meas-

Table 18.7.

Some properties of representative species of the genera of the **Purple Nonsulfur Bacteria**[a]

Genus and species	16S rRNA group[b]	rRNA superfamily[c]	Type of internal membrane structure[d]	Related cytochrome c_2 present[e]	HIPIP present[e]	Sulfonucleotide reduced during sulfate assimilation[f]	Ubiquinone[g]	Menaquinone[g]	Cosubstrate of GS/GOGAT[h]	D-Glucosamine	2,3-Diamino-2,3-dideoxy-D-glucose	3-OH-C-10	3-OH-C-14	3-OH-C-16	3-Oxo-C-14	Phosphate
Rhodospirillum rubrum	Ic	IVc	v	Lc_2		PAPS	10	−,*	NADPH	+	−	−	⊕	−	−	−
Rhodospirillum molischianum	Ic	nd	l	Sc_2		nd	9	9	NADH	+	−	−	⊕	+	−	−
Rhodospirillum fulvum	nd	nd	l	Sc_2		PAPS	9	9	NADH	+	−	−	⊕	−	−	−
Rhodocyclus purpureus	II	III	t	nd	nd	APS	8	8	NADH	+	−	⊕	−	−	−	+
Rhodocyclus gelatinosus	II	III	t	c_{551}	+	APS	8	8	nd	+	−	⊕	−	−	−	+
Rhodocyclus tenuis	II	III	t	c_{551}	+	APS	8	8	NADH	+	−	⊕	−	−	−	+
Rhodopseudomonas palustris	Ib	IVb	l	Lc_2		PAPS	10	−	NADPH	−	+	−	⊕	+	−	−
Rhodopseudomonas viridis	Ib	IVb	l	Sc_2		PAPS	9	9	nd	−	+	−	⊕	−	−	−
Rhodopseudomonas sulfoviridis	nd	nd	l	nd		−	*	*	nd	−	+	−	⊕	−	−	−
Rhodomicrobium vannielii	Ib	IVd	l	Sc_2	+	APS	10	−	NADH	+	−	−	+	⊕	−	−
Rhodopila globiformis	Ic	IVe	v	Sc_2	+	APS	*	*	NADH	nd	nd	nd	nd	nd	nd	nd
Rhodobacter capsulatus	Ia	IVa	v	Lc_2		PAPS	10	−	NADPH	+	−	+	⊕	−	⊕	+
Rhodobacter sphaeroides	Ia	IVa	v	Lc_2		PAPS	10	−	NADPH	+	−	+	⊕	−	+	+
Rhodobacter sulfidophilus	nd	IVa	v	Lc_2		PAPS	10	−	nd	+	−	+	⊕	−	−	+

[a] Symbols: −, component absent; +, component present; ⊕, amide-linked fatty acid; nd, not determined.

[b] According to Stackebrandt and Woese (1981).

[c] According to Gillis et al. (1982), the various subbranches of group IV are designated a, b, c, d and e; *Rhodomicrobium vannielii* and *Rhodopila globiformis* may be on the same subbranch.

[d] v, vesicles; l, lamellae; t, tubules.

[e] Cytochromes and high potential iron-sulphur proteins (HIPIP) according to Ambler et al. (1979). L, large; S, small.

[f] According to Imhoff (1982). PAPS, 3'-phosphoadenosine-5'-phosphosulfate; APS, adenosine-5'-phosphosulfate.

[g] According to Imhoff (1984b). Numbers indicate major isoprenoid chain length; *, *Rhodospirillum rubrum* has rhodoquinone-10; *Rhodopila globiformis* and *Rhodopseudomonas sulfoviridis* contain more than one component of ubiquinone and menaquinone in high proportion.

[h] According to the literature cited with the description of the genera. GS, glutamine synthetase; GOGAT, glutamate synthase.

[i] According to Weckesser et al. (1979) and the literature cited with the description of the genera.

urements) together with their physiological properties, and, in some instances, additional information on lipid and quinone compositions are sufficient to identify a known species.

Further Reading

Ambler, R.P., M. Daniel, J. Hermoso, T.E. Meyer, R.G. Bartsch and M.D. Kamen. 1979. Cytochrome c_2 sequence variation among the recognized species of purple nonsulfur bacteria. Nature *278:* 659–660.

Ambler, R.P., R.G. Bartsch, M. Daniel, M.D. Kamen, L. McLellan, T.E. Meyer and J. van Beeumen. 1981. Amino acid sequences of bacterial cytochromes c' and c-556. Proc. Natl. Acad. Sci. U.S.A. *78:* 6854–6857.

Biebl, H. and G. Drews. 1969. Das in-vivo-Spektrum als taxonomisches Merkmal bei Untersuchungen zur Verbreitung von *Athiorhodaceae*. Zentralbl. Bakteriol. Parasitenkd. Infektionskr. Hyg. Abt. II Orig. *123:* 425–452.

Clayton, R.K. and W.R. Sistrom (Editors). 1978. The Photosynthetic Bacteria. Plenum Press, New York.

Gibson, J., E. Stackebrandt, L.B. Zablen, R. Gupta and C.R. Woese. 1979. A phylogenetic analysis of the purple photosynthetic bacteria. Curr. Microbiol. *3:* 59–64.

Imhoff, J.F. 1981. Response of photosynthetic bacteria to mineral nutrients. *In* Mitsui and Black (Editors), CRC Handbook of Biosolar Resources. CRC Press, Boca Raton, Fla., pp. 135–146.

Imhoff, J.F. 1982. Occurrence and evolutionary significance of two sulfate assimilation pathways in *Rhodospirillaceae*. Arch. Microbiol. *132:* 197–203.

Imhoff, J.F., D.J. Kushner, S.C. Kushwaha and M. Kates. 1982. Polar lipids in phototrophic bacteria of the *Rhodospirillaceae* and *Chromatiaceae* families. J. Bacteriol. *150:* 1192–1201.

Imhoff, J.F., H.G. Trüper and N. Pfennig. 1984. Rearrangement of the species and genera of the phototrophic "purple nonsulfur bacteria." Int. J. Syst. Bacteriol. *34:* 340–343.

Künzler, A. and N. Pfennig. 1973. Das Vorkommen von Bacteriochlorophyll a_p

and a_{Gg} in Stämmen aller Arten der *Rhodospirillaceae*. Arch. Mikrobiol. *91:* 83–86.

Madigan, M., S.S. Cox and R.E. Stegeman. 1984. Nitrogen fixation and nitrogenase activities in members of the family *Rhodospirillaceae*. J. Bacteriol. *157:* 73–78.

Mandel, M., E.R. Leadbetter, N. Pfennig and H.G. Trüper. 1971. Deoxyribonucleic acid base composition of phototrophic bacteria. Int. J. Syst. Bacteriol. *21:* 222–230.

Pfennig, N. 1977. Phototrophic green and purple bacteria: a comparative systematic survey. Annu. Rev. Microbiol. *31:* 275–290.

Saunders, V.A. 1978. Genetics of *Rhodospirillaceae*. Microbiol. Rev. *42:* 357–384.

Silver, M., S. Friedman, R. Guay, J. Couture and R. Tanguay. 1971. Base composition of deoxyribonucleic acid isolated from *Athiorhodaceae*. J. Bacteriol. *107:* 368–370.

Stackebrandt, E. and C.R. Woese. 1981. The evolution of procaryotes. *In* Carlile, Collins and Mosely (Editors), Molecular and Cellular Aspects of Microbial Evolution. Cambridge University Press, Cambridge, England, pp. 1–31.

van Niel, C.B. 1941. The culture, general physiology, morphology and classification of the non-sulfur purple and brown bacteria. Bacteriol. Rev. *8:* 1–118.

Weckesser, J., G. Drews and H. Mayer. 1979. Lipopolysaccharides of photosynthetic procaryotes. Annu. Rev. Microbiol. *33:* 215–239.

Woese, C.R., E. Stackebrandt, W.G. Weisburg, B.J. Paster, M.T. Madigan, V.J. Fowler, C.M. Hahn, P. Blanz, R. Gupta, K.H. Nealson and G.E. Fox. 1984a. The phylogeny of purple bacteria: the alpha subdivision. Syst. Appl. Microbiol. *5:* 315–326.

Woese, C.R., W.G. Weisburg, B.J. Paster, C.M. Hahn, R.S. Tanner, N.R. Krieg, H.-P. Koops, H. Harms and E. Stackebrandt. 1984b. The phylogeny of purple bacteria: the beta subdivision. Syst. Appl. Microbiol. *5:* 327–336.

Woese, C.R., W.G. Weisburg, C.M. Hahn, B.J. Paster, L.B. Zablen, B.J. Lewis, T.J. Macke, W. Ludwig and E. Stackebrandt. 1985. The phylogeny of purple bacteria: the gamma subdivision. Syst. Appl. Microbiol. *6:* 25–33.

Key to the genera of the **Purple Nonsulfur Bacteria**

Unicellular bacteria, nonmotile or motile by means of flagella, containing bacteriochlorophyll *a* or *b* and various types of carotenoids, able to grow phototrophically under anaerobic conditions in the light.

1. Cells clearly spiral, 0.5–1.5 μm wide, motile by means of polar flagella; internal photosynthetic membranes as vesicles or lamella (Fig. 18.22, *A* and *B*) but not as small fingerlike intrusions of the cytoplasmic membrane (Fig. 18.23).

    Rhodospirillum

2. Cells spherical, 1.6–1.8 μm wide; cell division by binary fission; internal photosynthetic membranes as vesicles; containing bacteriochlorophyll *a* and special ketocarotenoids; optimal growth at acidic pH.

    Rhodopila

3. Cells spherical, ovoid or rod-shaped, 0.5–1.2 μm wide; cell division by binary fission; internal photosynthetic membranes as vesicles; containing bacteriochlorophyll *a* and carotenoids of the spheroidene series; slime production and chain formation common.

    Rhodobacter

4. Cells ovoid to rod-shaped, 0.5–1.3 μm wide, showing polar growth; multiply by budding; internal photosynthetic membranes as lamella lying parallel to the cytoplasmic membrane (Fig. 18.22C); containing bacteriochlorophyll *a* or *b* and various types of carotenoids.

    Rhodopseudomonas

5. Cells ovoid to rod-shaped, 1.0–1.2 μm wide; multiply by budding; perform a characteristic growth cycle with nonmotile stalked cells and peritrichously flagellated swarmer cells; internal photosynthetic membranes as lamella lying parallel to the cytoplasmic membrane; form exospores.

    Rhodomicrobium

6. Cells undulated to spiral or forming a half-circle to a circle, 0.3–0.7 μm wide, motile or nonmotile; internal photosynthetic membranes as small fingerlike intrusions of the cytoplasmic membrane (Fig. 18.23).

    Rhodocyclus

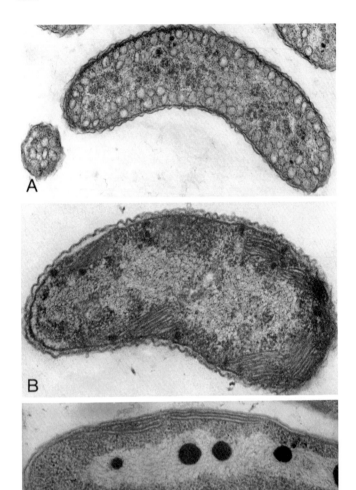

Figure 18.22. Fine structure of some Purple Nonsulfur Bacteria. *A*, *Rhodospirillum rubrum* strain FR1 grown anaerobically in the light. Note the vesicular structure of the intracytoplasmic membrane system. × 51,000. (Courtesy of G. Drews and R. Ladwig.) *B*, *Rhodospirillum molischianum* grown anaerobically in the light. Note the position and the lamellar stack type of the intracytoplasmic membrane system. × 90,000. (Courtesy of G. Drews.) *C*, *Rhodopseudomonas palustris* strain 11/1 grown semiaerobically in the dark. Note the position and type of intracytoplasmic membrane system. × 60,000. (Courtesy of H. D. Tauschel and R. Ladwig.)

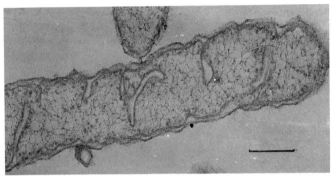

Figure 18.23. *Rhodocyclus gelatinosus* grown anaerobically at low light intensity. The intracytoplasmic membrane system consists of tubular intrusions of the cytoplasmic membrane. *Bar*, 0.2 µm. (Courtesy of W. E. de Boer.)

Genus **Rhodospirillum** *Molisch 1907, 24*[AL]

HANS G. TRÜPER AND JOHANNES F. IMHOFF

Rho.do.spi.ril′lum. Gr. n. *rhodos* the rose; M.L. dim. neut. n. *Spirillum* a bacterial genus; M.L. neut. n. *Rhodospirillum* red *Spirillum*.

Cells are spiral, 0.7–1.5 µm wide, and **motile by means of polar flagella;** divide by binary fission; and are Gram-negative. **Internal photosynthetic membranes are present as vesicles or as lamellae** lying parallel to the cytoplasmic membrane or forming a sharp angle to it. Photosynthetic pigments are bacteriochlorophyll *a* (esterified with phytol or geranylgeraniol) and carotenoids of the spirilloxanthin series with spirilloxanthin itself lacking in some species.

Growth occurs preferably photoheterotrophically under anaerobic conditions in the light but also occurs under microaerobic to aerobic conditions in the dark. Some species are very sensitive to oxygen; others grow equally well aerobically in the dark and, under phototrophic conditions, anaerobically in the light. Molecular hydrogen may be used as a photosynthetic electron donor during photoautotrophic growth. Polysaccharides, poly-β-hydroxybutyric acid and polyphosphates may be present as storage products.

The mol% G + C of the DNA is 60.5–65.8 (Bd) and 62.1–63.5 (T_m).

Type species: *Rhodospirillum rubrum* (Esmarch) Molisch 1907, 25.

Further Descriptive Information

All known representatives of *Rhodospirillum* clearly have spiral cells of varying width which are motile by means of polar flagella. The cell

wall of *R. salexigens* contains peptidoglycan and proteins but lacks glycolipids and lipopolysaccharides (Golecki and Drews, 1980).

Two different types of alcohols are esterified with the bacteriochlorophyll *a* of the *Rhodospirillum* species—phytol, as in most other PNSB, or geranylgeraniol with the major part of the bacteriochlorophyll *a* of *R. rubrum* and of some strains of *R. photometricum* (Brockmann and Knobloch, 1972; Künzler and Pfennig, 1973). Carotenoids of the spirilloxanthin series are present in all species, but the brown species are unable to synthesize the end product spirilloxanthin and accumulate intermediates of this pathway, such as lycopene and rhodopin. *R. photometricum* also contains anhydrorhodovibrin and rhodovibrin (Schmidt, 1978).

The brown species, *R. photometricum*, *R. molischianum* and *R. fulvum*, are very sensitive to oxygen and do not grow under aerobic conditions in the dark as the other species do (Pfennig, 1969b). They grow, however, under microaerophilic conditions in the dark, provided the oxygen tension is lower than 1.5 kPa for *R. fulvum*, 1.0 kPa for *R. molischianum*, and 0.5 kPa for *R. photometricum* (Lehmann, 1976). These bacteria are apparently unable to induce a second electron transport chain in the presence of oxygen and depend therefore on microaerobic conditions in which the internal membrane system and the light-driven electron transport chain are fully expressed. The cells are fully pigmented under these growth conditions (Lehmann, 1976). Only a few studies of taxonomic interest have been performed with the brown species (Pfennig et al., 1965; Sarkar and Banerjee, 1980; Lehmann, 1976), and the two halophilic species have been described only recently. Numerous investigations on the physiology and enzymology of *R. rubrum* have focused on metabolism under anaerobic or aerobic dark conditions, CO_2 fixation and ribulose-1,5-bisphosphate carboxylase, ATP generation and coupling-factor ATPase, and enzymes of the C_3 and C_4 metabolism.

R. rubrum can grow under photoheterotrophic conditions, but it can also grow under photoautotrophic conditions with molecular hydrogen (Klemme, 1968) or with sulfide at low concentrations (Hansen and van Gemerden, 1972) as electron donor. Autotrophic CO_2 fixation is well-documented and occurs via ribulose-1,5-bisphosphate carboxylase under autotrophic growth conditions (Anderson and Fuller, 1967a). This enzyme has been highly purified and is well-characterized (e.g. Tabita and McFadden, 1974a, b). Ribulose-1,5-bisphosphate carboxylase is derepressed only at low tensions of CO_2 (1.5–2.0% of the atmospheric tension) and, under such conditions, can make up about 50% of the total soluble protein of the cells (Sarles and Tabita, 1983). In the presence of malate or acetate, however, CO_2 is not assimilated via the reductive pentose phosphate cycle, but a number of other carboxylating reactions are involved. The first labeled phosphate ester with malate as additional carbon source was phosphoenolpyruvate (Anderson and Fuller, 1967b).

Various enzymes are active in the metabolism of C_8 compounds Pryruvate dehydrogenase is apparently responsible for the photoassimilation of pyruvate under photoheterotrophic growth conditions (Lüderitz and Klemme, 1977). The gluconeogenetic formation of phosphoenolpyruvate from oxaloacetate is catalyzed by a phosphoenolpyruvate carboxykinase, which is specifically activated by ATP in the direction of phosphoenolpyruvate formation but strongly inhibited by ATP in the reverse direction (Klemme, 1976). Under anaerobic dark conditions, the fermentation of sugars and pyruvate is possible (Kohlmiller and Gest, 1951; Gürgün et al., 1976; Gorrell and Uffen, 1977). Under these conditions, pyruvate is cleaved by pyruvate formate lyase, which is specifically induced at these growth conditions (Jungermann and Schön, 1974; Uffen, 1973). From formate, H_2 and CO_2 are formed by a CO-sensitive formic hydrogen lyase (Gorrell and Uffen, 1977). H_2, CO_2, acetate and, eventually, propionate are produced as fermentation products from pyruvate.

Like *Rhodobacter capsulatus*, *Rhodospirillum rubrum* also is able to perform an aerobic dark metabolism with DMSO and trimethylamine-N-oxide as electron acceptors (Schultz and Weaver, 1982). In the presence of these electron acceptors, an aerobic dark growth is also possible with succinate, malate and acetate as substrates; CO_2 and DMSO or trimethylamine are formed under these conditions (Schultz and Weaver, 1982).

With the exception of *Rhodospirillum salexigens* and *Rhodospirillum salinarum*, which depend on glutamate or complex nutrients, respectively, the species of this genus can grow with ammonia or dinitrogen as sole nitrogen source (Siefert, 1976; Madigan et al., 1984). Cultures of *R. salexigens* grown in the presence of 4 mM glutamate and dinitrogen formed readily detectable amounts of nitrogenase (Madigan et al., 1984). Ammonia assimilation is mediated by the glutamine synthetase/ glutamate synthase reactions, which are NADPH-dependent in *R. rubrum* but NADH-dependent in *R. molischianum* and *R. fulvum* (Brown and Herbert, 1977). An active transport system for ammonium has been found in *R. rubrum*. This system is repressed by high concentrations of ammonium (Alef and Kleiner, 1982). A nitrate reductase has been described, but the ability of *R. rubrum* to grow with nitrate as sole nitrogen source is not clear (Katoh, 1963; Taniguchi and Kamen, 1963; Ketchum and Sevilla, 1973; Klemme, 1979). Purines can be used as nitrogen source under anaerobic conditions in the light and under aerobic conditions in the dark (Aretz et al., 1978).

In *R. rubrum*, complete inhibition of growth occurs at penicillin concentrations of more than 1000 U/ml (Weaver et al., 1975), whereas in *R. photometricum*, complete inhibition occurs at penicillin concentrations of 10 U/ml and at streptomycin concentrations of 10 μg/ml. In *R. salexigens*, growth is inhibited by a number of antibiotics, e.g. tetracycline, chloramphenicol, penicillin, ampicillin, cycloserine, nisin, vancomycin and bacitracin, but it is not inhibited by oxacillin (Drews, 1981).

Enrichment and Isolation Procedures

Suitable and selective growth conditions for the different species of this genus are widely varying. The freshwater species grow on media suitable for most of the PNSB. Recipes for the media have been developed in many instances by various laboratories working with PNSB. In general, these recipes are only slightly modified in their mineral composition or in the organic carbon source used. Suitable media are given by Biebl and Pfennig (1981). A recipe for a mineral medium used in the authors' laboratory for cultivation of the great majority of the PNSB is given in the footnote below.* The two halophilic species need special media. The media used by Golecki and Drews (1980) for *R. salexigens* and by Nissen and Dundas (1984) for *R. salinarum* are given in the modification used in our laboratory. Both species grow well on a complex medium after Nissen and Dundas (1984).[†] *R. salexigens* is routinely grown on a modified medium of Golecki and Drews (1980).[‡]

Maintenance Procedures

Cultures of all species can be maintained by standard procedures in liquid nitrogen.

Differentiation of the genus **Rhodospirillum** from other genera

The spiral shape and the phototrophic capacity of the cells clearly distinguish species of *Rhodospirillum* from those of other genera. The species of the genus *Rhodocyclus*, which have also spiral-shaped cells, are thinner, have a simpler internal membrane system, and are also different in a number of structures of diagnostic valuable molecular cell constituents. Analyses of 16S rRNA show that *Rhodospirillum* species are separate from other PNSB. The DNA of *Rhodospirillum rubrum* shows some low homology to that of *Azospirillum brasilense* (Tarrand et al., 1978).

---

* The medium contains (per liter): 1.0 g KH_2PO_4, 0.5 g $MgCl_2 \cdot 6H_2O$, 0.1 g $CaCl_2 \cdot 2H_2O$, 1.0 g NH_4Cl, 3.0 g $NaHCO_3$, 0.7 g Na_2SO_4, 1.0 g NaCl, 1 ml sulfate-free trace element solution SLA (Imhoff and Trüper, 1977; see the footnote on page 1655) and 1 ml vitamin solution VA (Imhoff and Trüper, 1977). Organic carbon sources (routinely 10 mM sodium malate, sodium succinate or sodium pyruvate) and, for oxygen-sensitive strains, 0.5 g sodium ascorbate or 0.25 g thioglycolate are added separately. The initial pH is adjusted to 6.9. Vitamin solution VA in 100 ml of bidistilled water contains: 10 mg biotin, 35 mg niacin amide, 30 mg thiamine dichloride, 20 mg p-aminobenzoic acid, 10 mg pyridoxal hydrochloride, 10 mg calcium pantothenate and 5 mg vitamin B_{12}.

† The medium contain (per liter): 100 g NaCl, 3.5 g $MgCl_2 \cdot 6H_2O$, 0.3 g KH_2PO_4, 10 g sodium malate, 1.5 g yeast extract, 1.5 g peptone and 1 ml trace element solution SLA. The initial pH is adjusted to 7.0.

‡ The medium contains (per liter): 80 g NaCl, 0.4 g $MgCl_2 \cdot 6H_2O$, 0.1 g $CaCl_2 \cdot 2H_2O$, 0.5 g $(NH_4)_2SO_4$, 2.5 g KH_2PO_4, 1 g sodium acetate, 1 g sodium glutamate and 1 ml trace element solution SLA. The initial pH is adjusted to 7.0.

The Fe-protein component of the nitrogenase complex of *Azospirillum lipoferum* can be activated by the activating factor isolated from *Rhodospirillum rubrum* (Burris et al., 1977).

Taxonomic Comments

On the basis of DNA/rRNA hybridization data (Gillis et al., 1982), 16S rRNA oligonucleotide patterns (Gibson et al., 1979), cytochrome *c* amino acid sequences (Ambler et al., 1979) and a number of other properties (see Table 18.7), *Rhodospirillum tenue* Pfennig 1969b has been removed from this genus and is now treated as *Rhodocyclus tenuis* (Imhoff et al., 1984).

Differentiation of the species of the genus **Rhodospirillum**

Some of the major differentiating characteristics of the species are shown in Table 18.8. The species can easily be distinguished by their pigmentation (color of the cultures), size of the cells, and growth factor requirements. In addition, the brown species are very sensitive to oxygen and do not grow under aerobic conditions. *Rhodospirillum salexigens* and *Rhodospirillum salinarum* have a considerable and obligate requirement of sodium chloride, while the other species are freshwater bacteria. Very similar are *Rhodospirillum molischianum* and *Rhodospirillum fulvum*, which can be distinguished primarily by the cell size, the growth factor requirement (Table 18.8), and the utilization of benzoate (Table 18.9). With respect to their natural environment, salt requirement, cell morphology, and color of anaerobic and light-grown cultures, *R. salexigens* and *R. salinarum* are very similar. Both grow very well also under aerobic conditions in the dark. *R. salinarum* has, however, a complex nutrient requirement and could not be grown in the absence of substrate concentrations of yeast extract or peptone;

at reduced concentrations of these complex nutrients, only lactate was found to support growth. Glutamate is an obligate nitrogen source for *R. salexigens*. *R. salinarum* has internal photosynthetic membranes of the vesicular type, whereas *R. salexigens* has internal membranes of the lamellar type.

The cytochromes c_2 of *R. rubrum* and *R. photometricum* are most similar to each other, as are those of *R. fulvum* and *R. molischianum* (Ambler et al., 1979). The latter two species have a small type cytochrome c_2, as has been found in *R. salexigens* (Meyer, 1982), whereas the former two species have a large type cytochrome c_2. Similarities between the species have been found by comparison of amino acid sequences of the cytochromes *c'* (Ambler et al., 1981), by comparison of oligonucleotide patterns of 16S rRNA (Gibson et al., 1979; C. R. Woese, personal communication) and by analyses of their quinone compositions (Imhoff, 1984b).

List of species of the genus **Rhodospirillum**

1. **Rhodospirillum rubrum** (Esmarch) Molisch 1907, 25.[AL] (*Spirillum rubrum* Esmarch 1887, 230.)

rub'rum. M.L. neut. adj. *rubrum* red.

Cells are vibrioid-shaped to spiral, 0.8–1.0 μm wide; one complete turn of a spiral is 1.5–2.5 μm wide and 7–10 μm long (Fig. 18.24). Internal photosynthetic membranes are of the vesicular type. Anaerobic liquid cultures are pink to deep red, without a brownish tinge, under all conditions; under aerobic conditions, cells are colorless to light pink. Living cells show absorption maxima at 375–377, 510–517, 546–550, 590–595, 807–808 and 881–885 nm. Photosynthetic pigments are bacteriochlorophyll *a* (esterified with geranylgeraniol or phytol (minor component)) and carotenoids of the spirilloxanthin series with spirilloxanthin as the predominant component.

Photoautotrophic growth is possible with molecular hydrogen as electron donor. Cells preferably grow photoheterotrophically under anaerobic conditions in the light with various organic compounds as carbon and electron sources. Microaerobic to aerobic growth in the dark is possible. Fermentative metabolism with pyruvate under anaerobic dark conditions and "oxidant-dependent" anaerobic dark metabolism of sugars are also possible. The carbon sources utilized are shown in Table 18.9. Also used are alanine, asparagine and, by some strains, propanol. Ammonia, dinitrogen, several amino acids and, by some strains, nitrate, adenine, guanine, xanthin and uric acid may be used as nitrogen source. Sulfate can be used as sole sulfur source. Biotin is required as growth factor. Small amounts of yeast extract may be favorable. Growth occurs at pH 6.0–8.5 (optimum pH: 6.8–7.0) and at 30–35°C.

The mol% G + C of the DNA is 63.8–65.8 (Bd).

Type strain: DSM 467, ATCC 11170, NCIB 8255.

Table 18.8.
Differentiating characteristics of the species of the genus **Rhodospirillum**[a]

Characteristic	1. *R. rubrum*	2. *R. photometricum*	3. *R. molischianum*	4. *R. fulvum*	5. *R. salexigens*	6. *R. salinarum*
Cell diameter (μm)	0.8–1.0	1.1–1.5	0.7–1.0	0.5–0.7	0.6	0.8–0.9
Mol% G + C of DNA (Bd)	63.8–65.8	64.8–65.8	60.5–64.8	64.3–65.3	64	67.4
Color of cell suspensions	Red	Brown	Brown	Brown	Red	Red
Internal membrane system	Vesicles	Lamellar stacks	Lamellar stacks	Lamellar stacks	Lamellar stacks	Vesicles
Aerobic growth	+	−	−	−	+	+
Growth factors required	Biotin	Niacin	Amino acids	p-ABA[b]	None[c]	Complex nutrients
Salt requirement (%)	0	0	0	0	5–20	6–18

[a] Symbols: +, present; −, absent.

[b] p-ABA, *p*-aminobenzoic acid.

[c] Glutamate is, however, required as an organic nitrogen source.

Table 18.9.
Photosynthetic electron donors and carbon sources used by species of the genus **Rhodospirillum**[a]

Donor/source	1. R. rubrum	2. R. photometricum	3. R. molischianum	4. R. fulvum	5. R. salexigens	Donor/source	1. R. rubrum	2. R. photometricum	3. R. molischianum	4. R. fulvum	5. R. salexigens
Formate	−	−	o	o	o	Citrate	−	−	−	−	+
Acetate	+	+	+	+	+	Aspartate	+	±	±	±	o
Propionate	+	±	+	+	o	Arginine	+	+	−	−	−
Butyrate	+	+	+	+	o	Glutamate	+	−	o	o	+
Valerate	+	+	+	+	o	Benzoate	−	−	−	+	o
Caproate	+	−	+	+	o	Glucose	−	+	−	±	+
Caprylate	o	−	+	+	o	Fructose	±	+	−	−	−
Pelargonate	o	±	+	+	o	Mannitol	−	+	−	−	o
Glycolate	o	+	−	o	o	Glycerol	−	+	−	−	+
Pyruvate	+	+	+	+	+	Methanol	±	−	−	±	o
Lactate	+	+	±	−	−	Ethanol	+	+	+	+	o
Malate	+	+	+	+	o	Hydrogen	+	+	o	o	o
Succinate	+	+	+	+	+	Sulfide	+	−	−	−	−
Fumarate	+	+	+	+	o	Thiosulfate	−	−	−	−	−
Tartrate	−	−	−	o	o	Sulfur	−	−	−	−	−

[a] Symbols: −, substrate not utilized by most of the strains; o, not tested; +, substrate utilized by most of the strains; ±, substrate utilized by some strains.

2. **Rhodospirillum photometricum** Molisch 1907, 24.[AL]

pho.to.me′tri.cum. Gr. n. *phos* light; Gr. adj. *metricus* measuring; M.L. neut. adj. *photometricum* light-measuring.

Cells are spirals, 1.1–1.5 μm wide; one complete turn of a spiral is 2.5–4 μm wide and 4–7 μm long; cells 14–30 μm long are common (Fig. 18.25). Internal photosynthetic membranes consist of several lamellar stacks forming a sharp angle with the cytoplasmic membrane. Anaerobic liquid cultures are brown-orange to brown-red or dark brown. Photosynthetic pigments are bacteriochlorophyll *a* (esterified with phytol and, in some strains to a small extent, with geranylgeraniol) and carotenoids of the spirilloxanthin series. Spirilloxanthin is lacking, but the biosynthetic precursors lycopene and rhodopin are present as major components.

Cells grow preferably under anaerobic conditions in the light with various carbon compounds as carbon and electron sources and are unable to adapt to aerobic growth conditions. Microaerobic growth at very low oxygen tensions may be possible; under these conditions, cells are fully pigmented. Carbon sources utilized are shown in Table 18.8. Also used are asparagine, maltose, sucrose, raffinose, adonitol and dulcitol. Not used are cyclohexane carboxylate, mannose, galactose, xylose and inositol. Ammonia, dinitrogen, alanine, glutamate and asparagine are used as nitrogen source. Not used are nitrate, urea and arginine. Sulfate, thiosulfate, cysteine, thioglycolate and sulfide at low concentrations can be used as sulfur source. Nicotinic acid is required as growth factor. Ascorbic acid may be required as a reductant. Good growth occurs at pH 6.5–7.5 and at 25–30°C.

The mol% G + C of the DNA is 64.8–65.8 (Bd) and 63 (T_m).

Type strain: DSM 122, NTHC 132.

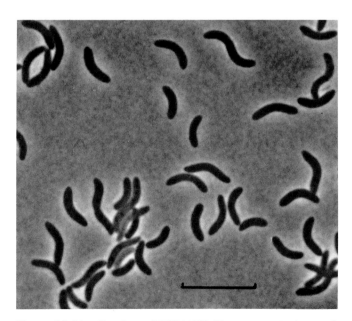

Figure 18.24. *R. rubrum* ATCC 11170. Phase-contrast micrograph. *Bar,* 10 μm. (Courtesy of N. Pfennig.)

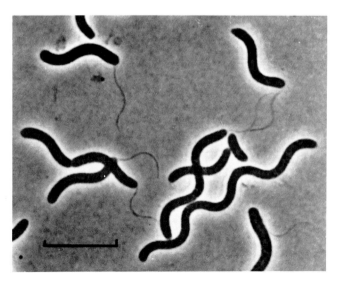

Figure 18.25. *R. photometricum* NTHC 132, cultured on malate-yeast extract medium. Phase-contrast micrograph. *Bar,* 10 μm. (Courtesy of N. Pfennig.)

3. **Rhodospirillum molischianum** Giesberger 1947, 142.[AL]

mo.li.schi.a′num. M.L. neut. adj. *molischianum* pertaining to Molisch; named for H. Molisch, an Austrian botanist.

Cells are vibrioid-shaped to spiral, 0.7–1.0 μm wide; one complete turn of a spiral is 1.5–2.5 μm wide and 4–6 μm long or even longer. Internal photosynthetic membranes are present as lamellar stacks forming a sharp angle to the cytoplasmic membrane. Anaerobic liquid cultures are brown-orange to brown-red or dark brown. Absorption maxima of living cells are at 375, about 465, 488–491, 520–528, 590–595, 803–807 and 850–855 nm. Photosynthetic pigments are bacteriochlorophyll *a* (esterified with phytol) and carotenoids of the spirilloxanthin series. Spirilloxanthin is lacking, but the biosynthetic precursors lycopene and rhodopin are present as major components.

Cells grow preferably under anaerobic conditions in the light with various carbon compounds as carbon and electron sources and are unable to adapt to aerobic growth conditions. Under very low oxygen tensions, microaerobic growth may be possible; under these conditions, cells are fully pigmented. Carbon sources utilized are shown in Table 18.9. Malonate is not used. Ammonia, dinitrogen and some amino acids are used as nitrogen source. Yeast extract and vitamin-free casamino acids stimulate growth considerably. For optimal development the addition of ascorbate or thioglycolate as a reductant may be necessary. Growth occurs at pH 6.0–8.5 (optimum pH: 7.3); good growth occurs at 30°C.

The mol% G + C of the DNA is 60.5–64.8 (Bd) and 62.1–62.6 T_m).

Type strain: DSM 120, ATCC 14031, NCIB 9957, NTHC 131.

4. **Rhodospirillum fulvum** van Niel 1944, 108.[AL]

ful′vum. M.L. neut. adj. *fulvum* deep or reddish yellow, tawny.

Cells are vibrioid-shaped to spiral, 0.5–0.7 μm wide; one complete turn of a spiral is 1.0–1.6 μm wide and about 3.5 μm long. Internal photosynthetic membranes are present as lamellar stacks forming a sharp angle to the cytoplasmic membrane. Anaerobic liquid cultures are deep brown. Photosynthetic pigments are bacteriochlorophyll *a* (esterified with phytol) and carotenoids of the spirilloxanthin series. Spirilloxanthin is lacking, but the biosynthetic precursors lycopene and rhodopin are present as major components.

Cells grow preferably under anaerobic conditions in the light with various carbon compounds as carbon and electron sources and are unable to adapt to aerobic growth conditions. At very low oxygen tensions, microaerobic dark growth may be possible; under these conditions, cells are fully pigmented. Carbon sources utilized are shown in Table 18.9. Ammonia and dinitrogen are used as nitrogen source. Sulfate can be used as sole sulfur source. Growth occurs at pH 6.0–8.5 (optimum pH: 7.3); good growth occurs at 25–30°C. As a growth factor, *p*-aminobenzoic acid is required; for optimal development the addition of ascorbate or thioglycolate as a reductant may be necessary.

The mol% G + C of the DNA is 64.3–65.3 (Bd) and 62.1–62.8 (T_m).

Type strain: DSM 113, ATCC 15798 (Pfennig 1360).

5. **Rhodospirillum salexigens** Drews 1982, 384.[VP] (Effective publication: Drews 1981, 327.)

sal.ex′i.gens. L. n. *sal* salt; L. part. adj. *exigens* demanding; *salexigens* salt-demanding.

Cells are rod-shaped to spiral, 0.6–0.7 μm wide; one complete turn of a spiral is 0.8–0.9 μm wide and 1–6 μm long. Internal photosynthetic membranes are present as lamellae lying parallel to the cytoplasmic membrane. Color of anaerobically grown liquid cultures is red. Absorption maxima of living cells are at 375, 485, 515, 550, 590, 800, 840 and 875 nm. Photosynthetic pigments are bacteriochlorophyll *a* (esterified with phytol) and carotenoids of the spirilloxanthin series with spirilloxanthin as the predominant component.

Cells grow under anaerobic conditions in the light with various carbon compounds as carbon and electron sources or under aerobic conditions in the dark. Carbon compounds assimilated are shown in Table 18.9; most amino acids are not used. Ammonia or dinitrogen cannot serve as sole nitrogen source; glutamate is required for growth; casein hydrolysate is used as carbon and nitrogen sources. Photoautotrophic growth with molecular hydrogen, sulfide or thiosulfate as electron donor is not possible. No growth factors are required. Growth occurs at pH 6.6–7.4, at 20–45°C (optimum temperature: 40°C) and at 5–20% NaCl.

The mol% G + C of the DNA is 64 $\pm$ 2 (Bd and T_m).

Type strain: DSM 2132 (Drews WS 68), ATCC 35888.

6. **Rhodospirillum salinarum** Nissen and Dundas 1985, 224.[VP] (Effective publication: Nissen and Dundas 1984, 255.)

sal.i.na′rum. L. fem. pl. n. *salinae* saltern or saltworks; *salinarum* of a saltern.

Cells are rod-shaped to spiral, 0.8–0.9 μm wide and about 2.0–3.5 μm long. Internal photosynthetic membranes are present as vesicles. Color of anaerobically grown cultures is red. Absorption maxima of living cells are at 380, 490, 520, 550, 595, 800 and 870 nm, indicating the presence of bacteriochlorophyll *a* (esterified with phytol) and carotenoids of the spirilloxanthin series with spirilloxanthin as the major component.

Growth occurs either under anaerobic conditions in the light or, even faster, under aerobic conditions in the dark. Cells have a complex nutrient requirement and do not grow in the absence of substantial amounts of yeast extract or peptone. At reduced concentrations of yeast extract and peptone, casamino acids and lactate support growth; acetate, citrate, fumarate, glutamate, malate, propionate, pyruvate, succinate, fructose, galactose, glucose, sorbose, sucrose, glycerol and mannitol do not support growth. Growth occurs at pH 7.5–8.0, at 20–45°C (optimum temperature: 42°C) and at 6–18% NaCl. Optimal growth under aerobic conditions in the dark occurs at 6–12% NaCl; optimal growth under anaerobic conditions in the light occurs at 12–18% NaCl; no growth has been noted at <2% NaCl.

The mol% G + C of the DNA is 67.4–68.1 (Bd and T_m).

Type strain: ATCC 35394.

Addendum

New species recently described by E. I. Kompantseva and V. M. Gorlenko (1984): *Rhodospirillum mediosalinum*.

Genus **Rhodopila** *Imhoff, Trüper and Pfennig 1984, 341*[VP]

Johannes F. Imhoff and Hans G. Trüper

Rho.do.pi′la. Gr. n. *Rhodos* the rose; M.L. fem. n. *pila* a ball or sphere; M.L. fem. n. *Rhodopila* red sphere.

Cells are spherical to ovoid, 1.6–1.8 μm in diameter under optimal growth conditions, and **motile by means of polar flagella** and divide by binary fission. Gram-negative. **The internal membrane system is of the vesicular type,** and photosynthetic pigments are bacteriochlorophyll and carotenoids.

Cells grow preferably photoheterotrophically under anaerobic conditions in the light. Cells are sensitive to oxygen but grow under microaerobic conditions in the dark and **prefer an acidic pH.**

The mol% G + C of the DNA is 66.3 (Bd).

Type species: *Rhodopila globiformis* (Pfennig 1974) Imhoff, Trüper and Pfennig 1984, 341.

Further Descriptive Information

Depending on the culture conditions, the diameter of the cells varies between 1.0 and 2.5 μm. After division, cells may be connected by a very short and thin filament. Cells appear single or, during cell division, paired.

Physiologically, *Rhodopila globiformis* is characterized by a number of peculiar properties: It is a photoheterotroph, not able to use most of the carbon substrates utilized by other PNSB. Good growth occurs only with ethanol, gluconate, mannitol and fructose (Pfennig, 1974). Ammonia is the best nitrogen source; dinitrogen, urea and a number of amino acids can also serve as sole nitrogen source. Peptone and yeast extract are utilized at low concentrations (0.05%) but are growth-inhibitory at higher concentrations. Nitrate is not utilized (Madigan and Cox, 1982). Ammonia is assimilated via the glutamine synthetase/glutamate synthase reaction (NADH-dependent). Glutamate dehydrogenase is not present, but low activities of an alanine dehydrogenase were found (Madigan and Cox, 1982). Growth with sulfate as sole sulfur source is possible at low concentrations, but with more than 1 mM sulfate, growth is inhibited. Sulfate is reduced via adenosine-5′-phosphosulfate (Imhoff, 1982). All enzymes necessary for sulfate assimilation are present; their activities, however, are misregulated (Hensel and Trüper, 1976; Imhoff et al., 1981), and this misregulation is taken as reason for the inhibitory effect of higher sulfate concentrations. Good sulfur sources are cysteine and thiosulfate. Some of the latter is assimilated, but most is oxidized in a dissimilatory process to tetrathionate (Then and Trüper, 1981). Sulfite and sulfide are growth-inhibitory even at low concentrations.

Rhodopila globiformis has unique aliphatic ketocarotenoids (Schmidt and Liaaen-Jensen, 1973), an unusual polar lipid composition (Imhoff et al., 1982) and a small type cytochrome c_2 and is among the few species of the PNSB that have readily detectable amounts of a high potential iron-sulfur protein (species of the genera *Rhodomicrobium* and *Rhodocyclus*, T. E. Meyer, personal communication).

Rhodopila globiformis has been isolated from a weak red layer of an acidic sulfur spring at Yellowstone National Park (U.S.A.) and is probably rare in nature.

Enrichment and Isolation Procedures

If samples from suitable natural habitats are available, *Rhodopila globiformis* can selectively be enriched in media with gluconate as carbon source, thiosulfate as sulfur source, and ammonia or dinitrogen as nitrogen source at acidic pH (4.8–5.0). Isolation can be achieved by standard procedures for phototrophic purple bacteria under strictly anaerobic conditions. A suitable medium for *R. globiformis* (after Pfennig, 1974) is given in the footnote below.*

Maintenance Procedures

Cultures are well-preserved in liquid nitrogen.

Differentiation of the genus **Rhodopila** from other genera

The genus *Rhodopila* is separated from the other genera of the PNSB by its outstanding physiological properties and some diagnostic valuable molecular cell constituents and their structures. Its cell shape and type of internal membranes distinguish *Rhodopila* from the genera *Rhodospirillum*, *Rhodopseudomonas*, *Rhodocyclus* and *Rhodomicrobium*. Vesicular internal membranes are also present in the genus *Rhodobacter*, which differs in carotenoid composition (Schmidt, 1978), pathway of sulfate assimilation (Imhoff, 1982), rRNA/DNA hybridization data (Gillis et al., 1982), 16S rRNA oligonucleotide catalogs (Gibson et al., 1979; C. R. Woese, personal communication), cytochrome c_2 structure (Dickerson, 1980) and polar lipid composition (Imhoff et al., 1982). All of these data separate *Rhodopila* from the other genera of the PNSB.

Taxonomic Comments

Description of this genus is based on a single species. Its outstanding characteristics, however, provide arguments for a treatment as a separate genus (Imhoff, Trüper and Pfennig, 1984). *Rhodopila globiformis* has formerly been included in the genus *Rhodopseudomonas* and was described as *Rhodopseudomonas globiformis* Pfennig 1974, 205.

List of species of the genus **Rhodopila**

1. **Rhodopila globiformis** (Pfennig, 1974) Imhoff, Trüper and Pfennig 1984, 341.[VP] (*Rhodopseudomonas globiformis* Pfennig 1974, 205.)

glo.bi.for′mis. L. n. *globus* sphere; L. n. *forma* shape; M.L. n. *globiformis* of spherical shape.

Cells are spherical to ovoid, diplococcus-shaped before cell division, 1.6–1.8 μm in diameter under optimal growth conditions, and motile by means of polar flagella. Internal photosynthetic membranes are of the vesicular type.

Color of cultures grown anaerobically in the light is intensively purple-red, and of microaerobically grown cells, is pink. Absorption spectra of living cells show maxima at 378, 594, 813 and 862 nm and a shoulder at 890 nm. Photosynthetic pigments are bacteriochlorophyll *a* (esterified with phytol) and so far unknown aliphatic ketocarotenoids.

Cells grow preferably as heterotrophs under anaerobic conditions in the light; growth is also possible microaerobically in the dark. Best growth is obtained with gluconate, mannitol, fructose or ethanol as carbon source. Glucose, tartrate, fumarate, malate, pyruvate and yeast extract at low concentration are also assimilated. No growth occurs with fatty acids, lactate, citrate, glycerol, mannose, sorbitol, amino acids and benzoate as carbon source. Ammonia is the best nitrogen source. Also used are dinitrogen, glutamate, glutamine, aspartate, arginine, urea, asparagine, alanine, and peptone and yeast extract at low concentrations; nitrate is not assimilated. Thiosulfate, cysteine or low concentrations of sulfate are the best sulfur sources; higher concentrations of sulfate are growth inhibitory. Methionine and tetrathionate can also be used, but sulfide and sulfite inhibit growth even at low concentrations. Biotin and *p*-aminobenzoic acid are required as growth factors. Growth occurs at pH 4.2–6.5 (optimum pH is 4.8–5.0 with mannitol and 5.6 with fumarate as carbon source). Optimum temperature is between 30 and 35°C. No growth has been noted at 40°C.

The mol% G + C of the DNA is 66.3 (Bd).

Type strain: ATCC 35887, DSM 161 (Pfennig 7950).

---

* The medium for *R. globiformis,* as given by Pfennig (1974), contains (per liter): 0.5 g KH_2PO_4, 0.4 g NH_4Cl, 0.4 g $MgSO_4·7H_2O$, 0.4 g NACl, 0.05 g $CaCl_2·2H_2O$, 0.2 g $Na_2S_2O_3·5H_2O$, 0.005 g ferrous citrate, 1.5 g mannitol, 0.5 g gluconate, 100 μg biotin, 200 μg *p*-aminobenzoic acid and 10 ml trace element solution 6 (Pfennig, 1974). The initial pH is adjusted to 5.0.

Genus **Rhodobacter** Imhoff, Trüper and Pfennig 1984, 342[VP]

JOHANNES F. IMHOFF

Rho.do.bac′ter. Gr. n. *rhodos* the rose; M.L. masc. n. *bacter* equivalent of Gr. neut. n. *bakterion* a rod; M.L. masc. n. *Rhodobacter* red rod.

Cells are ovoid or rod-shaped, 0.5–1.2 μm in diameter, and motile or nonmotile; motile forms have polar flagella. Cells divide by binary fission, **may produce capsules and slime, and may form chains of cells.** Gram-negative. **Internal photosynthetic membranes are present as vesicles.** Photosynthetic pigments are bacteriochlorophyll *a* (esterfied with phytol) and carotenoids of the spheroidene series.

Photoautotrophic growth is possible in the presence of sulfide as an electron donor and, in some species, with thiosulfate and molecular hydrogen. **Growth occurs photoheterotrophically under anaerobic conditions in the light with a great variety of organic compounds as carbon and electron sources.** Most species perform an oxidative metabolism and grow as chemoheterotrophs at the full oxygen tension of air in the dark.

The mol% G + C of the DNA is 64.4–73.2 (T_m).

Type species: *Rhodobacter capsulatus* (Molisch) Imhoff, Trüper and Pfennig 1984, 342.

Further Descriptive Information

Cells of all *Rhodobacter* species have similar shape and size but different tendencies to form capsules, slime or chains. Chain formation is also dependent on the growth conditions. Characteristic for *R. capsulatus* is the formation of zigzag chains, which is not observed in the other species. However, not all strains of this species form zigzag chains, and this phenomenon is best observed in mineral media. Most of the strains that form zigzag chains in mineral media form straight chains in complex media. Under these conditions, a marked tendency of spheroplast formation is observed, especially if the concentration of yeast extract is higher than 0.7% (Weaver et al., 1975). Pellerin and Gest (1983) report that cell division in *R. sphaeroides* may not occur by simple binary fission but that this species may have some sort of more complex life cycle.

Physiologically, *Rhodobacter* species are among the most versatile species of the PNSB and probably the most versatile bacteria of all. They can perform a number of different growth modes. All species grow well as photoheterotrophs under anaerobic conditions in the light with many different carbon compounds as carbon and electron sources. With the exception of *R. adriaticus*, they grow equally well under aerobic dark conditions at the full oxygen tension of air. Photoautotrophic growth is possible in the presence of growth factors with sulfide as electron donor by all species and with thiosulfate, elemental sulfur and molecular hydrogen by some species (see Table 18.10). Molecular hydrogen is an excellent electron donor for *R. capsulatus* and *R. sulfidophilus*; *R. sphaeroides* grows only slowly with hydrogen as electron donor (Klemme, 1968; Gest et al., 1983).

R. capsulatus can grow well under chemoautotrophic conditions aerobically in the dark with molecular hydrogen as electron donor (Madigan and Gest, 1979; Siefert and Pfennig, 1979). Under aerobic dark conditions, it can also use sulfide as electron donor (Kompantseva,

Table 18.10.
Differentiating characteristics of the species of the genus **Rhodobacter**[a]

Characteristic	1. *R. capsulatus*	2. *R. sphaeroides*	3. *R. sulfidophilus*	4. *R. adriaticus*	5. *R. veldkampii*
Cell diameter (μm)	0.5–1.2	0.7–4.0	0.6–0.9	0.5–0.8	0.6–0.8
Motility	+	+	+	−	−
Slime formation	±	±	±	+	−
DNA base ratio (T_m)	68.1–69.6	70.8–73.2	68.9–73.2	66.7	64.4–67.5
NaCl requirement	−	−	+	+	−
Growth factors required[b]	t	b, t, n	b, t, n, p-ABA	b, t	b, t, p-ABA
Sulfate assimilated	+	+	+	−	−
Sulfide oxidized to	Elemental S	Elemental S	Sulfate	Sulfate[c]	Sulfate[c]
Thiosulfate oxidized to	−	−	Sulfate[d]	Sulfate	Sulfate
Growth on H$_2$/CO$_2$	Excellent	Slow	Excellent	−	−
Aerobic dark growth	+	+	+	−	+
Nitrate assimilated	±	±	−	−	+
Utilization of					
Tartrate	−	±	−	−	−
Citrate	−	+	−	−	−
Mannitol	−	+	+	+	−
Glycerol	−	+	±	+	−
Ethanol	−	+	+	o	o
Gluconate	−	+	+	+	−
Sulfolipid present	−	+	+	−	−
Phosphatidylcholine	+	+	−	−	−

[a] Symbols: +, present or positive in most or all strains; −, absent or negative in most or all strains; ±, present or positive in some strains but absent or negative in other strains; t, thiamine; b, biotin; n, niacin; p-ABA, *p*-aminobenzoic acid; o, not determined.

[b] Some strains of *R. capsulatus* may require niacin and biotin in addition; niacin may be stimulatory to growth in *R. adriaticus*.

[c] Extracellular elemental sulfur is an intermediate in sulfate formation.

[d] Sulfite is formed as an intermediate.

1981). Under anaerobic dark conditions, pyruvate and sugars can be fermented (Gürgün et al., 1976; Schultz and Weaver, 1982). Sugars, as well as succinate, malate or acetate, can support anaerobic dark growth in *R. capsulatus* if DMSO or trimethylamine-*N*-oxide is present as electron acceptor (Yen and Marrs, 1977; Madigan and Gest, 1978; Schultz and Weaver, 1982). Molar growth yields from cultures grown anaerobically in the dark with fructose and DMSO were about 60% of the values obtained from aerobic respiratory growth with fructose (Schultz and Weaver, 1982) and about 4–5 times higher than those from cultures grown under anaerobic dark conditions without DMSO. Some strains of *R. sphaeroides* have the ability to grow under anaerobic dark conditions with nitrate as electron sink, as denitrifier (Satoh et al., 1974, 1976; Pellerin and Gest, 1983). Nitrate reductase-linked electron transport and membrane potential generation accompanied by nitrate reduction to nitrite have been found in strains of *R. capsulatus* (McEwan et al., 1983).

These different possibilities for the species to obtain energy from either light or oxidation of organic or inorganic compounds, with the implication of changes in carbon nutrition from predominantly reductive to oxidative processes, and the possible utilization of a great variety of carbon sources require that metabolic processes be under strong control. Light and partial pressure of oxygen are known as important regulators. In *R. capsulatus*, during transition from phototrophic growth under anaerobic conditions to chemotrophic growth under aerobic conditions, for example, respiratory activities such as α-ketoglutarate dehydrogenase and cytochrome *c* oxidase are significantly increased. This activation also takes place under phototrophic growth conditions if small amounts of oxygen (50 Pa) are present (Cox et al., 1983). Both *R. capsulatus* and *R. sphaeroides* have the capacity to degrade sugars via two different enzymatic pathways, depending on the sugar and the growth conditions. Glucose is degraded in both species via the Entner-Doudoroff pathway, irrespective of the growth conditions (Conrad and Schlegel, 1977a, b). Fructose is the preferred sugar in *R. capsulatus* and exerts catabolite repression on the enzymes of glucose degradation (Conrad and Schlegel, 1978b). It is transported via a fructose-specific phosphoenolpyruvate-phosphotransferase system (Saier, 1977) and specifically induces enzymes of the Embden-Meyerhof pathway (Conrad and Schlegel, 1978a). In contrast to exogenously applied fructose, fructose formed from sucrose inside the cells is metabolized, like glucose, via enzymes of the Entner-Doudoroff pathway (Conrad and Schlegel, 1978a).

On the basis of taxonomic studies on *R. capsulatus* (Weaver et al., 1975) and on *R. sphaeroides* (Pellerin and Gest, 1983), particularly with regard to their use of carbon compounds, a differentiation of the two species is possible by the utilization of tartrate, gluconate, mannose, glycerol, ethanol and citrate (see Table 18.11). However, as exemplified by these two species, when carbon source utilization is viewed as a diagnostic feature, care should be taken because strain-specific changes in the nutritional capacities occur rather easily and may be the result of a single mutation:

(i) Tartrate and gluconate are not used by all strains of *R. sphaeroides,* and some strains of *R. capsulatus* may use citrate and mannose.

(ii) Mutants have been obtained quite easily from *R. capsulatus,* which gained the ability to use glycerol as a carbon source, both anaerobically in the light and aerobically in the dark. The two enzymes glycerokinase and glycerophosphate dehydrogenase, which were absent from the wild type cells, were found in the mutant (Lueking et al., 1976).

(iii) In wild type strains of *R. capsulatus*, the first enzyme of the glyoxylate cycle, isocitrate lyase, is barely detectable (Albers and Gottschalk, 1976; Nielsen et al., 1979), and these strains grew poorly with acetate. Spontaneous mutants, which had high activities of isocitrate lyase, grew vigorously with acetate (Nielsen et al., 1979).

(iv) Furthermore, the utilization of a number of substrates largely depends on the growth conditions. This is particularly true for some fatty acids. Long chain fatty acids, which may be toxic for

Table 18.11.

Photosynthetic electron donors and carbon sources used by species of the genus **Rhodobacter**[a]

Donor/source	1. *R. capsulatus*	2. *R. sphaeroides*	3. *R. sulfidophilus*	4. *R. adriaticus*	5. *R. veldkampii*
Formate	+	−	+	+	−
Acetate	+	+	+	+	+
Propionate	+	+	+	+	+
Butyrate	+	+	+	−	+
Valerate	+	+	+	+	+
Caproate	+	+	+	+	+
Caprylate	+	+	+	o	+
Pelargonate	±	+	+	o	+
Pyruvate	+	+	+	+	+
Lactate	+	+	+	+	+
Malate	+	+	+	+	+
Succinate	+	+	+	+	+
Fumarate	+	+	+	+	+
Tartrate	−	+	−	−	−
Citrate	±	+	−	−	−
Aspartate	±	o	±	o	+
Arginine	o	o	−	o	o
Glutamate	+	+	+	o	+
Benzoate	−	−	−	−	−
Gluconate	−	+	±	o	o
Glucose	+	+	+	+	+
Fructose	+	+	±	−	−
Mannose	−	+	±	o	o
Mannitol	±	+	±	−	−
Sorbitol	±	+	±	o	−
Glycerol	−	+	+	+	−
Methanol	−	±	−	−	−
Ethanol	−	+	±	+	−
Propanol	+	o	±	−	−
Hydrogen	+	+	+	−	−
Sulfide	+	+	+	+	+
Thiosulfate	−	−	+	+	+
Sulfur	−	−	−	+	+

[a] All symbols are the same as those in Footnote *a*, Table 18.10.

certain strains at high concentrations, may be utilized if their concentration is sufficiently low. A significantly higher pH is required for methanol utilization than for utilization of other multicarbon sources (Quayle and Pfennig, 1975).

Besides ammonia and dinitrogen (Siefert, 1976; Madigan et al., 1984), among the nitrogen sources utilized by *Rhodobacter* species are nitrate (Klemme, 1979), purines (Aretz et al., 1978) and pyrimidines (Kaspari, 1979). Nitrogen fixation is possible not only under anaerobic conditions in the light but also under microaerobic to aerobic conditions in the dark (Siefert and Pfennig, 1980; Madigan et al., 1979) or under anaerobic denitrifying conditions in certain strains of *R. sphaeroides* (Kelley et al., 1982).

Ammonia is preferably assimilated via the glutamine synthetase/glutamate synthase (NADPH-dependent) reactions (Brown and Herbert, 1977) in *R. capsulatus* and *R. sphaeroides*. A nucleotide-unspecific glutamate dehydrogenase is present in *R. sphaeroides* (Engelhardt and Klemme, 1978). This enzyme is not present in *R. capsulatus* in which an alanine dehydrogenase was found, which acts, however, primarily in the catabolism of alanine (Johannson and Gest, 1976; Tolxdorff-Neutzling and Klemme, 1982).

Nitrate is assimilated under anaerobic conditions in the light by strains of *R. capsulatus*, *R. sphaeroides* (Klemme, 1979) and *R. veld-*

kampii (Hansen et al., 1975). The abilities to assimilate and dissimilate nitrate are not correlated to each other. Denitrifying strains of *R. sphaeroides* are unable to use nitrate as an assimilatory nitrogen source (Satoh et al., 1976) but have the capacity to fix dinitrogen derived from denitrification (Kelley et al., 1982).

Sulfate is assimilated via 3'-phosphoadenosine-5'-phosphosulfate in those species which are able to use sulfate as sole sulfur source (Imhoff, 1982). *R. adriaticus* and *R. veldkampii* lack this capability and depend on reduced sulfur compounds for growth. Sulfide is used as a photosynthetic electron donor in all species, and sulfide tolerance is remarkably high in *R. sulfidophilus*, *R. adriaticus* and *R. veldkampii* (Hansen and Veldkamp, 1973; Neutzling et al., 1984a; Hansen et al., 1975). The oxidation products of sulfide are either elemental sulfur, sulfate or both (Table 18.10). Those species which are able to oxidize sulfide to sulfate as final oxidation product can also use thiosulfate as electron donor.

Sensitivity towards penicillin is high in most species (Weaver et al., 1975; deBont et al., 1981; Hansen and Imhoff, 1985). With the exception of the *R. sulfidophilus* and *R. sphaeroides* strains, all species are inhibited completely by pencillin at 0.1 U/ml.

The species of this genus are particularly well-characterized by DNA/DNA hybridization studies (deBont et al., 1981). Different strains of the species *R. capsulatus*, *R. sphaeroides* and *R. sulfidophilus* showed intraspecies homology of 68 ± 6%, 71 ± 3%, and 59 ± 6%, respectively. Hybridization of DNA from strains of different species was generally below 30%. Among the 21 strains tested, 2 did not show a significant homology to any of the other strains, and 2 others were only homologous to each other (81%). These latter two strains are now recognized as the new species *R. veldkampii* (Hansen and Imhoff, 1985). The other two strains lacking homology to recognized species have tentatively been identified as *R. sulfidophilus* (Keppen et al., 1976; Imhoff, 1976), but their properties are not considered here, because of the lack of homology to recognized species.

In nature, species of this genus are widely distributed and found in freshwater as well as marine and hypersaline habitats.

Enrichment and Isolation Procedures

No special media or enrichment techniques are required for *Rhodobacter* species. In enrichment cultures set up for PNSB, usually members of this genus will grow faster than those of other PNSB species. In enrichments from marine sources, *R. sulfidophilus* may even successfully compete with *Chromatium* species, also in the presence of sulfide. For media and enrichment techniques, Biebl and Pfenning (1981) or the article on *Rhodospirillum* in this volume should be consulted.

Maintenance Procedures

Cultures can be preserved by standard procedures in liquid nitrogen or by lyophilization.

Differentiation of the genus **Rhodobacter** from other genera

Rhodobacter species are distinguished from other PNSB by their ovoid to rod-shaped morphology and the vesicular internal photosynthetic membrane system together with carotenoids of the spheroidene series. Though the latter property is shared by two other species, *Rhodocyclus gelatinosus* and *Rhodopseudomonas blastica*, these have different internal membrane structures. Although there are no physiological properties of *Rhodobacter* species which will not be found in other genera of the PNSB, these species have a greater versatility and higher capacity to adapt to different growth conditions than do most other PNSB.

The structures of some molecular cell constituents serve to separate this genus from other PNSB. All investigated species have a large type cytochrome c_2 (Ambler et al., 1979) and, as sole quinone component, Q-10 (Imhoff, 1984b). As far as they are able to assimilate sulfate, they use the pathway via 3'-phosphoadenosine-5'-phosphosulfate (Imhoff, 1982).

The lipopolysaccharides from *Rhodobacter capsulatus* and *Rhodobacter sphaeroides* have been analyzed (Omar et al., 1983; Strittmatter et al., 1983). Their lipid A moieties contain glucosamine as sole amino sugar and 3-OH-capric acid as the major fatty acid, together with 3-OH-myristic acid and, most characteristically, a 3-oxo-C-14 fatty acid not found in other PNSB. Significant amounts of phosphate (as in *Rhodocyclus* species) are also present. The lipid A structure is thus significantly different from those of other genera of the PNSB group (see Table 18.7, page 1660).

R. capsulatus and *R. sphaeroides* showed the highest similarity of all PNSB in their 16S rRNA oligonucleotide catalogs with an S_{AB} value of 0.7 (Gibson et al., 1979), being different from other PNSB species at an S_{AB} level of <0.5. Mature 23S rRNA is apparently lacking in *Rhodo*-*bacter capsulatus*, *Rhodobacter sphaeroides*, *Paracoccus denitrificans* and *Agrobacterium tumefasciens* (MacKay et al., 1979). These bacteria have 16S and 14S molecules instead, which are derived from a transient 23S species. Other PNSB, such as *Rhodopseudomonas viridis* and *Rhodopseudomonas palustris*, and most other bacteria do not have a cleaved 23S rRNA.

Taxonomic Comments

The species of this genus have, with the exception of *Rhodobacter veldkampii*, formerly been included in the genus *Rhodopseudomonas*. Their separation from the genus *Rhodopseudomonas* has been proposed by Imhoff et al. (1984). *Rhodobacter veldkampii* has been described quite recently (Hansen and Imhoff, 1985). The genus *Rhodobacter* can be regarded as the taxonomically best characterized genus of the PNSB. It is the sole genus in which DNA/DNA hybridization studies have been performed (with 12 strains in the five species). Most of the biochemical, biophysical and genetic research work with PNSB has been performed with either of the two species, *Rhodobacter capsulatus* and *Rhodobacter sphaeroides*.

The physiological and morphological properties of some denitrifying strains of *R. sphaeroides* are virtually identical to those of other strains of the species (Satoh et al., 1976; Pellerin and Gest, 1983). DNA/DNA hybridization showed no difference in homology between denitrifying and other strains of the species (deBont et al., 1981). I regard the ability to denitrify not sufficient to recognize respective strains separate from others as a subspecies, as proposed by Satoh et al. (1976), have treated them herein as ordinary strains of *R. sphaeroides*, and regard the ability to denitrify as a property of some of the strains of this species.

Differentiation of the species of the genus **Rhodobacter**

Despite the apparent morphological similarity, a very similar pigmentation, and rather great intraspecies variability regarding the utilization of carbon sources, the *Rhodobacter* species are clearly differentiated by a number of properties (Table 18.10). *R. sulfidophilus* and *R. adriaticus*, in contrast to the other species, are marine bacteria and require 1–7% NaCl for optimal development; attempts to isolate these species from freshwater sources have been unsuccessful. Characteristic also is the tolerance towards sulfide, which is considerably high in the two marine species and in *R. veldkampii*, and the oxidation products formed from sulfide. Other differentiating properties are the ability to assimilate sulfate as sole sulfur source, the utilization of molecular hydrogen as electron donor, sensitivity to oxygen, and utilization of some carbon sources, such as tartrate, citrate, gluconate, mannose, glycerol and ethanol (Table 18.11). Most species are very sensitive to penicillin, and growth is totally inhibited by 0.1 U/ml. Only *R. sulfi-dophilus* and *R. sphaeroides* are more resistant; more than 1000 U/ml and 1–100 U/ml are required, respectively, to inhibit growth of these species completely (Weaver et al., 1975; deBont et al., 1981; Hansen and Imhoff, 1985).

All strains of *R. capsulatus* are susceptible to lysis by at least 1 of 16 bacteriophages, which are species-specific and do not attack other PNSB (Wall et al., 1975). A differentiation of the *Rhodobacter* species is possible on the basis of their specific polar lipid composition (Kenyon, 1978; Imhoff et al., 1982; Imhoff, unpublished observations).

List of species of the genus **Rhodobacter**

1. **Rhodobacter capsulatus** (Molisch) Imhoff, Trüper and Pfennig 1984, 342.[VP] (*Rhodonostoc capsulatum* Molisch 1907, 23; *Rhodopseudomonas capsulata* (Molisch) van Niel 1944, 92.)

cap.su.la′tus. L. dim. n. *capsula* a small chest, capsule; L.M. masc. adj. *capsulatus* capsuled.

Cells are ovoid to rod-shaped, 0.5–1.2 μm in diameter, and 2.0–2.5 μm long or, sometimes, even longer. Spherical cells may occur in media below pH 7.0 and are often irregularly arranged in chains resembling streptococci. Ovoid and rod-shaped cells are characteristic in media above pH 7.0; above pH 8.0, irregular and pleomorphic cells appear and media become mucoid. Chains of cells in zigzag arrangement are typical, but in some strains these chains may be straight. Most strains that show zigzag arrangement in mineral media form straight chains in complex media. Capsules of varying thickness are formed. Cells are motile by means of polar flagella.

Cultures grown anaerobically in the light are yellowish brown to deep brown and, in some strains, greenish. When cultures are grown in the presence of oxygen, they are red to purple-red. Anaerobically grown cells change their color to distinct red when shaken with air for a few hours; light enhances the color change. Absorption spectra of living cells show maxima at 376–378, 450–455, 478–480, 508–513, 590–592, 802–805 and 860–863 nm. Photosynthetic pigments are bacteriochlorophyll *a* (esterified with phytol) and carotenoids of the spheroidene series, including spheroidene and hydroxyspheroidene. These two carotenoids are converted to the corresponding ketocarotenoids under aerobic conditions, which causes the color change to red.

Photoautotrophic growth is possible with sulfide or molecular hydrogen as electron source; such growth with hydrogen is excellent. Under photoheterotrophic anaerobic growth conditions in the light, a number of organic carbon compounds are used as carbon and electron sources. Aerobic growth in the dark is possible as a chemoheterotroph or, with molecular hydrogen, as an autotroph at the full oxygen tension of air. With sugars, anaerobic dark growth occurs in the presence of DMSO or trimethylamine-*N*-oxide as oxidant. Some strains may use nitrate as electron acceptor under similar conditions, reducing it to nitrite. Marginal growth is possible during fermentation of pyruvate or sugars. Carbon sources utilized are listed in Table 18.11. In addition, leucine and, by some strains, methanol may be used.

Good growth occurs with ammonia, dinitrogen and a number of amino acids as nitrogen sources; guanine, xanthine, uric acid, cytidine, uracil, thymine and adenine are used only under aerobic conditions. Nitrate can be used as nitrogen source by some strains. Sulfate can be used as sole sulfur source. Sulfide may serve as photosynthetic electron donor and is oxidized to elemental sulfur only; thiosulfate and elemental sulfur are not used. Thiamine is required as growth factor; some strains also require biotin or biotin and niacin. Growth occurs at pH 6.5–7.5 (optimum pH: 7.0); the optimum growth temperature is 30–35°C; the maximum temperature for the majority of the strains is above 36°C.

The mol% G + C of the DNA is 65.5–66.8 (Bd) and 68.1–69.6 (T_m).

Type strain: DSM 1710, ATCC 11166, NCIB 8286, van Niel ATH 2.3.1.

2. **Rhodobacter sphaeroides** (van Niel) Imhoff, Trüper and Pfen-342.[VP] (*Rhodopseudomonas sphaeroides* van Niel 1944, 95.)

sphae.ro′i.des. Gr. adj. *sphaeroides* spherical.

Cells have highly variable morphology, especially in media containing complex nutrients; morphology is more uniform in mineral salts media

(Fig. 18.26). Cells are spherical to ovoid and 0.7–4.0 μm wide; in sugar-containing media, cells are 2.0–2.5 μm wide and 2.5–3.5 μm long. Cells frequently occur in pairs or as a chain of beads which in many instances are connected by a thin filament and slightly unequal in size. As cultures age, they become viscous due to slime production, except when sugars serve as carbon source. Slime formation is enhanced in complex media. In young cultures, cells are motile by polar flagella; motility ceases in alkaline media.

Cultures grown under anaerobic conditions in the light are dirty greenish brown to dark brown. Cultures grown in the presence of air are red. The brown color of cells grown anaerobically in the light will change to red if cells are shaken with air; light stimulates this change. Absorption spectra of living cells have maxima at 372–375, 446–450, 474–481, 507–513, 588–590, 800–805, 850–852 and 870–880 nm. The relative absorbances at 850–880 nm vary greatly with the culture conditions. Photosynthetic pigments are bacteriochlorophyll *a* (esterified with phytol) and carotenoids of the spheroidene series, including spheroidene and hydroxyspheroidene, which are converted to their corresponding ketocarotenoids under aerobic conditions and thereby cause the color change to red.

Preferred growth mode is photoheterotrophic under anaerobic conditions with a number of organic compounds as carbon and electron sources. Photoautotrophic growth with molecular hydrogen or sulfide as electron donor is slow. Good growth is observed under aerobic conditions in the dark with a number of carbon sources. Anaerobic dark fermentative metabolism with pyruvate and sugars allows only marginal growth. Some strains are able to denitrify under anaerobic conditions in the dark.

The organic substrates utilized are shown in Table 18.11. Lower fatty acids are used at low concentrations. Higher fatty acids are toxic. Growth with glycerol depends on the presence of CO_2. Acids are produced in sugar-containing media under all conditions but disappear later. Ammonia, dinitrogen, alanine, glutamate and aspartate are used as nitrogen source; dinitrogen is also used under microaerobic to

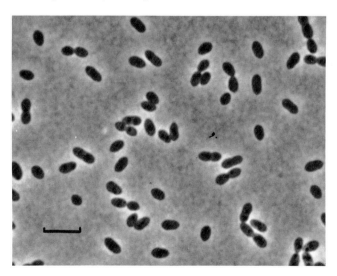

Figure 18.26. *R. sphaeroides* ATCC 17023 grown in mineral medium with 0.2% succinate and 0.05% yeast extract at pH 6.8, Phase-contrast micrograph. *Bar*, 5 μm. (Courtesy of N. Pfennig.)

aerobic growth conditions in the dark. Some strains use uric acid, guanine, xanthine, cytidine, uracil, thymine, adenine (only under aerobic conditions) and nitrate. Sulfate can be used as sole sulfur source. Sulfide is used as photosynthetic electron donor and oxidized to elemental sulfur; thiosulfate and elemental sulfur are not used. Thiamine, biotin and niacin are required as growth factors. Growth occurs at pH 6.0–8.5 (optimum pH: 7.0); the optimum growth temperature is 30–34°C.

The mol% G + C of the DNA is 68.4–69.9 (Bd) and 70.8–73.2 (T_m).

Type strain: DSM 158, ATCC 17023, NCIB 8253, van Niel ATH 2.4.1.

3. **Rhodobacter sulfidophilus** (Hansen and Veldkamp) Imhoff, Trüper and Pfennig 1984, 342.[VP] (*Rhodopseudomonas sulfidophila* Hansen and Veldkamp 1973, 55.)

sul.fi.do′phi.lus. Gr. adj. *philus* loving; M.L. adj. *sulfidophilus* sulfide-loving.

Cells are ovoid to rod-shaped, 0.6–0.9 µm wide and 0.9–2.0 µm long and do not form cell aggregates. Eventually, slime may be produced or short straight chains may be formed. Cells are motile by means of polar flagella.

Color of cell suspensions depends on the redox state of the culture and is from yellowish-green over yellowish-brown to dark brown and brown-red. In the presence of oxygen, cultures are red. Absorption spectra of living cells show maxima at 374–378, 451–455, 480–489, 508–512, 588–592, 800–805 and 850–855 nm. Photosynthetic pigments are bacteriochlorophyll *a* (esterified with phytol) and carotenoids of the spheroidene series with spheroidene and hydroxyspheroidene, which are converted to their corresponding ketocarotenoids under aerobic conditions and thereby cause the color change to red.

Sulfide, thiosulfate and molecular hydrogen are excellent electron donors for photoautotrophic growth. Photoheterotrophically under anaerobic conditions, a variety of organic compounds are used as carbon and electron source. Growth is also possible under aerobic conditions in the dark. Carbon sources utilized are shown in Table 18.11.

Ammonia and, by most strains, dinitrogen are used as nitrogen sources; nitrate is not used. Sulfate can be used as sole sulfur source under photoheterotrophic growth conditions or during growth with molecular hydrogen. Reduced sulfur compounds such as sulfite, thiosulfate, cysteine and reduced glutathione can be assimilated. During dissimilatory oxidative processes, sulfide and thiosulfate are oxidized to sulfate without intermediary accumulation of elemental sulfur; elemental sulfur is oxidized slowly. Sulfide tolerance is high, 5.2–6.3 mM in mineral media and 7–8 mM in the presence of 0.01% yeast extract. Biotin, niacin, thiamine and *p*-aminobenzoic acid are required as growth factors. Growth occurs at pH 6.5–8.0 if sulfide is the electron donor and at pH 5.0–7.5 if malate is the electron donor; the optimum growth temperature is 30–35°C; 1–6% NaCl is required for optimal growth.

The mol% G + C of the DNA is 68.9–73.2 (T_m).

Type strain: DSM 1374 (Hansen W4), ATCC 35886.

4. **Rhodobacter adriaticus** (Neutzling, Imhoff and Trüper) Imhoff, Trüper and Pfennig 1984, 342.[VP] (*Rhodopseudomonas adriatica* Neutzling, Imhoff and Trüper 1984b, 503.)

a.dri.a′ti.cus. M.L. masc. adj. *adriaticus* pertaining to the Adria, the Adriatic Sea.

Cells are ovoid to rod-shaped, 0.5–0.8 µm wide and 1.3–1.8 µm long, often occurring in short straight chains, form capsules, and produce slime.

Color of cell suspensions is yellowish-brown to dark brown. Absorption spectra of living cells show maxima at 374–378, 447–450, 475–480, 508–512, 588–590, 802–805 and about 869 nm. Photosynthetic pigments are bacteriochlorophyll *a* and carotenoids of the spheroidene series.

Good growth occurs under anaerobic conditions in the light with a variety of organic compounds as carbon and electron sources. Photoautotrophic growth is possible with sulfide, elemental sulfur and thiosulfate as electron donor. Molecular hydrogen is not used as electron donor. Sensitive to oxygen. Ascorbate stimulates phototrophic growth; microaerobic growth in the dark is possible. The carbon sources utilized are shown in Table 18.11. Ammonia, dinitrogen and some amino acids are used as nitrogen source; slow growth occurs with urea. Nitrate is not used but is reduced to nitrite. Sulfate is not used as sole sulfur source; cells depend on reduced sulfur sources such as sulfide, thiosulfate, cysteine and elemental sulfur. During oxidation of sulfide to sulfate, elemental sulfur is intermediately formed outside the cells. Biotin and thiamine are required as growth factors. Niacin has a stimulatory effect. Growth is observed at pH 6.9–8.5 (optimum pH: 6.5–7.0); the optimum growth temperature is 25–30°C; 2.5–7.5% NaCl is required for optimal growth.

The mol% G + C of the DNA is 66.7 (T_m).

Type strain: DSM 2781 (Imhoff 6II), ATCC 35885.

5. **Rhodobacter veldkampii** Hansen and Imhoff 1985, 115.[VP]

veld.kamp′i.i. M.L. gen n. *veldkampii* of Veldkamp; named for H. Veldkamp, a Dutch microbiologist.

Cells are ovoid to rod-shaped, 0.6–0.8 µm wide and 1.0–1.3 µm long, have pronounced tendency to form chains of cells under certain growth conditions, and do not produce slime.

Color of photosynthetically grown cells varies from yellowish-brown to dark brown and red. Aerobically grown cells are red. Absorption spectra of photosynthetically grown cells have maxima at 373, 448, 477, 510, 589, 803 and 855 nm, indicating the presence of bacteriochlorophyll *a* and carotenoids of the spheroidene series.

Good growth is possible under anaerobic conditions in the light with a variety of carbon compounds, sulfide, thiosulfate and elemental sulfur but not with hydrogen as electron donor. Aerobic growth in the dark is possible if a reduced sulfur source is provided. The carbon compounds utilized are shown in Table 18.11.

Ammonia, dinitrogen and nitrate can be used as nitrogen source. Reduced sulfur compounds are required for growth; sulfide, cysteine and cystine serve as sulfur source; sulfate, sulfite, thiosulfate and methionine are not used. During phototrophic growth with sulfide as electron donor, elemental sulfur is deposited outside the cells and oxidized further to sulfate after sulfide depletion in batch cultures. In sulfide-limited chemostat cultures, sulfate is the major oxidation product. Sulfide tolerance is high, about 5 mM at pH 7.3. Biotin, thiamine and *p*-aminobenzoic acid are required as growth factors; 0.01% yeast extract can replace the vitamin requirement. Optimal growth conditions for photoheterotrophic growth with succinate in the presence of cysteine are at pH 7.5, at 30–35°C and in the absence of NaCl.

The mol% G + C of the DNA is 64.4–67.5 (T_m).

Type strain: ATCC 35703 (Hansen 51).

Addendum

New species recently described by E. I. Kompantseva (1985): *Rhodobacter euryhalinus*.

Genus **Rhodopseudomonas** *Kluyver and van Niel in Czurda and Maresch 1937, 119*[AL]

HANS G. TRÜPER AND JOHANNES F. IMHOFF

Rho.do.pseu.do.mo′nas. Gr. n. *rhodos* the rose; M.L. fem. n. *Pseudomonas* a bacterial genus; M.L. fem. n. *Rhodopseudomonas* red *Pseudomonas*.

Cells are rod-shaped, 0.6–2.5 µm wide and 0.6–5.0 µm long, and motile by means of flagella or nonmotile; **show polar growth, budding and asymmetric cell division**; and are Gram-negative. **Internal photosynthetic membranes are present as lamellae under-**

lying and parallel to the cytoplasmic membrane. Photosynthetic pigments are bacteriochlorophyll *a* or *b* and various types of carotenoids.

Photoheterotrophic growth with a number of organic carbon compounds as carbon source and electron donor is the preferred mode of growth. Photoautotrophic growth may be possible under anaerobic conditions with hydrogen, thiosulfate or sulfide as electron donor. Chemotrophic growth under microaerobic to aerobic conditions is possible by some species. Various growth factors may be required.

The mol% G + C of the DNA is 61.5–71.4 (Bd and T_m).

Type species: *Rhodopseudomonas palustris* (Molisch) van Niel 1944, 89.

Further Descriptive Information

Cell morphology of the *Rhodopseudomonas* species is characterized by asymmetric cells during cell division. Most characteristic is the formation of tubes and rosettelike cell aggregates in *R. palustris* and *R. viridis*. With the exception of *R. blastica*, all known species are motile by means of flagella, which in most cases are located in a subpolar area of the cell. In *R. marina*, flagella also originate laterally.

R. sulfoviridis, *R. marina* and *R. blastica* show good growth on sugars and sugar alcohols, while *R. rutila* is characterized by the inability to grow with acetate and by poor growth on other fatty acids. *R. palustris* is the only species that utilizes benzoate as a carbon and energy source under phototrophic growth conditions. A reductive and oxygen-inhibited degradation of benzoate has been demonstrated by Dutton and Evans (1969) (see also Dutton and Evans, 1978). Citrate, which is used by some strains of *Rhodopseudomonas palustris*, is metabolized by citrate lyase, an enzyme similarly regulated as in *Rhodocyclus gelatinosus* (Giffhorn and Kuhn, 1980). During growth on methanol, *Rhodopseudomonas acidophila* assimilates its cell carbon via the ribulose-bisphosphate cycle and carboxylation reactions of C_3 fatty acids. There was no evidence for the operation of a reduced C_1 fixation sequence (Sahm et al., 1976). A slow fermentative metabolism may be a property of most *Rhodopseudomonas* species. Gürgün et al. (1976) quantitatively demonstrated the formation from pyruvate of CO_2, formate, acetate, lactate, butyrate and acetoin by *R. palustris* and of CO_2, formate, acetate, diacetyl, acetoin and butandiol by *R. acidophila*. Photoautotrophic growth with hydrogen has been found in *R. palustris* (Klemme, 1968), in *R. acidophila* (Pfennig, 1969a) and in *R. blastica* (Eckersley and Dow, 1980). *R. acidophila* also grows chemoautotrophically with hydrogen and utilizes methanol and formate under these conditions if the oxygen tension is kept at a low level (Siefert and Pfennig, 1979). The following amounts of oxygen are tolerated: with methanol, 16 kPa; with hydrogen, 3.33 kPa; and with formate, 1.3 kPa.

The utilization of reduced sulfur compounds as electron donor is found in *R. palustris*, *R. marina* and *R. sulfoviridis*. Sulfide is oxidized to elemental sulfur (Hansen, 1974), and thiosulfate is oxidized to sulfate (Rolls and Lindstrom, 1967) in cultures of *R. palustris*, whereas both are oxidized to sulfate in cultures of *R. sulfoviridis* (Keppen and Gorlenko, 1975). Sulfide oxidation by *R. marina* leads to thiosulfate

and elemental sulfur as the main oxidation products (Imhoff, 1983). The only species of this genus which is definitely unable to assimilate sulfate and depends on reduced sulfur compounds is *R. sulfoviridis* (Neutzling and Trüper, 1982). Although *R. viridis* and *R. palustris* assimilate sulfate via the 3′-phosphoadenosine-5′phosphosulfate pathway, *R. acidophila* assimilates sulfate via the adenosine-5′-phosphosulfate pathway (Imhoff, 1982).

Nitrogenase has been found in all species investigated (Madigan et al., 1984). In *R. palustris* (Zumpft and Castillo, 1978) and in *R. viridis* (Howard et al., 1983), nitrogenase shows a "switch-off" effect by ammonia and some organic nitrogen compounds. Although this effect is reversible in *R. palustris*, a recovery of the enzyme was not observed in *R. viridis*. Ammonia assimilation proceeds via glutamine synthetase and glutamate synthase in *Rhodopseudomonas palustris* (NADPH-linked) and *Rhodopseudomonas acidiphila* (NADH-linked) (Brown and Herbert, 1977; Herbert et al., 1978). A glutamate dehydrogenase present in the former species is lacking in the latter. Besides ammonia, *R. palustris* uses a great number of nitrogen sources: nitrate, dimethylamine and trimethylamine, azoguanine, L-histidine, L-glutamate, L-aspartate, L-arginine, L-cysteine, DL-methionine, DL-lysine, DL-alanine, DL-leucine, casein hydrolysate (Malofeeva and Laush, 1976), guanine, uric acid, xanthine (Aretz et al., 1978), cytidine and cytosine (Kaspari, 1979). Most strains of *R. palustris* are not able to use nitrate as a nitrogen source (Klemme, 1979). Three strains could be isolated, however, that were capable of dissimilatory nitrate reduction and able to grow under anaerobic dark conditions with nitrate as terminal electron acceptor (Klemme et al., 1980).

Enrichment and Isolation Procedures

Standard procedures are used for the isolation of *Rhodopseudomonas* species (see Biebl and Pfennig, 1981). A mineral medium which is suitable for most PNSB is, with some modifications, useful for the cultivation of all *Rhodopseudomonas* species (see the footnote on page 1663 for this medium). For selective enrichments, the preference for low pH values is used for cultures of *Rhodopseudomonas acidophila*. A succinate-mineral medium without growth factors with an initial pH of 5.2 is highly selective for *Rhodopseudomonas acidophila* (and also *Rhodomicrobium vannielii*) (Pfennig, 1969a). *Rhodopseudomonas palustris* is a very common species of the PNSB in nature, and many enrichments will end up with the development of a *R. palustris* strain. A selective advantage for this species would be the use of benzoate as carbon source in the enrichment cultures. *R. viridis* and *R. sulfoviridis* can selectively be enriched with appropriate light filters which allow only long wavelength radiation to penetrate, since both species, owing to their content of bacteriochlorophyll *b*, show absorption maxima above 1000 nm.

Maintenance Procedures

Cultures of all species can be maintained by standard procedures in liquid nitrogen.

Differentiation of the genus **Rhodopseudomonas** *from other genera*

The ability to perform a phototrophic mode of life, the rod shape of the cells, their asymmetric mode of growth and cell division, and the lamellar structure of internal membranes lying parallel and underlying the cytoplasmic membrane distinguish *Rhodopseudomonas* species from other genera.

Taxonomic Comments

Those species with vesicular intracytoplasmic membranes have been removed from the genus *Rhodopseudomonas* (Imhoff et al., 1984) and are now classified as *Rhodopila globiformis*, *Rhodobacter capsulatus*, *Rhodobacter sphaeroides*, *Rhodobacter sulfidophilus* and *Rhodobacter adriaticus*, respectively. This change has been supported by data on rRNA/DNA hybridization studies (Gills et al., 1982), 16S rRNA oligonucleotide catalog similarities (Gibson et al., 1979) and cytochrome

c amino acid sequences (Ambler et al., 1979). Oligonucleotide catalogs from 16S rRNA of *Rhodopseudomonas palustris* and *Nitrobacter winogradskii* showed a high degree of similarity (Seewaldt et al., 1982), and the lipid A structure of the lipopolysaccharide of *Nitrobacter* species contains the unusual 2,3-diamino-2,3-deoxy-D-glucose instead of glucosamine (Mayer et al., 1983, 1984). This sugar had so far been found only in *Rhodopseudomonas* species, namely *Rhodopseudomonas palustris*, *Rhodopseudomonas viridis* (see Weckesser et al., 1979). *Rhodopseudomonas sulfoviridis* (Ahamed et al., 1982) and, recently, *Pseudomonas diminuta* and *Pseudomonas vesicularis* (Mayer et al., 1983). Other *Rhodopseudomonas* species, such as *R. acidophila* and *R. blastica*, however, do contain glucosamine instead of 2,3-diamino-2,3-dideoxy-hexose in their lipid A (Werner et al., 1985). *Rhodopseudomonas blastica*, which, according to internal membrane structure and growth mode, is a member of this genus, has been found to belong to the rRNA superfamily IV subgroup a, together with *Rhodobacter* species and *Paracoccus denitrificans* (Gillis et al., 1982), but not to subgroup b, as do *Rhodopseudomonas palustris*, *Rhodopseudomonas viridis* and *Rho-* *dopseudomonas acidophila*. These data indicate that the criteria which are used to assign a species to this genus may need a thorough reinvestigation.

Differentiation of the species of the genus **Rhodopseudomonas**

Rhodopseudomonas species may well be differentiated on the basis of morphological and cultural characteristics. *R. viridis* and *R. sulfoviridis* are green due to their content of bacteriochlorophyll *b* and carotenoids and show long wavelength absorption maxima above 1000 nm. Although *R. viridis* is able to assimilate sulfate, *R. sulfoviridis* depends on reduced sulfur compounds for growth. *R. palustris* is morphologically indistinguishable from *R. viridis*, but cultures are red to brownish red as a consequence of the content of bacteriochlorophyll *a* and carotenoids of the spirilloxanthin series. *R. palustris* is the only species of this genus able to utilize benzoate. The cells of *R. acidophila* are larger than those of the other *Rhodopseudomonas* species, and *R. acidophila* is characterized by the preference for an acid pH (optimum pH: 5.5–6.0) and the lack of any growth factor requirement. *Rhodopseu-* *domonas marina* is, at present, the only true marine *Rhodopseudomonas* species and is further characterized by its low absorption maximum at 803 nm, which among the other PNSB is only found in *R. rubrum*. *R. blastica* is easily recognized by its brown color under anaerobic light conditions, which is the result of its content of carotenoids of the spheroidene series. Because of these carotenoids, however, it can be misidentified as belonging to the genus *Rhodobacter* if asymmetric cell growth and internal membrane structure are not recognized. The lack of growth with acetate and benzoate separates *R. rutila* from *R. palustris*. Both species have a different growth factor requirement. Some differentiating characteristics of the species of this genus are shown in Tables 18.12 and 18.13.

List of species of the genus **Rhodopseudomonas**

1. **Rhodopseudomonas palustris** (Molisch) van Niel 1944, 89.[AL] (*Rhodobacillus palustris* Molisch 1907, 14.)

pa.lus'tris. L. fem. adj. *palustris* marshy, swampy.

Individual cells are rod-shaped to ovoid, occasionally slightly curved, 0.6–0.9 μm wide and 1.2–2.0 μm long, and motile by means of subpolar flagella; reproduce by budding; and are Gram-negative. The mother cell produces a slender tube 1.5–2.0 times the length of the original cell at the pole opposite to that bearing the flagella. The end of the tube swells, and the daughter cell grows, producing a dumbbell-shaped organism (Fig. 18.27). Asymmetric division then takes place. Young individual cells are highly motile. The formation of rosettes and clusters in which the individual cells are attached to each other at their flagellated poles are characteristic in older cultures. In certain complex media, individual cells become up to 10 μm long and irregular in shape. Internal photosynthetic membranes are present as lamellae underlying and parallel to the cytoplasmic membrane; no lamellae are present in the tube. Color of cell suspensions is red to brownish-red. Living cells show absorption maxima at 375, 468, 493, 520–545, 589, 802 and 860–875 nm. Photosynthetic pigments are bacteriochlorophyll *a* (esterified with phytol) and carotenoids of the normal spirilloxanthin series.

Photoautotrophic growth is possible with hydrogen, sulfide and thiosulfate as electron donor in the presence of small amounts of yeast

Table 18.12.

Differentiating characteristics of the species of the genus **Rhodopseudomonas**[a]

Characteristic	1. *R. palustris*	2. *R. viridis*	3. *R. sulfoviridis*	4. *R. acidophila*	5. *R. blastica*	6. *R. rutila*	7. *R. marina*
Cell diameter (μm)	0.6–0.9	0.6–0.9	0.6–0.9	1.0–1.3	0.6–0.8	0.4–1.0	0.7–0.9
Motility	+	+	+	+	−	+	+
DNA base ratio (mol% G + C of DNA)	64.8–66.3	66.3–71.4	67.8–68.4	62.2–66.8	65.3	67.6–69.4	61.5–63.8
Color of cultures	Red to red-brown	Green	Olive green	Red to orange-brown	Brown	Red	Pink to red
Bacteriochlorophyll	*a*	*b*	*b*	*a*	*a*	*a*	*a*
Oxidation products of sulfide	S⁰	−	Sulfate	−	−	−	S⁰, thiosulfate
Sulfate assimilated	PAPS	PAPS	−	APS	+	+	+
H₂ as electron donor	+	−	nd	+	+	nd	nd
Major quinones	Q-10	Q-9, MK-9	Q-8, Q-10, MK-7, MK-8	Q-10, MK-10	Q-10	Q-10	Q-10, MK-10
Vitamins required	p-ABA (biotin)	p-ABA, biotin	p-ABA, biotin, pyridoxin	None	Thiamine, biotin, niacin, B₁₂	None	nd

[a] Symbols: +, present or positive; −, absent or negative; S⁰, elemental sulfur; PAPS, 3′-phosphoadenosine-5′-phosphosulfate; APS, adenosine-5′-phosphosulfate; nd, not determined; p-ABA, *p*-aminobenzoate; ( ), vitamin required by a few strains only. Data are from species descriptions and Hansen (1974), Imhoff (1982, 1984b), and Schmidt and Bowien (1983).

Table 18.13.
Photosynthetic electron donors and carbon sources used by species of the genus **Rhodopseudomonas**[a]

Donor/source	1. R. palustris	2. R. viridis	3. R. sulfoviridis	4. R. acidophila	5. R. blastica	6. R. rutila	7. R. marina	Donor/source	1. R. palustris	2. R. viridis	3. R. sulfoviridis	4. R. acidophila	5. R. blastica	6. R. rutila	7. R. marina
Formate	+	−	−	±	−	−	+	Aspartate	±	o	o	−	o	−	o
Acetate	+	+	+	+	+	−	+	Arginine	−	−	−	−	o	o	o
Propionate	+	−	−	+	+	±	+	Glutamate	+	+	o	−	+	+	o
Butyrate	+	−	+	±	+	o	+	Benzoate	+	−	−	−	−	−	−
Valerate	+	−	−	+	o	−	+	Gluconate	o	+	o	o	o	−	o
Caproate	+	−	o	±	o	+	+	Glucose	±	±	+	±	+	−	+
Caprylate	+	o	o	−	o	−	±	Fructose	±	−	+	−	+	+	+
Pelargonate	−	o	o	−	o	o	o	Mannitol	±	±	−	−	+	−	+
Glycolate	+	o	o	±	−	o	o	Sorbitol	+	+	+	o	+	o	+
Pyruvate	+	+	−	+	+	o	+	Glycerol	+	−	+	±	+	+	±
Lactate	+	±	+	+	+	+	±	Methanol	±	−	−	±	−	−	−
Malonate	+	−	−	±	o	+	o	Ethanol	±	+	+	+	−	+	±
Malate	+	+	+	+	+	+	+	Propanol	+	±	+	o	o	o	±
Succinate	+	+	+	+	+	+	+	Hydrogen	+	−	−	+	+	o	o
Fumarate	+	+	+	+	+	o	+	Sulfide	+	o	+	−	−	o	+
Tartrate	−	±	−	±	−	−	−	Thiosulfate	+	−	+	−	−	−	−
Citrate	±	−	−	±	+	±	±								

[a] Symbols: +, positive in most or all strains; −, negative in most or all strains; ±, positive in some strains but negative in other strains; o, not determined.

extract. Photoheterotrophic growth is possible with various organic substrates. Growth occurs in the dark under microaerobic to aerobic conditions and, with some substrates, under anaerobic conditions. Sulfate can be used as sole sulfur source. Ammonia, dinitrogen, some amino acids and, by a few strains, nitrate can be used as nitrogen source.

Growth factors required are *p*-aminobenzoate and, by some strains, biotin; yeast extract stimulates growth considerably. Optimal growth occurs at 30–37°C and pH 6.9 (pH range: 5.5–8.5).

The mol% G + C of the DNA is 64.8–66.3 (Bd).

Type strain: ATCC 17001, DSM 123 (van Niel ATH 2.1.6).

2. **Rhodopseudomonas viridis** Drews and Giesbrecht 1966, 261.[AL]

vi′ri.dis. L. adj. *viridis* green.

Cells are rod-shaped to ovoid, 0.6–0.9 μm wide and 1.2–2.0 μm long. Young cells are motile by means of subpolar flagella. Growth mode and

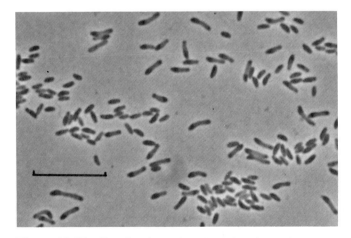

Figure 18.27. *R. palustris* strain 1850 grown in succinate-yeast extract medium. The budding type of reproduction can be recognized in a number of cells. Phase-contrast micrograph. *Bar,* 10 μm. (Courtesy of N. Pfennig.)

reproduction are very similar to the type species. Internal photosynthetic membranes are present as lamellae underlying and parallel to the cytoplasmic membrane. Anaerobic liquid cultures are yellowish green first, then green to olive-green. Aerobic cultures are colorless to light yellowish green. Photosynthetic pigments are bacteriochlorophyll *b* (esterified with phytol) and the major carotenoids 1,2-dihydroneurosporene and 1,2-dihydrolycopene. In vivo absorption spectra show characteristic maxima at 400, 420, 451, 483, 604, 835 and 1020 nm.

Cells grow photoheterotrophically under anaerobic conditions with various organic carbon sources or under microaerobic conditions in the dark. Photoautotrophic growth has not been demonstrated. Carbon sources used are acetate, pyruvate, malate, and succinate. Poor growth occurs in the presence of ethanol, glutamate, peptone, glucose and xylose. Higher fatty acids inhibit growth. Sulfide, thiosulfate and hydrogen cannot be used as electron donor. Sulfate can be used as sole sulfur source. Ammonia and dinitrogen are used as nitrogen sources; nitrate is not used. Most strains require biotin and *p*-aminobenzoate as growth factors; some strains require more or some require no growth factors. Optimal growth occurs at 25–30°C and pH 6.5–7.0.

The mol% G + C of the DNA is 66.3–71.4 (Bd).

Type strain: ATCC 19567, DSM 133 (Drews "F").

3. **Rhodopseudomonas sulfoviridis** Keppen and Gorlenko 1975, 258.[AL]

sul.fo.vi′ri.dis. L. neut. n. *sulphur* sulfur; L. adj. *viridis* green; *sulfoviridis* green and with sulfur.

Cells are rod-shaped to ovoid and form sessile buds and rosettes. Swarmer cells are motile by means of subpolar flagella. If cells age, they become immotile and encapsuled by slime. They are Gram-negative. Intracytoplasmic membranes are present as lamellae underlying and parallel to the cytoplasmic membrane. Color of cell suspensions is olive-green, sometimes with a brownish tinge. Photosynthetic pigments are bacteriochlorophyll *b* and carotenoids.

Growth is possible under anaerobic conditions in the light or under microaerobic conditions in the dark. A number of organic carbon sources, thiosulfate and sulfide are used as photosynthetic electron donor; sulfide and thiosulfate are oxidized to sulfate. Best growth occurs with the organic carbon sources glucose, fructose, maltose, sucrose, glycerol, propanol, fumarate and malate. Cystine, cysteine, sulfide and thiosulfate are used as sulfur source, but sulfate is not used. Ammonia and casein hydrolysate are used as nitrogen source, while arginine, glycine, alanine, asparagine and urea inhibit growth. Yeast extract or biotin, pyridoxin and p-aminobenzoate are required as growth factor. Growth occurs at 28–30°C and pH 7.0.

The mol% G + C of the DNA is 67.8–68.4 (chem. anal.).

Type strain: DSM 729 (Gorlenko P₁).

4. **Rhodopseudomonas acidophila** Pfennig 1969a, 601.[AL]

a.ci.do′phi.la. L. adj. *acidus* sour; M.L. neut. n. *acidum* an acid; Gr. adj. *philos* loving; M.L. fem. adj. *acidophila* acid-loving.

Cells are rod-shaped to elongate-ovoid, slightly curved, 1.0–1.3 μm wide and 2.0–5.0 μm long, motile by polar flagella, and Gram-negative. Daughter cells originate by polar growth as sessile buds at the pole opposite that bearing the flagella; there is no tube or filament between mother and daughter cells (Fig. 18.28). When the daughter cell reaches the size of the mother cell, cell division is completed by constriction. In the next cycle, both cells form buds at the poles of the former cell division. Under certain conditions, rosettes and clusters are formed that are similar to those of the type species. In media lacking calcium ions, cells are immotile. Internal photosynthetic membranes are present as lamellae underlying and parallel to the cytoplasmic membrane. Color of anaerobic liquid cultures is purple-red to orange-brown. Cells grown under aerobic conditions are colorless to light pink or orange. Absorption spectra of living cells show maxima at 375, 460, 490, 525, 590, 805, 855 and 890 nm. Photosynthetic pigments are bacteriochlorophyll *a* (esterified with phytol) and carotenoids of the spirilloxanthin series with glucosides of rhodopin and rhodopinal. The latter are characteristic of this species.

Photoheterotrophic growth with a number of organic carbon sources is the preferred growth mode. Photoautotrophic growth is possible with hydrogen as electron donor; sulfide and thiosulfate cannot be used. Cells grow under microaerobic to aerobic conditions in the dark, with hydrogen as electron donor autotrophically. The organic carbon sources used are acetate, propionate, butyrate, lactate, pyruvate, fumarate, malate, succinate, valerate, formate, methanol and ethanol. Not used are caprylate, pelargonate, glycerol, benzoate, sugars, sugar alcohols, glutamate and other amino acids. Sulfate can be used as sole sulfur source. Ammonia, dinitrogen and some amino acids are used as nitrogen source. Growth factors are not required; yeast extract or other complex nutrients do not increase the growth rate. Optimal growth occurs at 25–30°C and pH 5.5–6.0.

The mol% G + C of the DNA is 62.2–66.8 (Bd).

Type strain: ATCC 25092, DSM 137 (Pfennig 7050).

5. **Rhodopseudomonas blastica** Eckersley and Dow 1981, 216.[VP] (Effective publication: Eckersley and Dow 1980, 472.)

blas′ti.ca. Gr. adj. *blasticos* to bud: M. L. adj. *blastica* apt to bud.

Cells are ovoid to rod-shaped, 0.6–0.8 μm wide and 1.0–2.5 μm long, and nonmotile; reproduce by budding; form sessile buds and are Gram-negative. Although cells appear morphologically similar at cell division, they differ with regard to the time taken to reach the next division: The mother cell initiates cell growth immediately after division, whereas the daughter cell has to undergo an obligate period of maturation. In media containing yeast extract, abnormally swollen cells and spheroblasts are formed. Internal photosynthetic membranes are present as lamellae underlying and parallel to the cytoplasmic membrane. Cells grown under anaerobic conditions in the light are orange-brown; the color changes to red in the presence of oxygen. Cells grown under aerobic conditions in the dark are colorless to faint pink. Absorption spectra of living cells have maxima at 378, 418, 476, 506, 590, 795 and 862 nm. Photosynthetic pigments are bacteriochlorophyll *a* and carotenoids of the spheroidene series.

Cells grow preferably photoheterotrophically under anaerobic conditions with a wide range of organic carbon sources. Photoautotrophic growth with hydrogen as electron donor is possible; sulfide and thio-

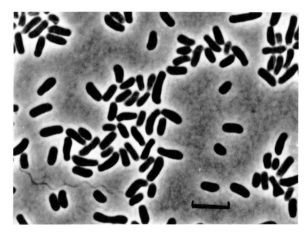

Figure 18.28. *R. acidophila* strain 2751. The shape of some of the cells is indicative of the polar type of cell growth. Tufts of detached flagella can be seen. Phase-contrast micrograph. *Bar,* 5 μm. (Courtesy of N. Pfennig.)

sulfate are not used as electron donors. Cells grow chemotrophically under aerobic dark conditions. Ammonia, dinitrogen, glutamate, aspartate, glutamine, alanine, ornithine, tyrosine, thymine and urea serve as nitrogen source; nitrate and nitrite are not used. In addition to thiamine and niacin, biotin and vitamin B₁₂ are required as growth factors (Schmidt and Bowien, 1983). Optimal growth occurs at 30–35°C and pH 6.5–7.5.

The mol% G + C of the DNA is 65.3 (Bd).

Type strain: NCIB 11576, ATCC 33485.

6. **Rhodopseudomonas rutila** Akiba, Usami and Horikoshi 1983, 555.[VP]

ru′ti.la. L. adj. *rutila* red, bloody.

Cells are rod-shaped, 0.4–1.0 μm wide and 1.5–3.0 μm long, and motile by means of polar flagella; reproduce by budding; and are Gram-negative. Internal photosynthetic membranes are present as lamellae underlying and parallel to the cytoplasmic membrane. Cells grown under anaerobic conditions in the light are red; cells grown under aerobic conditions in the dark are colorless to faint pink. Absorption maxima of living cells are at 375, 465, 490, 524, 590, 805 and 860 nm, indicating the presence of bacteriochlorophyll *a* and carotenoids.

Cells can grow photoheterotrophically under anaerobic conditions with various organic compounds as electron donors and carbon sources or chemoheterotrophically under aerobic conditions in the dark. Ammonia, dinitrogen and some amino acids are used as nitrogen source; nitrate is not used. Growth factors are not required, but yeast extract stimulates growth. Optimal growth occurs at 25–35°C and pH 6.0–7.0. Growth is inhibited by 3% NaCl.

The mol% G + C of the DNA is 67.6–69.4 (T_m).

Type strain: ATCC 33872 (Akiba R1).

7. **Rhodopseudomonas marina** Imhoff 1984c, 270.[VP] (Effective publication: Imhoff 1983, 519.)

ma.ri′na. L. fem. adj. *marina* marine.

Cells are ovoid to rod-shaped, 0.7–0.9 μm wide and 1.0–2.5 μm long, motile by flagella distributed at random, and Gram-negative. Internal photosynthetic membranes are present as lamellae underlying and parallel to the cytoplasmic membrane. Color of cell suspensions is pink to red. Absorption maxima of living cells are at 375, 483, 516, 553, 590, 803 and 883 nm. Photosynthetic pigments are bacteriochlorophyll *a* (esterified with phytol) and carotenoids of the spirilloxanthin series with spirilloxanthin as the dominant component.

Cells preferably grow photoheterotrophically under anaerobic conditions. Growth under microaerobic dark conditions and, with a few substrates such as fructose, under anaerobic dark conditions is possible. Under phototrophic growth conditions, a variety of organic carbon sources can be used, including alcohols, sugar alcohols, sugars and fatty acids. Sulfate, thiosulfate, tetrathionate, cysteine, methionine, glutathione, sulfite and sulfide at low concentrations are used as sulfur source. Yeast extract enhances growth and sulfide tolerance. Ammonia, glutamate, aspartate, alanine and urea serve as nitrogen source. Optimal growth occurs at 25–30°C, pH 6.9–7.1, and 1–5% NaCl.

The mol% G + C of the DNA is 61.5–63.6 (T_m).

Type strain: ATCC 35675, DSM 2698 (Imhoff 985).

Genus **Rhodomicrobium** Duchow and Douglas 1949, 415[AL]

JOHANNES F. IMHOFF AND HANS G. TRÜPER

Rho.do.mi.cro'bi.um. Gr. n. *rhodos* the rose; Gr. adj. *micros* small; Gr. n. *bios* life; M.L. neut. n. *Rhodomicrobium* red microbe.

Ovoid to elongate-ovoid bacteria showing polar growth and performing a characteristic vegetative growth cycle. This cycle includes the formation of peritrichously flagellated swarmer cells and nonmotile "mother cells" which form filaments from one to several times the length of the mother cell. Daughter cells originate as spherical buds at the end of the filaments and may undergo differentiation in various ways. Gram-negative. **Cells have intracytoplasmic membranes of the lamellar type and contain bacteriochlorophyll and carotenoids as photosynthetic pigments.**

Cells grow preferably photoheterotrophically under anaerobic conditions in the light with various organic substrates as carbon and electron sources; molecular hydrogen and sulfide at low concentrations may be used as photosynthetic electron donor. Cells are able to grow under microaerobic to aerobic conditions in the dark. pH values between 6 and 7 are preferred for growth.

The mol% G + C of the DNA is 61.8–63.8 (Bd).

Type species: *Rhodomicrobium vannielii* Duchow and Douglas 1949, 415.[AL]

Further Descriptive Information

Rhodomicrobium vannielii is the sole species of this genus. Its morphology and growth cycle resemble those of the nonphototrophic *Hyphomicrobium* species (Hirsch, 1974). The characteristic growth cycle has been the object of intensive studies (Whittenbury and Dow, 1977) and is given in detail in the species description. *Rhodomicrobium vannielii* grows best under anaerobic conditions in the light with a number of carbon sources at low light intensities and acidic pH (5.5–6.5). Dinitrogen and ammonia are the best nitrogen sources. Ammonia

is assimilated via glutamine synthetase/glutamate synthase (NADH-dependent); low activities of a glutamate dehydrogenase (NADPH-dependent) are also present (Brown and Herbert, 1977). Sulfate can be used as sole sulfur source and is assimilated via adenosine-5'-phosphosulfate (Imhoff, 1982). Sulfide is tolerated at 2–3 mM and oxidized exclusively to tetrathionate in sulfide-limited chemostat culture; in batch culture, sulfide may react with the tetrathionate formed, and under these conditions, thiosulfate and elemental sulfur are the major end products (Hansen, 1974).

Rhodomicrobium is commonly found in mud and water of ponds and lakes and in wastewater. About 50% of enrichment cultures with freshwater sediments proved to contain *Rhodomicrobium* species (Whittenbury and Dow, 1977). *Rhodomicrobium* has also been isolated from brackish water and seawater habitats (Hirsch and Rheinheimer, 1968).

Enrichment and Isolation Procedures

Enrichment, isolation and growth occur under conditions suitable for most of the other species of the PNSB group (see the article on *Rhodospirillum*) with organic acids or other organic substrates as carbon and electron sources. For selective enrichments, a succinate-mineral medium with an initial pH of 5.2–5.5 should be used, and growth factors should be omitted (Pfennig, 1969a).

Maintenance Procedures

Rhodomicrobium can be preserved by standard procedures in liquid nitrogen or by lyophilization.

Differentiation of the genus **Rhodomicrobium** from other genera

The lamellar structure of the internal membranes, the polar growth mode and the budding type of multiplication are, in particular, similar to the budding *Rhodopseudomonas* species. The filament formation and the characteristic growth cycle are the most obvious distinguishing features. The DNA from *Rhodomicrobium vannielii* is not homologous to that from *Hyphomicrobium* strains (Moore and Hirsch, 1972), but it shows a similar degree of homology (55%) to rRNA from *Hyphomicrobium* strain B-552, as does the DNA from *Hyphomonas polymorpha* (55–66%), *Caulobacter crescentus* (57%) or *Chromatium vinosum* (53%) (Moore, 1977). As in *Rhodopseudomonas viridis*, *Rhodopseudomonas acidophila* and *Rhodopila globiformis*, a cytochrome c' is absent from *Rhodomicrobium vannielii* or is expressed only at a very low level (Ambler et al., 1981). A high potential iron-sulfur protein is present, as in *Rhodopila globiformis*, *Rhodocyclus gelatinosus* and *Rhodocyclus tenuis* (T. E. Meyer, personal communication). Special similarities were found in the amino acid sequences of the small cytochromes c_2 and in the oligonucleotide pattern of the 16S rRNA to *Rhodopseudomonas viridis* and *Rhodopseudomonas acidophila*, respectively (Ambler et al., 1979; Gibson et al., 1979) As in *Rhodopila globiformis*, but unlike all other PNSB, high proportions of unusual aminolipids are present in *Rhodomicrobium vannielii* (Park and Berger, 1967; Imhoff et al., 1982). The fatty acid composition is characterized by an extremely high proportion of C (18:1), similar to strains of *Hyphomicrobium* species, *Pedomicrobium*

species, *Nitrobacter agilis* and *Nitrobacter winogradskii* (Auran and Schmidt, 1972; Eckhardt et al., 1979). According to rRNA/DNA hybridization studies (Gillis et al., 1982) and to its lipid A structure, *Rhodomicrobium* is not similar to *Rhodopseudomonas* and *Rhodobacter* species. The lipid A contains glucosamine as the sole amino sugar (not the 2,3-diamino-2,3-dideoxyglucose found in three of the budding *Rhodopseudomonas* species) and such fatty acids as myristic acid, 3-OH-myristic acid and, as major component, 3-OH-palmitic acid (Holst et al., 1981). A similar fatty acid spectrum has so far not been encountered in the lipid A of other PNSB.

Taxonomic Comments

According to similarities in 16S RNA oligonucleotide patterns, *Rhodomicrobium* appears particularly related to some species of the genus *Rhodopseudomonas*. The composition of the lipid A, dissimilarities based on rRNA/DNA hybridization stuides, polar lipid composition, filament formation and characteristic growth cycle are, however, significant distinguishing features. As pointed out by Imhoff et al. (1984), these factors provide strong argument for maintaining the genus *Rhodomicrobium*.

Further Reading

Gorlenko, V.M., N.N. Egorova, and A.N. Puchkov. 1974. Fine structure of exospores of nonsulfur purple bacterium *Rhodomicrobium vannielii*. Mikrobiologia *43:* 913–915.

Hirsch, P. 1974. Budding bacteria. Annu. Rev. Microbiol. *28:* 392–444.

Whittenbury, R. and C.S. Dow. 1977. Morphogenesis and differentiation in *Rhodomicrobium vannielii* and other budding and prosthecate bacteria. Bacteriol. Rev. *41:* 754–808.

List of species of the genus **Rhodomicrobium**

1. **Rhodomicrobium vannielii** Duchow and Douglas 1949, 415.[AL]

van.niel′i.i. M.L. gen. n. *vannielii* of van Niel; named for C. B. van Niel, an American microbiologist.

Mature cells are ovoid to lemon-shaped, 1.0–1.2 μm wide and 2.0–2.8 μm long, and multiply by polar growth and budding (Fig. 18.29). Cells perform a characteristic vegetative growth cycle; the motile, peritrichously flagellated swarmer cells, which loose their flagella during the further growth cycle, form a filament of about 0.3 μm in diameter, and a daughter cell arises as a spherical bud at the end of the filament. This daughter cell may separate from the filament and start a new cycle as a swarmer cell. After the swarmer cell is released, the pole of the filament is free for the formation of another bud. Alternatively, the daughter cell remains attached to the filament and forms another filament at the opposite pole. Branching of filaments may occur by lateral outgrowth of new filaments from the primary filament upon which the first daughter cell formed. A branched filament can only be formed on the most recently synthesized filament, and each daughter cell is accompanied by plug formation in its filament before that filament branches to form the next daughter cell. Only one daughter cell at a time is formed, and in any case, no more than four daughter cells are ever formed by one mother cell. Because cells tend to remain attached to the filament, aggregates containing large numbers of cells are usually formed. In addition, smaller cells, called exospores, may eventually be formed. These polyhedral cells are 1.0–1.5 μm in diameter. One to four such cells are formed sequentially as buds at a common branching point at the end of a filament (Fig. 18.29). The exospores are more resistant to dryness and heat than are normal vegetative cells.

Internal photosynthetic membranes are present as lamellae underlying and parallel to the cytoplasmic membrane; no lamellae are present in the filaments. Photosynthetic pigments are bacteriochlorophyll *a* (esterified with phytol) and carotenoids of the spirilloxanthin series with rhodopin as the major carotenoid and with small amounts of β-carotene. Color of cell suspensions is from salmon pink to deep orange-brown to red. Absorption spectra of living cells have maxima at 378, 461, 488–490, 522–525, 800–807 and 869–872 nm. Aerobically grown cells are colorless to pale orange-brown.

Cells grow preferably under photoheterotrophic conditions, anaerobically in the light, with a variety of organic substrates as carbon and electron sources. Addition of HOO_3^- is only essential when CO_2 cannot be generated from the organic carbon source. Substrates used are acetate, propionate, butyrate, valerate, caproate, caprylate, ethanol, propanol, butanol, lactate, pyruvate, malate, fumarate, succinate and malonate. Some strains also use methanol, formate, oxalacetate, β-OH-butyrate and glycerol. Not used are citrate, tartrate, fructose, glucose, mannose, mannitol, sorbitol, glycolate, oxalate, pelargonate, benzoate, aspartate, arginine and glutamate. Molecular hydrogen and sulfide may serve as electron donor for photoautotrophic growth. The latter is oxidized to tetrathionate in sulfide-limited continuous culture, but thiosulfate and elemental sulfur are formed as major oxidation products in batch culture. Ammonia and dinitrogen, as well as casamino acids and yeast extract, are used as nitrogen source. Some strains show poor growth with nitrate and urea. Sulfate can serve as sole sulfur source. No organic growth factors are required. Growth occurs at pH 5.2–7.5 (optimum pH: 6.0). Optimum growth temperature is 30°C.

The mol% G + C of the DNA is 61.8–63.8 (Bd).

Type strain: ATCC 17100, DSM 162.

Genus **Rhodocyclus** *Pfennig 1978, 285*[AL]

JOHANNES F. IMHOFF AND HANS G. TRÜPER

Rho.do.cy′clus. Gr. n. *rhodos* the rose; Gr. n. *cyclos* a circle; M.L. masc. n. *Rhodocyclus* red circle.

Cells are slender, curved or straight thin rods, 0.3–0.7 μm in diameter, motile by means of polar flagella or nonmotile, and multiply by binary fission. Gram-negative. **Internal photosynthetic membranes are present in the form of small, single fingerlike intrusions of the cytoplasmic membrane.** Photosynthetic pigments are bacteriochlorophyll *a* and carotenoids.

Photoautotrophic growth with molecular hydrogen is possible if growth factors are supplied. **Growth is preferably under anaerobic conditions in the light with different organic substrates as carbon and electron sources.** Growth is possible under microaerobic to aerobic conditions in the dark. Reduced sulfur compounds are not used as photosynthetic electron donors.

The mol% G + C of the DNA is 64.8–72.4 (Bd).

Type species: *Rhodocyclus purpureus* Pfennig 1978, 285.[AL]

Further Descriptive Information

This genus comprises three species, *Rhodocyclus purpureus, Rhodocyclus tenuis* (formerly *Rhodospirillum tenue*) and *Rhodocyclus gelatinosus* (formerly *Rhodopseudomonas gelatinosa*). With the exception of *Rhodocyclus purpureus,* which is nonmotile and grows as a half-circle or circle-shaped cells, cells of this genus are slender, slightly curved and fast-moving under opimal growth conditions.

Rhodocyclus gelatinosus occurs in two distinct morphological forms (Biebl and Drews, 1969). Form I cells are clearly curved 0.4–0.7 μm in diameter, and produce less slime during active growth. Form II cells are more or less straight rods, although they are sometimes also bent, and produce more slime during active growth, causing sedimentation of the cells in a gelatinous layer.

There is considerable variation in the nutritional requirements of the three species. Only a few carbon compounds can be assimilated by *Rhodocyclus purpureus.* Benzoate and cyclohexane carboxylate are both used, which may be indicative of the use of the same pathway for anaerobic benzoate degradation by *Rhodocyclus purpureus* and *Rhodopseudomonas palustris* (Dutton and Evans, 1969; Pfennig, 1978). Both of these carbon substrates, rarely used by the PNSB, are not utilized by the two other species which are, however, more versatile with respect to carbon nutrition (Table 18.14). Particularly characteristic of *Rhodocyclus gelatinosus* is the liquefaction of gelatin, which is catalyzed by an extracellular protease (Klemme and Pfleiderer, 1977). *R. gelatinosus* grows well with citrate as carbon source and, in this situation, excretes large amounts of acetate into the medium, which serve as carbon source after citrate is exhausted (Schaab et al., 1972). Citrate lyase, the key enzyme for growth on citrate, has been characterized in this species (Giffhorn et al., 1972; Beuscher et al., 1974). Isocitrate lyase is present in acetate-grown cells, but malate synthase could not be found and an alternate reaction sequence replacing the glyoxylate cycle with involvement of reactions of the serine pathway has been proposed (Albers and Gottschalk, 1976). *R. gelatinosus* can also be adapted to grow with CO as sole energy and carbon source under anaerobic conditions in the dark (Uffen, 1976). Under these conditions, activities of both enzymes of the serine pathway and ribulosebisphosphate carboxylase are enhanced (Uffen, 1983).

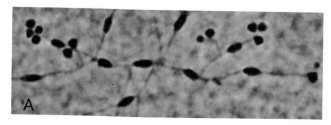

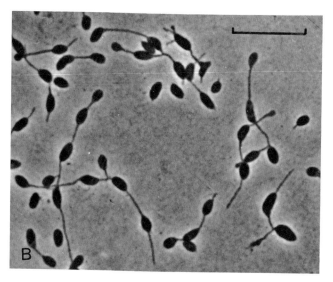

Figure 18.29. *R. vannielii* strain DSM 163. *A,* polyhedral exospores as buds at the ends of short filaments with common branching points. *B,* cells with filaments and buds of various sizes. Phase-contrast micrographs. *Bar,* 10 μm. (Courtesy of N. Pfennig.)

Exemplified by two strains from each of the morphological groups of *R. gelatinosus,* form I cells utilize a greater variety of carbon sources and have a much shorter doubling time than do form II cells (Weckesser et al., 1969).

R. purpureus and *R. tenuis* differ significantly in their nitrogen nutrition. Whereas the former species uses only ammonia and glutamine as nitrogen sources and is unable to fix dinitrogen (a property common to all other species of the PNSB group), the latter species utilizes a greater number of amino acids, urea, dinitrogen, yeast extract, peptone and casamino acids (Masters and Madigan, 1983). Masters and Madigan found alanine dehydrogenase absent from both species. Glutamate dehydrogenase (NADPH-dependent) is present in *R. purpureus* in unusually high activities under all growth conditions, and the glutamine synthetase inhibitor methionine sulfoximine exerts no growth inhibition. This may be taken as indication that the major route of nitrogen assimilation in *R. purpureus* is via glutamate dehydrogenase (unlike that in all other investigated PNSB). *R. tenuis* employs the glutamine synthetase/glutamate synthase (NADPH-dependent) pathway for the assimilation of ammonia (Masters and Madigan, 1983).

All three species are able to use sulfate as sole sulfur source and reduce it via adenosine-5'-phosphosulfate (Imhoff, 1982). The three species have a different requirement for growth factors. The requirement for vitamin B_{12}, which is unusual for PNSB, for the synthesis of 1 g cell dry weight is about 1 μg for *R. purpureus* (Pfennig, 1978; Siefert and Koppenhagen, 1982) and 0.2 μg for one strain of *R. tenuis* (Siefert and Koppenhagen, 1982).

R. gelatinosus is widely distributed in nature, and both *R. tenuis* and *R. gelatinosus* are found in habitats which are, in general, suitable for PNSB. *R. purpureus* was isolated from a swine waste lagoon in Ames, Iowa (U.S.A.), where it was the dominant phototrophic bacterium. It has not been observed in other localities and is probably a rare species.

Enrichment and Isolation Procedures

Media for enrichment, isolation and growth of *Rhodocyclus* species are those generally employed also for the other PNSB. For *R. purpureus,* the vitamin B_{12} requirement and its unusual carbon nutrition have to be considered. From a suitable habitat it should be selectively enriched with benzoic acid as carbon source and in the presence of vitamin B_{12} and the absence of reduced sulfur compounds, which could possibly serve as electron donors for other phototrophic bacteria. Citrate has been proven to be useful for the selective enrichment of

Table 18.14.
Differentiating characteristics of the species of the genus **Rhodocyclus**[a]

Characteristic	1. *R. purpureus*	2. *R. tenuis*	3. *R. gelatinosus*
Cell diameter (μm)	0.6–0.7	0.3–0.5	0.4–0.7
Cell shape	Half-circle to circle	Curved rod	Curved rod
Motility	−	+	+
Slime production	−	+	+
Major carotenoids	Rhodopin, rhodopinal	Rhodopin, rhodopinal, lycopene[b]	Spheroidene, OH-spheroidene, spirilloxanthin
Growth factors required	B_{12}, p-ABA, biotin	None[c]	Thiamine, biotin[d]
N_2 fixation	−	+	+
Gelatin liquefied	−	−	+
Benzoate utilized	+	−	−
Citrate utilized	−	−	+
Mol% G + C of DNA (Bd)	65.3	64.8	70.5–72.4

[a] Symbols: −, negative in most strains; +, positive in most strains; p-ABA, *p*-aminobenzoic acid.
[b] Some strains may contain carotenoids of the spirilloxanthin series and lack rhodopinal (Schmidt, 1978).
[c] Some strains may require vitamin B_{12} (Siefert and Koppenhagen, 1982).
[d] Some strains may also require pantothenate.

Rhodocyclus gelatinosus, even if some strains of a number of other species (*Rhodopseudomonas palustris*, *Rhodopseudomonas viridis*, *Rhodopseudomonas acidophila*, *Rhodobacter capsulatus* and *Rhodobacter sphaeroides*) also grow with citrate as sole carbon source.

Maintenance Procedures

Rhodocyclus species are well maintained by standard procedures in liquid nitrogen.

Differentiation of the genus **Rhodocyclus** from other genera

Rhodocyclus species are clearly distinguished from other phototrophic PNSB by their poorly developed internal photosynthetic membrane system, which consists of small, single, tubular or fingerlike intrusions. Their physiological properties are, in general, not significantly different from those of the other PNSB, although the utilization of citrate by *R. gelatinosus* and the utilization of benzoic acid by *R. purpureus* are not common among the PNSB, except in *R. gelatinosus*. A requirement found in species of the PNSB, except in *R. gelatinosus*. A requirement of vitamin B_{12} is also unusual among the PNSB and more common with the green and purple sulfur bacteria. Besides *Rhodocyclus purpureus*, only single strains of *Rhodocyclus tenuis* and *Rhodopseudomonas palustris* require vitamin B_{12}, i.e. about 0.8–0.9 µg, 0.20 µg, and 0.055 µg, respectively, for the synthesis of 1 g cell dry weight (Siefert and Koppenhagen, 1982).

The structures of some diagnostically valuable molecular cell constituents are not similar to those of other species of the PNSB: Cytochromes c_2 found in other genera of the PNSB are not present in *Rhodocyclus*. A smaller size cytochrome c_{551}, which is typically found in species of the *Chromatiaceae* and *Ectothiorhodospiraceae*, is present instead. Its amino acid sequence bears only a low degree of similarity to those of the cytochromes c_2 of other PNSB (Ambler et al., 1979).

The lipid A moiety of the lipopolysaccharide from all *Rhodocyclus* species contains significant amounts of phosphate (like that from the investigated *Rhodobacter* species) and, as sole amino sugar, glucosamine (as in most of the other PNSB). The fatty acid pattern of the lipid A is characterized by the absence of 3-OH-myristic acid, which is found in the lipid A structure of all other PNSB. Major fatty acids of all three species are myristic acid (14:0), 3-OH-capric acid (3-OH-C 10:0), and palmitic acid (C 16:0), which is replaced by lauric acid (C 12:0) in *R. gelatinosus* (Weckesser et al., 1975, 1977, 1983).

The oligonucleotide pattern of the 16S rRNA from *Rhodocyclus gelatinosus* and *Rhodocyclus tenuis* (and most probably also from *Rhodocyclus purpureus*) are different from those of the other PNSB at an S_{AB} level of about 0.3 (Gibson et al., 1979) and on a similar low level also from the *Chromataceae* (Fowler et al., 1984) and *Ectothiorhodospiraceae* (Stackbrandt et al., 1984).

All species of the PNSB except *Rhodocyclus* belong to the rRNA superfamily IV, while *Rhodocyclus* species are found in superfamily III (De Ley et al., 1978; Gillis et al, 1982). Unlike the other PNSB, but like the *Chromatiaceae* species, *Rhodocyclus* species contain Q-8 and MK-8 as quinone components (Imhoff, 1984b) and demonstrate *S*-sulfocysteine synthase activity (Hensel and Trüper, 1983).

A clear differentiation from the other genera of the PNSB on the basis of the above-mentioned molecular structures is obvious but is not reflected in the physiological properties.

Taxonomic Comments

All three species of *Rhodocyclus* are taxonomically poorly characterized and need thorough further investigation. The description of *R.*

purpureus is based on a single strain. Two morphological cell types of *R. gelatinosus* have been described (Biebl and Drews, 1969). The carbon sources utilized by two strains of each of these groups have been shown to be significantly different (Weckesser et al., 1969). Another strain of this species described by Klemme (1968) is, in carbon substrate utilization, intermediate to the two groups established by Weckesser et al. (1969). Furthermore, the lipopolysaccharides of *R. gelatinosus* show two different serotypes which do not cross-react with each other (Weckesser et al., 1975). Weckesser et al. give no information on the structural and nutritional type of the strains belonging to the different serotypes, and it seems that there is no correlation between serotype and morphological type.

A similar dichotomy has also been observed in *R. tenuis* strains on the basis of carotenoid composition (Schmidt, 1978), color of cell suspensions, and absorption spectra (Biebl, 1973). Some strains have carotenoids of the rhodopinal series, and others, of the spirilloxanthin series.

Further information is also required on the uniqueness of gelatin liquefaction by *Rhodocyclus gelatinosus*. Siefert et al. (1978) have identified about one half of the strains with this property as belonging to *Rhodobacter capsulatus*, while other strains with the morphology typical of *Rhodocyclus gelatinosus* did not liquefy gelatin.

Despite this intraspecies heterogeneity, the species are well-differentiated on the basis of work on representative strains. The binary similarity coefficient of 0.6 for the 16S rRNA of *Rhodocyclus tenuis* and *Rhodocyclus gelatinosus* (Gibson et al., 1979) appeared high, compared with those of other PNSB. Higher similarity coefficients were found only for the couples of *Rhodobacter capsulatus* and *Rhodobacter sphaeroides* and of *Rhodospirillum rubrum* and *Rhodospirillum photometricum* (Gibson et al., 1979; C. R. Woese, personal communication). On the other hand, on the basis of the same method, species of the *Chromatiaceae* family are similar to an S_{AB} value higher than 0.61 (Fowler et al., 1984), and the species of *Ectothiorhodospiraceae* are similar at an S_{AB} value of 0.49 (Stackebrandt et al., 1984). These data demonstrate the heterogeneity of the PNSB group. It seems, however, not appropriate to use certain S_{AB} values as the sole criterion and exclusion limit for association of taxa at a specific rank. Taking into account the heterogeneity of the PNSB group compared with the *Chromatiaceae* and *Ectothiorhodospiraceae*, we have proposed to recognize the three species of *Rhodocyclus* as a genus of the PNSB group and to avoid the further usage of the family name *Rhodospirillaceae* (Imhoff et al. 1984).

Further Reading

Pfennig, N. 1977. Phototrophic green and purple bacteria: a comparative systematic survey. Annu. Rev. Microbiol. *31:* 275–290.
Pfennig, N. and H.G. Trüper. 1983. Taxonomy of phototrophic green and purple bacteria: a review. Ann. Microbiol. (Inst. Pasteur) *134B:* 9–20.
Stackebrandt, E. and C.R. Woese. 1981. The evolution of procaryotes. *In* Carlile, Collins and Moseley (Editors), Molecular and Cellular Aspects of Microbial Evolution. Cambridge University Press, Cambridge, England, pp. 1–31.

Differentiation of the species of the genus **Rhodocyclus**

The major diagnostic properties of the species are listed in Table 18.14. Utilization of citrate and benzoate, gelatin liquefaction, growth factor requirement, carotenoid composition, and morphological properties enable a clear identification of the recognized species.

List of species of the genus **Rhodocyclus**

1. **Rhodocyclus purpureus** Pfennig 1978, 285.[AL]

pur.pu′reus. L. adj. *purpureus* purple or red-violet.

Cells are half-ring-shaped to ring-shaped before cell division and 0.6–0.7 μm wide. The diameter of a circle is 2.0–3.0 μm. A half-circle-shaped cell is about 2.7 μm long (Fig. 18.30). Under certain conditions, open or compact spirals or coils of variable length are formed. In sulfide-containing media, closely wound spirals are united in compact cell aggregates. Cells are nonmotile under all growth conditions.

The color of phototrophically grown cultures is purple-violet to violet. Aerobically grown cells are colorless to pale violet. Living cells demonstrate absorption maxima at 379, 408, 510, 535, 597, 813 and 866 nm; bacteriochlorphyll *a* (esterified with phytol) and carotenoids of the rhodopinal series with rhodopinal as major component are present as photosynthetic pigments.

Cells grow photoautotrophically with hydrogen as electron donor in the presence of growth factors. Photoheterotrophic growth occurs under anaerobic conditions in the light with a relatively small number of organic substrates as carbon and electron sources. Growth is also possible under microaerobic to aerobic conditions in the dark. Carbon sources utilized are listed in Table 18.15. In addition, cyclohexane carboxylate is used, but propanol, yeast extract and casamino acids are not utilized as sole carbon source. Photoheterotrophically grown cells use only ammonia and glutamine as nitrogen source; dinitrogen is not assimilated. Sulfate can be used as sole sulfur source. Vitamin B_{12}, *p*-aminobenzoic acid and biotin are required as growth factors. Growth with acetate occurs at pH 6.5–7.5 (optimum pH: 7.2). Optimum growth occurs at 30°C.

The mol% G + C of the DNA is 65.3 (Bd).

Type strain: DSM 168 (Ames 6770, Pfennig).

2. **Rhodocyclus tenuis** (Pfennig) Imhoff, Trüper and Pfennig 1984, 341.[VP] (*Rhodospirillum tenue* Pfennig 1969b, 619.[AL])

te′nu.is. L. masc. adj. *tenuis* slender, thin.

Cells are curved in a spiral of one to two complete turns, 0.3–0.5 μm wide and 1.5–6.0 μm long or, sometimes, even longer. One complete turn of a spiral is about 0.8–1.0 μm wide and 3 μm long (Fig. 18.31).

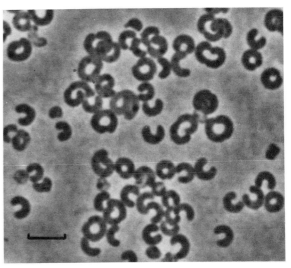

Figure 18.30. *R. purpureus* DSM 168. Phase-contrast micrograph. *Bar,* 5 μm (Courtesy of N. Pfennig.)

Cells tend to form a sticky sediment; they are motile by means of polar flagella.

The color of photosynthetically grown cells is brownish-red or purple-violet, depending on the strain; aerobically grown cells may be colorless or pigmented. Absorption maxima of brownish cells are at 378–380, 465, 492–495, 528, 592–594, 799–801 and 868–871 nm; these cells have carotenoids of the spirilloxanthin series. Absorption maxima of purple cells are at 377–378, 469, 495–500, 529–533, 590–592, 798–801 and 856–858 nm; carotenoids of the rhodopinal series occur in these cells. Both types of cells contain bacteriochlorophyll *a* esterified with phytol.

Photoautotrophic growth with molecular hydrogen is possible. Growth occurs preferably under anaerobic conditions in the light with

Table 18.15.

Photosynthetic electron donors and carbon sources used by species of the genus **Rhodocyclus**[a]

Donor/source	1. *R. purpureus*	2. *R. tenuis*	3. *R. gelatinosus*	Donor/source	1. *R. purpureus*	2. *R. tenuis*	3. *R. gelatinosus*
Formate	−	−	±	Aspartate	−	−	+
Acetate	+	+	+	Arginine	−	−	o
Propionate	−	±	±	Glutamate	−	−	+
Butyrate	+	+	±	Benzoate	+	−	−
Valerate	−	+	+	Glucose	−	−	+
Caproate	+	+	o	Fructose	−	−	+
Caprylate	−	±	o	Mannose	−	−	+
Pelargonate	−	+	o	Mannitol	−	−	−
Glycolate	−	−	o	Sorbitol	−	o	−
Pyruvate	+	+	+	Glycerol	−	−	−
Lactate	−	+	+	Methanol	−	−	±
Malonate	−	−	o	Ethanol	−	±	+
Malate	+	+	+	Hydrogen	+	+	+
Succinate	−	+	+	Sulfide	−	−	−
Fumarate	+	+	+	Thiosulfate	−	−	−
Tartrate	−	−	±	Sulfur	−	−	−
Citrate	−	−	+				

[a] Symbols: −, substrate not utilized by most strains; +, substrate utilized by most strains, ±, substrate utilized by some strains; o, not tested.

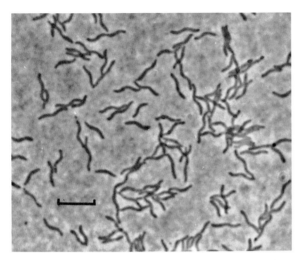

Figure 18.31. *R. tenuis* DSM 109. Phase-contrast micrograph. *Bar*, 5 μm. (Courtesy of N. Pfennig.)

numerous carbon substrates as carbon and electron sources. Growth is also possible under microaerobic to aerobic conditions in the dark. The organic substrates used are listed in Table 18.15. In addition, casamino acids and yeast extract are utilized, but cyclohexane carboxylate is not.

Good growth occurs with aspartate, glutamate, glutamine, ammonia and dinitrogen as nitrogen source; also utilized are casamino acids, peptone, yeast extract, alanine, arginine, lysine, methionine, serine, threonine and urea. Sulfate is used as sole sulfur source; sulfite, sulfide, thiosulfate, cysteine and reduced glutathione can also serve as assimilatory sulfur source. Growth factors are not required. Growth rate is increased in the presence of complex organic nutrients or yeast extract. Some strains may need vitamin B₁₂. Optimum growth occurs at pH 6.6–7.4 and 30°C.

The mol% G + C of the DNA is 64.8 (Bd).

Type strain: ATCC 19137, DSM 109 (Grünenplan).

3. **Rhodocyclus gelatinosus** (Molisch) Imhoff, Trüper and Pfennig 1984, 341.[VP] (*Rhodocystis gelatinosa* Molisch 1907, 22; *Rhodopseudomonas gelatinosa* (Molisch) van Niel 1944, 98.[AL])

ge.la.ti.no′sus. L. part. adj. *gelatus* frozen, stiffened; M.L. n. *gelatinum* gelatin, that which stiffens; M.L. masc. adj. *gelatinosus* gelatinous.

Cells are rod-shaped, straight or slightly curved, 0.4–0.7 μm wide and 1–3 μm long and, in older cultures, up to 15 μm long and irregularly curved. Most strains show abundant mucus production in all media, which causes the cells to clump together and appear immotile. In young cultures, cells are highly motile by means of polar flagella.

Cultures grown anaerobically in the light are pale peach to dirty yellowish brown; aerobically grown cells appear colorless to light yellowish brown. Cells contain bacteriochlorophyll *a* (esterified with phytol) and carotenoids of the spheroidene series with spheroidene, OH-spheroidene and spirilloxanthin as major components. Photoautotrophic growth is possible with hydrogen as electron source in the presence of growth factors. A variety of carbon compounds are used as electron and carbon sources under anaerobic conditions in the light. Growth is also possible under microaerobic to aerobic conditions in the dark. Some strains can adapt to grow anaerobically in the dark with CO as sole carbon and energy sources. Pyruvate is fermented anaerobically in the dark. The carbon sources utilized are listed in Table 18.15. In addition, a variety of amino acids, yeast extract and peptone can be used. Most characteristic is the liquefaction of gelatin. Fatty acids are utilized only at low concentrations. Suitable nitrogen sources are ammonia, dinitrogen and a number of amino acids; some strains may also utilize uracil, thymine, guanine, uric acid both anaerobically in the light and aerobically in the dark, and xanthine and adenine only under aerobic conditions. Sulfate can be used as sole sulfur source. Biotin and thiamine are required as growth factors; some strains also require pantothenate. Good growth occurs at pH 6.0–8.5 and at 30°C.

The mol% G + C of the DNA is 70.5–72.4 (Bd).

Type strain: ATCC 17011.

II. GREEN BACTERIA

GREEN SULFUR BACTERIA

NORBERT PFENNIG

Cells spherical, ovoid, straight or curved rod-shaped; multiplication by binary fission or binary plus ternary fission. In one genus (*Chloroherpeton*), cells unicellular filamentous, highly flexible and motile by gliding; all other genera nonmotile. Genera with or without gas vacuoles. Photosynthetic pigments located in the cytoplasmic membrane and the chlorosomes (former chlorobium vesicles; Cohen-Bazire et al., 1964; Staehelin et al., 1978) which underlie and are attached to the cytoplasmic membrane (Fig. 18.32).

The existing species exhibit one of two clearly distinguishable colors: cultures or cell material are either green (grass-green) or brown (chocolate-brown). All strains of the green species contain bacteriochlorophyll *c* or *d* as major component, in addition to small amounts of bacteriochlorophyll *a*; the major carotenoid of the green species is chlorobactene (group 5). All strains of the brown species contain bacteriochlorophyll *e* as major component, in addition to small amounts of bacteriochlorophyll *a* (Gloe et al., 1975); the major carotenoid of the brown species is isorenieratene (group 5) (Schmidt, 1978).

Strictly anaerobic and obligately phototrophic; capable of photolithoautotrophic growth with sulfide or sulfur as electron donor. If sulfide is oxidized, globules of elemental sulfur are formed outside the cells; sulfur is further oxidized to sulfate by most species. All genera are potentially mixotrophic and photoassimilate a number of simple organic substrates in the presence of both sulfide and bicarbonate.

Basically different from all purple bacteria, the green sulfur bacteria carry out autotrophic CO_2 assimilation by the reductive tricarboxylic acid cycle (Arnon cycle; Fuchs et al., 1980). Vitamin B₁₂ is required by most strains of all species (Pfennig and Lippert, 1966).

In nature, the green sulfur bacteria occur in the anaerobic and sulfide-containing parts of all kinds of aquatic environments, e.g. ditches, ponds, lakes, rivers, sulfur springs, estaurine and other marine habitats. The brown forms occur in sulfide-containing deeper layers of ponds and lakes and in the hypolimnion of meromictic lakes. Green or brown species with gas vacuoles are often found in stratified lakes in layers below the purple sulfur bacteria.

On the basis of the presence or absence of gas vacuoles and the selective advantage in enrichment cultures, two physiological-ecological subgroups can be differentiated among the green sulfur bacteria. The first group includes the species without gas vacuoles which have a selective advantage in liquid cultures with high sulfide concentrations (4–6 mM) and light intensities (1000 lx). The second subgroup includes the gas vacuole-containing species which compete successfully only at very low sulfide concentrations (1–2 mM), low light intensities (50–200 lx) and low incubation temperatures (10–20°C). The cells of the gas vacuole-containing species rise to the top of the culture bottles at low temperatures (4–10°C).

The mol% G + C of the DNA is 48.5–58.1 (Bd).

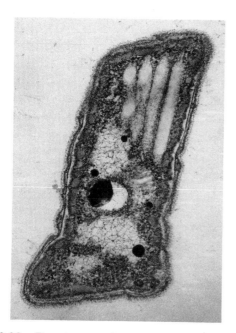

Figure 18.32. Fine structure of green sulfur bacterium *Pelodictyon clathratiforme* strain 1831. Note the chlorosomes (*dark gray area*) underlying and attached to the cytoplasmic membrane, the bundle of gas vesicles (*light gray areas with pointed ends*) in the upper part of the section, and the broadened end of the cell at the site of ternary fission. Electron micrograph (× 105,000). (Courtesy of G. Cohen-Bazire.)

Type genus: *Chlorobium* Nadson 1906, 190.

The major differentiating characteristics of the genera of the green sulfur bacteria are presented in Table 18.16. The consortium-forming symbiotic aggregates of green bacteria with colorless bacteria are given under "Addendum to the Green Sulfur Bacteria" (see page 1696). This appears justified in that the green or brown components of the consortia are morphologically similar to species of the green sulfur bacteria.

Further Comments

This subcategory of the phototrophic green bacteria comprises the family *Chlorobiaceae* Copeland 1956, 31 (Trüper and Pfennig, 1971) and the genus *Chloroherpeton* (Gibson et al., 1984). The latter genus comprises unicellular filamentous bacteria with highly flexible cells and gliding motility. According to 16S rRNA oligonucleotide catalogs, *Chloroherpeton* is phylogenetically more closely related to the genus *Chlorobium* of the green sulfur bacteria than to the multicellular filamentous gliding bacterium *Chloroflexus*. Nothing is known about the phylogenetic relationships of the species and genera of the green sulfur bacteria among themselves. The taxon *Chlorobiaceae* is not used here because an emended description of the family is required. Such a description should be based on nucleic acid analyses in order to avoid further rearrangements.

The present arrangement of genera and species of the green sulfur bacteria is based on simple phenotypic characteristics as used in the eighth edition of the *Manual* (Pfennig and Trüper, 1974). Nucleic acid studies for determining phylogenetic relationships are lacking so far.

Further Reading

Cohen-Bazire, G., N. Pfennig and R. Kunisawa. 1964. The fine structure of green bacteria. J. Cell. Biol. *22:* 207–225.

Fuchs, G., E. Stupperich and G. Eden. 1980. Autotrophic CO₂ fixation in *Chlorobium limicola.* Evidence for the operation of a reductive tricarboxylic acid cycle in growing cells. Arch. Microbiol. *128:* 64–71.

Gibson, J., N. Pfennig and J.B. Waterbury. 1984. *Chloroherpeton thalassium* gen. nov. et spec. nov., a non-filamentous, flexing and gliding green sulfur bacterium. Arch. Microbiol. *138:* 96–101.

Gloe, A., N. Pfennig, H. Brockmann, Jr., and W. Trowitzsch. 1975. A new bacteriochlorophyll from brown-colored *Chlorobiaceae.* Arch. Microbiol. *102:* 103–109.

Pfennig, N. and D. Lippert. 1966. Über das Vitamin B₁₂-Bedürfnis phtotropher Schwefelbakterien. Arch. Mikrobiol.

Staehelin, L.A., J.R. Golecki, R.C. Fuller and G. Drews, 1978. Visualization of the supramolecular architecture of chlorosomes (*Chlorobium*-type vesicles) in freeze-fractured cells of *Chloroflexus aurantiacus.* Arch. Microbiol. *119:* 269–277.

Trüper, H.G. and N. Pfennig. 1971. Family of phototrophic green sulfur bacteria: *Chlorobiaceae* Copeland, the correct family name; rejection of *Chlorobacterium* Lauterborn; and the taxonomic situation of the consortium-forming species. Int. J. Syst. Bacteriol. *21:* 8–10.

Table 18.16.

Differential characteristics of the genera of the **Green Sulfur Bacteria,** *a subcategory of* **Green Bacteria**[a]

Characteristic	Chlorobium	Prosthecochloris	Pelodictyon	Ancalochloris	Chloroherpeton	Consortia, symbiotic aggregates
Cultures and cells green	+	+	+	+	+	
Culture and cells brown	+	+	+	−	−	
Gas vacuoles	−	−	+	+	+	
Nonmotile	+	+	+	+	−	
Gliding motility	−	−	−	−	+	See "Addendum
Cells unicellular, filamentous, flexible	−	−	−	−	+	to the Green Sulfur Bacteria"
Cells starlike, with extrusions, prosthecae	−	+	−	+	−	
Cells spherical, ovoid or rod-shaped	+	−	+	−	−	
Cells curved, vibrioid-shaped, may form spirals	+	−	−	−	−	

[a]Symbols: +, positive or present; −, negative or absent.

Genus **Chlorobium** Nadson 1906, 190[AL]

NORBERT PFENNIG

Chlo.ro´bi.um. Gr. adj. *chloros* green, yellowish green; Gr. n. *bios* life; M.L. neut. n. *Chlorobium* green life.

Cells spherical, ovoid, straight or curved rod-shaped, 0.3–1.1 μm wide and 0.4–3 μm long or, sometimes, much longer. **Cells are often united in chains resembling streptococci or filaments; curved rod-shaped strains may form long spirals.** Multiplication by binary fission. **Nonmotile,** Gram-negative. The existing species exhibit one of two clearly distinguishable colors: **culture or cell material is either green** (grass-green) **or brown** (chocolate-brown). Significantly, these colors can also be recognized under the light microscope with brightfield illumination. **Photosynthetic pigments are located in the cytoplasmic membrane and the chlorosomes** (Staehelin et al., 1978) which underlie and are attached to the cytoplasmic membrane. Bacteriochlorophylls *c, d* or *e* occur as major photosynthetic pigments, in addition to small amounts of bacteriochlorophyll *a*. Chlorobactene is the major carotenoid component (Schmidt and Schiburr, 1970).

Obligately anaerobic and phototrophic. Photolithoautotrophic growth with sulfide or sulfur as electron donor. **During sulfide oxidation, globules of elemental sulfur are formed outside the cells; the sulfur may be further oxidized to sulfate.** In sulfide-reduced media, thiosulfate may be used as electron donor substrate. In the presence of reduced sulfur compounds and bicarbonate, a number of simple organic substrates can be photoassimilated. Ammonia is used as nitrogen source; molecular nitrogen is fixed by many strains. Growth temperature: 20–35°C. Storage materials are polyphosphate and polysaccharides (Sirevag and Ormerod, 1977). Habitat: hydrogen sulfide-containing mud and water of freshwater, brackish water and marine environments.

The mol% G + C of the DNA is 49.0–58.1 (Bd) (Mandel et al., 1971).

Type species: *Chlorobium limicola* Nadson 1906, 190.

Further Descriptive Information

The green or brown strains of the green sulfur bacteria included in the genus *Chlorobium* show essentially two types of cell morphology. One type is represented by strains with straight to slightly curved rod-shaped cells. In undisturbed stationary cultures, these strains may form long filaments of rod-shaped cells or, in the stationary phase of growth, chains of almost spherical cells resembling streptococci. Green, rod-shaped *Chlorobium* strains belonging to the species *C. limicola* can be isolated regularly from the sulfide-containing mud or sediment of all kinds of freshwater habitats. The brown, rod-shaped *Chlorobium* strains of the species *C. phaeobacteroides* are also typical freshwater bacteria; however, they thrive preferentially as planktonic forms in the sulfide-containing hypolimnion of lakes.

The second morphological type of the *Chlorobium* species is represented by strains with curved rod-shaped or C-shaped cells or vibrioid-

shaped to ringlike cells. Characteristically, the cell diameter of all strains of this morphological type is smaller than that of the rod-shaped strains. Depending on the culture conditions, the curved rod- or vibrioid-shaped cells may form C-shaped or ringlike chains of cells which may extend into coils or helical filaments. Both the green or brown strains of the curved rod-shaped cell type are isolated preferentially if anoxic water or mud samples from estuarine, brackish water or marine habitats are used as inoculum.

Depending on the culture conditions, the strains of all *Chlorobium* species tend to form soluble extracellular slime which turns the culture medium more or less viscous. This feature is particularly pronounced in the strains of *C. chlorovibrioides*.

Most strains of the *Chlorobium* species are able to use molecular hydrogen as an electron donor for CO_2 assimilation if reduced sulfur compounds are provided as a source of cell sulfur. Molecular nitrogen can be assimilated by most strains. Photosynthetic pigments of the green strains of all *Chlorobium* species are either bacteriochlorophyll *c* or *d*, together with the carotenoid chlorobactene or bacteriochlorophyll *e*, together with the carotenoid isorenieratene in the brown strains of all species. Small amounts of bacteriochlorophyll *a* are present in all species.

An outstanding characteristic of all green sulfur bacteria including the *Chlorobium* species is their capacity to grow reasonably well at light intensities of 5–10 lx which are too small to allow multiplication of any other phototrophic organisms including the purple bacteria (Biebl and Pfennig, 1978). Therefore, this feature can be used for the selective enrichment culture of *Chlorobium* strains from anoxic mud samples. In good agreement with this, *Chlorobium* is often found below the layers of other phototrophic organisms in muddy or sandy freshwater or marine sediments.

The pH range for growth of *Chlorobium* is fairly narrow, between 6.5 and 7.2, with an optimum at pH 6.8. Most strains require vitamin B_{12} for growth.

Enrichment and Isolation Procedures

Chlorobium species may be enriched and isolated from any anoxic water and mud samples of freshwater, brackish water, marine and saline habitats. The source and species composition of the inoculum is of primary significance for the results of enrichment experiments. In liquid enrichment cultures, however, strains or species may finally be obtained that were not directly detected in the original sample. A *Chlorobium* species which is the dominant type in a given natural habitat may be entirely outgrown by a species that occurs only incidentally in the habitat. When certain color or cell types that were detected microscopically in a given sample are to be isolated, agar shake dilution

---

* Defined medium for green sulfur bacteria is prepared in an Erlenmeyer flask with an outlet near the bottom at one side. Connected to the outlet is a silicon rubber tube with a pinchcock and a bell for aseptic distribution of the medium into bottles or tubes. The flask is closed by a silicon rubber stopper with an inlet and outlet for gas and a screw-capped glass tube through which additions or samplings can be made.

The defined basal medium has the following composition (per liter of distilled water): KH_2PO_4, 0.30 g; NH_4Cl, 0.34 g; KCl, 0.34 g; $CaCl_2 \cdot 2H_2O$, 0.15 g; NaCl (only for seawater medium), 20.0 g; $MgSO_4 \cdot 7H_2O$, 0.5 g (for seawater medium, 3.0 g); and trace element solution (see below), 1.0 ml. After the medium has been autoclaved and cooled under an atmosphere of 90% N_2 plus 10% CO_2, the following components (per liter of medium) are added aseptically from sterile stock solutions while access of air is prevented by continuous flushing with the gas mixture of 90% N_2 plus 10% CO_2: 15 ml of a 10% (w/v) solution of $NaHCO_3$ (saturated with CO_2 and autoclaved under a CO_2 atmosphere); 6 ml of a 10% (w/v) solution of $Na_2S \cdot 9H_2O$ (autoclaved under an N_2 atmosphere); and 1 ml of a vitamin B_{12} solution containing 2 mg of vitamin B_{12} in 100 ml of distilled water. The pH of the medium is adjusted to 6.7 with a sterile 2 M H_2SO_4 or 2 M Na_2CO_3 solution while the medium is magnetically stirred. The medium is then dispensed aseptically into sterile 100-ml bottles with metal screw tops containing autoclavable rubber seals. A small air bubble is left in each bottle to meet possible pressure changes.

The trace element solution contains (per liter): 25% (w/v) HCl, 10 ml; $FeSO_4 \cdot 7H_2O$, 2.0 g; $CoCl_2 \cdot 6H_2O$, 190 mg; $MnCl_2 \cdot 4H_2O$, 100 mg; $ZnCl_2$, 70 mg; $Na_2MoO_4 \cdot 2H_2O$, 36 mg; $NiCl_2 \cdot 6H_2O$, 24 mg; H_3BO_3, 6 mg; and $CuCl_2 \cdot 2H_2O$, 2 mg. Initially, the $FeSO_4$ is dissolved in the 10 ml of HCl; distilled water is then added, followed by the other components.

series should be prepared directly from the sample without prior use of liquid enrichments. The incubation conditions for the agar cultures should closely resemble the conditions to be used for liquid enrichment cultures of the particular species. The defined medium* has been found relatively nonspecific and useful for the cultivation of all green sulfur bacteria presently in pure culture. Other culture media useful for *Chlorobium* species were published by Larsen (1952), Sirevag and Ormerod (1977) and Pfennig and Trüper (1981). For the enrichment culture of *Chlorobium* species in the presence of large numbers of purple sulfur bacteria, advantage can be taken of the ability of *Chlorobium* to compete successfully with other phototrophic bacteria at growth-limiting light intensities between 5 and 50 lx. From other genera of the green sulfur bacteria, *Chlorobium* species may be selectively enriched by the application of high sulfide concentrations (4–6 mM) and high light intensities (500–1000 lx) at incubation temperatures of about 30°C.

The sulfide concentration that is initially provided in the fresh culture medium does not support much growth. To achieve reasonably high population densities in enrichment or pure cultures, repeated additions of neutralized sodium sulfide solution are necessary. Additions are made if the previously added sulfide is consumed and the transiently formed elemental sulfur is largely oxidized. The sulfide solution for feeding of cultures is prepared by neutralizing (pH to about 7.2) a stirred sodium sulfide solution (60 mM) with a certain amount of sterile 2 M sulfuric acid. The neutralized solution has to be applied immediately. Alternatively, a special device for preparation and storage of sterile neutral sulfide solution may be used (Siefert and Pfennig, 1984).

In agar shake dilution cultures, growth may be enhanced by the addition of 3.0–5.0 mM acetate to the defined medium. Pure cultures are obtained by repeated application of the agar shake dilution method. For this method, water agar is prepared with 3.3% (w/v) of repeatedly washed agar in distilled water. Depending on the salinity of the sample from nature or the enrichment culture medium, corresponding amounts of NaCl and $MgCl_2 \cdot 6H_2O$ are added per liter of water agar. The agar solution is dispensed in 3-ml amounts into test tubes, which are stoppered with cotton plugs and autoclaved. The agar tubes are kept molten in a water bath at 55°C. Ready, prepared defined culture medium is prewarmed to 40°C, and 6-ml amounts are added to the tubes of liquefied agar; exposure to air is minimized by dipping the tip of the pipette into the agar medium. Starting with a few drops of a sample from nature or an enrichment culture as inoculum and using 6–8 tubes, serial dilutions are made. All tubes are then hardened in cold water and immediately sealed with a sterile overlay consisting of 1 part paraffin wax and 3 parts mineral oil; the overlay should be 2 cm thick. The tubes are finally flushed with 90% N_2 plus 10% CO_2 and sealed with butyl rubber stoppers. The tubes are kept in the dark for 12 h and subsequently incubated at the desired light intensity and temperature. During the first 2 days of incubation, the paraffin overlay is gently reheated to achieve a complete sealing effect.

Well-separated yellowish green or brown colonies that occur in the higher dilutions can be removed with sterile Pasteur pipettes and without breaking the tube. The cells are suspended in 0.5–1.0 ml of anaerobic medium and used as the inoculum for subsequent agar shake cultures. The process is repeated until a pure culture is obtained.

When pure agar cultures are obtained, individual colonies are isolated and inoculated into liquid medium. It is advisable to start with small-size bottles or screw-capped tubes (10 or 25 ml) and then to scale up to the regularly used sizes. Purity is checked by use of both a microscope and an A-C medium (Difco) adjusted to the respective salinities.

Maintenance Procedures

Pure cultures of all species of the phototrophic green sulfur bacteria can be maintained in the defined mineral medium; 100-ml screw-capped bottles are preferentially used as culture vessels. The freshly grown cultures should just have used up the transiently formed elemental sulfur. At this stage, the stock cultures can be stored at 4°C for 3–4 months. After this time, the cultures keep well if they become supplemented with neutralized sulfide solution and put back to dim light at room temperature. After consumption of sulfide and sulfur, the cultures may be stored for another 3–4 months. Thereafter, the cultures are transferred to fresh culture medium

Long term preservation of green sulfur bacteria is successfully carried out by storage in liquid nitrogen. For this purpose, heavy cell suspensions of liquid cultures are supplemented with DMSO as a protective agent to a final concentration of 5%. Such suspensions are filled into 2-ml plastic ampuls, sealed, and freeze-stored.

Some *Chlorobium* strains were successfully preserved by lyophilization.

Differentiation of the genus **Chlorobium** from other genera

The differentiation of the *Chlorobium* species from the other genera of the green sulfur bacteria presents no problems. The genus *Chlorobium* comprises all green or brown strains with spherical to straight or curved rod-shaped cells that do not form gas vacuoles under any conditions of culture or storage at 4°C temperature. The cells of *Chlorobium* species never carry extrusions or prosthecae which are characteristic of the genera *Prosthecochloris* and *Ancalochloris*. In order to detect the prosthecae, high resolution phase-contrast microscope objectives (magnification: × 100, oil) should be used. *Chlorobium* strains are nonmotile under all conditions and, thus, are different from the unicellular filamentous gliding green sulfur bacterium *Chloroherpeton*.

Taxonomic Comments

The formation of species within the genus *Chlorobium* is entirely based on simple morphological and biochemical characteristics (photosynthetic pigments). In the two species *C. limicola* and *C. vibrioforme*, the forma specialis *thiosulfatophilum* was established for the thiosulfate-utilizing strains (Pfennig and Trüper, 1971). These strains contain an additional cytochrome c_{551} which is absent in the non-thiosulfate-using strains of the two species (Meyer et al., 1968; Steinmetz and Fischer, 1982) and which is supposed to be specifically involved in the thiosulfate metabolism. Although in the non-thiosulfate-using strains the first oxidation product of sulfide is elemental sulfur, the *thiosulfatophilum* strains form thiosulfate as the first product and release it into the medium. In a second step, thiosulfate is then further oxidized to elemental sulfur. These results indicate that the thiosulfate-using strains of the two species differ significantly from the other strains in their metabolism of sulfide. The wide variation of the DNA base ratios both within the genus and within single species indicates a marked genetic heterogeneity of the physiologically very homogeneous group. Nucleic acid studies, such as rRNA oligonucleotide cataloging and DNA/DNA hybridization are required to establish a genetically meaningful classification.

Differentiation of the species of the genus **Chlorobium**

The phenotypic traits that are presently used to differentiate the species of the genus *Chlorobium* are listed in Table 18.17.

Table 18.17.
Characteristics of the species of the genus **Chlorobium**[a]

Characteristic	1. *C. limicola*	1a. *C. limicola* f. sp. *thiosulfatophilum*	2. *C. vibrioforme*	2a. *C. vibrioforme* f. sp. *thiosulfatophilum*	3. *C. chlorovibrioides*	4. *C. phaeobacteroides*	5. *C. phaeovibroides*
Cells or cell suspensions green	+	+	+	+	+	−	−
Cells or cell suspensions brown	−	−	−	−	−	+	+
Cells rod-shaped to spherical	+	+	−	−	−	+	(+)
Cells curved rod- and vibrioid-shaped to ringlike	−	−	+	+	+	−	+
Cell diameter (μm)							
0.7–1.1	+	+	−	−	−	−	−
0.5–0.8	−	−	+	+	−	+	−
0.3–0.4	−	−	−	−	+	−	+
Thiosulfate used	−	+	−	+	−	−	−
NaCl requirement (%)	0	0	2	2	2–3	0	2
Mol% G + C of DNA	51–52	52.5–58	52–57	53.5	54	49–50	52–53

[a] Symbols: +, positive; −, negative.

List of species of the genus **Chlorobium**

1. Chlorobium limicola Nadson 1906, 190.[AL]

li.mi′col.la. L. n. *limus* mud; L. suff., verbal n. *cola* dweller; M.L. masc. n. *limicola* the mud dweller.

Cells straight or slightly curved rod-shaped, 0.7–1.1 μm wide, and 0.9–1.5 μm long or, sometimes, much longer (Fig. 18.33). Cells often united in chains resembling streptococci. Depending on the culture conditions, strains may produce slime. Color of individual cells light green, color of cell suspensions green. Major photosynthetic pigments are bacteriochlorophyll *c* (occasionally *d*) and carotenoid chlorobactene.

Photoautotrophic growth occurs with sulfide and sulfur; molecular hydrogen may be used as additional electron donor. In the presence of sulfide and bicarbonate, acetate or propionate are photoassimilated;

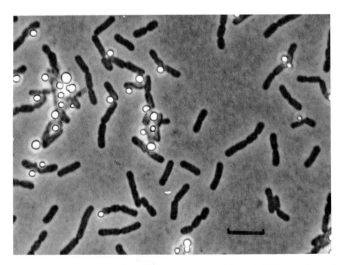

Figure 18.33. *C. limicola* f. sp. *thiosulfatophilum* DSM 249 cultured photoautotrophically with sulfide. Globules of elemental sulfur are outside the cells. Phase-contrast micrograph. *Bar*, 5 μm.

some strains may assimilate pyruvate, glutamate and fructose. Not utilized: thiosulfate, ethanol, succinate, butyrate or higher fatty acids. Nitrogen source: ammonium salts. Vitamin B_{12} may be required for growth. pH range: 6.5–7.0; optimum pH: 6.8. Growth temperature: 25–35°C. Habitat: mud and water of ditches, ponds and lakes with stagnant freshwater containing hydrogen sulfide and exposed to light.

The mol% G + C of the DNA of the neotype strain is 51.0 (Bd).

Neotype strain: DSM 245 (strain 6330, Gilroy Hot Spring).

1a. Chlorobium limicola f. sp. **thiosulfatophilum** (Larsen 1952) Pfennig and Trüper 1971, 14.

thi.o.sul.fa.to′phi.lum. M.L. n. *thiosulfatum* thiosulfate; Gr. adj. *philus* loving; M.L. adj. *thiosulfatophilum* thiosulfate-loving.

Description is the same as for *C. limicola*, except that thiosulfate is utilized as photosynthetic electron donor.

The mol% G + C of the DNA of the neotype strain is 58.1 (Bd).

Neotype strain: DSM 249 (strain 6230, Tassajara).

2. Chlorbium vibrioforme Pelsh 1936, 63.[AL]

vi.bri.o.for′me. L. v. *vibro* vibrate; M.L. n. *vibrio* that which vibrates, a generic name; L. adj. suff. *-formis* -like, of the shape of; M.L. neut. adj. *vibrioforme* of vibrio shape.

Cells curved rod-, C- or vibrioid-shaped, 0.5–0.7 μm wide and 1–2 μm long. In natural habitats and under unfavorable culture conditions, ringlike chains of cells occur which may extend into coils or helical filaments (Fig. 18.34). Color of individual cells light green, color of cell suspensions green. Major photosynthetic pigments are bacteriochlorophyll *d* (occasionally *c*) and carotenoid chlorobactene.

Photoautotrophic growth occurs with sulfide and sulfur; molecular hydrogen may be used as additional electron donor. In the presence of sulfide and bicarbonate, acetate or propionate may be photoassimilated. Not utilized: thiosulfate, ethanol, succinate and higher fatty acids. Nitrogen sources: ammonium salts. Most strains require vitamin B_{12} for growth and at least 1% NaCl. pH range: 6.5–7.3. Growth temperature: 25–35°C. Habitat: mud and stagnant water of anoxic marine and brackish water environments with hydrogen sulfide.

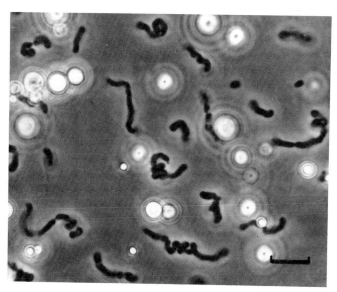

Figure 18.34. *C. vibrioforme* DSM 260 cultured photoautotrophically at high sulfide concentration (5 mM). The bacterium formed more or less coiled chains of cells; large extracellular sulfur globules are also seen. Phase-contrast micrograph. *Bar*, 5 μm.

The mol% G + C of the DNA of the neotype strain is 53.5 (Bd).
Neotype strain: DSM 260 (strain 6030, Moss Landing).

2a. Chlorobium vibrioforme f. sp. thiosulfatophilum (Larsen 1952) Pfennig and Trüper 1971, 14.

thi.o.sul.fa.to′phi.lum. M.L. n. *thiosulfatum* thiosulfate; Gr. adj. *philus* loving; M.L. adj. *thiosulfatophilum* thiosulfate-loving.

Description is the same as for *C. vibrioforme*, except that thiosulfate is utilized as photosynthetic electron donor.

The mol% G + C of the DNA of the type strain is 53.5 (Bd).
Type strain: DSM 265 (strain 1930, Sehestedt).

3. Chlorobium chlorovibrioides Gorlenko, Chebotarev and Kachalkin 1974, 908.[AL] (See also Puchkova and Gorlenko, 1982.)

chlo.ro.vi.bri.o.i′des. Gr. adj. *chlorus* green, greenish yellow; L. v. *vibro* vibrate; M.L. masc. n. *vibrio* that which vibrates, a generic name; Gr. n. *eidus* form, shape; M.L. adj. *chlorovibrioides* green, vibrioshaped.

Cells curved rod- or vibrioid-shaped, 0.3–0.4 μm wide and 0.4–0.8 μm long; in stationary phase, short rod-shaped to spherical. Color of cell suspensions bright green. Major photosynthetic pigments are bacteriochlorophyll *d* and carotenoid chlorobactene.

Photoautotrophic growth occurs with sulfide and sulfur. In the presence of sulfide and bicarbonate, formate, acetate and propionate are photoassimilated. Not utilized: thiosulfate, methanol, ethanol and glutamate. Ammonium salts are used as nitrogen source. NaCl of 2–3% is required for optimal growth. Vitamin B$_{12}$ is required. Optimum pH: 6.8. Growth temperature: 20–30°C. Habitat: The bacterium thrives planktonic in sulfide-containing stagnant water of meromictic Lake Repnoye, Lake Pomyaretskoye and others (U.S.S.R.).

The mol% G + C of the DNA of the type strain is 54 ± 0.3.
Type strain: DMS 1377 (strain PM-1, Pomyaretskoye).

4. Chlorobium phaeobacteroides Pfennig 1968, 225.[AL]

phae.o.bac.te.ro.i′des. Gr. adj. *phaeus* brown; Gr. neut. n. *bakterion* rod; Gr. n. *eidus* form, shape; M.L. adj. *phaeobacteroides* brown, rod-shaped.

Cells straight or slightly curved rod-shaped, 0.6–0.8 μm wide and 1.3–2.7 μm long or, sometimes, longer. Color of individual cells light yellowish brown, color of cell suspensions yellowish- to reddish-brown or chocolate-brown. Major photosynthetic pigments are bacteriochlorophyll *e* and carotenoid isorenieratene (Schmidt, 1978).

Photoautotrophic growth occurs with sulfide and sulfur; molecular hydrogen may be used as additional electron donor. In the presence of sulfide and bicarbonate, acetate or fructose are photoassimilated. Not utilized: thiosulfate, alcohols, pyruvate, propionate and higher fatty acids. Nitrogen source: ammonium salts. Strains from brackish water habitats may require at least 1% NaCl. Vitamin B$_{12}$ required for growth. pH range: 6.5–7.3. Growth temperature: 20–30°C. Habitat: hydrogen sulfide-containing stagnant water of ponds and lakes, frequently occurring in the upper hypolimnion of freshwater or meromictic lakes (Trüper and Genovese, 1968).

The mol% G + C of the DNA of the type strain is 49.0 (Bd).
Type stain: DSM 66 (strain 2430, Blankvann).

5. Chlorobium phaeovibrioides Pfennig 1968, 226.[AL]

phae.o.vi.bri.o′i.des. Gr. adj. *phaeus* brown; L. v. *vibro* vibrate; M.L. masc. n. *vibrio* that which vibrates, a generic name; Gr. n. *eidus* form, shape; M.L. adj. *phaeovibrioides* brown, vibrio-shaped.

Cells curved rod- to vibrioid-shaped, 0.3–0.4 μm wide and 0.7–1.4 μm long (Fig. 18.35). Under certain conditions, cells remain attached and grow into more or less wound coils and spirals. Color of cells light yellowish-brown, color of cell suspensions yellowish- to reddish-brown or chocolate-brown. Major photosynthetic pigments are bacteriochlorophyll *e* and carotenoid chlorobactene.

Photoautotrophic growth occurs with sulfide and sulfur; in the presence of sulfide and bicarbonate, acetate and propionate are photoassimilated. Not utilized: thiosulfate. Ammonium salts used as nitrogen source. Brackish water and marine strains require at least 1% NaCl. Vitamin B$_{12}$ required for growth. pH range: 6.5–7.3. Growth temperature: 20–30°C. Habitat: mud and stagnant water of anoxic marine and brackish water environments with hydrogen sulfide; hypolimnion of meromictic lakes.

The mol% G + C of the DNA of the type strain is 53.0 (Bd).
Type strain: DSM 269 (strain 2631, Langvikvann).

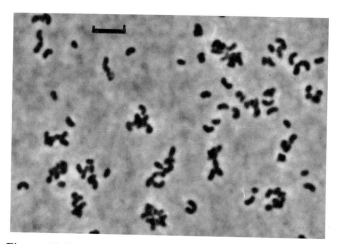

Figure 18.35. *C. phaeovibrioides* DSM 269 cultured photoautotrophically with sulfide. Vibrioid- and half-circle-shaped cells are present. Phase-contrast micrograph. *Bar*, 3 μm.

Genus **Prosthecochloris** Gorlenko 1970, 148[AL]

VLADIMIR M. GORLENKO

Pros.the′co.chlo′ris. Gr. n. *prostheca* appendage; Gr. adj. *chloros* green; M.L. fem. n. *Prosthecochloris* green (organism) with appendages.

Spherical to ovoid bacteria forming nonbranching prosthecae and multiplying by **binary fission** in various directions. When separation is incomplete, cells form groups and branched chains, the configuration of which depends on the direction of fissions. **Nonmotile.** Gram-negative. Cell suspensions appear green or chocolate-brown. Cells **contain bacteriochlorophyll *c, d* or *e*,** as the major bacteriochlorophyll component, **and carotenoids.** The photosynthetic apparatus includes antenna structures, **chlorosomes,** i.e. elongated-ovoid vesicles underlying and attached to the cytoplasmic membrane. Cells do not contain gas vacuoles.

Anaerobic. Capable of photosynthesis in the presence of hydrogen sulfide, during which they produce and deposit, as an intermediate oxidation product, **elemental sulfur in the form of globules outside the cells** in the medium.

The mol% G + C of the DNA is 50.0–56.1 (T_m, Bd).

Type species: *Prosthecochloris aestuarii* Gorlenko 1970.

Further Descriptive Information

Two known species, *P. aestuarii* (Gorlenko, 1968; Gorlenko, 1970) and *P. phaeoasteroidea* (Puchkova and Gorlenko, 1976), are identical morphologically (Figs. 18.36–18.38). Cells rigid, ovoid and 0.3–0.6 × 0.5–0.8 µm; form 10–20 prosthecae with rounded, occasionally thickened ends. Prosthecae are 0.1–0.16 µm wide and 0.07–0.3 µm long. Cells are enclosed in a thin slimy capsule. Considerable slime formation was reported in *P. aestuarii* (Gorlenko and Zhilina, 1968). Multiplication by binary fission. The daughter cell is sometimes considerably smaller than the mother cell. Mother and daughter cells remain connected for some time by one or two thin filaments which subsequently form prosthecae of new cells. The direction of fission is random. When separation is incomplete, cells form branched chains. The length of prosthecae in *P. phaeoasteroidea* was shown to depend on the light conditions of incubation; longer prosthecae are formed under low light intensities.

Ultrastructure of cells is typical of green sulfur bacteria (Gorlenko and Zhilina, 1968). The cell wall is of the Gram-negative type. The outer layer of the cell wall in *P. aestuarii* is assumed to take part in the excretion and holding of elemental sulfur near the cell. The chlorosomes underlie the cytoplasmic membrane and fill the prosthecae (Fig. 18.39). Gas vacuoles have never been observed.

In *P. aestuarii*, whose cell suspension appears green, the major pigment is bacteriochlorophyll *c* located predominantly in the chlorosomes (in vivo absorption maximum: 740–750 nm). Bacteriochlorophyll *a* (in vivo absorption maximum: 805 nm) is present in the reaction centers that are located in the cytoplasmic membrane. These centers also contain bacteriochlorophyll *c* and unidentified pigment P-665 which appears to be an unknown pheophytin. Since bacteriopheophytin *a* was not found in *P. aestuarii* (as distinct from *Chlorobium limicola*; Swarthof et al., 1982), P-665 instead of bacteriopheophytin *c* is assumed to serve as an acceptor in the photoreactions.

Green *P. aestuarii* strains contain two major carotenoids, chlorobactene (or its hydroxyl derivative) and rhodopin or lycopene (or its hydroxyl derivative). Three minor carotenoids are also present.

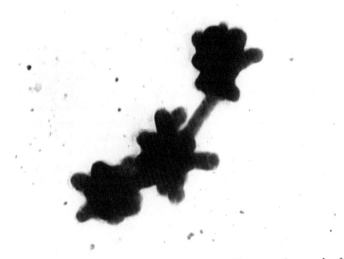

Figure 18.37. *P. aestuarii* strain SK-413. Electron micrograph of cells stained with phosphotungstic acid (× 20,000). (Reproduced with permission from N. N. Puchkova and V. M. Gorlenko, Mikrobiologiya *45:* 657, 1976.)

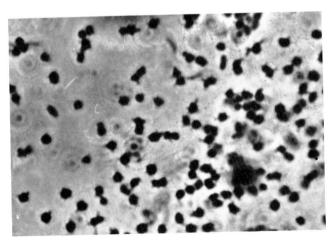

Figure 18.36. *P. aestuarii.* Phase-contrast micrograph (× 3500). (Reproduced with permission from N. N. Puchkova and V. M. Gorlenko, Mikrobiologiya *45:* 657, 1976.)

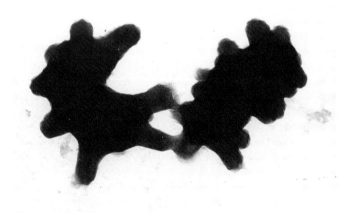

Figure 18.38. *P. phaeoasteroidea* strain MG-1. Electron micrograph of cells stained with phosphotungstic acid (× 22,000). (Reproduced with permission from N. N. Puchkova and V. M. Gorlenko, Mikrobiologiya *45:* 657, 1976.)

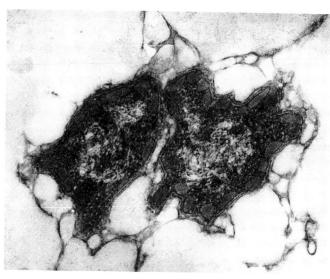

Figure 18.39. *P. aestuarii* strain SK-413. Electron micrograph of ultrathin section of cells fixed with OsO₄ (× 100,000). (Reproduced with permission from N. N. Puchkova, Mikrobiologiya *53:* 325, 1984.)

Brown *P. phaeoasteroidea* strains contain the major pigment bacteriochlorophyll *e* (in vivo absorption maximum: 713 nm) and the minor pigment bacteriochlorophyll *a* (in vivo absorption maximum: 805 nm). The major carotenoid is isorenieratene (in vivo absorption maximum: 523 nm; Puchkova and Gorlenko, 1976).

Species of the genus *Prosthecochloris* are strictly anaerobic and photolithotrophic. H_2S and S^0 are utilized as electron donors for photosynthesis. H_2S is oxidized to S^0 which is deposited extracellularly and then partly or fully oxidized to sulfate. Thiosulfate cannot be utilized as electron donor during photosynthesis. These cell cultures are capable of autotrophic growth with CO_2 (bicarbonate) as the sole carbon source and require vitamin B_{12}. In the presence of H_2S and CO_2, a number of organic compounds are assimilated; acetate and pyruvate are utilized by the majority of strains.

Since these cells are moderately halophilic, growth is possible with NaCl concentrations ranging from 0.2 to 10% NaCl (optimum salinity: 0.5–2% NaCl). Some strains of *P. aestuarii* are able to develop in the presence of up to 20% NaCl, with an optimum at 4% NaCl (Puchkova, 1984).

Subsurface colonies in 0.8% agar medium appear as uneven lumps, easily distinguishable from colonies of other species of green sulfur bacteria.

Ammonium salts are used as nitrogen source. Brown *P. phaeoasteroidea* also utilize glutamate or casein hydrolysate; nitrate and asparagine are not utilized.

The salt tolerance of *Prosthecochloris* strains correlates with their tolerance for sulfide (maximum: up to 2 g/l; optimum: 500–700 mg $Na_2S·9H_2O/l$) and their ability to live under high light intensities (up to

10,000 lx), i.e. they are eurysulfidophilic and euryphotophilic (Matheron and Baulaigue, 1972; Puchkova, 1984).

The two species occupy different ecological niches. Among the green *P. aestuarii*, benthic forms are typical inhabitants of shallow marine environments, whereas these forms are found less frequently in meromictic saline water bodies. The cells occur in microzones below purple sulfur bacteria under strictly anaerobic conditions up to 300 mg H_2S/l, pH 7.0–7.8, E_h −185 mV, 1.5–18% NaCl and 15–40°C. *P. aestuarii* has been isolated from different parts of the globe: a region of the White Sea, the Arkhangel'sk region, saline waters of the Crimean Peninsula, and coastal areas of France.

Among the brown *P. phaeoasteroidea*, the planktonic form develops in the metalimnion-hypolimnion of saline meromictic lakes of marine origin (Lake Mogil'noe, Island Kil'din, Barents Sea; Lake Faro, Sicily; Mediterranean Sea) (Gorlenko et al., 1976). Parameters of habitat: 10–40 mg H_2S/l, pH 6.5–7.5, E_h −50–240 mV, 3–3.5% NaCl, 10–15°C and a depth of occurrence of 10–13 m.

Enrichment and Isolation Procedures

P. aestuarii often occurs in the hydrogen sulfide-containing mud of shallow saline water bodies (Matheron and Baulaigue, 1972; Puchkova, 1984). It can be isolated by direct inoculation of a mud sample with dilutions into 0.8% agar medium of Pfennig (1965) (or the medium for *Chlorobium,* discussed on page 1684) containing the following: NaCl, 2%; $Na_2S·9H_2O$, 700–1500 mg/l; NH_4-acetate, 400 mg/l (instead of NH_4Cl, 330 mg/l); and vitamin B_{12}, 20 μg/l. Green colonies of *P. aestuarii* are: (a) lumpy, of typical olive green, with an uneven surface, and easily distinguishable from smaller diffuse colonies of *C. chlorovibrioides* and (b) brighter, flat, dense, often lens-shaped colonies of *C. vibrioforme.* Colonies of *P. luteolum* are distinguished from the latter by their greater transparency and emerald color.

Enrichment of *P. aestuarii* occurs when mud columns are exposed to diffused daylight. After growth of green bacteria in water or on the mud surface becomes evident, a sample is inoculated into agar medium of Pfennig. Isolated colonies are purified by repeated application of the agar shake dilution method. When a pure culture is obtained, a single colony is transferred into liquid medium of Pfennig and incubated in screw-capped glass bottles in a luminostat at 25–35°C and a light intensity of 500–2000 lx.

Brown *P. phaeoasteroidea* are enriched and purified in the same way as described for *P. aestuarii.*

In enrichment cultures containing brown strains of several species of green sulfur bacteria during prolonged storage in the dark, *Chlorobium phaeovibrioides* and *Pelodictyon phaeum* die out first, and thus a predominance of *Prosthecochloris phaeoasteroidea* can be obtained. Colonies of the latter in 0.8% agar are similar to those of *Prosthecochloris aestuarii* but appear dark brown. They are easily distinguishable by shape and color from other brown strains of green sulfur bacteria.

Maintenance Procedures

Prosthecochloris can be maintained in liquid cultures if transferred every 2–3 months. Grown cultures are stored at 4°C and very low light intensity.

Differentiation of the genus **Prosthecochloris** from other genera

The genus *Prosthecochloris* morphologically differs from other genera of green sulfur bacteria. The presence of short prosthecae with thickened ends and the absence of gas vacuoles differentiate it from the genera *Chlorobium, Pelodictyon* and *Ancalochloris.* The latter genus also possesses prosthecae, but the cells contain gas vacuoles. The shape and the number of prosthecae are different in *Ancalochloris* than in representatives of *Prosthecochloris.*

Taxonomic Comments

Studies on the genetic relationships of the species of *Prosthecochloris* with other green sulfur bacteria are lacking.

Differentiation of the species of the genus **Prosthecochloris**

Two species are recognized in the genus *Prosthecochloris*. The major differentiating characteristics are:

1. Cultures and cell material green, major photosynthetic pigments bacteriochlorophyll *c* and carotenoid chlorobactene.

                1. *P. aestuarii*

2. Cultures and cell material brown, major photosynthetic pigments bacteriochlorophyll *e* and carotenoid isorenieratene.

                2. *P. phaeoasteroidea*

List of species of the genus **Prosthecochloris**

1. **Prosthecochloris aestuarii** Gorlenko 1970, 148.[AL]

aes.tu.a′rii. L. n. *aestuarium* estuary; M.L. gen. n. *aestuarii* of the estuary.

Cells appear spherical after division and elongated before division, measuring 0.5–0.7 × 1.0–1.2 μm, and form 10–20 prosthecae/cell (Figs. 18.36 and 18.37). Ends of prosthecae are rounded and slightly thickened. Prosthecae are 0.1–0.17 μm wide; their length rarely exceeds the cell diameter and corresponds to 0.1– 0.25 μm. Cells are enclosed in slimy microcapsules.

Slimy strands are observed between divided cells. Multiplication is by binary fission; unequal division is possible. The direction of fission is random. Sister cells can be connected by one or more filaments which subsequently form new prosthecae. Incomplete separation results in formation of branched chains.

Strictly anaerobic, obligately phototrophic. Sulfide and elemental sulfur are utilized as electron donors for photosynthesis. Thiosulfate is not utilized. Cells photoassimilate simple organic compounds, acetate or pyruvate, only in the presence of sulfide and CO_2. Optimum pH: 6.7–7.0. Cells grow in 1–8% NaCl (optimum salinity: 2–5% NaCl). Color of liquid culture varies from intensive green to grayish-green. Following precipitation of elemental sulfur, the medium becomes milky turbid.

Vitamin B_{12} is required for growth. Sulfide is required as a sulfur source for biosynthesis.

The major photosynthetic pigment is bacteriochlorophyll *c*; the minor photosynthetic pigment is bacteriochlorophyll *a*. The carotenoids are chlorobactene, rhodopene or lycopene or their hydroxyl derivatives. Ammonium salts are utilized as nitrogen source.

Habitat: hydrogen sulfide-containing mud of shallow bodies of water with up to 18% NaCl.

The mol% G + C of the DNA is 52.0–56.1 (T_m, Bd).

Type strain: SK-413, INMI.

2. **Prosthecochloris phaeoasteroidea** Puchkova and Gorlenko 1976, 658.

phae′o.as.te.ro.i.de′a. Gr. adj. *phaeus* brown; Gr. adj. *asteroides* star-shaped; M.L. adj. *phaeoasteroidea* brown, star-shaped.

Morphology of the cells is similar to that of *P. aestuarii*; the size of the cell is 0.5–0.6 × 0.5–1.2 μm; the number of prosthecae are 10–20, and the prosthecae are 0.13–0.16 μm wide and 0.07–0.3 μm long. Slimy strands are absent (Fig. 18.38).

Color of cell suspensions varies from dark brown to chocolate-brown. Colonies in 0.8% agar are dark brown, lumpy and uneven.

The major pigment component is bacteriochlorophyll *e*; bacteriochlorophyll *a* is present in small amounts. The major carotenoid is isorenieratene.

Photoassimilate acetate, pyruvate, lactate, malate, fumarate, fructose, mannitol, glutamate and casein hydrolyzate in the presence of H_2S and CO_2. Do not utilize citrate, succinate, propionate, valerate, methanol, ethanol, glycerol, glucose, malonate, glycolate and asparagine.

Optimum pH for growth: 7.0; pH range: 6.0–7.5. Salinity range: 0.2–7.0% NaCl; optimum salinity: 0.5–2% NaCl.

Ammonium salts, casein hydrolysate or glutamate can be used as nitrogen source. Not utilized are nitrate and asparagine.

Habitat: the anoxic monimolimnion of meromictic saline lakes of marine origin. Depth of occurrence: 10–13 m; NaCl concentration: 3–3.5%; H_2S concentration: 10–40 mg/l.

The mol% G + C of the DNA is 52.2 (± 0.8) (chem. anal.).

Type strain: MG-1 (Lake Mogil'noe, Island Kil'din, Barents Sea), INMI.

Genus **Pelodictyon** Lauterborn 1913, 98 [AL]

NORBERT PFENNIG

Pe.lo.dic′ty.on. Gr. adj. *pelos* dark-colored; Gr. n. *dictyon* net; M.L. neut. n. *Pelodictyon* dark-colored net.

Cells rod-shaped to ovoid, occurring singly or in netlike or more or less spherical aggregates. Multiplication by binary fission. **Branching may occur as a result of ternary fission. Nonmotile. Gram-negative. Cells regularly contain gas vacuoles. Cultures or cell material is either green or brown. Photosynthetic pigments are located in the cytoplasmic membrane and the chlorosomes** which underlie and are attached to the cytoplasmic membrane. Bacteriochlorophyll *c*, *d* or *e* occurs as the major photosynthetic pigment, in addition to small amounts of bacteriochlorophyll *a*. Chlorobactene or isorenieratene is the major carotenoid component (Schmidt and Schiburr, 1970; Gorlenko, 1972).

Obligately anaerobic and phototrophic. Photoautotrophic growth with sulfide or sulfur as electron donor. During sulfide oxidation, globules of elemental sulfur are formed outside the cells; the sulfur may be further oxidized to sulfate. In the presence of reduced sulfur compounds and bicarbonate, a number of simple organic substrates may be photoassimilated. Growth temperature: 15–30°C. Habitat: hydrogen sulfide-containing water and mud of freshwater, brackish water and marine environments.

The mol% G + C of the DNA is 48.5–58.1 (Bd) (Mandel et al., 1971).

Type species: *Pelodictyon clathratiforme* (Szafer) Lauterborn 1913, 98.

Further Descriptive Information

The genus *Pelodictyon* was introduced by Lauterborn as a green sulfur bacterium that may form distinctive cell aggregate structures reminiscent of those found in the purple sulfur bacterium *Thiodictyon* and the green alga *Hydrodictyon*. In *Pelodictyon clathratiforme*, the rod-shaped cells are united into more or less large three-dimensional nets. Characteristically, the cells contain gas vacuoles which confer buoyancy to the cell aggregates. Two green strains of *P. clathratiforme* free of other phototrophic bacteria were obtained in laboratory cultures and characterized in detail (Pfennig and Cohen-Bazire, 1967). The microscopic study of various anoxic water samples collected from blooms of phototrophic sulfur bacteria in sulfide-containing ponds and lakes revealed the existence of a brown species with the same morphology as the green *P. clathratiforme* (Pfennig, 1977). So far, the brown strains have not been studied in pure culture.

Another gas vacuole-containing green sulfur bacterium which may form spherical or irregular round colonies (*Schmidlea luteola* Lauterborn 1913) was classified in the genus *Pelodictyon (P. luteolum)* by Pfennig and Trüper (1971). The third species of the genus *Pelodictyon* is a gas-vacuolate, brown sulfur bacterium, *P. phaeum* (Gorlenko, 1972). Thus, the genus *Pelodictyon* comprises the straight or curved rod-shaped, gas vacuole-containing green and brown species of the green sulfur bacteria group.

Although the species of the genera *Chlorobium* and *Pelodictyon* are physiologically and biochemically fairly similar, the possession of gas vacuoles in the latter genus is ecologically rather significant. The gas-vacuolated *Pelodictyon* species are buoyant because of their gas vesicles. Consequently, these species occur predominantly planktonic in sulfide-containing stagnant bodies of water in which they may exhibit a selective advantage over *Chlorobium* species.

Enrichment and Isolation Procedures

Enrichments for green or brown *Pelodictyon* species may be unsuccessful when liquid culture media are applied. Under laboratory conditions, such enrichments are readily outgrown by *Chlorobium* species. Isolations are more successful, therefore, if agar shake cultures are prepared directly from the natural sample in which cells of this genus

had been detected microscopically. Because of the presence of gas vacuoles, the colonies of *Pelodictyon* species maintain a chalky appearance (compared with that of *Chlorobium* colonies) even if the intermediarily formed elemental sulfur is consumed. The liquid culture medium and the agar shake dilution method are carried out in the same way as described for the isolation of *Chlorobium* species. Not more than 1.5-2 mM sulfide and 3 mM acetate are added to the medium; the light intensity should be limited to 50-200 lx from a tungsten lamp. The cultures are incubated at about 20°C (Pfennig and Cohen-Bazire, 1967). Before second agar shake dilution tubes are inoculated with suspensions of green or brown colonies isolated from the first dilution series, the cells are microscopically checked for the presence of gas vacuoles. Only cell suspensions of gas-vacuolated cells are cultivated further. The three-dimensional cell aggregates characteristic of some species may develop only in liquid culture media and dependent on the culture conditions.

Maintenance Procedures

The methods are the same as described for the genus *Chlorobium* (page 1684).

Taxonomic Comments

Our knowledge on the green sulfur bacteria presently grouped in the genus *Pelodictyon* is extremely limited. In order to establish a reliable taxonomy, the detailed study of more pure cultures is required. In addition, the genetic relationships within the genera of the green sulfur bacteria have to be established by RNA oligonucleotide catalogs as well as DNA/DNA hybridization studies.

Differentiation of the species of the genus **Pelodictyon**

The phenotypic traits presently used to differentiate the species of the genus *Pelodictyon* are listed in Table 18.18.

List of species of the genus **Pelodictyon**

1. **Pelodictyon clathratiforme** (Szafer 1911) Lauterborn 1913, 98.[AL] (*Aphanothece clathratiformis* Szafer 1911, 162.)

clath.ra.ti.for'me. L. part. adj. *clathratus* latticed; L. n. *forma* shape, form; M.L. neut. adj. *clathratiforme* latticelike.

Cells are rod-shaped, 0.7–1.2 μm wide and 1.5–2.5 μm long, although elongated cells up to 7 μm long may occur. Cells are characteristically united in three-dimensional nets which are formed as follows (Fig. 18.40): Successive binary fissions result in the formation of chains of cells. Occasionally, two adjacent cells in such a chain change their mode of growth. The contiguous poles start to branch simultaneously, resulting in the formation, in the middle of the chain, of two Y-shaped cells, in opposition at the ends of both arms of the Y. If these two cells do not separate, the ring structure between them enlarges, by subsequent cell elongation and binary fission, into a typical many-celled mesh. The arrangement of cells at the branch points of fully formed nets implies that these cells eventually undergo ternary fission to yield three daughter cells, all in apposition at one pole. The colonial structure of *P. clathratiforme* is therefore caused by its ability to perform both binary and ternary fissions (Pfennig and Cohen-Bazire, 1967).

Color of individual cells light green, of cell suspensions green. Major photosynthetic pigments are bacteriochlorophyll *c* and carotenoids of group 5.

Photoautotrophic growth occurs with sulfide and sulfur; in their presence, acetate is photoassimilated. Not utilized: thiosulfate, pyruvate, succinate and higher fatty acids. Ammonium salts serve as nitrogen source. pH range: 6.5–7.0. Growth temperature: 15–25°C. Only partially purified cultures exist.

2. **Pelodictyon luteolum** (Schidle 1901) Pfennig and Trüper 1971, 13.[AL] (*Aphanothece luteola* Schidle 1901, 179.)

lu.te'o.lum L. adj. *luteus* yellow; L. dim. adj. *luteolus* yellowish, somewhat yellow.

Cells straight or curved short rod-shaped, 0.6–0.9 μm wide and 1.2–2.0 μm long. Strains of larger cells (1.0–1.2 μm wide, 2–4 μm long) do occur. Pure cultures may contain free individual cells (Fig. 18.41); under certain conditions, the cells produce slime and are united into hollow spherical or irregular round colonies with the cells in a single layer (Fig. 18.42). The latter growth forms are occasionally observed in

Table 18.18.
Characteristics of the species of the genus **Pelodictyon**[a]

Characteristic	1. *P. clathratiforme*	2. *P. luteolum*	3. *P. phaeum*
Gas vacuoles	+	+	+
Cells or cell suspensions green	+	+	−
Cells or cell suspensions brown	−	−	+
Cells rod-shaped, binary and ternary fission, cells in netlike structures	+	−	−
Cells rod-shaped or ovoid, singly or in round colonies	−	+	−
Cells straight or curved rod-shaped, singly or in chains or aggregates	−	−	+

[a] Symbols: +, positive; −, negative.

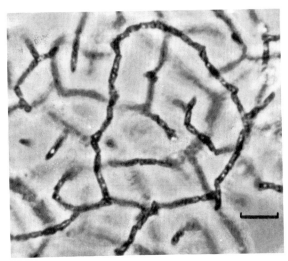

Figure 18.40. *P. clathratiforme* strain 1831 grown photoautotrophically with sulfide. Gas vacuole-containing cells are united in three-dimensional netlike structures. Phase-contrast micrograph. *Bar,* 5 μm.

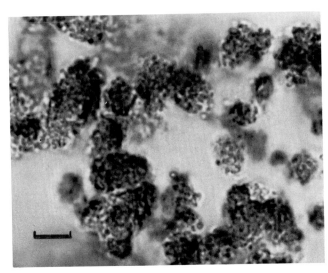

Figure 18.42. *P. luteolum* strain 2532 grown photoautotrophically with sulfide. Cells are united in irregular round colonies. Phase-contrast micrograph. *Bar,* 5 μm.

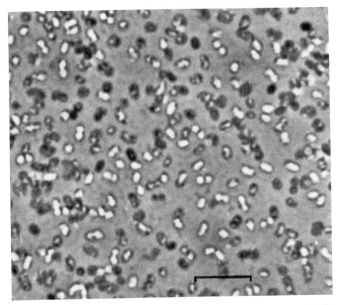

Figure 18.41. *P. luteolum* strain 2532 grown photoautotrophically with sulfide. The *light areas* inside the cells are the gas vacuoles. Phase-contrast micrograph. *Bar,* 5 μm.

mud samples or enrichment cultures. Color of cells or cell suspensions green. Major photosynthetic pigments are bacteriochlorophyll *c* or *d* and carotenoid chlorobactene (Schmidt and Schiburr, 1970).

Photoautotrophic growth with sulfide and sulfur. In the presence of sulfide and bicarbonate, acetate and propionate are photoassimilated. Not utilized: thiosulfate, pyruvate, succinate, higher fatty acids or peptone. Reduced sulfur compounds are required as a source of cell sulfur. Ammonium salts are used as nitrogen source. Strains from habitats with seawater require at least 1% NaCl in the medium. pH range: 6.5–7.0. Growth temperature: 15–25°C.

The mol% G + C of the neotype strain is 58.1 (Bd).

Neotype strain: DSM 273 (strain 2530, Polden).

3. **Pelodictyon phaeum** Gorlenko 1972, 370.[AL]

phae′um. Gr. adj. *phaeus* brown; M.L. neut. adj. *phaeum* brown.

Cells are straight or curved short rod-shaped, 0.6–0.9 μm wide and 1.0–2.0 μm long, and occur either as single cells or as coiled chains of cells or irregularly shaped cell aggregates embedded in slime. Color of cell suspensions is chocolate-brown. Major photosynthetic pigments are baceriochlorophyll *e* and carotenoid isorenieratene.

Photoautotrophic growth occurs with sulfide and sulfur; in their presence, acetate is photoassimilated. Not utilized: thiosulfate. Ammonium salts serve as nitrogen source. Vitamin B₁₂ required for growth. Optimum NaCl concentration: 3%. Optimum pH: 7.0. Growth temperature: 25°C.

Type strain: DSM 728 (strain WS-6, Lake Veisovo).

Genus **Ancalochloris** Gorlenko and Lebedeva 1971, 1038[AL]

VLADIMIR M. GORLENKO

An.ca′lo.chlo′ris. Gr. masc. n. *ancalos* arm; Gr. adj. *chloros* green; M.L. neut. n. *Ancalochloris* arm (-producing) green (microbe).

Bacteria of irregular shape, forming prosthecae of irregular length, wide at the base and pointed at the end (Fig. 18.43). The length of prosthecae can exceed the cell diameter. These bacteria **multiply by unequal fission** and form irregular chains of cells and typical perforated microcolonies. **Nonmotile. Gram-negative. Contain bacteriochlorophylls and carotenoid pigments.** The photosynthetic apparatus includes antenna structures of the **chlorosome** type and ovoid vesicles underlying and attached to the cytoplasmic membrane (Figs. 18.43 and 18.44). Cells **contain gas vacuoles.**

Anaerobic. Capable of photosynthesis in the presence of hydrogen sulfide. **Sulfur is deposited extracellularly.** Cell material and cultures appear **green or yellowish green** due to the photosynthetic pigments.

The mol% G + C of the DNA is not known.

Type species: *Ancalochloris perfilievii* Gorlenko and Lebedeva 1971, 1038.

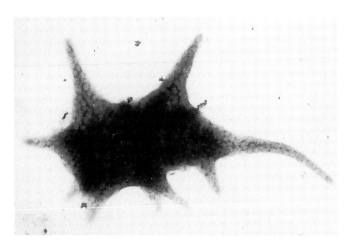

Figure 18.43. *A. perfilievii* from a water sample of the hypolimnion of meromictic Lake Bol'shoi, Kichier (U.S.S.R.). Electron micrograph of a single cell stained with phosphotungstic acid (× 30,000).

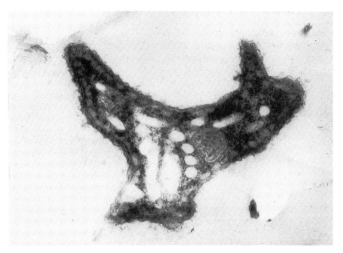

Figure 18.44. *A. perfilievii* from water samples of dimictic Lake Glukhaya Lamba. Electron micrograph of ultrathin section (× 50,000).

Further Descriptive Information

Cells are 0.5–1.0 μm wide, of irregular starlike shape due to the formation of several appendages with tapering ends (prosthecae) up to 2 μm long. Prosthecae are often as wide at the base as the cell but can also be of smaller diameter. Gas vacuoles are present in the central part of cells and consist of elongated gas vesicles measuring 40–80 × 230–360 nm.

These bacteria occur in nature as typical conglomerates consisting of 10–30 cells; less frequently, they have been observed as short chains of cells with long prosthecae. The length of the prosthecae depends on the growth conditions. The longer prosthecae are observed at low light intensity in the habitat of *Ancalochloris*.

Multiplication is unequal, division proceeds by constriction. Prosthecae between cells were not observed. Prosthecae are formed by local polar growth of the cell wall together with the cytoplasmic membrane. Additional chlorosomes are synthesized in emerging prosthecae. The process of prostheca formation resembles budding, but ultrathin sections of prosthecae do not reveal DNA filaments. Prosthecae may branch.

Ancalochloris is widely distributed in the anoxic hypolimnion of dimictic and meromictic freshwater lakes with low H_2S content (1–60 mg/l) at low light intensity at depths down to 10 m.

Enrichment and Isolation Procedures

Enrichment cultures can be obtained by using the same culture medium as described for *Chlorobium* (see page 1684) with a low H_2S content (300 mg $Na_2S \cdot 9H_2O$/l) (pH 6.8–7.0). Samples are incubated at low light intensity (100–200 lx) and at temperatures between 18 and 20°C. Vitamin B_{12} (20 μg/l) should be added. Pure culture isolation should be tried by dilution in liquid media, since *Ancalochloris* does not grow in agar shake dilution media.

Maintenance Procedures

Ancalochloris can be maintained in liquid cultures if transferred every 2–3 months. Grown cultures are stored at 4°C and very low light intensity.

Differentiation of the genus **Ancalochloris** from other genera

The genus *Ancalochloris* is characterized by the starlike shape of the cells and the possession of gas vesicles. The prosthecae differ from those of *Prosthecochloris* by their greater length and tapering ends.

Taxonomic Comments

The study of pure cultures is required to clarify the systematic position of *Ancalochloris* and its relationships to other genera of the green sulfur bacteria.

List of species of the genus **Ancalochloris**

1. **Ancalochloris perfilievii** Gorlenko and Lebedeva 1971, 1038.[AL]
per.fi'lie.vi.i. M.L. gen. n. *perfilievii* of Perfil'ev; named for B. V. Perfil'ev, a Russian microbiologist.

Cells of irregular starlike shape, 0.5–1 μm in diameter, without the prosthecae. One cell forms up to 6 prosthecae of varying length up to 2 μm long (Fig. 18.43). The length of prosthecae varies with the conditions of incubation. Prosthecae have tapering ends, 0.1 μm wide at the end and up to 0.7 μm wide at the base; sometimes, prosthecae are branched. Gas vacuoles are located in the center of the cells.

Multiplication by unequal fission. The direction of fission is random. Microcolonies are of irregular shape and comprise up to 30 cells. The peripheral cells of the microcolonies may have longer prosthecae than do cells in the center.

The chlorosomes of the photosynthetic apparatus are 70–85 nm long and 45–80 nm wide; they may occupy a large part of the prosthecae (Figs. 18.43 and 18.44).

Habitat: the anoxic metalimnion or hypolimnion of dimictic and meromictic lakes with low H_2S content.

Genus **Chloroherpeton** Gibson, Pfennig and Waterbury 1985, 223[VP] (Effective publication: Gibson, Pfennig and Waterbury 1984, 100)

J. GIBSON

Chlo.ro.her′pe.ton. Gr. adj. *chloros* green; Gr. n. *herpeton* a creeping organism; M.L. neut. n. *Chloroherpeton* green creeping organism.

Long rods, 8–20 × ~1 μm. Cells separate promptly after division, and no septa are seen in each unit (Figs. 18.45 and 18.46). Cells tend to grow in clumps and produce some extracellular slime. Gram-negative. **Gliding motility,** ~10 μm min⁻¹ at 20°C. **Cells flex** through up to 180°.

Cultures and cell material are green. **Photosynthetic pigments are located in the cytoplasmic membrane and chlorosomes** which underlie and are attached to the cytoplasmic membrane (Fig. 18.47);

bacteriochlorophyll *c* and γ-carotene are the main photosynthetic pigments.

Strictly anaerobic and obligately phototrophic. Sulfide and bicarbonate are required for growth. Growth yield slightly increased by acetate, propionate, malate, succinate or glutamate but not by glucose, fructose or casamino acids. During sulfide oxidation, **elemental sulfur is formed outside the cells** and only slowly oxidized further to sulfate. Optimum temperature: 25°C; maximum temperature: about 30°C. Optimum pH: 6.8–7.2.

The mol% G + C of the DNA is 45.0–48.2 (T_m).

Type species: *Chloroherpeton thalassium* Gibson, Pfennig and Waterbury 1985, 223.

Further Descriptive Information

The characteristic morphology of *Chloroherpeton* permits its identification in natural samples. It has been observed regularly on decaying vegetation and mud surfaces from littoral pools and channels on Cape Cod, Massachusetts (U.S.A.). Isolation has been achieved by repeated shake culture in medium containing 0.8% agar, which allows some cell gliding, so that the light green, fluffy colonies are clearly distinguishable from the smaller, darker and compact colonies of *Chlorobium* species. Specific enrichment conditions have not been found. *Chloroherpeton thalassium* isolates require 1–2% NaCl in the medium and do not tolerate more than 3 mM Na₂S; repeated sulfide additions must be made to obtain dense cultures in liquid medium. Vitamin B₁₂ is required for growth, and the culture appears yellow-orange instead of deep green after a single transfer without B₁₂ addition. Hydrogen can be used as electron donor, provided that small additions of sulfide are also made to serve as S source. Nitrogen fixation is indicated both by growth in the absence of ammonium and by acetylene reduction in suspensions incubated in light in the absence of NH₄⁺. The cells contain gas vesicles, which confer a characteristic banded appearance under phase-contrast optics. Electron micrographs of cross-sections or sagittal sections show chlorosomes of typical dimensions underlying the cytoplasmic membrane. The type species and four other isolates contain conical-ended gas vesicles; a single isolate (mol% G + C of 45.0) has never produced gas vesicles in culture.

The current isolates all contain bacteriochlorophyll *c* as the main light-harvesting pigment, together with a small quantity of bacteriochlorophyll *a* (*c:a* = ~50:1). More than 80% of the carotenoid is γ-carotene in the type species.

Acetate carbon appears in all cell fractions in proportions similar to

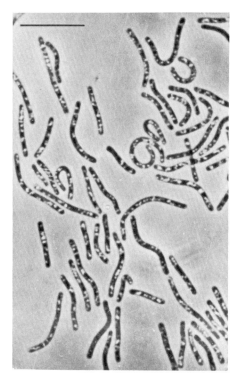

Figure 18.45. *C. thalassium* showing cell flexibility and refractive areas within the cells resulting from gas vacuoles. Phase-contrast photomicrograph. *Bar,* 10 μm. (Reproduced with permission from J. Gibson, N. Pfennig and J. B. Waterbury, Archives of Microbiology *138:* 96–101, 1984.)

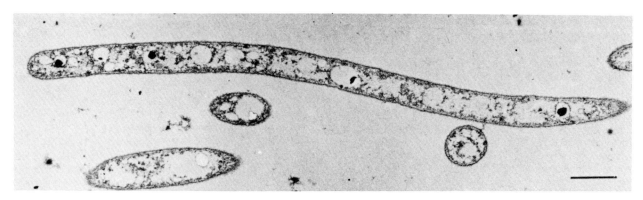

Figure 18.46. *C. thalassium* showing absence of cross-walls. Electron micrograph of a longitudinal thin section of a single cell. *Bar,* 1 μm.

(Reproduced with permission from J. Gibson, N. Pfennig and J. B. Waterbury, Archives of Microbiology *138:* 96–101, 1984.)

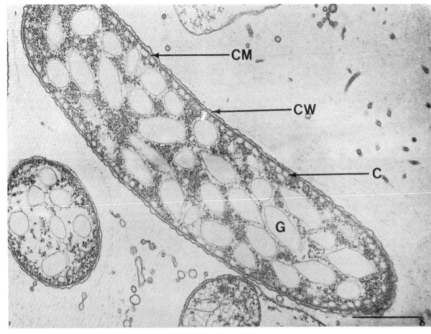

Figure 18.47. *C. thalassium.* Electron micrographs of thin cross-sections. *G*, vesicles: *C*, chlorosomes; *CW*, cell wall; *CM*, cytoplasmic membrane; *bar*, 0.5 μm. (Reproduced with permission from J. Gibson, N. Pfennig and J. B. Waterbury, Archives of Microbiology *138:* 96–101, 1984.)

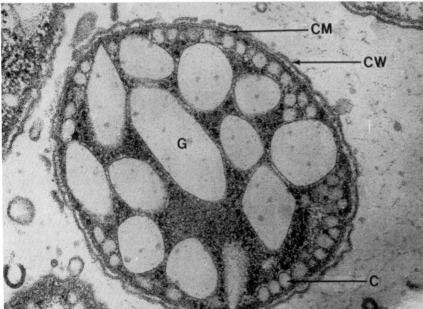

those found in *Chlorobium*. Ribulosebisphosphate carboxylase activity is not detectable (D. G. Nelson, personal communication), suggesting that the main carbon fixation reactions also correspond to those found in *Chlorobium* (Evans et al., 1966; Fuchs et al., 1980) rather than in *Chloroflexus* (Sirevåg and Castenholz, 1979).

Enrichment and Isolation Procedures

Samples of littoral marine muds·containing large quantities of decaying vegetation when brought into the laboratory and incubated in glass containers in dim light at 20–25°C will often develop green as well as red or purple patches on the container walls. *Chloroherpeton* may form a significant component of the microbial population of such green areas, especially those which appear first, and can be identified by its characteristic morphology. Isolation can be achieved by repeated shake cultures in medium that contains: NaCl, 170 mM; MgCl$_2$, 15 mM; KCl, 4 mM; CaCl$_2$, 1 mM; NH$_4$Cl, 5 mM; KH$_2$PO$_4$, 0.1 mM;

NaHCO$_3$, 30 mM; Na$_2$S, 2.5 mM; trace element mixture (Widdel and Pfennig, 1981); vitamin B$_{12}$, 0.05 μg 100 ml^{-1}; and 0.8% washed agar, pH 6.9. The inoculated tubes are sealed with a Vaseline:paraffin oil mixture (1:1) and incubated 50–100 cm from a 40-W incandescent lamp. Light green, fluffy colonies should appear within a week and are picked when they are 1–2 mm in diameter.

Maintenance Procedures

The cultures may be maintained illuminated in liquid culture as described above by additions of CO$_2$-neutralized Na$_2$S (pH 6.5–6.8) to a final concentration of 2 mM. Best growth is obtained if the cells are kept in suspension by magnetic stirring. Cultures should be transferred to fresh liquid medium once a month. Stab cultures in the agar medium used for isolation do not survive as well as liquid cultures. Long term preservation in liquid nitrogen is carried out with freshly grown cultures after addition of 5% DMSO.

Differentiation of the genus **Chloroherpeton** from other genera

Chloroherpeton differs from the multicellular filamentous green bacteria *Chloronema* (Dubinina and Gorlenko, 1975), *Oscillochloris* (Gorlenko and Pivovarova, 1977) and *Chloroflexus* (Pierson and Castenholz, 1974) in cell dimensions, in being unicellular rather than filamentous and in photosynthetic pigment composition. The differences to the other genera of the green sulfur bacteria are listed in Table 18.16, page 1683.

Taxonomic Comments

The physiology, pigmentation and fine structure of *Chloroherpeton* are similar to the green species of *Chlorobium*. A major difference lies in the flexing and gliding motility, which might suggest affinities with *Chloroflexus*. The 16S rRNA catalog, however, indicates that *Chloroherpeton* belongs with the green sulfur bacteria (*Chlorobiaceae*) (Gibson, 1980; Gibson et al., 1985), indicating that motility and flexing appear to be of lesser taxonomic importance than do the other characteristics. The possibility that more than one species has been isolated requires determination of mol% G + C of the DNA of more strains.

List of species of the genus **Chloroherpeton**

1. **Chloroherpeton thalassium** Gibson, Pfennig and Waterbury 1985, 223.[VP] (Effective publication: Gibson, Pfennig and Waterbury 1984, 100.)

tha.las′sium. Gr. n. *thalassa* the sea; Gr. adj. *thalassios* pertaining to the sea, marine; M.L. adj. *thalassius* marine.

The characteristics are the same as those described for the genus. Habitat: anoxic sulfide-containing marine littoral sediments, salt marshes and tidal inlets rich in rotting plant material.

The mol% G + C of the type strain is 47.8 (T_m).

Type strain: ATCC 35110 (strain GB-78).

Addendum to the **Green Sulfur Bacteria**

Norbert Pfennig

Phototrophic green sulfur bacteria living in consortia with other microorganisms.

The use of generic and species designations for the apparently stable complexes composed of two different microorganisms has been questioned (Buder, 1914; van Niel, 1957). According to the rules of bacterial nomenclature, the generic designations are not validly published (Trüper and Pfennig, 1971). Therefore, the generic and species designations with the addition of the term consortium are used here as laboratory names without taxonomic significance. It is possible that these consortia represent fortuitous combinations whose success depends on environmental factors. If so, the green components should be placed in the appropriate genera. The isolation of a green sulfur bacterium from the "*Chlorochromatium*" consortium by Mechsner (1957) was the first step in this direction. Unfortunately, this green sulfur bacterium was lost before detailed metabolic and taxonomic studies were made.

Only those consortia are included here that were repeatedly observed and described to thrive in water and mud samples collected in nature. Not one of the consortia has so far been isolated in pure culture. A schematic presentation is provided in Figure 18.48.

1a. "*Chlorochromatium aggregatum*" consortium Lauterborn 1906, 197. (*Chloronium mirabile* Buder 1914, 80.) (See also Pfennig, 1980.)

Barrel-shaped aggregates consisting of a rather large, colorless, polar flagellated bacterium as the center, which is surrounded by green bacteria arranged in 5–6 rows, ordinarily 2–4 cells long. The entire consortium behaves as a unit, is motile and is phototactically active. Multiplication occurs by the more or less simultaneous fission of the component cells; growth is dependent on both sulfide and light.

Cells of the green component are 0.5–1.0 μm wide and 1.0–2.5 μm long. Morphologically, the green cells resemble those of *Chlorobium limicola*. The central bacterium is usually surrounded by 12–24 green cells. The size of the entire motile barrel-shaped consortium is variable, generally 2.5–4.0 μm wide and 4–10 μm long.

The consortia usually occur together with other green and purple sulfur bacteria in the hypolimnion of stratified freshwater lakes or mud and sulfide-containing water of stagnant freshwater ponds exposed to light.

1b. "*Chlorochromatium glebulum*" (sic) consortium Skuja 1956, 36.

Cells of the green component are 0.5–0.6 μm wide and 0.7–1.0 μm long and contain gas vacuoles. Morphologically, the green cells resemble those of *Pelodictyon luteolum*. The curved central bacterium may be surrounded by 7–40 individual green cells. The size of the barrel-shaped motile consortium is 3–4 μm wide and 4–8 μm long. This kind of consortium was described as occurring in the hypolimnion of Swedish lakes.

2a. "*Pelochromatium roseum*" consortium Lauterborn 1913, 99 (see also Utermöhl, 1924; Gorlenko and Kusnezow, 1972; Pfennig 1980).

The morphology, multiplication and behavior of the "*Pelochromatium*" consortium resemble those of the "*Chlorochromatium*" consortium. Different from the latter, the phototrophic sulfur bacteria surrounding the colorless motile central bacterium morphologically resemble those of the brown *Chlorobium phaeobacteroides*.

Cells of the pinkish-brown component are straight or slightly curved rod-shaped, 0.6–1.0 μm wide and 1.2–2.5 μm long. The rod-shaped central bacterium may be surrounded by 10–20 individual brown cells. The size of the entire barrel-shaped motile consortium is variable, mostly 2.5–4.0 μm wide and 4–8 μm long.

The brown consortia have been observed most often in the sulfide-containing hypolimnion of stratified freshwater lakes. In these habitats, the consortia were found together with other green and purple sulfur bacteria.

2b. "*Pelochromatium roseo-viride*" consortium Gorlenko and Kusnezow 1972, 7.

The consortium represents a particular variation of the "*Pelochromatium roseum*" consortium. Instead of being surrounded by only one layer of a brown strain of green sulfur bacteria, the motile central bacterium of "*P. roseo-viride*" is covered by two layers of phototrophic bacteria. The inner layer consists of brown cells, as in "*P. roseum.*" The second, outer layer consists of rod-shaped green cells with gas vacuoles. The green cells are of about the same size as the brown cells and resemble *Pelodictyon luteolum*. The length of the entire motile barrel-shaped consortium is about 4 μm after division and 8 μm before division.

The brown plus green consortia consisting of three different kinds of bacteria occur in Lake Kononjer in the Mariji Republic of the U.S.S.R. The consortia were found to thrive together with "*Pelochromatium roseum*" in the sulfide-containing hypolimnion at a depth of 11.5 m.

3. "*Chloroplana vacuolata*" consortium Dubinina and Kusnezov 1976, 8 (see also Pfennig, 1980).

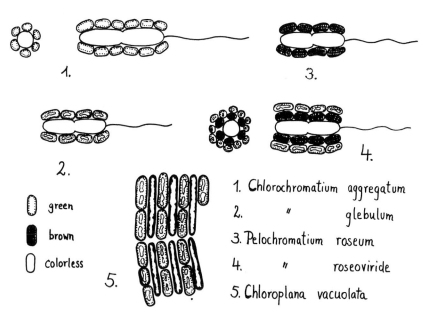

Figure 18.48. Schematic presentation of different kinds of symbiotic associations of phototrophic green sulfur bacteria with unknown chemotrophic bacteria. *1–4*, longitudinal and cross-sectional views through different consortia; *5*, top view of *"Chloroplana."* (Reproduced with permission from N. Pfennig. 1980. Anaerobes and Anaerobic Infections. Gustav Fischer Verlag, Stuttgart, p. 130.)

1. *Chlorochromatium aggregatum*
2. *"* *glebulum*
3. *Pelochromatium roseum*
4. *"* *roseoviride*
5. *Chloroplana vacuolata*

green

brown

colorless

Flat sheaths, lamellae or platelets composed of parallel rows of alternating green and colorless bacteria with gas vacuoles. The platelets are variable in size and may contain from a few to 300–400 green cells; consortia are nonmotile. Cells of the green bacteria are 0.6–0.8 μm wide and 1.2–2.0 μm long and resemble the gas-vacuolated green *Pelodictyon luteolum*. Cells of the gas vacuole-containing colorless rod-shaped bacterium are 0.35–0.45 μm wide and 3.0–6.0 μm long. By electron microscopy, the green cells were shown to contain chlorosomes, the typical light-harvesting structures of the green bacteria. The presence of bacteriochlorophyll *c* or *d* was inferred from the green fluorescence in reflected light.

The *"Chloroplana"* consortia were found in large numbers together with other green and purple sulfur bacteria in the anoxic sulfide-containing water of small forest lakes, Lesnaya Lamba, in southern Karelia (U.S.S.R.). The occurrence of these consortia in stagnant freshwater ponds has repeatedly been reported.

MULTICELLULAR FILAMENTOUS GREEN BACTERIA

Norbert Pfennig

Four genera of green bacteria capable of anoxygenic photosynthesis with bacteriochlorophylls in the light are, for morphological reasons, grouped under "Multicellular Filamentous Green Bacteria." The cells of all genera are uniseriately arranged in multicellular filaments that are capable of gliding motility. With the exception of *Heliothrix*, all other genera possess chlorosomes, the characteristic structural elements that are attached to the cytoplasmic membrane and house the light-harvesting bacteriochlorophylls.

Different from the green sulfur bacteria, all filamentous green bacteria are facultatively aerobic and preferentially utilize organic substances in their phototrophic or chemotrophic metabolism. Reduced sulfur compounds are not important electron donor substrates for laboratory cultures.

Based on 16S rRNA oligonucleotide catalogs, the genus *Chloroflexus* is related neither to the green sulfur bacteria nor to any other eubacteria (Stackebrandt and Woese, 1981). There is, however, evidence that the nearest genetic relatives to *Chloroflexus* are *Heliothrix* as well as the chemoorganotrophic flexibacterium *Herpetosiphon* (see under *Chloroflexus*, page 1702). This would support the view of Castenholz (1973) who considers the genera *Chloroflexus* and *Heliothrix* as phototrophic flexibacteria. Nothing is known about the genetic relationships of *"Oscillochloris"* or *Chloronema*.

The major differentiating characteristics of the genera of the filamentous green bacteria are presented in Table 18.19.

Table 18.19.

Differential characteristics of the genera of the uniseriately
Multicelluar Filamentous Green Bacteria, *a subcategory of*
Green Bacteria[a]

	Phototrophic flexibacteria		"Oscillochloris"	Chloronema
Characteristic	I. *Chloroflexus*	II. *Heliothrix*	III. *"Oscillochloris"*	IV. *Chloronema*
Optimum temperature for growth (°C)	20–25 or 50–60	40–55	10–20 or 20–35	3–15
Gas vacuoles	−	−	+	+
Gliding motility	+	+	+	+
Diameter of filaments (μm)				
0.5–1.0	+	−	−	−
1.0–1.5	−	+	+	−
1.5–2.5	−	−	−	+
4.5–5.5	−	−	+	−
Chlorosomes	+	−	+	+
Bacteriochlorophyll				
a	+	+	+	nt
c or *d*	+	−	+	+
Facultatively aerobic	+	+	+	+

[a] Symbols: −, negative; +, positive; nt, not tested.

Genus **Chloroflexus** *Pierson and Castenholz 1974a, 7*[AL]

RICHARD W. CASTENHOLZ

Chlo.ro.flex.'us. Gr. adj. *chloros* green; L. masc. n. *flexus* a bending; M.L. masc. n. *Chloroflexus* green bending.

Filaments of indefinite length; cells 0.5 to ~1.0 μm in diameter, 2 to ~6 μm in length; none differentiated (Fig. 18.49). Cell division by fission, no branching. No internal proliferations of cell membrane, except mesosomes; **chlorosomes present when anaerobically grown. Motile by gliding** (0.01–0.04 μm/s); no flagella. Gram-negative. Thin sheath sometimes present.

Anaerobic and facultatively aerobic (some). **Primarily photoheterotrophic,** secondarily photoautotrophic (probably not all strains) and chemoheterotrophic (not all strains). Several carbon sources utilized: e.g. acetate, glycerol, glucose, pyruvate and glutamate. Bacteriochlorophylls *a* and *c* present under anaerobic conditions; carotenoids include *β*- and *γ*-carotene and hydroxy- and oxo- derivatives and glycosides of both.

The mol% G + C of the DNA is 53.1–54.9.

Type species: *Chloroflexus aurantiacus* Pierson and Castenholz 1974a, 7.

Further Descriptive Information

Since only one species has been described, the generic limits may be subject to revision. Except for one published paper on a mesophilic variety, all work has been done on thermophilic strains of *C. aurantiacus*. In thermophilic *C. aurantiacus* (Pierson and Castenholz, 1974a) and "*C. aurantiacus* var. *mesophilus*" (Pivovarova and Gorlenko, 1977), transmission electron microscopy indicates a relatively simple cell interior with no invaginations of the cell membrane except for mesosomes which were more common and conspicuous in the mesophilic variety. The DNA area is centrally located; elongated chlorosomes are closely appressed to the cell membrane (Pierson and Castenholz, 1974a) (Fig. 18.50). More extensive work on the composition and development of these pigment-bearing sacs has been done (Schmidt, 1980; Schmidt et al., 1980; Sprague et al., 198lb; Feick et al., 1982; Staehelin et al., 1978).

Poly-*β*-hydroxybutyric acid granules, polyphosphate granules and, possibly, glycogen bodies may be seen by use of transmission electron microscopy (Pierson and Castenholz, 1974a) (Fig. 18.50). Polyglucose was present in cells under certain conditions (Sirevåg and Castenholz, 1979).

Pigments and Lipids

The bulk bacteriochlorophyll *a* has in vivo absorbance maxima at 802 and 865 nm, unlike the single maximum at about 810 nm in *Chlorobium* (Pierson and Castenholz, 1974a). Gloe and Risch (1978), however, found that the bacteriochlorophyll *c* from *Chloroflexus aurantiacus* (four thermophilic strains) was unique in possessing a stearyl alcohol "tail." Also, bacteriochlorophyll c_s is not a mixture of isomeric, homologous molecules, as are bacteriochlorophylls *c, d,* and *e* of the green bacteria. In addition, there is a "baseplate" bacteriochlorophyll a_{792} located in the chlorosome adjacent to the point of attachment to the cell membrane (Schmidt et al., 1980; Betti et al., 1982).

As in the case of other studied anoxygenic bacteria, the synthesis of bacteriochlorophyll *a* is controlled by both light intensity and O_2. Bacteriochlorophyll *c* synthesis is also controlled by these factors, but the responses were differential, suggesting independent regulation of the two pigments (Pierson and Castenholz, 1974b; Sprague et al., 1981a; Feick et al., 1982; Schmidt et al., 1980). The green bacteria per se are generally inhibited by even low O_2; and pigment regulation by O_2, if any exists, is therefore obscured.

Carotenoids of phototrophic cells consisted largely of monocyclic *γ*-carotene and the bicyclic *β*-carotene (Halfen et al., 1972; Schmidt et al., 1980) and OH-*γ*-carotene glucoside. Aerobic, heterotrophic cells contained largely 4-oxo-*β*-carotene (echinenone) and 4-oxo-*γ*-carotene glucoside (myxobactone) (K. Schmidt, personal communication). Unlike the weak response or lack of carotenoid synthesis under aerobic

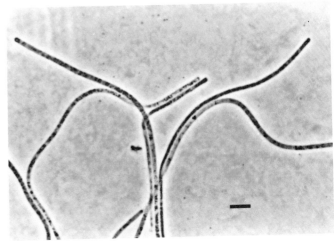

Figure 18.49. *C. aurantiacus* strain OK-70-fl. The transverse septa are not apparent. Phase-contrast photomicrograph. *Bar,* 5 μm.

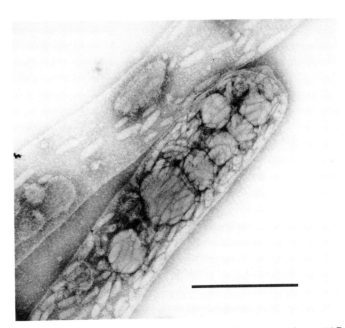

Figure 18.50. *C. aurantiacus* strain J-10-fl grown at about 45°C under low light intensity (incandescent, ~320 lx). Samples were negatively stained with 1% phosphotungstic acid on a carbon-stabilized Formvar grid and viewed with a Siemens Elmiskop operating at 80 kV. Numerous chlorosomes may be seen. The large granules are probably poly-*β*-hydroxybutyric acid. Transmission electron micrograph. *Bar,* 0.5 μm. (Courtesy of M. Broch-Due.)

conditions in the purple bacteria, *Chloroflexus* shows greatly enhanced synthesis of some carotenoids (Pierson and Castenholz, 1974b).

Recently, the reaction center of *Chloroflexus* has been characterized independently by two research groups (Pierson and Thornber, 1983; Pierson et al., 1983; Bruce et al., 1982). It appears that the reaction center resembles that of the Purple Nonsulfur Bacteria far more than the green bacterial component.

All three examined strains possessed both monogalactosyl- and digalactosyl-diglyceride lipids (Kenyon and Gray, 1974). Phosphatidylethanolamine and cardiolipin were absent (Knudsen et al., 1982). Phosphatidylglycerol and phosphatidylinositol were also present in substantial amounts, as were single wax esters (unusual in bacteria) (Knudsen et al., 1982). Waxes ranged from C_{28} to C_{38}, with fully saturated C_{36} being the major species. Longer chain fatty acids (C_{17} and C_{18-20}) predominated with a high degree of saturation, although monenoic (16:1, 17:1, 18:1, 19:1, 20:1) acids occurred (Kenyon and Gray, 1974; Knudsen et al., 1982). *C. aurantiacus* also contains four unsaturated fatty alcohols (C_{16-19}) (Knudsen et al., 1982).

Physiology

The versatility of *Chloroflexus* in using various carbon sources has not been well-documented, since growth in complex medium is superior in terms of both of rate and yield. Yeast extract, sometimes with added casamino acids, has so far resulted in the most rapid growth rates and greatest yields under photoheterotrophic or aerobic chemoheterotrophic conditions. Pierson and Castenholz (1974a) found that in strain J-10-fl, 80–90% of the expected yeast extract yield could be achieved with glycerol and 60–70% could be achieved with acetate if either was supplemented with "growth factor" concentrations of yeast extract. Lower yields occurred with glucose, pyruvate, glutamate or lactate with the same yeast extract supplement. Ethanol, succinate, malate and butyrate were not adequate substrates. Madigan et al. (1974), using the same and different strains, had both similar and different results. Yields were estimated, not quantified. Without supplemental yeast extract but with a vitamin mixture, Madigan et al. (1974) found consistently good growth with glucose in all four strains and good growth with glycerol, pyruvate, glutamate or aspartate in a few strains only—all under anaerobic conditions in the light. Only moderate to low yields were achieved under these conditions with use of acetate, lactate, succinate, malate, butyrate, citrate, ribose, galactose, ethanol, mannitol or glycylglycine. Aerobic dark growth occurred with most of the substrates already mentioned, but most strains rejected ethanol and citrate, all strains rejected glycylglycine, and 1 of 4 strains did not grow on acetate, butyrate or glycerol. Inorganic carbon was present under all conditions described.

Løken and Sirevåg (1982) found that acetate supported substantial growth of strain OK-70-fl in the absence of CO_2; however, the key enzymes of the glyoxylate cycle, isocitrate lyase and malate synthase, were present. A normal tricarboxylic acid cycle appears to operate under other conditions (Sirevåg and Castenholz, 1979).

Although Bartsch (1978), on the basis of some work, suggested that *C. aurantiacus* possessed only a cytochrome *c*, Pierson (1979) has found cytochrome *c* and *b* types, as in other phototrophic anoxygenic bacteria. When *C. aurantiacus* is grown under aerobic conditions, the presence of an *a* type cytochrome with an γ peak near 596 nm has also been substantiated.

Some strains of *C. aurantiacus* lack the ability to grow aerobically in darkness (S. Giovannoni, personal communication). Although O_2 is tolerated (and even consumed), growth does not resume until light is applied (if bacteriochlorophyll is still present). If pigment is low, semianaerobic conditions are necessary for synthesis to occur before growth resumes.

CO_2 may serve as sole carbon source in at least one strain (OK-70-fl) (Madigan et al., 1974; Madigan and Brock, 1975; 1977). Sulfide-dependent photoautotrophic growth is slow in the laboratory (Madigan and Brock, 1977; Castenholz, 1973). It is apparent, however, that this mode of growth operates under some field conditions to the probable exclusion of photoheterotrophy (Castenholz, 1973; and S. Giovannoni, personal communication). Although the use of CO_2, mainly via entry into the reductive tricarboxylic acid cycle is likely, low activities of ribulose-1,5-bisphosphate and phosphoribulokinase were detected even in photoheterotrophically grown *Chloroflexus* (Sirevåg and Castenholz, 1979).

Growth factor requirements have not been thoroughly investigated. Madigan (1976) reported that folic acid and thiamine were required by the two strains tested.

Ammonium and some amino acids will serve as nitrogen source; nitrate and N_2 will not (Madigan, 1976; Brock, 1978).

There is little known of the genetics of *Chloroflexus*. So far no plasmids have been reported and no viruses (specific or nonspecific) are known. A number of mutants have been obtained. These are strains lacking colored carotenoid pigments or deficient in bacteriochlorophyll *c* as a result of mutagenesis (Pierson et al., 1984b). All strains showed frequent reversion of the latter mutation.

The optimum temperature (~52–60°C) is known for a few strains of *C. aurantiacus*. The strains originally isolated and those used in the original description were all thermophiles from hot springs. The upper limit was between 65 and 70°C in the laboratory (Pierson and Castenholz, 1974a). The lower limit was between 30 and 35°C. At temperatures below 40°C, the filaments formed aggregates and often adhered to culture vessel walls (Pierson and Castenholz, 1974a). In strain J-10-fl, these observations were more systematically confirmed by Oelze and Fuller (1983). The optimum pH of the holotype (J-10-fl) was 7.6–8.4, and growth was severely limited below pH 7.0 (Pierson and Castenholz, 1974a).

The mesophilic variety "*C. aurantiacus* var. *mesophilus*" Pivovarova and Gorlenko, 1977) showed a temperature range for growth of 10–40°C, with an optimum at about 20–25°C (Gorlenko, 1975). The optimum pH (7.0–7.2) was also lower for the mesophilic strains than for the thermophilic strains in culture. It appears that the mesophilic strains are no longer available, at least as axenic cultures (V. M. Gorlenko, personal communication).

Natural Populations

Populations of *Chloroflexus* in their native habitats have been studied extensively (reviewed by Brock, 1978; Castenholz, 1984). Almost all such studies have necessarily been of hot spring habitats, since verification of *Chloroflexus* populations elsewhere is lacking. Gorlenko (1975) suggests that mesophilic *Chloroflexus* populations are common in the anaerobic portions of freshwater lakes. Likewise, mesophilic *Chloroflexus*-like organisms from shallow, marine microbial mats have been reported, but the necessary culture isolations have not been made (see Castenholz, 1984). Confirmed and massive *Chloroflexus* populations occur worldwide in neutral to alkaline pH hot springs forming gel-like, orange-pink-reddish mats generally under a thin (~1 mm) surface layer of cyanobacteria. *Chloroflexus* trichomes may be seen microscopically mixed with the cyanobacteria to about 70–72°C in North America but become the predominant undermat-forming organism below about 68–69°C. Such mats may persist to temperatures of 30–40°C in hot spring outflows.

These populations appear to be primarily (a) heterotrophic or (b) photoheterotrophic if the usual anaerobic conditions of undermat have allowed bacteriochlorophyll synthesis. The organic carbon is, at least, ultimately derived from the cyanobacteria (Ward et al., 1984). Being dependent on cyanobacteria restricts major development of heterotrophic populations to the temperature range of the cyanobacteria. In western North America, cyanobacteria commonly can be found in temperatures with upper limits of 73–74°C. In most of the rest of the world, upper limits for cyanobacteria are about 63–64°C, thus setting a lower upper limit for *Chloroflexus*. Whenever sufficient sulfide (H_2S, HS^-, S^{2-}) is present in source waters, however, the dependence of *Chloroflexus* on cyanobacteria is relieved, and a switch to sulfide-dependent photoautotrophy occurs. In that case, *Chloroflexus* can commonly be found in temperatures extending to about 66°C, forming essentially pure mats (see Castenholz, 1973). This is seen even in North America, since sulfide inhibits and excludes the cyanobacterial species otherwise found above 57°C in nonsulfide waters (Castenholz, 1973; Revsbech and Ward, 1984). The organic substrates for heterotrophic growth of *Chloroflexus* in hot springs are not verified, but fermentation products in the undermat (e.g. acetate, lactate, propionate and butyrate) from decomposing cyanobacteria may be used (Ward et al., 1984).

Apparently, similar mats occur in shallow marine lagoons and tidal flats. *Chloroflexus*-like filaments have been identified by transmission electron microscopy (i.e. chlorosome-containing filaments) (Stolz, 1984; Cohen, 1984). However, no cultures have yet been reported from these sources.

Enrichment and Isolation Procedures

Gorlenko (1975) reported a successful enrichment of a freshwater, mesophilic variety of *C. aurantiacus* in lake-bottom water and sediment columns to which mineral salts, trace elements, Na_2SO_4 (0.6 g/l), $Na_2S \cdot 9H_2O$ (0.1 g/l), yeast extract (0.025 g/l) and casein hydrolysate (0.025 g/l) have been added. He used a low light intensity (<3 klx) and a temperature of 25–30°C (Castenholz and Pierson, 1981).

The thermophilic varieties of *C. aurantiacus* have not been enriched for with great success. However, co-enrichment with cyanobacteria is an extremely simple and usually foolproof method of obtaining the common physiological types of *Chloroflexus*, i.e. those that will grow under aerobic or semiaerobic conditions. Cyanobacterial samples from hot spring mats (pH 5–11) will almost always contain *Chloroflexus*, even if it is not obvious. The cyanobacteria (one or more strains) may be enriched for simply by inoculating a small sample into a common cyanobacterial, liquid medium and incubating this at an appropriate temperature (e.g. 45–55°C) under the low intensity light (1–3 klx) provided by fluorescent or incandescent bulbs (Castenholz and Pierson, 1981). A mixed culture or a monoculture of cyanobacteria will develop, and trichomes of *Chloroflexus* and other heterotrophs will be carried along. It is essentially impossible to rid this enrichment of *Chloroflexus*.

Thermophilic *Chloroflexus* may be isolated from a cyanobacterial enrichment or directly from hot spring mats by placing small (4–16 mm²) pieces of cyanobacteria or sample on agar-solidified (1.5% w/v) cyanobacterial medium and incubating for one to a few days. Commonly, some of the cyanobacteria will spread extensively by gliding motility. *Chloroflexus*, a much slower glider, may be carried along to some extent but will form its own wisps of gliding trichomes which will commonly spread away from central or radiating masses of less motile or nonmotile cyanobacteria (Fig. 18.51). These wisps of *Chloroflexus* may then be picked up by cutting out the minute piece of agar on which they rest, inverting it on a new plate which contains some yeast extract (e.g. 0.02–0.2 g/l), and streaking, smearing or dragging the trichomes over the virgin agar. By repeatedly picking trichomes from the tips of spreading wisps, an axenic culture can be established. More details of this procedure are given by Pierson and Castenholz (1974a) and Castenholz and Pierson (1981).

Clones of the 1.0-μm-diameter trichomes may be established by the manual picking of individual trichomes spread on an agar surface. Presumptive clones of these and the narrower diameter trichomes (0.5–0.7 μm) may be established by streaking. Units of <20 μm long can be prepared by short term (10–20 s) ultrasonic disruption, followed by plating in a thin overlay of 0.7% (w/v) agar medium (Pierson et al., 1984b).

For thermophilic varieties of *Chloroflexus* that do not grow in the continued presence of oxygen, anaerobic techniques need to be applied. However, the other aspects of the procedure are similar. *Chloroflexus* samples directly from hot spring mats are placed or streaked on agar plates which have been stored previously under anaerobic conditions. For samples that contain cyanobacteria, approximately 10^{-5} M 3-(3,4,-dichlorophenyl)-1,1-dimethylurea should be used in the medium to prevent oxygenic photosynthesis. Incubation and growth in gas packs containing H_2 plus CO_2 have resulted in strains that are obligately phototrophic but that can tolerate O_2 without lethal effects for at least several hours (S. Giovannoni, personal communication).

Maintenance of Cultures

Cultures may be maintained under anaerobic or semianaerobic conditions in liquid or agar-solidified medium. Presumably, a variety of

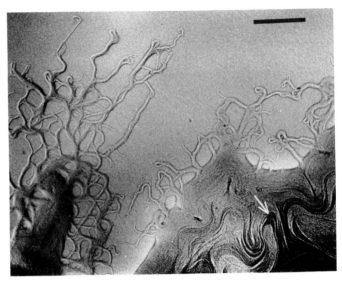

Figure 18.51. *C. aurantiacus* strain J-10-fl grown on agar plate in co-culture with the unicellular cyanobacterium *Synechococcus* species seen as dark streaks (*white arrow*). The growth temperature was 45°C. *Bar*, about 50 μm.

media would suffice, but the author and several others have used medium D (Table 18.20) with the chelator nitrilotriacetic acid (0.1 g/l) and the buffer glycylglycine (0.8 g/l) (e.g. Castenholz and Pierson, 1981). Yeast extract (2–3 g/l) or 1 g yeast extract plus casamino acids (2 g/l) are used as principal substrates. Screw-capped tubes or flasks nearly filled with hot sterile medium provide sufficiently anaerobic conditions for massive pigment synthesis and photoheterotrophic growth. Incandescent lamps provide good growth at low intensities (1–3 klx). Cultures may be maintained easily at 45–60°C. Cultures must be transferred every 7–14 days (Castenholz and Pierson, 1981).

Pigment-containing trichomes of the common forms of *Chloroflexus* will develop on agar plates in incubators (45–55°C) with or without an overlay procedure. Plate cultures richer in bacteriochlorophylls require incubation in anaerobic conditions. These cultures must be transferred every 7–14 days. Agar shake or stab cultures may also be used.

A third system, which requires less frequent transferring, is the use of a co-culture with a known pure strain of cyanobacterium (in this case a thermophilic unicell, *Synechococcus lividus*, strain OH-53-s). In such cultures, no yeast extract or casamino acids are used, and organic carbon for *Chloroflexus* is provided by the cyanobacterium. Although this process is essentially aerobic, under low light intensity, bacteriochlorophyll will be present in the co-culture. When pure *Chloroflexus* is required, separate wisps (Fig. 18.51) may be manually removed and transferred to organic medium. In the co-culture presently used, the cyanobacterium has a lower temperature tolerance than does the *Chloroflexus* and can be eliminated by raising the temperature in liquid cultures to 60–62°C for 4–5 days.

Chloroflexus may be kept in ampul at −196°C (liquid N_2) for a few years, but results have been variable. Dense, but not aged, cultures should be used, suspended in their own medium.

More details on maintenance are given by Castenholz and Pierson (1981).

Table 18.20.

Media for cultivation of phototrophic **C. aurantiacus**[a]

Medium D[b]		Micronutrient solution	
Double distilled water	1000 ml	Double distilled water	1000 ml
Nitrilotriacetic acid	0.1 g	H_2SO_4 (conc.)	0.5 ml
Micronutrient solution	0.5 g	$MnSO_4 \cdot H_2O$	2.28 g
$FeCl_3$ solution (0.29 g/l)	1.0 ml	$ZnSO_4 \cdot 7H_2O$	0.50 g
$CaSO_4 \cdot 2H_2O$	0.06 g	H_3BO_3	0.50 g
$MgSO_4 \cdot 7H_2O$	0.10 g	$CuSO_4 \cdot 5H_2O$	0.025 g
NaCl	0.008 g	$Na_2MoO_4 \cdot 2H_2O$	0.025 g
KNO_3	0.10 g	$CoCl_2 \cdot 6H_2O$	0.045 g
$NaNO_3$	0.70 g		
Na_2HPO_4	0.11 g		
Additions[c]			
Glycylglycine	0.8 g		
NH_4Cl	0.2 g		
Yeast extract (Difco)	1.0–2.0 g		
Vitamin-free casamino acids (Difco)	2.0 g		

[a] The medium is prepared (in order of listing) as a 20-fold concentrated stock that is stored unautoclaved in darkness at 4°C. The micronutrients and $FeCl_3$ solutions are included in the 20-fold stock. The pH is adjusted to 8.2 with 2 M NaOH after medium dilution. Agar (15 g/l), if used, is added after pH adjustment.

[b] Values are in final concentrations.

[c] Before pH adjustment.

Differentiation of the genus **Chloroflexus** from other genera

Chloroflexus may not be easily distinguished by morphological criteria from the other three genera considered to be related. Ultrastructural and biochemical characteristics are required (Table 18.21). All are filamentous. The much larger trichome diameter and the abundance of chlorosomes on complete and incomplete septa seem sufficient to separate *Oscillochloris* (Gorlenko and Pivovarova, 1977) from *Chloroflexus*, although *Oscillochloris* has not been isolated in axenic culture. The possession of gas vesicles, a characteristic so erratically spread through the eubacteria and archaeobacteria, should probably not be used as a character to distinguish genera. Characteristics of the genus *Chloronema* (Dubinina and Gorlenko, 1975), i.e. gas vesicles, trichome diameters of 2.0–2.5 μm (*Chloronema giganteum*) or 1.5–2.0 μm (*Chloronema spiroideum*), and the presence of a conspicuous sheath, are not necessarily adequate for erecting a genus separate from *Chloroflexus*. The probable presence of bacteriochlorophyll *d* rather than of bacteriochlorophyll *c* is also not a good distinguishing characteristic, since

bacteriochlorophylls *c* and *d* occur in different species of *Chlorobium*. Bacteriochlorophyll *c* mutants can be recovered from bacteriochlorophyll *d* clones of *Chlorobium* under low light intensity (Broch-Due and Ormerod, 1978). Again, neither species of *Chloronema* has been grown in culture, other than as enrichments.

Heliothrix, on the other hand, is a thermophilic, filamentous type only slightly broader in diameter than *Chloroflexus* (1.5 vs. <1.0 μm), but *Heliothrix* does not possess chlorosomes nor the accessory bacteriochlorophyll *c* or *d* that would be associated with these structures (Pierson et al., 1984a, 1985) (see under *Heliothrix* in this volume). The known aerobic tolerance or possible aerobic requirements of *Heliothrix* are not at this time adequately defined. *Chloroflexus*, en masse, may be green to orange. *Heliothrix*, en masse, is always orange or orange-red. Sequence data obtained from the 5S rRNA indicates that *Heliothrix* should be regarded as related to *Chloroflexus* but not so closely related as to be considered the same genus (Pierson et al., 1985). *Heliothrix*,

Table 18.21.

Characteristics of **Chloroflexus** *and gliding organisms of similar appearance*[a]

Genus	Bacteriochlorophyll	Carotenoid	Color	Cell diameter (μm)	Sheath	Gas vesicles	Chemoheterotrophy
Chloroflexus	*a, c*	β- + γ-Carotene; OH- γ-carotene glucoside; oxo-γ-carotene and glucosides; echinenone	Orange-green	0.5–1.0	±	−	±
Chloronema	*a, d*	?	Green	1.5–2.5	+	+	?
"*Oscillochloris*"	*a, c*	?	Green	4.5–5.5	−	+	?
Heliothrix	*a*	Oxo-γ-carotene and glucosides	Orange	1.5	−	−	?
Herpetosiphon	−	γ-Carotene and glucosides	Orange-red	0.5–1.5	−	−	+
Chloroherpeton	*a, c*	γ-Carotene (<80%)	Light green	1.0	−	±	−

[a] Symbols: ±, present or absent; −, absent; +, present; and ?, unknown.

although not in axenic culture, is currently in co-culture with the chemoheterotrophic bacterium *Isosphaera pallida* (see under this genus and species in this volume).

Flexibacteria, particularly *Herpetosiphon*, are aerobic filamentous bacteria of dimensions and color which are similar to orange *Chloroflexus* but which lack chlorophylls of any type (Soriano, 1973). Some carotenoids (e.g. γ-carotene, and carotenoid glucosides) are similar to those of *Chloroflexus* (Kleinig and Reichenbach, 1977), and 16S rRNA oligonucleotide sequence catalogs indicate a relatively close relationship to *Chloroflexus* (C. R. Woese, personal communication). *Chloroherpeton thalassium* (Gibson et al., 1984) is an elongate unicell (8–30 μm long, 1 μm wide) that resembles a short *Chloroflexus* trichome. However, there are no transverse septa, and *Chloroherpeton* is an obligate sulfide-dependent photoautotroph. Furthermore, 16S catalog data indicate that *Chloroherpeton* fits more closely with the *Chlorobium* "branch" than with *Chloroflexus* (Gibson et al., 1984). *Heliobacterium*, recently described by Gest and Favinger (1983), is a gliding cell containing bacteriochlorophyll *g* which resembles the rod-shaped myxobacteria more than it does *Chloroflexus*.

Additional Taxonomic Comments

Chloroflexus, when first cataloged with respect to the base sequence of 16S rRNA oligonucleotides, stood alone among all other eubacteria as the deepest branch on the phylogenetic tree (Stackebrandt and Woese, 1981). Even the division between it and *Chlorobium* is deep. This has led to speculation that *Chloroflexus* may represent a very ancient branch of the eubacteria. Henderson et al. (1983) confirmed, however, that the ribosomal 30S subunit was structurally typical of eubacteria and lacked the archaeobacterial "bill." Recently, Pace and co-workers (N. Pace, personal communication) have compared the complete sequence of the 5S rRNA subunits of *Chloroflexus* with over 100 other bacteria. These results also support the great separateness of *Chloroflexus* from all other eubacteria tested, with the exception of *Heliothrix* (Pierson et al., 1985) and *Herpetosiphon*. Although the extent of relatedness among these three genera is not yet clear, it is certain, at least, that each should be regarded as a distinct genus.

The proposal by Trüper (1976), that *Chloroflexus* be separated formally from the green bacteria (*Chlorobiaceae*) as the family *Chloroflexaceae*, is still valid, but the definition of this family should be revised as discoveries occur. At this time the family should include *Heliothrix*, and therefore, the requirement for chlorosomes and bacteriochlorophyll *c, d* or *e* needs to be dropped. It seems appropriate now that the photosynthetic members be called the "photosynthetic flexibacteria," as was suggested earlier (Castenholz, 1973).

List of species of the genus **Chloroflexus**

1. **Chloroflexus aurantiacus** Pierson and Castenholz 1974, 7.[AL]
au.ran.ti´a.cus. M.L. neut. n. *aurantium* specific name of the orange; M.L. adj. *aurantiacus* orange-colored.

The characteristics are the same as those described for the genus. The type species is thermophilic and grows in the temperature range of 40–66°C with an optimum at about 52–60°C. Optimum pH: 7.6–8.4.

The mesophilic variety of *C. aurantiacus* (var. "*mesophilus*"; Gorlenko, 1975) grows in the temperature range of 10–40°C with an optimum at about 20–25°C. Optimum pH: 7.0–7.2.

The mol% G + C of the type strain is 54.9 (Bd).

Type strain: ATCC 29366 (strain J-10-fl).

Genus **Heliothrix** Pierson, Giovannoni, Stahl and Castenholz 1986, 354[VP] (Effective publication: Pierson, Giovannoni, Stahl and Castenholz 1985, 164)

R. W. CASTENHOLZ AND B. K. PIERSON

He´li.o.thrix. Gr. masc. n. *helios* sun; Gr. fem. n. *thrix* hair; M.L. fem. n. *Heliothrix* sun hair.

Clearly septate filaments of indefinite length, unbranched and undifferentiated. Cells about 1.5 μm in diameter, much longer than broad (Fig. 18.52). Thin sheath present or not. Cell division by fission, in one plane only. **Gliding motility, no flagella.** Cells granular, poly-β-hydroxybutyric acid inclusions present; gas vacuoles unknown. Cells stain Gram-negative. **Bacteriochlorophyll *a* present, but no accessory bacteriochlorophylls or chlorosomes. Filaments orange; carotenoids abundant.** Internal membranous structures unknown.

Aerotolerant; anaerobic growth uncertain; probably mainly **photoheterotrophic metabolism**, light-dependent uptake of acetate. Temperature range: ~35–56°C; optimum temperature: 40–55°C (for acetate uptake).

Type species: *Heliothrix oregonensis* Pierson, Giovannoni, Stahl and Castenholz 1986, 354.

Further Descriptive Information

Only the type species has been described. The gliding rate is 0.1–0.4 μm/s (Pierson and Castenholz, 1971). Electron microscopy revealed no conspicuous or identifiable internal inclusions except granules of poly-β-hydroxybutyric acid (Pierson et al., 1984a). En masse, *H. oregonensis* is bright orange. Bacteriochlorophyll *a* was identified by characteristic absorption spectra of cavitated cells and of methanolic extracts (Pierson and Castenholz, 1971). Oxygenated derivatives of γ-carotene and glycosides of γ-carotene are the predominant carotenoids (K. Schmidt, personal communication; Pierson et al., 1984a).

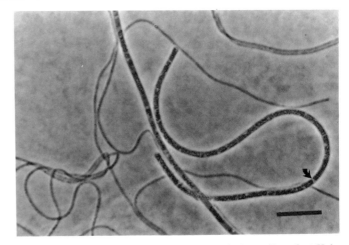

Figure 18.52. *H. oregonensis* from a population collected at Kahnee-ta Hot Springs, Warm Springs, Oregon (U.S.A.). A cross-wall is indicated by an *arrow*. The narrower filaments are *C. aurantiacus* (J-10-fl) added to the collection for comparison. Phase-contrast micrograph. *Bar*, 10 μm. (Reproduced with permission from B. K. Pierson, S. J. Giovannoni, D. A. Stahl and R. W. Castenholz, Archives of Microbiology *142*: 164–167, 1984b.)

Enrichment and Isolation Procedures

H. oregonensis grows in a relatively few hot springs in Oregon where it forms a conspicuous orange mat, a few millimeters in vertical thickness, which generally overlies a greenish layer composed of several cyanobacteria (Pierson et al., 1984a; Castenholz, 1984a, b). The pH is about 8.5. In these springs, the population constitutes a spectacular enrichment, of which *H. oregonensis* may comprise >95%. The masses of filaments are commonly found as a "puffy" upper layer which can easily be collected by a syringe with a 17- or 18-gauge needle. Since the filaments also aggregate rapidly, the collected material can be washed and allowed to aggregate repeatedly, thus further purifying the material by washing out unicellular cyanobacteria and other bacteria (Pierson et al., 1984a).

H. oregonensis has been brought into co-culture with *Isosphaera pallida*, an aerobic, chemoheterotrophic bacterium (Giovannoni and Castenholz; see page 1959 of this volume). A single, axenic filament of *H. oregonensis* is manually removed from an agar plate, on which filaments have been gliding, and transferred to the edge of a colony of axenic. *I. pallida* growing in the light at 45°C on IMC medium (Giovannoni and Castenholz; see page 1960 of this volume; Pierson et al., 1984a). Numerous attempts to grow *H. oregonensis* axenically have failed.

Maintenance Procedures

Co-cultures of *H. oregonensis* and *I. pallida*, as well as axenic cultures of *I. pallida*, are maintained by monthly transfers on slants or plates of agar-solidified IMC medium (pH 8.1). They are incubated at 45°C and under a moderate light intensity (~3 klx, coolwhite fluorescent lamps) in an atmosphere of 95% air and 5% CO_2. It is not known whether the co-culture survives lyophilization or storage at the temperature of liquid nitrogen.

Differentiation of the genus **Heliothrix** from other genera

The genus *Heliothrix* may be distinguished from the filamentous genus *Chloroflexus* in that *Heliothrix* possesses bacteriochlorophyll *a* only and no accessory light-harvesting bacteriochlorophyll or chlorosomes. In the one species of *Heliothrix* known, the filament diameter is also greater (1.5 μm) and the septa (cross-walls) may be seen easily in *Heliothrix* with phase-contrast microscopy (Fig. 18.52). Flexibacteria of indefinite filament length (e.g. *Herpetosiphon*) also may strongly resemble the genus *Heliothrix* morphologically (Reichenbach and Golecki, 1975). However, among the flexibacteria there are no bacteriochlorophylls, although the carotenoids may be somewhat similar (see under *Chloroflexus*, page 1701).

Taxonomic Comments

The complete nucleotide sequence of the 5S rRNA of *H. oregonensis* indicates a homology of 0.767 compared with that of *Chloroflexus aurantiacus* (see Pierson et al., 1985). Although these two organisms are not very closely related, they are more closely related to each other than either is to any of about 100 other bacteria (see Pierson et al., 1985). However, 5S sequence data from members of the genus *Herpetosiphon* were not available for comparison. It appears, however, that *Herpetosiphon* is related to *Chloroflexus* (and presumably *Heliothrix*) when 16S rRNA oligonuleotide catalogs are used for comparison (Stackebrandt et al., 1984).

It is probable that organisms of the genera *Chloroflexus*, *Heliothrix* and *Herpetosiphon* had a common ancestor. Whether, in the case of *Heliothrix*, chlorosomes and accessory chlorophylls were initially possessed and then lost is completely speculative at this time. If *Herpetosiphon* is a *close* relative of *Chloroflexus*, however, it would appear that this obligate aerobe evolved from a *Chloroflexus*-like ancestor by loss of the ability to synthesize chlorophyll.

List of species of the genus **Heliothrix**

1. **Heliothrix oregonensis** Pierson, Giovannoni, Stahl and Castenholz 1986, 354.[VP] (Effective publication: Pierson, Giovannoni, Stahl and Castenholz 1985, 164.)

o.re.gon.en'sis. M.L. adj. *oregonensis* pertaining to Oregon, state in the U.S.A.

The characteristics are the same as those described for the genus. Habitat: orange top layer over cyanobacterial mats in relatively few hot springs in Oregon (U.S.A.).

Type strain: strain IS/F-1 (Pierson et al. 1985).

Genus "Oscillochloris" Gorlenko and Pivovarova 1977, 406

VLADIMIR M. GORLENKO

Os.cil'lo.chlo'ris. L. n. *oscillans* oscillating; Gr. adj. *chloros* green; M.L. fem. n. *Oscillochloris* oscillating green (bacterium).

Cells arranged in uniseriately multicellular flexible filaments with gliding motility. Trichomes uniformly wide throughout their length, length variable, **nonbranching, without sheath.** Trichomes are morphologically similar to cyanobacteria of the genus *Oscillatoria*; however, occasionally a differentiated end cell is present which produces attaching material. **Trichomes multiply by hormogonia. Cells contain gas vacuoles.** Gram stain may be positive or negative. **Trichomes appear green or yellow-green. Contain bacteriochlorophylls *c* and *a* as well as carotenoids.** The light-harvesting structures of the photosynthetic apparatus are **chlorosomes. Phototrophic under anaerobic conditions**; may be capable of chemoorganotrophic growth under aerobic conditions in the dark.

The mol% G + C of the DNA was not determined.

Type species: "*Oscillochloris chysea*" Gorlenko and Pivovarova 1977, 406.

Further Descriptive Information

Width of trichomes varies considerably in the two existing species: 1.0–1.4 μm in "*O. trichoides*" and 4.5–5.5 μm in "*O. chrysea*." Individual cells of the trichomes may be flat or elongated. In "*O. chrysea*," multiple incomplete septa are typical, consisting of the cytoplasmic membrane and peptidoglycan layers. Cell walls are formed by diaphragm-like narrowing and closing of cell septa and subsequent formation of the other components of the cell wall. Formation of porous thick cell septa results in the breakage of the trichome and its multiplication. Short sections of trichomes, hormogonia, may separate at the end of a filament, or the entire filament may break up into hormogonia. Long trichomes as well as hormogonia possess gliding motility. The rate of gliding varies in the two species from 0.1 to 7 μm/s. Trichomes are capable of phototactic and chemotactic reactions. The cell wall consists of multiple layers and is of the Gram-negative type. In "*O. chrysea*," the outer membrane is poorly pronounced, while trichomes stain Gram-positive.

Cells contain bacteriochlorophyll c as the predominant pigment and small amounts of bacteriochlorophyll a. In "O. trichoides," oxygen suppresses the synthesis of bacteriochlorophyll c, while the synthesis of carotenoids is unaffected.

Under anaerobic phototrophic conditions, cell suspensions appear green or olive-green. Colonies of "O. trichoides" grown at low oxygen concentrations either in the dark or in the light appear orange or pink. Oxygen does not repress the synthesis of bacteriochlorophylls in "O. chrysea" (field observations).

Cells are capable of photosynthesis under anaerobic conditions, utilizing organic compounds or H_2S as electron donor. Growth in the dark under aerobic (microaerobic) conditions is possible.

"Oscillochloris" organisms are typical benthic forms, occurring in algobacterial mats formed on the surface of anaerobic mud sediments. "O. trichoides" often occurs in warm springs with temperatures up to 45°C (Lenkoran' (Azerbaijan), Dagestan (Caucasus), Kamchatka), in areas with high H_2S content or in microzones below the purple sulfur bacteria *Chromatium* or *Thiocapsa*. "O. chrysea" preferably develops in water bodies with high content of organic matter (e.g. domestic effluents). "Oscillochloris" organisms occur together with filamentous cyanobacteria and *Beggiatoa*.

Enrichment and Isolation Procedures

"O. trichoides" was isolated from algobacterial mats by serial dilutions in test tubes with the modified agar medium used for green sulfur bacteria (see page 1684) which contains: additional anhydrous Na_2SO_4, 330 mg/l; Difco yeast extract, 25 mg/l; tryptone, 25 mg/l; vitamin B_{12}, 20 µg/l; trace elements; agar, 0.2–0.4%; and $Na_2S·9H_2O$, 300 mg/l, at pH 7.5. Inocula were incubated at a light intensity of 2000 lx and at a temperature of 20–35°C. Isolated colonies (green or yellow-green, of irregular fuzzy shape) were isolated from the highest dilutions and purified by further dilution series. Thus, associated phototrophic bacteria (mainly purple nonsulfur bacteria) were removed after 3–4 dilution series. Monocultures still contained (a) facultative anaerobic fermenting bacteria producing H_2 from lactate and (b) sulfur- and sulfate-reducing bacteria.

Good growth of cultures free of other phototrophic bacteria was obtained in the medium described above. The concentration of cell material increased 10- to 20-fold.

"O. chrysea" did not grow in semisolid agar media. Therefore, it was not possible to obtain purified cultures.

Maintenance Procedures

Cultures of "O. trichoides" may be stored in a refrigerator at 4°C in liquid medium for 1–2 months at low light intensity.

Differentiation of the genus "Oscillochloris" from other genera

The major differentiating characteristics of "Oscillochloris" in comparison with the other genera of multicellular filamentous green bacteria are given in Table 18.19, page 1697.

Taxonomic Comments

Mesophilic representatives of the multicellular filamentous green bacteria have been studied so far in monoculture or in samples from the mass development in nature (Lauterborn, 1915; Gicklhorn, 1921; Gorlenko and Pivovarova, 1977; Gorlenko and Korotkov, 1979). Further information based on pure culture studies is required in order to obtain additional differentiating features and to establish the genetic relationships.

List of species of the genus "Oscillochloris"

1. **"Oscillochloris chrysea"** Gorlenko and Pivovarova 1977, 406. (*Oscillatoria coerulescens* Gicklhorn 1921.)

chry.se′a. L. adj. *chryseus* gold-shining; M.L. fem. n. *chrysea* gold-shining.

Trichomes yellow-green, multicellular, flexible, 4.5–5.5 µm wide and up to 2.5 mm long. Individual cells vary in length from 3.5 to 7.0 µm but may be shorter (Figs. 18.53 and 18.54). Trichomes carry multiple transverse striae because of complete and incomplete cell septa. The terminal cells of trichomes are smaller in diameter and possess a thicker cell envelope. Occasionally, the ends of trichomes carry slimy dome-shaped structures for the attachment to solid particles. Division and formation of septa occur by centripetal infolding of the cytoplasmic membrane and inner peptidoglycan layer of the cell wall. The cell wall has no pronounced outer membrane and contains a thicker nonuniform peptidoglycan layer (up to 25.2 nm). Trichomes have no sheath but are surrounded by a microcapsule 25–30 nm thick. Stain Gram-positive. Motile by gliding at a rate of about 7 µm/s. Multiplication of trichomes by hormogonia. More frequently, the end section of trichomes 15 µm or more long is separated, or trichomes break up in the middle. Less frequently, trichomes break up into short sections of 15–30 µm. Some cells contain a few gas vacuoles localized along the cell septa.

Individual trichomes appear yellow-green, irrespective of the presence or absence of oxygen. Cell suspension appears dark green. Trichomes appear blue if observed under the microscope in reflected light.

Chlorosomes, the photosynthetic structures, are localized on the cytoplasmic membrane along complete and incomplete septa (Fig. 18.54). Chlorosomes are absent from the cytoplasmic membrane parallel to the long axis of the filaments.

The major photosynthetic pigment is bacteriochlorophyll c; bacteriochlorophyll a is present in smaller amounts. Carotenoid pigments are present.

Physiology: phototrophic, tolerant of hydrogen sulfide (500 mg/l $Na_2S·9H_2O$), probably capable of aerobic dark metabolism. Storage materials: poly-β-hydroxybutyrate, glycogen, polymetaphosphates. Habitat: surface of hydrogen sulfide-containing mud of freshwater bodies. Development at pH 7.5–8.5 and at 10–20°C. The following other bacteria were observed in the same habitat: *Oscillatoria* species, flexibacteria, *Beggiatoa alba* and, occasionally, *Amoebobacter roseus*, *Thiodictyon bacillosus* and *Chlorobium limicola*.

2. **"Oscillochloris trichoides"** Gorlenko and Korotkov, 1979, 855. (*Oscillatoria trichoides* (Szafer) Lauterborn 1915, 436.)

tri.cho′i.des. L. fem. adj. *trichoideus* hairlike; M.L. fem. adj. *trichoides* hairlike (bacteria).

Trichomes straight or wavy, yellow-green and 1.0–1.4 µm wide (Figs. 18.55 and 18.56). Individual cells in a filament vary in length from 2.3 to 3.8 µm. There is no sheath, but trichomes are surrounded by a thin slime layer (microcapsule). Cells are motile by gliding at a rate of 0.2 µm/s and multiply by separation of a short section of the filament (hormogonium) or of an individual cell from the mother trichome. At some stages of development, gas vacuoles are formed which are localized along the cell septa (Fig. 18.56). The photosynthetic structures are chlorosomes. Trichomes deposit poly-β-hydroxybutyrate inside the cells. Sulfur is not accumulated inside the cells. Globules and crystals of sulfur are present outside the cells in the immediate proximity of the trichomes. Cell suspensions appear dark green if grown under

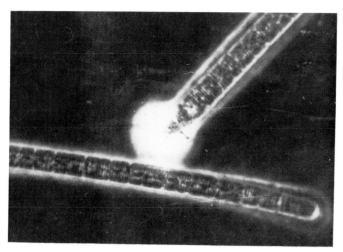

Figure 18.53. *"O. chrysea"* from a mud-water sample from a creek contaminated with domestic effluents. Phase-contrast light micrograph of section with India ink (× 2,000). (Reproduced with permission from V. M. Gorlenko and N. N. Pirovarova, Izvestiya Akademii Nauk S.S.S.R. Seriya Biologicheskaya (Moskva) *23:* 406, 1977.)

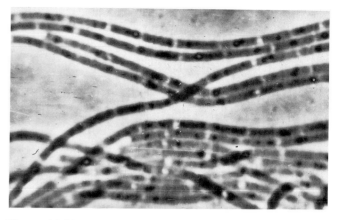

Figure 18.55. *"O. trichoides"* strain SR-1. Phase-contrast light micrograph (× 2,500). (Reproduced with permission from V. M. Gorlenko and S. A. Kozotkov, Izvestiya Akademii Nauk S.S.S.R. Seriya Biologicheskaya (Moskva) *6:* 855, 1979.)

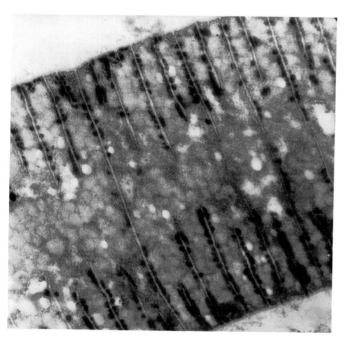

Figure 18.54. *"O. chrysea"* from a mud-water sample from a creek contaminated with domestic effluents. Electron micrograph of ultrathin section fixed with KMnO₄ (× 20,000). (Reproduced with permission from V. M. Gorlenko and N. N. Pirovarova, Izvestiya Akademii Nauk S.S.S.R. Seriya Biologicheskaya (Moskva) *23:* 406, 1977.)

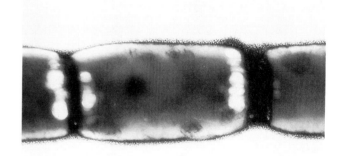

Figure 18.56. *"O. trichoides"* strain SR-1. Electron micrograph of section stained with phosphotungstic acid (× 25,000). (Reproduced with permission from V. M. Gorlenko and S. A. Kozotkov, Izvestiya Akademii Nauk S.S.S.R. Seriya Biologicheskaya (Moskva) *6:* 855, 1979.)

anaerobic conditions in the light and appear orange if grown under aerobic conditions. In stab cultures grown in agar medium in the light, dark green colonies are formed; colonies in the upper part of the tube may appear orange. The major photosynthetic pigment is bacteriochlorophyll *c;* a small amount of bacteriochlorophyll *a* is also present. The major carotenoids are γ- and β-carotene; the amount of γ-carotene is about twice that of β-carotene.

Photoheterotrophic, but capable of photoautotrophic development. Tolerant to sulfide, with an optimum initial concentration of sulfide of 500 mg Na₂S·9H₂O/l. Utilizes sulfide as electron donor for photosynthesis and oxidizes it to elemental sulfur. Optimum development at pH 7.5. Mesophilic. Growth factor requirements are satisfied by yeast extract.

Habitat: mats on the surface of freshwater mud containing hydrogen sulfide. These bacteria occur together with the following other phototrophic organisms: *Chlorobium limicola, Chromatium* species, cyanobacteria *Oscillatoria* species and *Pseudanabaena* species.

Type strain: Not in pure culture. Strain SR-1 (free from other phototrophic bacteria) was obtained from mats in Lake Sernoe (Kuibyshev region of U.S.S.R.). Stored in the collection of the Institute of Microbiology, Academy of Sciences of the U.S.S.R., Department of Geological Activity of Microorganisms.

Genus **Chloronema** Dubinina and Gorlenko 1975, 515[AL]

VLADIMIR M. GORLENKO

Chlo.ro.ne′ma. Gr. adj. *chloros* green; Gr. n. *nema* thread; M.L. neut. n. *Chloronema* green filament.

Cells cylindrical, combined in a trichome surrounded by a sheath. Trichomes **straight or spiral,** appear **yellow-green** (Fig. 18.57). Cells multiply by separation of sections of trichomes (**hormogonia**) of varying length. **Gliding motility.** The major pigment is **bacteriochlorophyll *d*;** also contain bacteriochlorophyll *c*. The photosynthetic structures are **chlorosomes.** Cells are capable of **anoxygenic photosynthesis.**

The mol% G + C of the DNA has not been studied.

Type species: *Chloronema giganteum* Dubinina and Gorlenko 1975, 515.

Further Descriptive Information

Descriptive information is based on the study of *Chloronema* in natural water bodies (Dubinina and Gorlenko, 1975; Dubinina and Kuznetsov, 1976; Gorlenko and Lokk, 1979). Cells of *C. giganteum*, 2–2.5 × 3.5–4.5 μm, form straight or spiral trichomes 75–250 μm long. Trichomes are surrounded by a slimy sheath of varying thickness. In lakes containing iron salts, sheaths of *Chloronema* contain iron oxides, occasionally in considerable amounts. In this case, sheaths appear brown. Bacteria multiply by separation of a short end section of trichomes or of an individual cell, which separate from the sheath by gliding. The rate of gliding is about 10 μm/s. *Chloronema* organisms rapidly attach themselves to solid surfaces, e.g. glass slides, and move by gliding.

The sheath is filamentous, clearly delimitated on the inside. The trichome and the sheath are separated by a vacant space. The cell wall is of the Gram-negative type. Bacteria stain Gram-negative. The cytoplasmic membrane forms multiple invaginations of the mesosome type. Chlorosomes are located predominantly in the periphery of cells but also occur along the cell septa and are associated with the membrane invaginations. During division of cells, the cytoplasmic membrane extends to the inner portion of the cell, and then a cell septum is formed which is similar to the cell wall. The central part of each cell is filled with elongated gas vesicles (Fig. 18.58).

Analysis of natural samples from zones of mass development of *C. giganteum* revealed the presence of bacteriochlorophyll *d* (in vivo absorption maximum: 720 nm). *Chloronema* occurs in dimictic freshwater lakes of the mesohumous type, with high ferrous iron content and only traces of H_2S. *C. giganteum* occurs predominantly below the chemocline under anaerobic conditions.

Observations at natural habitats indicate that *Chloronema* is capable of anoxygenic photosynthesis. *C. giganteum* exhibits positive aerotaxis in the dark, indicating a capacity for aerobic chemotrophic metabolism.

Enrichment and Isolation Procedures

Chloronema requires low light intensity and low temperature (4–15°C). Trichomes may accumulate on glass slides immersed in water samples rich in *Chloronema* filaments. Growth has not been obtained in liquid or solid media.

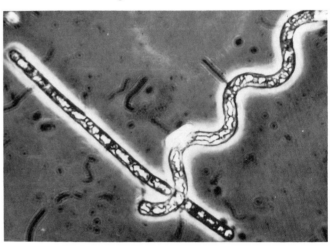

Figure 18.57. *C. giganteum* from a water sample of dimictic Lake Lesnaya Lamba. Phase-contrast light micrograph (× 2000).

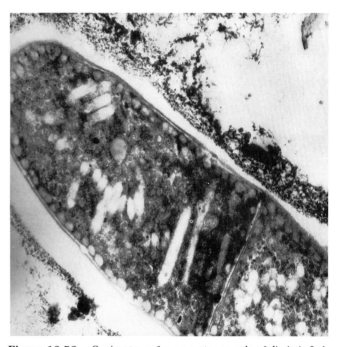

Figure 18.58. *C. giganteum* from a water sample of dimictic Lake Lesnaya Lamba. Electron micrograph of ultrathin section fixed with OsO_4 and glutaraldehyde (× 20,000).

Differentiation of the genus **Chloronema** from other genera

The major differentiating characteristics of *Chloronema* in comparison with the other genera of multicellular filamentous green bacteria are given in Table 18.19, page 1697.

List of species of the genus **Chloronema**

1. Chloronema giganteum Dubinina and Gorlenko 1975, 515.[AL]

gi.gan.te′um. Gr. neut. adj. *giganteum* gigantic.

Cells are cylindrical, 2–2.5 × 3.5–4.5 μm, and contain large centrally located gas vacuoles. Cells are combined in trichomes surrounded by a sheath (Fig. 18.57). Iron oxides may be accumulated in the sheath, sometimes in considerable amounts. Trichomes, together with the sheath, are 3–4 μm wide and up to 250 μm long. Waves in spiral trichomes are 15–20 μm long.

Motile by gliding. Multiplication of trichomes by separation of a part of the trichome (hormogonium) from the mother filament. Hormogonia actively separate themselves from the sheath. Bacteria are capable of phototaxis and chemotaxis.

Filaments appear yellowish green. Contain bacteriochlorophyll *d*. The photosynthetic structures are chlorosomes which are underlying and attached to the cytoplasmic membrane (Fig. 18.58).

Habitat: the metalimnion and upper hypolimnion of stratified freshwater lakes with high ferrous iron content and no or low concentrations of H_2S. This species occurs together with many other species of the purple and green sulfur bacteria.

Other organisms belonging to the genus Chloronema

Chloronema spiroideum Dubinina and Gorlenko 1975, 516.[AL]

Placement with the green bacteria is doubtful as the presence or absence of chlorosomes and bacteriochlorophylls was not determined.

III. GENERA INCERTAE SEDIS

Genus Heliobacterium Gest and Favinger 1985, 223[VP] (Effective publication: Gest and Favinger 1983, 15)

HOWARD GEST AND JEFFREY L. FAVINGER

He.li.o.bac.te′ri.um. Gr. n. *helios* sun; Gr. neut. n. *bakterion* a small rod; M.L. neut. n. *Heliobacterium* sun bacterium

Rod-shaped cells that are **frequently slightly bent,** Gram-negative, and **obligately anaerobic and photoheterotrophic,** and show gliding motility. Contain **bacteriochlorophyll *g**** as the major photosynthetic pigment. Extensively developed intracytoplasmic membranes of the kind produced by most anoxygenic photosynthetic bacteria are not observed. **Cells do not contain chlorosomes or gas vacuoles.**

The mol% G + C of the DNA of the type strain is 52 (T_m).

Type species: *Heliobacterium chlorum* Gest and Favinger 1985, 223.

Further Descriptive Information

Mature cells are typically ~1 μm wide and of variable length (4–10 μm or longer) (Fig. 18.59); occasionally, short filaments observed. Colonies on medium 112[†] agar have irregular margins because of wavy protrusions of cell masses in palisade formations, typical of gliding bacteria (no motility is apparent in direct microscopic observations of wet mounts). Paper chromatography of acid hydrolysates of purified cell wall preparations of *H. chlorum* revealed the presence of muramic acid, glucosamine, alanine, glutamic acid and diaminopimelic acid (S. Woeste, personal communication); the peptidoglycan is sensitive to lysozyme. It appears, however, that the architecture of the cell envelope may have unusual features. Thus, the organism shows a strong tendency to form spheroplasts and lyse; nutritional factors that influence the extent of spheroplast formation (some observed to be quite high) have still not been identified.

The type strain grows readily as an anaerobic photoheterotroph in medium 112 and can also be grown in several synthetic media that contain organic carbon sources, *d*-biotin (a required growth factor), and ammonium ions as nitrogen source (Gest and Favinger, 1983). The sulfur requirement for growth is satisfied by sulfate (sulfide is not required). Attempts to grow *H. chlorum* photoautotrophically with either H_2 or sulfide as electron donor have given negative results.

H. chlorum is very sensitive to molecular oxygen. To ensure growth, transfers are made in an anaerobic hood (atmosphere: ~85% N_2 plus 10% H_2 plus 5% CO_2), and other stringent anaerobic techniques are employed. Media free of O_2 are supplemented with 0.04% sodium thioglycolate, sodium ascorbate, or Ti^{3+} citrate. Inoculated cultures are exposed to incandescent illumination and must either be well-sealed, so as to prevent air leakage, or be incubated within an illuminated anaer-

obic jar. In contrast to many other kinds of anoxygenic photosynthetic bacteria, *H. chlorum* cannot grow aerobically in darkness.

The *in vivo* absorption spectrum of *H. chlorum* is characterized by a major peak at 788 nm and relatively small peaks at 575 and 670 nm. It appears that even low concentrations of O_2 cause irreversible alterations in the structure of bacteriochlorophyll *g*; in organic solvents (pyridine or acetone:methanol), the peak in the infrared disappears rapidly in the presence of light and air. The color of masses of cells, either on agar or in liquid media, is brownish-green in young cultures and tends to become emerald-green as cultures age. It is noteworthy that in contrast to other anoxyphototrophs, *H. chlorum* has a low carotenoid content.

Growth occurs over a temperature range of 20–45°C and is optimal at 35–42°C. *H. chlorum* fixes N_2 readily, a characteristic observed in virtually all procaryotic anoxyphototrophs.

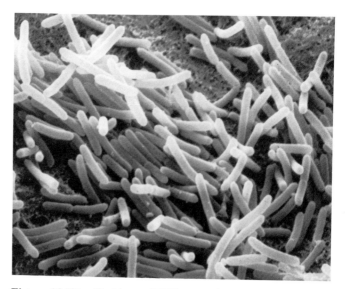

Figure 18.59. *H. chlorum* ATCC 35205. Scanning electron micrograph (× 5000). (Prepared by F. R. Turner, Indiana University.)

---

* The photosynthetic pigment was originally designated bacteriochlorophyll g_{G_g}, with G_g indicating geranylgeraniol as the esterifying alcohol (Brockmann and Lipinski, 1983). Further study has identified the alcohol as farnesol (Michalski et al., 1987).

†In our modification of ATCC medium 112, deionized water is used in place of tap water. The medium contains (per liter of water): K_2HPO_4, 1 g; $MgSO_4$, 0.5 g; and yeast extract, 10 g. The pH is adjusted to 7.0. For preparation of plates and stabs, 2% agar is used.

Enrichment and Isolation Procedures

H. chlorum was first observed in an enrichment culture designed (Gest et al., 1983) for selection of phototrophic anaerobes capable of using (a) N_2 as the major or sole source of cellular nitrogen, (b) light as the energy source and (c) certain organic acids as carbon sources. Ordinarily, a low concentration of NH_4Cl is added to provide nitrogen for *initiation* of growth, but in this instance ammonium sulfate was inadvertently used in place of chloride salt. Because of the presence of sulfate, the medium became strongly reducing, owing to generation of sulfide by sulfate reducers, and *H. chlorum* developed as a patch of dark green "slimy" mat. Organisms from the latter were subcultured once more in the liquid enrichment medium and then streaked on medium 112 agar plates (incubations under anaerobic photosynthetic conditions). Isolated colonies showing greenish pigmentation were re-streaked repeatedly, eventually yielding pure cultures of *H. chlorum*.

Maintenance Procedures

The ATCC has successfully stored *H. chlorum* at liquid N_2 temperature (for at least 6 months) in medium 112 supplemented with 10% glycerol. In our laboratory, we have observed good viability in medium 112 agar stabs stored either in the anaerobic hood at ambient temperature and room light or at $-20°C$ (in darkness). Growth in fresh agar stabs (medium 112) was recently demonstrated by using inocula from 16-month-old stabs stored as noted (the stored stabs were incubated in the light cabinet overnight before subculture).

Differentiation of the genus **Heliobacterium** *from other genera*

Heliobacterium shows superficial similarities with representatives of certain genera of *Rhodospirillaceae*, *Chloroflexaceae* and *Chlorobiaceae* but is readily distinguished on the basis of morphological, physiological and other properties. Although *Rhodopseudomonas gelatinosa* can resemble *Heliobacterium* in gross morphology, it differs in numerous other respects. Typical organisms of the green bacteria contain the photosynthetic pigments and accessory catalysts in chlorosomes, but these subcellular structures are absent from *Heliobacterium*. *Chloroflexus* has a high carotenoid content and can grow aerobically in darkness; on the other hand, *Heliobacterium* has a low carotenoid content and is an obligate photoanaerobe. The physiological character of *Chlorobium* is primarily photoautotrophic, whereas *Heliobacterium* is photoheterotrophic. The presence of bacteriochlorophyll *g*, with its unique in vivo absorbancy maximum at 788 nm, distinguishes *Heliobacterium* from all known genera of photosynthetic procaryotes.

List of species of the genus **Heliobacterium**

1. **Heliobacterium chlorum** Gest and Favinger 1985, 223.[VP] (Effective publication: Gest and Favinger 1983, 15.)

chlo′.rum. Gr. adj. *chloros* green.

The characteristics are the same as those described for the genus. Habitat: The type strain was isolated from surface soil.

The mol% G + C of the DNA of the type strain is 52 (T_m). *Type strain:* ATCC 35205.

Genus **Erythrobacter** *Shiba and Simidu 1982, 215*[VP]

HANS G. TRÜPER

E.ryth′ro.bac.ter. Gr. adj. *erythros* red; M.L. masc. n. *bacter* rod; M.L. masc. n. *Erythrobacter* red rod.

Cells are ovoid to rod-shaped, multiply by binary fission, and are Gram-negative. **Motile by means of subpolar flagella.** Cell suspensions and colonies orange or pink. **Contain bacteriochlorophyll *a* and carotenoids.**

Growth is aerobic, chemoorganoheterotrophic. Cultures do not grow anaerobically in the light and do not grow chemoautotrophically with H_2. **Metabolism is predominantly respiratory.** Under microaerobic conditions, small amounts of acid are produced from a wide range of carbohydrates.

Methanol is not utilized. Voges-Proskauer and methyl red tests are negative. Gelatin is hydrolyzed; some strains also hydrolyze alginate and Tween 80. Oxidase- and catalase-positive. Biotin is required for growth; some strains may also require thiamin, nicotinic acid and pantothenate. Susceptible to penicillin, chloramphenicol and tetracycline, not to nalidixic acid.

The mol% G + C of the DNA is 60-64 (T_m).

Type species: *Erythrobacter longus* Shiba and Simidu 1982, 216.

Further Descriptive Information

Since 1978, several bacteria have been reported to contain bacteriochlorophyll *a*, although they were incapable of anaerobic phototrophic growth (Harashima et al., 1978; Sato, 1978; Shiba et al., 1979; Nishimura et al., 1981). Only one new genus and species, however, has been described in which these properties are taxonomically important features: *Erythrobacter longus* Shiba and Simidu, 1982.

The distribution of *Erythrobacter*-like bacteria in aerobic marine environments was assessed by Shiba et al. (1979). Shiba and Simidu (1982) have recognized three different clusters of strains but have named only one of these, *E. longus*. They apparently consider the other two clusters to be different species to be further studied before these species should be legitimately named. Harashima et al. (1982) found reversible photooxidation of cytochromes, reversible photobleaching of bacteriochlorophyll, and light-inhibited O_2 uptake by cells of *Erythrobacter* species. They also observed vesicular intracytoplasmic membranes. Biosynthesis of bacteriochlorophyll a_p and carotenoids was found to be stimulated by oxygen (Harashima et al., 1980). Shiba (1984) showed that *Erythrobacter* species OCh 114 utilizes light energy in the aerobic environment. He found with this species, in comparison with dark controls, (a) increased intracellular ATP levels under light, (b) strongly increased survival times in the light in the absence of an organic energy source, and (c) enhancement of CO_2 incorporation by light as well as by oxygen.

Enrichment and Isolation Procedures

Enrichment of *Erythrobacter* strains has been done from marine beach sand, surface seawater and several seaweeds. The samples are diluted 10-fold with seawater and spread on agar plates of "PPES-II" medium (Taga, 1968) containing (per liter): 2 g polypeptone (Daigo Co.). 1 g proteose-peptone no. 3 (Difco), 1 g Bacto soytone (Difco), 1 g Bacto yeast extract (Difco), 0.1 g ferric phosphate "soluble" (Merck), 100 ml marine mud extract, 900 ml aged seawater and 15 g agar (Wako). The pH is adjusted to 7.6–7.8. Shiba et al. (1979) used a slightly modified version of this medium omitting the mud extract and replacing ferric phosphate with 0.1 g of ferric citrate. The agar plates are incubated at 20°C. Characteristic pink or orange colonies are streaked out on further agar plates by using the usual aerobic techniques. Thus pure cultures are easily obtainable.

Taxonomic Comments

Sato (1978) reported the occurrence of bacteriochlorophyll *a* in the facultatively methylotrophic aerobic bacteria *"Protaminobacter ruber"* den Dooren de Jong 1926, 159 and *"Pseudomonas AM-1"* (Peel and Quayle, 1961). These bacteria are not listed in the Approved Lists of Bacterial Names nor in the eighth edition of the *Manual.* Sato and Shimizu (1979) showed that in *"P. ruber,"* bacteriochlorophyll *a* formation was stimulated by exposure to light during early growth stages and that the presence of oxygen was needed. Continuous illumination, however, prevented pigment formation. A more detailed study by Sato et al. (1981) showed that a change from light to darkness in early growth stages stimulated pigment synthesis. Although the cells possessed vesicular intracytoplasmic membrane structures, the specific pigment-protein complexes typical for anaerobic phototrophic bacteria (e.g. *Rhodobacter sphaeroides*) were lacking. Nishimura et al. (1981) observed the occurrence of bacteriochlorophyll formation in *Pseudomonas radiora* Ito and Iizuka 1971, 1566,[AL] compared *P. radiora* with *Pseudomonas AM-1* (Peel and Quayle, 1961), and came to the conclusion that these bacteria do not belong in the same species. As the taxonomic position of *"Protaminobacter ruber"* and *"Pseudomonas AM-1"* is rather insecure (Leadbetter, 1974), detailed studies are necessary to clarify whether these organisms and, in addition, *Pseudomonas radiora* are similar or even related to *Erythrobacter* or to anaerobic phototrophic nonsulfur bacteria. Harashima et al. (1982) have considered the *Erythrobacter* group "aerobic photosynthetic bacteria."

List of species of the genus **Erythrobacter**

1. **Erythrobacter longus** Shiba and Simidu 1982, 216.[VP]

lon'gus. L. adj. *longus* long.

Cells rod-shaped and 0.5×1.0–$5.0 \ \mu m$. Contain vesicular intracytoplasmic membrane system. Pigments are bacteriochlorophyll *a* (esterified with phytol) and carotenoids. Metabolism is aerobic chemoorganotrophic, never anaerobic phototrophic. The carbon sources utilized are: glucose, acetate, pyruvate, glutamate and butyrate; not utilized are: citrate, malate, succinate, glycolate, lactate, formate and methanol. Optimal growth temperature: 25–30°C. Optimal salinity of media: 1.7–3.5% NaCl. Optimal pH: 7.0–8.0. Biotin required for growth. Phosphatase, catalase and oxidase present. Some strains reduce nitrate to nitrite. H_2S not produced. Indole produced; gelatin and Tween 80 and, by some strains, alginate are hydrolyzed. Susceptible to chloramphenicol, penicillin, tetracycline and fusidic acid but not to streptomycin, polymyxin B or nalidixic acid. Habitat: oxic marine environments, predominantly on seaweeds.

The mol% G + C of the DNA is 60–64 (T_m) (type strain: 60.7 (T_m).

Type strain: 0Ch 101; Institute for Fermentation, Osaka, Japan, (IFO) no. 14 126.

SECTION 19

Oxygenic Photosynthetic Bacteria

The oxygenic photosynthetic procaryotes comprise two separate groups. The most thoroughly studied and understood group is the cyanobacteria. This is a widely distributed and diverse collection of unicellular to multicellular photosynthetic bacteria that possess chlorophyll *a* and carry out oxygenic photosynthesis.

A more recently discovered group of oxygenic photosynthetic procaryotes is placed in the order *Prochlorales*. These bacteria share many features with the cyanobacteria, but they also contain chlorophyll *b* as well as chlorophyll *a,* lack phycobilin pigments, and differ in some other features. This group appears to be phylogenetically related to the cyanobacteria on the basis of 16S rRNA data, but their exact position has not yet been determined. A special glossary for these organisms has been included.

Key to the **Oxygenic Photosynthetic Bacteria**

I. Contain chlorophyll *a* and have phycobilins
>> Group I. Cyanobacteria, p. 1710
II. Contain both chlorophylls *b* and *a* and lack phycobilins
>> Group II. *Prochlorales*, p. 1799

Glossary to the **Oxygenic Photosynthetic Bacteria**

Baeocyte: a small cell formed internally by multiple fissions in parent cells of Subsection II (*Pleurocapsales*).

False branch: a branch formed by a slipping to one side of a section or loop of trichome through the sheath; a branch not formed by lateral division of a cell (see Figs. 19.7 and 19.49).

Filament: a chain of cells together with an investing sheath (in cyanobacteria).

Gas vacuole: an area in cells that refracts light, during observation under light microscopy, because of its gaseous nature, often appearing red; composed of numerous gas vesicles.

Gas vesicle: a subunit of a gas vacuole; each subunit is a cylindrical structure with conical ends (as seen with transmission electron microscopy), composed of a single protein envelope (~2 nm thick), impervious to water and containing gas.

Geminate: to become doubled or paired; arranged in pairs.

Hormocyst: a hormogoniumlike short chain of cells enveloped or encapsulated by a thick outer envelope or sheath.

Hormogonium: a fragmented, short segment of trichome that is motile and apparently functions as a disseminule.

Lectotype: an element subsequently designated or selected from among syntypes to serve as the definitive type.

Meristem: a localized region of cell division.

Multiseriate: arranged with more than one row of cells, as a result of cells in trichome dividing in more than one plane.

Necridial cell: a localized dead or dead-appearing cell of a trichome; the possible result of regulated differentiation and lysis; the cell at which trichome fragmentation occurs.

Syntype: any of two or more elements used as types by the author of a name, whether or not it is designated as such by the author.

Thallus: a plantlike body composed of many cells or filaments; the thallus may have a definite shape but lacks internal differentiation.

Thylakoid: the intracellular membrane system that includes the reaction center, chlorophyll *a* (and *b* in *Prochlorales*), and some carotenoid pigments.

Trichome: a chain of cells without an investing sheath (in cyanobacteria).

True branch: a branch formed by lateral or oblique division of a cell in a trichome.

Tychoplankton: floating or free-living organisms in shallow water of a lake, intermingled with attached vegetation and periphyton, usually near shore.

Uniseriate: arranged in a single row or series of cells, such as in a branched or unbranched trichome.

GROUP I. **CYANOBACTERIA**

Preface

R. W. Castenholz and John B. Waterbury

HISTORICAL BACKGROUND

Nucleotide base sequence data from 16S and 5S rRNA place blue-green procaryotes within the eubacteria, a group distinct and apart from the archaeobacteria and eucaryotes. For this reason alone they should now be given extended treatment in this manual of systematic bacteriology. There are, however, considerable obstacles in the way of describing this group in the same manner as most other procaryotes. The problem is the great array of existing genera and species that were described solely on the basis of morphological characteristics obtained from field-collected samples, and the difficulty of relating these to living populations growing as clones in axenic culture. The cyanobacteria or blue-green algae were traditionally treated as algae, i.e. a group that could be defined by broad morphological/cytological/chemical features and separated into distinct divisions, classes, orders, and lower categories on the basis of morphological distinctions. There was ample reason to proceed in this manner from early in the past century to the middle of the present century, since cytological data were limited to impressions from light microscopy and only relatively crude chemical data were available. There were reasons to connect the blue-greens with bacteria, but the evidence was not overwhelming. By late in the past century (see Fritsch, 1945) it had been realized that blue-green algae were unique and lacked the traditional nucleus and chloroplasts of the green and other algae. However, the morphological characteristics of the blue-green algae and their ecological niches were so similar to those of many microalgae that few investigators doubted their place as the base or a branch of a true algal phylogeny (Fritsch, 1945). Cohn, however, concluded that the blue-green algae and bacteria were closely related and proposed that the blue-greens (*Schizophyceae*) and bacteria (*Schizomycetes*) be grouped in the one division *Schizophyta* (Cohn, 1872, 1875).

The size of the blue-green cell ranges from <1 μm to >100 μm in diameter, a range also spanned by the eucaryotic green algae (division *Chlorophyta*). However, wide-diameter cells are invariably short (discoid). Demoulin and Janssen (1981) speculate that this may not be fortuitous but may be related to the typically short-lived mRNA in procaryotes. The complexity of simple multicellular and branched filaments and even multiseriate and thalliform "macrophytes" among the blue-greens would also lead most casual observers to the conclusion that these were "algae," not "bacteria." Pigments, although they could not be ascribed to chloroplasts in blue-green algae, nevertheless, include phycobilins extremely similar to those of the red algae (division *Rhodophyta*). The phycobiliproteins of both groups were fairly well-defined chemically as early as the 1930s (see Strain, 1951). The possession of water-soluble phycobiliproteins but the lack of membrane-bounded nuclei and chloroplasts led most investigators to set aside the blue-greens as a separate class (*Myxophyceae* Wallroth 1833 (Gr. fem. n. *myxa* slime or mucus), *Cyanophyceae* Sachs 1874 (Gr. n. *kyanos* blue); hence, blue-green algae—Eng.; Blaualgen—Ger.; Algues bleues—Fr.).

The building of the current morphology-based taxonomy of blue-greens began in earnest with Bornet and Flahault (1886–1888) and Gomont (1892). Under the International Code of Botanical Nomenclature, the starting point for the valid publication of names of nonheterocystous, filamentous blue-green algae (family *Oscillatoriaceae*) is with Gomont (1892), and that for the heterocystous forms is with Bornet and Flahault (1886–1888). Otherwise, the starting point is with Linnaeus (1753), as for almost all algal groups. The gathering of genera and species was continued, culminating with Geitler (1932) who produced a comprehensive treatise which recognized approximately 1300 species, 145 genera, 20 families, and 3 orders. This treatise, although regional in intent, in practice is worldwide. However, freshwater forms are more completely treated than marine forms. A similarly comprehensive treatise was published by Elenkin (1936, 1938, 1949) in Russian, but because of the language barrier for most phycologists, it was less used. Other major gatherings of blue-green species on a regional basis are those of Tilden (1910), Borzi (1916–1917), Frémy (1929–1933), Huber-Pestalozzi (1938), Hollerbach et al. (1953), Komárek (1958), Desikachary (1959) and Starmach (1966). Bourrelly (1970, 1985) reorganized the freshwater blue-greens at the familial and generic level. All followed a classification similar to that of Geitler (1932); this has become known as the "Geitlerian" system. In recent years, most blue-green specialists and nonspecialists have followed this organization. However, beginning with Drouet and Daily (1956), a major revision and consolidation of blue-green names was initiated (Drouet, 1968, 1973, 1978, 1981). The "Drouet" system, although gradually modified during the course of his work, resulted in an enormous reduction in the profusion of recognized generic and species names. Over 2000 species in over 140 genera were eventually reduced to 62 species in 24 genera. This system was not accepted by most "blue-green" taxonomists. However, several "blue-green" biochemists and physiologists have used the Drouet system because of its simplicity and the relative ease with which a binomial could be allocated.

A large number of species and genera had been described over the years on the basis of a single difference, such as trichome width, presence or nature of sheath, number of trichomes per sheath, color, and other features which later have been shown to have a great flexibility within clonal populations of some species, particularly when environmental conditions vary (e.g. Pearson and Kingsbury, 1966). However, some cyanobacterial clones in culture are quite conservative morphologically (Stam, 1978; Stulp, 1982; Stulp and Stam, 1982). Drouet presumed that relatively few cyanobacterial genotypes existed but that there were many phenotypes expressed in different environments (ecophenes). His decisions, however, were based mainly on his appreciation of the group through the microscopic examinations of an extremely large number of collected specimens. No matter how much material is examined, decisions of this type are, of necessity, more arbitrary and less likely to reflect true relationship than decisions based on manipulations of clonal strains in culture. No clonal cultures were established by Drouet; no physiological, biochemical or genetic information was included. The incorrectness of several decisions by Drouet has now been established by various means, including DNA/DNA hybridization and DNA base composition comparisons, by Stam and associates (Stam and Holleman, 1975, 1979; Stam and Venema, 1977; Stam, 1980). For a more exhaustive critique of Drouet's system, see Komárek (1983).

By the early 1970s, Stanier and associates had begun the development of a taxonomy of cyanobacteria which was based on information that could be used to address essentially the same profusion of names that Drouet had wished to correct (e.g. Stanier et al., 1971; Waterbury and Stanier, 1978; Rippka et al., 1979, 1981b). This system is based on the use of axenic, clonal cultures only and some of their morphological, cytological, genetical, chemical and physiological characteristics. At this time, however, mainly generic distinctions have been formulated, and the problem of species has largely been avoided.

The morphological and cytological data used by Stanier's group to distinguish genera were based on characteristics observable with light microscopy, except in the case of the presence or absence of thylakoids for which electron microscopy is required. The main characteristics include: the type of cellular division and the plane of subsequent divisions; the formation of baeocytes ("endospores" of the older blue-green algal terminology); the formation and structure of hormogonia; the presence and type of sheath or glycocalyx; the shape and dimensions of cells and the presence of constrictions between adjacent cells of trichomes; the nature of trichomes (helical or straight, unbranched, false branched or true branched, tapered or not); the presence and location of heterocysts and resting spores (akinetes); and the presence and location of gas vacuoles.

Chemical, genetical and physiological characteristics include: motility and phototaxis; base composition (mol% G + C) of the DNA; chemoheterotrophic and photoheterotrophic capability and substrate specificity; vitamin requirements; aerobic and anaerobic N_2-fixation ability; types of phycobilin pigments; temperature and salt tolerance or requirement; and sensitivity to lysis by specific cyanophages.

The comparison of base sequence catalogs of oligonucleotides of 16S rRNA indicate that cyanobacteria represent a moderately deep phylogenetic unit within the Gram-negative eubacteria and that chloroplasts of eucaryotes, most particularly those of the red alga *Porphyridium*, fall into this unit (see Stackebrandt and Woese, 1981).

Through all of the developments and controversies of blue-green taxonomy, there has seldom been a dispute about whether a particular organism (collected or in culture) was a blue-green or not, but the use of the term "cyanobacteria" in place of "blue-green algae" has offended many. The objections to the term "cyanobacteria" seem to be based on tradition as well as on ecological and physiological grounds. Stanier and van Niel (1962) assumed that the term "bacterium" was regarded as synonymous with procaryote. Others have believed that the term "bacterium" should be relegated to the group traditionally known by that name and that the term "blue-green alga" should be retained. They have argued that in cell size and morphological complexity the blue-greens more closely resemble the green algae and other microalgae than the other bacteria and that their dual photosystems were almost identical with that of the eucaryotic algae and higher green plants rather than with anything known in the anoxygenic photosynthetic bacteria. Most of the blue-greens occur as primary producers in aerobic environments, alternating or interspersed with the eucaryotic algae as plankton, tychoplankton and periphyton. From the ecological point of view, it was much easier to think of the blue-greens as algae, and this remains so for many biologists.

In the late 18th century, the term "algae" was introduced by Roth as representing a taxonomic group. During the first half of the 19th century, the heterogeneity of this group became evident (see Nägeli, 1849). Cohn (1872) pointed out that the "algae" was an artificial group, taxonomically. By the end of the past century, the use of the term "algae" as a taxonomic unit virtually disappeared from botanical classifications. "Algae" remained, however, as a general term for the assemblage of all photosynthetic organisms with a level of differentiation less than that characteristic of archegoniate plants. This definition appears satisfactory, as it admits that the term "algae" represents a biological grouping of taxonomically and phylogenetically widely divergent organisms. A comparable situation exists in the case of "Protozoa," "Flagellatae," and "Protista," biologically useful terms without taxonomic implications, since they include both "algae" and animallike groups. Similarly, there seems to be no reason why the term "algae" could not continue to include both eucaryotes and the oxygenic procaryotes. From the definition of "algae" above, it follows that *"Cyanophyceae"* and "blue-green algae" are proper, alternative terms to "cyanobacteria" and "blue-green bacteria," since they have only a biological, not taxonomic, implication.

However, the use of the terms *"Cyanophyta"* or "cyanophytes" should be discouraged, since it implies that the blue-greens are plants (Gr. n. *phyton* plant). The term *"Cyanophyceae"* merely indicates that they are algae (Gr. n. *phykos* algae).

Bacteria (like "plants" but unlike "algae") form a taxonomic group; at least individually the "eubacteria" and "archaeobacteria" do. The term "bacteria" is presently defined by bacteriologists as synonymous with "procaryotes." From this it follows that the term "cyanobacteria" is a taxonomically correct name for the blue-greens, although it has no official standing. Both "cyanobacteria" and "blue-green algae" (*Cyanophyceae*) should be considered usable and compatible names. The first refers to a phylogenetic/taxonomic relationship and certainly will be preferred by bacteriologists and many others, while the second refers to the ecological/biological nature of the group and will probably be used by many, but not all, botanists.

PROBLEMS OF NOMENCLATURE

Stanier et al. (1978) proposed that cyanobacteria be placed under the rules of the International Code of Nomenclature of Bacteria (ICNB), removing them from the jurisdiction of the Botanical Code. In addition, the proposed date for the publication of approved names for these procaryotes was set at January 1, 1985. This proposal was not adopted by the International Union of Microbiological Societies (IUMS) in Munich in 1978. The proposal resulted in many objections from the "botanical community" (e.g. Bourrelly, 1979; Geitler, 1979; Golubic, 1979; Lewin, 1979). The "botanists" were concerned that if such a proposal had force, a rich array of names of uncultured blue-green algae would be unrecognized and perhaps lost. Many ecological studies for which identification of field specimens is necessary could come into disrepute because of the lack of names recognized by the "bacteriological community." At present, the names of cyanobacteria, which are based on cultures, are often inapplicable to field material because of the loss of numerous morphological and cytological characteristics under common culture conditions. There is reason for optimism, however, since it is becoming a more common practice to vary culture conditions to the extent that these characteristics are often exhibited (e.g. Evans et al., 1976; Jeeji-Bai, 1976; Sinclair and Whitton, 1977a, b; Stulp, 1982; Stulp and Stam, 1984a; Douglas et al., 1986). However, most cyanobacterial cultures that are used extensively have little or no attendant information on the natural population and habitat from which they were originally isolated. There is also concern that a type culture, being mutable, may change with time and no longer resemble the original material from which it came. A type culture, therefore, in some ways is less adequate than a type specimen.

From the traditional bacteriologist's point of view, a preserved type specimen (as demanded by the Botanical Code) is unsatisfactory in lieu of a type culture. One of the particular objections is that when microorganisms are involved, feral samples may contain hundreds or thousands of individuals and genetic heterogeneity is very likely. There is also apprehension about descriptions of species based on observations of the morphology of field samples where considerable phenotypic variation could result from environmental variables. The present chaotic state of blue-green taxonomy is based primarily on morphology; thus, some biologists would prefer a new start, thereby discarding the older system entirely.

There is no doubt that both "botanical" and "bacteriological" taxonomists will continue to describe new taxa and reorganize older taxa of blue-greens, following the rules of the Botanical and the Bacteriological Code, respectively. Some working agreement is absolutely required in order to avoid the extremely confusing situation in which there are two names for each organism.

A recent change in the Rules of Botanical Nomenclature (Recommendation 9A.1.) states that whenever practicable a living culture should be prepared from the holotype material of a new taxon of algae (or fungi) and deposited in a reputable culture collection. This does not replace the need for the preserved holotype specimen (Article 9.5).

In addition, Article 45.4 of the Botanical Code states in part (Voss, 1983): "If the taxon is treated as belonging to the algae, any of its names need satisfy only the requirements of the pertinent non-botanical code for status equivalent to valid publication under the Botanical Code." Thus, a cyanobacterium described correctly under the rules of the Bacteriological Code would be recognized as valid by botanists.

Nevertheless, it is necessary that a complete compromise become legitimized. The problems were addressed during the 1981 Eighth International Botanical Congress. The following excerpt is from Friedmann and Borowitzka (1982):

"On August 25, 1981, an informal discussion group (L. J. Borowitzka, Michael A. Borowitzka (Sydney, AUSTRALIA), V. Demoulin, E. I. Friedmann, Mark A. Mackay (Sydney, AUSTRALIA), V. May, Roseli Ocampo-Friedmann (Tallahassee, FL, USA), W. T. Stam, R. Townsend, J. B. Waterbury) agreed on the following compromise Proposal:

1. Blue-green algae (Cyanobacteria) may be described following either the Botanical or the Bacteriological Code, with nomenclatural types chosen according to the Rule of each Code. It is understood that the different type concepts which are intrinsic to each Code are not affected by this proposal.
2. According to Article 9 of the Botanical Code, the type of a species is a preserved specimen (or, in absence of such, a description or a figure). It is recommended that, when describing a blue-green alga, all efforts should be made to obtain a living pure culture which then should be deposited in a permanently established culture collection. Whenever possible, physiological and genetic characteristics of the cultured material should be determined. The new name, to-

gether with reference to the type and effectively published description, should be published in the *International Journal of Systematic Bacteriology,* in accordance with Appendix 7 of the International Code of Nomenclature of Bacteria.

3. According to Rule 18A of the Bacteriological Code, the type of a species is, whenever possible, a designated strain made up of living cultures of an organism which are descended from a strain designated as the nomenclatural type (or, if unculturable, a description, a preserved specimen, or an illustration). It is recommended that, when describing a cyanobacterium, a large sample of the type culture should be preserved (preferably as a dry specimen) which then should be deposited in a permanent institution (herbarium) and that the description be accompanied by photomicrographs or drawings in accordance with Article 39 of the International Code of Botanical Nomenclature. Whenever possible, the specimen from which the type culture was obtained should be preserved and information about environmental conditions recorded.

4. The starting date for the Approved List of Bacterial Names for Cyanobacteria is indefinitely postponed.

5. Names of Cyanophyta validly published under the Bacteriological Code as Cyanobacteria are valid according to the Botanical Code.

6. Names of Cyanobacteria validly published under the Botanical Code as Cyanophyta are valid according to the Bacteriological Code."

Points 2 and 5 have already been addressed by the Botanical Code. The following recommendation was approved by the International Committee on Systematic Bacteriology (ICSB) in 1986:

"The Subcommittee for the Taxonomy of Phototrophic Bacteria of the ICSB proposes that names of cyanobacteria described and validly published as blue-green algae under the International Code of Botanical Nomenclature are recognized as having been validly published under the International Code of Nomenclature of Bacteria [(ICNB)].

"The immediate goal of this proposal is to avoid a possibly chaotic situation resulting from the introduction of new names for already existing and recognizable taxa.

"The Subcommittee recommends that, when cyanobacteria are described under the ICNB, in addition to depositing a living type culture in at least one permanently established culture collection (Recommendation 30a, ICNB), a preserved sample of the type culture (preferably as a dry specimen) be deposited in a permanent institution (herbarium) and that the description be accompanied by photomicrographs or drawings in accordance with Article 39 of the . . . [ICNB]. Whenever possible the specimen from which the type culture was obtained should be preserved and information about environmental conditions recorded. The new name, together with reference to the type and effectively published description, should be published in the *International Journal of Systematic Bacteriology* in accordance with Appendix 7, ICNB."

This recommendation is being processed by the Rules Revision Committee and will then be formally proposed and voted upon at the International Congress for Microbiology in 1990. The acceptance of this proposal by the bacteriologists would establish the reciprocity that is needed for compromise and should allow a climate of cooperation for the naming of blue-green procaryotes.

The above proposal recognizes that priority, with regard to names, rests with the Botanical Code. Stanier's group (Rippka et al., 1979) has proceeded in this manner, using previously recognized botanical names throughout. However, it is important that bacteriologists not regard the names used by Rippka et al. (1979) as an unofficial starting point for cyanobacterial names. The limited number of names used was determined by the limited number of cultures available. If more taxa had been represented, other names from the botanical literature would have been used. If correspondence is lacking between a novel organism in culture and the generic categories established by Rippka et al. (1979) or those used in this chapter, a preexisting botanical name, if any exist that are recognizable as the same taxon, should be chosen. There are numerous, clearly defined genera of blue-greens named in the botanical literature that would have been used by Rippka et al. (1979) if representatives had been studied in culture. Many of these are described later in this chapter.

A new date for establishing an "Approved List of Names" may never occur as a unilateral action of "bacteriologists," but it may be done as a cooperative venture with "botanists." It may be highly desirable, however, to eventually produce such a list. The use of Linnaeus (1753) as a starting point for some groups is not very useful. The publication of Geitler (1932) represents a reasonable and practical point of departure.

One problem will continue for several years. When botanical names are used, they are expected to be used according to their strict (e.g. "Geitlerian") meaning unless they are subsequently redefined. The generic names used in this publication (sensu Castenholz or Waterbury) are nearly always interpreted differently. In order to avoid confusion, it should be indicated whether the names are used "sensu Geitler," "sensu Rippka et al.," "sensu Drouet," etc. Eventually, different interpretations may be merged as more information becomes available, and the distinctions could be dropped.

In the foreseeable future, the two systems for the classification of cyanobacteria will exist. This may not cause difficulties if these two systems run in parallel and do not diverge without control. This is best achieved by developing the bacteriological system from the existing botanical assemblage of names, whenever such taxa are recognizable. It is also important that scientists following the Botanical Code try, to a greater extent, to expand the descriptions of new taxa beyond that of morphological characteristics to additional physiological and genetic characteristics obtained from the use of cultures. Persons following either code should provide much more ecological information than has generally been customary.

CHARACTERISTICS AND CRITERIA FOR NEW SPECIES DESCRIPTIONS

New taxa may be described by fulfilling the requirements of both the Bacteriological and the Botanical Code without much difficulty.

For "Bacteriologists"

If a taxon is described according to the Bacteriological Code, *in addition:*

1. Describe and illustrate the feral sample.
2. Indicate the specific location of the collection.
3. Preserve the feral sample ("herbarium" specimen), deposit it in a recognized institution (e.g. herbarium), and indicate the place of deposition.
4. Preserve the dry sample of culture, deposit it in a recognized institution, and indicate the place of deposition.
   (Note: Latin diagnosis is not required!)

For "Botanists"

If a taxon is described according to the Botanical Code, *in addition:*

1. Isolate the clonal culture (preferably axenic; at least no other blue-green), deposit it in recognized culture collection, and indicate the place of deposition.
2. Submit the name and the relevant reprint to the *International Journal of Systematic Bacteriology.*

Although there are as yet no legalized, minimal requirements for the description of a new species of cyanobacteria under the Bacteriological Code, the following list of desirable information ("Guidelines for Characterization of the Cyanobacteria") may be of help. This list is similar to that currently proposed for phototrophic bacteria by the Subcommittee on the Taxonomy of the Phototrophic Bacteria (ICSB of the IUMS). Minimal standards may eventually be legalized in the Bacteriological Code.

It is difficult to separate *desirable* and *required* or *absolutely minimal* information. Obviously, the more characteristics known, the more rigorous the description will be. Describers should consider sending out cultured material to specialists who are willing to apply their techniques. Some characteristics are more important for certain groups of cyanobacteria than for others. Whenever possible, characteristics from both cultures and field specimens should be used, with the sources indicated.

Similar criteria should be used for redescribing poorly characterized cyanobacteria that were previously named under the Bacteriological or the Botanical Code. The following list ("Guidelines") includes some characteristics that may be applicable only to restricted groups of cyanobacteria. The accounts of individual cyanobacterial sections include more specific characteristics. Whenever possible, statistically significant quantitative information should be gathered. Some authors have proposed numerical coding systems of characters that can be computerized (e.g. Whitton et al., 1979; Griffiths, 1984; Stulp and Stam, 1984b).

The protocol of precedence for reporting on all the characters listed below are spread over numerous references, many of which will be cited in a succeeding section which is a general description of cyanobacteria.

There will be many difficulties and tasks concerned with the description and naming of cyanobacteria over the next few decades. For persons approaching this work from a bacteriological background, an Advisory Panel on Cyanobacterial Nomenclature has been established by the Subcommittee on the Taxonomy of Phototrophic Bacteria of the ICSB. All members of the "phototrophic subcommittee" concerned with cyanobacterial taxonomy are automatically members, and other interested persons have been added. Currently, John B. Waterbury is the Advisory Panel Chairman.

The tasks of the Advisory Panel are:

1. To offer assistance to editorial boards of microbiological journals to whom manuscripts are submitted that newly describe and name cyanobacterial taxa under the rules of the Bacteriological Code. The panel will then quickly advise if the new name is appropriate. If it appears not to be because of a similar taxon previously described as a blue-green alga, the chairman will send appropriate references to the journal editor, along with advice on the use of the name, for transmittal to the author or authors.

2. To offer assistance and information directly to workers who wish to describe and name new cyanobacterial taxa. To avoid the use of a new name for a "Geitlerian" genus or species that is already adequately delineated by the botanical system, authors are encouraged to approach the panel before submitting manuscripts of this type to journals. It is the author's ultimate responsibility to find out whether the "name" corresponds to a previous name; this procedure, however, should hasten the process and may avert the later rejection of the new names by reason of synonymy.

3. To inform "botanists" (phycologists, planktonologists) about what is necessary for a description of cyanobacteria under the ICNB, by periodic publication of that information in the journals *Taxon* and *Phycologia*.

4. To compile a list of cyanobacterial strains in axenic culture and keep this updated. The list will be circulated among the members of the "phototrophic subcommittee" and the Advisory Panel.

Guidelines for Characterization of the Cyanobacteria

Cell Morphology	*Physiology/Biochemistry*
• Cell shape, polarity • Cell dimensions (diameter, length) • Number and regularity of planes of fission or of budding • Color of cells and cell suspension *If present:* • Sheath or glycocalyx description • Location of "chromatoplasm" • Gas vacuoles (location) • Baeocyte ("endospore") description • Heterocyst and akinete description (dimensions, shape, etc.)	• Absorption spectrum ("in vivo") • Types of phycobilin pigments present • Capacity for chromatic adaptation • Temperature optimum and upper limit • Capacity for dark chemoheterotrophy (aerobic vs. anaerobic) and photoheterotrophy (with DCMU); substrates used • Motility (speed, rotation, smoothness) • Growth and/or acetylene reduction in aerobic or anaerobic conditions free of combined nitrogen and in light • Salinity tolerance • Vitamin requirements • Morphological responses to deficiencies of phosphate and combined nitrogen • Sensitivity to soluble sulfide; sulfide-dependent anoxygenic photosynthetic capacity • Calcium carbonate deposition
Ultrastructure	
• Thylakoid arrangement • Cell wall structural appearance • Cell inclusion types (identification of storage granules) • Sheath structure	
Colony or Trichome Morphology	*Culture Conditions*
• Colony or thallus shape, arrangement and symmetry • Trichome type: tapered, straight or helical; constricted at septa; false or true branching; shape of terminal cell; terminal hair formation; dimensions and characteristics of hormogonia • Location and pattern of heterocysts and akinetes • Akinete germination patterns	• Specifics of medium, temperature, light intensity, isolation method, strain history, and conservation of cultures including the type strain
Genetic Characteristics	*Habitat/Ecology*
• DNA base composition (mol% G + C) • DNA/DNA or DNA/RNA hybridization data with other species • Partial or complete sequence data for 16S rRNA • Complete sequences for 5S rRNA	• General description of habitat (e.g. marine, brackish water, freshwater, terrestrial; eutrophic, oligotrophic; flowing or static waters; temperature; depth; aerobic or anaerobic; high or low light intensity; associated organisms; possible symbiotic situations) • Growth habit (planktonic: fascicles, clusters, nonaggregated; attached: streamers, tufted, crustose, nodular, etc.)

CULTURES OF CYANOBACTERIA

At present, a small (perhaps minuscule) percentage of cyanobacteria are in culture, either axenically or with one or more heterotrophic bacteria. This paucity reflects relatively few attempts to isolate blue-greens from some habitats and also a very real difficulty in growing a large variety of forms by using present culture methods. For example, some cyanobacteria appear to be sensitive to high nutrient concentrations; others appear not to tolerate the contaminants in even reagent grade chemicals (e.g. Morel and Rueter, 1979). Tables 19.1 and 19.2 are arranged so that the media of lower nutrient concentration are given in the columns on the left side. The sensitivity of some cyanobacteria to high or even moderate light intensities is well-known but rarely documented (see Rippka et al., 1981a).

The task of bringing all or most cyanobacteria into culture will take many decades, but it will undoubtedly be pursued actively, and a taxonomy based on the cultured material will continue to expand. Many difficulties exist at present in relating culture strains to blue-greens in their native habitats, but for ecological and taxonomic reality this must become a goal with high priority. The normally rich nutrient concoction of the average batch culture medium in which cyanobacteria are maintained does not allow the expression of many morphological and physiological characteristics which are seen in the native habitat (see Tables 19.1–19.3). For example, hair differentiation at the tips of some species of the *Rivularia/Calothrix* group may be suppressed by high phosphate concentration (Sinclair and Whitton, 1977a; Wood et al., 1986); hetero-cyst differentiation and nitrogenase synthesis as well as trichome taper and other morphological features are suppressed by high ammonia or nitrate concentrations in the medium (e.g. Sinclair and Whitton, 1977a; Stewart, 1980). Cell diameter, pigment content, sheath formation and pigmentation, colony formation, typical branching and many other characteristics are sometimes altered by the commonly used culture conditions (e.g. Evans et al., 1976). Cultures need not be maintained or studied under only one condition; and there is certainly reason for optimism, since many investigators continually produce the equivalent of natural population morphology in their culture isolates. More culturists should make this effort. If one is certain of the source of the isolate and can match culture and field populations, the goal is always in sight, and morphological and physiological observations can be cross-matched.

Bergey's is intended as a manual of the characteristics of procaryotes in pure culture. However, several noncultured bacteria that are known to exist because of repeated observations or because of vivid, nonconfusing characteristics are included in the eighth edition of the *Manual* as well as in the first edition of *Bergey's Manual® of Systematic Bacteriology*. Volume 3, includes a detailed description of only a few outstanding cyanobacterial genera which lack representatives in culture.

There is no reason to exclude information from clonal cultures of cyanobacteria that include one or more heterotrophic bacteria. Although much biochemical and physiological data cannot be obtained from such cultures, the requirement of axenic cultures should not become a dogma.

Table 19.1.

Composition of freshwater media for **Cyanobacteria**[a]

Ingredient	CHU no. 10 (modified)	Gerloff et al. (1950)	BG-11[b]	D medium[c]	Allen and Arnon	Kratz and Myers
Na$_2$-EDTA			1[d]		4[e]	
NTA				100		
Citric acid	3	3	6			165[f]
NaNO$_3$		41	1500[g]	700		
KNO$_3$				100	2020	1000
Ca(NO$_3$)$_2$·4H$_2$O	40–60					25
K$_2$HPO$_4$·3H$_2$O	13		40		456	1000
Na$_2$HPO$_4$		8		110		
MgSO$_4$·7H$_2$O	25	15	75	100	246	250
CaSO$_4$·2H$_2$O				60		
MgCl$_2$·6H$_2$O		21				
CaCl$_2$·2H$_2$O		36	36		74	
KCl		9				
NaCl				8	232	
Na$_2$CO$_3$(·H$_2$O)	20	20	20			20 (optional)
Ferric ammonium citrate			6			
Ferric citrate	3	3				
	or					
FeCl$_3$	3			0.3[h]		
Fe$_2$(SO$_4$)$_3$·6H$_2$O						4
Micronutrients	i	i	1 ml[j]	0.5 ml[k]	i	1 ml[j]
Vitamin mix	i	i	i	i	i	i

[a]Unless otherwise indicated, concentrations are in mg l^{-1} of double-distilled or deionized water. (Modified from R. W. Castenholz, Methods in Enzymology *167*: 81, 1988, ©Academic Press, New York.)

[b]pH 7.4 after cooling.

[c]Prepared as a 20-fold concentrated stock, stored at 4°C. Micronutrients and FeCl$_3$ are included in the stock. pH is adjusted to 8.2 with NaOH before autoclaving. After cooling and clearing, pH is about 7.5.

[d]Na$_2$Mg-EDTA is generally used.

[e]13% FeNa-EDTA.

[f]Na$_3$ citrate·2H$_2$O.

[g]The nitrate concentration is often lowered.

[h]Sometimes, 2–4 times this amount is used. A stock solution of 0.29 g l^{-1} is kept at 4°C.

[i]Micronutrients and vitamins are optional; if they are used, they should be 0.5–1.0 ml of any mixture in Table 19.3.

[j]The medium generally uses "A5 + Co" (see Table 19.3).

[k]D-micro (see Table 19.3).

Table 19.2.
Composition of marine and hypersaline media for **Cyanobacteria**[a]

Ingredient	"Grund"[b]	"f/2"[b]	"MN"[c]	Ong et al.[d]	ASP-M[e]	"Aquil"[f]	"Erdschreiber's"[b]	Yopp et al.[g]
Na_2-EDTA	2	10[h]	0.5	5	0.8[h]		10[h]	5[h]
Citric acid			3					
$NaNO_3$	40	90	750	750	40–170	8.5	150	
$Ca(NO_3)_2 \cdot 4H_2O$								1000
Na_2HPO_4	4						40	
$NaH_2PO_4 \cdot H_2O$		5–20	20	15	7–14	0.5		65
$MgSO_4 \cdot 7H_2O$			38		4,920			10,000
$MgCl_2 \cdot 6H_2O$					4,040	11,030		10,680
$CaCl_2 \cdot 2H_2O$	10		18		1,270	1,000–1,350		
$Na_2CO_3(\cdot H_2O)$			20					
$NaHCO_3$					168	200		
Na_2SO_4						4,090		
NaCl					23,200	24,360		117,000
KCl					740	695		2,000
KBr						10		
NaF						3		
$Fe_2(SO_4)_3 \cdot 6H_2O$	0.2							
Na_2SeO_4 (0.01 mM stock)	1 ml							
$NiSO_4(NH_4)_2SO_4 \cdot 6H_2O$ (0.1 mM stock)	1 ml							
Micronutrients	0.2 ml[i]	1 ml[j]	1 ml[k]	1 ml	1 ml[l]	0.5 ml[m]		1 ml[n]
Ferric ammonium citrate			3					
Vitamin mix	0.5 ml[o]	1 ml[o]		1–2 ml	1 ml[p]	0.5–1.0 ml[q]	0.5 ml[q]	
Natural or artificial seawater	1000 ml	1000 ml	750 ml	877 ml			950 ml	
Distilled/deionized H_2O			250 ml	120 ml	1000 ml	1000 ml		1000 ml
Soil extract							50 ml[r]	

[a]Unless otherwise indicated, concentrations are in mg l⁻¹ of natural or artificial seawater or distilled H_2O. (Modified from R. W. Castenholz, Methods in Enzymology *167:* 84–85, 1988, ©Academic Press, New York.)

[b]Data are from McLachlan (1973). The present version has been modified by R. W. Castenholz.

[c]Data are from Rippka et al. (1979).

[d]Data are from Ong et al. (1984).

[e]See Footnote *a*; in addition to the ingredients listed, glycylglycine at 660–1320 mg l⁻¹ may be added as buffer for axenic cultures.

[f]See Ohki et al. (1986) and Castenholz (1988); H_3BO_3 at 30 mg l⁻¹ and $SrCl_2 \cdot 6H_2O$ at 17 mg l⁻¹ are also added.

[g]See Waterbury and Stanier (1981); glycylglycine at 500 mg l⁻¹ is used as buffer.

[h]13% FeNa-EDTA

[i]A5 + Co" or "D-micro" is generally used (see Table 19.3).

[j]Optional, but if it is used, Fe-EDTA should be eliminated from the original formula.

[k]A5 + Co" (see Table 19.3).

[l]See Footnote *a* for suggested micronutrient addition; however, "f/2" should be adequate (see Table 19.3).

[m]Use "PIV" or "f/2" (see Table 19.3).

[n]Sheridan and Castenholz solution (see Table 19.3).

[o]Optional. The mix of Ong et al. (1984) would generally be adequate (Table 19.3).

[p]S-3 mix (see Table 19.3).

[q]Use Ong et al. (see Table 19.3).

[r]See Castenholz (1988) for preparation.

Cyanobacteria (and eucaryotic microalgae) dominate autotrophic media and generally do not become overgrown or eradicated by the heterotrophs except by the unusual cyanolytic types. Many cyanobacteria are presently cultured with much greater ease and in an obviously more healthy condition with other bacteria than without them. Much information can be obtained from such cultures, including some physiological data and nucleotide sequences from various rRNA fractions—certainly more information than from nonviable, preserved specimens alone.

The media used in the culturing of cyanobacteria are numerous (Tables 19.1–19.3). The most pertinent references are: Carr et al. (1973); Allen (1973); Fogg et al. (1973); Castenholz (1981, 1988); Rippka et al. (1981a); and Waterbury and Stanier (1981). Most are autotrophic media containing organic compounds only in the form of chelator (EDTA or NTA) and an organic buffer which is often omitted (Tables 19.1–19.3). Generally, cotton-plugged or foam rubber-plugged Erlenmeyer flasks or test tubes are used for maintenance cultures in liquid or agar-solidified medium, and quite often the only source of inorganic carbon is that of the atmosphere. Although many cyanobacteria grow well in rich medium (e.g. isolates from hot springs), many should probably be treated as "oligotrophs." For example, the successful culturing of two species of planktonic, marine *Trichodesmium* took place only after the severe lowering of nutrient content, which could also have been influenced by the dilution of toxic metal contaminants (Ohki and Fujita, 1982; Ohki et al., 1986) (see Table 19.2, "Aquil" medium). These cyanobacteria appear to be suppressed by phosphate concentrations of >30 µM and, when trace metal contamination is not removed, by even lower concentrations. On the other hand, additional Ca^{2+} (7.5 mM) must be added to provide active growth in some cases (see Ohki et al., 1986). The stimulation or allowance of growth by 0.3–2 mM Na_2SO_3 has been noted (Parker, 1982; J. B. Waterbury, unpublished data). The beneficial effect may be related to the lower

Table 19.3.

Composition of micronutrient solutions[a] and vitamin mixes[b]

Micronutrients (g l^{-1})						Vitamins (mg ml^{-1})[c]			
Ingredient	"A5 + Co"[d]	D-micro[e]	Sheridan and Castenholz[f]	"PIV"[g]	"f/2"[h]	Ingredient	"DN"[i]	S-3[h]	Ong et al.[j]
H$_2$SO$_4$ (conc.)		0.5 ml				Nicotinic acid	0.100	0.1	
HCl (conc.)			3 ml			p-Aminobenzoic acid	0.010	0.10	
H$_3$BO$_3$	2.86	0.5	0.5			Biotin	0.001	0.001	0.001
MnSO$_4$·H$_2$O		2.28				Thiamine	0.200	0.5	2.0
MnCl$_2$·4H$_2$O	1.81		2.0	0.041	0.177	Cyanocobalamin	0.001	0.001	0.001
ZnNO$_3$·6H$_2$O			0.5			Folic acid	0.001	0.002	
ZnSO$_4$·7H$_2$O	0.22	0.5			0.018	i-Inositol	0.001	5.0	
ZnCl$_2$				0.005		Thymine		3.0	
CuCl$_2$·2H$_2$O			0.025			Ca-pantothenate	0.100	0.10	
CuSO$_4$·5H$_2$O	0.08	0.025			0.010				
Na$_2$MoO$_4$·2H$_2$O	0.39	0.025	0.025	0.004	0.007				
Co(NO$_3$)$_2$·6H$_2$O	0.049		0.025						
CoCl$_2$·6H$_2$O		0.045		0.002	0.011				
VOSO$_4$·6H$_2$O			0.025						
FeCl$_3$·6H$_2$O				0.097	1.90				
Na$_3$-EDTA				0.75 (add first)	4.35				

[a]Ni and Se should be included in all micronutrient solutions, e.g. NiSO$_4$(NH$_4$)$_2$SO$_4$·6H$_2$O at 10 mg l^{-1} and N$_2$Na$_2$SeO$_4$ at 2 mg l^{-1}.

[b]Modified from R. W. Castenholz, Methods in Enzymology *167*: 84–85, 1988, ©Academic Press, New York.

[c]Concentrations are designed for additions of usually 1 ml l^{-1}. Vitamin mixes are generally filter-sterilized and added after the medium is autoclaved. No cyanobacteria have been shown to have a complex vitamin requirement. Most have none at all.

[d]Values are from Rippka et al. (1979).

[e]Values are from Castenholz (1981).

[f]Values are from Waterbury and Stanier (1981).

[g]Values are from Starr (1978).

[h]Values are from McLachlan (1973).

[i]Values are from Nelson et al. (1982).

[j]Values are from Ong et al. (1984).

redox potential and/or a protection against photooxidative damage. Fluorescent lamps are generally used instead of incandescent lamps, since they provide wavelengths almost entirely within the "visible" range, also the range of the various pigments of cyanobacteria. Although continuous light is usually used, the damaging effect of higher light (photoinhibition) may be partially avoided by a light/dark cycle. In most cases, an intensity of 500–2000 lx is acceptable (Castenholz, 1981), but <500 lx is strongly recommended for many cyanobacteria (Rippka et al., 1981a).

The conservation of cultures in a nongrowing state has been successful via several methods. The most universally applicable method is to freeze dense culture material that has passed the exponential growth phase in liquid N$_2$ (−196°C) (e.g. Castenholz, 1981, 1988; Malik, 1984). Cryogenic protective agents such as dimethyl sulfoxide (5–10%) or glycerol (10–15%) may enhance survival in some cases, but there have been few quantitative, survival experiments with comparisons of different media. The newer plastic ampuls with screw caps are much preferable to the glass ampuls formerly in use. With gas-vacuolate cyanobacteria, gas vesicles must be collapsed (e.g. by hand pressure increase in closed syringe) before placing in liquid N$_2$.

A dense sludge of cyanobacteria in 15% glycerol with freezing and storage at from −70° to −90°C has worked very well for some cyanobacteria (C. P. Wolk, personal communication). Lyophilization also works well for many strains. Corbett and Parker (1976) had most success with use of lamb serum as the suspending agent. Some cyanobacteria are extremely

tolerant and survive air drying at room temperature; others (particularly some strains of *Oscillatoria* from various habitats) have failed to survive all types of conservation (R. W. Castenholz, unpublished data). In general, sheathed filamentous forms survive drying better than do other forms.

Few cyanobacteria grown at moderate to high temperatures survive storage well at refrigerator temperatures (3–5°C), probably because of irreversible membrane damage (see Brand et al., 1979).

Methods of isolation and culture have been described by various authors (e.g. Allen, 1952; Allen, 1973; Meffert and Chang, 1978; Castenholz, 1981, 1988; Rippka et al., 1981a; Walsby, 1981; Waterbury and Stanier, 1981) and will not be described in detail here. However, a few aspects should be mentioned: manual methods (i.e. manipulation with watchmaker's forceps or glass needles under a dissecting microscope) are used far more extensively than with other bacteria because of the generally greater size of cells, colonies, filaments or thalli of the blue-greens. Gliding motility of most filamentous and some unicellular forms allows self-isolation methods to be used on agar plates, even when the only motile stages are hormogonia produced under restricted environmental conditions. Although initial manual or self-isolation techniques may result in axenic cultures, quite often heterotrophic bacteria may remain.

Many large-diameter, sheathed filamentous cyanobacteria are immotile (e.g. *Stigonema*) and grow much slower than small-diameter species which, as contaminants, tend to overgrow the larger organism. The larger forms are, therefore, quite difficult to isolate. Zehnder (1985) successfully demonstrated the isolation of such a recalcitrant type by the use of filter paper growth supports which contact the medium on one edge only.

Isolation by micromanipulation (or self-isolation) is generally preferred over any method that involves enrichment, since the isolated strain may then be more easily related to the natural population from the field collection.

A number of special methods have been used to rid cultures of heterotrophic bacteria; none are foolproof. Since cyanobacteria are procaryotes, antibiotics are usually useless in purifying cultures. However, the use of some bacterial antibiotics may act differentially in the dark as suggested by Whitton (1968), since most cyanobacteria are obligate phototrophs. Rippka et al. (1981a) have found that starving the cyanobacteria before adding ampicillin (or penicillin) and organic medium in

the dark greatly reduces the contaminants upon subsequent dilution.

For the most part, the special methods have been applied to only a few genera or strains, and many have not been tested extensively. Carmichael and Gorham (1974) used 0.3% (v/v) phenol in the dark for 4–6 h to reduce the population of heterotrophic bacteria. This was followed by washing of cells on a membrane filter, followed by plating. McCurdy and Hodgson (1974) used a blending and dilution technique associated with two platings on agar. Heaney and Jaworski (1977) have successfully used a washing/filtering technique with rather large pore size (8.0-μm) polycarbonate "Nuclepore" filters. Fitzsimmons and Smith (1984) also successfully used a filtration procedure to produce a high trichome-to-bacteria ratio and a subsequent serial dilution. They also warn that in some species, growth of the cyanobacterium may be poor in the absence of the bacteria.

CULTURE COLLECTIONS

The need for permanent culture collections of cyanobacteria and microorganisms, in general, is very great. Most isolations of feral strains require an enormous effort, and a gene bank of mutant forms can never be replaced. Nevertheless, there are only a few collections today that maintain, by either transfers or storage, strains of cyanobacteria, and most of these have neither the work force nor the financial resources to add many more strains to the collections.

The problems are multiple. Some cyanobacterial strains need special handling; growth and storage conditions cannot be uniform for all. Most smaller collection facilities, even if funded, may have only one culture-handling person, and this person may change every few years.

Many of the collection institutes have difficulty in honoring requests, particularly if they are frequent. Many cultures are sent in a nonviable condition or die in transit, requiring multiple mailings.

There is, at present, a great need for at least one internationally acknowledged, well-funded culture collection for cyanobacteria.

The American Type Culture Collection (ATCC) (12301 Parklawn Drive, Rockville, Maryland 20852) will conserve cyanobacteria, but this institution is primarily interested in accepting type strains.

The principal collection of cyanobacteria is that of the Institut Pasteur (PCC) (Unité de Physiologie Microbienne, Dept. Biochimie et Génétique Moléculaire 75724, Paris Cedex 15), which now maintains over 350 strains, many of which were included in the taxonomic analysis

of Rippka et al. (1979, 1981b).

The Culture Collection of Algae at the University of Texas (UTEX) (Austin, Texas 78712) possesses many cyanobacteria (blue-green algae), but many of the strains bear names which may be taxonomically incorrect, since the cultures were sent to the collection by a great diversity of workers over many years.

The Culture Centre of Algae and Protozoa (CCAP) in Cambridge, England, has been closed, and culture strains have been moved to the Freshwater Biological Association, The Ferry House, Ambleside, Cumbria, LA22 0LP, U.K. (for freshwater cultures), and the Scottish Marine Biological Association, Dunstaffnage Research Laboratory, P.O. Box 3, Oban, Argyll, PA34 4AD, U.K. (for marine cultures). The culture collection of the Institute of Applied Microbiology (IAM), University of Tokyo, Bunkyo-ku, Tokyo, Japan, also contains cyanobacteria.

There are, in addition, many smaller collections at institutions which are often the responsibility of one person, the founder of the collection. Most of these are listed and annotated, along with the number of strains of each genus, in Komárek (1973). However, some of these collections no longer exist or have been greatly altered.

More recent lists of general bacterial culture collections that may include cyanobacteria are available (McGowan and Skerman, 1982; see "List of Culture Collections," pp. 1629–1630).

GENERAL CHARACTERISTICS OF THE CYANOBACTERIA

Besides sharing the basic cellular features of other eubacteria, the cyanobacteria possess several unique and diagnostic characteristics. Several reviews of general cyanobacterial characteristics are available (e.g. Stanier and Cohen-Bazire, 1977; Stewart, 1980; Wolk, 1980; Fay, 1983). The book, *Biology of Cyanobacteria* (Carr and Whitton, 1982), provides a more comprehensive review.

Cell Envelope

The cell wall is of a Gram-negative type, but in some the structural, peptidoglycan layer (LII) is considerably thicker than in other eubacteria (e.g. Halfen and Castenholz, 1971; Lang, 1977; Drews and Weckesser, 1982; Guglielmi and Cohen-Baxire, 1982b; Vaara, 1982; Gantt et al., 1984; Büdel and Rhiel, 1985). This thickness is usually 1–10 nm, but it reaches 200 nm in the case of *Oscillatoria princeps* (Fig. 19.1). The thicker walls, as in this species, are partially perforated by numerous incomplete pore pits (~70 nm in diameter) extending from the cell interior and carrying the cytoplasmic membrane outward to contact the outer lipopolysaccharide (LPS) "outer membrane" (Halfen and Castenholz, 1971) (Fig. 19.1). But in one example (Lang, 1977), the pore pit extends

from the outside inward to the cytoplasmic membrane. Small-diameter pores (5–13 nm) are present in regular or scattered order in the walls of all cyanobacteria, but the arrangement varies greatly. For example, in filamentous forms the peripheral (longitudinal) wall may be perforated by pores over most of the surface or only by a ring or rings of pores subtending the cross-walls (junctional pores) (Fig. 19.1). The cross-wall (transverse septum) may be perforated by a single minute central pore or by numerous pores (microplasmodesmata) (Fig. 19.2), sometimes within a conspicuous "synapsis" (e.g. Giddings and Staehelin, 1981; Couté, 1982; Drews and Weckesser, 1982; Guglielmi and Cohen-Bazire, 1982b). Although lipophilic photosynthetic pigments are localized in the thylakoids of the cell interior, a major fraction of the cell's carotenoids may be in the cell envelope, particularly in the cytoplasmic membrane (Omata and Murata, 1984). Large quantities of distinct carotenoids may also occur in the LPS "outer membrane" (Resch and Gibson, 1983).

Numerous unicellular, colonial and filamentous cyanobacteria possess an "envelope" outside of the LPS "outer membrane" (Figs. 19.2 and 19.3). This is variously called the sheath, glycocalyx, or capsule or, merely, gel, mucilage, or slime, depending on the consistency. Occasionally, if tough

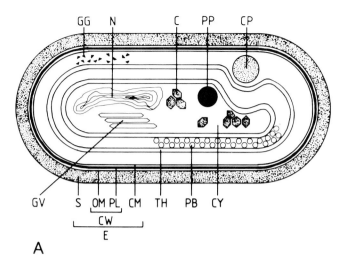

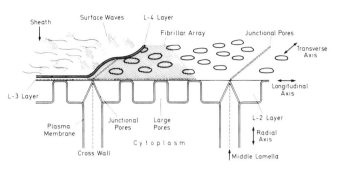

A

B

Figure 19.1. *A,* schematic diagram of a cyanobacterial vegetative cell. *S,* external layer (slime or sheath); *OM,* outer membrane; *PL,* peptidoglycan layer; *CM,* cytoplasmic membrane; *CW,* cell wall; *E,* cell envelope; *TH,* thylakoid; *PB,* phycobilisome; *CY,* cytoplasm; *GV,* gas vesicle; *GG,* glycogen granules; *N,* nucleoplasmic region; *C,* carboxysome; *PP,* polyphosphate granule; *CP,* cyanophycin granule. (Reproduced with permission from L. J. Stal. 1986. Nitrogen-fixing Cyanobacteria in a Marine Microbiol Mat. Littmann-Druck, Oldenburg.) *B,* diagram of the cell wall of *Oscillatoria princeps.* (Reproduced with permission from L. N. Halfen. 1979. Gliding movements. *In* Haupt and Feinleib (Editors), Physiology of Movements. Encyclopedia of Plant Physiology N.S. Vol. 7. Springer-Verlag, Berlin, pp. 268–309.)

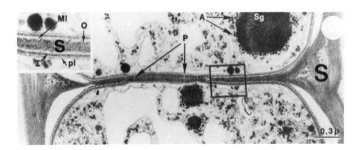

Figure 19.2. Electron micrograph of a stage of cell division and sheath formation in a branch filament of *Fischerella.* Cell division is almost complete. *P,* pores (microplasmodesmata) in the remaining septum. *A,* alpha granules (glycogen granules); *Sg,* structured granule (cyanophycin in granule); *S,* sheath. *Insert:* enlargement of septum showing two walls separated by sheath(s). *Pl,* plasmalemma; *Ml,* middle layer; *I,* inner layer (peptidoglycan layer); *O,* outer membrane; *S,* sheath. (Reproduced with permission from E. L. Thurston and L. O. Ingram, Journal of Phycology 7: 203–210, 1971, ©Phycological Society of America.)

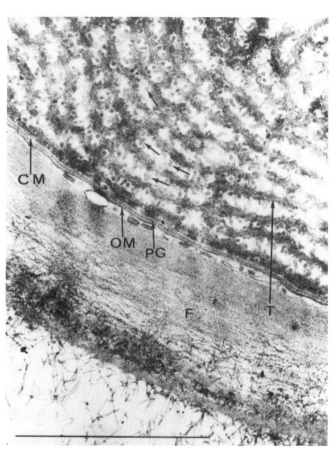

Figure 19.3. Electron micrograph of a thin section of part of a large vegetative cell of *Dermocarpa* (PCC 7302). *F,* fibrous outer wall layer, 750 nm thick and of variable density; *OM,* outer membrane; *PG,* peptidoglycan wall layer; *CM,* cytoplasmic membrane; *T,* thylakoids; *arrows,* glycogen granules. *Bar,* 1.0 μm. (Reproduced with permission from J. B. Waterbury and R. Y. Stanier, Microbiological Reviews *42:* 2–44, 1978, ©American Society for Microbiology.)

and fibrous, the equivalent envelope is referred to as an outer wall layer (see Drews and Weckesser, 1982). Many sheaths show a microfibrillar substructure, the microfibrils being parallel and oriented in the thin elastic sheaths shed by motile *Oscillatoria* trichomes. Some sheaths thicken (to several micrometers) with the aging of the inhabiting trichome and have distinct laminations. The sheaths of cyanobacteria are predominantly polysaccharide, but >20% of the weight may be polypeptides, and depending on the species, many types of sugar residues may be involved (Drews and Weckesser, 1982; Schrader et al., 1982). In *Chlorogloeopsis,*

the major sheath polysaccharide is composed of glucose, arabinose and xylose; the minor polysaccharide mainly contains galactose (Schrader et al., 1982). In some marine forms, fucose, arabinose, rhamnose or galacturonic acid may be the predominant monomer (J. Bauld, personal communication). In firm sheaths of some colonial and filamentous cyanobacteria, yellow, red or blue pigments may accumulate and mask the color of the cells. The chemistry and the function of these pigments are unknown, but protection from high light intensity (particularly UV) has been suggested for the yellow pigments (Rambler et al., 1977; Muehlstein and Castenholz, 1983).

Cell Division

Most unicellular and colonial cyanobacteria and some filamentous forms undergo binary fission by a constrictive type of division in which all envelope layers (often including sheath) grow inward until cell separation is complete or nearly complete (see Drews and Weckesser, 1982) (Fig. 19.4). In some filamentous types, firm sheath material grows inward, eventually separating cells of older trichomes (Nierzwicki et al., 1982b). In others, particularly the oscillatorian types lacking constrictions at the cross-walls, the LPS "outer membrane" (and sheath) is continuous and not involved in division, but rather the cytoplasmic membrane and peptidoglycan layer invaginate. In some actively growing trichomes, different stages of ingrowth may be seen simultaneously, anticipatory to one to three future divisions (Fig. 19.5). In most cyanobacteria, binary fission results in a central division of each cell into two equal daughter cells. In *Chamaesiphon,* however, reproduction is similar to a budding process, but in some cases, at least, it is an asymmetric constrictive division of a polarly differentiated unicell or "exospore" (Waterbury and Stanier, 1978; Rippka et al., 1979; Komárek et al., 1985). In Subsection II (*Pleurocapsales*), reproduction occurs by an internal multiple fission, usually in addition to the potential for binary fission (Waterbury

and Stanier, 1978; Rippka et al., 1979) (Fig. 19.6). The resulting minute cells (baeocytes, formerly "endospores"), when released from the mother cell wall, may in some cases show slow gliding motility. No comparable process of cell division is known in the other eubacteria or in the archaeobacteria.

Binary fission in cyanobacteria results in unicellular populations when constrictive separation is complete and when no sheath holds daughter cells together. When fission regularly alternates the plane of division to two or three, and when sheath or gel retains cells together, orderly or disorderly colonies of many cells result. When fission is normally in one plane only and separation is incomplete, short or long chains of cells occur (trichomes). In sheathed trichomes (trichome + sheath = filament), local weaknesses in the sheath may allow the bulging out of trichomes or the breaking out of single trichome fragments within a sheath (false branching; see Fig. 19.7). In some genera (e.g. *Gardnerula*), orderly "branches" occur in the thick sheaths that harbor multiple trichomes. In Subsection V (*Stigonematales*), branches of sheathed trichomes occur when the plane of division changes about 90° in some cells of the trichome. This results in "true branching" (Fig. 19.8).

Cell Exterior and Motility

Fimbriae (pili) occur abundantly in many cyanobacteria, with a great variety of patterns (Guglielmi and Cohen-Bazire, 1982a). Although bacterial type flagella have never been demonstrated in cyanobacteria, a swimming type of motility has recently been described in a small unicellular type (Waterbury et al., 1985). A gliding (sliding) type of motility is known in a large variety of cyanobacteria but mainly in filamentous forms. The mechanism for this type of propulsion is not yet clear (see Halfen, 1979; Castenholz, 1982). In the case of oscillatorian cyanobacteria, continuous, proteinaceous, microfibrillar bands associated with the wall or periplasmic space may be responsible. Gliding motility in diverse procaryotes may be due to several different mechanisms.

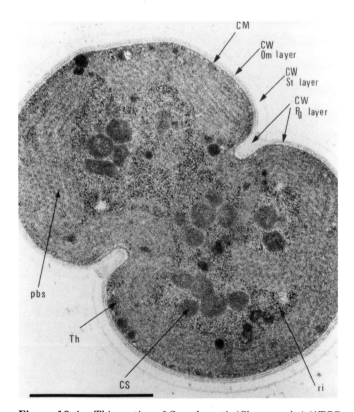

Figure 19.4. Thin section of *Synechocystis* (*Chroococcales*) (ATCC 27178) in the course of division. The cell membrane (*CM*) is surrounded by a wall (*CW*) composed of three layers: the peptidoglycan (*Pg*) layer, the outer membrane (*Om*) layer, and an additional structured (*St*) layer. The regularly spaced thylakoids (*Th*) bear rows of phycobilisomes (*pbs*) attached to both surfaces. *CS,* carboxysome; *ri,* 70S ribosome. *Bar,* 1 μm. (Reproduced with permission from R. Y. Stanier, Carlsberg Research Communications *42:* 77–98, 1977, ©Carlsberg Laboratoriet.)

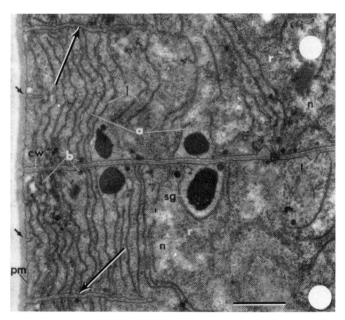

Figure 19.5. Electron micrograph of longitudinal thin section of *Symploca muscorum* (*Oscillatoriales*), showing a complete cross-wall (*cw*) and two stages of developing cross-walls (*arrows*). *l,* lamellae (thylakoids); *n,* "nucleoplasm"; *r,* ribosomes; *t,* local thickening of cross-wall; *sg,* structured granules (cyanophycin granule); *a,* organic glycogen; *b,* β granules; *pm,* plasma membrane. *Bar,* 0.4 μm. (Reproduced with permission from H. S. Pankratz and C. C. Bowen, American Journal of Botany *50:* 387–399, 1963, ©Botanical Society of America.)

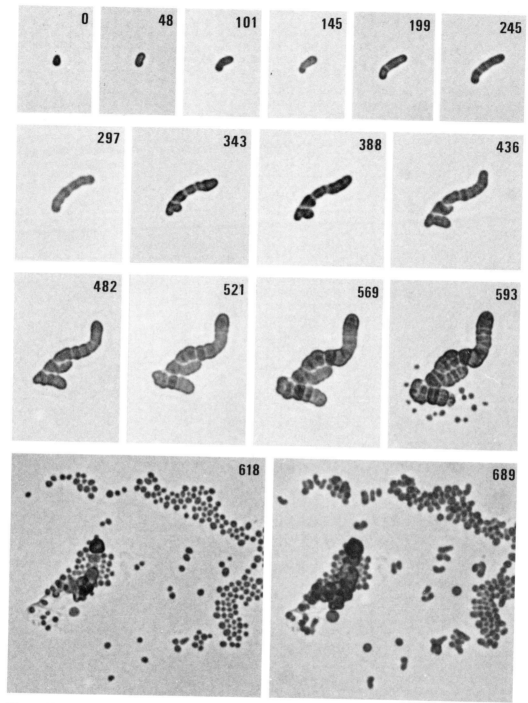

Figure 19.6. Development of a member of a *Pleurocapsa*-like cyanobacterium (PCC 7516) in a Cooper dish culture. The *number* on *each photomicrograph* indicates the elapsed time in hours. A total of 593 hours elapsed from the time of observation of the initial baeocyte to the first release of new baeocytes. × 500. (Reproduced with permission from J. B. Waterbury and R. Y. Stanier, Microbiological Reviews *42:* 2–44, 1978, ©American Society for Microbiology.)

Cell Interior

The most obvious internal feature distinguishing cyanobacteria from other eubacteria, including the anoxygenic purple phototrophic bacteria, is the type of pigment-bearing apparatus. In almost all cases, it consists of a series of thylakoid membranes which appear mainly independent of the cytoplasmic membrane. Although thylakoids in cyanobacteria do not appear to be invaginations of the cytoplasmic membrane, nevertheless,

there are orderly "attachment points" or "thylakoid centers" associated with the periphery of the cytoplasm or the cytoplasmic membrane (Kunkel, 1982; Nierzwicki-Bauer et al., 1983). The thylakoids of cyanobacteria, whether concentrically or spirally arranged (Fig. 19.9, *A* and *B*) around a central thylakoid-free area ("centroplasm") or seemingly interspersed in another manner (Fig. 19.9*C*), do not show the accordionlike pleating or the obvious, frequent cytoplasmic membrane connections so

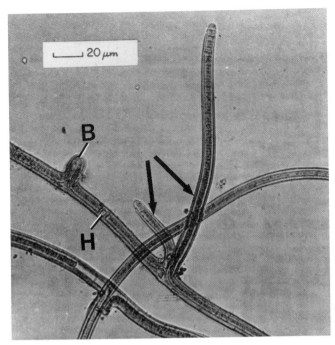

Figure 19.7. *Scytonema* species showing geminate (double) false branching. An initial bulge (*B*) breaks, with the two ends then growing out separately (*arrows*). A heterocyst (*H*) is indicated. (Reproduced with permission from G. E. Fogg, W. D. P. Stewart, P. Fay and A. E. Walsby. 1973. The Blue-Green Algae. Academic Press, London, p. 18.)

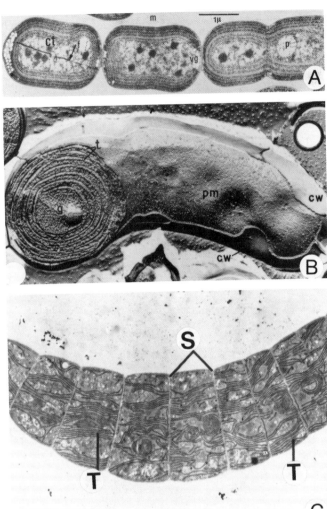

Figure 19.9. *A*, electron micrograph of *Pseudanabaena* (PCC 6901). *ct*, terminal cell; *vg*, gas vesicles; *f*, "filament"; *p*, polyphosphate granule; *m*, mucous sheath. (Reproduced with permission from G. Guglielmi and G. Cohen-Bazire, Protistologica *20*: 377–391, 1984, ©Editions du CNRS.) *B*, electron micrograph of a freeze-etched cell of *Synechococcus*, showing views of cross and longitudinal fractures. *t*, thylakoids; *g*, nuclear region; *pm*, plasma membrane; *cw*, cell wall. (Reproduced with permission from S. C. Holt and M. R. Edwards, Canadian Journal of Microbiology *18*: 175–181, 1972, ©National Research Council of Canada.) *C*, electron micrograph of a longitudinal section of *Arthrospira (Spirulina) platensis. T*, thylakoid; *S*, septum (cross-wall). (Reproduced with permission from G. Hedenskog and A. W. von Hofsten, Physiologia Plantarum *23*: 209–216, 1970, ©Munksgaard International.)

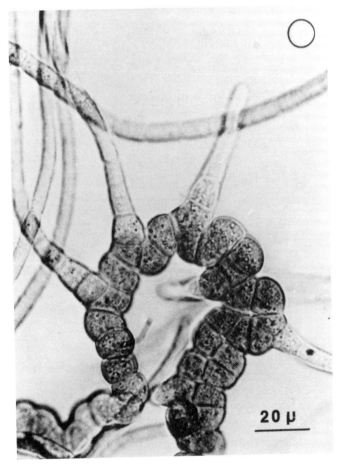

Figure 19.8 (left). Photomicrograph of multiseriate filament of *Fischerella* with true branches. (Reproduced with permission from E. L. Thurston and L. O. Ingram, Journal of Phycology *7*: 203–210, 1971, ©Phycological Society of America.)

characteristic of purple bacteria. Fingerlike, tubular thylakoids and open vesicular types are absent, at least in healthy cells (see Golecki and Drews, 1982). However, thylakoids probably cannot be distinguished easily from those of the *Prochlorales* via electron microscopy (see in this volume; and Burger-Wiersma et al., 1986), the single other known group of oxygenic procaryotes. Cyanobacteria (again with one known exception) possess upright hemidiscoidal or hemispherical phycobilisomes which are complex protein-pigment aggregates arranged in orderly rows on both surfaces of the thylakoids. The size of these structures (20–70 nm in diameter) is greater than the thickness of the double thylakoid membrane, so that with proper preparation (high phosphate buffering) they are retained for electron microscopy (Fig. 19.10). Neither the *Prochlorales* nor the anoxygenic phototrophs possess these structures. However, among the cyanobacteria, *Gloeobacter* lacks thylakoids, with the cytoplasmic membrane used as the chlorophyll-bearing vehicle. Instead of discrete, individual phycobilisomes, *Gloeobacter* possesses rows of phycobilisome type rods standing perpendicular to the cytoplasmic membrane (see Guglielmi et al., 1981).

The thylakoids of cyanobacteria consist of two "unit type" membranes of about 7 nm in thickness, separated by an electron-transparent intrathylakoidal space of about 3–5 nm. However, they may be more closely appressed or separated by a greater gap (~10 nm). They are similar in most respects to the thylakoid membranes of chloroplasts, particularly those of the red algae. In some cyanobacteria, the thylakoids contain

about 130–140 light-harvesting chlorophyll *a* molecules per P-700 photosystem I (PS I) reaction center, and 20–50 light-harvesting chlorophyll *a* molecules per P-680 photosystem II (PS II) reaction center (see Glazer, 1983). Thus, the antennal chlorophyll proportions associated with the two photosystems differ from those of green algae or higher green plants. The phycobilisomes are attached to the outside of both thylakoid membranes in orderly rows (Fig. 19.10). Attachment is by a portion of allophycocyanin (APC), the basal biliprotein, to PS II particles (exoplasmic fracture face particles of 10 nm in diameter) of the thylakoid membrane (see Cohen-Bazire and Bryant, 1982; Glazer, 1983; Allen, 1984). The phycobilisome of most cyanobacteria is hemidiscoidal in general shape but consists of a series of rods composed of disks of biliprotein spread out as a fan centering in the core which is composed of stacks of biliprotein in trimeric disks laid on their sides (Fig. 19.11) (see Nies and Wehrmeyer, 1981; Cohen-Bazire and Bryant, 1982; Wehrmeyer, 1983; Glazer, 1984; Guglielmi and Cohen-Bazire, 1984b). The phycobilisome comprises the major light-harvesting complex of most cyanobacteria. The death of a cell usually results in the early release into the medium of these water-soluble phycobiliproteins following the disaggregation of the structures.

The pigments comprising the phycobilisome are APC in the core (including APC-B) and phycocyanin (PC) in the rods, at least in the basal trimers (Fig. 19.11). Phycoerythrocyanin (PEC) or phycoerythrin (PE), if present, occurs as outer disks of the rods. The phycobilisomes constitute an efficient energy-focusing system (see Glazer, 1984). Absorbance maxima and fluorescence emission maxima for major cyanobacterial pigments are summarized in Table 19.2.

There are many other common components and "inclusions" in the cytoplasm of cyanobacteria (see Allen, 1984; Jensen, 1985), most of which can be visualized readily via various preparative techniques for electron microscopy (Figs. 19.1*A* and 19.4). They include:

(a) *Glycogen* (polyglucose) granules which are ovoid or elongate and rod-shaped, usually between the thylakoids (not in the intrathylakoidal space). Poly-β-hydroxybutyrate granules are apparently absent in most cyanobacteria.

(b) *Cyanophycin* granules which are polymers of arginine and aspartic acid. These "structured granules" are recognizable with a radiating

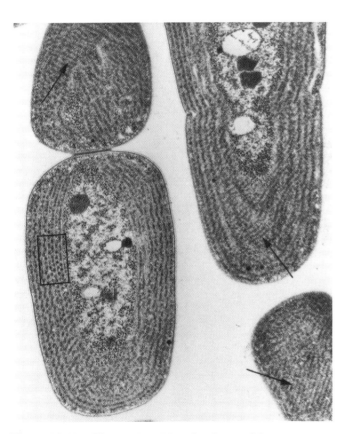

Figure 19.10. Thin section of *Pseudanabaena* PCC 7408. The rows of phycobilisomes are seen in cross-section, longitudinal section and tangential section. In tangential sections, the rows of closely packed phycobilisomes appear as electron-dense cords running at an angle to the long axis of the cells (*arrows*). When the rows of phycobilisomes are cut in cross-section, they are seen in face view (e.g. in *box*). They alternate with one another on the apposing stromal surfaces of thylakoids. (Reproduced with permission from G. Cohen-Bazire and D. A. Bryant. 1982. Phycobilisomes: composition and structure. *In* Carr and Whitton (Editors), The Biology of Cyanobacteria. Blackwell, Oxford, p. 147.)

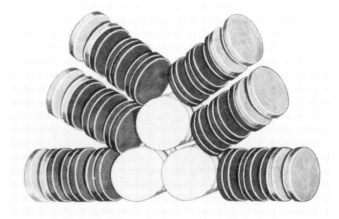

Figure 19.11. Model of hemidiscoidal phycobilisome of *Mastigocladus laminosus* (*Fischerella*).Two disks of phycoerythrocyanin (*gray*) lie at the distal end of each of the six rods. Each rod also contains five disks of phycocyanin (*dark*) which lie proximal to the allophycocyanin core (*light*). Each disk symbolizes a trimeric biliprotein aggregate including the uncolored proteins. (Reproduced with permission from M. Nies and W. Wehrmeyer, Archives of Microbiology *129*: 374–379, 1981, ©Springer-Verlag.)

substructure pattern and are often large enough to be recognizable with light microscopy (~500 nm). They are apparently unique to cyanobacteria, although a few strains lack them. Functionally, they serve as reserves of nitrogen.

(c) *Carboxysomes* (polyhedral bodies) which are also large but which are more angular structures composed largely of ribulosebisphosphate carboxylase protein, apparently serving as reserves of this carboxylating enzyme or possibly as a site of CO_2 fixation. It appears that all autotrophic procaryotes utilizing the reductive pentose phosphate cycle for CO_2 fixation contain carboxysomes under appropriate conditions (Allen, 1984).

(d) *Polyphosphate* (volutin) granules reaching 0.1–0.3 μm in diameter. With transmission electron microscopy they appear as spherical, electron-dense or porous structures, depending on fixation and staining.

(e) *Gas vacuoles* which are composed of many elongate, cylindrical *gas vesicles* which are polyhedral in cross-section. Gas vesicles are constructed of a 2-nm-thick protein coat and contain gases, being completely impervious to water. They occur in most planktonic and some other cyanobacteria (Fig. 19.12).

Ribosomes are typically most abundant in the nucleoplasmic region of eubacteria. The nucleoplasm of cyanobacterial cells is a lighter pigmented "centroplasm" as seen in light microscopy or less dense when viewed with transmission electron microscopy. The DNA fibrils are in a complex, folded and helical arrangement, but if unfolded, each is circular (Herdman, 1982). The range in total molecular weight for a cyanobacterial genome is between 1.6 and 8.6×10^9. Multiple or "excess" DNA occurs in the more complex, filamentous types. Unicellular forms, however, have sizes usually below 4×10^9 daltons, which is similar to those known for procaryotes other than cyanobacteria. The genome size of two types of "cyanelles" (cyanobacteria serving as "chloroplasts" in unicellular, eucaryotic hosts) is very small ($\sim 1 \times 10^9$ daltons), presumably too small to allow autonomy (e.g. Herdman and Stanier, 1977). More unusual, cytoplasmic inclusions in cyanobacteria are reviewed by Jensen (1985).

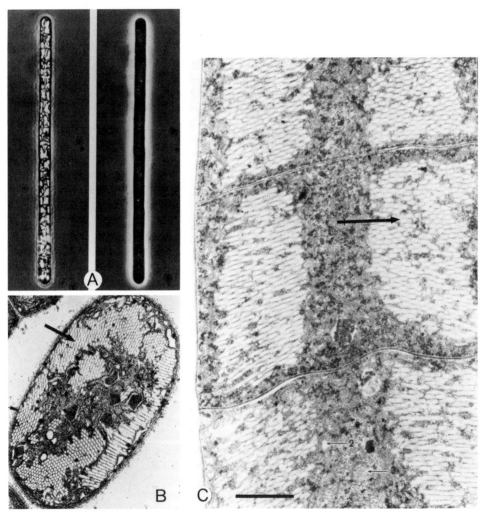

Figure 19.12. *A,* photomicrograph of *Oscillatoria agardhii* with gas vesicles (left-hand trichome). The right-hand trichome was subjected to a pressure of 12 atm, and the gas vesicles have collapsed. (Reproduced with permission from A. E. Walsby, Scientific American *237* (2): 90–97, 1977, ©Scientific American, Inc.) *B,* electron micrograph of a section of a vegetative cell of *Anabaena circinalis,* a planktonic form, with most of the cell volume occupied by gas vesicles (*arrow*). (Reproduced with permission from M. J. Daft and W. D. P. Stewart, New Phytologist *72:* 799–808, 1973, ©Academic Press.) *C,* electron micrograph of a median longitudinal section through a trichome of *Trichodesmium erythraeum,* showing the concentric arrangement of gas vesicles (*arrow*). *Bar,* 1.0 μm. (Reproduced by permission from C. Van Baalen and R. M. Brown, Jr., Archiv für Mikrobiologie *69:* 79–91, 1969, ©Springer-Verlag.)

Specialized Cells

Heterocysts

Members of the *Nostocales* and *Stigonematales,* Subsections IV and V, respectively (Rippka et al., 1979), produce heterocysts at intervals in trichomes through the differentiation of vegetative cells, usually only after the concentration of combined inorganic nitrogen in the surrounding medium has been lowered. Heterocysts are unique to cyanobacteria. With light microscopy, they can be recognized by their pale color, thicker wall, and refractive polar nodules (one if the heterocyst is terminal) (Fig. 19.13). Obvious cytoplasmic granulation is generally absent. The structure, development and function of heterocysts have been studied extensively (see Fay, 1980; Stewart, 1980; Adams and Carr, 1981; Wolk, 1982; Fay, 1983). In brief, vegetative cells differentiate by usually adding a multilayered wall to the outside of the normal envelope and by forming a synaptic pore channel between the cell and the adjacent vegetative cell or cells. The polar wall together with a plug of cyanophycin (later) form the "polar nodules." In addition, the thylakoidal membrane system is "reorganized," and cyanophycin granules and phycobilisomes (usually) are degraded. Functionally, PS II (oxygenesis) and ribulosebisphosphate carboxylase activity is lost, PS I activity is retained and enhanced (including cyclic photophosphorylation), and with high rates of endogenous respiration, reducing conditions are attained. Nitrogenase synthesis then proceeds. Heterocyst spacing is regulated by inhibitory substances emanating as gradients through the trichome, from heterocysts or proheterocysts (see Adams and Carr, 1981). Heterocysts are sustained by mobile carbohydrates and/or organic acids from vegetative cells, while combined nitrogen is supplied in organic form from heterocysts to vegetative cells.

Akinetes

Akinetes of the type produced by cyanobacteria in the *Nostocales* (sensu Castenholz) appear to be unlike any cells of other procaryotes. Many (but not all) of the heterocystous cyanobacteria produce akinetes ("resting spores") from vegetative cells, particularly under conditions of nutrient deficiency and/or light limitation (see Adams and Carr, 1981; Nichols and Adams, 1982). Akinetes differentiate from vegetative cells, grow, and acquire a thick wall surrounding the old. Akinetes are quite granular, accumulating cyanophycin, glycogen, lipids, and carotenoid pigments. Polyphosphates disappear but the RNA content increases. Photosynthetic capacity decreases greatly or ceases altogether. The pattern of akinete formation is generally related to the location of heterocysts. Akinetes usually succeed heterocyst formation, and their positioning is either adjacent to heterocysts or the greatest distance from them (Fig. 19.13A). In one genus, at least, an akinete-promoting substance has been related to the presence of heterocysts (Hirosawa and Wolk, 1979a, b). Akinetes are often in long series. Those of planktonic cyanobacteria lose their gas vesicles and sink, often after detachment. They tolerate drying, freezing, and long term storage in anaerobic sediments but apparently do not require a resting period before germination. A light-dependent emergence occurs in most types after one or more cell divisions and the localized dissolution of a polar wall (see Nichols and Adams, 1982).

Terminal Cells and Hairs

In some filamentous cyanobacteria, the terminal cells of trichomes are usually differently shaped than intercalary cells. When trichomes fragment, the new terminal cells of the trichomes "balloon" out to some ex-

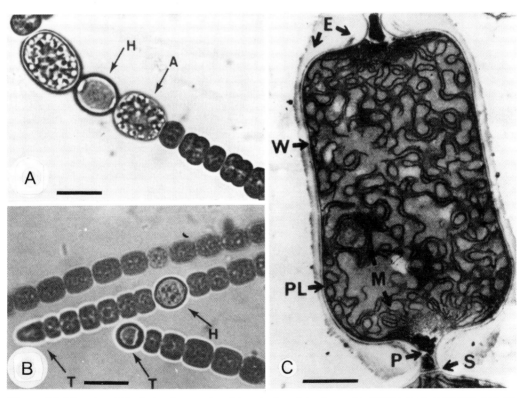

Figure 19.13. *A* and *B,* photomicrographs of two strains of *Anabaena* (*A,* UTEX 1616; *B,* UTEX 377). *H,* heterocyst; *A,* akinete; *T,* terminal cell or terminal heterocyst. *Bar,* 10 μm. (Reproduced with permission from B. K. Stulp and W. T. Stam, Archiv für Hydrobiologie Supplementband *63:* 35–52, 1982, ©E. Schweizerbart'sche.) *C,* electron micrograph of a longitudinal section of a heterocyst of *Anabaena. W,* cell wall; *E,* additional outer walls; *M,* membrane system; *P,* pore channel; *S,* septum with microplasmodesmata. *Bar,* 1 μm. (Reproduced with permission from P. Fay and N. J. Lang, Proceedings of the Royal Society Series B *178:* 185–192, 1971.)

tent, and this appears to be accompanied by increased wall thickening and growth until a typical apical cell morphology is achieved. In most cases, this is probably little different from the shape expected as a result of cell turgor and wall resistance. However, many species develop very characteristic shapes, ranging from long and tapered to conical, capitate or blunt. The differentiated apical cells, in most cases, do not divide again.

The most extreme differentiation, however, is the metamorphosis of a long, terminal, multicellular and tapered hair in some tapered members of the *Nostocales* (Subsection IV) (see Wood et al., 1986; Whitton, 1987). A narrowing of cell widths, along with a great increase in length, results in a large increase in cell surface area. Pigments, granular inclusions and much of the cytoplasm is lost. Hair formation is correlated with a phosphorus or, sometimes, an iron deficiency in the medium (see Whitton, 1987).

Hormogonia

Although a hormogonium is simply a short chain of cells, the cells are often quite different from the vegetative cells of the trichome. Although they may not be easily distinguished in the *Oscillatoriales* (Subsection III), within the heterocystous types hormogonia are often defined 5–15-cell chains with a cell diameter less that of the vegetative trichomes. They may also form in specific regions of the parent organism, such as below the terminal hair in *Calothrix* (*Nostocales*) (Subsection IV) and at the end of lateral branches in some of the *Stigonematales* (Subsection V).

The formation and liberation of hormogonia appears to be a timed process associated with environmental conditions (e.g. phosphorus repletion) or with particular stages of a morphogenetic cycle.

Physiology and Biochemistry

The chief physiological/biochemical characteristic of cyanobacteria, distinguishing them from all other procaryotes except the *Prochlorales,* is the dual photosystem allowing the use of H_2O as photoreductant and the consequent liberation of O_2. This is associated with chlorophyll *a*, both as a light-harvesting pigment and as a reaction center pigment, as in the chloroplasts of green algae and more advanced green plants. Even some of the carotenoids are common to the eucaryotic green line (e.g. zeaxanthin, β-carotene), while certain types are mainly restricted to the cyanobacteria (e.g. myxoxanthophyll, echinenone, oscilloxanthin and others) (see Goodwin, 1980). There are, of course, some consistent differences between the structure, components and biochemistry of the cyanobacterial and eucaryotic (chloroplastidic) photosystems, but these will not be discussed here (e.g. see Glazer, 1983).

The phycobilin pigments of the phycobilisome may often constitute the major light-harvesting pigments in cyanobacteria. Under low light intensity the cell content of light-harvesting chlorophyll *a* may be relatively low, compared with that of phycobilin components. CO_2 reduction involves the reductive pentose phosphate cycle.

The typically oxygenic photosynthesis of cyanobacteria can be altered in an adaptive response to the presence of free sulfide, where photosystem II is inhibited and electrons derived from sulfide enter the photosynthetic electron transport system and result in CO_2 reduction (anoxygenic photosynthesis) (Cohen et al., 1986). Not all cyanobacteria are capable of tolerating or adapting to sulfide in this way.

Respiration in all cyanobacteria may involve the use of portions of the electron transport system of the photosystem; thus, terminal O_2 reduction is associated with the thylakoid network. The production of reduced FAD/NAD/NADP does not involve the oxidative TCA cycle, since this operative cycle is lacking in cyanobacteria (see Fay, 1983). However, low levels of enzymes of the glyoxylate shunt are present. Most of the reductant generated in the dark is reduced NADP through the oxidative pentose phosphate cycle (see Smith, 1982). The dark period, for most cyanobacteria, is one of protein synthesis and maintenance with the degradation and oxidation of glycogen accumulated during bright daylight. Most cyanobacteria are obligate photoautotrophs, since dark catabolic rates are often not increased by external substrates, either because of set, low or negligible uptake rates or because of unenhanceable endogenous

rates of NADP reduction or respiration. A relatively small number, however, can grow as aerobic dark heterotrophs at much slower rates than as photoautotrophs, mainly at the expense of glucose, sucrose or fructose (Smith, 1982). Artificially, at least, heterotrophic growth rates can be enhanced in the light with PS II inhibited (photoheterotrophy). At higher light intensities, low CO_2 concentration and high O_2 values, photorespiration occurs (as in eucaryotic algae and green plants), but this involves only the oxidative cleavage of ribulose bisphosphate into 3-phosphoglycerate and phosphoglycolate and not a useful energy gain. Anaerobic metabolism in the dark is usually limited to maintenance, but lactate fermentation is known; in at least one species, dark survival is greatly enhanced when aerobic conditions are changed to anaerobic, with appropriate substrate and low redox environment (Richardson and Castenholz, 1987).

Cyanobacteria regulate enzymes in manners similar to other eubacteria. The synthesis of several enzymes, such as nitrogenase, nitrate reductase, and alkaline phosphatase, is inducible and controlled by repression and derepression (see Doolittle, 1979).

Cyanobacterial generation times (when growth is exponential) are often >12 h and, commonly, 24 h or more, even in culture with unlimited nutrients and a saturating intensity of continuous light. There are at least a few unicellular and oscillatorian strains in culture that have generation times of 4 h or less.

Although growth or reproduction in cyanobacteria consists of cell division, some species undergo a complex morphogenetic life cycle which may involve nongrowth hormogonial dispersal phases, an aseriate stage, the process of filamentation (the joining of cells to produce trichomes) and the differential growth of certain portions of filaments (e.g. Lazaroff, 1973; Fay, 1983; Whitton, 1987). Phases of some cycles are controlled by light through one or more photoreversible phytochromelike pigments (see Björn, 1979).

The photobiology of cyanobacteria, in addition to photosynthesis and photomorphogenesis, involves the control of phycobilin synthesis (chromatic adaptation), again via a photoreversible phytochromelike pigment. For example, many cyanobacteria cease synthesis of phycoerythrin when light is enhanced in the red wavelengths rather than in the green portion of the spectrum.

Phototaxis (+ and −) and photophobic reactions are also well-documented in the cyanobacteria. Many cyanobacteria move up light gradients (positive phototaxis) because of a cessation of reversals when trichomes become oriented parallel to the light gradient (see Häder, 1979, 1987; Castenholz, 1982; Gabai, 1985), while others are quite capable of steering or turning movements when light is unidirectional (Nultsch and Wenderoth, 1983). Photophobic reactions are known in some of the same species that exhibit phototaxis. Step-down responses have been documented more commonly than step-up responses; these result in retaining filamentous cyanobacteria in illuminated niches.

Endogenous rhythms, although previously unknown in procaryotes, have tentatively been demonstrated for nitrogen fixation in one strain of a unicellular cyanobacterium (Grobbelaar et al., 1986).

Ecology

The occurrence and predominance of cyanobacteria in a vast array of habitats is a result of several general characteristics and of some features characterizing certain cyanobacterial species clusters. It is presumed that cyanobacteria per se evolved in the Precambrian well before the Paleozoic boundary, and this is borne out by microfossils of the late Proterozoic that are nearly identical morphologically to some living cyanobacteria (see Schopf and Walter, 1982; Knoll, 1985).

Planktonic dominance by several filamentous forms today is probably related strongly to the possession of gas vesicles and the ability to regulate buoyancy (see Van Liere and Walsby, 1982). However, in eutrophic lakes, N_2 fixation capability following depletion of combined nitrogen and/or the ability to efficiently utilize a very low photon flux density is thought to enhance the success of some cyanobacteria (Gibson and Smith, 1982; Van Liere and Walsby, 1982; Mur, 1983). In oligotrophic marine or fresh waters, the N_2-fixing ability may also be of primary importance (e.g. *Trichodesmium* species). The minute picoplanktonic unicells of *Synechococcus* may thrive in deep-mixing, oligotrophic waters because of their efficient absorption of a low photon flux (Glover, 1986). Extracellular excretions of substances such as hydroxymates, which may inhibit the growth of potential competitors, have been suggested as contributing to cyanobacterial success (see Gibson and Smith, 1982). It has also been suggested that siderochrome (trihydroxymate) excretion by planktonic cyanobacteria in iron-poor waters may aide in sequestering iron. In addition, several planktonic cyanobacteria produce potent toxins of two types: alkaloid neurotoxins and peptide hepatotoxins (Skulberg et al., 1984).

Cyanobacterin, an effective inhibitor of other cyanobacteria and some eucaryotic algae, is a diaryl-substituted γ-lactone with a chlorine substitution on one of the aromatic rings. It is produced by the nonplanktonic cyanobacterium *Scytonema hofmanni* (Gleason and Baxa, 1986). On the other hand, cyanobacterial populations are sometimes controlled by attacks of specific cyanophages or by lytic myxobacters or aquatic fungi.

The temperature optimum for growth of many or most cyanobacteria is higher by at least several degrees than for most eucaryotic algae. This tendency may also play an important role in the notable summertime dominance of cyanobacteria in temperate latitudes, but this tendency is extended to even higher temperatures for some species of hot springs (up to 74°C), tropical pools, and intertidal habitats where eucaryotic phototrophs are inhibited or excluded. Cyanobacteria may also predominate at low and freezing temperatures due to the exclusion of most other phototrophs, but in those cases the actual temperature optimum may be considerably higher (Vincent and Howard-Williams, 1986). Extensive freshwater and terrestrial microbial mats of the Antarctic are composed mainly of cyanobacteria for which dominance may be achieved through the ability to tolerate alternating freezing and thawing or freeze-drying.

The ability of many cyanobacteria to tolerate high salinity (Borowitzka, 1986) results in blue-green predominance in many hypersaline marine lagoons and inland saline lakes (Bauld, 1981). Cyanobacteria may also be especially tolerant of specific substances at higher concentrations. Free sulfide is tolerated and sometimes utilized by cyanobacteria at levels much higher than those tolerated by eucaryotic algae (Padan and Cohen, 1982).

Most of the adaptations mentioned above apply also to various members of the anoxygenic phototrophic bacteria, especially sulfide, salinity, and high temperature tolerance, but dominance in this group is less obvious because of general relegation to "out of sight," anoxic environments.

Cyanobacteria have an especially great tolerance of desiccation which is the basis for the prevalence of extensive cyanobacterial mats in sabkhas, desert and tropical soils, and terrestrial or subaerial habitats in numerous tropical or subtropical regions. Cyanolichen associations are very common, in various climatic regions. Nitrogen-fixing cyanobacteria may form the single photosynthetic partner with the fungus or the nitrogen-fixing partner in a tripartite association where a green alga provides the photosynthate (e.g. Ahmadjian, 1982; Stewart et al., 1983).

Other symbioses include cyanobacteria that serve as functional "chloroplasts" in a variety of eucaryotic "hosts" or simply as nitrogen-fixing "factories" in several unrelated types of green plants (Stewart et al., 1983). Most of these are intercellular and capable of independent growth.

"Cyanelles" are functional intracellular "chloroplasts" in a few restricted unicellular host eucaryotes. They are suspected of being unicellular cyanobacteria that, through a long term symbiosis in the host cell, have lost the potential for autonomy (Trench, 1982). The loss of the cyanobacterial wall is nearly complete, but remnants of peptidoglycan are retained (Scott et al., 1984).

Taxa of the Cyanobacteria
R. W. CASTENHOLZ AND JOHN B. WATERBURY

The classification of organisms into various taxa has as "one of its main aims the division of the existing organisms (which are the result of an evolutionary process) in such a way that one can take one's bearings among them, ..." (Komárek, 1983). The usual unit which is basic to the traditional system of taxonomy is the species. In all groups it is represented by a narrow or widely distributed assemblage of populations which characterize a delimited habitat. Within procaryotic populations there is a range of genetic variability expressed as features that can be recorded and evaluated, often statistically. Distinct and stable differences, whether merely quantitative or more obvious, can be used to delimit species, particularly wherever clear discontinuities occur in the distribution of traits. However, it is not always clear that a discontinuity occurs between cyanobacterial taxa that represent, statistically, two different species (Anagnostidis and Komárek, 1985).

The extent or existence of genetic recombination or lateral transfer of genetic elements in feral cyanobacterial populations is unknown at present. The clonal spread of mutants when selection is favorable may be presumed to be the first event in speciation.

Recently, two courses for the delimitation of genera have been followed by blue-green specialists: (a) to retain "small" genera (Anagnostidis and Komárek, 1985) or (b) to gather many species into fewer genera (Bourrelly, 1970, 1985). It appears that the first course may be the more practical of the two and that small clusters of species within more unambiguously defined genera will result. However, at this time we believe that there is insufficient information, based on cultures, to pursue this course. Therefore, the "larger" genera used here are, in most cases, meant as temporary vehicles for various groups of species, ecotypes or strains.

The wisdom of this tactic at present is borne out by recent results (Giovannoni et al., 1988) in which the sequences of 800–900 consecutive nucleotides of 16S rRNA were compared in over about 30 strains of cyanobacteria, spanning Subsections I–V (Rippka et al., 1979). A preliminary interpretation of these results indicates that the five strains of Subsection IV that were analyzed (*Nostocales*), the three strains of Subsection II (*Pleurocapsales*), and the two strains of Subsection V (*Stigonematales*) were phylogenetically coherent but that the remaining representatives of Subsections I (*Chroococcales*) and III (*Oscillatoriales*), for the most part, did not cluster according to the expectations of section groups or of generic designation (sensu Rippka et al., 1979). Thus, considerably more sorting will be required.

At this time, a modest revision of the temporary scheme published by Rippka et al. (1979) will be used. Generic names will usually be given without species epithets. It is possible, at least by the time of the next revision of this manual, that enough monographic work with pure cultures will have been done to warrant the use of species names.

The subsections of Rippka et al. (1979) are here given names of ordinal rank which is more in accord with botanical practice. Familial names for each subsection would give them very different meanings from the same names in botanical usage. The inclusiveness of each order is, at least, close to that accepted by some authorities, namely Golubic (1976). However, broader meaning is commonly given to orders. For example, Drouet (1981) merely differentiated between unicellular (order *Chroococcales*) and filamentous types (order *Hormogonales*). Geitler (1932) included the order *Chamaesiphonales*.

The key to the subsections of cyanobacteria which follows is simple and is merely a modification of the table-key used by Rippka et al. (1979). The generic descriptions included within each subsection (order) are based largely on cultured material. It should be understood that only a small number of genera of cyanobacteria have representatives in axenic culture and many of these have not been studied extensively enough to be used for characterization. In addition, many of the cultured strains have not been grown under conditions which elicit the various morphological features generally ascribed to them. Consequently, the degree of detail used in generic descriptions will vary considerably, depending on the thoroughness of recent studies. Thus, the classification system and genera included here will, by need, go through a long process of revision and expansion in the future.

Diagnostic key to the "subsections" or orders of Cyanobacteria (Group II)

A. Unicellular or nonfilamentous aggregates of cells held together by outer walls or a gellike matrix (colonies) ....B

A. Filamentous; trichome of cells branched or unbranched, uniseriate or multiseriate......................................C

B. Binary fission in one, two or three planes, symmetric or asymmetric; or by budding
Subsection I. Order *Chroococcales*, p. 1728

B. Reproduction by internal multiple fissions with production of daughter cells smaller than the parent; or by multiple and binary fission
Subsection II. Order *Pleurocapsales*, p. 1746

C. Binary fission in one plane only giving rise to uniseriate, unbranched trichomes, although false branching may occur (see "General Characteristics of the Cyanobacteria") ....D

C. Binary fission periodically or commonly in more than one plane, giving rise to multiseriate trichomes or trichomes with true branches or both (see "General Characteristics of the Cyanobacteria")
Subsection V. Order *Stigonematales*, p. 1794

D. Trichomes composed of cells which do not differentiate into heterocysts or akinetes
Subsection III. Order *Oscillatoriales*, p. 1771

D. One or more cells of each trichome differentiate into a heterocyst, at least when concentration of combined nitrogen is low; some also produce akinetes
Subsection IV. Order *Nostocales*, p. 1780

SUBSECTION I. ORDER **CHROOCOCCALES** WETTSTEIN 1924, EMEND. RIPPKA ET AL., 1979

JOHN B. WATERBURY and ROSMARIE RIPPKA

Chro.o.coc.cal′es. M.L. masc. n. *Chroococcus* genus of order; *-ales* to denote an order; M.L. fem. pl. n. *Chroococcales* the *Chroococcus* order.

Unicellular cyanobacteria that reproduce by binary fission or budding. Cells are coccoid to rod-shaped and vary in size from 0.5 to 30 μm in diameter. Division occurs in one, two or three successive planes at right angles to one another or in irregular planes, resulting in **cells occurring singly or in aggregates of varying size.** Cell aggregate form and cohesiveness depend on the planes and regularity of division and the presence or absence of extracellular slime or structured sheaths to hold the cells together. Division by budding occurs in the genus *Chamaesiphon.*

Further Descriptive Information and Taxonomic Comments

The ordinal definition used here corresponds to "Section I" of Rippka et al., 1979. It differs from traditional botanical definitions by the inclusion of unicellular cyanobacteria that divide by budding (e.g. *Chamaesiphon*). The budding cyanobacteria have traditionally been included in the order *Dermocarpales* (synonym, *Chamaesiphonales*) along with the unicellular cyanobacteria that reproduce by multiple fission.

In traditional botanical field taxonomic treatments of the cyanobacteria, genera have been defined almost exclusively by structural characteristics. Similarly, when studied in pure culture, morphological and developmental features are sufficiently distinct that they currently form the basis for generic definitions in four of the five orders of cyanobacteria. In contrast, many of the unicellular members of the *Chroococcales*, when studied in pure culture, lack adequate morphological and developmental complexity to permit genera to be defined by these criteria alone.

Stanier et al. (1971), in their early monograph on pure culture studies of unicellular cyanobacteria, recognized that genera defined by using structural features, such as cell size and shape, planes of division, and the presence or absence of a well-defined sheath, often resulted in heterogeneous assemblages of strains exhibiting large spans in their DNA base ratios. Use of additional phenotypic characteristics such as ultrastructural properties and physiological and chemical characteristics has in some instances provided sufficient additional information to enable genera to be clearly defined (Rippka et al., 1979). Generic and species assignments, used here, have been correlated as closely as possible with existing descriptions from the botanical "Geitlerian" system of classification.

In some instances, even the additional phenotypic information has proven insufficient to enable clear generic boundaries to be established, resulting in large heterogenous strain clusters provisionally treated here as "groups." In these groups, genetic analyses, such as partial sequence analysis of 16S rRNA and DNA/DNA homology studies, will be necessary for clear delineation of generic and specific boundaries. Once taxa have been defined genetically, it is anticipated that characteristic, readily determinable phenotypic properties will be identified that will permit strains to be assigned to genera and species. The potential for and, in some instances, the inevitability of divergence between botanical and bacteriological systems of classification for cyanobacteria is greatest within the *Chroococcales*. Successful delineation of genera and species in this order will require, in addition to structural and ecological characteristics, the use of phenotypic and genetic properties that were unavailable to traditional systematists.

Two major structural and developmental properties of unicellular cyanobacteria warrant comment. The presence or absence and characteristics of cell aggregates and the number and regularity of the planes of division are major characteristics used to delineate genera and "groups" of unicellular cyanobacteria in culture and to describe genera in the traditional botanical literature.

Cell aggregates in the *Chroococcales* are held together either by multilaminated sheath material or by amorphous slime or capsular material. The possession of extracellular sheath layers has proven to be a stable feature of many cyanobacterial groups in culture and is a primary character used in the description of several unicellular groups including: *Gloeobacter, Gloeothece* and the *Gloeocapsa*-group. Other unicellular cyanobacteria, primarily some members of the *Synechocystis*-group, occur in cell aggregates in nature and, more rarely, in culture that are held together by amorphous slime or capsular material. Slime production has proven to be an unreliable taxonomic characteristic because its production in culture is affected by the growth phase of the cyanobacteria and the conditions under which they were grown.

Members of the *Chroococcales* reproduce by transverse binary fission or budding. Binary fission occurs in one, two or three successive planes at right angles to one another or in irregular planes. The number and regularity of the successive planes of division are stable features of individual cyanobacteria that should, in principle, be readily determinable from cultured material. In practice, however, it is often difficult to determine the number of successive planes of division, with the distinction between division in two or three planes being especially problematical. Examination of batch cultures growing either in liquid or on solid media usually is insufficient to unequivocally provide this information. Ideally, it should be possible to grow individual strains in slide culture and to document the planes of division by time lapse photography along with light microscopy. This has not been done for many of the strains currently in pure culture, with the result that some of the loosely defined groups, particularly the *Synechocystis*-group, contain some strains that divide in two successive planes and some that divide in three successive planes.

Most traditional botanical taxonomic treatments of the *Chroococcales* (Fritsch, 1945; Desikachary, 1959; Bourrelly 1970, 1985) follow the system of Geitler (1925, 1942, 1960). In that system, the order *Chroococcales* contains two families. The first family, *Chroococcaceae*, includes the unicellular cyanobacteria that conform to the ordinal definition used here, except that Geitler did not include the budding forms (e.g. *Chamaesiphon*). The second family, the *Entophysalidaceae*, is a poorly defined group whose members form vegetative cell aggregates resulting from binary fission in irregular planes. The cell aggregates often resemble those produced by members of the *Pleurocapsales*. They are distinguished

from members of that group because multiple fission and baeocyte formation have not been observed. It is probable that future studies will show that many entophysalidacean forms are actually members of the *Pleurocapsales*.

The most recent taxonomic treatment of the unicellular cyanobacteria is that of Komárek and Anagnostidis (1986). It is a significant departure from the Geitlerian system that places all the chroococcalean and pleurocapsalean cyanobacteria in one order (the *Chroococcales*) that contains seven families. The unicellular forms included in the *Chroococcales* by Geitler are placed in three families by Komárek and Anagnostidis. The family *Microcystaceae* contains unicellular cyanobacteria that divide in one, two or three planes at right angles to one another. The family *Chroococcaceae* contains unicellular forms that divide in three irregular planes, and the family *Entophysalidaceae* corresponds to the Geitlerian definition. The distinction between the latter two families is based on the presence of "thallus polarity" in the *Entophysalidaceae*.

Drouet and Daily (1956), in their revision of the coccoid *Myxophyceae* (unicellular cyanobacteria), drastically reduced the number of chroococcalean genera and species. Their system, based primarily on the examination of many preserved specimens, has not proven successful for the identification of unicellular cyanobacteria in the field or in pure culture (Stanier et al., 1971).

Further Reading

Geitler, L. 1932. *Cyanophyceae. In* Kolkwitz (Editor), Kryptogamenflora von Deutschland, Osterreich und der Schweiz. Akademische Verlagsgesellschaft, Leipzig, Vol. 14, pp. 1–1196.

Komárek, J. and K. Anagnostidis. 1986. Modern approach to the classification system of cyanophytes. Arch. Hydrobiol. Suppl. *73:* 157–226.

Rippka, R., J. Deruelles, J.B. Waterbury, M. Herdman and R.Y. Stanier, 1979. Generic assignments, strain histories and properties of pure cultures of cyanobacteria. J. Gen. Microbiol. *111:* 1–61.

Rippka, R., J.B. Waterbury and R.Y. Stanier. 1981. Provisional generic assignments for cyanobacteria in pure culture. *In* Starr, Stolp, Trüper, Balows and Schlegel (Editors), The Prokaryotes. A Handbook on Habitats, Isolation, and Identification of Bacteria. Springer-Verlag, Berlin, pp. 247–256.

Key to the genera and groups of the order **Chroococcales** *(Subsection I)*

A. Reproduction by binary fission ....B

A. Reproduction by repeated budding from the apical pole of the cell; cells ovoid; thylakoids present
        1. Genus I. *Chamaesiphon,* p. 1730

B. Thylakoids present C

B. Thylakoids absent; division in one plane; cells rod-shaped; sheath present
        2. Genus II. *Gloeobacter,* p. 1731

C. Division in one plane ....D

C. Division in two or three planes ....F

D. Cell diameter of >3 μm; capable of aerobic N_2 fixation or nitrogenase produced anaerobically ....E

D. Cell diameter of <3 μm
        3. *Synechococcus*-group, p. 1731

E. Cells rod-shaped; sheath present
        4. Genus III. *Gloeothece,* p. 1738

E. Cells rod-shaped; sheath absent
        5. *Cyanothece*-group, p. 1739

F. Cells coccoid to hemispherical, held together in aggregates by multilaminated sheath material
        6. *Gloeocapsa*-group, p. 1741

F. Cells coccoid, occurring singly, in pairs, or in aggregates held together by amorphous capsular material
        7. *Synechocystis*-group, p. 1742

DESCRIPTION OF THE GENERA AND "GROUPS"

1. Genus I. **Chamaesiphon** Braun and Grunow 1865, emend. Geitler 1925

Cha.mae.si′phon. Gr. adv. *chamai* dwarf; Gr. masc. n. *siphon* tube; M.L. masc. n. *Chamaesiphon* microbial tube.

Unicellular cyanobacteria that reproduce exclusively by budding. The small spherical buds are produced in succession at one pole of the mother cell. This mode of reproduction confers an intrinsic polarity on the cell.

Type species (Botanical Code): *Chamaesiphon confervicola* A. Braun 1865.

Reference strain: Pasteur Culture Collection (PCC) 7430 (ATCC 29397). Isolated from a freshwater stream, Sarka Valley near Prague, Czechoslovakia, 1963 by J. Komárek and F. Hindák.

Further Descriptive Information

The developmental cycle of *Chamaesiphon* is shown schematically in Figure 19.14. The bud enlarges and elongates during *period A*. During *period B*, unequal binary fission (budding) produces an apical bud and a larger basal cell. The second generation bud forms from the reproductive pole (*r*) of the primary basal cell during *period C*. The future reproductive pole (*r′*) of the bud has been demonstrated for only one strain (PCC 6605) (Waterbury and Stanier, 1977). A batch culture of strain PCC 7430 is illustrated in Figure 19.15.

In nature, members of the genus *Chamaesiphon* typically develop as epiphytes and epiliths in freshwater streams and lakes. The cells are at-

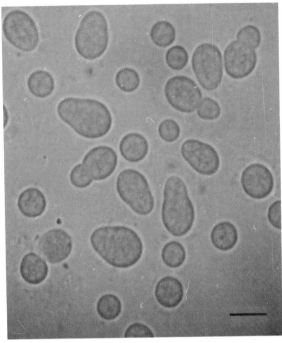

Figure 19.15. Light micrograph of *C. subglobosus* (strain PCC 7430) grown in liquid medium BG-11. Phase contrast. *Bar,* 5.0 μm. (Reproduced with permission from J. B. Waterbury and R. Y. Stanier, Archives of Microbiology *115:* 249–257, 1977, ©Springer-Verlag.)

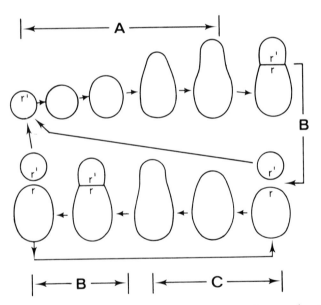

Figure 19.14. Schematic representation of the developmental cycle of *Chamaesiphon* strains PCC 6605 and PCC 7430. See text for explanation and description. (Reproduced with permission from J. B. Waterbury and R. Y. Stanier, Archives of Microbiology *115:* 249–257, 1977, ©Springer-Verlag.)

tached to the substrate by the nonreproductive (basal) pole and are often partly enclosed by a distinct sheath layer, although this structure is not always present. Newly formed buds may be liberated shortly after the completion of division or may remain attached to one another, forming a short chain of spherical cells that adhere to the reproductive (apical) pole of the mother cell.

Taxonomic Comments

Chamaesiphon as defined here conforms to the botanical description of the genus, except for differences in terminology. In the botanical literature the smaller daughter cell (bud) resulting from unequal binary fission is termed an "exospore," and the structured sheath (lacking in the two strains in pure culture) is termed the "pseudovagina."

Further Reading

Kann, E. 1972. Zur Systematik und Ökologie der Gattung *Chamaesiphon* (Cyanophyceae). 1. Systematik. Archiv Hydrobiol. Suppl. 41, Algological Studies 7: 117–171.

Waterbury, J.B. and R.Y. Stanier. 1977. Two unicellular cyanobacteria which reproduce by budding. Arch. Microbiol. *115:* 249–257.

List of species of the genus **Chamaesiphon** represented in pure culture

The properties of the two strains of *Chamaesiphon* from the Pasteur Culture Collection are shown in Table 19.4. Strain PCC 6605 conforms to the botanical description of *C. minutus* (sensu Kann 1972) and strain PCC 7430 conforms to the description of *C. subglobosus* (sensu Kann 1972).

Table 19.4.
Properties of the strains of **Chamaesiphon**[a, b]

Characteristic	C. minutus PCC 6605 ATCC 27169	C. subglobosus PCC 7430 ATCC 29397	Characteristic	C. minutus PCC 6605 ATCC 27169	C. subglobosus PCC 7430 ATCC 29397
Morphology (μm)			Chromatic adaptation	+	−
Diameter of mother cell	3–3.5	5	PUFA content		
Length of mother cell	5	6–7	High	+	+
Diameter of bud	2.5–3	3	Low		
Motility	−	−	Source: freshwater	+	+
Facultative photoheterotrophy	−	+	Maximum temperature permitting growth (°C)	30	27
Glucose	NA	+	Mol% G + C of DNA		
Fructose	NA	+	T_m	46.9	46.7
Sucrose	NA	+	Bd	46.9	
Nitrogenase: synthesis in anaerobiosis	−	−			
Pigment system: synthesis of C-PE	+	−			

[a]Data are from Waterbury and Stanier (1977).

[b]Symbols and abbreviations: −, negative; +, positive; NA, not applicable; C-PE, c-phycoerythrin; and PUFA, polyunsaturated fatty acids.

2. Genus II. **Gloeobacter** Rippka et al. 1974

Gloe.o.bac'ter. Gr. adj. *gloios* sticky; Gr. n. *bakterion* (dim. of *baktron*) small rod; M.L. n. *Gloeobacter* sticky bacterium.

Unicellular cyanobacteria that possess **oval to rod-shaped cells that divide by transverse binary fission in a single plane. Cells occur in irregular aggregates held together by multilayered sheath material. Intracellular photosynthetic thylakoids are lacking;** the photosynthetic apparatus is associated with the cytoplasmic membrane.

The mol% G + C of the DNA is 64 (T_m) from a single strain, PCC 7421.
Holotype species: *Gloeobacter violaceus* Rippka et al. 1974.

Further Descriptive Information and Taxonomic Comments

The genus *Gloeobacter* can be differentiated from other genera of unicellular cyanobacteria by its lack of photosynthetic thylakoids. This is a character not discernible in the field but readily recognizable in thin sections of fixed material examined by transmission electron microscopy. Before it was known that these cyanobacteria lacked photosynthetic thylakoids, they were placed in the genus *Gloeothece*. They resemble *Gloeothece* morphologically by having rod-shaped cells that divide in one plane and that are held together in cell aggregates by a multilayered sheath.

This genus is currently represented by a single species, *Gloeobacter violaceus*. Two strains are available in pure culture (PCC 7421 and PCC 8105), both of which were isolated from the same location during different years.

Further Reading

Rippka, R., J. Waterbury and G. Cohen-Bazire. 1974. A cyanobacterium which lacks thylakoids. Arch. Microbiol. *100:* 419–436.

Differentiation of the species of the genus **Gloeobacter** (**Gloeobacter violaceus** Rippka et al. 1974 (**Gloeothece coerulea** Geitler 1927))

General features of *Gloeobacter violaceus* are found in the generic description. Individual cells are approximately 1.5×2.0–3.0 μm. A striking feature of the cells is the large refractile granules, typically located near each cell pole (Fig. 19.16). These granules stain metachromatically and appear to be composed of polyphosphate, an interpretation supported by their appearance in electron micrographs. Single cells appear colorless, but cell aggregates, dense liquid cultures, and colonies on solid media possess a characteristic violet color. Colonies on solid media remain small and compact, with entire edges. Growth in liquid cultures results in a mixture of single cells and aggregates of widely varying size, resulting in a clumpy and heterogenous appearance.

G. violaceus contains chlorophyll *a* as its primary photosynthetic pigment and both phycocyanin and phycoerythrin in a ratio of 3:2, respectively, as its major light-harvesting pigments. The phycoerythrin is unusual for a terrestrial cyanobacterium, in that it possesses both phycoerythrobilin and phycourobilin that absorb at 564 and 498 nm, respectively. *G. violaceus* is incapable of chromatic adaptation. The phycobiliproteins are present in a cortical layer 50–70 nm thick that immediately underlies the cytoplasmic membrane.

G. violaceus is an obligate photoautotroph incapable of using organic compounds as sole sources of cell carbon. Dinitrogen is not fixed, nor has it been possible to induce nitrogenase activity anaerobically. Growth rates are slow, a mean doubling time of 73 h (strain PCC 7421) was achieved in continuous light (50 fc) at 25°C. Growth does not occur at 37°C.

G. violaceus is known from the European Alps, where it occurs on calcareous rocks. Both strains currently in culture (PCC 7421 and PCC 8105) were isolated from calcareous rocks near Kastanienbaum, Vierwaldstättersee, Switzerland, in 1972 and 1981, respectively.

The mol% G + C of the DNA is 64 (T_m) from strain PCC 7421.
Type strain: ATCC 29082 (PCC 7421).

3. Synechococcus-group

The *Synechococcus*-group is a provisional assemblage which can be loosely defined as unicellular coccoid to rod-shaped cyanobacteria that divide by binary fission in a single plane. The cells are <3 μm in diameter, contain photosynthetic thylakoids located peripherally, and lack structured sheaths.

Further Descriptive Information

In culture, the members of this group are deceptively similar morphologically. However, the true extent of heterogeneity within the group is manifested by the span of their DNA base ratios which range from 39 to 71 mol% G + C, a span almost as broad as that for all procaryotes.

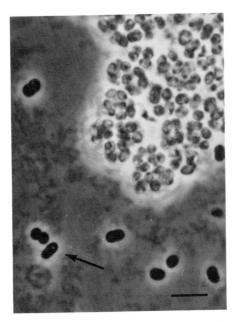

Figure 19.16. Light micrograph of *Gloeobacter violaceus* (strain PCC 7421) grown in liquid medium BG-11. Both characteristic cell aggregates and individual cells released from aggregates during slide preparation are visible. Polyphosphate granules located in the poles of cells are faintly visible in some cells (*arrow*). Phase contrast. *Bar,* 5.0 μm.

Discontinuities in the DNA base ratios resulting in distinct strain clusters within the *Synechococcus*-group became apparent as the collection of pure cultures grew, providing what appeared to be logical break-off points for subdivision of the group. Stanier et al. (1971) recognized two strain clusters, one from 45 to 56 mol% G + C and another from 66 to 71 mol% G + C. In the monograph of Rippka et al. (1979), three DNA base ratio clusters with spans of 39–43, 47–56 and 66–71 mol% G + C were recognized. Rippka and Cohen-Bazire (1983) proposed that these three clusters be given generic status, assigning *Cyanobacterium, Synechococcus* and *Cyanobium* to the low, medium and high DNA base ratio clusters, respectively. Recently, a large number of marine strains have been isolated that can be assigned to the *Synechococcus*-group (Waterbury et al., 1986). The DNA base ratios of this group of strains span from 55 to 64 mol% G + C, effectively filling the gap between the medium and the high DNA base ratio strain clusters and obscuring the basis for the subdivision of the *Synechococcus*-group by DNA base ratio discontinuities.

By using morphological, physiological and chemical properties, in addition to the DNA base ratios, it has been possible to subdivide the *Synechococcus*-group phenotypically into six "strain-clusters" (Table 19.5). These clusters are equivalent to genera but have not been formalized because they are based on an incomplete data set, with a relatively limited number of phenotypic properties used. In some cases (e.g. the *Synechococcus*-cluster), further subdivision at the generic level may be warranted. Thus, formal delineation of genera and species will have to await further phenotypic and genetic analyses.

A brief description of each strain cluster within the *Synechococcus*-group follows.

a. Cyanobacterium-Cluster. This cluster contains two strains, one isolated from an alkaline pond and the other from an acidic peat bog. The cells range in diameter from 1.7 to 2.3 μm, slightly larger than the majority of strains in the *Synechococcus*-group, and are nonmotile (Fig. 19.17). They contain phycocyanin as their major light-harvesting pigment, phycoerythrin is absent, and all are obligate photoautotrophs incapable of using organic compounds as sole sources of cell carbon.

The mol% G + C of the DNA ranges from 39 to 40.

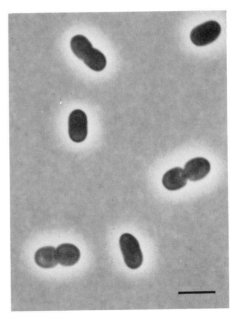

Figure 19.17. Light micrograph of strain PCC 7202, reference strain of the *Cyanobacterium*-cluster of the *Synechococcus*-group, grown in liquid medium BG-11. Phase contrast. *Bar,* 5.0 μm.

Reference strain: PCC 7202 (ATCC 29140). Isolated from an alkaline pond, Chad, 1963 by M. Lefévre.

b. Synechococcus-Cluster. This cluster is represented by 10 strains, some isolated from freshwater (Fig. 19.18) and some from hot springs (Fig. 19.19). The cells range in diameter from 1 to 2 μm and are usually nonmotile. Strain PCC 6910 is larger (3.0 μm in diameter) and is the only strain in the *Synechococcus*-group capable of gliding motility. All of the strains in this cluster contain phycocyanin as their major light-harvesting pigment, phycoerythrin is absent, and all are obligate photoautotrophs incapable of using organic compounds as sole sources of cell carbon. Three strains (PCC 6715, PCC 6716 and PCC 6717) were isolated from hot springs, are thermophilic, and probably are independent isolates of the same species. Five other strains (PCC 6301, PCC 6311, PCC 6908, PCC 7942 and PCC 7943) are also similar, with three (6301, 7942 and 7943) showing a high degree of DNA/DNA homology (Wilmotte and Stam, 1984), and are independent isolates of a single species.

The mol% G + C of the DNA for the entire cluster ranges from 48 to 56.

Reference strain: PCC 6301 (ATCC 27144). Isolated from freshwater, Texas, 1952 by W. A. Kratz.

Reference strain (thermophile): PCC 6715 (ATCC 27149). Isolated from a hot spring, Yellowstone National Park, 1961 by D. L. Dyer.

c. Marine-Cluster C. This cluster contains five strains isolated from coastal marine or brackish waters. Cells range in diameter from 1.2 to 2.0 μm and are nonmotile (Fig. 19.20). Four of the five strains contain phycocyanin as their major light-harvesting pigment. One strain (PCC 7335) produces c-phycoerythrin and is capable of chromatic adaptation. This strain is also remarkable in being the only strain in the entire *Synechococcus*-group capable of synthesizing nitrogenase under anaerobic conditions. Four of the five strains in this cluster are capable of photoheterotrophic growth (PCC 7117 is not) and are the only strains in the *Synechococcus*-group possessing this property. Two of the five strains (PCC 7335 and PCC 7003) have elevated salt requirements for growth, whereas the other three strains are merely halotolerant.

The mol% G + C of the DNA ranges from 47 to 50.

Reference strain: PCC 7002 (ATCC 27264). Isolated from a marine sediment sample, Puerto Rico, 1961 by C. Van Baalen.

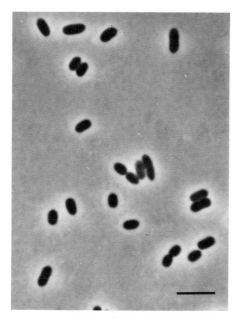

Figure 19.18. Light micrograph of strain PCC 6301, reference strain of the *Synechococcus*-cluster of the *Synechococcus*-group, grown in liquid medium BG-11. Phase contrast. *Bar,* 5.0 μm.

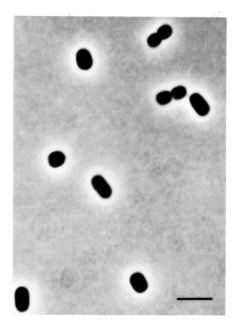

Figure 19.20. Light micrograph of strain PCC 7002, reference strain of Marine-cluster C of the *Synechococcus*-group, grown in liquid medium SN. Phase contrast. *Bar,* 5.0 μm.

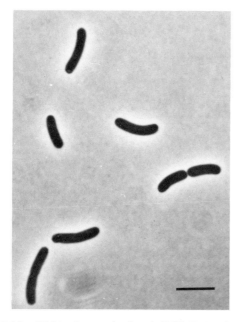

Figure 19.19. Light micrograph of strain PCC 6716, a thermophilic strain of the *Synechococcus*-cluster of the *Synechococcus*-group, grown in liquid medium BG-11. Phase contrast. *Bar,* 5.0 μm.

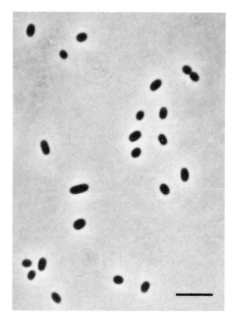

Figure 19.21. Light micrograph of strain WH 8103, reference strain of Marine-cluster A of the *Synechococcus*-group, grown in liquid medium SN. Phase contrast. *Bar,* 5.0 μm.

d. **Marine-Cluster A.** This cluster is represented here by 15 strains isolated from both coastal waters and the open ocean. Cells range in diameter from 0.6 to 1.7 μm and are either nonmotile or capable of swimming (Fig. 19.21). This novel form of motility has not been reported in any other group of cyanobacteria but is common in the open ocean isolates of this strain cluster (Waterbury et al., 1986). All the strains of this cluster contain phycoerythrin as their major light-harvesting pigment but are incapable of classical chromatic adaptation. There is a consider-

able spectral diversity of phycoerythrins in this strain cluster, resulting primarily from the presence or absence of phycourobilin and the ratio of phycoerythrobilin to phycourobilin chromophores contained in the individual phycoerythrins.

The strains in this cluster are all obligate photoautotrophs incapable of using organic compounds as sole sources of cell carbon. All the strains have elevated growth requirements for NA^+, Cl^-, Mg^{2+} and Ca^{2+} that reflect the chemistry of seawater.

Table 19.5.
Properties of the strains of the **Synechococcus-group**[a,b]

Characteristic	Cyanobacterium-cluster		Synechococcus-cluster									
	PCC 7202 / ATCC 29140	PCC 7502 / ATCC 29172	PCC 6312	PCC 6910	PCC 6715	PCC 6716	PCC 6717	PCC 6301 / ATCC 27144	PCC 6311 / ATCC 27145	PCC 6908 / ATCC 27146	PCC 7942 R-2	PCC 7943
Morphology: cell diameter (μm)	1.7–2.3	1.8–2.0	1.3–1.5	3.0	1.2–1.4	1.2–1.4	1.2–1.4	1–1.2	1–1.2	1–1.2	1–1.2	1–1.2
Motility												
Gliding	–	NA	NA	+	–	–	–	NA	–	NA	–	NA
Swimming	–	NA	NA	+	NA	NA	NA	NA	NA	NA	NA	NA
Facultative photoheterotrophy												
Fructose	NA	NA	NA	NA	NA	NA	NA	NA	NA	NA		
Glycerol	NA	NA	NA	NA	NA	NA	NA	NA	NA	NA		
Nitrogenase: synthesis in anaerobiosis	–	–	–	–	–	–	–	–	–	–		
Pigment system												
Phycoerythrin	–	NA	–	–	–	–	–	–	–	NA		
A495/A545[c]	NA	NA	–	–	–	–	–	NA	NA	NA		
Chromatic adaptation	NA	NA	–	–	–	–	–	NA	NA	NA		
PUFA content[e]												
High	+			+								
Low			+		+	+	+	+	+			
LPS type[f]			II	III				III	III	III		
Source												
Freshwater			+	+				+	+			
Acid bog		+										
Alkaline pond	+											
Hot spring					+	+	+					
Brackish water											+	
Marine												
Salt requirements for growth[g]: elevated requirements for Na+, Cl–, Mg2+, Ca2+	–		–	–	–	–	–	–	–	–	–	–
Maximum temperature for growth (°C)	39.0		37	39	>53	>53	>53	43	43	43		
Mol% G + C of DNA[h]												
T_m				47.5				55.1	54.8	56.0		
Bd	40.5		50.2	48.0	53.6	53.6	52.0	55.1	55.1	55.6	55.0	

[a] Data are from Stanier et al. (1971), Rippka et al. (1979), Rippka and Cohen-Bazire (1983) and Waterbury et al. (1986).

[b] Symbols and abbreviations: PCC, Pasteur Culture Collection; ATCC, American Type Culture Collection; WH, Woods Hole Culture Collection; [/], strains bracketed together are probably independent isolates of the same species; –, negative; +, positive; NA, not applicable; No PUB, no phycourobilin; and PUFA, polyunsaturated fatty acid.

[c] A495/A545 is the ratio of absorbance at 495 nm and 545 nm that is related to the bilin chromophore content of the phycoerythrin. Phycourobilin absorbs near 495 nm, and phycoerythrobilin absorbs near 545 nm.

[d] The chromophore ratio varies with light intensity.

[e] Data are from Kenyon et al. (1972).

[f] Data are from Schmidt et al. (1980).

[g] Obligately marine strains have elevated growth requirements for Na+, Cl–, Mg2+, and Ca2+.

[h] Data are from Herdman et al. (1979).

Table 19.5.—continued

Characteristic	Marine-cluster C					Marine-cluster A						
	PCC 7335	PCC 7003	PCC 7002	PCC 7109	PCC 7117	WH 7805	WH 8010	WH 8018	WH 8110	WH 8105	WH 7802	WH 8003
Morphology: cell diameter (μm)	1.9–2.1	1.8–2.0	1.2–1.5	1.2–1.5	1.2–1.5	1.0–1.2	1.2–1.3	1.2–1.5	1.1–1.4	0.9–1.4	0.9–1.2	0.6–1
Motility												
Gliding	−	−	NA	NA	NA	NA	NA	NA	NA	NA	NA	NA
Swimming	−	−	NA	NA	NA	NA	NA	NA	NA	NA	NA	NA
Facultative photoheterotrophy												
Fructose	+	+	+	+	NA	NA	NA	NA	NA	NA	NA	NA
Glycerol	+	−	−	+	NA	NA	NA	NA	NA	NA	NA	NA
Nitrogenase: synthesis in anaerobiosis	−	−	−	−	−	−	−	−	−	−	−	−
Pigment system												
Phycoerythrin	+	−	−	−	−	+	+	+	+	+	+	+
A495/A545[c]	No PUB	NA	NA	NA	NA	No PUB	No PUB	No PUB	No PUB	0.6	0.4	0.4
Chromatic adaptation	+	NA	NA	NA	NA	−	−	−	−	−	−	−
PUFA content[e]												
High	+	+										
Low			+									
LPS type[f]												
Source												
Freshwater												
Acid bog												
Alkaline pond												
Hot spring												
Brackish water		+										
Marine	+	+	+	+	+	+	+	+	+	+	+	+
Salt requirements for growth[g]: elevated requirements for Na+, Cl−, Mg2+, Ca2+	+	+	−	−	−	+	+	+	+	+	+	+
Maximum temperature for growth (°C)		39	43			30	30	30	30	30	30	30
Mol% G + C of DNA[h]												
T_m	47.4	49.3	49.1	49.0								
Bd	49.5	49.5	49.0	48.5	48.5	60	59	58	57	55	58	59

[a] Data are from Stanier et al. (1971), Rippka et al. (1979), Rippka and Cohen-Bazire (1983) and Waterbury et al. (1986).

[b] Symbols and abbreviations: PCC, Pasteur Culture Collection; ATCC, American Type Culture Collection; WH, Woods Hole Culture Collection; [/], strains bracketed together are probably independent isolates of the same species; −, negative; +, positive; NA, not applicable; No PUB, no phycourobilin; and PUFA, polyunsaturated fatty acid.

[c] A495/A545 is the ratio of absorbance at 495 nm and 545 nm that is related to the bilin chromophore content of the phycoerythrin. Phycourobilin absorbs near 495 nm, and phycoerythrobilin absorbs near 545 nm.

[d] The chromophore ratio varies with light intensity.

[e] Data are from Kenyon et al. (1972).

[f] Data are from Schmidt et al. (1980).

[g] Obligately marine strains have elevated growth requirements for Na+, Cl−, Mg2+, and Ca2+.

[h] Data are from Herdman et al. (1979).

Table 19.5.—continued

Characteristic	Marine-cluster A (continued) WH 8005	WH 7803	WH 6501	WH 8011	WH 8103	WH 8102	WH 8112	WH 8113	Marine-cluster B WH 8007	WH 8101	WH 5701	PCC 7001
Morphology: cell diameter (µm)	0.9–1.3	0.9–1.2	0.7–0.9	0.9–1.1	0.9–1.1	0.9–1.4	0.9–1.7	1.0–1.5	0.9–1.1	1.1–1.2	1.2–1.4	0.8
Motility												
Gliding	NA	NA	NA	–	–	–	+	+	NA	NA	NA	NA
Swimming	NA	NA	NA	+	+	NA	+	+	NA	NA	NA	NA
Facultative photoheterotrophy												
Fructose	NA	NA	NA	NA	NA	NA	NA	NA	NA	NA	NA	NA
Glycerol	NA	NA	NA	NA	NA	NA	NA	NA	NA	NA	NA	NA
Nitrogenase: synthesis in anaerobiosis	–	–	–	–	–	–	–	–	–	–	–	–
Pigment system												
Phycoerythrin	+	+	+	+	+	+	Variable^d	+	NA	NA	NA	NA
A495/A545^c	0.4	0.4	0.4	0.8	2.4	2.0	Variable^d	Variable^d	NA	NA	NA	NA
Chromatic adaptation	–	–	–	–	–	–	–	–	NA	NA	NA	NA
PUFA content^e												
High												+
Low												
LPS type^f												
Source												
Freshwater												
Acid bog												
Alkaline pond												
Hot spring												
Brackish water	+	+	+	+	+	+	+	+	+	+	+	+
Marine	+	+	+	+	+	+	+	+	+	–	–	–
Salt requirements for growth^g: elevated requirements for Na$^+$, Cl$^-$, Mg^{2+}, Ca^{2+}												
Maximum temperature for growth (°C)	30	30	30	30	30	30	30	30				41
Mol% G + C of DNA^h												
T_m	59	61	62	59	59	60	60	61	63	64	66	69.5
Bd												69.4

^{a}Data are from Stanier et al. (1971), Rippka et al. (1979), Rippka and Cohen-Bazire (1983) and Waterbury et al. (1986).

^{b}Symbols and abbreviations: PCC, Pasteur Culture Collection; ATCC, American Type Culture Collection; WH, Woods Hole Culture Collection; [/], strains bracketed together are probably independent isolates of the same species; –, negative; +, positive; NA, not applicable; No PUB, no phycourobilin; and PUFA, polyunsaturated fatty acid.

^{c}A495/A545 is the ratio of absorbance at 495 nm and 545 nm that is related to the bilin chromophore content of the phycoerythrin. Phycourobilin absorbs near 495 nm, and phycoerythrobilin absorbs near 545 nm.

^{d}The chromophore ratio varies with light intensity.

^{e}Data are from Kenyon et al. (1972).

^{f}Data are from Schmidt et al. (1980).

^{g}Obligately marine strains have elevated growth requirements for Na$^+$, Cl$^-$, Mg^{2+}, and Ca^{2+}.

^{h}Data are from Herdman et al. (1979).

Table 19.5.—continued

Characteristic	Cyanobium-cluster							
	PCC 6307	PCC 6907	PCC 6911	PCC 6713	PCC 6904	PCC 7009	PCC 6603	PCC 6710
Morphology: cell diameter (µm)	0.8–1	0.8–1	0.8–1	0.8–1	0.8–1	0.8–1	1.2–1.4	1.2–1.4
Motility:								
Gliding	NA	NA	NA	NA	NA	NA	NA	NA
Swimming	NA	NA	NA	NA	NA	NA	NA	NA
Facultative photoheterotrophy:								
Fructose	NA	NA	NA	NA	NA	NA	NA	NA
Glycerol	NA	NA	NA	NA	NA	NA	NA	NA
Nitrogenase: synthesis in anaerobiosis	–	–	–	–	–	–	–	–
Pigment system								
Phycoerythrin	–	–	–	–	–	–	–	–
A495/A545[c]	NA	NA	NA	NA	NA	NA	NA	NA
Chromatic adaptation	NA	NA	NA	NA	NA	NA	NA	NA
PUFA content[e]								
High								
Low	+	+	+		+	+	+	
LPS type[f]	I	I	I				II	
Source								
Freshwater	+	+	+	+	+		+	
Acid bog								
Alkaline pond								+
Hot spring								
Brackish water								
Marine						+		
Salt requirements for growth[g]: elevated requirements for Na⁺, Cl⁻, Mg²⁺, Ca²⁺	–	–	–	–	–	–		–
Maximum temperature for growth (°C)	35–37	35–37	35–37	35–37			35	35
Mol% G + C of DNA[h] — Tₘ	69.7	71.4	66.3	69.4	67.8	66.6		
Bd							65.7	68.4

[a] Data are from Stanier et al. (1971), Rippka et al. (1979), Rippka and Cohen-Bazire (1983) and Waterbury et al. (1986).

[b] Symbols and abbreviations: PCC, Pasteur Culture Collection; ATCC, American Type Culture Collection; WH, Woods Hole Culture Collection; [/], strains bracketed together are probably independent isolates of the same species; –, negative; +, positive; NA, not applicable; No PUB, no phycourobilin; and PUFA, polyunsaturated fatty acid.

[c] A495/A545 is the ratio of absorbance at 495 nm and 545 nm that is related to the bilin chromophore content of the phycoerythrin. Phycourobilin absorbs near 495 nm, and phycoerythrobilin absorbs near 545 nm.

[d] The chromophore ratio varies with light intensity.

[e] Data are from Kenyon et al. (1972).

[f] Data are from Schmidt et al. (1980).

[g] Obligately marine strains have elevated growth requirements for Na⁺, Cl⁻, Mg²⁺, and Ca²⁺.

[h] Data are from Herdman et al. (1979).

The mol% G + C of the DNA ranges from 55 to 62.

Reference strain: Woods Hole (WH) 8103 (ATCC 53061). Isolated from surface waters, Sargasso Sea (28°N, 67°W), 1981 by J. B. Waterbury.

e. Marine-Cluster B. This cluster contains four strains isolated from coastal marine samples. Cells range in diameter from 0.8 to 1.4 μm and are nonmotile (Fig. 19.22). All contain phycocyanin as their major light-harvesting pigment, phycoerythrin is absent, and all are obligate photoautotrophs incapable of using organic compounds as sole sources of cell carbon. One strain (WH 8007) has elevated salt requirements for growth, whereas the other three strains are merely halotolerant.

The mol% G + C of the DNA ranges from 63 to 69.

Reference strain: WH 5701. Isolated from Long Island Sound, U.S.A., 1957 by R. R. L. Guillard.

f. Cyanobium-Cluster. This cluster contains eight strains, seven of freshwater origin and one (PCC 7009) isolated from brackish water. Cells range in diameter from 0.8 to 1.4 μm and are nonmotile (Fig. 19.23). All contain phycocyanin as their major light-harvesting pigment, phycoerythrin is absent, and all are obligate photoautotrophs incapable of using organic compounds as sole sources of cell carbon.

The mol% G + C of the DNA ranges from 66 to 71.

Reference strain: PCC 6307 (ATCC 27147). Isolated from freshwater, Wisconsin, U.S.A., 1949 by G. C. Gerloff.

Taxonomic Comments

In the traditional botanical literature, the unicellular cyanobacteria that divide in a single plane are placed in a number of genera that are described by using structural and ecological properties. The descriptions of many of the genera are based on colonial morphology which is a feature that is poorly manifested in cultures. As a consequence, it is difficult in many instances to correlate the strain clusters described here with traditionally described genera. Eventual resolution of this problem will require the isolation of cultures from carefully described and documented natural samples.

Further Reading

Komárek, J. 1976. Taxonomic review of the genera *Synechocystis* Sauv. 1892, *Synechococcus* Näg. 1849, and *Cyanothece* gen. nov. (Cyanophyceae). Arch. Protistenk. Bd. *118:* 119–179.

Rippka, R. and G. Cohen-Bazire. 1983. The *Cyanobacteriales:* a legitimate order based on the type strain *Cyanobacterium stanieri?* Ann. Microbiol. (Inst. Pasteur) *134B:* 21–36.

Stanier, R.Y., R. Kunisawa, M. Mandel and G. Cohen-Bazire, 1971. Purification and properties of unicellular blue-green algae (order *Chroococcales*). Bacteriol. Rev. *35:* 171–205.

Waterbury, J.B., S.W. Watson, F.W. Valois and D.G. Franks. 1986. Biological and ecological characterization of the marine unicellular cyanobacterium *Synechococcus.* Can. Bull. Fish. Aquat. Sci. *214:* 71–120.

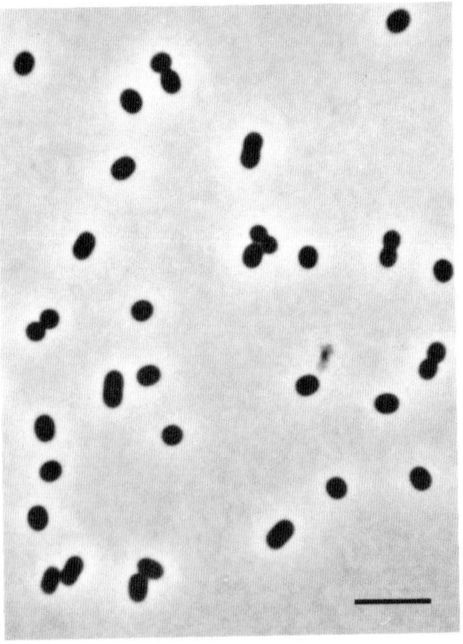

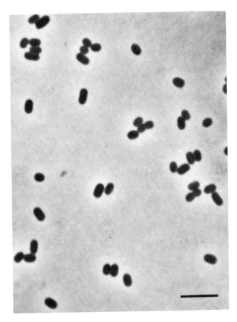

Figure 19.22. Light micrograph of strain WH 5701, reference strain of Marine-cluster B of the *Synechococcus*-group, grown in liquid medium SN. Phase contrast. *Bar,* 5.0 μm.

Figure 19.23. Light micrograph of strain PCC 6307, reference strain of the *Cyanobium*-cluster of the *Synechococcus*-group, grown in liquid medium BG-11. Phase contrast. *Bar,* 5.0 μm.

4. Genus III. **Gloeothece** *Nägeli 1849*

Gloe.o.the′ce. Gr. adj. *gloios* sticky; Gr. fem. n. *theke* case, envelope; M.L. fem. n. *Gloeothece* gelatinous sheath.

Unicellular rod-shaped cyanobacteria that divide by transverse binary fission in a single plane. Cells occur in aggregates that are held together by well-defined sheath layers.

Type species (Botanical Code): *Gloeothece linearis* Nägeli 1849.

Reference strain: PCC 6501 (ATCC 27151), isolated from freshwater, California, U.S.A., 1965 by M. M. Allen.

Further Descriptive Information

Three characteristics are used here to distinguish numbers of the genus *Gloeothece* from other unicellular cyanobacteria. Possession of well-defined sheath layers separates *Gloeothece* from members of both the *Synechococcus*-group and the *Cyanothece*-group. Division by binary fission in a single plane distinguishes *Gloeothece* from members of the *Gloeocapsa*-group, and the possession of photosynthetic thylakoids dispersed throughout the cytoplasm of the cell distinguishes *Gloeothece* from *Gloeobacter*.

Cell orientation within the aggregates of *Gloeothece* can be misleading. The juxtaposition of the cells gives the impression that division has occurred in three planes at right angles to one another, an interpretation that led to the early misidentification of pure cultures of this cyanobacterium as members of the genus *Gloeocapsa* (Stanier et al., 1971). In reality, the cell axes, not the planes of division, of the daughter cells shift following cell division. This shift is the result of cell movement caused by tension exerted on the cells by their surrounding sheath layers.

Gloeothece is presently represented by six strains isolated from a variety of freshwater sources. All six strains are phenotypically very similar and can be assigned to a single species, *Gloeothece membranacea*.

Taxonomic Comments

Gloeothece as defined here conforms to the traditional botanical descriptions of the genus (Geitler, 1932; Desikachary, 1959; Bourrelly, 1970, 1985; Komárek and Anagnostidis, 1986). The treatise of Geitler (1932) contains 16 species in the genus, including *G. coerulea* which is now placed in the genus *Gloeobacter*.

Further Reading

Rippka, R., J. Deruelles, J.B. Waterbury, M. Herdman and R.Y. Stanier. 1979. Generic assignments, strain histories and properties of pure cultures of cyanobacteria. J. Gen. Microbiol. *111*: 1–61.

Rippka, R. and G. Cohen-Bazire. 1983. The *Cyanobacteriales*: a legitimate order based on the type strain *Cyanobacterium stanieri?* Ann. Microbiol. (Inst. Pasteur) *134B*: 21–36.

Differentiation of the species of the genus Gloeothece (Gloeothece membranacea Bornet 1892)

The six strains assigned to *G. membranacea* are very similar. Many of their features are contained in Table 19.6 and in the generic description. The cells are ovoid to rod-shaped and are 5–6 μm in diameter and 6–10 μm in length. They occur in aggregates that are held together by concentric sheath layers (Fig. 19.24). Individual cells, colonies on solid media, and liquid cultures appear dark blue-green as a result of the presence of both phycocyanin, as the major light-harvesting phycobiliprotein, and phycoerythrin, which contains both phycoerythrobilin and phycourobilin chromophores. No strain is capable of chromatic adaptation. All strains are obligate photoautotrophs incapable of using organic compounds as sole sources of cell carbon. The most striking feature of this species is the ability of all the strains to fix dinitrogen in the presence of atmospheric concentrations of oxygen.

The species has a wide geographic distribution and has been isolated from freshwater, acid bogs and alkaline caves.

The mol% G + C of the DNA ranges from 40.8 to 42.7 (T_m, Bd).

Suggested neotype strain: ATCC 27151 (PCC 6501).

5. Cyanothece-group

The *Cyanothece*-group is a provisional assemblage of strains that is loosely defined as unicellular coccoid to rod-shaped cyanobacteria that divide by transverse binary fission in a single plane. The cells are 3 μm or greater in diameter, contain photosynthetic thylakoids, and lack structured sheaths.

Reference strain: PCC 7424 (ATCC 29155), isolated from a rice paddy, Senegal, 1972 by P. Roger.

Further Descriptive Information

The *Cyanothece*-group is superficially distinguished from the *Synechococcus*-group by cell size and from *Gloeothece* and *Gloeobacter* by the absence of well-defined sheath layers.

In addition to morphological similarities (Fig. 19.25), partial characterization of the seven strains included in this group reveals that with one

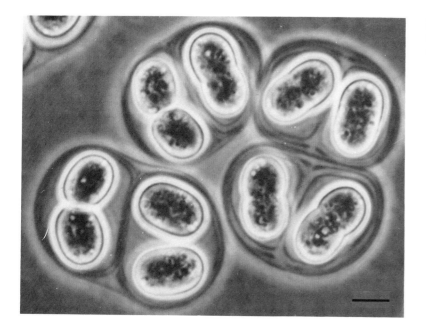

Figure 19.24. Light micrograph of *G. membranacea*, strain PCC 6501, grown in liquid medium BG-11. Phase contrast. *Bar*, 5.0 μm.

Table 19.6.

Properties of strains of **Gloeothece** *and the* **Cyanothece-group**[a, b]

Characteristic	*G. membranacea* PCC 6501 ATCC 27151	*G. membranacea* PCC 6909 ATCC 27152	*G. membranacea* PCC 7109 ATCC 29163	*G. membranacea* PCC 73107 ATCC 29116	*G. membranacea* PCC 73108 ATCC 29164	*G. membranacea* PCC 8302	RF-1[c]	PCC 7425	PCC 7424 ATCC 29155	*Aphanothece halophytica*[d]	PCC 7418 ATCC 29534	BG 43511[e]	BG 43522[e]
Morphology													
Cell diameter (μm)	5–6	5–6	5–6	5–6	5–6		3	3–3.5	5–6	3.5	4–5	4–5	4–5
Sheath formation	+	+	+	+	+	+	−	−	−	−	−	−	−
Planes of division	1	1	1	1	1	1	1	1	1	1	1	1	1
Facultative heterotrophy	−	−	−	−	−	−	−				−		
Nitrogen fixation													
Fixation under aerobic conditions	+	+	+	+	+	+	+			−	+	+	+
Synthesis of nitrogenase in anaerobiosis	NA	NA	NA	NA	NA	NA	NA	+	+		+	NA	NA
Pigment system													
Phycoerythrin	+	+	+		+		−	+		−	−		
PUB present	+	+	+		+		NA	−		NA	NA		
Chromatic adaptation	−	−	−		−								
Salt requirements for growth													
Halophilic[f]										+			
Marine and halotolerant[g]											+		
Marine[h]												+	+
Freshwater	+	+	+	+	+	+	+	+	+				
Source													
Freshwater	+					+[i]							
Acid bog				+	+								
Limestone cave			+										
Rice field							+	+	+				
Mangrove algal mat												+	+
Brine pond										+	+		
Maximum temperature (°C)	39	35								43	35		
Mol% G + C of DNA													
T_m	41.7	41.5	42.0	40.4	42.7			48.6	41.2		42.4		
Bd	40.8	41.3											

[a]Symbols and abbreviations: +, positive; −, negative; NA, not applicable; and PUB, phycourobilin.

[b]Data are from Rippka et al. (1979) and Rippka and Cohen-Bazire (1983), except as otherwise noted.

[c]Data are from Huang and Chow (1986).

[d]Data are from Yopp et al. (1978).

[e]Data from Mitsui et al. (1986).

[f]Optimal growth occurs at 2 M NaCl; the minimum requirement to support growth is 0.7 M NaCl; elevated concentrations of Ca^{2+} and Mg^{2+} are also required.

[g]Optimal growth occurs between 0.7 and 1.0 M NaCl, but a concentration of 3 M NaCl is tolerated; elevated concentrations of Ca^{2+} and Mg^{2+} are also required.

[h]Isolated from seawater; absolute salt requirements are unknown.

[i]Isolated from a drinking fountain, Voges, France by R. Rippka.

possible exception (*Aphanothece halophytica*), members of this group are either capable of dinitrogen fixation at atmospheric oxygen concentrations or capable of synthesizing the enzyme nitrogenase under anaerobic conditions (Table 19.6). By contrast, only one strain (PCC 7335) in the large *Synechococcus-group* is capable of nitrogenase synthesis under anaerobic conditions.

In other respects the seven strains included in the *Cyanothece-group* are a diverse assemblage. Three strains (RF-1, PCC 7424, PCC 7425) were isolated from rice paddies, two were isolated from marine coastal algal mats (BG 43511, BG 43522), and two were isolated from coastal solar evaporation ponds (PCC 7418, *A. halophytica*). Their major ionic requirements for growth reflect their origins. Strains RF-1, PCC 7424 and PCC 7425 grow well in freshwater media. The actual salt requirements of strains BG 43511 and BG 43522 are not known, but they grow well in media made with a seawater base. Strain PCC 7418 grows optimally at NaCl concentrations between 0.7 and 1.0 M. Like many marine strains it also has elevated requirements for Ca^{2+} and Mg^{2+} but differs from typical marine strains by tolerating salinities as high as 3 M NaCl. The *A. halophytica* strain of Yopp et al. (1978) is remarkable in being the only truly halophytic cyanobacterium in culture. It grows optimally in 2 M NaCl, has a minimum requirement of 0.7 M NaCl, and requires elevated concentrations of Mg^{2+} and Ca^{2+}.

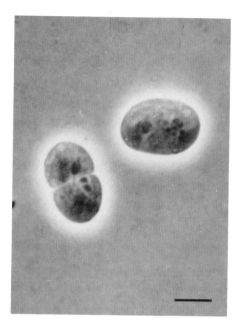

Figure 19.25. Light micrograph of strain PCC 7424, reference strain for the *Cyanothece*-group, grown in liquid medium BG-11. Phase contrast. *Bar,* 5.0 µm.

Taxonomic Comments

In the traditional taxonomic treatments of the cyanobacteria the strains included in the *Cyanothece*-group would have been assigned to a variety of genera including *Cyanothece, Aphanothece* and *Synechococcus*. Future studies of this group will probably show it should be subdivided into several genera.

Further Reading

Huang, T.C. and T.J. Chow. 1986. New type of N₂-fixing cyanobacterium (blue-green alga). FEMS Microbiol. Lett. *36:* 109–110.
Komárek, J. 1976. Taxonomic review of the genera *Synechocystis* Sauv. 1892; *Synechococcus* Näg. 1849, and *Cyanothece* gen. nov. (Cyanophyceae). Arch. Protistenkd. *118:* 119–179.
Mitsui, A., S. Kumazawa, T. Takahashi, H. Ikemoto, S. Cao and T. Arai. 1986. Strategy by which nitrogen-fixing unicellular cyanobacteria grow photoautotrophically. Nature *323:* 730–732.
Rippka, R. and G. Cohen-Bazire. 1983. The *Cyanobacteriales:* a legitimate order based on the type strain *Cyanobacterium stanieri?* Ann. Microbiol. (Inst. Pasteur) *134B:* 21–36.
Yopp, J.H., D.R. Tindall, D.M. Miller and W.E. Schmid. 1978. Isolation, purification and evidence of the obligate halophilic nature of the blue-green alga *Aphanothece halophytica* Frenig (Chroococcales). Phycologia *17:* 172–177.

6. Gloeocapsa-group

The *Gloeocapsa*-group is a provisional assemblage which is loosely defined as unicellular cyanobacteria that divide by binary fission in two or three successive planes at right angles to one another. The cells occur in aggregates that are held together by multilaminated sheath material.

Reference strain: PCC 73106 (ATCC 27928), isolated from an acidic bog, Switzerland, 1971 by R. Rippka.

Further Descriptive Information and Taxonomic Comments

The six strains assigned to the *Gloeocapsa*-group are a heterogenous assemblage that in the traditional botanical literature would be assigned to either *Gloeocapsa* or *Chroococcus* (Figs. 19.26 and 19.27 and Table 19.7). Cell shape and the characteristics of the extracellular sheath layers are the primary characteristics used in the botanical literature to distinguish between the two genera. Immediately following division, *Chroococcus* possesses hemispherical cells that are surrounded by tightly appressed sheath layers. *Gloeocapsa* has spherical cells that are held loosely together by their surrounding sheath layers. However, distinction between the two genera in field material and in laboratory cultures with reference to the two primary structural characteristics can be problematic due to transitional stages.

In culture, individual strains often contain both rounded and hemispherical postdivisional cells (Rippka et al., 1979). Even in strains N-41 and S-24, which conform well to the description of *Chroococcus* (Fig. 19.27), the hemispherical postdivisional cells become spherical when released from their sheath layers (Potts et al., 1983). These observations indicate that the postdivisional shape of the cells in these two genera depend on the degree of compression applied to the cells by their surrounding sheath layers. Thus, the primary characteristics of cell shape and sheath morphology appear to be inadequate criteria for the differentiation of the two genera.

Other phenotypic properties may provide a basis for defining clusters within the *Gloeocapsa*-group. Division in both *Chroococcus* and *Gloeocapsa* is reported to occur in three successive planes at right angles to one another, but this fundamental property has not yet been verified in the strains now in culture. Morphologically, strains S-24 and N-41 conform to the description of *Chroococcus turgidus* but differ physiologically by having elevated salt requirements for growth.

Further Reading

Potts, M., R. Ocampo-Friedmann, M.A. Bowman and B. Tözün. 1983. *Chroococcus* S-24 and *Chroococcus* N-41 (cyanobacteria): morphological, biochemical and genetic characterization and effects of water stress on ultrastructure. Arch. Microbiol. *135:* 81–90.

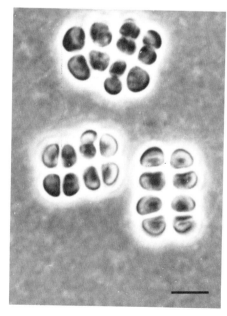

Figure 19.26. Light micrograph of strain PCC 7428, member of the *Gloeocapsa*-group, grown in liquid medium BG-11. Phase contrast. *Bar,* 5.0 µm.

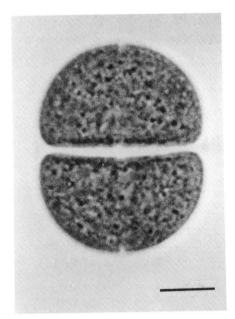

Figure 19.27. Light micrograph of strain N-41, member of the *Gloeocapsa*-group, grown in liquid medium MN. *Bar,* 10.0 μm. (Reproduced with permission from M. Potts, R. Ocampo-Friedmann, M. A. Bowman and B. Tözön, Archives of Microbiology *135:* 81–90, 1983, ©Springer-Verlag.)

Table 19.7.

Properties of strains of the **Gloeocapsa-group**[a]

Characteristic	PCC 7428	ATCC 29159[b]	PCC 7512	ATCC 29115[b]	PCC 7501	ATCC 29113[b]	PCC 73106	ATCC 27928[b]	S-24[c]	N-41[c]
Morphology: cell diameter (μm)	3					6.5		<30 ± 2	25 ± 3	
Gliding motility	−		−		+		+		+	+
Facultative heterotrophy										
Glucose	+		−		+		−		−	−
Fructose	+		−		−		−		−	−
Ribose	+		−		−		−		−	−
Sucrose	+		−		−		−		+	+
Glycerol	−		−		−		−		−	−
Nitrogenase: synthesis in anaerobiosis	−		−		−		−		+	+
Pigment system										
Phycoerythrin	−		+		+		+		−	−
PUB present	NA		−		+		−		NA	NA
Chromatic adaptation	NA				−				NA	NA
Source										
Hot Spring	+									
Terrestrial			+		+					
Acid bog							+			
Desert										+[d]
Marine intertidal									+[d]	
Mol% G + C of DNA										
T_m	46		39.8		40.9		41.7			
HPLC									48.9	47.1

[a]Symbols and abbreviations: −, negative; +, positive; PUB, phycourobilin; NA, not applicable; and HPLC, high pressure liquid chromatography.
[b]Data are from Rippka et al. (1979).
[c]Data are from Potts et al. (1983).
[d]Require elevated concentrations of NA+, Cl−, Ca2+ and Mg2+ for growth.

7. Synechocystis-group

The *Synechocystis*-group is a provisional assemblage that is loosely defined as unicellular cyanobacteria that divide by binary fission in two or three successive planes at right angles to one another. The cells typically occur singly or in pairs in culture; but in nature and, rarely, in culture, some can also occur in aggregates held together by amorphous slime material.

Further Descriptive Information

By using morphological, physiological and chemical properties, including DNA base ratios, the *Synechocystis*-group has been subdivided into four "strain clusters" (Table 19.8). These clusters are equivalent to genera but have not been formalized because their characterization is based on an incomplete data set, with a relatively limited number of phenotypic properties used. Brief descriptions of each strain cluster within the *Synechocystis*-group follow:

a. **Marine-cluster.** This cluster is represented by two strains, both isolated from the tropical Atlantic Ocean. The cells are spherical, occur singly or in pairs, divide in two planes at right angles to one another, and are nonmotile (Fig. 19.28). Neither cell aggregates nor amorphous capsular material is produced. Both strains are obligate photoautotrophs incapable of using organic compounds as sole sources of cell carbon. They are unique within the *Synechocystis*-group by being capable of fixing dinitrogen under atmospheric concentrations of oxygen. Photosynthesis and dinitrogen fixation are separated temporally. Dinitrogen fixation occurs during the dark at the expense of glycogen reserves accumulated in the light. They contain phycoerythrin high in phycourobilin content as their primary light-harvesting pigment and are incapable of chromatic adaptation. They have a very restricted temperature range, growth occurs between 26 and 32°C, which restricts their distribution to the equatorial oceans. They are obligately marine with elevated growth requirements for Na+, Cl−, Mg2+ and Ca2+.

The mol% G + C of the DNA ranges form 30 to 32.

Reference strain: WH 8501, isolated from the tropical Atlantic Ocean (28°S, 43°W), 1984 by S. Watson and F. Valois.

b. **Low GC-cluster.** This cluster is represented by five strains isolated from freshwater. They possess spherical to oval cells ranging from 3 to 7 μm in diameter (Fig. 19.29 and Table 19.8). The planes of division have only been determined for one strain. PCC 6808 divides in two planes at

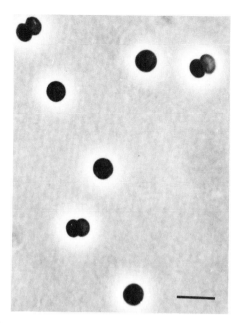

Figure 19.28. Light micrograph of strain WH 8501, reference strain of the Marine-cluster of the *Synechocystis*-group, grown in liquid medium SN. Phase contrast. *Bar,* 5.0 μm.

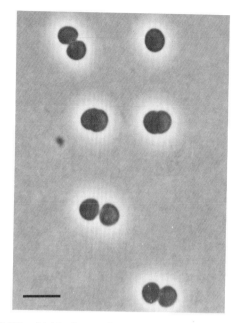

Figure 19.29. Light micrograph of strain PCC 6308, reference strain of the low GC-cluster of the *Synechocystis*-group, grown in liquid medium BG-11. Phase contrast. *Bar,* 5.0 μm.

right angles to one another and, if grown without agitation, is capable of forming flat sheets of regularly arranged cells. Amorphous capsular material is produced by strains PCC 6711 and PCC 6804. Three of the five strains (PCC 6711, PCC 6804, PCC 6808) are capable of gliding motility. The strains of this cluster are all obligate photoautotrophs incapable of using organic compounds as sole sources of cell carbon. Three of the five strains (PCC 6701, PCC 6711, PCC 6808) produce phycoerythrin that contains only phycoerythrobilin chromophores. Strains PCC 6701 and PCC 6808 are capable of type II chromatic adaptation (Tandeau de Marsac, 1977). The strains of the cluster are all low in polyunsaturated fatty acid content. They are mesophiles with maximum temperatures permitting growth between 37 and 39°C.

The mol% G + C of the DNA ranges from 35 to 37.

Reference strain: PCC 6308 (ATCC 27150), isolated from a freshwater lake, Wisconsin, U.S.A., 1949 by G. Gerloff.

c. **High GC-cluster.** This cluster contains 11 strains isolated from freshwater, brackish water, and terrestrial sources. They possess spherical to oval cells ranging from 2 to 3 μm in diameter (Fig. 19.30 and Table 19.8). The planes of division have only been determined for one strain. PCC 6906, when first isolated, produced cubical cell aggregates, indicating that binary fission had occurred in three planes at right angles to one another in this strain. The production of amorphous capsular material has been observed in one strain (PCC 6714). Gliding motility has been reported in 4 of the 11 strains (PCC 6803, PCC 6905, PCC 7201, PCC 6902). Nine of the 11 strains in this cluster are capable of photoheterotrophic growth on a limited number of organic compounds (Table 19.8); strains PCC 6902 and PCC 7008 appear to be obligate photoautotrophs. Phycocyanin is the major light-harvesting pigment in this cluster; phycoerythrin does not occur. The five strains that have been examined for cellular fatty acid composition were all high in polyunsaturated fatty acids. The maximum temperature permitting growth ranged from 37 to 39°C for the five strains examined to date.

The mol% G + C of the DNA ranges from 42 to 48.

Reference strain: PCC 6714 (ATCC 27178), isolated from freshwater, California, U.S.A., 1967 by R. Kunisawa.

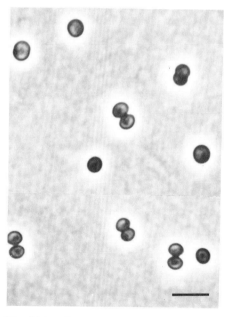

Figure 19.30. Light micrograph of strain PCC 6714, reference strain of the high GC-cluster of the *Synechocystis*-group, grown in liquid medium BG-11. Phase contrast. *Bar,* 5.0 μm.

d. **Microcystis-cluster.** This cluster contains seven strains isolated from freshwater. Cells are spherical to oval and vary from 3 to 8 μm in diameter (Fig. 19.31). In culture, five of the seven strains occur singly or in pairs. However, two strains (C3-9 and P1-15) have retained the ability to form loose cell aggregates, held together by amorphous capsular material, that are characteristic of natural populations of *Microcystis.* Char-

Table 19.8.

Properties of strains of the **Synechocystis-group**[a,b]

Characteristic	Marine-cluster		Low GC-cluster					High GC-cluster									
	WH 8501[c]	WC 8502[c]	PCC 6308 ATCC 27150	PCC 6701 ATCC 27170	PCC 6711 ATCC 27175	PCC 6804 ATCC 27185	PCC 6808 ATCC 27189	PCC 6702 ATCC 27171	PCC 6714 ATCC 27178	PCC 6803 ATCC 27184	PCC 6805 ATCC 27186	PCC 6806 ATCC 27187	PCC 6905 ATCC 29109	PCC 7201 ATCC 29152	PCC 6902 ATCC 29108	PCC 6906 ATCC 27266	PCC 7008 ATCC 29110
Morphology																	
Cell diameter (μm)	2.5–4	2.5–4	4–5	3–4	3–4	7	6–7	2–3	2–3	2–3	2–3	2–3					
Planes of division	2	2					2									3	
Aggregate formation	−	−	−	−	−	−	+[h]							−[i]		+[j]	
Capsule production				+	+				+								
Gas vacuoles	−	−	−	−	−	−	−	−	−	−	−	−	−	−	−	−	−
Gliding motility	−	−	−	−	+	+	+	−	−	+	−	−	+	+	+	−	−
Facultative heterotrophy	−	−	−	−	−	−	−	+	+	+	+	+	+	+	−	+	−
Glucose	NA	NA	NA	NA	NA	NA	NA	+	+	+	+	+	+	+	NA	(+)	NA
Sucrose	NA	NA	NA	NA	NA	NA	NA	−	−	−	−	−	−	−	NA	−	NA
Glycerol	NA	NA	NA	NA	NA	NA	NA	−	−	−	−	−	−	−	NA	+	NA
Nitrogen fixation																	
Fixation under aerobic conditions	+	+	−	−	−	−	−	−	−	−	−	−	−	−	−	−	−
Synthesis of nitrogenase in anaerobiosis	+	+	−	−	−	−	−	−	−	−	−	−	−	−	−	−	−
Pigment system																	
Phycoerythrin	+	+	−	+	+	−	+	−	−	−	−	−	−	−	−	−	−
PUB present[h]	+	+	NA	−	−	NA	−	NA	NA	NA	NA	NA	NA	NA	NA	NA	NA
Chromatic adaptation	−	−	+[k]				+[k]	NA	NA	NA	NA	NA	NA	NA	NA	NA	NA
PUFA content																	
Low			+	+	+	+	+										
High								+	+	+	+	+					
Production of β-cyclocitral[f]																	
Toxin production[e]																	
Source																	
Freshwater			+	+	+	+	+	+	+	+	+	+					+
Terrestrial														+			
Saline lake																+	
Brackish water													+		+		
Marine	+	+															
Maximum temperature for growth (°C)	32	32	37	39	37	37	39	39	39	39	39	37					
Mol% G + C of DNA																	
T_m	30.5	31.7		35.8	36.7	36.9	36.0		47.9	47.5		46.6					
Bd			35	35.7	37.0	36.2	35.7	47.4	47.4	47.4	48.0	46.4	47.1	46.1	42.1	46.9	44.9

[a]Symbols and abbreviations: −, negative; +, positive; NA, not applicable; (+), weakly positive; PUB, phycourobilin; and PUFA, polyunsaturated fatty acid.

[b]Data are from Stanier et al. (1971) and Rippka et al. (1979), except as otherwise noted.

[c]Data are from J. B. Waterbury, unpublished information.

[d]Data are from R. Rippka, unpublished information.

[e]Data are from Codd and Carmichael (1982).

[f]Data are from Jüttner (1984).

[g]Data are from Parker (1982).

[h]Forms sheets of cells when grown without agitation.

[i]Occurred as a macroscopic hemispherical colony in nature.

[j]When newly isolated, formed cubical packets of cells.

[k]Type II chromatic adaptation (Tandeau de Marsac, 1977).

Table 19.8.—*continued*

	High GC-cluster *(continued)*		Microcystis-cluster					
Characteristic	PCC 7509 ATCC 29235	NRC-1[d,e] PCC 7941	PCC 7806[d,f]	PCC 7820[d,e]	PCC 7005[b,f] ATCC 27153	C3-9[g]	P1-15[g]	C5-34[g]
Morphology								
Cell diameter (μm)				3–4	4	6–8		4–5
Planes of division								
Aggregate formation		−	−	−	−	+	+	
Capsule production								
Gas vacuoles	−	+	+	+	−	+	+	+
Gliding motility	−							
Facultative heterotrophy	+				−			
Glucose	−				NA			
Sucrose	+				NA			
Glycerol	+				NA			
Nitrogen fixation								
Fixation under aerobic conditions					−			
Synthesis of nitrogenase in anaerobiosis					−			
Pigment system								
Phycoerythrin	−				−			
PUB present[h]	NA							
Chromatic adaptation	NA							
PUFA content								
Low								
High					+			
Production of β-cycocitral[f]			+		+			
Toxin production[e]		+		+				
Source								
Freshwater		+	+	+	+	+	+	+
Terrestrial	+							
Saline lake								
Brackish water								
Marine								
Maximum temperature for growth (°C)					35			
Mol% G + C of DNA								
T_m								
Bd	42.5				45.4			

[a]Symbols and abbreviations: −, negative; +, positive; NA, not applicable; (+), weakly positive; PUB, phycourobilin; and PUFA, polyunsaturated fatty acid.

[b]Data are from Stanier et al. (1971) and Rippka et al. (1979), except as otherwise noted.

[c]Data are from J. B. Waterbury, unpublished information.

[d]Data are from R. Rippka, unpublished information.

[e]Data are from Codd and Carmichael (1982).

[f]Data are from Jüttner (1984).

[g]Data are from Parker (1982).

[h]Forms sheets of cells when grown without agitation.

[i]Occurred as a macroscopic hemispherical colony in nature.

[j]When newly isolated, formed cubical packets of cells.

[k]Type II chromatic adaptation (Tandeau de Marsac, 1977).

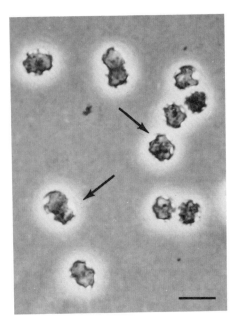

Figure 19.31. Light micrograph of strain PCC 7820, reference strain of the *Microcystis-cluster* of the *Synechocystis-group,* grown in liquid medium BG-11. Note the light refractile gas vacuoles (*arrows*). Phase contrast. *Bar,* 5.0 μm.

acterization of the cluster is tentative because of a very limited data set. The possession of three characteristics—gas vacuoles, toxin production, and β-cyclocitral production—by some of the strains forms the basis for separating them from the high GC-cluster (Table 19.8). Six of the seven strains possess gas vacuoles; strain PCC 7005, originally designated as *Microcystis aeruginosa,* does not. However, gas-vacuolated strains have been observed to lose these organelles in culture (Rippka, 1982), raising the possibility that strain PCC 7005 may have originally possessed gas vacuoles. Jüttner (1984) has shown that strains of *Microcystis,* including strains PCC 7005 and PCC 7806, liberate large amounts of β-cyclocitral, whereas its production has not been demonstrated in other cyanobacteria including *Synechocystis.* Finally, members of the genus *Microcystis*

are often associated with toxic blooms in nature (Gibson and Smith, 1982). Codd and Carmichael (1982) have demonstrated toxin production in strains PCC 7941 and PCC 7820.

Reference strain: PCC 7820, isolated from a freshwater lake, Forfar, Scotland, 1976 by R. Stewart.

Taxonomic Comments

In the traditional botanical literature (Geitler, 1932; Desikachary, 1959; Bourrelly, 1970, 1985), the strains included in the *Synechocystis*-group would be assigned to five principal genera: *Synechocystis, Aphanocapsa, Microcystis, Merismopedia* and *Eucapsis.* Geitler (1932) places unicellular cyanobacteria that possess spherical cells that do not occur in aggregates in the genus *Synechocystis.* Unicellular spherical to oval cyanobacteria that formed cell aggregates held together by amorphous capsular material were placed in the genera *Aphanocapsa* and *Microcystis.* The two genera were distinguished by the presence of gas vacuoles in *Microcystis.* These definitions from Geitler (1932) did not include the number and planes of successive divisions. More recently, Komárek (1976) and Komárek and Anagnostidis (1986) described division in these genera as occurring in two planes at right angles to one another in *Synechocystis* and *Aphanocapsa* and in three planes at right angles to one another in *Microcystis.* The genera *Merismopedia* and *Eucapsis* in the Geitlerian literature are described as coccoid unicellular cyanobacteria that occur in cell aggregates. *Merismopedia* forms flat cell plates of regularly arranged cells resulting from synchronous division in two planes at right angles to one another. *Eucapsis* forms cubical cell aggregates resulting from synchronous binary fission in three planes at right angles to one another.

Generic and specific assignments for the low GC-cluster, high GC-cluster, and *Microcystis*-cluster will have to await further phenotypic and genotypic characterization. However, the strains of the marine cluster are a novel group of cyanobacteria that differ significantly from the other members of the *Synechocystis*-group. The two strains are very similar and will be assigned to a new genus and species.

Further Reading

Komárek, J. 1976. Taxonomic review of the genera *Synechocystis* Sauv. 1892, *Synechococcus* Näg. 1849, and *Cyanothece* gen. nov. (*Cyanophyceae*). Arch. Protistenkd. *118S:* 119–179.
Parker, D. 1982. Improved procedures for the cloning and purification of *Microcystis* cultures (*Cyanophyta*). J. Phycol. *18:* 471–477.
Stanier, R.Y., R. Kunisawa, M. Mandel, and G. Cohen-Bazire. 1971. Purification and properties of unicellular blue-green algae (order *Chroococcales*). Bacteriol. Rev. *35:* 171–205.

SUBSECTION II. ORDER **PLEUROCAPSALES** GEITLER 1925, EMEND. WATERBURY AND STANIER 1978

JOHN B. WATERBURY

Pleur.o.cap.sa′les. M.L. fem. n. *Pleurocapsa* genus of order; *-ales* suffix to denote order; M.L. fem. pl. n. *Pleurocapsales* the order containing the genus *Pleurocapsa.*

Cyanobacteria that reproduce by the formation of small, spherical cells (baeocytes) produced through multiple fission of a vegetative cell and released through rupture of the fibrous outer wall of the parental cell. Enlargement of vegetative cells is always accompanied by progressive thickening of the fibrous outer wall layer. **Unicellular genera of the order divide exclusively by multiple fission. In other genera, cell aggregates are produced by binary fission,** after which **some or all of the cells composing the aggregate undergo multiple fission** and release baeocytes.

Further Descriptive Information

Members of this order reproduce by multiple fission, a feature that distinguishes them from all other cyanobacteria. Three primary features contribute to the different developmental patterns that occur in the

Pleurocapsales: the relative roles of multiple and binary fission, the planes of successive vegetative divisions, and the changes in the structure of the cell envelope that occur during the cell cycle.

The process of multiple fission is initiated by the rapid successive cleavage of a vegetative cell into at least four (and often many more) spherical daughter cells termed baeocytes. During the course of multiple fission there is no significant increase in cell volume following each successive cleavage. Consequently, the volume of each daughter cell is a quarter or less than that of the parental cell. This marked diminution in cell size that accompanies multiple fission distinguishes it from a series of binary fissions during which each round of division is followed by cell growth.

In the botanical literature, the small vegetative cells that are the product of multiple fission are termed "endospores" or nannocytes. The term "endospore" is widely used and has a precise definition in the botanical literature, but it is confusing when used in a procaryotic context, since the pleurocapsalean "endospore" differs from the bacterial endospore in its mode of formation, structure and development. The term nannocyte has been used botanically to describe unusually small cells produced by cyanobacteria (Geitler, 1932; Fritsch, 1945; Bourrelly, 1970, 1985; Komárek and Anagnostidis, 1986). However, the term has never been precisely defined and has been applied to small cells in cyanobacterial groups that never undergo multiple fission, notably the *Chroococcales* (Geitler, 1932, 1942, 1960; Fritsch, 1945; Komárek and Anagnostidis, 1986). The term *baeocyte* was introduced by Waterbury and Stanier (1978) to avoid both a dual meaning of the term endospore in the procaryotic literature and the confusion that would have resulted from a re-definition of the term nannocyte.

In unicellular members of the *Pleurocapsales (Dermocarpa and Xenococcus)*, cell division occurs solely by multiple fission. In these genera, the baeocyte enlarges into a spherical vegetative cell that subsequently undergoes multiple fission and releases baeocytes that again enlarge into the next generation of vegetative cells. In other members of the group, baeocyte enlargement is followed by binary fission to produce an aggregate of vegetative cells. In *Dermocarpella*, only one to three binary fissions intervene before the onset of multiple fission. In other genera, binary fission is more extensive, with the gross form of the aggregate produced being determined by the planes of successive binary fissions. Regular binary fission in three planes at right angles to one another results in cubical packets of cells, characteristic of *Myxosarcina* and *Chroococcidiopsis*. In the *Pleurocapsa*-group, the planes of successive binary fissions are less regular, and the aggregate consists of a mass of vegetative cells, sometimes bearing filamentous extensions, either branched or unbranched. Some or all of the cells that compose the vegetative aggregates eventually undergo multiple fission and release baeocytes.

In addition to the Gram-negative cell wall layers, the wall of vegetative cells in pleurocapsalean cyanobacteria is always surrounded by a third external layer that structurally resembles the sheath of other cyanobacteria. Electron micrographs of thin sections show that this wall layer has a fibrous structure of varying thickness and density and is usually closely appressed to the outer membrane layer of the Gram-negative wall (Fig. 19.32). During growth and enlargement of vegetative cells, the peptidoglycan and outer membrane layers of the cell wall maintain a constant thickness. In contrast, the fibrous outer wall layer thickens progressively throughout the vegetative cell cycle and may reach a thickness of 1000 nm.

In pleurocapsalean cyanobacteria, existing fibrous outer wall layers do not participate in cell cleavage during either binary or multiple fission. Thus, in binary fission the transverse wall is formed through the ingrowth of the two layers of the Gram-negative cell wall. Following the completion of transverse wall formation, synthesis of new fibrous outer wall material is initiated over the entire surfaces of the two daughter cells. Daughter cells are thus pushed apart by the synthesis of new fibrous outer wall material which continues to thicken progressively until the onset of the following division, but these cells remain enclosed by a common fibrous outer wall layer synthesized by the parental cell. Successive layers of fibrous outer wall material serve to hold vegetative cell aggregates together and to maintain their characteristic topology (Fig. 19.33). In some of the more developmentally complex members of the *Pleurocapsales* the cell aggregates produce "filamentous" appendages. However, these "filamentous" aggregates of cells (pseudofilaments) differ structurally from the filaments in the *Oscillatoriales* and *Nostocales*. In these latter groups the fibrous outer wall layers (sheath) do not intercalate between adjacent cells.

The synthesis of the fibrous outer wall material during multiple fission follows two distinct patterns. In some pleurocapsalean genera, the cleavage products, each surrounded by a Gram-negative cell wall, immediately initiate the synthesis of fibrous outer wall material following each successive division of multiple fission. In these genera, baeocytes, at the time of their release, are consequently surrounded by the Gram-negative wall layers as well as a thin fibrous outer wall layer. Thus, cell wall synthe-

sis during multiple fission in these subgroups follows the same pattern as that of binary fission; the resulting baeocytes can be distinguished from vegetative cells by their size, but not by wall structure.

In the majority of pleurocapsalean subgroups, the synthesis of the fibrous outer wall material is completely suppressed during the course of multiple fission, resulting in baeocytes that are surrounded only by a Gram-negative cell wall at the time of their release.

Baeocytes are released shortly after the completion of multiple fission. As they initiate vegetative growth, their increase in volume causes the fibrous outer wall layer of the parental cell to rupture, presumably as the result of physical stress (Fig. 19.34).

The vegetative cells of all pleurocapsalean cyanobacteria are permanently nonmotile. In members of the *Pleurocapsales*, where the synthesis of the fibrous outer wall layer is suppressed during multiple fission, the resulting baeocytes are capable of gliding motility for a short period (6–24 h) immediately following their release. Motile baeocytes react phototactically in a light gradient, moving toward or away from the light source, depending on its intensity (Fig. 19.35). Loss of motility appears to coincide with the onset of synthesis of the fibrous outer cell wall material that occurs as the baeocytes begin to enlarge into vegetative cells. Baeocytes of the members of the *Pleurocapsales* that are surrounded by a thin fibrous outer wall layer at the time of their release have never been observed to move.

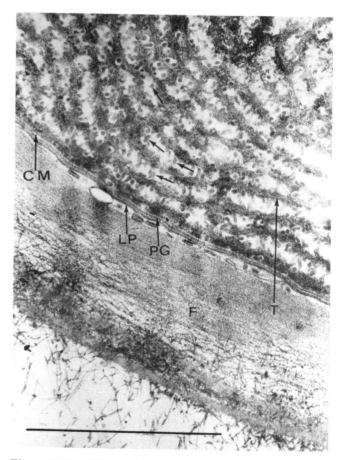

Figure 19.32. Electron micrograph of a thin section of part of a large vegetative cell of *Dermocarpa* (PCC 7302). *F*, fibrous outer wall layer, 750 nm thick and of variable density; *LP*, lipopolysaccharide wall layer; *PG*, peptidoglycan wall layer; *CM*, cytoplasmic membrane, *T*, thylakoids; *arrows*, glycogen granules. *Bar*, 1.0 μm. (Reproduced with permission from J. B. Waterbury and R. Y. Stanier, *Microbiological Reviews 42*: 2–44, 1978, ©American Society for Microbiology.)

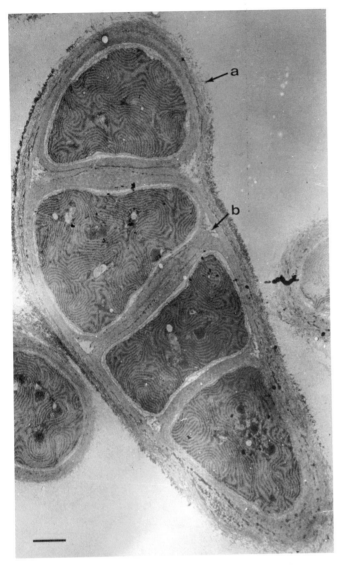

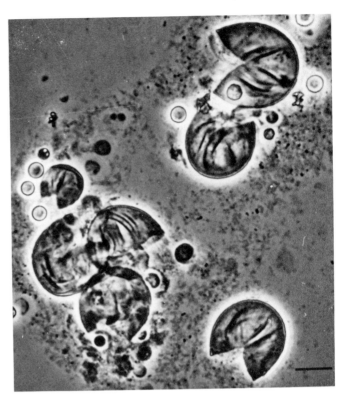

Figure 19.34. Fibrous outer wall layers of parental cells, emptied of their baeocytes, in a liquid culture of *Dermocarpa* (PCC 7437). Phase contrast. *Bar,* 10.0 μm. (Reproduced with permission from J. B. Waterbury and R. Y. Stanier, Microbiological Reviews *42:* 2–44, 1978, ©American Society for Microbiology.)

Figure 19.33. Electron micrograph of a thin section of *Pleurocapsa* (PCC 7314) grown in an agar overlay. Each cell is enclosed by individual peptidoglycan, outer membrane and fibrous outer wall layers. The group of cells is also enclosed by additional fibrous outer wall layers synthesized during previous generations. As cell volume increases, the outermost layers of fibrous wall material become either stretched (*a*) or torn (*b*). *Bar,* 1.0 μm. (Reproduced with permission from J. B. Waterbury and R. Y. Stanier, Microbiological Reviews *42:* 2–44, 1978, ©American Society for Microbiology.)

In nature, members of the *Pleurocapsales* grow attached to solid substrates. Observations made on laboratory cultures suggest that attachment occurs at the baeocyte stage. The firmness of attachment appears to be enhanced during subsequent vegetative growth, as synthesis of fibrous outer wall material causes this layer of the cell wall to flare out around the base of the developing vegetative cell, enlarging the area in contact with the substrate.

Methods for the study of growth and development of members of this family are given in Waterbury and Stanier (1978). The developmental cycles of pleurocapsalean cyanobacteria, in culture, can take several weeks to complete as a result of both slow growth and the complexity and size of the cell aggregates attained before the onset of multiple fission. The Cooper dish culture technique (Waterbury and Stanier, 1978) was designed to sustain growth and permit semicontinuous observations of development over long periods of time. The technique has proven extremely useful for the elucidation of developmental patterns in members of the *Pleurocapsales* but does have severe optical limitations restricting its utility to relatively large-celled cyanobacteria. The optical limitations are imposed by the thickness of the agar layer employed, the thickness of the plastic in the Cooper dishes, and the relatively low power of the objective (× 16) necessary to achieve a sufficiently long working distance. Additional information on isolation and purification is also given in Rippka et al. (1981a).

Pleurocapsalean cyanobacteria have a wide natural distribution, occurring as attached forms in terrestrial, freshwater, and marine environments. The marine intertidal zone contains a particularly abundant and diverse population of these organisms, which grow as epiphytes on other algae and as epiliths on rocks and the shells of marine invertebrates. Some are endoliths that in nature are capable of penetrating calcareous substrates, where they develop in microscopic tunnels formed through dissolution of calcium carbonate. Members of some genera are very cosmopolitan. *Chroococcidiopsis,* for example, occurs in both freshwater and terrestrial habitats, as chasmoendoliths in both cold and hot deserts and as symbionts in lichens.

Taxonomic Comments

The ordinal and generic definitions used here are those proposed by Waterbury and Stanier (1978). They are based on developmental patterns determined on axenic cultures by use of light and electron microscopy. Semicontinuous light microscopic observations of development were made throughout entire developmental cycles, starting with individual baeocytes. These observations were supplemented by electron mi-

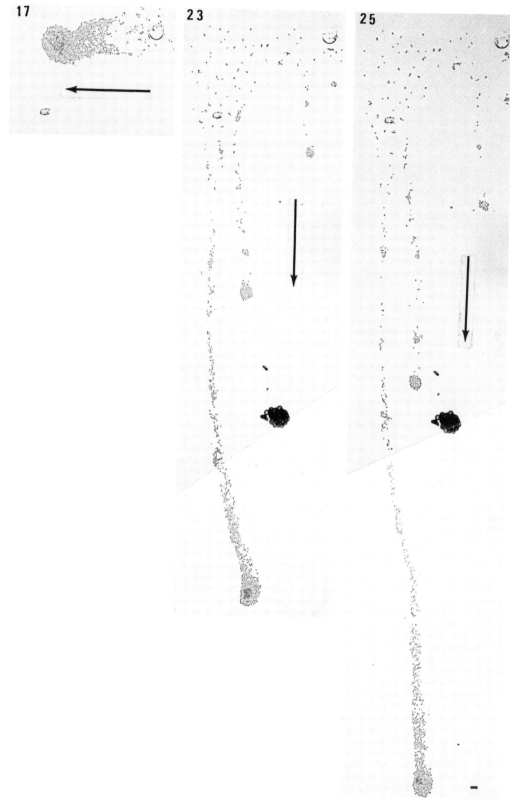

Figure 19.35. Phototactic response of baeocytes liberated from a parental cell of *Dermocarpa* (PCC 7302) which had been placed in a Cooper dish culture and illuminated laterally with unidirectional light. Successive light micrographs of the same field, taken 17, 23, and 25 h after the preparation was made. *Arrows* indicate the direction of illumination, which was changed at 17 h. Note the remnants of the parental fibrous outer layer in the upper right-hand corner of each micrograph. *Bar,* 10.0 µm. (Reproduced with permission from J. B. Waterbury and R. Y. Stanier, Microbiological Reviews *42:* 2–44, 1978, ©American Society for Microbiology.)

croscopic examination of thin sections of cultures fixed at various growth stages. The resulting six developmental groups were correlated as closely as possible with existing generic descriptions from the botanical "Geitlerian" system of classification. In some instances, the botanical definitions were modified to incorporate new properties and the reinterpretation of features from the botanical descriptive literature that were documented during the study of developmental cycles in culture.

Most botanical taxonomic treatments of pleurocapsalean cyanobacteria (Fritsch, 1945; Desikachary, 1959; Bourrelley, 1970, 1985) follow the system of classification originally proposed by Geitler (1925, 1942), although at least two other systems exist (Drouet and Daily, 1956; Komárek and Anagnostidis, 1986).

Geitler assigned the pleurocapsalean cyanobacteria to two orders, the *Pleurocapsales* and the *Dermocarpales* (synonym, *Chamaesiphonales*), and included within the latter order the genus *Chamaesiphon* whose members reproduce by budding (exospore formation in the botanical literature). Members of both orders reproduce by multiple fission (with the exception of *Chamaesiphon* and related genera) and are distinguished by two primary differences: members of the *Dermocarpales* are unicellular and display polarity, and members of the *Pleurocapsales* are "multicellular" and do not display polarity. Waterbury and Stanier (1978), by analyzing the developmental patterns revealed in pure cultures, showed that of the genera Geitler included in the *Dermocarpales*, *Chamaesiphon* possesses both ordinal properties: it is unicellular, and the cells possess a well-defined apical-basal polarity, but it differs from all pleurocapsalean cyanobacteria in its mode of reproduction, i.e. budding. However, none of the other genera in the *Dermocarpales* conforms to the ordinal definition. *Dermocarpa* is unicellular, but the cell is devoid of the polarity. *Dermocarpella* displays polarity, but it is not, in strict terms, unicellular, since its development always leads to the formation of a two- to four-celled aggregate. *Chroococcidiopsis* is not unicellular, always developing as a many-celled aggregate, and does not display polarity; it thus possesses neither of the defining properties of the order *Dermocarpales* but conforms fully to Geitler's definition of the *Pleurocapsales*. Of the genera Geitler included in the *Pleurocapsales*, all lack polarity, and all, with one exception, form many-celled aggregates. With the exception of *Xenococcus* and the inclusion of *Chroococcidiopsis*, the *Pleurocapsales*, as defined by Geitler, can be justified as a higher taxon. The *Dermocarpales*, on the other hand, remains a heterogeneous assemblage. Waterbury and Stanier (1978) concluded that all cyanobacteria that reproduce by multiple fission with the production of baeocytes could be placed in a single order: the *Pleurocapsales*.

Approximately 25 genera of pleurocapsalean cyanobacteria have been described in the "Geiterlerian system," based on the examination of field material. Of these, five genera plus the heterogeneous *Pleurocapsa*-group have been recognized and redefined on the basis of differences in structure and development established through studies on pure cultures (Waterbury and Stanier, 1978). Of the remaining "Geitlerian genera," some have not yet been successfully cultured, while others will almost certainly be combined as the extent of environmentally induced variation is documented within this group.

Drouet and Daily (1956), in their revision of the coccoid *Myxophyceae* (unicellular cyanobacteria), reduced the pleurocapsalean cyanobacteria to a few genera and species. Their system, based primarily on the examination of many preserved specimens, has neither proven successful for the identification of field material, nor has it been useful in evaluating the developmental patterns revealed by pure cultures.

In the recent revision of the unicellular cyanophytes by Komárek and Anagnostidis (1986), both chroococcalean and pleurocapsalean cyanobacteria are placed in one order: the *Chroococcales*, comprising seven families. These authors do not believe that a distinction should be made between simple binary fission and multiple fission, arguing that multiple

fission is, in principle, a variant of binary fission. Komárek and Anagnostidis divide the pleurocapsalean cyanobacteria (sensu Waterbury and Stanier 1978) into four families.

1. The family *Chamaesiphonaceae* (sensu Komárek and Anagnostidis 1986) contains cyanobacteria that display apical-basal polarity and that reproduce by the production of exocytes (synonyms, exospores or buds). Included in this family is the genus *Chamaesiphon* that reproduces by the formation of single terminal exocytes through a process homologous with budding. Also included is a new genus *Chamaecalyx* that is synonymous with the genus *Dermocarpella* (sensu Waterbury and Stanier 1978), a cyanobacterium that divides initially by binary fission to form a sterile basal cell and an apical reproductive cell, that subsequently cleaves into baeocytes following multiple fission.

2. The family *Dermocarpellaceae* (sensu Komárek and Anagnostidis 1986) contains pleurocapsalean genera that are unicellular, that may or may not possess polarity, and that divide exclusively by multiple fission. Included are the genera *Cyanocystis* (synonym, *Dermocarpa* sensu Waterbury and Stanier 1978) that displays apical-basal polarity, a new genus *Stanieria* (synonym, *Dermocarpa* sensu Waterbury and Stanier 1978) that possesses spherical cells (no polarity), and the genus *Dermocarpella* (sensu Komárek and Anagnostidis 1986) that possesses polarity and cleaves entirely into baeocytes. It differs from *Cyanocystis* by reputedly having the first several divisions, during multiple fission, occurring in one plane perpendicular to the plane of polarity rather than in alternating planes, as is usually observed during the cleavage sequence in multiple fission.

3. The family *Xenococcaceae* (sensu Komárek and Anagnostidis 1986) contains pleurocapsalean genera that form tightly clustered aggregates of cells through successive vegetative binary fissions; filamentous appendages are lacking. Some or all of the vegetative cells eventually undergo multiple fission. Included are the genera *Chroococcidiopsis* and *Myxosarcina* whose circumscription corresponds closely to the descriptions of Waterbury and Stanier (1978). The genus *Xenococcus* is used in the traditional Geitlerian sense, which defines it as possessing both vegetative divisions and multiple fission, rather than as redefined by Waterbury and Stanier (1978) who consider this genus to be unicellular, dividing exclusively by multiple fission.

4. The family *Hydrococcaceae* (sensu Komárek and Anagnostidis 1986) contains the pleurocapsalean genera that make cell aggregates with "filamentous" appendages produced through binary fissions in irregular planes. Some of the cells in the aggregates subsequently undergo multiple fission and release baeocytes. This family corresponds to the heterogeneous *Pleurocapsa*-group of Waterbury and Stanier (1978).

The treatment of the pleurocapsalean cyanobacteria by Komárek and Anagnostidis (1986) has yet to be critiqued by the botanical community, but rather than clarifying and simplifying the traditional botanical treatment of these cyanobacteria, it seems to introduce yet another degree of complexity and ambiguity into their taxonomy.

Further Reading

Geitler, L. 1932. *Cyanophyceae. In* Kolkwitz (Editor), Kryptogamenflora von Deutschland, Osterreich und der Schweize. Akademische Verlagsgesellschaft, Leipzig, vol. 14, pp. 1–1196.

Komárek, J. and K. Anagnostidis. 1986. Modern approach to the classification system of cyanophytes. Arch. Hydrobiol. Suppl. *73:* 157–226.

Rippka, R., J. Deruelles, J.B. Waterbury, M. Herdman and R.Y. Stanier. 1979. Generic assignments, strain histories and properties of pure cultures of cyanobacteria. J. Gen. Microbiol. *111:* 1–61.

Rippka, R., J.B. Waterbury and R.Y. Stanier. 1981. Isolation and purification of cyanobacteria: some general principles. *In* Starr, Stolp, Trüper, Balows and Schlegel (Editors), The Prokaryotes. A Handbook on Habitats, Isolation, and Identification of Bacteria. Springer-Verlag, Berlin, pp. 212–220.

Waterbury, J.B. and R.Y. Stanier. 1978. Patterns of growth and development in pleurocapsalean cyanobacteria. Microbiol. Rev. *42:* 2–44.

Key to the genera of the order **Pleurocapsales** (Subsection II)

A. Cell division solely by multiple fission ....B
A. Cell division by a combination of binary and multiple fission C
 B. Baeocytes motile
> 1. Genus I. *Dermocarpa*, p. 1751

 B. Baeocytes nonmotile
> 2. Genus II. *Xenococcus*, p. 1751

C. Baeocyte development leads to the formation of a vegetative cell that undergoes one to three binary fissions, to produce a single apical cell which divides by multiple fission and releases baeocytes; the basal cell subsequently enlarges and repeats the cycle.
> 3. Genus III. *Dermocarpella*, p. 1754

C. Baeocyte development followed by repeated binary fissions, to produce cell aggregates of varying size and complexity ....D

 D. Binary fissions occur in three planes at right angles to one another, producing a cubical aggregate of cells, all of which normally undergo multiple fission. ....E

 D. Binary fissions occur in many different planes, to produce irregular, sometimes filamentous aggregates of cells. Some or all of the cells in the aggregate undergo multiple fission.
> 6. *Pleurocapsa*-group, p. 1762

 E. Baeocytes motile
> 4. Genus IV. *Myxosarcina*, p. 1758

 E. Baeocytes nonmotile
> 5. Genus V. *Chroococcidiopsis*, p. 1758

1. Genus I. **Dermocarpa** Crouan 1858, emend. Waterbury and Stanier 1978

Der.mo.car′pa. Gr. n. *derma* skin; Gr. n. *karpos* fruit; M.L. fem. n. *Dermocarpa* fruit in skin, or cells within coating.

Unicellular cyanobacteria that reproduce exclusively by multiple fission leading to the formation and release of motile baeocytes. The baeocyte enlarges into a vegetative cell that is intrinsically spherical, showing no polarity, but may become pyriform or cleavate when development occurs under crowded conditions. The successive cleavage stages of multiple fission are not normally detectable by light microscopy.

Type species (Botanical Code): *Dermocarpa violacea* Crouan 1858.
Reference strain: PCC 7301 (ATCC 29367, CCAP 1416/1, UTEX 1635); isolated from marine aquarium, Scripps Institute of Oceanography, La Jolla, California, U.S.A., 1964, by R. A. Lewin.

2. Genus II. **Xenococcus** Thuret 1880, emend. Waterbury and Stanier 1978

Xe.no.coc′cus. Gr. n. *xenos* stranger, foreigner; Gr. n. *kokkos* a grain or kernel; M.L. masc. n. *Xenococcus* strange (spherical) cell.

Unicellular cyanobacteria that reproduce exclusively by multiple fission, leading to the formation and release of nonmotile baeocytes. The baeocyte enlarges into a spherical vegetative cell. The successive cleavage stages of multiple fission are readily detectable by light microscopy.

Type species (Botanical Code): *Xenococcus schousboei* Thuret 1880.
Reference strain: PCC 7305 (ATCC 29373); isolated from marine aquarium, Scripps Institute of Oceanography, La Jolla, California, U.S.A., 1971, by R. A. Lewin.

Further Descriptive Information on **Dermocarpa** *and* **Xenococcus**

The developmental patterns of these two genera are similar, differing in the timing of the onset of outer cell wall synthesis during the cleavage process of multiple fission. In *Dermocarpa*, the synthesis of the fibrous outer wall material is suppressed during multiple fission; consequently, the cleavage stages during multiple fission are not visible by light microscopy, and the baeocytes are motile for a short period following their release. In *Xenococcus*, the synthesis of fibrous outer wall material occurs during the cleavage process of multiple fission, resulting in nonmotile baeoctyes and the ability to resolve by light microscopy the successive division stages of multiple fission.

Superficially, mass cultures of *Dermocarpa* and *Xenococcus* appear very similar when examined with light microscopy (Figs. 19.36, *A* and *B*). The photomicrographs contain spherical, internally homogeneous cells ranging from 2 to 30 µm in diameter. Some of the larger cells have undergone multiple fission and are filled with baeocytes. Mass cultures of *Xenococcus* differ strikingly in one respect from those of *Dermocarpa*. Cultures of *Xenococcus* often contain cells that appear to be dividing by binary fission but that are, in fact, cells in the process of multiple fission. The division stages that are evident in Figure 19.36*B* are visible because of the refractile nature of the fibrous outer wall material which in *Xenococcus* is synthesized during the cleavage process (Fig. 19.38*B*).

The developmental patterns of *Dermocarpa* and *Xenococcus* are indistinguishable at the level of resolution of the Cooper dish culture technique (Fig. 19.37). The baeocytes enlarge symmetrically into spherical vegetative cells which increase in size until the onset of multiple fission.

The structural basis for the distinction between the two genera is apparent when thin sections of vegetative cells in the process of multiple fission are examined by transmission electron microscopy (Fig. 19.38). The baeocytes of *Dermocarpa* (Fig. 19.38*A*) are surrounded only by a Gram-negative cell wall, whereas the baeocytes of *Xenococcus* have, in addition, a thin fibrous outer wall layer (Fig. 19.38*B*).

In these two genera, the baeocytes of individual strains are nearly uniform but may vary in size between strains (Table 19.9), whereas the size of the vegetative cells at the onset of multiple fission can vary widely within each strain. Since the size of the vegetative cells of individual strains at the onset of multiple fission varies, while the size of the baeocytes at the time of their release is constant, it follows that the number of baeocytes produced from a single parental cell is variable. It is not unusual for a strain to produce 10–1000 baeocytes per parental cell. If a culture in the stationary phase of growth is transferred to fresh medium,

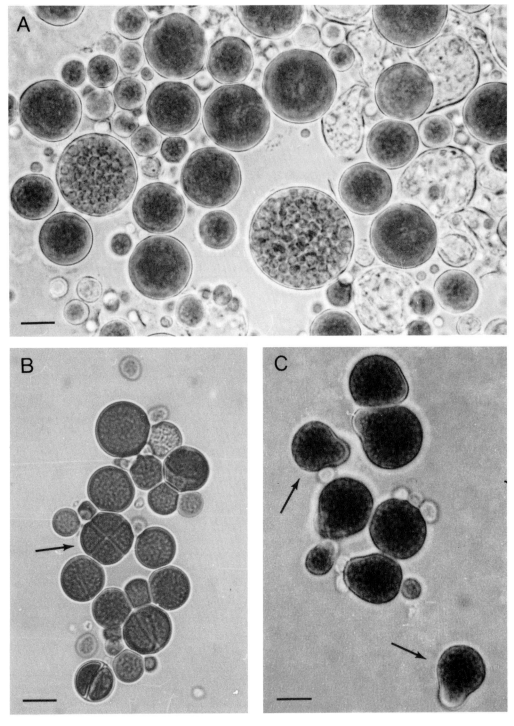

Figure 19.36. *A*, light micrograph of a mass culture of *Dermocarpa* (PCC 7437), revealing spherical cells of varying size that appear either homogeneous or filled with baeocytes. *B*, light micrograph of a mass culture of *Xenococcus*, showing that the cleavage stages during multiple fission are visible by light microscopy (*arrow*). *C*, light micrograph of *Dermocarpa* (PCC 7302), showing pyriform cells (*arrows*) produced through mutual compression when developing under crowded conditions attached to a substrate. Preparation is from a culture grown in an unagitated flask of mineral medium where many cells grow in dense masses attached to the wall of the flask. *Bars*, 10 μm. (Reproduced with permission from J. B. Waterbury and R. Y. Stanier, Microbiological Reviews *42:* 2–44, 1978, ©American Society for Microbiology.)

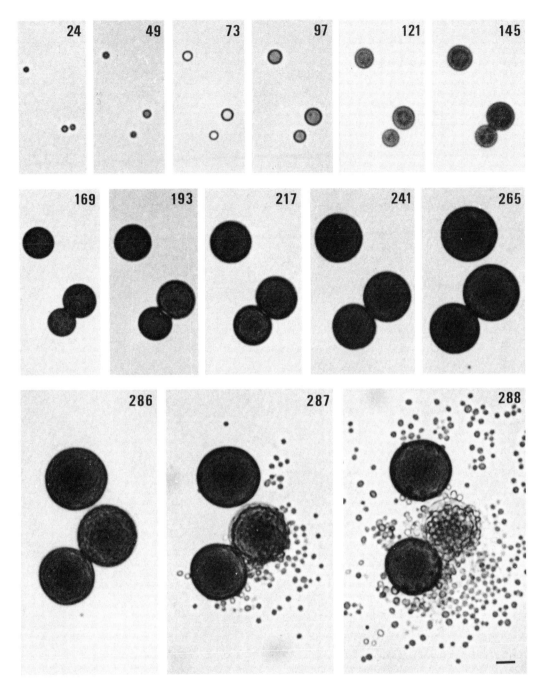

Figure 19.37. Development of *Dermocarpa* (PCC 7302) in a Cooper dish culture. *Numbers* in the upper right-hand corners of the micrographs in Cooper dish cultures indicate the elapsed time, in hours, following the initial observation. *Bar*, 10 µm. (Reproduced with permission from J. B. Waterbury and R. Y. Stanier, Microbiological Reviews *42:* 2–44, 1978, ©American Society for Microbiology.)

a large fraction of the vegetative cells, irrespective of size, will cleave and release baeocytes within 12–24 h, suggesting that environmental factors strongly affect the onset of multiple fission. If Cooper dish cultures are followed for more than one generation, typically more baeocytes are produced per parental cell in each successive generation as the cells become crowded and the growth conditions less favorable, thus inferring that favorable growth conditions lead to early cleavage.

The vegetative cells in all strains of *Dermocarpa* and *Xenococcus,* now in culture, are intrinsically spherical (Figs. 19.36, *A* and *B,* and 19.37). However, the shape of vegetative cells can be markedly modified by environmental factors. When populations of baeocytes attach in dense clusters to a common substrate (e.g. the glass wall of a culture vessel), the enlarging vegetative cells are subjected to mutual compression and assume a pyriform or clavate shape (Fig. 19.36*C*). Cells of this form are frequently observed in natural populations of *Dermocarpa,* leading to the commonly held view in the botanical literature that vegetative cells of *Dermocarpa* possess an intrinsic polarity.

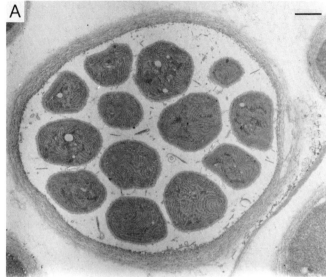

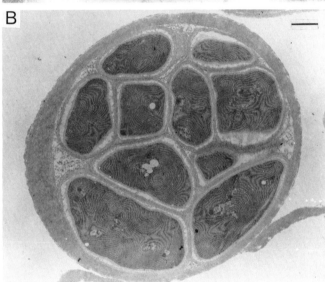

Figure 19.38. Electron micrographs of thin sections of parental cells that have completed multiple fission and are filled with baeocytes. *A, Dermocarpa* (PCC 7304). *B, Xenococcus* (PCC 7307). *Bars,* 1.0 μm. (Reproduced with permission from J. B. Waterbury and R. Y. Stanier, Microbiological Reviews *42:* 2–44, 1978, ©American Society for Microbiology.)

3. Genus III. **Dermocarpella** Lemmermann 1907

Der.mo.car.pel'la. L. suffix-*ella* diminutive; M.L. fem. n. *Dermocarpella* small *Dermocarpa*.

Cyanobacteria that undergo binary fission to form an ovoid aggregate consisting of a large apical cell and from one to three smaller basal cells. The cell aggregate possesses an intrinsic apical-basal polarity. **Multiple fission of the apical cell then occurs, followed by the release of motile baeocytes. The baeocytes enlarge asymmetrically into ovoid vegetative cells before initiating binary fission.** After the initial round of multiple fission, the remaining basal cells enlarge asymmetrically, undergo binary fission to form apical reproductive cells and smaller basal cells, and initiate multiple fission in the apical cells.

Type species (Botanical Code): *Dermocarpella incrassata* Lemmermann 1907.

Reference strain: PCC 7326 (ATCC 29376); isolated from snail shell, intertidal marine, Puerto Penasco, Mexico, 1971, by J. B. Waterbury.

Further Descriptive Information on **Dermocarpella**

Dermocarpella is the simplest pleurocapsalean cyanobacterium whose developmental cycle incorporates division by both binary and multiple fissions. Characteristic developmental stages of *Dermocarpella* are shown in the photomicrographs of Figure 19.39.

The distinctions between binary and multiple fission in pleurocapsalean cyanobacteria are revealed with particular clarity in the electron micrographs of thin sections illustrating the division stages of *Dermocarpella* (Figs. 19.40 and 19.41). The ovoid parental cell first undergoes transverse binary fission, producing a small basal vegetative cell and a much larger apical reproductive cell (Fig. 19.40*A*). The Gram-negative cell wall of the basal vegetative cell remains closely appressed to the fibrous outer wall layer of the parental cell both during and after cell division. Contrastingly, the Gram-negative wall layers of the apical reproductive cell begin to retract from the fibrous outer wall layer of the parental cell even before separation from the basal vegetative cell is complete. Immediately after the completion of transverse division, the basal vegetative cell begins to synthesize new fibrous outer wall material over its entire surface. If the basal vegetative cell undergoes further binary fissions (Figs. 19.40*B* and 19.41), new fibrous outer wall material is intercalated between them and continues to thicken throughout the vegetative cell cycle. Multiple fission of the large reproductive cell occurs through rapid successive cleavage of the entire cell contents (Figs. 19.40*B* and 19.41*A*), producing a large number of baeocytes (Fig. 19.41*B*). Synthesis of fibrous outer wall material is suppressed during the cleavage process,

Table 19.9
Properties of strains of **Dermocarpa, Xenococcus** *and* **Dermocarpella**[a]

Characteristic	Dermocarpa					Xenococcus			Dermocarpella
	D. violacea PCC 7301 ATCC 29367	*Dermocarpa* sp. PCC 7302 ATCC 29368	*Dermocarpa* sp. PCC 7303 ATCC 29369	*D. cyanosphaera* PCC 7437 ATCC 29371	*D. cyanosphaera* PCC 7438 ATCC 29372	*Xenococcus* sp. PCC 7305 ATCC 29373	*Xenococcus* sp. PCC 7306 ATCC 29374	*Xenococcus* sp. PCC 7307 ATCC 29375	*D. incrassata* PCC 7326 ATCC 29376
Morphology									
Baeocyte diameter (μm)	3–4	1.5–2	1.5–2	3–4	3–4	2–3	2–3	2–3	2
Maximum diameter of vegetative cells (μm)	30	30	30	30	20	15	25	10–15	10–13
Facultative photoheterotrophy with									
Glucose	+	–	–	+	+	–	–	+	+
Fructose	+	–	–	–	+	–	–	–	+
Sucrose	+	–	–	+	–	–	–	+	+
Nitrogenase: synthesis in anaerobiosis	+	–	+	–	–	+	–	–	–
Pigment system									
Synthesis of									
C-PE	+	+	+	+	–	–	–	–	+
X-PE	–	–	–	–	+	+	+	+	–
Chromatic adaptation	–	+	+	+	+	+	+	+	+
Source[b]									
Freshwater	–	–	–	+	+	–	–	–	–
Marine[c]	+	+	+	–	–	+	+	+	+
Maximum temperature (°C) permitting growth	37	35	37	44	44	35	30	35	35
Vitamin B$_{12}$ requirement	+[d]	+[e]	+[e]	–	–	–	–	–	–
Mol% G + C of DNA (T_m)	44.0	42.9	43.6	40.7	ND	44.2	ND	43.4	45.1

[a]Symbols and abbreviations: +, positive; –, negative; PCC, Pasteur Culture Collection; ATCC, American Type Culture Collection; C-PE, c-phycoerythrin; X-PE, phycoerythrin containing both phycoerythrobilin and phycourobilin; and ND, not determined.
[b]See Rippka et al. (1979) for details of isolation and strain histories.
[c]Requires elevated concentrations of Na$^+$, Cl$^-$, Ca^{2+} and Mg^{2+} for growth.
[d]Obligate requirement for vitamin B$_{12}$.
[e]Vitamin B$_{12}$ stimulates growth but is not an obligate requirement.

resulting in baeocytes that are surrounded only by the layers of the Gram-negative cell wall.

Contrary to the situation in *Dermocarpa* and *Xenococcus,* the number of baeocytes produced per individual cell in *Dermocarpella* is not greatly influenced by environmental factors. The relative constancy of the size of the ovoid parental cell at the onset of division restricts the number of baeocytes produced per reproductive cell; typically 60–120 baeocytes are formed.

Dermocarpella is unique among the pleurocapsalean cyanobacteria now in culture because of its intrinsic polarity. This polarity results from the asymmetric enlargement of the baeocyte to produce an ovoid vegetative cell and from the characteristic division plane of the first transverse fission. This polarity of development is not determined by the site of attachment of baeocytes to their substrates. Electron micrographs of thin sections of *Dermocarpella,* which had developed from baeocytes attached to a sheet of dialysis membrane deposited on the surface of an agar plate, show that the planes of elongation and division are completely unrelated to the plane of the underlying substrate (Waterbury and Stanier, 1978).

Taxonomic Comments on **Dermocarpa,** **Xenococcus** and **Dermocarpella**

Currently, there is disagreement and confusion within the botanical literature concerning the structural and developmental differences between the genera *Dermocarpa, Xenococcus* and *Dermocarpella.* This is due in part to the inherent difficulty of inferring developmental cycles from isolated observations on field material or mass cultures and is exacerbated by the practice of describing new taxa rather than amending existing ones to incorporate new or reinterpreted properties. In contrast, comparative studies of these three genera in pure culture have shown that each genus is characterized by a specific structure and pattern of development and constitutes a readily recognizable taxonomic entity, albeit with some modification of the original botanical definitions.

Dermocarpa as originally described by Crouan (1858) included unicellular forms possessing either spherical or pyriform cells in which the entire contents of the parental cell divided by multiple fission; vegetative division was lacking. *Xenococcus* as described by Thuret (1880) included forms composed of solitary spherical or irregularly shaped cells that following growth became clustered into cell aggregates, typically one cell

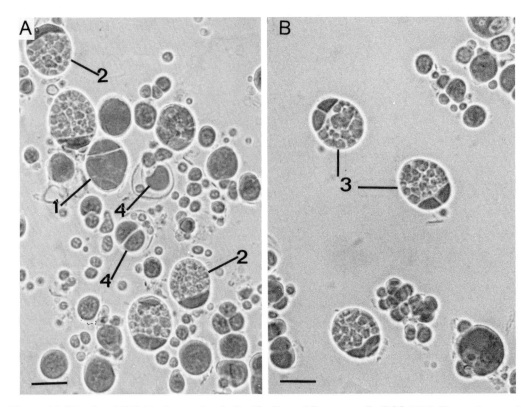

Figure 19.39. *A* and *B*, light micrographs of a liquid culture of *Dermocarpella* (PCC 7326). These micrographs show various division stages which cannot be resolved in Cooper dish culture: *1,* an individual which has just undergone binary transverse fission to form a small basal and a large apical cell; *2,* individuals containing a single basal cell and an apical cell which has completed multiple fission; *3,* individuals containing a pair of basal cells and an apical cell which has completed multiple fission; and *4,* individuals in which baeocytes have been released from the apical cell, revealing the outline of a parental fibrous outer wall layer which also encloses the basal cell or cells. *Bars,* 10 μm. (Reproduced with permission from J. B. Waterbury and R. Y. Stanier, Microbiological Reviews *42:* 2–44, 1978, ©American Society for Microbiology.)

layer in thickness. Two types of division were thought to be present in *Xenococcus:* (a) vegetative division (repeated binary fission), resulting in the formation of cell aggregates, and (b) multiple fission of some of the cells within the aggregate to form "endospores" (baeocytes). As a consequence of the presumed existence of two modes of division, *Xenococcus* has traditionally been placed with the cell aggregate-forming members of the *Pleurocapsales* (e.g. *Myxosarcina, Pleurocapsa, Hyella*). *Dermocarpella* as originally described by Lemmermann (1907) and verified by Ginsburg-André (1966) corresponds to the definition of Waterbury and Stanier (1978).

The confusion concerning these three genera in the botanical literature stems from the interpretation of the types of division that occur and the presence or absence of cell polarity. A reexamination of the type material of *Dermocarpa violacea* (Feldmann and Feldmann, 1953) showed what appeared to be cells undergoing vegetative division (binary fission). This observation, if correct, indicated that the type of *D. violacea* corresponded to and represented an earlier synonym for *Xenococcus* Thuret 1880. Bourrelly (1970) confirmed the observations by Feldmann and Feldmann and proposed that *Cyanocystis* Borzi 1882 be used to replace *Dermocarpa* and that *Dermocarpa* be used as an earlier synonym for *Xenococcus*. Komárek and Anagnostidis (1986) proposed an additional change, dividing *Cyanocystis* (sensu Bourrelly 1970) and reserving *Cyanocystis* for species displaying apical-basal polarity and placing species with spherical cells in a new genus *Stanieria*.

The situation is complicated further by the position of *Dermocarpella*. As originally described by Lemmermann (1907) and verified by Ginsburg-André (1966) and Waterbury and Stanier (1978), this genus consti-

tutes a readily recognizable taxonomic entity. However, Geitler (1932, 1942, 1967) doubted its validity and made it synonymous with *Dermocarpa* (sensu Crouan 1858). He argued that in nature, species of *Dermocarpa* were observed in which some individuals divided their entire cell contents by multiple fission, while in others, large segments of the parental cell did not undergo cleavage. This phenomenon has also been infrequently observed in cultured strains of *Dermocarpa* (Waterbury and Stanier, 1978), where it was interpreted as an error in division, since the undivided portion was never observed to retain viability. Geitler considered these division errors as normal properties of certain species and concluded that *Dermocarpella* merely represented the extreme of variability within *Dermocarpa*. Finally, Komárek and Anagnostidis (1986) place cyanobacteria with the developmental pattern of *Dermocarpella* (sensu Waterbury and Stanier 1978) in a new genus *Chamaecalyx* and reserve *Dermocarpella* for cyanobacteria with the same developmental pattern as *Cyanocystis* (sensu Komárek and Anagnostidis 1986) but distinguished from it by having the initial cleavages of multiple fission in one plane perpendicular to the plane of cell polarity (a division pattern which has never been observed in cultures).

Establishment of the structural and developmental characteristics defining these pleurocapsalean genera requires the resolution of the following problems:

1. Vegetative divisions in *Xenococcus* (sensu Thuret 1880; and subsequent Geitlerian literature)
2. Vegetative divisions in the type material of *Dermocarpa violacea* (Feldmann and Feldmann, 1953; Bourrelly, 1970)

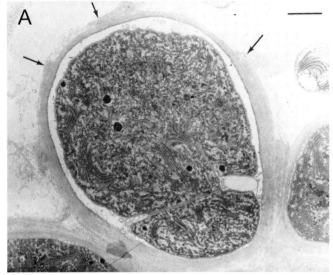

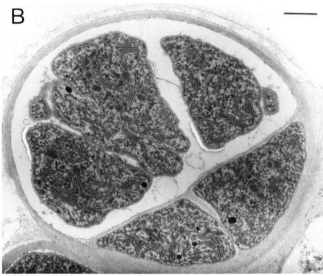

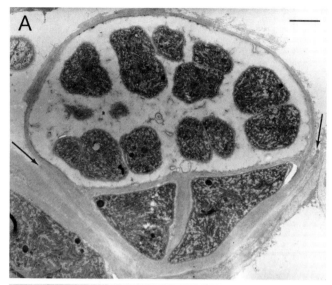

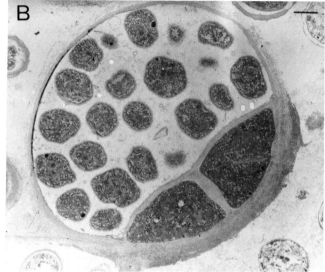

Figure 19.40. Electron micrographs of thin sections of *Dermocarpella* (PCC 7326) grown on agar plates. *A*, an individual which has just completed the binary fission which separates the apical cell from the basal cell. *B*, an individual which has undergone a second binary fission to form two basal cells. The apical cell has begun to undergo multiple fission, producing cleavage products which are initially not of equal size. The basal cells have begun to synthesize new fibrous outer wall layer material over their entire surfaces, but no new synthesis of fibrous outer wall layer material has occurred around the dividing cells of the apical portion. *Bar*, 1.0 μm. (Reproduced with permission from J. B. Waterbury and R. Y. Stanier, Microbiological Reviews *42*: 2-44, 1978, ©American Society for Microbiology.)

Figure 19.41. Electron micrographs of thin sections of *Dermocarpella* (PCC 7326) from the same preparation as the cells illustrated in Figure 19.40. *A*, an individual nearing completion of multiple fission. The fibrous outer wall layer surrounding the basal cells is markedly thicker than in the earlier developmental stage shown in Figure 19.40. No fibrous outer wall layer material surrounds the cleavage products in the apical cell. *B*, an individual which has completed multiple fission and is filled with baeocytes. *Bars*, 1.0 μm. (Reproduced with permission from J. B. Waterbury and R. Y. Stanier, Microbiological Reviews *42*: 2-44, 1978, ©American Society for Microbiology.)

3. Incomplete division in *Dermocarpa* (Geitlerian literature; Komárek and Anagnostidis, 1986)

4. Polarity in *Dermocarpa* (Geitlerian literature; Komárek and Anagnostidis, 1986)

5. Polarity in *Dermocarpella* (Komárek and Anagnostidis, 1986)

1. Vegetative Divisions in *Xenococcus*. The definitions and illustrations of members of the genus *Xenococcus* (sensu Thuret 1880) found in the Geitlerian literature show the presence of "vegetative division." Mass cultures of axenic strains of *Xenococcus* also contain cells that ap-

pear to be dividing vegetatively (Fig. 19.36*B*) but which are, in fact, in the process of multiple fission. The cleavage process of multiple fission is readily visible by light microscopy because of the synthesis of the fibrous outer cell wall layer during multiple fission. These observations led Waterbury and Stanier (1978) to emend the definition of *Xenococcus* to: unicellular forms dividing exclusively by multiple fission, resulting in the production of nonmotile baeocytes.

2. Vegetative Divisions in Type Material of *D. violacea*. The problem of the type material of *D. violacea* apparently containing cells undergoing vegetative division (Feldmann and Feldmann, 1953; Bourrelly, 1970) can be explained by analogy with *Xenococcus*. During multiple fission the individual cleavage products are not normally visible by light microscopy in pure cultures of *Dermocarpa* (Fig. 19.36*A*), which is consistent with the original description of Crouan (1858). However, it is quite possible that the division stages now visible in the type material are the result of dehydration and subsequent rehydration of the 100-year-old type specimen. Instead of the fibrous outer wall material being intercalated between the individual cleavage products, spaces left by incomplete rehydration might have caused the individual cleavage stages to be visible in the type material. Waterbury and Stanier (1978) chose to define *Dermocarpa* according to the original description rather than to accept the analyses of the reexamined type material.

3. Incomplete Division in *Dermocarpa*. As previously described, the incomplete division of *Dermocarpa* observed in some natural specimens by Geitler (1932, 1942, 1967) has also been observed in culture. Waterbury and Stanier (1978) interpreted these as division errors rather than as a regular feature of development, since the resulting uncleaved portion of the parental cells were observed to be nonviable.

4. Polarity in *Dermocarpa*. The possession of apical-basal polarity

has been a consistent feature of the Geitlerian definition of *Dermocarpa*. Illustrations of many of the botanically described species made from observations of natural material show clumps of pyriform cells. By contrast, all of the cultured strains of *Dermocarpa* and *Xenococcus* are intrinsically spherical throughout their development (Figs. 19.36, *A* and *B*, 19.37 and 19.38). However, the shape of the parental cell in *Dermocarpa* can be markedly modified when many baeocytes attach to a common substrate in close proximity to one another. Subsequent development under crowded conditions results in the formation of pyriform or clavate-shaped parental cells (Fig. 19.36*C*). Thus polarity in *Dermocarpa* appears to be an environmentally induced trait, not an inherent developmental feature.

5. Polarity in *Dermocarpella*. In contrast to *Dermocarpa* and *Xenococcus*, *Dermocarpella* possesses an intrinsic polarity expressed by the asymmetric enlargement of the vegetative cell, by its subsequent asymmetric division and by the different fate of the cells produced (Figs. 19.39–19.41).

Differentiation of the species of the genera **Dermocarpa, Xenococcus** and **Dermocarpella** in pure culture

The properties of the strains of *Dermocarpa*, *Xenococcus* and *Dermocarpella* from the Pasteur Culture Collection (PCC) are shown in Table 19.9.

Dermocarpa strain PCC 7301 is of marine origin and closely resembles the botanical type species in developmental characteristics, size, pigmentation and source and could be assigned to *D. violacea* and designated the holotype of the type species. Strains PCC 7302 and PCC 7303 are also marine but distinct from PCC 7301. They were isolated from the same locality, closely resemble one another, and should probably be assigned to a new species. Strains PCC 7437 and PCC 7438 are freshwater

isolates described as *Stanieria cyanosphaera* by Komárek and Anagnostidis (1986) but here placed in *D. cyanosphaera*.

Xenococcus strains PCC 7305, PCC 7306 and PCC 7307 are each distinct. They have not been assigned to species because of the lack of sufficient strains to set species boundaries and because of the difficulty of correlating the properties of the strains in pure culture with existing botanical descriptions.

Dermocarpella is represented by a single strain (PCC 7326). Of the botanically described species, it most closely resembles the types species *D. incrassata*.

4. Genus IV. **Myxosarcina** Printz 1921, emend. Waterbury and Stanier 1978

Myx.o.sar'ci.na. Gr. fem. n. *myxa* slime, mucus; L. n. *sarcina* bundle or packet; M.L. fem. n. *Myxosarcina* slime bundle, or packet of cells in slime.

Cyanobacteria that undergo repeated binary fission in three planes to form more or less cubical aggregates of cells. Multiple fission occurs simultaneously in most cells of the aggregate and is followed by the massive release of motile baeocytes. The baeocyte initiates growth by enlarging symmetrically into a spherical vegetative cell that, just prior to the onset of binary fission, **attains a size that is characteristic and constant for any given strain.**

Type species (Botanical Code): *Myxosarcina concinna* Printz 1921.

Reference strain: PCC 7312 (ATCC 29377), isolated from snail shell, intertidal marine, Puerto Penasco, Mexico, 1971, by J. B. Waterbury.

5. Genus V. **Chroococcidiopsis** Geitler 1933, emend. Waterbury and Stanier 1978

Chro.o.coc'ci.di.op'sis. Gr. fem. n. *chroa* skin; Gr. n. *kokkidios* presumed diminutive of *kokkos* small seed or grain; Gr. fem. n. *opsis* appearance; M.L. fem. n. *Chroococcidiopsis* small cells appearing in skin or coating.

Cyanobacteria that undergo repeated binary fission in three planes to produce more or less regular cubical cell aggregates. Multiple fission occurs simultaneously in most cells of the aggregate and is followed by the massive release of nonmotile baeocytes. The baeocyte initiates growth by enlarging symmetrically into a spherical vegetative cell that, just before the onset of binary fission, attains a size that is characteristic and constant for any given strain.

Type species (Botanical Code): *Chroococcidiopsis thermalis* Geitler 1933.

Reference strain: PCC 7203 (ATCC 27900, CCAP 1451/1), isolated from soil sample near Greifswald, DDR, 1962 (Komárek, 1972).

Further Descriptive Information on **Myxosarcina** *and* **Chroococcidiopsis**

The developmental patterns of these two genera are similar, differing only in the pattern of synthesis of the fibrous outer cell wall layer during

multiple fission. The baeocytes of *Myxosarcina* do not possess a fibrous outer wall layer at the time of their release and, as a consequence, are motile, whereas the baeocytes of *Chroococcidiopsis* are surrounded by a thin fibrous outer cell wall layer at the time of their release and are nonmotile.

Photomicrographs of mass cultures of these two genera are very similar; typically they show cubical or somewhat irregularly shaped cell aggregates that vary considerably in size (Figs. 19.42 and 19.43). Binary fission resulting in the production of large cell aggregates plays a dominant role in the developmental patterns of *Myxosarcina* and *Chroococcidiopsis*, whereas binary fission is lacking or plays a minor role in the developmental patterns of *Dermocarpa*, *Xenococcus* and *Dermocarpella*.

The developmental patterns of *Myxosarcina* and *Chroococcidiopsis*, examined at the level of resolution of Cooper dish cultures, are virtually indistinguishable. A marine strain (PCC 7312) of *Myxosarcina* is illustrated in Figure 19.44. The spherical baeocyte enlarges symmetrically into a vegetative cell that subsequently begins to divide by binary fission.

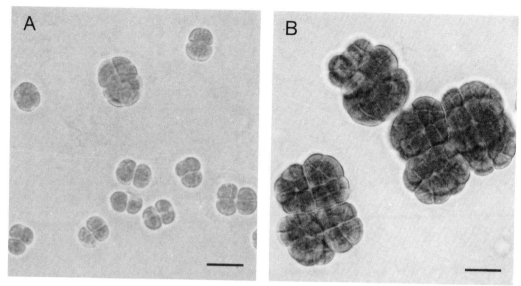

Figure 19.42. Light micrographs of *Myxosarcina* (PCC 7312) grown on an agar plate. *A*, young aggregates showing the uniformity of cell size and the regularity of the planes of successive divisions. *B*, older aggregates showing the maintenance of fairly regular cubical packets of cells. *Bars*, 10 μm. (Reproduced with permission from J. B. Waterbury and R. Y. Stanier, Microbiological Reviews *42*: 2–44, 1978, ©American Society for Microbiology.)

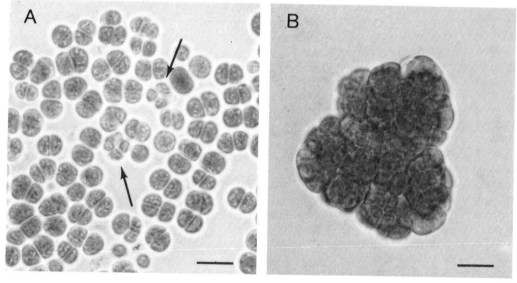

Figure 19.43. Light micrographs of mass cultures of *Chroococcidiopsis* grown on agar plates. *A*, dispersed cells from a crushed cell aggregate of strain PCC 6712, showing the regularity of cell size. Some of the cells (*arrows*) have undergone multiple fission, producing 4 baeocytes/parental cell. *B*, characteristic cell aggregates of strain PCC 7431. *Bars*, 10 μm. (Reproduced with permission from J. B. Waterbury and R. Y. Stanier, Microbiological Reviews *42*: 2–44, 1978, ©American Society for Microbiology.)

The sizes of the baeocytes and of the vegetative cells prior to the onset of binary fission are constant for a particular strain but may vary between strains (Table 19.10). Repeated binary fission occurs in three alternating planes at right angles to one another, to produce a large, approximately cubical cell aggregate. Multiple fission, when it occurs, is massive; almost all cells in the aggregate undergo cleavage simultaneously and release many baeocytes.

Baeocytes of *Chroococcidiopsis* are nonmotile, implying that synthesis of the fibrous outer cell wall layer occurs during the course of multiple fission. Because of their similarity in size, the distinction between baeocytes and vegetative cells, as revealed by either light or electron microscopy, is particularly difficult to make in this genus and rests entirely on the relatively small differences in cell size (Figs. 19.43 and 19.45). Electron micrographs of thin sections of *Chroococcidiopsis* aggregates are illustrated in Figure 19.45. Figure 19.45A is a section of a two-celled aggregate which Waterbury and Stanier (1978) interpreted as having just undergone binary fission. The individual cells are of approximately the same dimensions as the cells of this strain seen in Cooper dish cultures

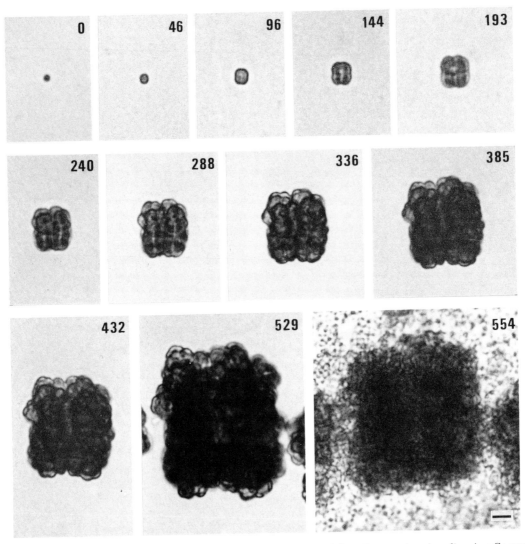

Figure 19.44. Development of a single baeocyte of *Myxosarcina* (PCC 7312) on a mineral medium in a Cooper dish culture. *Numbers* in the upper right-hand corner of each micrograph indicate hours following the initial observation. *Bar*, 10 µm. (Reproduced with permission from J. B. Waterbury and R. Y. Stanier, Microbiological Reviews *42:* 2–44, 1978, ©American Society for Microbiology.)

following the first binary fission. The cell aggregate in Figure 19.45*B* is similar in size to the two-celled aggregate in Figure 19.45*A* but contains many more cells. This was interpreted as a two-celled aggregate in which both cells were in the process of multiple fission. The cleavage products are individually surrounded by fibrous outer wall material, in accordance with the observation that free baeocytes in *Chroococcidiopsis* are never motile.

The baeocytes of *Myxosarcina* and *Chroococcidiopsis* do not differ markedly in size from their vegetative cells, which indicates that a rather small (and probably constant) number of baeocytes is produced from each vegetative cell following multiple fission. Although baeocyte counts are difficult to determine, the strains examined appear to produce 4 baeocytes/vegetative cell, except for one marine strain of *Myxosarcina* (PCC 7325) that produces between 8 and 16 baeocytes/vegetative cell.

Environmental factors influence the developmental patterns of *Myxosarcina* and *Chroococcidiopsis* by affecting the number of vegetative binary fissions that occur prior to the onset of multiple fission. Thus, the size of the cell aggregate rather than the number of baeocytes produced per vegetative cell is affected.

Taxonomic Comments on **Myxosarcina** *and* **Chroococcidiopsis**

Myxosarcina as defined here conforms well to botanical descriptions of the genus (Printz, 1921; Geitler, 1932; Desikachary, 1959; Bourrelly, 1970, 1985; Komárek and Anagnostidis, 1986).

The definition of *Chroococcidiopsis* also agrees well with current botanical descriptions (Komárek and Anagnostidis, 1986). However, earlier diagnoses of this genus, based both on observations of field material and on development inferred from mass cultures, incorporated many of the characteristic developmental stages of *Chroococcidiopsis* but were unclear about how these stages were linked together to form the complete developmental cycle (Geitler, 1933; Friedman, 1961; Komárek, 1972; Komárek and Hindak, 1975).

Myxosarcina and *Chroococcidiopsis* not only resemble one another but may also be confused with other cyanobacteria. Unicellular forms such as *Gloeocapsa* (sensu Rippka et al. 1979), which possess extracellular sheath layers and divide by binary fission in three planes, may produce cell aggregates that closely resemble the vegetative cell aggregates of *Myxosarcina* and *Chroococcidiopsis*.

Table 19.10.

Properties of strains of **Myxosarcina** *and* **Chroococcidiopsis**[a]

	Myxosarcina		Chroococcidiopsis							
Characteristic	*Myxosarcina* sp. PCC 7312 ATCC 29377	*Myxosarcina* sp. PCC 7325 ATCC 29378	*C. thermalis* PCC 7203 ATCC 27900	*C. thermalis* PCC 7431 ATCC 29379	*C. thermalis* PCC 7432 ATCC 29380	*C. thermalis* PCC 7433 ATCC 29381	*C. thermalis* PCC 7436 ATCC 29383	*C. thermalis* PCC 7439 ATCC 29384	*C. thermalis* PCC 7434 ATCC 29382	*Chroococcidiopsis* sp. PCC 6712 ATCC 27176
Morphology										
Baeocyte diameter (μm)	2	3	3	3	3	3	3	3	3	4
Diameter of cell at time of first vegetative division (μm)	5	8–10	5	5	5	5	5	5	5	6.3
Probable number of baeocytes produced per vegetative cell	4	>4	4	4	4	4	4	4	4	4
Facultative photoheterotrophy with										
Glucose	−	+	+	+	+	+	+	+		+
Fructose	−	−	+	+	+	+	+	+	+	+
Sucrose	+	+	+	+	+	+	+	+	+	+
Nitrogenase: synthesis in anaerobiosis	+	−	+	+	+	+	+	+	+	+
Pigment system										
Synthesis of										
PEC	−	+	+	+	+	+	+	+	−	−
X-PE	+	−	−	−	−	−	−	−	−	+
Chromatic adaptation	+	+	−	−	−	−	−	−	−	+
Source[b]										
Freshwater	−	−	+	+	+	+	+	+	+	+
Marine[c]	+	+	−	−	−	−	−	−	−	−
Maximum temperature (°C) permitting growth	39	35	ND	44	44	40	40	40	40	39
Mol% G + C of DNA (T_m)	44.0	42.7	45.8	45.9	45.9	46.4	46.4	46.3	45.8	40.2

[a]Symbols and abbreviations: −, negative; +, positive; PCC, Pasteur Culture Collection; ATCC, American Type Culture Collection; PEC, phycoerythrocyanin; X-PE, phycoerythrin containing both phycoerythrobilin and phycourobilin; and ND, not determined.

[b]See Rippka et al. (1979) for details of isolation and strain histories.

[c]Requires elevated concentrations of Na^+, Cl^-, Ca^{2+}, and Mg^{2+} for growth.

A more complex situation also occurs in which growth conditions in the laboratory and presumably also in nature can lead to instances in which developmental features are not recognized, are not completely expressed, or are severely altered. The following two examples are furnished to illustrate these points.

Strain PCC 6712, now recognized as a *Chroococcidiopsis*, was for many years thought to divide solely by binary fission and was consequently placed in the *Chroococcales* (Stanier et al., 1971). Its ability to reproduce by multiple fission was not recognized until its development was fol-

lowed in Cooper dish cultures (Waterbury and Stanier, 1978).

The developmental cycle of strain PCC 7322, a member of the *Pleurocapsa*-group, can be dramatically altered by growth conditions. When it is grown photoautotrophically, it develops into cell aggregates that have pseudofilamentous appendages (Fig. 19.46A), whereas when it is grown photoheterotrophically with sucrose, it produces cubical cell aggregates (Fig. 19.46B) that cannot be distinguished from those of *Myxosarcina* and *Chroococcidiopsis*.

Differentiation of the species of the genera **Myxosarcina** *and* **Chroococcidiopsis** *in pure culture*

Myxosarcina and *Chroococcidiopsis* are now distinguished from one another by the presence or absence of baeocyte motility. This feature of their development was not incorporated into earlier botanical diagnoses of the genera; consequently, the assignment of cultured strains to botanically described species is somewhat arbitrary.

The properties of the strains of *Myxosarcina* and *Chroococcidiopsis* from the Pasteur Culture Collection are shown in Table 19.10. The two

strains of *Myxosarcina* (PCC 7312 and PCC 7325) are marine isolates that have elevated salt requirements for growth, a property that distinguishes them from species described in the botanical literature. They also differ sufficiently from each other, both morphologically and physiologically, to be assigned to separate new species. The botanical type species, *M. concinna*, closely resembles strain PCC 7312 morphologically but is of terrestrial origin. It would presumably, therefore, not have elevated salt requirements for growth, indicating that the marine strain PCC 7312 should not be assigned to the botanical type species.

The strains of *Chroococcidiopsis* from the Pasteur Culture Collection fall into two groups. Seven strains (PCC 7203, PCC 7431, PCC 7432, PCC 7433, PCC 7434, PCC 7436 and PCC 7439) show a high degree of internal homogeneity in structural, developmental and physiological properties (Table 19.10). These same seven strains, when analyzed morphologically in bacterized batch cultures, were assigned to three species: strains PCC 7203, PCC 7431, PCC 7432 and PCC 7433 were assigned to *C. thermalis;* strains PCC 7434 and PCC 7436, to *C. cubana;* and strain PCC 7439, to *C. doonensis* (Komárek and Hindak, 1975). However, the high degree of similarity between the seven strains when characterized in pure culture indicates that they should be placed in a single species. On the basis of morphology and development they could be assigned to the botanical type species, *C. thermalis,* with strain PCC 7203 (ATCC 27900) becoming the holotype of the type species.

Strain PCC 6712 differs from the seven strains assigned to *C. thermalis* and should be placed in another species.

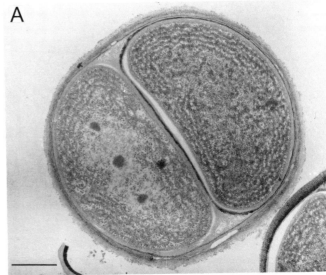

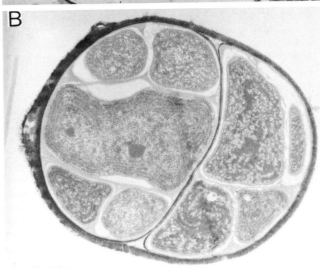

Figure 19.45. Electron micrographs of thin sections of *Chroococcidiopsis* (PCC 7436) grown on an agar plate. *A,* two vegetative cells produced by binary fission. *B,* a pair of cells that have undergone multiple fission after one binary fission; note the small size of the cells and the thinness of their individual fibrous outer cell wall layers. *Bars,* 1 μm. (Reproduced with permission from J. B. Waterbury and R. Y. Stanier, Microbiological Reviews *42:* 2–44, 1978, ©American Society for Microbiology.)

6. Pleurocapsa-group *sensu Waterbury and Stanier 1978*

The *Pleurocapsa*-group is a provisional assemblage which can loosely be defined as cyanobacteria that undergo repeated binary fissions in many different planes to produce cell aggregates that are diverse in size and form. They range from small, compact masses of cells to complex structures consisting of a central mass of cells from which radiate more or less extensive pseudofilamentous appendages. Multiple fission occurs in some cells of the aggregate and is followed by the release of motile baeocytes. The group can be split into two distinct subgroups by their mode of baeocyte enlargement. In subgroup I, the baeocyte enlarges symmetrically into a spherical vegetative cell before the onset of binary fission. In subgroup II, the baeocyte enlarges asymmetrically into an elongated vegetative cell before the onset of binary fission.

Reference strains: subgroup I—PCC 7319 (ATCC 29388), isolated from a snail shell, intertidal marine, Puerto Penasco, Mexico, 1971, by J. B. Waterbury; and subgroup II—PCC 7516 (ATCC 29396), isolated from a rock chip, marine intertidal zone, l'Ile Riou, Marseille, France, 1974, by T. Le Campion-Alsumard.

Further Descriptive Information on **Pleurocapsa-group**

The cyanobacteria placed in the *Pleurocapsa*-group by Waterbury and Stanier (1978) are an internally diverse strain cluster (Table 19.11). The primary characteristic that distinguishes members of this group from *Myxosarcina* is the irregularity of successive planes of binary fission, even early in vegetative growth. The diversity of cell aggregate size and arrangement is illustrated by light micrographs of mass cultures of representative strains (Figs. 19.47–19.49).

The two modes of baeocyte enlargement are illustrated in Figures 19.49 and 19.50. Figure 19.50 shows the development of strain PCC 7319 in a Cooper dish culture. The baeocyte initially enlarges symmetrically, then divides in many irregular planes to produce a complex cell aggregate with prominent pseudofilamentous appendages. Multiple fission then occurs in some of the cells in the aggregate, resulting in the release of motile baeocytes. Characteristic growth stages of a strain belonging to subgroup II (PCC 7516) are shown in Figures 19.49 and 19.6. The baeocyte

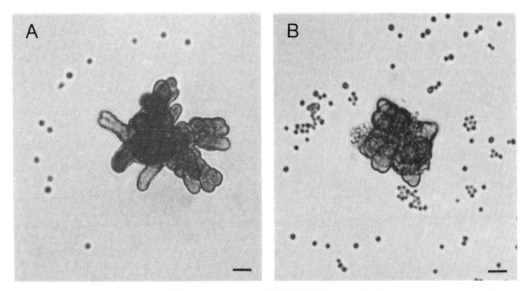

Figure 19.46. Cell aggregates of *Pleurocapsa*-group (PCC 7322). Some cells in the aggregate have undergone multiple fission and released baeocytes. Grown in the light, on an agar plate in mineral medium (*A*) and on an agar plate in a mineral medium supplemented with sucrose (*B*). *Bars*, 10 μm. (Reproduced with permission from J. B. Waterbury. 1979. *In* Parish (Editor), Developmental Biology of Prokaryotes, Vol. 1: Studies in Microbiology. ©Blackwell Scientific Publications, Palo Alto.)

Table 19.11.

Properties of strains of the **Pleurocapsa-group**[a]

Characteristic	Subgroup I					Subgroup II		
	PCC 7317 ATCC 29387	PCC 7320 ATCC 29389	PCC 7322 ATCC 29391	PCC 7319 ATCC 29388	PCC 7324 ATCC 29392	PCC 7314 ATCC 29386	PCC 7321 ATCC 29390	PCC 7516 ATCC 29396
Morphology								
Enlargement of baeocyte								
Symmetric	+	+	+	+	+			
Asymmetric						+	+	+
Baeocyte diameter (μm)	2–2.5	2	2–3	2.5	3	2.5–3	2.5–3	2.5–3
Diameter of cell at onset of vegetative division (μm)	5–7	6	6–8	6–8	5	NA	NA	NA
Formation of filamentous appendages	−	+	+	+	Rarely	+	+	+
Diameter of filamentous appendages (μm)	NA	6–7	6–10	6–10	NA	6–10	5–8	6–10
Probable number of baeocytes produced per vegetative cell	ND	30	16	14–32	4	8–16	ND	8
Faculative photoheterotrophy with								
Glucose	+	+	+	−	−	−	−	−
Fructose	−	+	+	+	−	+	−	−
Sucrose	−	+	+	+	−	+	+	+
Nitrogenase: synthesis in anaerobiosis	−	+	+	−	+	+	+	+
Pigment system								
Synthesis of								
C-PE	+	−	+	−	+	+	−	+
X-PE	−	+	−	+	−	−	+	−
Chromatic adaptation	−	+	+	+	−	+	−	ND
Maximum temperature (°C) permitting growth	30	39	37	39	39	37	37	ND
Mol% G + C of DNA (T_m)	45.4	43.0	43.0	43.2	43.3	43.3	43.0	ND

[a]Symbols and abbreviations: +, positive; −, negative; PCC, Pasteur Culture Collection; ATCC, American Type Culture Collection; NA, not applicable; ND, not determined; C-PE, c-phycoerythrin; and X-PE, phycoerythrin containing both phycoerythrobilin and phycourobilin.

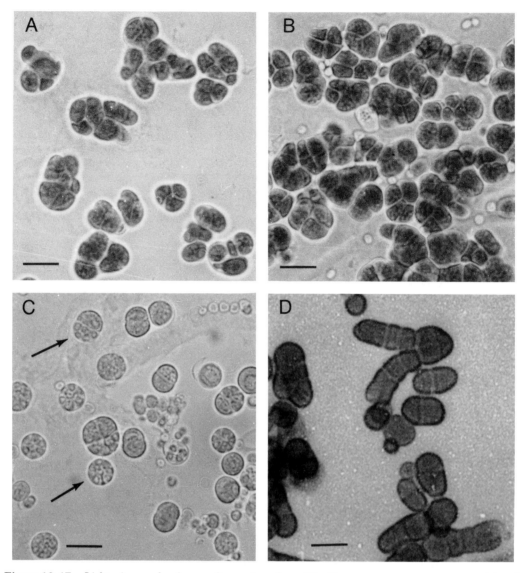

Figure 19.47.   Light micrographs of mass cultures of members of the *Pleurocapsa*-group grown on agar plates. *A* and *B*, small cell aggregates of strain PCC 7317. *C*, strain PCC 7320 showing cells (*arrows*) that have undergone multiple fission at the one- or two-celled stage. *D*, small branched cell aggregates typical of strain PCC 7320. *Bars*, 10 μm. (*A* is reproduced with permission from J. B. Waterbury and R. Y. Stanier, Microbiological Reviews *42:* 2–44, 1978, ©American Society for Microbiology.)

elongates and enlarges asymmetrically before the onset of binary fission (Fig. 19.49, *A* and *B*). Binary fission in irregular planes results in a cell aggregate with pseudofilamentous appendages. Aggregate formation is followed by multiple fission of some of the vegetative cells to form motile baeocytes (Fig. 19.49*D*).

Environmental factors affect the developmental patterns of strains belonging to the *Pleurocapsa*-group in two ways. As in *Myxosarcina* and *Chroococcidiopsis,* the number of binary fissions that precede the onset of multiple fission is not fixed. Multiple fission occurs earlier under favorable growth conditions. Indeed, some strains that normally produce pseudofilamentous appendages may undergo multiple fission after only one or two binary fissions (Fig. 19.47, *C* and *D*).

In contrast to *Myxosarcina* and *Chroococcidiopsis,* the planes of successive binary fission that determine the three-dimensional configuration of vegetative cell aggregates may be altered by environmental factors in most strains of the *Pleurocapsa*-group. As a result, the range of mor-

phological and developmental variation within individual strains of this group can be extensive, as illustrated by the following examples.

The differences in developmental expression caused by growth under photoautotrophic and photoheterotrophic conditions have been illustrated for strain PCC 7322 (Fig. 19.46). Under photoheterotrophic conditions cubical cell aggregates that can be confused with those of *Myxosarcina* are produced (Fig. 19.46*B*), whereas under photoautotrophic conditions cell aggregates with pseudofilamentous appendages are produced (Fig. 19.46*A*) (Waterbury, 1979).

In strain PCC 7319, the addition of sucrose to the growth medium does not change the gross structure of the aggregate. Instead, the pseudofilamentous outgrowths, which are uniserate at their tips when grown photoautotrophically, become multiserate throughout their entire length when grown photoheterotrophically (Fig. 19.48, *A* and *B*) (Waterbury, 1979).

Strain PCC 7324, like the other strains of subgroup I, is characterized

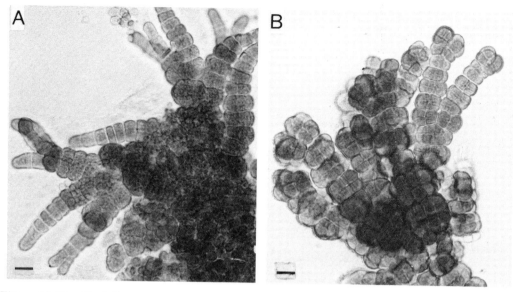

Figure 19.48. The influence of sucrose on the development of a member of the *Pleurocapsa*-group (PCC 7319). *A*, strain PCC 7319 grown on an agar plate in a mineral medium in the light; note the uniseriate, branched filaments. *B*, strain PCC 7319 grown on an agar plate in a mineral medium supplemented with 0.3% sucrose in the light; note the multiseriate structure of the filaments. *Bars*, 10 μm. (Reproduced with permission from J. B. Waterbury. 1979. *In* Parish (Editor), Developmental Biology of Prokaryotes, Vol. 1: Studies in Microbiology. ©Blackwell Scientific Publications, Palo Alto.)

by symmetrical baeocyte enlargement but is unusual in several other respects. Binary fission occurs predominantly in two planes, forming relatively flat cell aggregates which may reach considerable size before undergoing multiple fission (Fig. 19.51*D*). Nearly all the cells in the aggregate undergo multiple fission simultaneously, a property not possessed by any other strain which we have assigned to the *Pleurocapsa*-group. In liquid cultures of strain PCC 7324 that are several months old, some cells of the population become embedded in a mass of extracellular material which has the form of dichotomously branched threads with a diameter slightly less than that of the contained cells. The cells associated with this material are widely dispersed and are typically located at the apices of the threads (Fig. 19.51*E*). Such forms, present only in old and presumably senescent cultures of this strain, are striking because they display the principal diagnostic feature that distinguishes members of the subfamily *Solentioideae* (Komárek and Anagnostidis, 1986) from the three other subfamilies of the family *Hydrococcaceae* (Komárek and Anagnostidis, 1986), a family that encompasses the *Pleurocapsa*-group as defined here. Cells of strain PCC 7324, when growing under favorable conditions, occasionally become covered by an amorphous precipitate (Fig. 19.51*C*), giving them an appearance characteristic of natural populations of *Entophysalis,* a genus currently placed in the *Chroococcales* in the botanical literature.

Pleurocapsa and *Hyella,* two of the principle botanical genera that fall into the *Pleurocapsa*-group, are distinguished solely by their growth habits in natural environments. Members of *Pleurocapsa* are epiphytes or epiliths, whereas members of *Hyella* are endoliths that penetrate calcareous substrates. It is generally believed that the ability to penetrate calcareous substrates is an inherent property possessed by some cyanobacteria and that the mechanism of penetration, while not known, follows a pattern suggestive of chemical dissolution of the substrate (Golubic, 1973).

The eight marine strains of the *Pleurocapsa*-group (Table 19.11) were all isolated from mollusk shells or rock chips and could, in principle, have been either epiliths or endoliths. Except for PCC 7516, observed to be endolithic in its natural habitat, the relations of these strains to their natural substrates were not determined at the time of their isolation.

Following purification, several of these strains (PCC 7314, PCC 7319, PCC 7321, PCC 7322 and PCC 7324) were grown on oyster shell chips that were transferred frequently in a liquid growth medium for a period of 2 years. All grew profusely on the surface of the oyster shell chips, but none penetrated the surface, indicating that all five strains were epiliths. A similar experiment performed with strain PCC 7506 prior to purification showed definite penetration of the oyster shell chips after 4 months, suggesting that penetration of calcareous substrates might depend on the activity of associated acid-producing bacteria. This hypothesis was tested by isolating acid-producing, aerobic, chemoheterotrophic bacteria from the impure culture of strain PCC 7506. One of the strongest acid-producing bacterial isolates was grown with strains of the *Pleurocapsa*-group (PCC 7440 and PCC 7516, with the latter known to be endolithic under natural growth conditions) in two-membered cultures on oyster shell chips in a mineral medium in the light. After 2 months, PCC 7440 and PCC 7516, when grown together with the acid-producing bacterium, penetrated the oyster shell chips, whereas the controls containing pure cultures of the cyanobacteria showed no penetration of the substrate (Fig. 19.52). This demonstration indicates that associated chemoheterotrophic bacteria can play a role in facilitating the penetration of calcareous substrates by members of the *Pleurocapsa*-group. Additional studies will be required to determine whether the ability of cyanobacteria to grow endolithically always requires the presence of chemoheterotrophic bacteria or whether growth conditions can be established that will permit the cyanobacteria to penetrate calcareous substrates by themselves. However, the effects of chemoheterotrophic bacteria on the expression of the endolithic habit by cyanobacteria, whether obligate or facultative, limits the utility of endolithy as a major taxonomic character for the differentiation of genera within the *Pleurocapsa*-group.

Taxonomic Comments on **Pleurocapsa-group**

Cyanobacteria that display the general developmental features described for the *Pleurocapsa*-group are placed in a variety of genera in the botanical literature, including: *Pleurocapsa, Hyella, Myxohyella, Radaisia, Radaisiella, Solentia, Hormathonema* and *Cyanostylon.* The dis-

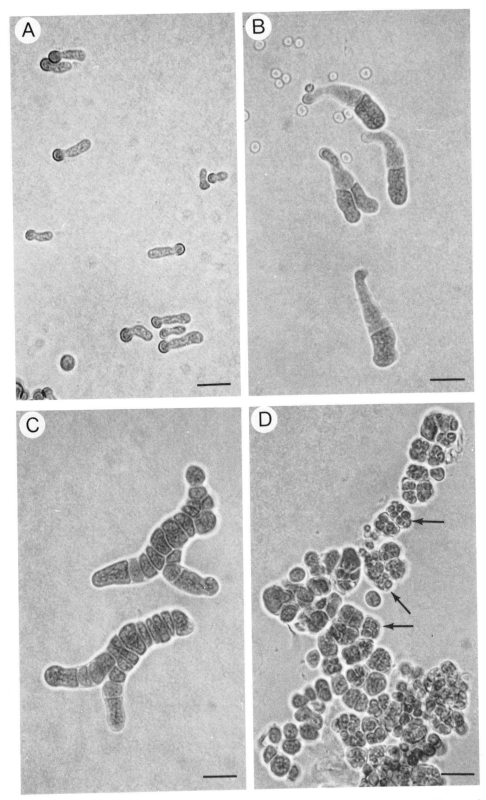

Figure 19.49.   Light micrographs of wet mounts of *Pleurocapsa*-group strain PCC 7516 prepared by sampling an agar plate culture at various intervals after inoculation. *A*, initial outgrowth of baeocytes. *B*, asymmetric enlargement and initial vegetative divisions in young aggregates. *C*, pseudofilamentous cell aggregate. *D*, large cell aggregate containing cells that have undergone multiple fission and are filled with baeocytes. *Bars*, 10 μm.

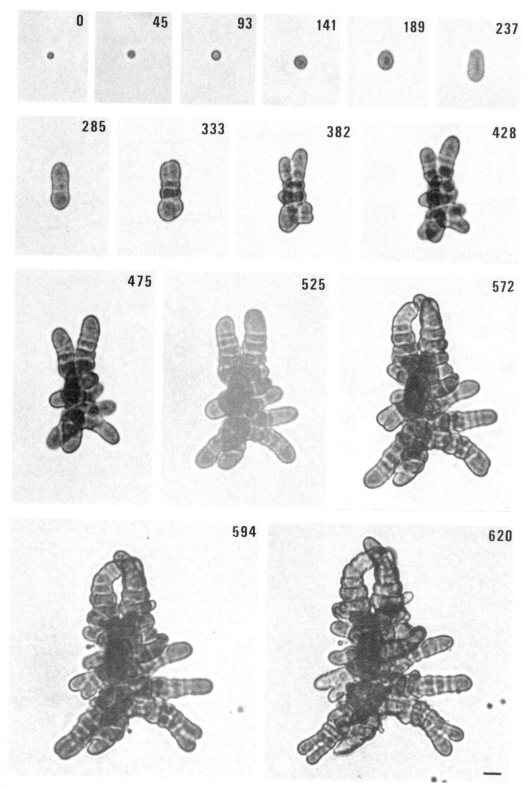

Figure 19.50. Development of a member of subgroup I (PCC 7319) of the *Pleurocapsa*-group in a Cooper dish culture. *Numbers* in the upper right-hand corner of each micrograph indicate hours following the initial observation. *Bar*, 10 μm. (Reproduced with permission from J. B. Waterbury and R. Y. Stanier, Microbiological Reviews *42:* 2–44, 1978, ©American Society for Microbiology.)

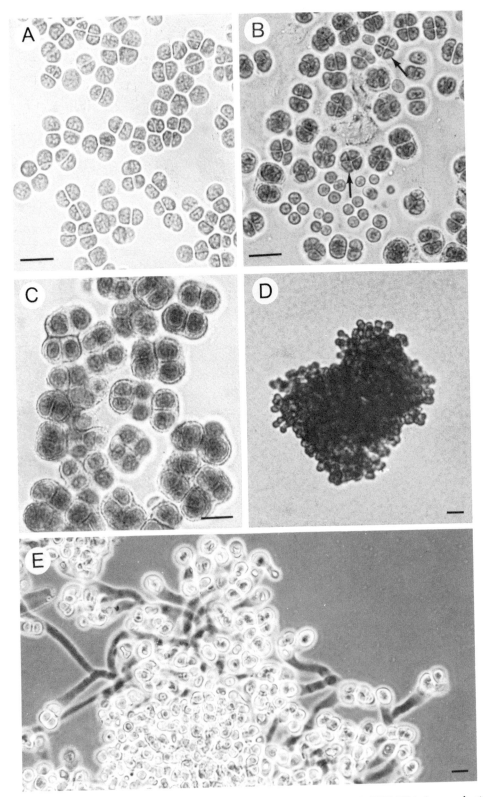

Figure 19.51. Light micrographs of mass cultures of *Pleurocapsa*-group strain PCC 7324. *A*, an early stage of vegetative growth from an agar plate culture. *B*, a later stage of development from an agar plate culture showing aggregates, some of which have undergone multiple fission and contain baeocytes (*arrows*). *C*, cell aggregates from a liquid culture showing groups of cells covered with an amorphous precipitate. *D*, a large aggregate on an agar plate. *E*, a phase-contrast micrograph of a 2-month-old liquid culture, showing threads of extracellular material in which isolated clumps of cells are embedded. *Bars*, 10 μm.

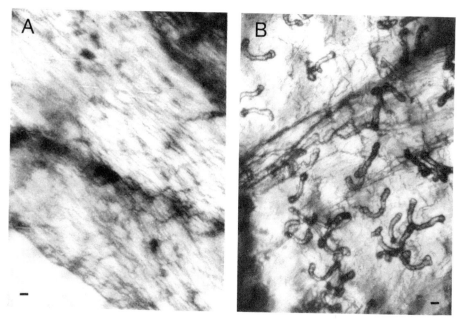

Figure 19.52. Light micrographs of *Pleurocapsa*-group strain PCC 7440 growing on fragments of oyster shell immersed in a mineral medium and incubated in the light. Prior to photography, the oyster shells were scraped to remove the surface growth. *A,* appearance of the oyster shell chip after incubation for 2 months with the pure culture of the cyanobacterium. Penetration of the substrate did not occur. *B,* appearance of the oyster shell after incubation for 2 months with both an acid-producing chemoheterotrophic bacterium and the cyanobacterium. Penetration of the oyster shell chip by the two-membered culture is clearly evident. *Bars,* 10 μm.

tinctions between these genera are made on the basis either of characteristics not easily determinable with cultures or of characteristics that appear not to be inherent properties of the cyanobacteria themselves but of ramifications of the interaction of the cyanobacteria with their environment, both physical and biological. It was therefore concluded by Waterbury and Stanier (1978) that the characterization of this group was insufficient to permit even generic boundaries to be established for the strains in pure culture. A resolution of the problem of setting generic and species boundaries in this heterogeneous group will require the direct isolation, purification and characterization of strains from field specimens that have been well characterized by using the botanical (Geitlerian) system of classification.

Schematic Representation of Pleurocapsalean Developmental Cycles

Figure 19.53 presents a schematic summary of the similarities and differences among the seven developmental groups established within the *Pleurocapsales* through the study of pure cultures.

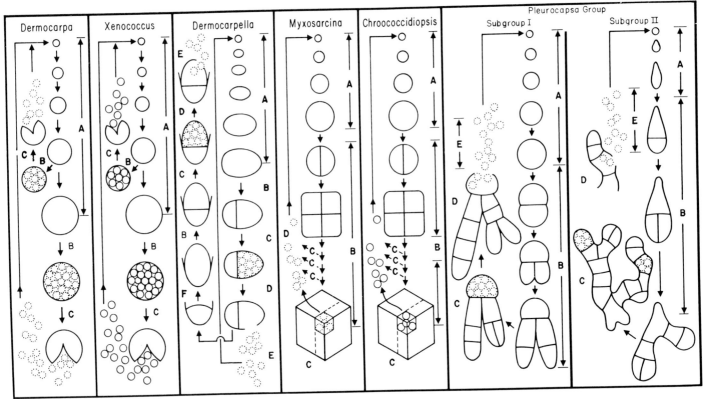

Figure 19.53. Diagrammatic comparison of pleurocapsalean developmental cycles. *Dotted circle,* baeocytes that are not surrounded by a fibrous outer cell wall layer at the time of release and are consequently motile; *solid circles,* baeocytes that are surrounded by a fibrous outer cell wall layer; *A–F,* developmental stages defined below. (Reproduced with permission from J. B. Waterbury and R. Y. Stanier, Microbiological Reviews *42:* 2–44, 1978, ©American Society for Microbiology.)

Genus	Developmental stage					
	A	B	C	D	E	F
Dermocarpa and *Xenococcus*	Symmetric baeoctye enlargement	Multiple fission	Release of baeocytes[a]			
Dermocarpella	Asymmetric baeocyte enlargement	Binary fission	Multiple fission of apical cell	Baeocyte release	Baeocyte motility	Basal cell enlargement
Myxosarcina and *Chroococcidiopsis*	Symmetric baeocyte enlargement	Repeated binary fission in three planes	Multiple fission of nearly all cells, and baeocyte release	Baeocyte motility[b]		
Pleurocapsa subgroups I and II	Baeocyte enlargement[c]	Binary fission in many irregular planes	Multiple fission of some cells	Baeocyte release	Baeocyte motility	

[a]Baeocytes are motile in *Dermocarpa* and nonmotile in *Xenococcus.*
[b]*Myxosarcina* only; *Chroococcidiopsis* baeocytes are not motile.
[c]Symmetric in subgroup I; asymmetric in subgroup II.

SUBSECTION III. ORDER **OSCILLATORIALES**

R. W. Castenholz

Os.cil.la.to′ri.al′es. M.L. fem. n. *Oscillatoria* genus of order; -*ales* to denote an order; M.L. fem. pl. n. *Oscillatoriales* the *Oscillatoria* order.

Included are all **filamentous cyanobacteria that undergo binary fission in a single plane and** that **produce "vegetative" cells only. Heterocysts and akinetes do not occur. Trichome diameters** may range **from about 0.4 to** (rarely) well **over 100 μm.** The terminal cell of some species may be distinctly shaped but is apparently still capable of photosynthesis. **Sometimes the terminal cell is tapered** and with a cap or calyptra, but in a few forms **the taper may include several subterminal cells** as well. Generally within a strain the **trichome diameter varies little** (<10%) in contrast to some other orders of cyanobacteria. As a rule, all cells retain the ability to divide; in practice, certain portions of a trichome may be more active meristematically than terminal regions. The terminal cell in some strains may never divide. Trichomes may be flexible or semirigid. In some cases, the entire trichome is wound into a loose or tight spiral; in others, only terminal portions of the trichome may be openly spiraled.

An apparent **sheath may be present,** but even species without an easily visible sheath leave behind at least a very thin, gossamer sheath when moving by gliding. Those species that commonly produce a thickened (even laminated) sheath may move only slightly and occasionally within this confinement (Fig. 19.54). When short fragments of a few cells separate from the remainder of the trichome near the free, open end of a sheath, these free trichomes (i.e. terminal hormogonia) may glide out, eventually forming new sheaths. Although trichomes without apparent sheaths also fragment, a separable, migrating, hormogonial phase is difficult to distinguish, since all lengths of trichome are generally motile. **Gliding motility occurs on solid to semisolid substrates in all genera** known. Movement forward or backward may or may not be accompanied by a right- or left-handed rotation of the trichome. Fragmentation of trichomes occurs in some forms where a cell loses much of its contents and dies. In some cases, there appears to be an orderly sacrificial death of these cells (necridial cells) which determine the sites of trichome breakage (Lamont, 1969; Ciferri, 1983).

The range in **mol% G + C** of the DNA is large **(40–67)** (Herdman et al., 1979a). The range of genome sizes is also great (2.14–5.19 × 10⁹ daltons), but all sizes are generally less than those in the *Nostocales* or *Stigonematales* (Herdman et al., 1979b).

The range in DNA base composition and in genome size indicates a probable artificiality in the grouping *Oscillatoriales,* a conclusion further supported by the degree of disparity in some sequences of 800–900 con-

tinuous nucleotides of 16S rRNA from 11 strains of 7 genera of this grouping (Giovannoni et al., 1988). The triviality of some generic distinctions used here should also be emphasized. Often only one (but convenient) characteristic is used, a characteristic that may be the result of a slight difference in genetic code.

In the "Geitlerian" system, generic distinction in the *Oscillatoriales* is based primarily on the diversity of sheaths or their absence. Although still used as a characteristic in the present system, knowledge of physiology, biochemistry, and nucleotide base sequence homologies will eventually determine degrees of relatedness.

Members of the *Oscillatoriales* occur in an enormous diversity of habitats: freshwater and marine, both as plankton, mats, and periphyton. Terrestrial crusts, mats, and turfs are also common. Hot spring mats of some oscillatorian cyanobacteria develop up to temperatures of about 62°C (Castenholz, 1969). Intimate symbiotic relationships are rare in this family.

Taxonomic Comments

The *Oscillatoriales* is being used in a context similar to Geitler's usage of the family *Oscillatoriaceae* (Geitler, 1932), although Geitler included a number of additional genera. Drouet (1968) also defined this family in much the same way but reduced the 25 genera of Geitler to 6. Bourrelly (1970) recognized 11 genera and conceded that several others may be considered separable (Bourrelly, 1985). Also, the order has been extensively revised by Anagnostidis and Komárek (1988). Rippka et al. (1979) used three genera in this group (designated Subsection III). Several "Geitlerian" genera were excluded because distinctions were based on the consistency of the sheath (or slime), i.e. the "LPP group" (Rippka et al., 1979) which included *Lyngbya* Agardh 1824, *Phormidium* Kützing 1843 and *Plectonema* Thuret 1875. This characteristic was considered variable in culture. *Plectonema*, which exhibits occasional or regular false branching, was excluded from the *Oscillatoriaceae* by Geitler (1932); it was included by Drouet (1968) but was suppressed into other generic names. Drouet (1968) included many unicellular rod-shaped cyanobacteria that divide in one plane (e.g. *Synechococcus*) in the genus *Schizothrix* Kützing 1843, which is also a filamentous member of the *Oscillatoriaceae*.

Oscillatoria (sensu Castenholz) is somewhat broader than interpreted by Rippka et al. (1979, 1981b) and includes some of the "LPP group." *Oscillatoria* is no longer being restricted to trichomes with disk-shaped cells lacking constrictions at cross-walls. Thus, it is similar to the inclusive genus as seen by Geitler (1932). The genus *Lyngbya* is used for "LPP" strains that produce and retain readily visible persistent sheaths, even under a variety of culture conditions. The genus *Pseudanabaena* (sensu Castenholz) also incorporates some strains of the "LPP group."

A number of genera were described that included more than one trichome in a common, persistent sheath or mucilage (e.g. *Schizothrix* Kützing 1843, *Microcoleus* Desmazières 1823, *Sirocoleus* Kützing 1849, and *Hydrocoleum* Kützing 1843). In some cultures, the multiple groupings of the trichomes disappears, and the use of these names for cultures should wait for additional work. The fact that *Microcoleus chthonoplastes* (Mertens) Zandardini is a very distinctive and ubiquitous marine species speaks for the retention of this genus (Fig. 19.55). *Porphyrosisphon notarisii* Kützing 1849 is an extremely abundant tropical subaerial cyanobacterium. Although occasionally with >1 trichome/sheath, it is known primarily for a single trichome within a red to red-brown, laminated sheath. At this time, the characterization of this genus has not been based on cultures.

The genus *Isocystis* Borzi was included by Geitler (1932) in the *Oscillatoriales* and later was classified with the yeasts (Geitler, 1955, 1963). One species, *I. pallida*, has recently been isolated in axenic culture, recharac-

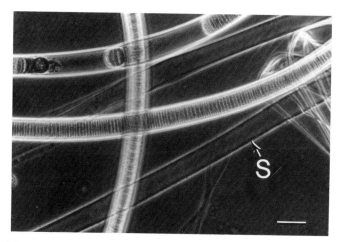

Figure 19.54. Photomicrograph (phase contrast) of *Lyngbya* cf. *aestuarii.* Culture University of Oregon WH-82-L. *S,* sheath. *Bar,* 20 μm.

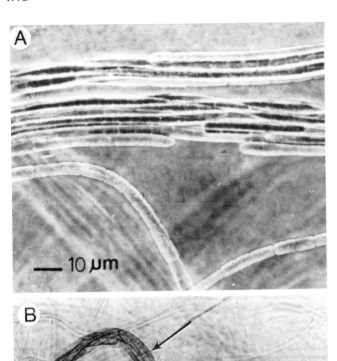

Figure 19.55. *A*, culture of *M. chthonoplastes* showing bundles of trichomes. (Reproduced with permission from B. J. Javor and R. W. Castenholz, Geomicrobiology Journal *2:* 237–273, 1981, ©Taylor & Francis). *B*, collection of *Microcoleus* cf. *chthonoplastes* from hypersaline microbial mat. Trichome bundle (*arrow*) within common sheath. *Bar*, 20 μm. Both *A* and *B* are from mats in Guerrero Negro lagoons, Baja, California, Mexico.

terized, and renamed *Isosphaera pallida* (Woronichin) Giovannoni et al. (1987); also Giovannoni and Castenholz (1988: this volume). It is an aerobic, chemoheterotrophic and nonphotosynthetic eubacterium. However, it is possible that some of the remaining species of the genus *Isocystis* are cyanobacteria.

Other genera that may be regarded as separable but that claim few or no axenic cultures at present are: *Borzia* Cohn 1882 (see Bicudo, 1985), *Palikiella* Claus 1962, and *Crinalium* Crow 1927 (see Bourrelly, 1985, for details).

The proposal by Guglielmi and Cohen-Bazire (1982b) to divide Subsection III into three tribes is based primarily on the type and arrangements of wall perforations and pores. Although pore criterion cannot be used for identification with a light microscope, it can certainly be applied to any serious work when cultures are available.

The tribe "*Oscillatoriae*" includes organisms in which only one circle of pores occurs in close proximity to the cross-wall (junctional pores). In the context of extant cultures available, this criterion encompasses strains called *Oscillatoria*, *Arthrospira*, and at least one member of the "LPP group." The tribe "*Spirulinae*" includes strains (genus *Spirulina*) in which pores are distributed as patches in the concave region of each turn in the spiral. The tribe "*Pseudanabaenae*" comprises many strains in which cross-wall constrictions are prominent and in which wide rings of pores are distibuted near cell poles (Guglielmi and Cohen-Bazire, 1982b). There still remain many strains, placed in the "LPP group" by Rippka et al. (1979), that cannot with confidence be given a generic name.

Again, it should be emphasized that all generic categories included or excluded here are provisional. In some cases, only a single known criterion is used to separate genera. Separation is particularly difficult and arbitrary when gradations exist. Some generic names, therefore, merely emphasize "pinnacles" in what appears to be a continuum of character changes.

Key to the order **Oscillatoriales** *(Subsection III)*

Subsection III includes some genera not fully characterized from cultures.

A. Trichomes cylindrical...C
A. Trichomes not cylindrical (flattened or triradiate in cross-section)...B
  B. Trichomes flattened, i.e. elliptical in cross-section
      Genus VII. *Crinalium*,* p. 1779
  B. Trichomes triradiate in cross-section
      Genus VI. *Starria*, p. 1779
  C. Trichomes straight or sinuous for portion of length...E
  C. Trichomes helically coiled (open or closed), usually for entire length..D
    D. Pitch of trichome helix is <45° (from transverse axis); cross-walls are thin and usually invisible with the light microscope; with the electron microscope, pores near cross-walls appear in semicircular patches on concave side of coil.
        Genus I. *Spirulina*, p. 1773
    D. Pitch of trichome helix is >45° (from transverse axis); cross-walls are visible with the light microscope; with the electron microscope, circular rows of junctional pores are visible near cross-walls.
        Genus II. *Arthrospira*, p. 1774

---

*Not characterized from axenic cultures.

E. Trichomes are usually immobile in a persistent sheath (hormogonia may, at times, migrate out from sheaths) ....F

E. Trichomes are usually motile; and there is no persistent sheath (trichomes when gliding may leave a nearly transparent, thin, sheathlike trail) ....G

F. Common sheath regularly harbors two or more trichomes (side by side or overlapping).
    Genus VIII. *Microcoleus*,* p. 1780

F. Single trichome per sheath; in some, the sheath may be confluent, resulting in a mat or a colonial structure.
    Genus IV. *Lyngbya* (incl. *Porphyrosiphon* and *Phormidium*), p. 1777

G. Constrictions are absent at cross-walls or are feeble, not exceeding ⅛ of trichome diameter.
    Genus III. *Oscillatoria* and *Trichodesmium** (also some of "LPP" group (Rippka et al., 1979)), p. 1775

G. Constrictions at cross-walls are strong to moderate, exceeding ⅛ of trichome diameter.
    Genus V. *Pseudanabaena* (also some of "LPP" group (Rippka et al., 1979)), p. 1778

Genus I. **Spirulina** *Turpin 1829*

Spi.ru.li′na. L. n. *spira* a coil; L. n. *linea* a line; M.L. fem. n. *Spirulina* coiled filament.

Filamentous organisms that divide exclusively by binary fission and in one plane but that **grow in the form of a** tight to nearly tight coiled right- or left-handed **helix. The cross-walls are thin** and are invisible or nearly so with light microscopy (Holmgren et al., 1971) (Fig. 19.56). Originally characterized as being a long unicellular thread. **No sheath is visible** under light microscopy, and "healthy" **trichomes are in constant motion.** Gliding motility consists of a "turning of the screw," thus with great transverse movement and little forward motion. The trichome does not truly rotate but moves along the outer surface of the helix. Free ends not in contact with substrate may oscillate wildly as the coil turns. The **terminus of the trichome is either blunt or pointed.** In different species the **width of the trichome may be from**

<1 μm to about 5 μm. In the latter case, the width of the tight helix may be as great as 12 μm. **Color is variable, blue-green to red;** some marine strains are extremely red, containing phycoerythrin as the major light-harvesting pigment. Variations in the tightness of the trichome helix occur in both *Spirulina* and *Arthrospira* (Jeeji-Bai and Seshadri, 1980; Lewin, 1980; Hindák, 1985). Several strains in culture have lost much of their coiled structure, so care needs to be taken when considering *Spirulina* in culture collections (Jeeji-Bai, 1985).

In four strains, Guglielmi and Cohen-Bazire (1982b) found patches of pores at cross-walls on only the inner concave surfaces of the helix (Fig. 19.57). This feature may become a good diagnostic feature of a natural taxonomic unit. In addition, Guglielmi and Cohen-Bazire (1982a) found

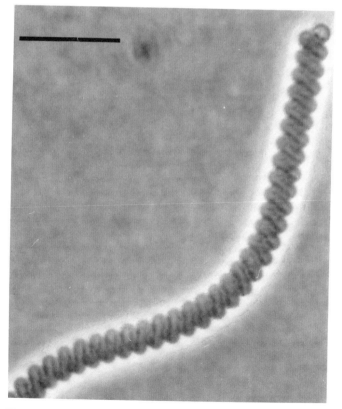

Figure 19.56. Photomicrograph (phase contrast) of *Spirulina* cf. *labyrinthiformis*, a moderately thermophilic strain isolated from Mammoth Springs, Yellowstone National Park, U.S.A. *Bar*, 10 μm. (Reproduced with permission from R. W. Castenholz, Microbial Ecology *3:* 79–105, 1977, ©Springer-Verlag.)

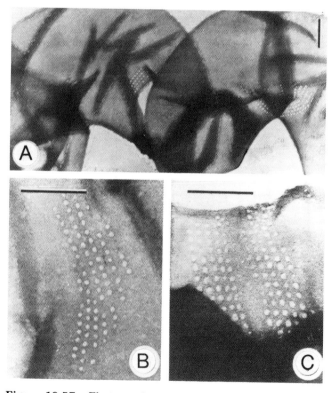

Figure 19.57. Electron micrograph of sacculus of *Spirulina* (PC 6313) treated with sulfuric acid. *A*, spiral envelope showing distribution pores. *B*, pores marking an incomplete transverse septum. *C*, pores disposed on both sides of a complete transverse septum. *Bar*, 200 nm. (Reproduced with permission from G. Guglielmi and G. Cohen-Bazire, Protistologica *18:* 151–165, 1982, ©Editions du CNRS.)

distinctive periodic tufts of fimbriae extending out from the walls of the one *Spirulina* strain examined.

The mol% G + C of the DNA of the reference strain (PCC 6313) is 54, and the genome size is 1.53×10^9 daltons (Herdman et al., 1979a, b).

The members of this genus have a known **worldwide distribution in freshwater, marine, and brackish waters.** Species are **also seen in inland saline lakes and in some hot springs at temperatures as high as 50°C** (Castenholz, 1977, 1978). They are commonly **tolerant of free sulfide** in many habitats. They are aquatic and uncommon in terrestrial habitats subjected to periodic drying. They are also unknown as intimate endosymbionts or exosymbionts.

Little is known of the physiology of *Spirulina* (excluding *Arthrospira* (*Spirulina*) *platensis* and related species). Strain PCC 6313 is a strict photoautotroph and is able to synthesize nitrogenase anaerobically. Some red (shade-adapted) marine strains require "oligotrophic" medium and grow very slowly (R. W. Castenholz, unpublished data). A thermophilic strain (cf. *S. labyrinthiformis*) is capable of sulfide-dependent anoxygenic photosynthesis (Castenholz, 1977).

The best isolation procedures involve self-isolation by gliding motility, but because of poor forward progress on agar, isolation on glass or plastic surfaces in liquid medium is often more successful (see Castenholz, 1981).

Reference strain: PCC 6313 (ATCC 29542), isolated from brackish water, Berkeley, California, 1963 (see Rippka et al., 1979).

Type species (Botanical Code): *Spirulina major* Kützing ex Gomont 1892 (lectotype).

Taxonomic Considerations

Spirulina has, in the opinions of various authors, included the genus *Arthrospira* (e.g. Geitler, 1932). Bourrelly (1970, 1985), considering that the degree of coiling showed a gradual transition from one extreme to the other, included both *Spirulina* and *Arthrospira* in *Oscillatoria*.

Spirulina (sensu Castenholz) has a continuous helical coil with thin (invisible) cross-walls and, possibly, a distinctive pore pattern. *Arthrospira* Stizenberger 1852 (e.g. *A. platensis*, PCC strain 7345) is a spirally arranged trichome in which cross-walls are clearly visible via light microscopy. The species of *Arthrospira* described on the basis of morphology have open coils. Some coils are so open that these organisms could easily be regarded as species of *Oscillatoria*, many of which are sinuous or with a very open helix near the terminus of the trichome. Since the strain of *Arthrospira* (PCC 7345) included by Rippka et al. (1979) in *Spirulina* has visible cross-walls, an open coil, a mol% G + C of the DNA (44%) unlike that of the *Spirulina* reference strain (54%), and a single row of junctional pores and fimbrial arrangements similar to the several strains of *Oscillatoria*, it and others like it are here regarded as *Arthrospira*. Rippka has subsequently agreed with this position (R. Rippka, personal communication). According to a tentative phyletic tree based on a sequence of 800–900 nucleotides of 16S rRNA, the reference strain of *Spirulina* falls in a cluster of Subsection I and II strains, quite distant from other filamentous cyanobacteria (Giovannoni et al., 1988).

To separate *Spirulina* from the other coiled *Oscillatoriales* on the basis of degree of visibility of cross-wall alone is not intended, but this characteristic may be correlated with the tightness of the coil and the unique pore patches.

Genus II. **Arthrospira** *Stizenberger 1852*

Ar.thro.spi′ra. Gr. n. *arthron* a joint; L. n. *spira* a coil; M.L. fem. n. *Arthrospira* jointed coil.

Filamentous organisms that divide exclusively by binary fission and in one plane. The entire **trichome is arranged as an open helix** in which **transverse walls may be seen** via light microscopy (Fig. 19.58). Cells are generally shorter than broad to quadrate but are occasionally elongate. Constrictions at cross-walls may be present or absent. A single circle of junctional pores occurs, and fimbriae are closely appressed along the trichome. **Persistent sheaths are not produced. Gliding motility** is evident **in most strains. Trichome widths vary from about 3 to 12 μm** in a variety of forms. The helix is an open spiral with diameters ranging from about 35 to 60 μm (Ciferri, 1983; Ciferri and Tiboni, 1985). On solid medium, the helix undergoes a transition to a "flat spiral." Considerable variation occurs in degree of helix pitch within some strains, and culture variants occur that are nearly straight (Jeeji-Bai, 1985).

The **mol% G + C of the DNA of the reference strain (PCC 7345) is 44.3** (Herdman et al., 1979a).

The physiology of some strains has been studied extensively (see Ciferri, 1983). PCC strain 7345 is a gas-vacuolate marine organism with 16-μm-wide trichomes (Rippka et al., 1979). It is an **obligate photoautotroph,** as are all other known strains, and it is unable to synthesize nitrogenase anaerobically. It contains c-phycocyanin, allophycocyanin, and c-phycoerythrin (C-PE). Many strains, however, also lack C-PE (Ciferri, 1983). PCC strain 7345 corresponds to *Arthrospira* (*Spirulina*) *maxima* Setchell and Gardner. Much attention has been paid to this and another species, *A.* (*Spirulina*) *platensis* (Nordst.) Gomont, as sources of human protein (Ciferri, 1983).

The "life cycle" of *Arthrospira* in laboratory culture involves the breaking up of trichomes at the sites of a necridium (lysing cell) at intervals of every 4–6 cells (Ciferri, 1983). The resulting short and uncoiled hormogonia form a migratory phase. Each hormogonium then undergoes cell division, growing into a new helical trichome.

This group with spirally formed trichomes and visible cross-walls, known interchangeably as *Spirulina* or *Arthrospira*, has been found in **marine, brackish water, and saline lake environments of tropical and semitropical regions.** Many culture isolates have been made for use in **aquaculture. Some forms are planktonic and gas-vacuolate, others are benthic and without gas vacuoles.** They often dominate the plankton of warm lakes high in carbonate and/or bicarbonate with pH levels as high as 11.

Reference strain: PCC 7345 (ATCC 29408), as *Arthrospira platensis*, isolated from saline marsh, Del Mar Slough, California, 1969 (Rippka et al., 1979).

Type species (Botanical Code): *Arthrospira jenneri* (Hass.) Stizenberger.

Taxonomic Considerations

Arthrospira has commonly been submerged in the genus *Spirulina* (Geitler, 1932) or in *Oscillatoria* along with *Spirulina*, by Bourrelly (1970, 1985). On the basis of ultrastructural work (Guglielmi and Cohen-Bazire, 1982a, b) it appears that the smaller, more tightly coiled *Spirulina* strains that lack easily discernible cross-walls may constitute a real taxonomic unit. Similar information on junctional pores and fimbriae in *Arthrospira* indicates a strong relationship to *Oscillatoria*. Since *Oscillatoria* spp. show various degrees of spiraling near the trichome termini, it might be correct to include *Arthrospira* in that genus. At this point, however, it seems justified to preserve the distinctiveness of these forms in the genus *Arthrospira*.

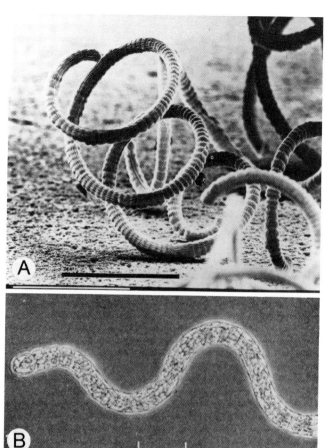

Figure 19.58. *A*, Scanning electron micrograph of a trichome of axenic *Arthrospira (Spirulina) platenis. Bar,* 40 μm. (Reproduced with permission from O. Ciferri, Microbiological Reviews *47:* 551–578, 1983, ©American Society for Microbiology.) *B, Arthrospira (Spirulina)* PC 7345. *Bar,* 20 μm. (Reproduced with permission from R. Rippka et al., Journal of General Microbiology *111:* 1–61, 1979, ©Society for General Microbiology.)

Genus III. **Oscillatoria** *Vaucher 1803*

Os.cil.la.to′ri.a. L. v. *oscillare* to swing; L. adj. suffix *-torius* belonging to; M.L. fem. n. *Oscillatoria* (filament) that swings.

Filamentous organisms that divide exclusively by binary fission and in one plane. The **trichomes are straight to loosely sinuous** near apices; flexible or semirigid. **Transverse septa are generally visible** under light microscopy (Fig. 19.59). Constrictions may or may not occur at cross-walls, but the total indentation never exceeds one eighth of the trichome diameter. Generally, the transverse septum (cross-wall) is thinner than the longitudinal wall. During fission the cytoplasmic membrane invaginates, with a thinner peptidoglycan layer separating the new membranes of the daughter cells (Fig. 19.5). This characteristic applies to the genera *Spirulina, Arthrospira,* and *Lyngbya* in addition to *Oscillatoria.*

Cells may be much shorter than broad (appearing as stacked disks) to a few times longer than broad (Fig. 19.59). The **trichome diameters range from about 1 μm to occasionally >100 μm.** Invariably in **broader trichomes** (>15 μm in diameter) **the cells are shorter than long.** The **trichome is** usually **motile and rotates** in either a left- or right-handed manner with respect to the direction of movement. If terminal regions are not in contact with substrate, the free end may appear to oscillate as the trichome rotates, particularly if the free end is curved. **Rates of movement range from <1 to about 11 μm/s** (Halfen and

Castenholz, 1971). Usually, **sheaths are nearly invisible,** gossamer **tubes that are shed as flattened trails when the trichome moves on solid substrates.** Occasionally, more visible sheath may build up on some trichomes, particularly during periods of immobility in liquid culture (Chang, 1977). Trichomes are solitary, but if clustered or in fabriclike mats they are not surrounded by a morphologically distinct common sheath. Copious amounts of gellike matter, however, may be produced, particularly in liquid culture.

The terminal cell of many species of *Oscillatoria* is differentiated to the extent of developing a shape distinct from the simple bulging of an unattended cross-wall, which occurs immediately after trichome fragmentation. Species-consistent shapes include round, blunt, truncate, conical, prolonged-attenuate, and capitate. In addition, some terminal cells acquire an outside thickening of the outer cell wall termed the calyptra. Trichomes may be attenuated as well, but only for the length of a few to several cells near the terminus. The terminus of recently fragmented trichomes will generally appear different from those allowed to differentiate. The terminus of many species may be bent (whether tapered or not), and this may extend for the length of several cells. Further cell divisions may not be possible in the differentiated terminal cell.

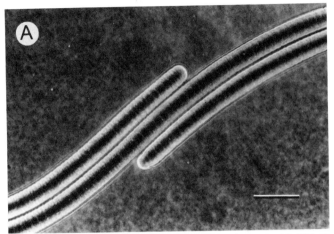

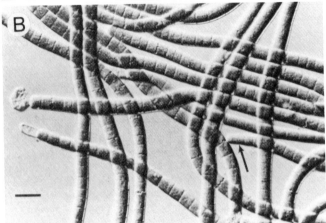

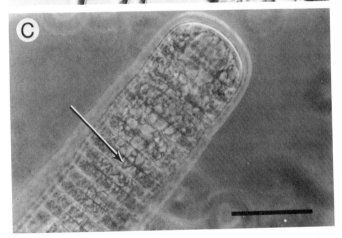

Figure 19.59. *A, Oscillatoria* cf. *margaritifera,* a marine form isolated from intertidal mats. Cells are much shorter than broad. *Bar,* 40 μm. *B, O. terebriformis* (culture University of Oregon OH-51-Ot, Clone 1) from hot springs. Nomarski interference contrast optics. Normal trichome tip. (*arrow*). Photograph by D. C. Nelson. *Bar,* 10 μm. (Reproduced with permission from R. W. Castenholz, Mitteilungen Internationale Vereinigung für Limnologie *21:* 296–315, 1978, ©Schweizerbart'sche Verlag.) *C, Oscillatoria* species. A large diameter marine form with "cytoplasmic strands" forming reticulum (*arrow*) through "sap vacuole" as in *O. borneti. Bar,* 40 μm.

The **color is variable, ranging from bright blue-green to deep red.** Several species show "chromatic adaptation" (Tandeau de Marsac, 1977). **Some species, almost black in color,** contain abundant C-PE

and c-phycocyanin. Phycoerythrin with a large absorption maximum of 493–495 nm in addition to the maximum of 543–546 nm occurs in some shade-inhabiting species of *Oscillatoria* (R. W. Castenholz, unpublished information) and in the marine planktonic *Trichodesmium* (*Oscillatoria* of some authors) (Fujita and Shimura, 1974). This represents a phycourobilin-containing phycoerythrin similar to rhodophycean phycoerythrin (r-PE).

Guglielmi and Cohen-Bazire (1982b) found that the junctional pores occurred in a single circular row near each cross-wall in strains designated *Oscillatoria* or *Arthrospira* (PCC 7345) and in at least one "LPP" strain (PCC 7105). Midcell and cross-wall perforations varied among strains. In addition, *Oscillatoria* and *Arthrospira* produced fimbriae that appeared closely appressed along the trichome, almost forming an envelope (Guglielmi and Cohen-Bazire, 1982a).

In the Pasteur Culture Collection, the mol% G + C of the DNA of strains included in *Oscillatoria* ranged from about 40 to 50, and the genome size ranged from 2.50 to 4.38 × 10⁹ daltons (Herdman et al, 1979a, b).

The species of *Oscillatoria* have a **worldwide distribution in freshwater, marine, and brackish waters. They also occur in inland saline lakes, and a few species tolerate temperatures as high as 56–60°C in some hot springs** (Castenholz, 1969). Some species are known as mat-formers in streams. **A number of species are planktonic in freshwater** (e.g. *O. agardhii, O. rubescens, O. borneti*) **and warmer marine waters** (e.g. *Trichodesmium* species) (Figs. 19.12 and 19.59). **These almost invariably contain gas vesicles** (exception: *O. borneti*). Several species are known as motile (gliding) components of microbial mats. Species of *Oscillatoria* are known commonly in other anaerobic, sulfide-containing habitats such as sediments in stratified eutrophic lakes. A few species occur in terrestrial habitats subjected to severe drying or in a shallow, ephemeral freshwater in polar regions where freeze-drying accompanies winter.

The physiology of some species of *Oscillatoria* has been studied, including several of the planktonic forms (e.g. Van Liere and Walsby, 1982; Mur, 1983; Ahlgren, 1985). In the Pasteur Culture Collection, none were able to grow as dark chemoheterotrophs, but some showed photoheterotrophic potential (Rippka et al., 1979). A few strains were capable of synthesizing nitrogenase when the medium was purged of O₂. **Marine planktonic forms** (*Trichodesmium* species) **fix N₂ when growing as clusters in nature.** All species are capable of **photoautotrophic** growth; **some are obligate photoautotrophs.** One species (*O. terebriformis*) is capable of a very slow growth under dark anaerobic conditions with fructose or glucose (Richardson and Castenholz, 1987). Sulfide-dependent anoxygenic photosynthesis is known in several species of oscillatorian cyanobacteria. In *O. amphigranulata* (thermophilic strain) only reduced nitrogen compounds can be used (R. W. Castenholz, unpublished observation).

Isolation can usually be done by "self-isolation" on agar, with the sometimes-rapid gliding rates used (Castenholz, 1981, Rippka et al., 1981a). However, many species are extremely refractory to present culture techniques. These have included a large number of apparently oligotrophic marine forms, including the species of *Trichodesmium*. However, Ohki et al. (1986) have now successfully cultured two species of *Trichodesmium*.

Reference strains: PCC 7515 (ATCC 29209) with C-PE, isolated from a greenhouse water tank, Stockholm, Sweden, 1972 (Rippka et al., 1979); and PCC 6506 (ATCC 29081, UTEX 1547) without phycoerythrin, from an unknown source (Rippka et al., 1979).

Type species (Botanical Code): *Oscillatoria princeps* Vaucher 1803.

Taxonomic Considerations

Oscillatoria Vaucher 1803, *Lyngbya* Agardh 1824, *Phormidium* Kützing 1843, *Microcoleus* Desmazières, *Symploca* Kützing 1843, and *Schizothrix* Kützing 1843 are common genera that are nearly identical in the sense that a similar range of cell and trichome types have been described within each genus. The boundaries of these and a few other genera have been based on what may be a superficial characteristic, the presence or absence of a firm or diffluent sheath and on the number of trichomes within each sheath. These characteristics are variable in some strains and are possibly controlled by only very slight genomic differences. Moreover, *Oscillatoria,* when gliding, also produces a very thin sheath casing. Thus, there appears to be a cline from extremely thin to thicker and even laminated sheaths but with a similar range of oscillatorian cell types within each sheath type.

Rippka et al. (1979) were unable to establish good generic boundaries within the culture strains that possessed sheaths, and they established a temporarily expedient grouping, the "LPP group," representing the former generic categories of *Lyngbya, Phormidium* and *Plectonema* as well as others. *Plectonema* Thuret 1875 was included because the occasional false branching which originally distinguished this genus appeared to be simply a result of the irregular consistency of the sheath. However, the "LPP group" also included trichomes with isodiametric or cylindrical cells (i.e. longer than broad) and with variable degrees of constriction between adjacent cells (Rippka et al., 1979).

The genus *Oscillatoria* is not considered in such restrictive terms as those used by Rippka et al. (1979). Nevertheless, 16S rRNA sequence data indicate a great disparity among some species of this genus (Giovannoni et al., 1988). *Oscillatoria* here includes strains with isodiametric or elongated cells (not just those with shortened disklike cells) and those which show slight to moderate constrictions at the cross-walls but less than one eighth of the diameter of the trichome (Fig. 19.59). Admittedly, the latter breakoff point is arbitrary, but with the data available, the more restrictive definition was also arbitrary. The criteria of Guglielmi and Cohen-Bazire (1982a, b) on pore patterns and arrangement of fimbriae may better define the taxonomic unit when more strains are examined. The species of the genus *Trichodesmium* are regarded as species of *Oscillatoria* by many cyanobacteriologists (Geitler, 1932; Sournia, 1968), but this easily identified cluster of marine, planktonic organisms may show enough distinctive cytological and other features to warrant separation from *Oscillatoria* (Gantt et al., 1984).

Genus IV. **Lyngbya** Agardh 1824

Lyng′by.a. M.L. fem. n. *Lyngbya* Lyngbye; named after H. C. Lyngbye, Danish botanist, 1782–1837.

Filamentous organisms that share the entire range of cellular types with *Oscillatoria* but **which produce a distinct and persistent sheath. The sheath may be thin but can be seen with phase-contrast optics,** particularly where it extends beyond the terminal cell of the trichome (Fig. 19.54). The **trichome diameters range from about 1 μm to about 80 μm. Cell features are the same as** for the description of **Oscillatoria, including coloration.**

Trichomes are usually nonmotile within the sheath, **but short sections of trichome (hormogonia) sometimes move slowly** when placed on new agar-solidified medium. Some strains produce many hormogonia which glide free of the sheaths and appear as *Oscillatoria* until new sheath production again immobilizes them. In some cases, rapid growth extends trichomes out of old sheaths, and terminal portions appear sheathless.

The mol% G + C of the DNA is 43.4 (Herdman et al., 1979a) in the reference strain (PCC 7419, ATCC 29346), **and the genome size is about 4.58 × 10⁹ daltons** (Herdman et al., 1979b). However, with the present concept of *Lyngbya,* others of the "LPP group" would also fall within this generic boundary, since most have at least thin sheaths (see Table 15 in Rippka et al., 1979).

Stam (1980) included several sheathed "oscillatorian" forms in his DNA/DNA hybridization studies. The mol% G + C of the DNA in these was from about 42 to 49.

The sheaths of some strains, including PCC 7419, are quite prominent and strong, so that an entire entangled mass of filaments in liquid culture will hold together if attempts are made to remove only a small part with forceps. Laminated sheaths occur commonly in the large diameter species, in both freshwater and marine forms. A yellow pigment ("scytonemin") commonly occurs in the sheaths of some marine mat-forming species, giving the whole filament a brownish color. Although little is known about this pigment, the broad absorption maximum lies in the near UV, violet, and blue regions of the spectrum (Muehlstein and Castenholz, 1983). In some species, intense purple to red pigments occur in multilayered sheaths (i.e. *Porphyrosiphon* Kützing 1849).

Lyngbya, as here defined, has a **worldwide distribution.** In contrast to *Oscillatoria,* **however, few species are planktonic. Gasvacuolate forms are uncommon** (Walsby, 1981). As an additional contrast, *Lyngbya* (including *Symploca* and *Porphyrosiphon*) forms turflike terrestrial mats. *Lyngbya* (including *Phormidium*) also forms fabriclike mats in shallow marine (including intertidal) and freshwater habitats.

In general, the thicker-sheathed species of *Lyngbya* are more difficult to isolate in culture than are *Oscillatoria* species. On agar the production of motile hormogonia is not assured, and the older sheaths sometimes carry a heavy burden of attached, contaminating microorganisms. Growth rates of the thicker-sheathed species also appear commonly to be about an order of magnitude slower than those of most *Oscillatoria* species known in culture.

The first reference strain below (PCC 7419) was separated by Rippka et al. (1979) from the "LPP group" as the single member of LPP-A, and is characterized by having a thick and persistent sheath, wide trichome (15–16 μm) and short disklike cells.

Since *Lyngbya* as a distinct taxonomic unit is still uncertain, little can be said regarding the physiology of the group. In reference strain PCC 7419, a marine mat-forming type, nitrogenase was synthesized under sustained anaerobic conditions (Rippka et al., 1979).

Reference strains: PCC 7419 (ATCC 29346), isolated from salt marsh, Woods Hole, Massachusetts, 1974 (Rippka et al., 1979); and UTEX 1566, as *Oscillatoria tenuis* Agardh, from an unknown source Stam and Holleman, 1979; Stam, 1980).

Type species (Botanical Code): *Lyngbya confervoides* Agardh 1824.

Taxonomic Considerations

The retention of the genus *Lyngbya* Agardh 1824 for those oscillatorian forms with persistent sheaths will still not eliminate the "LPP group," although a number of strains would fall under *Lyngbya.* The ambiguity will still remain in cases where sheaths are very thin or develop only in aging cultures or are simply variable as to whether they are present or not (Rippka et al., 1979; Stam and Holleman, 1979; Stam, 1980). Some of these thin-sheathed forms and those with more gelatinous, diffluent sheaths would have fallen into the genus *Phormidium* Kützing 1843 or *Symploca* Kützing 1843 (Geitler, 1932). Bourrelly (1970, 1985) also considers the boundaries between these genera too slight to demarcate and therefore recognizes only *Lyngbya* by right of priority. *Plectonema,* also in the "LPP group," with more frequent false branching than other sheathed types, may also fit into *Lyngbya* if the value of the false branching is discounted at the generic level. Bourrelly (1970, 1985), however, considers members of this genus to be heterocyst-less members of the *Scytonemataceae* (part of Subsection IV) (Rippka et al., 1979). *Porphyrosiphon* Kützing 1849 another genus similar to *Lyngbya* but is separated from it by having a multilaminated sheath with a red or brown pigment (Bourrelly, 1985). However, a greater problem comes with the several genera described that have multiple, unbranched trichomes within a common sheath. These are *Microcoleus* Desmazières 1823, *Hydrocoleum* Kützing 1843, *Schizothrix* Kützing 1843, and others less well known (see Geitler, 1932). Rippka et al. (1979) have included two strains designated *Microcoleus* in the LPP-B group, since multiple trichomes were not present in common sheaths in culture and even the presence of sheath was variable. Some cultures of *Microcoleus* have been maintained, however, in which consistent multiple trichomes grew in a common sheath, as in field material. Consequently, with future culture refinements, at least one of these generic names may be used for culture strains.

Genus V. **Pseudanabaena** *Lauterborn, 1916*

Pseu′da.na.baen′a. Gr. adj. *pseud* false; *anabaena* (cf. *Anabaena*); M.L. fem. n. *Pseudanabaena* false *Anabaena*.

Filamentous organisms that divide exclusively by binary fission in one plane and **that have conspicuous constrictions at the cross-walls;** in most strains, constriction cuts into about one half or more of the diameter of the trichome (Fig. 19.60). In a few strains, the constriction is less but is still more than one eighth the diameter (Guglielmi and Cohen-Bazire, 1984a). **Cells are longer than broad to isodiametric and are often barrel-shaped.** The **diameter of trichomes** of strains characterized in culture **ranges from about 1 to 3 μm.** The transverse septum involves a partial centripetal ingrowth of all wall layers. In some cases, the remaining connection appears quite narrow, as if the cells were strung as beads. The structural (peptidoglycan) layer of the cross-wall is 3–6 times thicker than that layer surrounding the rest of the cell (Guglielmi and Cohen-Bazire, 1984a) (Figs. 19.9*A*, 19.10 and 19.61). The **trichomes are usually straight and** quite frequently **short**, consisting of only a few to several cells (see genus *Borzia*). **Single, detached cells are frequent** in most culture populations. **Gliding motility occurs in trichomes and unicells,** probably without rotation. Gliding motility has apparently been lost in a few culture strains (Guglielmi and Cohen-Bazire, 1984a).

In one species, *Pseudanabaena* cf. *galeata* (University of Oregon strain OL-75-Ps), gliding aggregates of many trichomes develop and usually move at rates greater than those of individual trichomes (Castenholz, 1982) (Fig. 19.38).

Many strains have polar gas vacuoles, but this characteristic is commonly not expressed under all culture conditions and in some clones seems to have been lost permanently. Although similar in appearance to some forms of *Anabaena* in the "*Nostocaceae*," *Pseudanabaena* as here defined is **incapable of producing** specialized cells such as **heterocysts or akinetes.**

Terminal cells of trichomes are not differentiated with respect to shape, as in many species of *Oscillatoria* and *Lyngbya,* and they do not acquire a calyptra. Guglielmi and Cohen-Bazire (1982b) found that *Pseudanabaena* strains and some LPP-B strains that had the appearance of *Pseudanabaena* possessed rings (400–500 nm wide) of multiple pores (300–500) near the cell poles, thus differing from the single ring of pores found in strains of *Oscillatoria* (also see Guglielmi and Cohen-Bazire, 1984a) (Fig. 19.61).

The color of *Pseudanabaena* may be blue-green to red, depending of the presence or absence of C-PE. Electrophoretic patterns of phycobilin and the ultrastructure of phycobilisomes have shown a uniformity for culture stains comprising "phenon" A, which further supports the redefinition of the genus *Pseudanabaena* by Guglielmi and Cohen-Bazire (1984b).

The mol% G + C of the DNA ranges from about 42 to 47 (Herdman et al., 1979a; Guglielmi and Cohen-Bazire, 1984a), **and the genome size is from 2.14 to 5.19 × 10⁹ daltons.**

The distribution of *Pseudanabaena* is worldwide. It is seen in collections from **hot springs** (probably not above 55°C) and in **marine and freshwater muds.** It is particularly **common in anaerobic, sulfide-containing sediments.** Some forms are known in freshwater plankton and include those in the mucilage of other planktonic cyanobacteria.

All strains known are **obligate photoautotrophs.** Some are capable

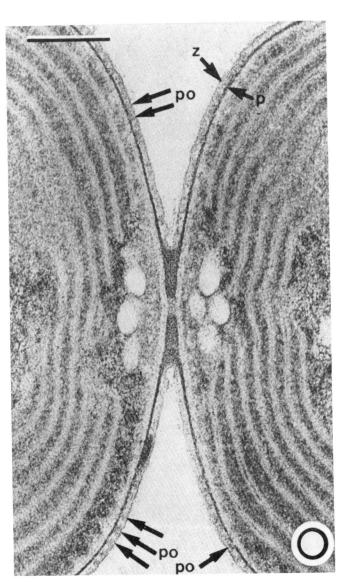

Figure 19.61. Longitudinal section of *Pseudanabaena* species (PCC 7367) at point of constricted cross-wall. *p,* peptidoglycan layer of cell wall; *po,* multiple pores restricted to cell pole region. Gas vesicles are seen at both cell poles. Bar, 200 nm. (Reproduced with permission from G. Guglielmi and G. Cohen-Bazire, Protistologica *18*: 167–177, 1982, ©Editions due CNRS.)

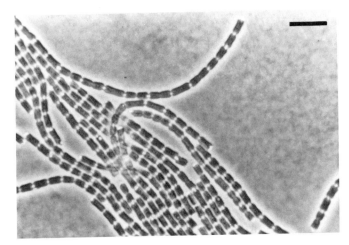

Figure 19.60. *Pseudanabaena* cf. *galeata* (culture University of Oregon OL-75-Ps) showing gas vesicle clusters at poles of cells (*light areas*). Also see Figures 19.9*A* and 19.61. *Bar,* 10 μm.

of synthesizing nitrogenase when cultures are kept anaerobic (Rippka et al., 1979).

Culture isolation can usually be done by using gliding self-isolation (see Castenholz, 1981; Rippka et al., 1981a).

Reference strains: PCC 7429 (ATCC 29536), without phycoerythrin and without nitrogenase under anaerobiosis, with polar gas vacuoles, isolated from a *Sphagnum* bog near Vierwaldstättersee, Switzerland, 1974 (Rippka et al., 1979); and PCC 7408 (ATCC 29344, UTEX 425, CCAP 1464/1), grown near the Thames River, England, 1940 (Rippka et al., 1979).

Type species (Botanical Code): *Pseudanabaena catenata* Lauterborn 1916.

Taxonomic Considerations

The genus *Pseudanabaena,* as here defined, is not as restrictive as that proposed by Rippka et al. (1979) but corresponds closely to the redefinition of this genus by Guglielmi and Cohen-Bazire (1984a, b). Gliding motility of *Pseudanabaena* was used in 1979 to distinguish *Pseudanabaena* (including unicells) from certain strains or species of the unicellular genus *Synechococcus* which sometimes forms short chains in addition to unicells. The criterion is imperfect, since some strains of *Pseudanabaena* have lost gliding ability and some strains of *Synechococcus* do move (e.g. PCC 6910 (Stanier et al., 1971)). In contrast to the criterion applied by Rippka et al. (1979), the possession of polar gas vesicles is no longer considered a valid characteristic, since they are lost in some cultures and have been seen in terminal cells of *Oscillatoria,* lacking constrictions at cross-walls. On the other hand, populations of apparent *Synechococcus* from hot springs sometimes possess polar gas vacuoles (R. W. Castenholz, unpublished observations).

The genus *Pseudanabaena* as redefined by Guglielmi and Cohen-Bazire (1984a, b) now includes the following strains, some which were placed earlier in the "LPP-B group": PCC 6903, PCC 7402, PCC 7429, PCC 7955, PCC 6901, PCC 7408 and PCC 7409. Strains PCC 6802, PCC 7403, PCC 7367 and PCC 6406, included in *Pseudanabaena* by Rippka et al. (1979), are now excluded from this genus.

The comparative sequences of 800–900 nucleotides of 16S rRNA for two strains of *Pseudanabaena,* as here defined, place these together but quite distant from other members of Subsections III, IV and V (Giovannoni et al., 1988).

Genus VI. **Starria** *Lang 1977*

Star′ri.a. M.L. fem. n. *Starria* Starr; named after R. C. Starr, U.S. phycologist.

This nonbranching, **filamentous cyanobacterium** is unique in that the **short trichomes in cross-section are triradiate** (Lang, 1977). The **trichomes are straight to helically twisted, about 15 μm in diameter. The cells are short (1–2 μm).** The triradiate form usually has broad, armlike projections 120° apart, separated by U-shaped depressions (Fig. 19.62). The pigmentation is concentrated in the arms. **A thin sheath (3 μm thick) covers the trichome.** Cross-walls are as in the genus *Oscillatoria,* with an invagination of the peptidoglycan layer but not of the outer LPP envelope. The relatively thick peptidoglycan layer of longitudinal walls is characterized by evenly distributed pits 70 nm in diameter, as in some species of *Oscillatoria,* e.g. *O. princeps* (Halfen and Castenholz, 1971; Guglielmi and Cohen-Bazine, 1982b).

This organism is known from a **single strain isolated from a soil sample** in Zimbabwe. Growth occurred on common cyanobacterial medium with soil extract added. Low light intensity was recommended.

Little is known about the physiology or biochemistry of this organism, but its very unusual structure has been documented by light and electron microscopy (Lang, 1977).

Reference strain: UTEX 1754, isolated from depressions in granite rocks, Zimbabwe, 1969.

Type species (Botanical Code): *Starria zimbabweënsis* Lang 1977.

Taxonomic Considerations

Although morphological variants were derived from the wild type, all possessed a distinct semblance to the triradiate feature. The only slightly similar genera are *Gomontiella* Teodoresco 1901 (Bourrelly, 1985) and *Crinalium* Crow 1927 (see below).

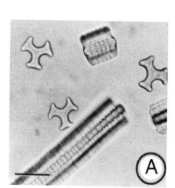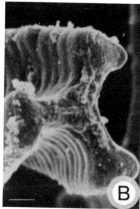

Figure 19.62. *Starria zimbabweënsis* in culture. *A,* longitudinal and cross-sectional views, with the latter showing projecting arms with slightly broadened extremities. *Bar,* 20 μm. *B,* enlarged cross-section. *Bar,* 2.0 μm. (Both *A* and *B* are reproduced with permission from N. J. Lang, Journal of Phycology *13:* 288–296, 1977, ©Phycological Society of America.)

ADDENDUM TO SUBSECTION III

A number of genera, some with numerous "species," have not been included above because they have not yet been cultured or cultures have not been maintained or used for detailed study. A few of the genera follow (see Geitler (1932), Desikachary (1959)' and Bourrelly (1985) for additional generic names). Those included are because of unusual morphological features or because of extensive work on field material.

Genus VII. **Crinalium** *Crow 1927*

Cri.na′li.um. L. adj. *crinalis* of hair; Gr. suff. *-ion* diminutive; M.L. neut. n. *Crinalium* small hairlike (filament).

An oscillatorianlike **trichome** which **is flattened to elliptical in cross-section** rather than cylindrical or triradiate. The cross-walls are delicate and difficult to see. A **thin sheath** exists.

Little is known about this organism, since it has **not yet** been **cultured.** However, the two species have been seen in a few collections (see Desikachary, 1959; Bourrelly, 1985).

Genus VIII. **Microcoleus** Desmazières 1823

Mi.cro.co′le.us. Gr. adj. *mikros* small; Gr. n. *koleos* sheath; M.L. masc. n. *Microcoleus* small sheath.

These oscillatorian type **trichomes are characterized by** the presence of **a common, homogeneous sheath. It surrounds several parallel trichomes** that are often spirally and tightly interwoven (Fig. 19.55). Several **species from marine and freshwater** have been described (Geitler, 1932), and one species in particular has been studied extensively but mainly as feral material from intertidal mats (*M. chthonoplastes* Thuret). Although cultures (including axenic) have been used at times (Pearson et al., 1979, 1981; Javor and Castenholz, 1981), little characterization of *Microcoleus* has come from work with cultures.

In axenic culture, some workers have found that **the common sheath disappears,** e.g. PCC 7420 (Rippka et al., 1979). **In other cultures** (see Javor and Castenholz, 1981), fascicles of **trichomes were maintained with thin common sheaths,** particularly under unidirectional light (Pearson et al. 1979).

No reference strain was designated.

Taxonomic Considerations

There are other genera with a habit similar to that of *Microcoleus*. In *Schizothrix* Kützing 1843, the common sheath is often branched toward the termini, and the sheath is usually laminated. In *Hydrocoleum* Kützing 1843, there are fewer trichomes per sheath than in *Microcoleus*. Other genera included, based primarily on variations of sheath and trichome numbers, are: *Sirocoleus* Kützing 1849; *Polychlamydum* West and West 1879; and *Dasygloea* Thwaites 1848 (see Geitler, 1932).

SUBSECTION IV. ORDER **NOSTOCALES**

R. W. Castenholz

Nos.to.cal′es. M.L. fem. n. *Nostocaceae* family of the order; *-ales* suffix to designate order; M.L. fem. pl. n. *Nostocales* the order containing the family *Nostocaceae*.

Members of the *Nostocales* (Subsection IV, sensu Rippka et al. 1979) are distinguished from all other cyanobacteria by being **filamentous organisms dividing exclusively by binary fission in one plane only** (some with the possibility of "false branching") *and* **having the potential to produce heterocysts.** Some possess heterocysts under almost all conditions. In others, heterocyst differentiation occurs only when ammonium (and nitrate) nitrogen concentration in the medium is low. There are also a few genera that may have lost the ability to produce heterocystous genera but still resemble heterocystous genera enough in other ways to be considered, at this time, related. **False branching** (described in the "Preface" to "Group I. Cyanobacteria") **may occur** frequently in some genera (e.g. *Scytonema*), but this does not involve division in more than one plane.

Further Descriptive Information

It seems natural to divide the broad *Nostocales*, as here defined, into three well-circumscribed families: *Nostocaceae*, *Scytonemataceae* and *Rivulariaceae*. The traditional use of these families is defended by the following distinguishing criteria:

A. Within the *Nostocaceae* ("Subsection IV, Family I"), all vegetative cells possess the capacity to divide; both heterocysts and akinetes are formed, although the latter are rare in some species or strains. In essentially all cases, heterocysts are formed under lowered concentrations of combined nitrogen, and the location and spacing of these specialized cells is used as a distinguishing generic characteristic. Heterocysts precede akinete formation (Fig. 19.63), and the location of the latter appears to be determined to a large extent by the location of the heterocysts. A sporulation-stimulating substance associated with the presence of heterocysts has been identified in a *Cylindrospermum* (Hirosawa and Wolk, 1979a, b). In the *Nostocaceae*, **trichomes are composed of vegetative cells of uniform diameter (the trichomes do not taper), and false branching does not occur** or, if the organism is sheathed, occurs only rarely.

B. In the *Scytonemataceae* ("Subsection IV, Family II"), **false branching is prevalent in all genera, tapered trichomes seldom occur,** and cell divisions are not diffuse within the trichome; instead, a variety of specific "meristematic" regions develop (usually subapical) which often result in a trichome breaking out of a sheath, thus forming a false branch (see Fig. 19.7). Heterocysts are sometimes frequent and usually associated with a false branch, but akinetes are lacking.

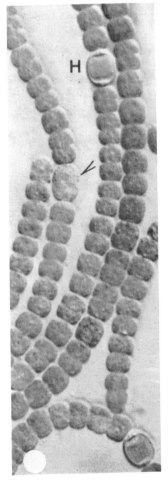

Figure 19.63. *Anabaena variabilis.* Trichome with heterocysts (*H*) and developing akinete (*arrow*). No scale given. (Reproduced with permission from W. Braune, Archives of Microbiology *126:* 257–261, 1980, ©Springer-Verlag.)

C. The *Rivulariaceae* ("Subsection IV, Family III") are characterized by **tapered trichomes; i.e. trichomes are polar with base and apex, with the tapered apex often ending in a long, colorless multicellular hair. The "meristematic" zone is restricted to a basal or intercalary region of the trichome. A heterocyst is usually the basal cell of each trichome,** at least when NH_4^+ and NO_3^- are limiting (Fig. 19.64). Heterocysts may sometimes differentiate in intercalary positions. When an akinete differentiates, it is adjacent to the heterocyst in this family. False branching may also occur within the *Rivulariaceae*.

Within the *Rivulariaceae* and *Scytonemataceae* the distribution of intercalary "meristematic" zones and the position of heterocysts often determine the points of false branch formation via trichome breakage. The heterocyst "holds" the trichome inside the sheath while localized growth pressure accompanying cell divisions causes the trichome to rupture the sheath and grow outward.

Within the *Nostocaceae* ("Subsection IV, Family I") motility occurs essentially at all times for free trichomes (e.g. *Anabaena*, *Nodularia*, *Cylindrospermum*, *Aphanizomenon*), but in others (e.g. *Nostoc*), trichomes are immobile in a viscous matrix of gel, and motility is restricted to the few-celled, small-cell-diameter hormogonia (without heterocysts) which are formed and released under specific conditions. In the *Rivulariaceae* and *Scytonemataceae*, vegetative trichomes are usually bounded by persistent sheaths and are often arranged in macromultitrichome thalli. These trichomes are not motile. In both groups, however, a hormogonium of short cells is differentiated in the subterminal zone and may, in some cases, be released only after the terminal portion of the trichome (e.g. hair) has been shed (in the *Rivulariaceae*).

Trichome diameter may range from 1 to 30 μm in various species with untapered trichomes. In tapered types (e.g. *Rivulariaceae*), the basal heterocyst may be as large as 25 μm, whereas the terminal hair cells may be only 1 μm in diameter.

Many members of Subsection IV produce gellike or mucilagelike sheaths or extracellular matrices which may range in consistency from firm and leathery (e.g. some *Nostoc* species) to very soft and slimy. The most conspicuous sheaths, however, are those which form in the *Rivulariaceae*: some are thick and laminated and nearly always exclude the basal heterocyst. The "branching" sheaths of such genera as *Dichothrix* and *Gardnerula* form some of the most orderly and morphologically complex thallus structures in the cyanobacteria.

Gliding motility in the vegetative trichomes of members of the *Nostocaceae* is commonly an order of magnitude slower (i.e. <1.0 μm/s) than the faster-moving trichomes of some of the *Oscillatoriales* (Subsection III). The trichomes are not known to rotate as they do in the *Oscillatoriales* (Nultsch and Wenderoth, 1983).

The mol% G + C of the DNA in many strains (35) in Subsection IV (*Nostocales*) are somewhat similar, ranging only from 38.3 to 46.7 (Herdman et al., 1979a). The genome sizes, however, are quite different, ranging from 3.17 to 8.58×10^{-9} daltons (Herdman et al., 1979b). The results of sequencing 800–900 consecutive nucleotides in single strains of five different genera covering the three subsections shows that there is a greater degree of relatedness among members of Subsection IV than with any members outside, with the exception of the *Stigonematales* (Subsection V), a heterocystous group exhibiting true branches (Giovannoni et al., 1988).

Members of the *Nostocales* may occur in a greater diversity of habitats than members of the *Oscillatoriales*, perhaps because of the more common ability to fix N_2 and enter into symbiotic associations. Several species of *Anabaena*, *Nodularia*, *Aphanizomenon* and *Gloeotrichia* (the latter of "Subsection IV, Family III") are planktonic and form major blooms in lakes, particularly in warmer lakes or, during summer and fall, in temperate lakes. *Nodularia* forms major blooms in saline lakes and in brackish waters such as the Baltic Sea. All of the planktonic members produce gas vesicles. Certain species of *Anabaena* and *Aphanizomenon* are known worldwide for their blooms in eutrophic lakes. Many species of most genera are also commonly attached in freshwater and marine habitats: species of *Calothrix* and the separable genera *Gloeotrichia*, *Rivularia*, *Dichothrix*, and *Gardnerula*, form firm to gelatinous cushions on solid substrates; some species are commonly encrusted by $CaCO_3$ deposition. *Nostoc* forms firm spherical to amorphous gelatinous colonies ranging from microscopic to the size of bowling balls. *Calothrix*, *Scytonema*, and related genera are better known than others for subaerial habitats, particularly in moist or tropical climates. Many, however, are capable of seemingly complete desiccation. *Nostoc*, like some members of Subsection III, is well-known to form terrestrial mats which dry seasonally and also in Antarctic streams where freezing and thawing is frequent and where freeze-drying occurs each year (Vincent and Howard-Williams, 1986). No members of this subsection occur at very high temperatures in hot springs; a temperature of 52–54°C is the maximum for the most thermophilic strain known (*Calothrix* species, Wickstrom and Castenholz, 1978).

Planktonic forms in nonbrackish marine habitats are rare, although *Richelia* occurs in planktonic cells of some centric diatoms.

Members of this subsection are very well known as endosymbionts and exosymbionts, in some cases serving as the source of fixed carbon and nitrogen. In other associations, they appear to be utilized by the host strictly as a source of fixed nitrogen. Symbiotic associations are nearly restricted to species of *Nostoc* and *Anabaena*. The most common associations occur in lichens but also in green plants such as liverworts, hornworts, ferns and cycads and in a genus of angiosperms, *Gunnera*. For further information see Stewart (1980) and Stewart et al. (1983).

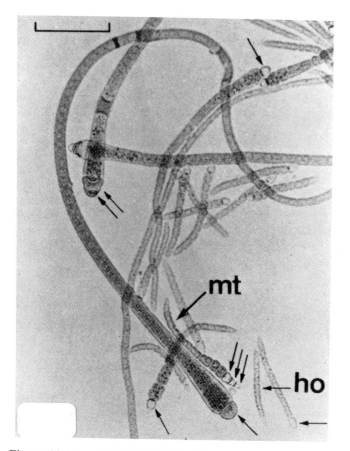

Figure 19.64. *Calothrix* PCC 7103. Note taper of trichomes with basal heterocyst or heterocysts (*arrows*). Hormogonia (*ho*) do not bear a heterocyst, but one is differentiated early in further development (*lowest right-hand arrow*). *mt*, maturing trichome. *Bar*, 50 μm. (Reproduced with permission from R. Rippka et al., Journal of General Microbiology *111*: 1–61, 1979, ©Society for General Microbiology.)

Taxonomic Comments

In general, the visual, microscopic identification of members of Subsection IV is considerably easier than that of Subsection III. The heterocyst is the key mark for most genera. Therefore, its presence is indicative, but its absence is not conclusive. Heterocysts are rare in some feral populations or, in culture, often must be induced. Also, some genera possibly related to other tapered members of the *Rivulariaceae* lack heterocysts under all known conditions. The seven genera described under *Nostocales* can be distinguished by morphological criteria alone. Rippka et al. (1979) described six of these genera. Drouet (1981) had reduced these six genera to four and added a fifth. Bourrelly (1985), on the other hand, recognized 22 genera, and Geitler (1932), over 33 genera.

One of the major problems in determining degree of relatedness by morphological, physiological and biochemical criteria is how to evaluate the inability to differentiate heterocysts. There are filamentous cyanobacteria with frequent false branches but which fail to produce heterocysts seemingly under any conditions and which fail to fix N$_2$ in culture, except sometimes when continually purged of O$_2$. These (e.g. genus *Plectonema*) have for now been included in Subsection III and submerged within the genus *Lyngbya* (see Subsection III). Breaking out of a weak or thin sheath to form a false branch when localized cell divisions occur may be an occasional and accidental occurrence in a wide variety of sheathed cyanobacteria.

There are numerous cyanobacteria included, with such generic names as *Homoeothrix, Amphithrix, Leptochaete, Tapinothrix* and *Hammatoidea,* that have tapered trichomes similar to those of *Calothrix* but which lack heterocysts. Since these have not been studied in culture, it is impossible to evaluate the lack of heterocysts vs. the presence of taper. In some cases (e.g. some populations of *Homoeothrix*), the lack of a heterocyst could be nothing more than the genetic loss of the ability to differentiate a heterocyst in a strain of *Calothrix*.

Another current problem in evaluation of morphological characteristics is the multiplicity of trichomes in common sheaths, a problem also discussed in relation to Subsection III, the *Oscillatoriales.* In many tapered trichomes that individually could not be distinguished from strains of *Calothrix*, false branching and concomitant "branching" of the sheaths produce brushlike cushions (e.g. *Dichothrix sensu* Geitler), and elaborate dichotomies of branches occur to form sturdy thalli several centimeters in height (e.g. *Gardnerula = Polythrix*). A common gel binds filaments of *Rivularia* and *Gloeothrichia* into dense colonies. Since the typical macromorphology is lost under some culture conditions, the significance of these arrangements may seem trivial, yet they are probably of key importance for survival in natural populations, and the use of several generic names to describe these forms in nature will continue.

A similar problem exists in evaluating the multiplicity of *Anabaena*-like trichomes in a common gellike or leathery matrix (e.g. *Nostoc*). Rippka et al. (1979) found that this characteristic was lost in culture, and their separation of *Anabaena* and *Nostoc* was based on the specialized hormogonia produced periodically by the latter genus. But hormogonial release is probably a necessary consequence of the growth form of *Nostoc* as a gel-bound colony, and some cultures now exist in which normal colony formation occurs.

The only practical solution to the problem of relatedness with present methodology is to address the genetic basis for these differences. For major differences the techniques of sequencing large samples of the nucleotides of rRNA (e.g. 16S fraction) seem most useful (Olsen et al., 1986). For more closely related organisms, comparisons of DNA base compositions, DNA/DNA reassociation rates, the thermal stability values of DNA/DNA hybrids, and the electrophoretic behavior of various enzymes have proven to be excellent criteria to establish species boundaries among strains of the genus *Anabaena* (e.g. Stulp and Stam, 1982; 1984a, b; 1985). In these and other studies (see later under genus *Anabaena*), it was determined that the species categories determined by these means usually matched well with the traditional morphological species-determining characteristics that were stable over a wide range of environmental conditions.

Key to the order **Nostocales** *(Subsection IV)*

Heterocysts are potentially present in all genera included in this key.

A. Trichomes that reproduce by diffuse cell divisions and trichome breakage (do not produce hormogonia) and are motile by gliding motility...B

A. Trichomes that reproduce by diffuse or localized cell divisions but are not motile except for short chains of cells that lack heterocysts (i.e. hormogonia)...E

B. Heterocysts intercalary and often terminal as well; position of akinetes (if present) variable C

B. Heterocysts are exclusively terminal, usually on one end but sometimes on both ends; akinete or akinetes form adjacent to heterocyst.

         Genus IV. *Cylindrospermum,* p. 1787

C. Vegetative cells are spherical, ovoid or cylindrical-elongated...D

C. Vegetative cells are shorter than broad and may be disk-shaped.

         Genus III. *Nodularia,* p. 1786

D. Vegetative cells are cylindrical; at the ends of the trichome, cells are more elongate and mainly colorless.

         Genus II. *Aphanizomenon,* p. 1786

D. Vegetative cells are cylindrical, ovoid or spherical, reproducing by trichome fragmentation only.

         Genus I. *Anabaena,* p. 1783

         (in key, includes *Anabaenopsis* and *Cyanospira*)

E. Trichomes are polarly tapered and with sheaths; a heterocyst (when present) at least forms a basal cell at the wide end of the trichome; hormogonia (composed of *narrow* cells) form a basal heterocyst when motility ceases.

         Genus I. *Calothrix,* p. 1791

         (in key, includes *Rivularia, Gloeotrichia* and others)

E. Trichomes are untapered and with sheathes; false branches usually occur at site of intercalary heterocyst; hormogonia are composed of cells of *normal* diameter which form a basal heterocyst when motility ceases.

         Genus I. *Scytonema,* p. 1790

         (in key, includes *Tolypothrix*)

E. Trichomes are without taper and without false branching. Common gell surrounds many trichomes, at least in nature; hormogonia of normal or narrow diameter form a terminal heterocyst, usually at both ends, when motility ceases.

         Genus V. *Nostoc,* p. 1788

FAMILY I. **NOSTOCACEAE**

R. W. Castenholz

Nos.to.ca′ce.ae. M.L. fem. n. *Nostoc* a genus of the family; -*aceae* ending to denote a family; M.L. fem. n. *Nostoca-ceae* the *Nostoc* family.

In culture, this family is known primarily for strains that fit under the generic names *Anabaena, Nostoc, Nodularia, Cylindrospermum* and *Aphanizomenon*. All except *Aphanizomenon* are genera that lack polarity in terms of tapered trichomes; they also lack false or true branching.

The general distinguishing characteristics are:

1. **Trichomes uniseriate without false or true branches**
2. Trichomes **not tapered** (except sometimes for terminal cell alone)
3. **Cell divisions diffuse** (not restricted to certain portions of trichome)
4. Vegetative trichomes motile or nonmotile
5. Hormogonia (specialized short motile trichomes) formed only in *Nostoc*
6. Sheaths (mucilaginous) common around individual trichomes in some strains
7. Common sheath (mucilaginous or firm, leathery) forming multi-trichome colonies (of various shapes) but not always under culture conditions and only in genus *Nostoc*
8. Trichomes seldom attached to substrates individually, colonies of *Nostoc* attached or free; most members of other genera planktonic or tychoplanktonic, commonly with gas vesicles
9. **Heterocysts terminal and intercalary in some genera, terminal only in others** (genera: *Cylindrospermum* and some species of *Anabaena,* traditionally referred to as genus *Anabaenopsis*)
10. Akinetes produced in most but not all members of this family, with position varying with species

Some of the other genera, not completely described here, that have been included in the botanical family *Nostocaceae* (or *Microchaetaceae*)

by Geitler (1932), Desikachary (1959) and Bourrelly (1985) are:

Richelia J. Schmidt 1901—an unbranched and untapered short trichome with the heterocyst polar when present. It occurs intracellularly in planktonic marine diatoms, mainly *Rhizosolenia* species, not in culture.

Wollea Bornet and Flahault 1888—a genus differentiated from *Nostoc* by saclike gelatinous thalli in which the trichomes are arranged in parallel fashion; one species described.

Anabaenopsis (Woloszynska) V. Miller 1923—a genus possibly distinct from *Anabaena* (and *Cylindrospermum*). The principal criteria are that heterocysts are terminal (intercalary and in pairs during differentiation just before separation) and that akinetes are formed as distally as possible from heterocysts (thus, unlike *Cylindrospermum*). Since species of *Anabaenopsis* sometimes have single intercalary heterocysts, there seems to be insufficient reason at this point to argue for the separation of *Anabaenopsis,* although future information from cultures may prove otherwise. The genus *Cyanospira* Florenzano, Sili, Pelosi and Vincenzini 1985 probably fits into this group (see "Genus I. *Anabaena*").

Hormothamnion Grunow 1867—a genus well-known from marine specimens which form bushlike tufts of false-branching filaments. Heterocysts are intercalary only.

Aulosira Kirchner 1878—a genus with several common species in tropical freshwaters; similar to *Anabaena* but with persistent sheath. Heterocysts are intercalary; and akinetes are often in series. Bourrelly (1985) includes it in the *Nodularia*.

Raphidiopsis Fritsch and Rich 1929—Bourrelly (1985) includes this genus in the *Nostocaceae,* although no heterocyst is formed, only a centrally located akinete in a trichome tapered at both ends (see also "Subsection IV, Family III, *Rivulariaceae*").

Genus I. **Anabaena** *Bory de St. Vincent 1822*

A.na.bae′na. Gr. adj. *ana* up again; Gr. v. *baino* to walk, to step; M.L. fem. n. *Anabaena* to step up again, repeating line of units (cells).

Trichomes are untapered with conspicuous constrictions at cross-walls. Trichomes may be straight, curved or helically (spirally) formed. The cells are cylindrical, spherical or ovoid (barrel-shaped) and not shorter than broad (or only slightly so), usually ranging in width from about 2 to 10 μm but in some species to over 20 μm (Desikachary, 1959). The terminal cells may be rounded, tapered or conical in shape. **Heterocysts are intercalary or terminal or both** (Fig. 19.13). Intercalary heterocysts are nearly spherical to cylindrical with rounded ends; terminal heterocysts are similar or sometimes conical. Akinetes are usually formed, and their position in trichomes differs with the species. **A firm individual sheath is absent,** but a soft mucilaginous covering is often present.

Trichomes, when free of adhesive mucilage, are normally motile (usually <1 μm/s), and **colonies are not formed. Reproduction is by fragmentation of "parental" trichomes into shorter trichomes indistinguishable in cell dimensions from the former trichome. Gas vesicles occur in many species;** however they occur mainly in those that are planktonic. Many species are known worldwide as major components of the freshwater plankton and also of many saline lakes. Others occur as tychoplankton, and a few are symbiotic (e.g. *Anabaena azollae* of the aquatic fern *Azolla*), although in association with host species it is often difficult to distinguish *Anabaena* and *Nostoc*. Most of the symbiotic strains are ascribed to the genus *Nostoc*. Surprisingly, *Anabaena* is not known as a major component of marine plankton, although combined nitrogen is often the limiting nutrient. There are at

least 15 gas-vacuolate species in freshwater, and *A. spiroides, A. circinalis* and *A. flos-aquae* are the most common in the plankton. Instead, nitrogen-limited pelagic marine environments are dominated primarily by the oscillatorian genus *Trichodesmium,* a gas-vacuolate nitrogen fixer which lacks heterocysts, and possibly by some minute unicellular forms. *Anabaena flos-aquae,* however, has invaded brackish marine environments such as the low-salinity portions of the Baltic Sea.

The physiology and biochemistry of *Anabaena* strains has been studied with respect to numerous facets. It is beyond the scope of this treatment to go into detail. The most extensive studies of cyanobacterial nitrogen fixation and of heterocyst structure and differentiation have used *Anabaena* (Stewart, 1980; Wolk, 1989). The most detailed studies of nitrogen fixation gene organization in cyanobacteria have also been with *Anabaena* (see Haselkorn, 1986; and the general characteristics of cyanobacteria in this chapter).

Seven strains in the Pasteur Culture Collection were judged to be obligate phototrophs (Rippka et al., 1979). All contained phycoerythrocyanin in addition to phycocyanin, but species exist that are reddish, i.e. containing phycoerythrin and phycocyanin. Some culture strains of *Anabaena* are well known as facultative heterotrophs (Wolk, 1980). The mol% G + C of the DNA of 19 strains ranged from about 35 to 47 (Herdman et al., 1979a; Stulp and Stam, 1984b; Florenzano et al., 1985). The genome size of six strains ranged from 3.17 to 3.89 × 10^{-9} daltons (Herdman et al., 1979b).

Differentiation of the genus **Anabaena** *from other genera*

Rippka et al. (1979), on the basis of culture strains alone, differentiate *Anabaena* from *Nostoc* primarily on the basis of motility. In *Anabaena*, all vegetative trichomes are normally motile, and any fragmented shorter trichomes appear no different from the "parental" trichome. In *Nostoc*, on the other hand, vegetative trichomes are nonmotile. *Nostoc* appears identical with *Anabaena* in essentially all morphological aspects, but motility is restricted to hormogonia, short chains of cells (lacking heterocysts) often of lesser width than normal vegetative trichomes. Typically, when motility ceases, a terminal heterocyst is differentiated at each end of the new trichome. However, in culture, commonly all motility is lost, in which case *Nostoc* is still distinguished by the production of short, heterocyst-free trichomes which are often narrower than typical trichomes (Rippka et al., 1979). Quite commonly these "hormogonia" possess gas vesicles, even when the parental trichomes do not.

Nostoc is traditionally distinguished from *Anabaena* by forming large or small gelatinous colonies, often of distinctive shape. In some cultures, however, colony growth does not occur. Therefore, the above criteria of Rippka et al. (1979) must be applied. Colonies do form in some axenic cultures (Lazaroff, 1973), however, and this feature in nature is well-correlated with the immotility stage, followed by the dispersal of motile hormogonia. In the case of *Nostoc muscorum*, the "coming-to-rest" of hormogonia is followed by terminal heterocyst differentiation, then by gel formation accompanied by continued cell division (filamentous or aseriate), resulting in a globoid colony from each hormogonium (Lazaroff, 1973). Since colony formation in feral *Nostoc* correlates well with the production of hormogonia which are distinguishable from the parental vegetative trichome, colony formation should continue to be a usable criterion to distinguish *Nostoc* from *Anabaena* as it has been in the past (Geitler, 1932; Bourrelly, 1985).

Anabaena (sensu Castenholz) is here differentiated from *Nodularia*, although the bases for this may be trivial. *Nodularia* has cells which are easily seen to be shorter than broad and usually disklike. Like *Anabaena*, no distinguishable hormogonia are formed, and the vegetative trichomes are motile. *Anabaena* is also distinguished from the well-known genus *Aphanizomenon* by one main characteristic, although other features are also associated with the few species known in the latter genus. In *Aphanizomenon*, the cells are longer than broad, but the last few to several cells at the extremities of the trichomes become gradually more elongate, narrower and essentially hyaline. Other specific features of *Aphanizomenon* are given under the description of that genus.

Anabaena is easily distinguished from *Cylindrospermum* which is characterized (initially) by a single terminal heterocyst which eventually subtends a subterminal, adjacent akinete. Again, no specialized hormogonia are formed, and the vegetative trichomes are normally motile. Commonly, when trichomes of *Cylindrospermum* elongate enough to fragment medially, another terminal heterocyst (and sometimes adjacent akinete) will form on the opposite terminus, either before or after trichome fragmentation.

Florenzano et al. (1985) recently proposed that *Cyanospira*, on the basis of two species isolates, be considered a new genus. These authors separated their material from *Anabaena* on the basis of *Cyanospira* trichomes retaining a characteristic helical pattern even when in culture. Although none of the seven *Anabaena* strains of Rippka et al. (1979) retained a helical shape, it was not the intention of Rippka et al. (1979) to exclude from *Anabaena* those that did. Booker and Walsby (1979) have shown that helical mutants of *Anabaena flos-aquae* may arise from straight trichome clones (Fig. 19.65). Some of the best known species of *Anabaena* have helical trichomes. The 1979 publication of Rippka et al. was intended to begin a tentative definition of *Anabaena* on the basis of seven culture strains, and further extensions were anticipated. Naming new genera because they do not appear exactly as in Rippka et al. (1979) circumvents the entire aim of the "Stanier" system which is to utilize, whenever possible, generic names that have existed previously in the "Geitlerian" tradition and to base these names on an ever-expanding culture collection.

Anabaenopsis Miller 1923 is a genus which, for now, may best be included in *Anabaena* but which may eventually warrant separate status. Most species are curved or helically arranged, but heterocysts occur only terminally, except when trichomes have elongated and double heterocysts form at midlength, with the trichome finally fragmenting between the two, which results again in terminal heterocysts. Although both species of *Cyanospira*, described by Florenzano et al. (1985), had intercalary as well as terminal heterocysts, they appear very similar in other respects to two traditionally described species of *Anabaenopsis*, also known from alkaline African lakes (see Jeeji-Bai et al., 1977).

Cultures

The isolation of *Anabaena* strains by using washing (Carmichael and Gorham, 1974) or self-isolation-by-gliding methods (see this chapter) works, as with many filamentous, gliding cyanobacteria, but here, at least, prior enrichment with or general use of medium free of combined nitrogen has positive selective value. Heterocysts will be formed (if not already present) and nitrogen fixation will occur within a couple of days, often following an initial yellowing (nitrogen-free) period. For the maintenance of cultures, nitrogen-free or nitrogen-depleted medium should also be used for "normal" development and appearance of trichomes.

Reference strains: PCC 7122 (ATCC 27899; CCAP 1403/2a; UTEX 629) as *Anabaena cylindrica* Lemm. (see Stulp and Stam, 1982, 1984b); and UTEX 1616 as *Anabaena sphaerica* Bornet and Flahault (Stulp and Stam, 1982, 1984b).

Type species (Botanical Code): *Anabaena oscillarioides* Bory 1822.

Additional Taxonomic Comments

Anabaena has received more monographic treatment on the basis of axenic cultures than has any other genus in Subsection IV: only *Anabaena* strains have had the benefit of numerous comparisons on the basis of DNA/DNA hybridizations. The major analysis of *Anabaena* has been of Stulp (1983) and Stulp and Stam (1982; 1984a, b; 1985). Sixteen cul-

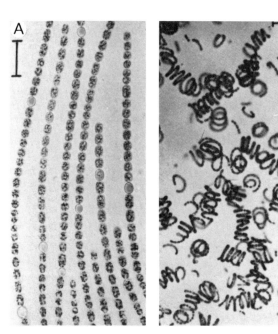

Figure 19.65. *Anabaena flos-aquae* strains. *A,* Gas-vesiculate wild type with straight trichomes (CCAP 1403/13f). *Bar,* 20 µm. *B,* helical mutant (CCAP 1403/13e). *Bar,* 20 µm. (Reproduced with permission from M. J. Booker and A. E. Walsby, British Phycological Journal *14:* 141–150, 1979, ©Academic Press for the British Phycological Society.)

ture strains which could be identified morphologically as falling into previously described species were compared with respect to their DNA base composition, their DNA/DNA reassociation rates, the thermal stability values of DNA/DNA hybrids, and the electrophoretic behavior of five different enzymes. A comparison of these criteria was made with a numerical analysis of morphological traits (Stulp and Stam, 1984b). The results confirmed in almost all cases that most traditionally used morphological criteria used for species distinction reflected genetic and biochemical differences of a similar order of magnitude.

As expected, the mol% G + C of the DNA of all strains was not a useful criteria for separation of species, since all were similar, ranging between 39.0 and 42.6 (Stulp and Stam, 1984b, 1985). The results of DNA/DNA hybridization experiments are given in Table 19.12. The relative binding (%RB) of a heteroduplex (TT) was calculated as:

$$\frac{\text{renaturation rate heteroduplex}}{\text{renaturation rate homoduplex}} \times 100$$

The thermal elution midpoint ($T_{m(e)}$) was determined as the temperature of 50% elution. The $\Delta T_{m(e)}$ value for the heteroduplex is:

$$T_{m(e)} \text{ homoduplex} - T_{m(e)} \text{ heteroduplex}$$

It may be seen that $\Delta T_{m(e)}$ values of intergeneric crosses (i.e. *Anabaena variabilis* × *Nodularia* and *A. variabilis* × *Nostoc*) yielded relative high values for $\Delta T_{m(e)}$ of 11.2 and 12.0°C, respectively. *Intra*specific hybrids of different strains (i.e. *A. cylindrica* × *A. cylindrica* and *A. variabilis* × *A. variabilis*), on the other hand, gave low values for $\Delta T_{m(e)}$, ranging from −0.1 to 2.2°C, and %RB values of 96–108 (Stulp and Stam, 1984b). It is apparent from Table 19.12 that all *inter*specific crosses (species determined by morphological criteria) had relatively high $\Delta T_{m(e)}$ values (4.8–8.8°C) and relatively low %RB values (20.7–53.5). The morphological criteria used in the numerical analysis were: color, trichome shape, vegetative cell shape, heterocyst shape, akinete shape, position of akinetes, shape of terminal cell, and germination pattern. Various alternatives were used for all these criteria (Stulp and Stam, 1984b). The following criteria were each scored as a morphological difference if the mean values

differed by > 10%: vegetative cell length and cell width, heterocyst length and width, and akinete length and width. The clustering of 20 strains based on the numerical analysis of morphological characteristics was in good agreement with identification of the strains to species by Geitler (1932) or most other descriptive treatises (Stulp, 1983; Stulp and Stam, 1982). On this basis, strains showing similarities of >60% were regarded as one species; different species had similarities of 22% or less (Stulp and Stam, 1984b, 1985).

The combined results showed that culture strains of *Anabaena* could be identified as species by using several criteria including morphological characteristics. These characteristics were also shown to be hardly influenced by a wide range of light intensities (350–4000 1x) and by a temperature range of 15°C (Stulp, 1982). In addition, 21 freshwater strains of *Anabaena* were tolerant of medium containing 50% seawater, without morphological change, but 100% seawater greatly affected the morphology of some strains that survived this treatment (Stulp and Stam, 1984a).

The morphologically defined species which stood the scrutiny of the DNA hybridization and other tests were: *Anabaena cylindria* Lemm., *A. variabilis* Kützing, *A. sphaerica* Bornet and Flahault, *A. randhawae*, *A. torulosa* (Carm.) Lagerh. and, to a somewhat lesser extent, *A.* cf. *subtropica* Gardner, *A.* cf. *verrucosa* Boye-Petersen, and *A.* cf. *flos-aquae* (Lyngb.) Bréb. out of as many species. It is, of course, possible that many or most of the remaining species of *Anabaena* described previously by conventional means may also remain after similar tests. The work of Stulp and Stam illustrates that the reduction by Drouet (1978) of *Anabaena* species to only two was one of overskepticism, whereas the compilation of 100 species names for *Anabaena* was probably also quite unrealistic (Stulp, 1983).

A numerical taxonomic study of several species of *Anabaena* and *Nostoc* was undertaken by McGuire (1984) using 28–30 morphological characteristics. No DNA/DNA hybridization was attempted. Of the 10 species of *Anabaena* separated, only 3 (*A. subtropica*, *A. verrucosa* and *A. cylindrica*) were the same as those used by Stulp and Stam (1984b). Therefore, little meaningful comparison can be made at this time. Nevertheless, McGuire (1984) agreed that a separation between the genera *Nostoc* and *Anabaena* was warranted.

Table 19.12.

%RB and $\Delta T_{m(e)}$ values of intraspecific and interspecific hybridizations with DNA from strains[a] of **Anabaena** *and two other genera[b]*

Species names	Strain nos.	%RB	$\Delta T_{m(e)}$
A. cylindrica × *A. cylindrica*	1609 × 1403/2a	108	0.9
A. cylindrica × *A. cylindrica*	1611 × 1446/1a		0.2
A. variabilis × *A. variabilis*	1617 × 1403/8	102	
A. variabilis × *A. variabilis*	1403/12 × 1403/4b		1.2
A. cf. *subtropica* × *A.* cf. *subtropica*	1613 × 1618		7.3
A. cf. *subtropica* × *A.* cf. *subtropica*	1613 × 103		5.1
A. cylindrica × *A. variabilis*	1446/1a × 1403/12	32	7.7
A. cylindrica × *A. variabilis*	1609 × 1403/12		7.1
A. cylindrica × *A. sphaerica*	1611 × 1616		8.8
A. cylindrica × *A.* cf. *flos-aquae*	1611 × 1403/13a	20.7	
A. cylindrica × *A.* cf. *flos-aquae*	1609 × 1403/13a		9.4
A. cylindrica × *A.* cf. *verrucosa*	1611 × 1619	53.5	4.8
A. cylindrica × *A.* cf. *subtropica*	1611 × 1613		8.8
A. cylindrica × *A. randhawae*	1611 × 1823	23.1	
A. cylindrica × *A. torulosa*	1609 × 106	34.2	
A. variabilis × *A.* cf. *flos-aquae*	1403/12 × 1403/13a	34.1	
A. variabilis × *A. randhawae*	1403/8 × 1823	34.3	
A. variabilis × *A. torulosa*	1403/8 × 106	38.6	6.0
A. randhawae × *A. sphaerica*	1823 × 1616	28.3	
A. variabilis × *Nodularia*	1403/8 × 2091		11.2
A. variabilis × *Nostoc*	1403/12 × 382		12.0

[a]Strain numbers of 3 and 4 digits are from UTEX; others are from CCAP.
[b]Data are from Stulp and Stam (1984b, 1985).

Genus II. **Aphanizomenon** Morren 1838

A.pha.ni.zo′me.non. Gr. v. *aphanizo* to disappear; Gr. neut. pass. part. *aphanizomenon*; M.L. neut. n. *Aphanizomenon* obscure thing.

Trichomes are straight and often slightly tapered at both ends; the cells near the termini are also more elongate and more hyaline (low pigment content), appearing vacuolate (Fig. 19.66). Other characteristics include the **arrangement of trichomes into flakelike fascicles (bundles), typically planktonic. The individual trichomes glide against others of the fascicle. Heterocysts are intercalary,** often infrequent and more elongate than the vegetative cells but not much broader. **Akinetes are distant from heterocysts, extremely elongate,** and somewhat wider than vegetative cells. **Gas vesicles** are normally abundant in vegetative cells.

This genus is best known worldwide for the **abundant planktonic species,** *A. flos-aquae* Ralfs ex Bornet and Flahault and *A. gracile* Lemm. which characterize many **mesotrophic and eutrophic lakes** in temperate climates, particularly in late summer and fall. *Aphanizomenon* also occurs in **brackish waters** of the Baltic Sea along with *Nodularia spumigena.*

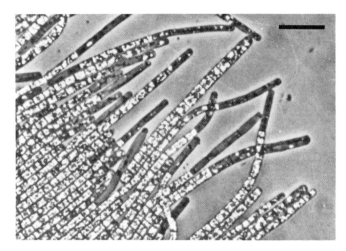

Figure 19.66. *Aphanizomenon flos-aquae* showing empty-appearing cells of terminal portion of trichomes. Light, refractile areas in other cells are masses of gas vesicles. *Bar,* 20 µm. (Reproduced with permission from A. E. Walsby. 1981. Cyanobacteria: planktonic gas-vacuolate forms. *In* Starr, Stolp, Trüper, Balows and Schlegel (Editors), The Prokaryotes. A Handbook on Habitats, Isolation, and Identification of Bacteria. Springer-Verlag, Berlin.)

Differentiation of the genus **Aphanizomenon** from other genera

The special features of *Aphanizomenon* which probably warrant its continuance as a genus apart from *Anabaena* are: (a) the hyaline, elongate cells comprising the trichome termini; and (b) the persistence, at least in nature, of trichomes in fascicular bundles.

Cultures

As yet, little work of a taxonomic nature has been done with pure cultures of *Aphanizomenon.* Problems of isolation and maintenance of this important cyanobacterium are discussed by O'Flaherty and Phinney

(1970), Heaney and Jaworski (1977), McLachlan et al. (1963), and Gentile and Maloney (1969). In unicyanobacterial cultures, normal flake bundle formation was easily maintained if sufficient iron was available (O'Flaherty and Phinney, 1970).

Reference strain: CCAP 1401/1 as *Aphanizomenon flos-aquae* (Lyngb.) Ralfs (see Heaney and Jaworski, 1977).

Type species (Botanical Code): *Aphanizomenon flos-aquae* (Lyngb.) Ralfs (*Byssus flos-aquae* Lyngb.) designated as lectotype.

Genus III. **Nodularia** Mertens 1822

Nod.u.la′ri.a. L. adj. *nodulus* diminutive of nodus, small and knotty, knobby; L. n. *arium* place; M.L. fem. n. *Nodularia* knobby microbial filament.

Nodularia has **vegetative cells, akinetes and heterocysts** that are **shorter than broad and often referred to as discoid or disklike** (Fig. 19.67). Cell **breadth is constant the entire length of the trichome.** The compressed **heterocysts are intercalary,** with equally compressed **akinetes** (often in series) **forming usually distant from heterocysts.** *Nodularia* shows **slow gliding** motility under most conditions.

The mean mol% G + C of the DNA of the one strain analyzed in axenic culture is 40.5 (Herdman et al., 1979a), and the genome size is 3.89×10^9 daltons (Herdman et al., 1979b). The same strain is a facultatively aero-

bic chemoheterotroph using glucose, fructose or sucrose (Rippka et al., 1979).

This genus, particularly *N. spumigena,* is known worldwide as a **planktonic, gas-vesiculate** organism which is often dominant **in inland saline lakes** (Nordin and Stein, 1980) **and in brackish marine waters** such as the Baltic Sea (Östrom, 1976). Salinity appears to be the key factor in the distribution of *Nodularia.* Isolates have generally been made from waters of 3–67°/$_{oo}$ (Nordin and Stein, 1980). Optimum growth occurred in 5–20°/$_{oo}$ (NaCl). *Nodularia* populations are also characteristic of waters with pH values of 8.2–10.0.

Differentiation of the the genus **Nodularia** from other genera

Like *Aphanizomenon,* *Nodularia* is distinguished from *Anabaena* by essentially one characteristic and few species. *Nodularia* has compressed cells, i.e. shorter than broad. Cells of *Anabaena* are longer than broad or more or less spherical. The use of this characteristic for possibly only two species may or may not be sufficient to maintain *Nodularia* as a separate

genus unless future research reveals additional differences. In one test, however, the thermal stability value of a DNA/DNA hybrid between *Nodularia* (UTEX 2091) and *Anabaena variabilis* (CCAP 1403/8) indicates that differences worthy of generic rank may exist between these two strains (Table 19.12).

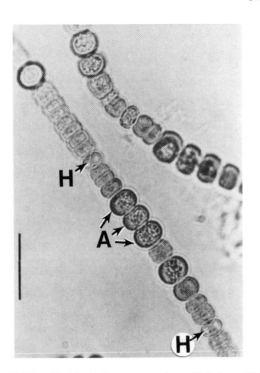

Figure 19.67. *Nodularia harveyana* culture N-8 from Wallender Lake, British Columbia. Cultured at 25°C, pH 9 and 1.6⁰/₀₀. *H,* heterocyst; *A,* akinete. *Bar,* 10 μm. (Reproduced with permission from R. N. Nordin and J. R. Stein, Canadian Journal of Botany *58:* 1211–1224, 1980, ©National Research Council of Canada.)

Cultures

The reference strains have been cultured in medium BG-11 (Rippka et al., 1979) and may be cultured in the culture medium of Hughes et al. (1958) as modified by Booker and Walsby (see Walsby, 1981). Rippka et al. (1979) noted that aerobic growth of PCC 73104 at the expense of N_2 was slow. The range of 25–30°C is usually optimal for growth.

Reference strains: PCC 73104 (ATCC 29167) as *Nodularia harveyana,* isolated from an alkaline saline lake in British Columbia, Canada (UTEX culture 2093, Nordin and Stein, 1980); and UTEX 2091 as *N. spumigena* (Nordin and Stein, 1980).

Type species (Botanical Code): *Nodularia spumigena* Mertens ex Bornet and Flahault.

Additional Taxonomic Comments

Nordin and Stein (1980), on the basis of unicyanobacterial cultures and collected material, have judged that only two species of *Nodularia* exist, *N. spumigena* Mertens ex Bornet and Flahault 1886 and *N. harveyana* (Thwaites) Thuret 1875 emend.

Genus IV. **Cylindrospermum** *Kützing 1843*

Cy.lin.dro.sper′mum. Gr. n. *kylindros* roller, cylinder; Gr. n. *sperma* seed; M.L. neut. n. *Cylindrospermum* (filament) cylinder of seedlike cells.

Trichomes are untapered with a single terminal heterocyst (Fig. 19.68). However, when trichome length increases beyond a certain point, a heterocyst will form at the other end, followed eventually by mid-trichome breakage. **A single akinete or series of akinetes form adjacent to the heterocyst** (Hirosawa and Wolk, 1979a, b). *Cylindrospermum* is **slowly motile and does not produce specialized hormogonia.** Individual sheaths are not produced, but a confluent mucilage holding **many trichomes together** is common.

The mean mol% G + C of the DNA of three strains ranges from 42.1 to 46.7 (Herdman et al., 1979a) with genome sizes of 5.71–6.15 × 10⁹ daltons for two strains (Herdman et al., 1979b).

Of the three strains included by Rippka et al. (1979), all produce phycoerythrocyanin, two are obligate photoautotrophs, and one strain (PCC 7417) is a facultative aerobic chemoheterotroph that grows on fructose or sucrose.

Cylindrospermum is best known as nonplanktonic, i.e. as a part of the **tychoplankton or periphyton of freshwaters.** Some species also occur in **moist subaerial (terrestrial) habitats.**

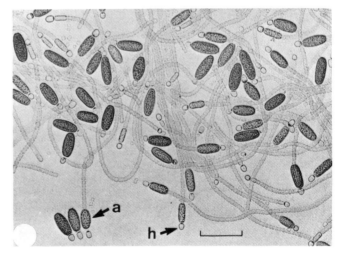

Figure 19.68. *Cylindrospermum* PCC 73101. *h,* heterocyst; *a,* akinete. *Bar,* 50 μm. (Reproduced with permission from R. Rippka et al., Journal of General Microbiology *111:* 1–61, 1979, ©Society for General Microbiology.)

Differentiation of the genus **Cylindrospermum** from other genera

Cylindrospermum, because of the polarity of its trichomes with respect to heterocysts, may be most easily confused with *Calothrix* or some other member of the *Rivulariaceae* ("Subsection IV, Family III"). Since *Calothrix,* when grown in a nitrogen-rich medium, often lacks taper as well as the terminal heterocyst, it may be confused with *Cylindrosper-* *mum* or other genera under those conditions. However, cells of "young" *Cylindrospermum* trichomes are more rectangular than those of *Calothrix* when viewed from the side. It is best to grow material under nutrient restrictive conditions in order to distinguish genera that have trichome polarity.

Cultures

The reference strain is cultured in medium BG-11 (Rippka et al., 1979) (Table 19.1). As with other heterocystous cyanobacteria, *Cylindrospermum* strains are capable of growth in the absence of combined nitrogen.

Reference strain: PCC 7417 (ATCC 29204) as *Cylindrospermum*, isolated from soil in a greenhouse, Stockholm, Sweden (Rippka et al., 1979).

Type species (Botanical Code): *Cylindrospermum stagnale* (Kützing) Bornet and Flahault.

Genus V. **Nostoc** *Vaucher 1803*

Nos′toc. M.L. n. *Nostoc* (origin uncertain, probably invented name).

The **trichomes are untapered** with conspicuous constrictions at cross-walls. The **cells are cylindrical, spherical or ovoid (barrel-shaped)** and are not shorter than broad. **Heterocysts are intercalary** under most circumstances. In general, the description of individual trichomes of *Nostoc* is covered by the description of *Anabaena* ("Family Nostocaceae, Genus I").

Nostoc (sensu Geitler) **is characterized by a confluent gel holding masses of trichomes together, often in the form of a massive thallus which may be spherical, ovoid or of a less discernible shape.** Some colonies or thalli take the form of flattened disks or large sheets or may be soft and amorphous. In many cases, the outer layer of the colony is firm and contains most of the trichomes, while the interior layer is a soft gel with few trichomes which may be radially arranged (Fig. 19.69). The size of colonies range from microscopic (originating from a single hormogonium come to rest) to over 20 cm in diameter.

However, Rippka et al. (1979) consider the formation of a gelatinous colony to be a secondary character, since in culture, **some strains do not form gel and a thallus.** *Nostoc* is, therefore, distinguished (in the absence of colony formation) by the presence of a **developmental cycle.** In *Nostoc,* vegetative trichomes are not capable of gliding motility. However, short chains of cells **(hormogonia) are formed** and released. These, **usually motile** trichomes are initially located adjacent to a heterocyst or between two heterocysts but **lack heterocysts** themselves. The **hormogonia cease movement after a period of "migration," at which time two terminal heterocysts are differentiated. Cell division and growth then resume; this is accompanied by gel formation** under feral and some culture conditions (Lazaroff, 1973). The cell width of hormogonia is commonly less than that of the vegetative trichomes; **often hormogonia are gas-vesiculate and buoyant when the vegetative trichomes are not.** These latter characteristics may be sufficient to distinguish this stage (hormogonium) even when motility is not apparent (as in some culture strains).

The mol% G + C of the DNA for 13 strains of *Nostoc* ranges from **39 to 45** (Herdman et al., 1979a), although several species are probably represented by this assortment. The genome size of 11 of these strains ranges from 4.00 to 6.42×10^9 daltons (Herdman et al., 1979b).

Of the 13 strains examined by Rippka et al. (1979), only 3 were unable to grow as photoheterotrophs. Several species and strains of *Nostoc* grown elsewhere are known to grow slowly as dark chemoheterotrophs (Lazaroff, 1973). Of the 13 strains referred to above, 4 synthesized c-phycoerythrin in addition to phycocyanin. Seven of the others synthesized phycoerythrocyanin instead of phycoerythrin. A few have apparently lost the ability to fix nitrogen aerobically despite the presence of heterocysts. In 10 strains akinetes were capable of being induced. In 2 strains, trichomes of old cultures commonly break up into unicells. Detached unicells commonly occur in masses in developing colonies or in symbiotic associations as well.

Gas vesicles occur in the vegetative cells of several species of *Nostoc*, although few colonies are buoyant enough to be planktonic. Various species of *Nostoc* are known from **benthic habitats in freshwater lakes and springs.** In many cases, the semispherical colonies are not attached but rest lightly on firm or unconsolidated sediments. **Some species are attached to solid substrate in lakes or streams.** Many species of *Nostoc* occur as **amorphous sheets or masses of gel-bound**

trichomes in freshwater or in moist terrestrial locations. As such, *Nostoc* is known to form thick, soft mats in polar regions where presumably it is a major contributor of fixed nitrogen. As a symbiont, *Nostoc* is the the major phycobiont in cyanolichens, but it also occurs as the N_2-fixing symbiont in tripartite, cephalodiate lichens and in several embryophytes such as bryophytes, cycads, and the angiosperm genus *Gunnera* (Stewart et al., 1983).

McGuire (1984), using numerical taxonomy, has distinguished several species of *Nostoc* on the basis of 30 morphological characteristics.

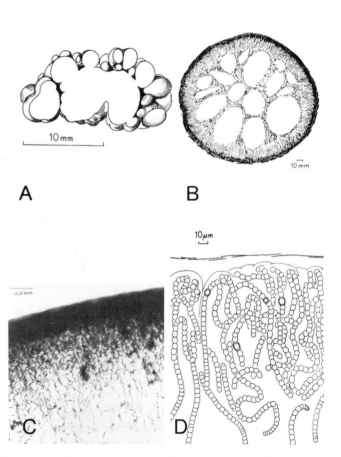

Figure 19.69. *A,* section of proliferating colony of *Nostoc pruniforme. B,* section of spherical colony of *N. pruniforme* with some areas devoid of trichomes in the interior. *C, N. linckia,* showing orientation of trichomes within colony. *D,* diagram of *N. pruniforme,* showing trichome orientation in colony in more detail. (*A, B* and *D* are reproduced with permission from D. Mollenhauer, Abhandlungen der Senckenbergischen Naturforschenden Gesellschaft *524:* 1–80, 1970, ©Waldemar Kramer & Co. *C* is reproduced with permission from P. Bourrelly. 1985. Les Algues d'Eau Douce. Les Algues Bleues et Rouges, Les Eugleniens, Peridiniens et Cryptomonadines. H. Boubée, Paris.)

Differentiation of the genus **Nostoc** from other genera

The principal criterion used for differentiation by Rippka et al. (1979) is the presence of a developmental cycle in *Nostoc* that usually involves nonmotile vegetative trichomes and motile and often morphologically distinct hormogonia. *Anabaena*, the genus most closely resembling *Nostoc*, is distinguished by generally being motile in the vegetative state and lacking a developmental cycle which involves differentiated hormogonia. Rippka et al. (1979) found that hormogonia of *Nostoc* are distinct from vegetative trichomes even when motility was apparently lost (as in some culture strains). Hormogonia of some species of *Nostoc* are very similar microscopically to trichomes of *Pseudanabaena* (Subsection III), including the polar gas vacuoles (Figs. 19.60 and 19.70). However, hormogonia will eventually develop into the nonmotile, thickened and heterocystous trichomes of *Nostoc* with or without gel formation.

The criterion of a developmental cycle in *Nostoc* is recognized by the older, botanical treatments of this genus as well, but the formation of a gelatinous colony or thallus is considered the principal criterion distinguishing this genus. This criterion certainly applies to feral populations but also applies to several culture strains.

Stulp and Stam (1984b) report that the $\Delta T_{m(e)}$ of the heteroduplex (DNA/DNA hybrids) of *Anabaena variabilis* (CCAP 1403/12) and *Nostoc* (UTEX 382) is great enough (12.0°C) to warrant generic separation (see Table 19.12).

Cultures

The reference cultures at the Pasteur Institute are routinely grown in medium BG-11 without the $NaNO_3$, the medium for nitrogen-fixing freshwater cyanobacteria (Table 19.1). However, many species and strains of *Nostoc* exist, and many cyanobacterial culture media are suitable. Since motile or buoyant (gas-vesiculate) hormogonia are produced by *Nostoc*, the isolation of new strains usually employs the recovery of these on agar or liquid surfaces after freshly collected material (or aged crude cultures) are placed on or in nutrient-replete medium.

Reference strains: PCC 73102 (ATCC 29133), isolated from a section of root of the cycad *Macrozamia* (Australia) (Rippka et al., 1979), which contains c-phycoerythrin; and PCC 7107 (ATCC 29150), isolated from a

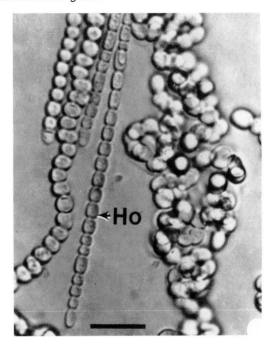

Figure 19.70. *Nostoc muscorum A.* Aseriate stage in early development on *right. Ho*, hormogonium without heterocysts. *Bar*, 10 μm. (Reproduced with permission from N. Lazaroff and W. Vishniac, Journal of General Microbiology *35:* 447–457, 1964, ©Society for General Microbiology.)

shallow pond, Point Reyes Peninsula, California (Rippka et al., 1979), which contains phycoerythrocyanin.

Type species (Botanical Code): *Nostoc commune* Vaucher.

FAMILY II. **SCYTONEMATACEAE**

R. W. Castenholz

Scy.to.ne.ma.ta′ce.ae. M.L. fem. n. *Scytonema* a genus of the family; -aceae ending to denote a family; M.L. fem. n. *Scytonemataceae* the *Scytonema* family.

The family is characterized by the following:

1. **Trichomes, uniseriate,** usually **untapered, and sheathed.**
2. **False branching,** single or double (geminate), frequent or infrequent.
3. **Meristematic regions** instead of diffuse cell divisions usually develop near the apex of the trichome while cell degeneration progresses from the base.
4. **Heterocysts** are predominantly **intercalary** and are often associated with false branches.
5. Akinetes are absent or rare.
6. **Non-heterocyst-containing hormogonia** may be formed (usually terminally) and released. Although a distinctive short chain of cells, hormogonia are the same cell width as the parent trichome.
7. Hormogonia, after coming to rest, differentiate a single terminal heterocyst.
8. Organisms are usually attached, aquatic (freshwater or marine) or terrestrial, often forming macroscopic tufts, cushions or entangled masses.

Geitler (1932) considered that there were 12 genera within this group. Bourrelly (1985) recognized six or seven. Few strains of any genus within this group have been studied in culture for the purposes of taxonomic characterization. Although several genera are described briefly for the purposes of general recognition, only *Scytonema* is characterized here in any detail. Although Geitler (1932), Desikachary (1959) and Bourrelly (1985) include *Plectonema* within this group, it has been mentioned earlier as a part of Subsection III. The lack of heterocysts under any conditions should exclude it from Subsection IV, the order *Nostocales* (sensu Castenholz). *Plectonema* is essentially a sheathed "lyngbyan" trichome that exhibits frequent to infrequent false branching.

Partial list of the genera of the family **Scytonemataceae**

Some genera of the *Scytonemataceae* are briefly described below; others are mentioned by Geitler (1932), Desikachary (1959) and Bourrelly (1970, 1985):

A. *Scytonema* C. A. Agardh 1824—single trichome per sheath and false branches double (geminate), with occasional single false branches; false branching often associated with a heterocyst

B. *Tolypothrix* Kützing 1843—single trichome per sheath and false branches single and generally associated with a single or double heterocyst

C. *Hydrocoryne* Schwabe 1827—a few to several trichomes within one sheath, false branches single, long and lying close to the main filament

D. *Coleodesmium* Borzi 1879 (*Desmonema* Berkeley and Thwaites 1849)—a few to several trichomes within one sheath, false branches single, forming a thallus with pseudodichotomous branching pattern

E. *Scytonematopsis* Kisselewa 1930—single trichome per sheath, false branches usually single, sometimes double (geminate), with the single characteristic separating this genus from *Scytonema* being trichomes that are somewhat tapered at the termini

---

Genus I. **Scytonema** *C. A. Agardh 1824*

Scy.to.ne′ma. Gr. n. *skytos* leather; Gr. n. *nema* thread; M.L. neut. n. *Scytonema* leather thread.

Trichomes are uniseriate and sheathed, with **false branches** double (geminate), sometimes multiple or single, meristematic region near apex (Figs. 19.7 and 19.71). If *Tolypothrix* is included in *Scytonema* (e.g. as a subgenus) or excluded, geminate false branching is absent or rare in that taxon.

Cells may be longer or shorter than broad (Geitler, 1932; Desikachary, 1959; Bourrelly, 1985).

In the reference strain, **hormogonia are formed** which have the same lateral dimensions as vegetative trichomes. **When the period of motility ends, a single terminal heterocyst is formed before cell division and growth resumes** (Rippka et al., 1979).

The mol% G + C of the DNA of the reference strain **is 44.4** (Herdman et al., 1979a). The **genome size is 7.40 × 10⁹ daltons, the largest of all cyanobacteria tested, with the exception of some strains of** *Calothrix* (Herdman et al., 1979b).

The reference strain (cultured in BG-11 medium, Table 19.1) possesses phycoerythrocyanin in addition to phycocyanin and allophycocyanin. It is a facultative aerobic chemoheterotroph, growing in the dark on glucose, fructose or sucrose (Rippka et al., 1979). On agar-solidified medium, upright, aerial growth is conspicuous. Results of studies of *Scytonema stuposum* in nonaxenic, unicyanobacterial cultures showed that the degree of geminate, multiple or single false branching is positively related to heterocyst frequency and, therefore, inversely to the nutrient concentration (e.g. combined nitrogen) of the medium (Jeeji-Bai, 1976). The most typical *Scytonema*-like appearance occurred in the low-nutrient medium. False branching often occurred when immobile heterocysts appear to restrict further growth of the trichome, thus resulting in the bulging and breaking out of trichomes through the sheath.

Reference strain: PCC 7110 (ATCC 29171), subaerial (moist terrestrial), isolated from Crystal Cave, Bermuda, 1971 (see Rippka et al., 1979).

Type species (Botanical Code): *Scytonema hofmanni* Agardh.

Taxonomic Comments

In future revisions, there may be reasons to retain *Tolypothrix* and some other genera as separate entities if *single* false branching develops into a reliable characteristic that is substantiated by *genetic* criteria (e.g. DNA/DNA hybridization tests). *Tolypothrix tenuis* is well-known for axenic culture studies of chromatic adaptation (Diakoff and Scheibe, 1973), but few taxonomic evaluations have been made.

That the type of culture medium (presumably nutrient concentration) can in some cases determine whether single or geminate false branches occur suggests that there may not be a clear generic boundary between *Scytonema* and *Tolypothrix* (Jeeji-Bai, 1976).

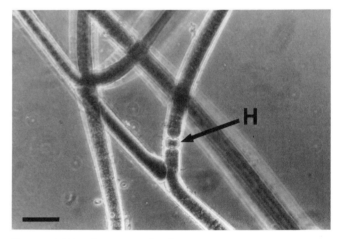

Figure 19.71. *Scytonema* cf. *polycystum* from tropical marine mangrove "lake." *H,* heterocyst above single false branch. *Bar,* 40 μm.

FAMILY III. **RIVULARIACEAE**

R. W. Castenholz

Ri.vu.la.ri.a′ce.ae. M.L. fem. n. *Rivularia* a genus of the family; *-aceae* ending to denote a family; M.L. fem. n. *Rivulariaceae* the *Rivularia* family.

In culture, the family *Rivulariaceae* is best known by strains most easily classified in the genus *Calothrix*. The key characteristic is trichome polarity as seen by taper at one end. However, the polar (basal) heterocyst under appropriate environment may be an even more reliable criterion of true relatedness.

The general distinguishing characteristics are:

1. **Trichome is uniseriate, false branching is rare to common** (no true branching); **trichome is tapered,** although not under all culture conditions.

2. **Heterocysts are terminal** and single-pored, at widened end (base) under appropriate conditions of low combined nitrogen (intercalary heterocysts may also be present).

3. **Cell divisions are usually intercalary** and localized.
4. **Tapered end of the trichome commonly extends into long, pale multicellular hair** (particularly with phosphorus deficiency).
5. **Hormogonia**, short lengths of cells **smaller in diameter than the larger cells of the trichome,** are formed in culture in response to phosphate repletion, following depletion. **After** a period of **gliding, hormogonia** come to rest, **produce a basal heterocyst, and begin tapered growth.**
6. Trichomes are usually attached to substrates individually or in groups forming hemispherical or subspherical "cushions." Colonial planktonic forms (*Gloeotrichia*) with radially arranged trichomes forming spheres also contain gas vesicles, as do hormogonia of many sessile members of this group.

A large number of "traditional" genera have been included in the family *Rivulariaceae. Calothrix* and, to a lesser extent, *Gloeotrichia* and *Rivularia* have been studied extensively in culture, but only *Calothrix* has been studied with mainly taxonomic considerations in mind. Therefore, only *Calothrix* is described in detail. Several species of *Gloeotrichia* and *Rivularia*, however, are well-known as field populations.

Partial list of genera, with heterocysts, of the family **Rivulariaceae**

Many of the "traditional" interpretations of genera of the family *Rivularicaceae* are noted below. Others are described by Geitler (1932), Desikachary (1959) and Bourrelly (1985).

Calothrix C. A. Agardh 1824—basal heterocysts, multicellular terminal hair sometimes absent, akinetes rare, may form adjacent to heterocyst. Sheath or gelatinous mucilage may be present, or aggregates of filaments may occur.
Gloeotrichia C. A. Agardh 1824—similar to *Calothrix* but radially arranged, with sheathed trichomes (filaments) forming a spherical or hemispherical colony. Some species are planktonic; akinete is formed in the later growth phase, adjacent to the heterocyst.
Rivularia C. A. Agardh 1824—similar to *Gloeotrichia.* Gelatinous or crustose hemispherical colonies of *Calothrix*-like filaments are attached, but no akinetes are formed.
Sacconema Borzi 1882—colonial. Sheath is soft, thick and somewhat confluent between *Calothrix*-like trichomes.
Isactis Thuret 1875—crustose expanse of *Calothrix*-like filaments.
Dichothrix Zanardini 1858—*Calothrix*-like trichomes forming false branches. A few to many trichomes in a common sheath, forming brushlike macrothalli, in some cases.
Gardnerula deToni 1936 (*Polythrix* Zanardini 1872)—an elaboration of *Dichothrix.* The attached thallus branches subdichotomously, reaching heights of 1–3 cm.
Microchaete Thuret 1875 (*Fremyella* deToni 1936)—in Geitler (1932) and elsewhere included in the family *Microchaetaceae.* However, it differs from *Calothrix* only by having less taper in the trichome, no terminal hair and a greater number of intercalary heterocysts.

Partial list of genera, without heterocysts, of the family **Rivulariaceae**

Several genera have been described in which trichomes consistently taper, as in *Calothrix;* however, no heterocyst is seen. Since the induction of heterocyst differentiation is usually dependent on external concentrations of ammonium or nitrate, these genera can only be evaluated when they have been critically studied in culture. The following is a partial list of these genera:

Homoeothrix (Thuret) Kirchner 1898—a polarly tapered trichome, but no heterocyst known, with the lack of a heterocyst not merely being considered an environmental effect in at least one study (Whitton, 1987)

Leptochaete Borzi 1882, *Amphithrix* Kützing 1843 and *Tapinothrix* Sauvageau 1892—three polarly tapered genera considered synonymous with *Homoeothrix* (Komárek and Kann, 1973)
Hammatoidea West and West 1897 (or *Ammotoidea* (see Bourrelly, 1985))—a trichome tapered at both ends
Raphidiopsis Fritsch and Rich 1929—a trichome tapered at both ends but producing centrally located akinete or akinetes

The above genera are grouped here in the family *Rivulariaceae* solely on the basis of trichome taper. Whether this is a basic characteristic indicating relatedness or whether it is trivial is unknown.

Genus I. **Calothrix** *Agardh 1824*

B. A. WHITTON

Ca′lo.thrix. Gr. adj. *kalos* beautiful; Gr. n. *thrix* hair; M.L. fem. n. *Calothrix* beautiful filament.

Mature trichome with a tapered morphology, a basal, one-pored heterocyst, and a sheath which is open at the apical end and is usually laminated (Fig. 19.42). **Tapered trichomes range in diameter in their basal region from ~2.5 to 18 μm, with the filaments (i.e. trichome plus sheath) sometimes reaching 30 μm.** *Calothrix* has been discussed in some detail in a review on the *Rivulariaceae* (Whitton, 1987), where references can be found to the literature on which most of the present account is based.

Further Descriptive Information

The principal features used to delimit the various species which have been recognized (80+) are:

1. Trichome width
2. Whether the basal region of trichome is swollen
3. Whether a mature trichome ends in a colorless, multicellular hair
4. Whether intercalary heterocysts occur in addition to the basal one
5. Whether the mature sheath is brown or colorless
6. Whether the trichomes are aggregated into tufts
7. Whether akinetes are formed (*C. stagnalis* Gomont only)

All of these features can be influenced by environmental factors to a greater or lesser extent within individual strains, so the recognition of species by morphological criteria is often difficult. There are, however, considerable differences in the maximum trichome diameter which different strains can attain, so cell dimensions are of some value for taxonomic purposes.

The trichomes of all the species and strains which have been studied critically undergo a somewhat similar "cycle" of morphological changes when grown in culture medium lacking a source of combined nitrogen. In most strains, tapered trichomes and the basal heterocyst develop only when the medium is deficient in combined nitrogen (Sinclair and Whitton, 1977b) (Fig. 19.72). Under phosphorus-rich conditions the apical region of the trichome gives rise to hormogonia usually some 8–10 cells long. These hormogonia are often gas-vacuolate and buoyant. They are sometimes very narrow—perhaps only one quarter of the width of a ma-

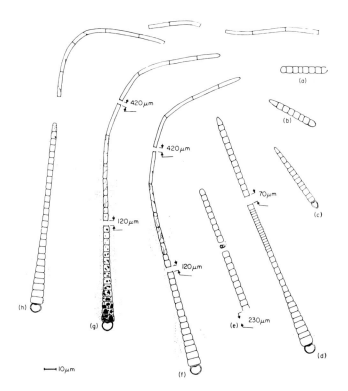

Figure 19.72. Morphological changes in batch culture of *C. parientina* grown to phosphorus deficiency (*a–f*), followed by subsequent changes after addition of further phosphate (*g–h*). Granular inclusions are illustrated only in *g; dotted lines* indicate sheath. *a*, stage I, hormogonium. *b*, stage I, asymmetrical hormogonium. *c*, stage II, heterocyst formation. *d*, stage II, trichome before hair formation. *e*, stage II, hormogonium release from stage II trichome. *f*, stage III, trichome with hair. *g*, stage IV, formation of polyphosphate bodies on the addition of phosphate. *h*, stage IV, hair cells breaking away from trichome, prior to release of hormogonia (stage I). (Reproduced with permission from D. Livingstone and B. A. Whitton, British Phycological Journal *18:* 29–38, 1983, ©Academic Press for the British Phycological Society.)

ture trichome—and can easily be mistaken for *Oscillatoria*. In at least some cases, the width of the hormogonium appears to be influenced by the width of the terminal part of the trichome from which it was derived. The gas-vacuolate condition has a relatively short existence—seldom much more than a day. The hormogonia often have a marked tendency to aggregate into subspherical clumps or ropes, with motility playing an important role at this stage. In *C. kossinskajae* Poljansky, this morphology persists into the mature form, but in most species it is lost, although there is a marked tendency for the trichomes to grow together in clumps. In related "traditional" genera the aggregations of hormogonia persist and ultimately give rise to macroscopic colonies. A terminal cell of each hormogonium differentiates into a single-pored heterocyst; where critical observations have been made, this heterocyst is derived from what was the most basal cell in the parent trichome, thus retaining the original polarity (Fig. 19.72). The developing heterocyst rapidly becomes much paler than adjacent vegetative cells. There is usually only one heterocyst at the base of a trichome, but under conditions in which certain nutrients (especially iron and molybdenum) are limiting, a new one-pored heterocyst may develop from the basal vegetative cell, while the previous heterocyst collapses (Fig. 19.64).

The trichome increases in length by an increase in cell size and cell division. Cell division is restricted to the basal part, although differences occur between strains in the extent to which this is localized. Where

localization of division is marked, some authors refer to this region as a meristematic zone. A taper develops because basal cells increase in width and apical cells decrease in width. If the phosphate content of the trichome remains high enough, a hormogonium develops at the apex, and in some species, it appears that formation of new hormogonia can take place indefinitely. At least in some cases (Wood et al., 1986), each hormogonium is separated from the rest of the trichome by a necridial cell, which is detached when the next hormogonium to form glides out of the sheath (Fig. 19.72).

Hormogonium formation ceases when the phosphorus content of the trichome drops sufficiently low. In some cases, the end of the trichome then starts to differentiate into a multicellular hair. No new cells are involved, merely a further narrowing of cell width combined with great increase in length, resulting in an overall increase in cell surface. The cells lose their pigment, granular inclusions and most of the cytoplasm. Much of the interior of a mature hair cell consists of one or more intrathylakoidal "vacuoles." Although hairs are a typical feature of many of the commonest species of *Calothrix*, some forms never develop a hair in the field or the laboratory.

When inorganic or organic phosphate is added (under conditions favorable for metabolic activity) to trichomes with hairs, polyphosphate bodies form rapidly in vegetative cells, often being visible with the optical microscope in cells of the basal region of the trichome in <5 min (Sinclair and Whitton, 1977a). Sometime later the most apical region of the vegetative cells, below the hair, differentiates into a hormogonium (without any cell division), and the hair falls off. In the laboratory, hairs can sometimes also form under conditions of iron deficiency (Sinclair and Whitton, 1977a; Douglas et al., 1986), although it is unclear whether this has any functional importance in nature. Such hairs do not reach the same lengths as those formed under conditions of phosphorus deficiency.

Many strains of phycoerythrin-containing *Calothrix* show "chromatic adaptation." There is a tendency for some heterocysts of many tropical species to be blue, a tendency which has been noted by Fritsch (1945) for tropical *Rivulariaceae* (*sensu* Rabenhorst 1865) as a whole. The blue, which is associated with the phycocyanin of phycobilisomes of the thylakoids, is not persistent from the original vegetative cell, as was suggested by Fritsch, but arises afresh in mature heterocysts (Whitton et al., 1987).

Considerable differences occur in the arrangement and structure of the sheath, although, as with other cyanobacteria, little is known of its possible significance. Colored sheaths range from golden brown to very dark brown. The color is usually obvious only in cultures which are becoming nutrient-limited. The sheath seldom covers the basal heterocyst, whereas in most cases it reaches only to the most basal vegetative cell. Freshly released hormogonia sometimes orientate themselves in particular ways within or adjacent to one part of the sheath of a mature trichome, and complex arrangements sometimes result in the formation of a thallus with a characteristic appearance. This effect is most pronounced in the "traditional" genus *Dichothrix* Zanardini, which is separated from *Calothrix* in most botanical treatments (e.g. Geitler, 1932; Desikachary, 1959).

Results of a study by Herdman et al. (1979a) of the DNA base composition of a wide range of cyanobacteria showed that all 11 *Calothrix* strains fell within a narrow span (mol% G + C of the DNA is 39.8–44.4). The genome sizes of 10 of these strains studied by Herdman et al. (1979b) fell into two groups: 7 ranged from 5.07×10^9 to 5.46×10^9 daltons and 3 ranged from 7.75×10^9 to 8.58×10^9 daltons. However, a division of the genus on this basis is not consistent with any other known phenotypic properties (Rippka et al., 1979). Hybridization of three different nitrogen fixation genes from *Anabaena* species to DNA of *Gloeothece* species and *Calothrix* species PCC 7601 showed that the *Calothrix* was more like *Anabaena* than *Gloeothece* (Kallas et al., 1983).

Culture

Most species of *Calothrix* are easily brought into culture. Those which commonly grow in nature in alternating wet-dry environments, such as

C. parietina at the margins of lakes, ponds and streams and *C. crustacea* on marine shores, are particularly robust. The production of clonal isolates can, in most cases, be regarded as a routine procedure. The best method is to induce the formation of hormogonia on agar by adding phosphate to phosphate-deficient material under conditions favorable for metabolic activity, such as a suitable temperature and light. This can often be done directly by dissecting out portions of a mixed population which includes *Calothrix* and continuing growth in the laboratory for a few days in a low-phosphate enrichment culture. After phosphate is added, the culture should be observed with a dissecting microscope every couple of hours in order to remove a hormogonium as soon as possible after it has moved out of the parent sheath. The procedure can also be carried out in liquid culture, when gas-vacuolate hormogonia will tend to float to the surface; however, under these conditions it is impossible to be certain which was the parent trichome of a particular hormogonium. It is usually possible to obtain bacteria-free cultures by letting the hormogonia grow to form a mature culture, repeat the above procedure, and make subcultures from a number of carefully chosen hormogonia.

Although most *Calothrix* strains appear to form easily in a range of laboratory media, care is needed if the organism is to develop a morphology similar to that typical of its growth in nature. The most important requirements are to use a medium with a low phosphate and low combined nitrogen content. At least for preliminary studies, phosphate-P in the medium should not be allowed to rise above 1 mg l^{-1}, and batch cultures should always be grown to moderate phosphorus deficiency. Under such conditions, the bulk of the culture should appear healthy, lacking anomalous swellings or contorted hairs. Strains which have been subcultured in a high-phosphate medium for a long time often develop strange morphologies, even if they grow rapidly (B. A. Whitton, unpublished data). It is unclear whether such changes involve irreversible genetic change, but it is recommended that strains in older culture collections should be avoided for most research purposes, unless their previous cultivation history is known.

Reference strain: Durham Culture Collection 550.

Details of the stream from which this strain was isolated have been given by Holmes and Whitton (1981) and Livingstone and Whitton (1984), and details of its growth in the laboratory have been given by Livingstone et al. (1983), Livingstone and Whitton (1983) and Wood et al. (1986).

Mature trichomes of this strain are mostly 8–10 µm wide near the base, occasionally reaching 12 µm. The basal region of the trichome is not swollen, so the trichome tapers gradually. Phycoerythrin is not formed when this strain is grown in green light. Hormogonia are gas-vacuolate initially; they soon show a marked tendency to aggregate, forming long ropes if sufficient numbers of hormogonia at a similar stage in development come into contact with each other. A terminal (one-pored) heterocyst is formed when the hormogonium is grown in the absence of combined nitrogen; this heterocyst shows no tendency for a secondary development of blue color; intercalary heterocysts are rare. A multicellular hair develops under conditions of moderate phosphate deficiency, eventually becoming many times the length of the vegetative trichome with increasing phosphate deficiency; an older hair cell usually contains only one large intrathylakoidal vacuole. Shorter hairs are formed under conditions of iron deficiency. Akinetes are not formed, nor is there any tendency for pseudodichotomous branching or groups of trichomes to originate within a single sheath. Phosphorus can be supplied as inorganic phosphate or as a variety of organic forms. Cultures grown on a light-dark cycle show nitrogenase activity during both light and dark parts of the cycle, although activity is much reduced in the dark. When sucrose is used, this strain is capable of prolonged growth in the dark, providing conditions are otherwise very favorable; such growth is much slower than that of many other cyanobacteria grown in the dark, although it is considerably better in the presence of ammonia than in the absence of combined nitrogen; when this strain is grown in the dark, the sheath is a particularly dark brown.

Taxonomic Considerations

Results of two types of biochemical study suggest possible differences separating *Calothrix* and related genera from most other cyanobacteria, and these genera merit further study. Four strains of cyanobacteria, referred to as the "*Calothrix* type" by Kenyon et al. (1972), all possess a tetra-unsaturated fatty acid (octodecatetraenoic acid), a feature found in only one strain belonging to other groups. Brominated substances have been reported from a *Calothrix* (Pedersen and DaSilva, 1973) and two different species of *Rivularia* (Pedersen and DaSilva, 1973; Norton and Wells, 1982; Maehr and Smallheer, 1984).

A number of other genera resemble *Calothrix,* in that the typical trichome form is a tapered one. Examples of the most important genera have been brought into culture, but studies are too fragmentary for them to receive a full treatment here. *Homoeothrix,* which includes tapered forms lacking a heterocyst, has been the subject of a detailed taxonomic and ecological study with classical botanical approaches used (Komárek and Kann, 1973). At least superficially, some species look somewhat like a tapered *Lyngbya,* whereas others look much like species of *Calothrix* lacking a heterocyst. Where critical studies have been made, it has been shown that the lack of a heterocyst is not merely an environmental effect.

Growth of *Calothrix* strains in the presence of combined nitrogen usually results in profound morphological changes (Sinclair and Whitton, 1977b). Heterocyst formation is suppressed, and in most cases the trichomes lack tapering. If tapering does occur, it may take place in only one direction (thus resembling the genus *Homoeothrix*) or in both directions (resembling *Hammatoidea*).

Rivularia and *Gloeotrichia* form macroscopically visible colonies, usually hemispherical or subspherical. These genera have tapered trichomes which have orientated such that the heterocysts are toward the inside of the colony. Colonies almost always develop from an aggregation of many hormogonia (Whitton, 1987). Almost all species in these genera have the ability to form long hairs, and this is the typical condition in which they occur in nature. *Rivularia* lacks the ability to form akinetes, whereas *Gloeotrichia* forms them. Although species within these genera have been brought into culture, in general this is more difficult to do than with *Calothrix,* and in many cases, trichome morphology in culture has proved to be different from that in nature. There are indications that these genera may differ from typical species of *Calothrix* by more than just the ability to form colonies.

Ultrastructural studies have been made of species of *Gloeotrichia* (Miller and Lang, 1971; Cmiech et al., 1984), and there is some indication that they may differ from species of *Calothrix,* particularly with respect to hair structure (Guglielmi, 1975; Wood et al., 1986). Fliesser and Jensen (1982) have described a range of cell inclusions from strains of *Calothrix* and related genera, several of which have so far not been recorded from other cyanobacteria. To establish what use these inclusions are for taxonomic purposes will, however, require further study.

There are considerable advantages in retaining the generic names *Gloeotrichia* and *Rivularia* for descriptive purposes in habitats such as rice fields. It is therefore suggested that they be reserved as separate genera, at least until they have been subjected to detailed study using modern criteria. On the other hand, there seems little justification in retaining *Dichothrix* as a separate genus. Here the trichome shows subdichotomous branching, and several trichomes originate from within a single sheath at each branching point. Some 25+ species of *Dichothrix* have been recognized. There are several other genera which include forms which appear to provide a continuum with forms included in *Calothrix.* The rivularian type most widely used in the physiological research has been *Microchaete* Thuret 1875 (synonym *Fremyella* deToni 1936), some species of which differ from a non-hairforming *Calothrix* in little more than a lesser tendency to taper and a greater tendency to form intercalary heterocysts. In spite of this similarity, *Microchaete* has seldom been included, even within the family *Rivulariaceae.* Some species of *Tolypothrix* (see "Subsection IV, Family II. *Scytonemataceae*") have a developmental stage which appears rather like a filament of *Calothrix.*

SUBSECTION V. ORDER **STIGONEMATALES**

R. W. CASTENHOLZ

Stig′o.ne.ma.tal′es. M.L. fem. n. *Stigonema* genus of order; -*ales* ending denoting order; M.L. fem. pl. n. *Stigonematales* the *Stigonema* order.

Genera of the order *Stigonematales* exhibit the **highest degree of morphological complexity and differentiation within the cyanobacteria. Pitlike synapses or pore channels occur between cells** of trichomes in some of these genera. **Longitudinal and oblique cell divisions occur** in addition to transverse cell divisions. This **results in periodic true branching in all genera and in multiseriate trichomes (two or more rows of cells) in some genera.** False branching also occurs in some genera. **Heterocysts are both intercalary and terminal.** Although reproduction occurs by random breakage of trichomes, **hormogonia are also formed in most strains. Akinetes are produced in some** genera.

In most cases, **the width of trichomes varies greatly even within a single clone,** since narrower *secondary* trichomes, arising as branches of thickened primary trichomes, occur as a regular phenomenon, even in uniseriate species.

The **mol% G + C of the DNA ranges only from 41.9 to 46.3** for the nine strains examined (Herdman et al., 1979a). However, these represent only two genera and probably two species as well. The **genome size**

of the same two genera (six strains in all) **ranges from 3.62 to 5.24 × 10⁹ daltons** (Herdman et al., 1979b).

The **best known aquatic forms** in culture are the various isolates of *Fischerella (Mastigocladus laminosus)* which **typify flowing waters of hot springs,** at least below temperatures of 57–58°C. However, **a large number** of uncultured or poorly studied stigonematalean cyanobacteria **are known from slightly acidic, oligotrophic lakes and from fast-flowing streams.** An equally large number occur in **moist subaerial environments.**

Only two genera have been recharacterized from axenic culture strains, *Fischerella* and *Chlorogloeopsis.* However, it is certain from field observations that several other genera exist and have not yet been cultured. Bourrelly (1985) recognizes six families and 35 genera within the *Stigonematales.* Geitler (1932), not recognizing the order, nevertheless, includes four families and most of the genera. Because of the large number of genera and species, few of which are known in culture, only four genera are described here. The following simplified key includes relatively few of the genera considered by Bourrelly (1985) and others.

Key to the selected genera of the order **Stigonematales** *(Subsection V)*

A. True branching dichotomous or subdichotomous ....B
A. True branching lateral, irregular or filamentous habit indistinct C
B. Calcareous deposits surrounding filaments
      Genus IV. *Geitleria* Friedmann 1955 (described in text), p. 1798
B. Noncalcareous
      Genus *Loriella* Borzi 1892
C. Heterocysts as distinct lateral cell, or terminal on short lateral branches, but not intercalary
      Genus *Nostochopsis* Wood 1869
    Or, if marine, endolithic in carbonates
      Genus *Mastigocoleus* Lagerheim 1886
C. Heterocysts intercalary, sometimes terminal ....D
D. Produces *hormocysts* and hormogonia, trichomes uniseriate
      Genus *Westiella* Borzi 1907
D. Hormogonia may be produced; trichomes uniseriate or multiseriate, or semiamorphous ....E
E. True branches, if distinguishable, not different in cell type from main axis ....F
E. True branches with cells different from those of main axis (including *Mastigocladus* Cohn 1862)
      Genus II. *Fischerella* Gomont (described in text), p. 1795
F. Trichome uniseriate throughout
      Genus *Hapalosiphon* (Näg.) Kützing
F. Trichome multiseriate, at least in part
      Genus III. *Stigonema* Agardh (described in text), p. 1798
F. Mature trichomes divide in more than one plane but fragment into irregular *Gloeocapsa*-like aggregates.
      Genus I. *Chlorogloeopsis* Mitra and Pandey (described in text), p. 1794

Genus I. **Chlorogloeopsis** *Mitra and Pandey 1966*

Chlor′o.gloe.op′sis. Gr. adj. *chloros* green; Gr. adj. *gloios* sticky; Gr. n. *opsis* appearance, hence resemblance; M.L. fem. n. *Chlorogloeopsis* (cyanobacterium) resembling alga *Chlorogloea* Mitra.

The **filamentous nature** of this organism is **often unclear, except in hormogonia. Hormogonia** are composed of **short chains of cylindrical or barrel-shaped cells which, after ceasing motility, enlarge to become spherical cells** (Fig. 19.73). **Heterocysts develop in both intercalary and terminal positions** when levels of combined nitrogen are low. Growth continues with cell divisions in more than one plane (Fig. 19.73), so that **multiseriate trichomes** develop. The filamentous nature of the organism is usually lost, however, since the **growing mass of cells commonly fragments into clusters or amorphous aggregates of cells,** generally within a mucilaginous sheath (Rippka et al., 1979) (Fig. 19.73). **Hormogonia arise from such aggregates. Uneven (asymmetric) divisions of vegetative cells**

occur; small heterocysts occur when strains are deprived of combined nitrogen (Foulds and Carr, 1981). **Masses of vegetative cells may also enlarge to form thicker-walled cells (akinetes). Akinete germination** takes place with division **in several planes** and the shedding of the extra wall layers (Rippka et al., 1979). Synaptic "pore channels," common in many genera in Subsection V, are not present.

The **mol% G + C of the DNA of two strains are 42.1 and 42.9** (Herdman et al., 1979a). The **genome sizes are 4.20 and 5.24 × 10⁹ daltons** (Herdman et al., 1979b). Both strains included by Rippka et al. (1979) are **facultative, aerobic chemoheterotrophs** utilizing sucrose best but also glucose, fructose and ribose. **Phycoerythrocyanin** is synthesized by both strains.

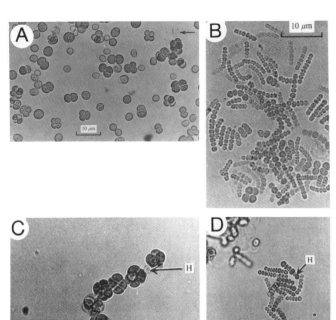

Figure 19.73. *Chlorogloeopsis fritschii* (CCAP 1411/1). *A,* photoheterotrophic growth after growth in solid medium. *arrow,* discarded sheath material. *B,* photoautotrophic growth, after transfer from photoheterotrophic conditions. Many hormogonia are present. *C,* photoheterotrophic growth in liquid medium lacking combined nitrogen. *H,* heterocyst. *D,* earlier stage of growth as depicted in *C,* with heterocysts (*H*) sometimes differentiating in hormogonia. (Reproduced with permission from E. H. Evans, I. Foulds and N. G. Carr, Journal of General Microbiology *92:* 147–155, 1976, ©Society for General Microbiology.)

Differentiation of the genus **Chlorogloeopsis** *from other genera*

There is a close resemblance of *Chlorogloeopsis* to phases of the developmental cycle of some species of *Nostoc.* The aseriate stages of *Nostoc* are hardly distinguishable from similar phases of *Chlorogloeopsis.* The motile hormogonia are also similar. However, in *Chlorogloeopsis* there are very clearly divisions in more than one plane, in hormogonia that have come to rest and in the "unicellular" and cluster phases (see Fig. 19.73). In *Nostoc* during aseriate stages, cells become detached and disoriented, but two or more planes of division are not discernible.

Cultures

Chlorogloeopsis is one of the cyanobacteria most easily grown as a chemoheterotroph. A common growth medium used is that of Kratz and Myers (1955) supplemented with NaHCO₃ (0.1%) (Table 19.1). Sucrose at 10 mM concentration is included when necessary (Evans et al., 1976). Under photoautotrophic conditions (after inoculation), there is a progression from short trichomes or hormogonia (Fig. 19.73) to multiseriate trichomes, to aseriate clusters or aggregates (Fig. 19.73). Growth in the light in the presence of sucrose, however, did not allow the development of trichomes. Unicells or small groups of cells (Fig. 19.73*A*) gave rise to larger spherical clusters of cells and eventually to larger aseriate aggregates (Fig. 19.73). Dark chemoheterotrophic growth on sucrose maintained aseriate clusters of cells and again no trichome formation (Evans et al., 1976).

Reference strain: PCC 6912 (ATCC 27193, CCAP 1411/1). This culture was first isolated from the soil of India by A. K. Mitra as *Chlorogloea fritschii.*

Type species (Botanical Code): *Chlorogloeopsis fritschii* Mitra and Pandey 1966.

Additional Taxonomic Considerations

Although there are few criteria besides morphological characteristics to use at present, the thermophilic cyanobacterium referred to recently as "high temperature form (HTF) *Mastigocladus*" appears to resemble *Chlorogloeopsis* in most respects (Castenholz, 1978). It occurs in hot springs worldwide up to temperatures of 63–64°C. Similar hormogonia are formed by both aseriate and essentially unicellular cultures (Fig. 19.74).

The mol% G + C of the DNA in three strains of "HTF *Mastigocladus*" are 43.2, 43.5 and 44.8 (R. Rippka, personal communication).

Earlier authors observing forms in nature similar to "HTF *Mastigocladus*" have simply referred to these as forms or varieties of *Mastigocladus* (or *Hapalosiphon*) *laminosus* (e.g. Frémy, 1936; Schwabe, 1960). *Mastigocladus laminosus* (sensu stricto), which displays true branches, is here included in the genus *Fischerella* as in Rippka et al. (1979).

Genus II. **Fischerella** *Gomont 1895*

Fisch.er.el'la. M.L. fem. n. *Fischerella* Fischer; probably named for B. Fischer, botanical bacteriologist, 1852–1915.

The **true branches** of this organism are **uniseriate and composed of cells** that are **generally longer than broad,** particularly those distal from the base. **The axis (primary trichome)** from which they arise is **mainly uniseriate** as well **but may become multiseriate** in part, with divisions in more than one plane. The axis in these regions, however, is seldom more than 2–3 cells in thickness. In addition, the cells of the axes become enlarged, often semispherical in shape. The older cells of a

main axis may become separated from each other by sheath material and may act as akinetes (Martin and Wyatt, 1974). Most of the widened cells of the axial trichome, however, possess a true filamentous nature with only a peptidoglycan septum separating cells (Nierzwicki et al., 1982b; Balkwill et al., 1984). **The main axis forms when a hormogonium comes to rest, cells enlarge, and some cell divisions begin that are parallel to the long axis** or diagonal (oblique); **some of the resulting**

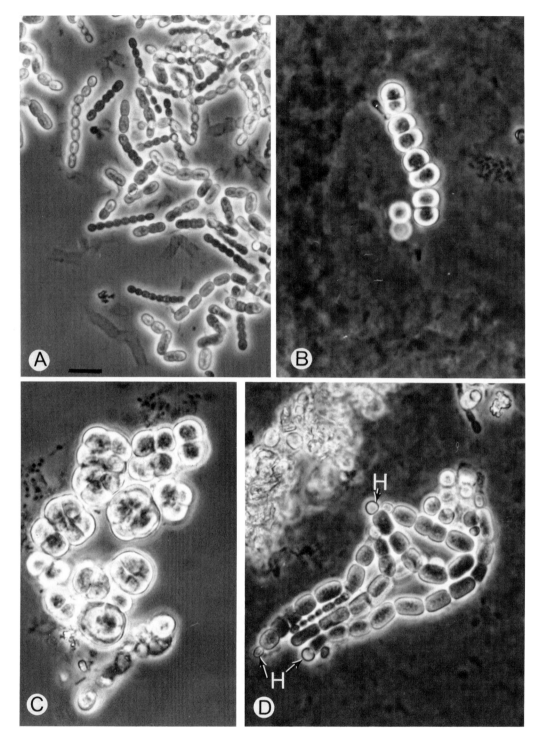

Figure 19.74.   HTF *Chlorogloeopsis* (culture University of Oregon I-15-HTF, clone 1). *A*, motile hormogonia in nitrate-replete medium (45°C). *Bar*, 10 μm. *B*, later stage under the same conditions. *C*, later amorphous phase. *D*, trichomes in medium lacking combined nitrogen. *H*, heterocyst. For *B–D*, the same scale as in *A* applies.

cells elongate to form branches (secondary trichomes) (Balkwill et al., 1984; Nierzwicki-Bauer et al., 1984) (Fig. 19.75).

These narrow secondary trichomes (which may taper) become progressively longer with cell elongation and transverse divisions. In field populations of *Fischerella (Mastigocladus laminosus)* in flowing hot springs, almost the entire mass is composed of tufts or streamers of secondary trichomes several centimeters in length, and no branching is seen except in the prostrate attached mass or primary trichomes (main axes). In culture, at least, secondary trichomes of thermophilic *Fischerella* may eventually differentiate series of spherical, thick-walled cells that are akinetelike. Typical cyanobacterial akinete types are not easily recognizable. In some cases, the widened cells may divide in a second plane and form new branches (i.e. secondary trichomes).

The **hormogonium is a gliding, rotating trichome composed of**

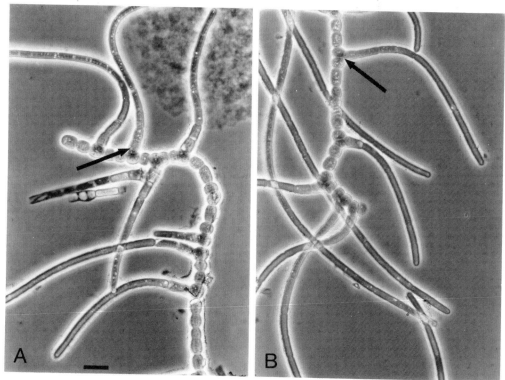

Figure 19.75. *Fischerella (Mastigocladus laminosus)* culture University of Oregon I-S₅-M, clone 5, growing in replete medium at 45°C. *A*, showing true branching (*arrow*) from uniseriate primary trichome (main axis). *Bar*, 10 μm. *B*, showing "inverted v" branching (*arrow*) (see Castenholz, 1972). For *B*, the same scale as in *A* applies.

few (~11–16), **narrow, morphologically uniform cells that are cylindrical or slightly barrel-shaped** (Hernández-Muñiz and Stevens (1987)) (Fig. 19.76). They are formed as the distal portion of branches. No heterocysts differentiate until after hormogonia have ceased motility. **Heterocysts** of *Fischerella (Mastigocladus laminosus)* **are elongate, spherical or even compressed (shorter than broad) and are lateral, terminal or intercalary.** Heterocysts of thermophilic strains are, at least, different from typical heterocysts of the *Nostocales,* in that they possess only one additional wall layer (homogeneous type) and have densely stacked lamellar membranes (Nierzwicki-Bauer et al., 1984).

Most of the information on *Fischerella* from culture has been from the thermophilic species, which is common in neutral pH and alkaline hot springs throughout the world (Castenholz, 1978). However, Martin and Wyatt (1974) have compared the physiology of six strains of stigonematalean cyanobacteria, including five strains of three species of *Fischerella,* none of which were thermophilic. Besides the true branching habit, the great diversity of form as described by Frémy (1936), Schwabe (1960), Rippka et al. (1979) and Balkwill et al. (1984) for *Fischerella (Mastigocladus laminosus)* also applies to these nonthermophilic representatives. In the nonthermophilic strains, hormogonia were not always formed under the expected conditions, and sometimes the multiseriate condition of the axis was rare or lacking.

Thurston and Ingram (1971) have also studied the morphology and fine structure of another nonthermophilic species of *Fischerella* in which they show details of synaptic connections, with microplasmodesmata joining adjacent cells in the branch trichomes (Fig. 19.2).

All seven strains of *Fischerella* examined by Rippka et al. (1979) synthesize phycoerythrocyanin (see also Füglistaller et al., 1981). All strains were capable of **photoheterotrophic and dark chemoheterotrophic** growth, utilizing glucose, fructose or sucrose and, in two cases, ribose.

The mol% G + C of the DNA of the seven strains ranged from 41.9 to 46.3 (Herdman et al., 1979a). The genome size of four strains ranged from 3.62 to 4.75 × 10⁹ daltons (Herdman et al., 1979b).

Although *Fischerella (Mastigocladus laminosus)* forms dominant, almost monotypic, populations in many **hot springs,** species of nonthermophilic *Fischerella* are generally not as conspicuous and often occur in **moist subaerial habitats.** Marine forms are rare or lacking.

Differentiation of the genus **Fischerella** from other genera

The complex variety of forms or developmental stages taken by *Fischerella,* which may include primary and secondary trichomes, hormogonia, unicells and amorphous cell aggregates, makes identifying any single stage difficult. *Fischerella,* however, is most easily confused with the genera, *Stigonema* and *Hapalosiphon.* In *Stigonema,* the main axis and the branches become multiseriate or multicellular; however, the growing tips are usually uniseriate, and this condition may extend for some distance. *Fischerella,* on the other hand, has secondary trichomes (branches) with more elongate and narrower cells than those of the primary trichome (main axis). The main axis may be multiseriate in part.

Hapalosiphon (not described here) is defined as being uniseriate throughout with branches similar to the main axis. The limits separating these three genera are not clear-cut for all species described (see Desikachary, 1959; Geitler, 1932; Bourrelly, 1985).

Cultures

The several strains used for the description of *Fischerella* by Rippka et al. (1979) were all thermophiles ascribed to the genus *Mastigocladus.* Cultures are easily maintained in a variety of media with or without combined nitrogen, e.g. BG-11 (Rippka et al., 1979), medium B (Stevens et al., 1973), and D medium (Castenholz, 1981) (Table 19.1). When mature cultures are inoculated on agar-solidified medium, motile hormogonia are readily formed. Although thermophilic forms are the cosmopolitan "weeds" of hot springs, medium with a high content of ammonium (i.e. >2 mM) is usually inhibitory. Nonthermophilic species of *Fischerella* have been grown in CG-10 medium (Thurston and Ingram, 1971) and ASM-1 medium (Gorham et al., 1964; Carr et al., 1973; Martin and Wyatt, 1974).

Reference strains: PCC 7115 (ATCC 27929), isolated from Tassajara Hot Springs, California (Rippka et al., 1979) as *Mastigocladus* species H₂; and PCC 7522 (ATCC 29539, Oregon NZ-86-m), isolated from a hot spring, Whakarewarewa, New Zealand (Rippka et al., 1979) as *Mastigocladus laminosus*.

Type species (Botanical Code): *Fischerella thermalis* (Schwabe) Gomont.

Additional Taxonomic Considerations

For the present, there appears to be insufficient reason to separate the genus *Mastigocladus* from *Fischerella*. The original description (*Mastigocladus* Cohn 1862) gave insufficient information, and subsequent redefinitions have attempted to use the possession of inverted "V" branches in addition to true and false branches to distinguish *Mastigocladus* from *Fischerella* (Schwabe, 1960) or to establish *Mastigocladus laminosus* as *Hapalosiphon laminosus* (Frémy, 1936). Although such modified false branches ("V" type) do occur in some strains (see Fig. 19.75B), this characteristic does not warrant separation of *Mastigocladus* as a separate genus until further study is completed.

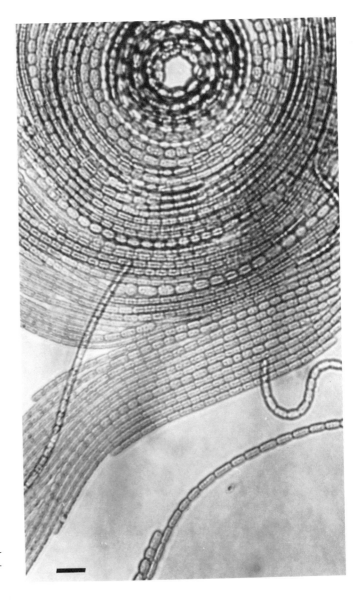

Figure 19.76. *Fischerella (Mastigocladus laminosus)* culture NZ-69-M, clone 1, showing the circling of motile hormogonia on an agar surface at 45°C. *Bar,* 10 μm.

Genus III. **Stigonema** Agardh 1824

Sti.go.ne′ma. Gr. n. *stigeus* one who marks; Gr. n. *nema* thread; M.L. fem. n. *Stigonema* segmented filament.

Many species of this genus are **extreme examples of multicellular complexity** in the cyanobacteria. **Main axes with numerous branches may reach thicknesses of 1 mm** (Fig. 19.77). **Pore channels (synapses of microplasmodesmata) occur between all cells derived by divisions** (Fig. 19.78). Branches, although initially simpler than the main axis, eventually become as complex. Tips of branches may be uniseriate for a considerable distance.

Only *Stigonema minutum* (Agardh) Hass. has been isolated in culture (unicyanobacterial), but taxonomic studies have not been made (Zehnder, 1985).

Stigonema is a **freshwater or subaerial (terrestrial) genus found commonly on moist rocks or soil or in oligotrophic, slightly acidic lakes and** in some **streams.** Conspicuous tufted benthic mats of *Stigonema* occur in some oligotrophic lakes.

Genus IV. **Geitleria** Friedmann 1955

Geit.ler′i.a. M.L. fem. n. *Geitleria* Geitler; named after L. Geitler, Austrian botanist and specialist in blue-greens, 1899–.

Branching is pseudodichotomous, dichotomous and lateral (Fig. 19.78). The **sheath becomes heavily calcified,** and only the **cells near the tips of trichomes** are able to **give rise to a lateral branch** or, when an apical cell undergoes an oblique division followed by further divisions of both cells, to a false dichotomy (Friedmann, 1955). The ultrastructure of decalcified specimens, including that of pore channels

(i.e. "pit connections") has been studied by Couté (1982, 1985) (Fig. 19.78B). **No cultures** of this genus have been established.

Geitleria calcarea is a **calcified cyanobacterium of limestone caves,** together with *Scytonema julianum* (Friedmann, 1955; Couté, 1985).

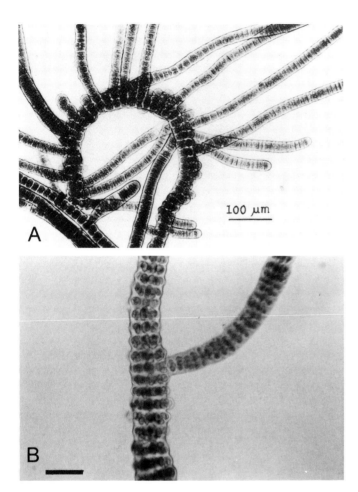

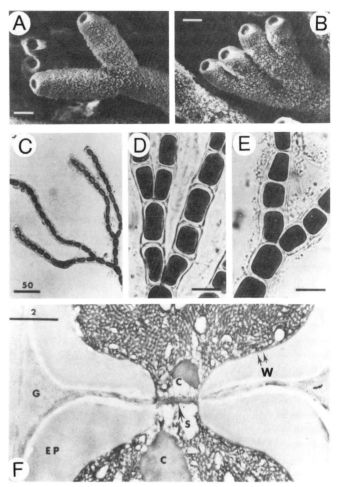

Figure 19.77. *A, Stigonema minutum.* Young culture showing multi-seriate axis and primarily uniseriate branches. (Reproduced with permission from A. Zehnder, Archives of Hydrobiology Supplement *71:* 281–289, 1985, ©E. Schweizerbart'sche Verlag.) *B, Stigonema* species with multiseriate axis and branch. *Bar,* 20 μm.

Figure 19.78. *Geitleria calcarea. A* and *B,* scanning electron micrographs of apical ramifications of filaments with CaCO₃-encrusted sheath. *Bars,* 10 μm. *C, D* and *E,* photomicrograph of material decalcified with the aid of EDTA. Various views of branching system. *Bars,* 10 μm except for *C. F,* electron micrograph of section of decalcified material, showing pore channel ("pit connection") between two cells of a trichome. *S,* synapsis which contains microplasmodesmata; *C,* cyanophycin granules; *W,* cell wall; *EP,* parietal (additional) wall; *G,* sheath. *Bar,* 2 μm. Patterns of phycobilisomes on thylakoids can be seen, particularly in the upper cell. (Reproduced with permission from A. Couté, Hydrobiologia *97:* 255–274, 1982, ©Dr. W. Junk Publishers.)

GROUP II. ORDER **PROCHLORALES*** LEWIN 1977, 216 ^{VP†}

Ralph A. Lewin

Pro.chlo.ra′les. M.L. fem. n. *Prochloron* type genus of the order; *-ales* ending to denote an order; M.L. fem. pl. n. *Prochlorales* the *Prochloron* order.

Unicellular or filamentous, branched or unbranched procaryotes resembling cyanophytes, i.e. **cyanobacteria,** from which they differ in that they **form chlorophylls** *a* **and** *b* **and lack accessory red or blue bilin pigments.**

*Editorial note: The scientific names of the organisms originally described in this order by Lewin (1977) were validly published under the Botanical Code. Later, Florenzano et al. (1986) validly published the names in the *International Journal of Systematic Bacteriology* under the rules of the Bacteriological Code. For purposes of the treatment of the cyanobacteria in this volume, and until such time as there is better resolution of the nomenclatural problems of which code should cover these names, we will ascribe the names to Lewin, the original describer.
†*VP* denotes that this name, although not on the Approved Lists of Bacterial Names, has been validly published in the official publication, *International Journal of Systematic Bacteriology.*

Key to the order **Prochlorales** *(Group II)*

A. Unicellular

           Family I. *Prochloraceae,* p. 1800

B. Filamentous

           Genus *"Prochlorothrix,"* p. 1805

FAMILY I. **PROCHLORACEAE** LEWIN 1977, 216[VP]

R ALPH A. L EWIN

Pro.chlo.ra′ce.ae. M.L. fem. n. *Prochloron* type genus of the family; *-aceae* ending to denote a family; M.L. fem. pl. n. *Prochloraceae* the *Prochloron* family.

Unicellular, not encapsulated (or encapsulated, though none are yet known with capsules) procaryotes.

Further Comments

So far, only one genus is known: *Prochloron* q.v.

Genus **Prochloron** *Lewin 1977, 216[VP]*

R ALPH A. L EWIN

Pro.chlo′ron. Gr. prefix *pro-* primitive; Gr. adj. *chloros* green; M.L. neut. n. *Prochloron* primitive green (cell).

Unicellular, spherical, without evident mucilaginous **sheath.** Only form of reproduction so far observed: binary division, by equatorial constriction. So far, found **almost exclusively** associated as **extracellular symbionts of colonial ascidians** (chiefly didemnids) on subtropical or tropical marine shores.

Type species: *Prochloron didemni* (Lewin 1975) Lewin 1977, 216 (*Synechocystis didemni* Lewin 1975).

Further Descriptive Information

The type species was described on the basis of cells with diameters of 8–14 µm, growing as facultative symbionts on colonies of *Didemnum* (*candidum*?). *Prochloron* cells up to 30 µm in diameter are also found as obligate symbionts inside colonies of other genera and species of didemnids. Cells on the surface or inside colonies of host animals, and cells freed from such a host, are illustrated in Figures 19.79–19.83. A tabulation of cell sizes in various host associations has been published by Lewin et al. (1984). Whether these are conspecific has not been established, since they have not been grown in laboratory culture; the subject is discussed by Griffiths and Thinh below. A report of limited growth of *Prochloron* from *Diplosoma virens* (Patterson and Withers, 1982) has not been followed up or confirmed elsewhere, despite considerable efforts by other investigators. Information has therefore had to be obtained from cells grown in nature on or in various species of host didemnids, mostly studied after being frozen and/or freeze-dried.

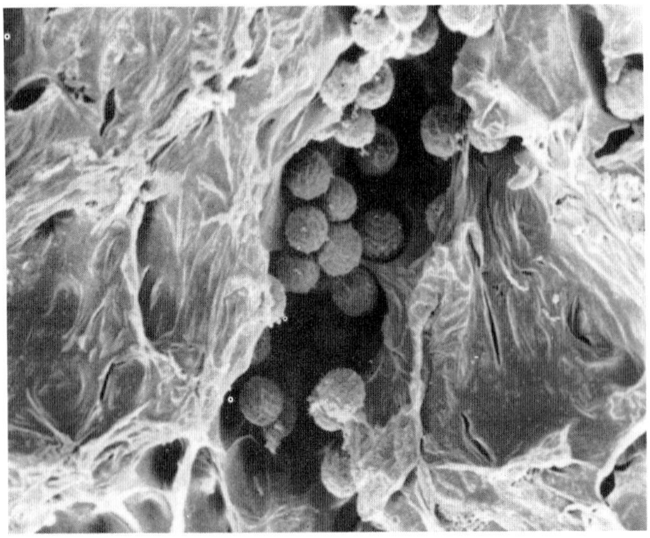

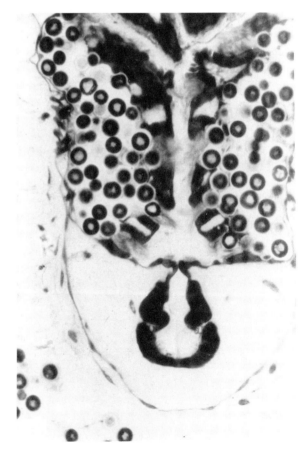

Figure 19.79. Scanning electron micrograph of *Prochloron* cells, 8 µm in diameter, in the perioral groove on the upper surface of a colony of *Didemnum candidum.* (Reproduced with permission from L. Cheng.)

Figure 19.80. Section of *Prochloron* cells in peripharyngial atria of *Diplosoma virens.* (Reproduced with permission from N. D. Holland.)

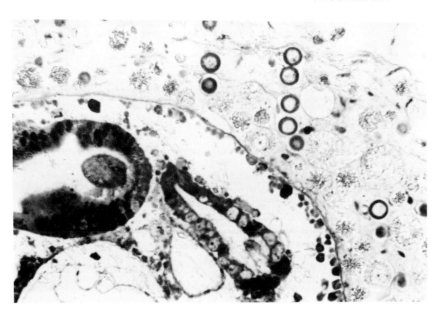

Figure 19.81. Section of *Prochloron* cells embedded in test of *Lissoclinum punctatum.* (Reproduced with permission from L. Cheng.)

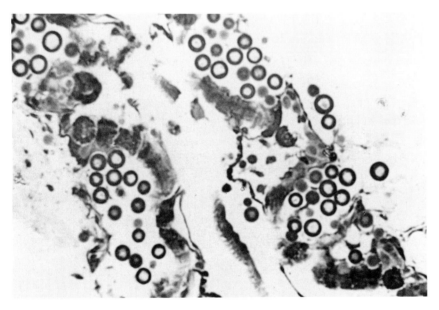

Figure 19.82. Section of *Prochloron* cells in cavities of test of *Lissoclinum patella.* (Reproduced with permission from L. Cheng.)

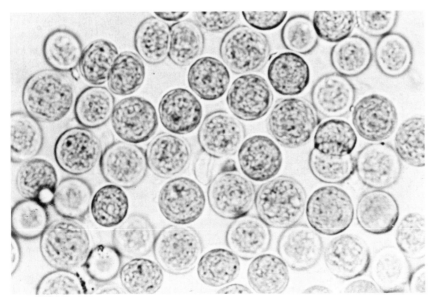

Figure 19.83. Photomicrograph of *Prochloron* cells rinsed from surface of *Didemnum candidum.* (Reproduced with permission from R. W. Hoshaw.)

The cells have several nuclear bodies that stain with 4′, 6-diamidino-2-phenylindole (DAPI). The genome size is 3.6×10^9 daltons. The mol% G + C of the DNA is 41. The rRNA has 5S, 16S and 23S moieties in which nucleotide sequence data indicate phylogenetic affinities with certain filamentous cyanophytes. The cell walls are composed of peptidoglycan and muramic acid. The lipids comprise glycerides with low proportions of polyunsaturated fatty acids, phosphatidylglycerol (but no phosphatidylcholine or phosphatidylethanolamine), and small amounts of steroids. Carbohydrates, including branched and unbranched 1,4α-polyglucose, have been demonstrated, but no cyanophycin [poly (*N*-arginyl-aspartic acid)] or poly-β-hydroxybutyric acid. Gas vacuoles have not been observed.

The thylakoids tend to be paired or stacked; phycobilisomes (and phycobilin pigments) are absent. The predominant green pigments are chlorophylls *a* and *b* associated with β-carotene and a variety of xanthophylls including echinenone, β-cryptoxanthin, mutachrome and isocryptoxanthin. Chlorophyll *a*/*b* ratios in various hosts range from 3.1 to 8.8 (Lewin et al., 1984) or from 1.8 to 19.7 (Paerl et al., 1984), with the data depending somewhat on the extraction methods employed. CO_2 is fixed by illuminated cells; some of the photosynthate escapes and may be taken up by the cells of the animal symbionts (hosts). Acetylene reduction—indicating an ability to fix N_2—has been reported in one association (Paerl, 1984).

Almost all of the literature on *Prochloron* (to the end of 1983) has been reviewed in two articles (Lewin, 1981, 1984). Accumulating evidence (Table 19.13) now prompts a few informed guesses about the origin of *Prochloron*. (The subject has been discussed more fully by Lewin (1983, 1986).) It could conceivably be a descendant of ancestral chlorophytes or of the postulated free-living ancestor of chloroplasts. Alternatively, it could be a deviant cyanophyte. It might have arisen, perhaps in the Jurassic, from a pink cyanophyte such as *Synechocystis raspaigallae* that somehow developed the ability to synthesize chlorophyll *b*. This could have occurred as a mutation or a series of mutations; or by interspecific transfer of requisite genes from a chlorophyte (as a plasmid, perhaps in a viral vector); or as a consequence of protoplasmic fusion between cells of a chlorophyte and a cyanophyte, possibly in an animal's gut. One consequence of a 2-chlorophyll system might have been the ad-

Table 19.13.

Differential characteristics indicating predominant affinities between **Prochloron** *and either* **Chlorophyta** *or* **Cyanophyta**[a,b]

Prochloron characteristic	Predominant affinities with	
	Chlorophyta	*Cyanophyta*
Nucleus type (procaryotic)	−	+
Thylakoids (paired or stacked)	+	−
Chlorophylls (*a* and *b*)	+	−
Phycobilins (absent)	+	−
Cell wall (peptidoglycan type)	−	+
Fatty acids and steroids (low contents)	−	+
Types of carotenoids	−	+
Types of other lipids	−	+
Sucrose (absent)	−	+
Nucleotide sequence		
5S rRNA	−	+
16S rRNA	−	+

[a]Data are from Lewin (1986).

[b]Symbols: −, 90% or more of strains are negative; +, 90% or more of strains are positive.

hesion of thylakoids in pairs or stacks, as we now find them in *Prochloron*. Another might have been the evolutionary elimination of the less efficient light-harvesting system involving phycobilins, which are now lacking from *Prochloron*. Some of these hypotheses could now be subject to experimental tests.

The recent discovery of another prochlorophyte, with dissimilar features (Burger-Wiersma et al., 1986), opens up further experimental possibilities, particularly because, unlike *Prochloron*, it can be grown reproducibly in laboratory culture. This genus, "*Prochlorothrix*," may be unrelated to *Prochloron:* the prochlorophytes may prove to be polyphyletic. We shall soon see.

Current status of the taxonomy of the genus **Prochloron**

D. J. GRIFFITHS AND LUONG-VAN THINH

Although *P. didemni* is the only formally described species, a number of different types of *Prochloron* have been recognized, largely on the bases of ultrastructural evidence and the nature of their association with the ascidian host. Establishing the distinct taxonomic status of each of these different types is hindered by the failure, thus far, of all attempts to obtain viable cultures of *Prochloron* free of the host.

In all published work on *Prochloron* the alga has therefore been identified by reference to the host species (generally ascidian), the taxonomy of which, at least in the Indo-West Pacific region, is now well-established (Kott, 1980, 1982). On this basis, three major types of *Prochloron* may be recognized, and these are described below. Since they share the common characteristics of a procaryotic ultrastructure, with chlorophylls *a* and *b* but no accessory phycoblin pigments, only those features that help to distinguish the three types will be described.

1. The apparently specific symbiont in the common cloaca of **Didemnum molle.** This symbiont has been described by Newcomb and Pugh (1975) and by Thorne et al. (1977) (the host being at that time known as *Didemnum ternatanum*) and by Cox and Dwarte (1981). Newcomb and Pugh differentiated the isolate of *Didemnum molle* from that of two other hosts (*Diplosoma virens* and *Lissoclinum punctatum*, which was then named *L. molle*), since it lacked a clear central region when viewed in section. This feature of the *Didemnum molle* alga has since been confirmed by others, as also has the relatively large size of the cells (~20 μm in diameter).

Apart from a generally greater tendency for the paired thylakoids to be further aggregated into stacks, the major diagnostic feature in the ultrastructure of *Prochloron* from *Didemnum molle* concerns its cellular inclusions. The most prominent of these are electron-dense, almost spherical bodies, ranging in diameter from 0.6 to 2.1 μm (Fig. 19.84). They have been variously described as osmiophilic globules (Newcomb and Pugh, 1975; Thorne et al., 1977) or polyhedral bodies (Cox and Dwarte, 1981). Thinh et al., (1985) showed that they differ in size, shape and electron-staining characteristics from the polyhedral bodies which are a common feature of all *Prochloron*, cyanobacteria and autotrophic bacteria (Shively, 1974). They stain with Nile blue sulfate, as do lipoproteins, and are thought to be storage bodies (Thinh et al., 1985).

2. Nonobligate symbionts on the surface of certain didemnids and holothurians. This kind of symbiont, first reported by Lewin and Cheng (1975) as epizoic on various *Didemnum* species along the shores of the Gulf of California, was more fully described by Lewin (1975) and by Schultz-Baldes and Lewin (1976). It was originally identified as a cyanophyte, *Synechocystis didemni* but was later renamed *Prochloron didemni* as the type species for the *Prochlorophyta* (Lewin, 1977).

The cells are spherical, 8–14 μm in diameter, considerably smaller than those of the *Prochloron* from the cloacal cavity of *Didemnum molle* but, like the latter, with no clear central region when viewed in section (Fig. 19.85). Many of the thylakoids form aggregates of more than 20 double lamellae. Although in some cells, presumed to be older cells, there are

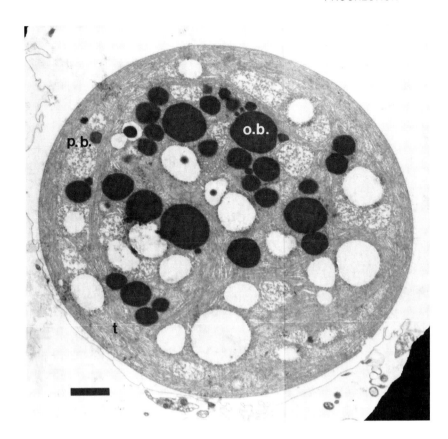

Figure 19.84. Section of *Prochloron* from the common cloaca of *Didemnum molle,* showing thylakoids (*t*), prominent electron-dense osmiophilic bodies (*o.b.*) and polyhedral bodies (*p.b.*) distributed throughout the cytoplasm which fills the cell. Fixed in 4% glutaraldehyde in filtered seawater, postfixed in 1% osmium tetroxide in filtered seawater, dehydrated, and embedded in Spurr's resin for sectioning and staining with uranyl acetate and lead citrate. *Bar,* 2 μm. (Reproduced with permission from D. J. Griffiths and Luong-Van Thinh.)

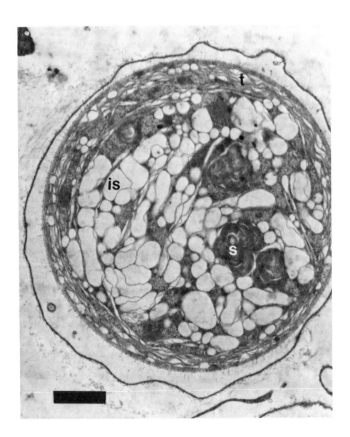

Figure 19.85. Section of *Prochloron didemni* epizoic on *Didemnum* aff. *candidum,* showing the peripherally arranged stacked thylakoids (*t*), large intrathylakoidal spaces (*is*) and storage bodies (*s*). Preparation is the same as in Figure 19.84 but with decalcification in 2% ascorbic acid in filtered seawater. *Bar,* 2 μm. (Reproduced with permission from L-V. Thinh, D. J. Griffiths and H. Winsor, Botanica Marina *XXVIII:* 167–177, 1985, Walter de Gruyter & Co.)

many lipid globules disposed closely under the cell wall, these are appreciably smaller and less numerous than the osmiophilic bodies described for the *Prochloron* of *Didemnum molle.*

Schultz-Baldes and Lewin's description of *P. didemni* was the first to include speculation on the site of the genome, which was presumed to be represented by fine fibrillar material in otherwise electron-transparent regions distributed throughout the cell. Fluorescence microscopy of cells stained with 4′,6-diamidino-2-phenylindole later indicated that the DNA occurs as 15–20 irregularly shaped aggregates up to 5 μm long, scattered among the thylakoids around the periphery of the cell (Coleman and Lewin, 1983).

Also reported by Schultz-Baldes and Lewin (1976) was the four-layered cell envelope, since recognized as typical of the genus (Fig. 19.86), and the polyhedral bodies, another feature common to all *Prochloron* preparations so far examined (see Fig. 19.87). Among the most prominent cellular inclusions of *P. didemni* are what Lewin (1975) identified as "structured granules," ∼1–1.5 μm in diameter, which did not stain with iodine. Thinh et al. (1985) have confirmed the presence of these bodies in *P. didemni* and their absence from *Prochloron* cells in other hosts. They resemble starch grains, with regularly arranged concentric lamellae, but in electron micrographs they stain differently from starch (Fig. 19.85).

Other kinds of *Prochloron* have been reported epizoic on the "tests" (organic skeletons) of species of *Cystodytes* and *Aplidium* (family *Polycitoridae*) (Lewin, 1978; Kott et al., 1984), *Trididemnum cerebriforme* and *Didemnum membranaceum* (family *Didemnidae*) (Kott et al., 1984) and a species of holothurian, *Synaptula lamperti* (Cheng and Lewin, 1984). The only isolates unequivocally identified as *P. didemni* occur in nonobligate association on the outer surface of the test of ascidians. There are some nonobligate symbionts, however, which cannot be identified as *P.*

didemni. Thus, Kott et al. (1984) report that *Prochloron* cells which occur sporadically on some *Aplidium* species more closely resemble those normally embedded in the test of *Trididemnum miniatum.*

3. Obligate symbionts in the common cloacal system and test of other didemnid ascidian species. The first *Prochloron* of this type to be described at the ultrastructural level was that from *Diplosoma virens* (Newcomb and Pugh, 1975). *Prochloron* cells from *Diplosoma virens* have since been described by Thorne et al. (1977), Whatley (1977), Thinh (1978), Withers et al. (1978) and Giddings et al. (1980). The cells are relatively small (6–14 μm in diameter) with a prominent electron-transparent central body. In addition to peripheral paired thylakoids (some of which may be loosely stacked), the cytoplasm contains osmiophilic globules, polyphosphate granules and polyhedral bodies. The algal symbiont of *Diplosoma similis* is ultrastructurally indistinguishable from that of *Diplosoma virens* (our unpublished observations). *Diplosoma multipapillata* contains algal symbionts in the same size range (Kott, 1982), although their identity as *Prochloron* has not yet been confirmed.

Crystalline and paracrystalline inclusions (other than polyhedral bodies), although occurring sporadically in *Prochloron* cells from various hosts (see below), have not been found in the algae from *Diplosoma virens* or *Diplosoma similis* (Thinh et al., 1985).

Prochloron from the cloacal cavity of *Trididemnum cyclops* has many of the features of the *Diplosoma* algae described above, including a similar size range and the presence of a large electron-transparent central

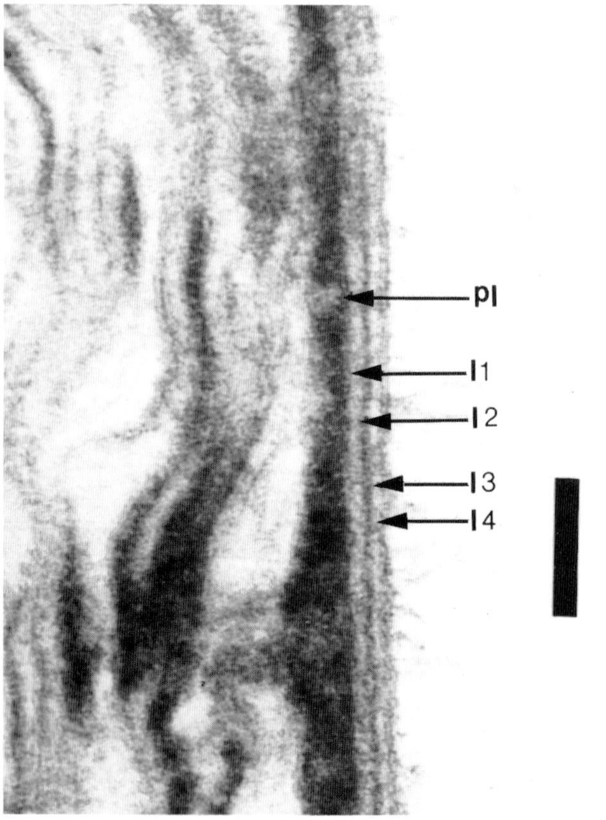

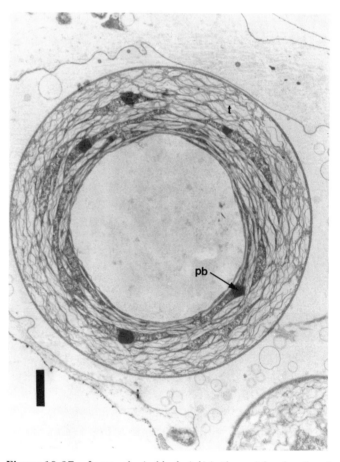

Figure 19.86. Profile of cell envelope of *Prochloron* from *Lissoclinum patella,* showing the plasmalemma (*pl*) and cell wall layers (*l1–l4*). Preparation is the same as in Figure 19.85. *Bar,* 0.1 μm. (Reproduced with permission of D. J. Griffiths and L-V. Thinh.)

Figure 19.87. Large spherical body (*pb*) in the peripheral region of the cell of *Prochloron* from *Trididemnum cyclops.* Preparation is the same as in Figure 19.85. *t,* thylakoids. *Bar,* 1 μm. (Reproduced with permission from D. J. Griffiths, L-V. Thinh and H. Winsor, Botanica Marina *XXVII*: 117–128, 1984, Walter de Gruyter & Co.)

body (Thinh, 1979) (Fig. 19.87). Other similarities with the *Prochloron* from *Diplosoma virens,* including pigment composition and photosynthetic characteristics (Thinh and Griffiths, 1977), led Thinh (1979) to conclude that *Diplosoma virens* and *T. cyclops* probably harbor the same species of alga.

However, the *Prochloron* symbiont of *T. cyclops* differs from those of *Diplosoma virens* and *Diplosoma similis* in often containing crystalline and paracrystalline cellular inclusions (Thinh et al., 1985). These include large crystals (resembling protein crystals of higher-plant chloroplasts) spherical bodies (thought to be a different form of these large crystals) and paracrystalline arrays (often found in close association with polyhedral bodies) (Griffiths et al., 1984). The *Prochloron* symbionts of *T. miniatum,* which occur both in the common cloacal cavity and in the test, have crystalline inclusions resembling those in *T. cyclops.* The *Prochloron* symbionts of *T. paracyclops* are similar in size (Kott, 1982) but have not yet been described in detail.

The didemnid genus *Lissoclinum* has four species known to harbor *Prochloron.* Kott (1982) has reported that while *Prochloron* cells from *L. patella* and *L. punctatum* reach diameters up to 10 μm, those from *L. bistratum* and *L. voeltzkowi* do not exceed 15 μm. All share common ultrastructural features such as an electron-transparent central body and characteristic paracrystalline inclusions (Newcomb and Pugh, 1975; Thinh et al., 1985).

Comparative analyses of the 16S rRNA of *Prochloron* from *Diplosoma virens, Trididemnum cyclops, Lissoclinum patella* and *L. voeltzkowi* gave almost identical oligonucleotide catalogs (Stackenbrandt et al., 1982).

Moreover, studies of DNA/DNA reassociation have indicated a close genotypic relationship between *Prochloron* from *L. patella, Diplosoma similis* and another unnamed didemnid ascidian host (but only a distant relationship with a strain of the cyanobacterium *Synechocystis*) (Stam et al., 1985). In both these studies, the ascidian hosts were collected from a relatively restricted geographical area (the latter albeit extending over at least 3000 km). It is yet to be established, therefore, whether the apparent conspecificity suggested by these studies is also valid for *Prochloron* from other, more widely separate localities.

Concluding Comments

Although we have some criteria for distinguishing *Prochloron* types from different hosts, the evidence is too fragmentary to create new species. The nonobligate epizoic species associated with *Didemnum* and described as *P. didemni* differs in many respects from the algae found in the common cloacal cavity of *Didemnum molle,* as well as from those found in similar associations with other didemnid hosts.

Further, more detailed work, especially at the molecular level is needed. This requires viable pure cultures to provide the necessary genetic material and to test the reliability as taxonomic criteria of the ultrastructural features described above.

Acknowledgments

Our work on *Prochloron* is supported by the Australian Research Grants Committee. Expert assistance was provided by Heather Winsor.

OTHER TAXA

Genus "**Prochlorothrix**" *Burger-Wiersma, Veenhuis, Korthals, van de Wiel and Mur 1986*

T. BURGER-WIERSMA AND L. R. MUR

Pro.chlo′ro.thrix. Gr. pref. *pro-* before; Gr. adj. *chloros* green; Gr. n. *thrix* hair; M.L. n. *prochlorothrix* early green filament.

Unbranched trichomes of indefinite length. No cell differentiation. Gram-negative. **Photosynthetic membranes lack phycobilisomes.** Cells contain **chlorophylls *a* and *b*. Phycobilin pigments absent.** Oxygen evolving photoautotrophs with respiratory oxygen uptake in the dark.

The mol% G + C of the DNA is 53 (one species, one strain).

Type species: "*Prochlorothrix hollandica*" Burger-Wiersma, Veenhuis, Korthals, van de Wiel and Mur 1986.

Further Descriptive Information

Thus far, "*Prochlorothrix hollandica*" has been the only documented species in this genus. The cylinder-shaped cells are 3–15 μm long and have a diameter of 0.5–3 μm, depending on growth conditions and the phase-in cell division cycle (Fig. 19.88). The cells are arranged in trichomes of 2 to >100 cells. The trichomes are straight, not branched, and have no special end cells, and a sheath is absent. Hitherto, no cell differentiation has been observed. There is no evidence that this strain forms hormogonia. No motility was observed when the strain was grown on agar.

The cell wall organization of "*P. hollandica*" is comparable to that of cyanobacteria, i.e. the peptidoglycans are of the A1 type of peptidoglycan classification and show a high degree of cross-linkage (Jürgens and Burger-Wiersma, in press).

The ultrastructure of "*P. hollandica*" is very similar to that of cyanobacteria (Burger-Wiersma et al., 1986). The absence of phycobilisomes on the thylakoid membranes is the most striking difference with cyanobacteria.

"*P. hollandica*" can be grown in liquid cultures in a mineral medium described by Van Liere and Mur (1978) or in BG-11 (Stanier et al., 1971). The organism can be cultivated on aerobic plates on the basis of these

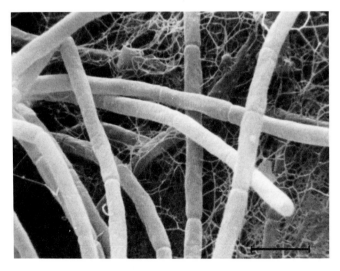

Figure 19.88. Scanning electron micrograph of "*Prochlorothrix hollandica.*" Note the difference in cell length due to the difference in the phase of cell division. Cells were grown in a mineral medium at a growth-saturating light intensity (60 μE m^{-2} s^{-1}). Fixation in 4% glutaraldehyde in phosphate buffer. After dehydration, the samples were critical point-dried and gold-sputtered. *Bar,* 3 μm. (Micrograph is from Sabine Seufer, courtesy of Prof. Dr. W. E. Krumbein, University of Oldenburg, F.R.G.)

media as well, but the growth potential decreases with increasing agar concentration. Optimum growth was obtained by using 0.5% agar in medium BG-11. "*P. hollandica*" forms a one-layered film of trichomes; the color is bright or yellowish green.

Attempts to grow "*P. hollandica*" in medium deprived of combined nitrogen failed, indicating the incapability of aerobic nitrogen fixation. This was confirmed by the absence of any nitrogenase activity (Burger-Wiersma, Stal and Mur, submitted for publication).

Optimum growth occurred between 20 and 30°C and at pH 8.4, which was the pH in turbidostat cultures without external pH adjustment.

Thus far, "*P. hollandica*" has only been identified in samples of shallow, eutrophic freshwater lakes that originate from peat mining.

Isolation Procedure

"*P. hollandica*" can be isolated by micromanipulation into a mineral medium or after growth on plates of 0.5% agar in a mineral medium. Plates or liquid cultures are incubated at (40–100 µE m^{-2} s^{-1}) and 20°C for 2–6 weeks. No selective isolation procedure is known.

Maintenance Procedure

"*P. hollandica*" cultures maintained in mineral medium (Stanier et al., 1971; Van Liere and Mur 1978) at 10°C are transferred every 4–6 weeks. Cell suspensions in mineral medium with 5% dimethyl sulfoxide are kept at −70°C. After defrost, suspensions are inoculated on solid mineral medium (0.5% agar). "*P. hollandica*" does not survive the lyophilization procedure.

Differentiation of the genus "**Prochlorothrix**" from *the genus* **Prochloron**

The genus "*Prochlorothrix*" is distinguished from the genus *Prochloron* by its morphology, i.e. the cells are arranged in trichomes. Differences between "*P. hollandica*" and *Prochloron* species are summarized in Table 19.14.

Taxonomic Comments

"*Prochlorothrix*," like *Prochloron*, is separated from the cyanobacteria by the lack of phycobilisomes. Instead of phycobilin pigments, the organisms contain chlorophyll *b* in addition to chlorophyll *a*, a combination commonly found in chloroplasts. There is both physiological and biochemical evidence of a functional role of chlorophyll *b* in "*P. hollandica*." The chlorophyll *b* content of cells changes independently from chlorophyll *a* upon a change in light intensity (Burger-Wiersma and Post, in preparation). Native and denaturing gel electrophoresis revealed similarity of the chlorophyll-protein complexes of *Prochloron* species and "*P. hollandica*." The chlorophyll *a*-binding proteins of the cores of photosystems I and II appeared to be immunologically related to those of cyanobacteria and chloroplasts. The antenna complex, which serves to funnel the light energy toward the reaction center, is completely different from that found in cyanobacteria because of the lack of phycobilisomes. However, the chlorophyll *a/b*-binding proteins are also distinct from the analogous light-harvesting complex in higher plants, as was indicated by: (1) the lack of immunological cross-reactivity, (2) the higher *a/b* ratio, (3) deviating molecular mass estimates (Bullerjahn et al., 1987) and (4) lack of negative deflection in the circular dichroism spectrum below 650 nm, indicating a difference in the molecular organization of chlorophyll *b* (H. C. P. Matthijs, personal communication).

The 16S rRNA sequence, determined by using the reverse transcriptase method (Olsen et al., 1986), revealed that "*P. hollandica*" falls within the cyanobacterial line of descent, as do green plant chloroplasts. However, within this line of descent, "*P. hollandica*" is a deeply branching member not directly related to these chloroplasts. Because the RNA data on *Prochloron* were derived from partial RNA sequence determination (Seewaldt and Stackebrandt, 1982), no conclusions can be drawn on the evolutionary distance between "*P. hollandica*" and the *Prochloron* species.

Table 19.14.
Characteristics differentiating **"Prochlorothrix hollandica"** *and the* **Prochloron species** *(as obtained from the literature)*[a]

Characteristic	"*Prochlorothrix hollandica*"	*Prochloron* sp.
Pigments		
Chlorophyll *a/b* ratio	>7	>4
Echinenon	−	+
Morphology		
Unicellular	−	+
Filamentous	+	−
Spherical cells	−	+
Cylindrical cells	+	−
Habitat		
Freshwater	+	−
Marine	−	+
Free living	+	−
Symbiotic	−	+
Growth conditions		
Mineral medium	+	−
Host needed	−	+
N$_2$ fixation	−	+
Temperature (°C)	20–30	>25
Mol% G + C of DNA	53	31–41

[a]Symbols: −, 90% or more of strains are negative; +, 90% or more of strains are positive.

Characterization of "**Prochlorothrix hollandica**"

"**Prochlorothrix hollandica**" Burger-Wiersma et al., 1986.

hol.lan′di.ca. M.L. fem. adj. *hollandica* Holland, part of The Netherlands.

Straight, sheathless trichomes of variable length. The trichomes are not motile on agar. The cylinder-shaped cells are 3–15 µm long and 0.5–3 µm in diameter. Ultrastructure studies revealed the presence of gas vacuoles at the polar ends of the cells (U. J. Jürgens, personal communication). Zeaxanthin and β-carotene were shown to be the major carotenoids (Burger-Wiersma et al., 1986). The nitrogen source is nitrate or ammonium salt; no N$_2$ fixation or nitrogenase activity could be shown. "*P. hollandica*" appeared to be explicitly sensitive to NaCl, since 25 mM of

this salt severely inhibit growth.

The mol% G + C of the DNA is 53 (T_m).

Acknowledgments

The authors are indebted to Dr. S. Turner and Prof. N. R. Pace (Indiana University, Bloomington, Indiana, U.S.A.), Dr. L. J. Stal (University of Oldenburg, F.R.G.), Dr. Gy. Garab (National Academy of Science of Hungary, Szeged, Hungary) and Dr. H. C. P. Matthijs (University of Amsterdam, The Netherlands) for making results available prior to publication. Thanks are also due to Andien van den Heuvel, Robert Baard and Geertjan Niemeijer for technical assistance. T. B-W. is financially supported by the Dutch Ministry of Public Housing, Physical Planning and the Environment.

Aerobic Chemolithotrophic Bacteria and Associated Organisms

The bacteria included in this section are Gram-negative eubacteria that, if motile, have flagella. Most of these bacteria, in particular the nitrifiers, the genus *Hydrogenobacter*, and many of the colorless sulfur bacteria, are able to derive energy by aerobic respiration of reduced inorganic compounds. A few can oxidize inorganic energy sources by anaerobic respiration (e.g. *Thiobacillus denitrificans* if nitrate is available). Bacteria that are able to obtain energy from the oxidation of inorganic compounds are called chemolithotrophs.

Many of the bacteria discussed in this section can utilize carbon dioxide as a sole or principal source of carbon and are therefore termed autotrophs. All of the organisms included in this section whose autotrophic metabolism has been studied utilize the reductive pentose phosphate (Benson-Calvin) cycle for carbon dioxide fixation and therefore have the enzyme ribulose-1,5-bisphosphate carboxylase.

Not all of the bacteria treated in this section are true chemolithotrophs. For example, members of the genus *Acidiphilium*, which are commonly found growing in association with members of the genus *Thiobacillus*, can oxidize reduced sulfur compounds but do not derive energy from the process. Thus they are really heterotrophs but are included in this section until more is known about their proper classification. In addition, many of the chemolithotrophs discussed in this section are able to utilize organic compounds and are therefore not entirely dependent upon carbon dioxide as sole source of carbon. Thus, there is a gradation in physiological types treated within this section, from obligate chemolithotrophic, autotrophic (chemolithoautotrophic) bacteria to heterotrophic bacteria. The colorless sulfur bacteria are a particularly diverse group. Table 20.16 defines the terms that are used to describe the nutritional and physiological types of chemolithotrophic bacteria and associated organisms.

Many bacteria included in other sections and volumes of the *Manual* are able to obtain energy from the oxidation of molecular hydrogen (H_2). Furthermore, some of these bacteria can utilize the Benson-Calvin cycle for carbon dioxide fixation. However, these bacteria also utilize organic sources of carbon for growth. The only known obligately chemolithotrophic hydrogen bacteria are found in the genus *Hydrogenobacter*.

The iron- and manganese-oxidizing and depositing bacteria are, in general, a less well understood group within the chemolithotrophs. Many have not yet been isolated in pure culture. The only known chemolithotrophic iron and manganese bacteria are found in the genera *Gallionella* (Section 21) and *Thiobacillus* (i.e. *T. ferrooxidans*). The iron and manganese bacteria are included in this section for deterministic purposes, with the full understanding that their ultimate classification has yet to be determined.

Key to the identification of groups

I. Reduced inorganic nitrogen compounds (ammonia and nitrite) can be used as energy sources for growth.
   A. Nitrifying Bacteria, p. 1808
II. Reduced inorganic sulfur compounds can be oxidized, and most organisms can utilize this as sole source of energy.
   B. Colorless Sulfur Bacteria, p. 1834
III. Hydrogen gas (H_2) is used as the energy source for growth.*
   C. Obligately Chemolithotrophic Hydrogen Bacteria, p. 1872
IV. Iron and/or manganese oxides are produced or deposited on or within the cells.
   D. Iron- and Manganese-Oxidizing and/or Depositing Bacteria, p. 1873

---

*Many bacteria can use molecular hydrogen as an alternative energy source but will use organic compounds if they are available. *Hydrogenobacter* is not known to use organic sources of carbon.

A. NITRIFYING BACTERIA

FAMILY **NITROBACTERACEAE** BUCHANAN 1917, 349, EMEND. MUT. CHAR. STARKEY 1948, 69; WATSON 1971a, 262[AL][†]

STANLEY W. WATSON, EBERHARD BOCK, HEINZ HARMS, HANS-PETER KOOPS AND ALAN B. HOOPER

Ni.tro.bac.te.ra´ce.ae. M.L. masc. n. *Nitrobacter* type genus of the family; *-aceae* ending to denote a family; M.L. fem. pl. n. *Nitrobacteraceae* the *Nitrobacter* family.

A diverse group of rods, vibrios, cocci and spirilla having in common the ability to **utilize ammonia or nitrite** as a major source of energy and carbon dioxide as the chief source of carbon. With the exception of *Nitrobacter* species, all others are **obligate chemolithotrophs,** but some can grow mixotrophically.

Gram-negative. Many but not all strains possess a complex arrangement of intracytoplasmic membranes which usually form flattened vesicles or tubes within the cell. All strains are **aerobic,** but some may be grown in low oxygen concentrations.

The mol% G + C of the DNA ranges from 45 to 62.

Type genus: *Nitrobacter* Winogradsky 1892, 127.

Further Descriptive Information

The organisms in this family, commonly referred to as nitrifying bacteria, are composed of two physiological groups of bacteria which are not phylogenetically related (Woese et al., 1984a, b). Species in one group oxidize ammonia to nitrite, while those in the second group oxidize nitrite to nitrate. No single species yet found oxidizes ammonia to nitrate. It should be noted that the names of genera of nitrite oxidizers have the prefix *Nitro-*, whereas those of ammonia oxidizers have the prefix *Nitroso-*. Strains are assigned to genera primarily on their morphological characteristics. Although strains in a given species are phenotypically similar or identical, they may vary genotypically.

Cells are rod-shaped, ellipsoidal, spherical, spirillar and lobular without endospores. Most, but not all, species have a typical Gram-negative multilayered cell wall. Many, but not all, of the nitrifying bacteria possess intracytoplasmic membranes which may occur as flattened lamellae or randomly arranged tubes. Cells are motile or nonmotile; when cells are motile, flagella are polar to lateral or peritrichous. In nature and in enrichment cultures, many of the nitrifying bacteria occur in cell aggregates referred to as zoogloeae or cysts. Zoogloeae are composed of loosely associated cells embedded in a soft slime layer, while cysts (Fig. 20.1) are comprised of closely packed cells embedded and surrounded by a firm slime layer. Selected characteristics permitting the differentiation of the genera included in the family *Nitrobacteraceae* are given in Table 20.1.

Habitat and Ecological Importance of Nitrifying Bacteria

Nitrifying bacteria are found in most aerobic environments where organic matter is mineralized. They are widely distributed in soils, freshwater, brackish water, seawater, and sewage disposal systems. In nature, they frequently can be found in suboptimal environments. For example, nitrifying bacteria are aerobes, yet they can be isolated from sewage disposal systems and from marine sediments which have extremely low oxygen tensions. They can also be isolated from soils having a pH of 4 (Walker and Wickramasinghe, 1979), from deep oceans where the temperature is <5°C, and from deserts and hot springs where the temperatures can be 60°C or more (Golovacheva, 1976). However, obligate psychrophilic or thermophilic nitrifying bacteria have never been isolated. In sewage disposal systems and, possibly, other environments, nitrifying bacteria have a proclivity to attach to surfaces and to grow in tight clusters of cells, forming structures called cysts (Fig. 20.1).

In nature, chemolithotrophic nitrifying bacteria are the only important group of organisms producing nitrite and nitrate from ammonia, although many heterotrophic bacteria and fungi are reported to produce nitrite and/or nitrate. However, the heterotrophic nitrifiers produce only low levels of nitrite and nitrate and often use organic sources of nitrogen rather than ammonia (Focht and Verstraete, 1977).

Ammonia, nitrite and nitrate are chemically stable, and their transformations in nature are usually biologically catalyzed. Both nitrite and nitrate can serve as terminal electron acceptors for many bacteria under low oxygen tensions or anaerobic conditions. Nitrate serves as the chief source of inorganic nitrogen for plant growth in soils. In the terrestrial environment, ammonia liberated during mineralization of organic matter is complexed with soil particles and often cannot reach the root zone of many plants. When nitrifying bacteria oxidize ammonia, the products are solubilized and become available for plant growth. Nitrite and nitrate leaching from soil can penetrate ground and surface waters. High concentrations of nitrite are toxic to fish and other vertebrates. In oceanic waters, over 70% of all combined nitrogen is in the form of nitrate (Vaccaro, 1962) which serves as a major source of nitrogen for plant growth in that environment.

Under favorable conditions, nitrifying bacteria have been found on concrete surfaces such as in cooling towers. If these bacteria reach high concentrations, corrosion occurs due to the release of nitric acid. Nitrification is one of the major biological processes in sewage disposal systems. Both N_2O and NO are produced during ammonia oxidation, thus nitrifying bacteria may be a major source of these atmospheric gases.

Taxonomic Comments

Early knowledge concerning nitrifying bacteria stems chiefly from the classical work of Sergej and Helene Winogradsky. The taxonomic

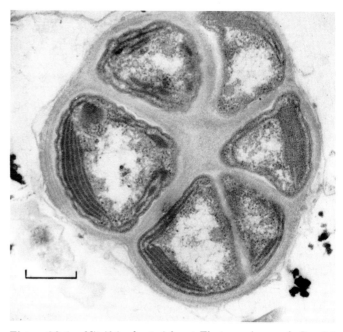

Figure 20.1. Nitrifying bacterial cyst. Electron micrograph. *Bar*, 0.5 μm.

[†]*AL* denotes inclusion of this name on the Approved Lists of Bacterial Names (1980).

Table 20.1.

Differentiation of the genera of the family **Nitrobacteraceae**[a]

Characteristic	1. Nitrobacter	2. Nitrospina	3. Nitrococcus	4. Nitrospira	5. Nitrosomonas	6. Nitrosococcus	7. Nitrosospira	8. Nitrosolobus	9. "Nitrosovibrio"
Oxidation of									
$NH_3 \rightarrow NO_2^-$	−	−	−	−	+	+	+	+	+
$NO_2^- \rightarrow NO_3^-$	+	+	+	+	−	−	−	−	−
Cell shape									
Straight rod	+	+	−	−	+	−	−	−	−
Coccus	−	−	+	−	−	+	−	−	−
Helical	−	−	−	+	−	−	+	−	−
Curved rod	−	−	−	−	−	−	−	−	+
Lobed	−	−	−	−	−	−	−	+	−
Reproduction									
Binary fission only	−	+	+	+	+	+	+	+	+
Budding (autotrophically); budding or binary fission (heterotrophically)	+	−	−	−	−	−	−	−	−
Motility	D	−	+	−	D	+	D	+	+
Cytomembranes present	+	−[b]	+	−	+	+	−	+	−[c]
Nature of cytomembranes									
Peripheral	+[d]	−	−	−	+	D[e]	−	−	−
Randomly arranged	−	−	+	−	−	−	−	−	−
Central	−	−	−	−	−	D[e]	−	−	−
Tubular	−	−	+	−	−	−	−	−	−
Lamellar	+	−	−	−	+	D[e]	−	−	−
Internal, compartmentalizing the cell	−	−	−	−	−	−	−	+	−
Capable of facultatively chemoheterotrophic growth	D	−	−	−					
Mol% G + C of DNA	60–62	58	51	50	45–54	48–51	53–55	53–56	54

[a]Symbols: −, 90% or more of strains are negative; +, 90% or more of strains are positive; and D, different reactions in different taxa.

[b]Only occasional bleblike invaginations of the plasma membrane into cytoplasm.

[c]Occasional invagination of plasma membrane.

[d]Only at polar region of cell.

[e]Occur as a centrally located parallel bundle or in a peripheral lamellar arrangement. For other symbols, see standard definitions.

categorization of this group of organisms in the seventh edition of the *Manual* (Starkey, 1957) was based primarily on the Winogradskys' early studies (S. Winogradsky, 1890a, b, 1891, 1892, 1904, 1930, 1931, 1935; S. and H. Winogradsky, 1933; H. Winogradsky, 1935a, b, 1937). In that edition, the organisms in the family *Nitrobacteraceae* were categorized into 14 species with the following seven genera: *Nitrobacter, Nitrocystis, Nitrosomonas, Nitrosococcus, Nitrosospira, Nitrosocystis* and *Nitrosogloea*. Watson (1971a), in revising this family, accepted the genera *Nitrobacter, Nitrosomonas, Nitrosococcus* and *Nitrosospira* but combined *Nitrocystis* with *Nitrobacter*, placed *Nitrosocystis* and *Nitrosogloea* as *genera incertae sedis*, and added the following three new genera: *Nitrospina, Nitrococcus* and *Nitrosolobus*. More recently, Harms et al. (1976) described a new genus, "*Nitrosovibrio*," of the ammonia-oxidizing bacteria, and Watson et al. (1986) described a new genus, *Nitrospira*, of the nitrite-oxidizing bacteria.

In the past, the systematic categorization of members of the *Nitrobacteraceae* has been difficult because classification was based primarily on morphological characteristics. Most investigators limited their studies to only two genera, *Nitrosomonas* and *Nitrobacter*. In the eighth edition of the *Manual* (Watson, 1974), only two species were listed in the genus *Nitrosococcus*, and only one species was listed in each of the remaining genera.

Investigations have shown that it may be possible to utilize the DNA homology technique for assigning the nitrifying bacteria to different species and, possibly, to different genera. Watson and Mandel (1971) recognized that there were three species in the genus *Nitrosomonas*; this was later confirmed by Dodson et al. (1983). More recently, Koops and Harms (1985) presented data showing that each genus of ammonia-oxidizing bacteria was composed of two or more species.

These preliminary taxonomic studies must be expanded by using additional techniques, especially the 16S rRNA sequence technique. Initial data obtained by use of the latter method (Woese et al., 1984a, b) revealed that it should be possible to develop a detailed outline of phylogenetic relationships among the nitrifying bacteria and their possible phylogenetic relationships to other groups of bacteria. Present results indicate that several strains categorized in the same species have divergent genotypic characteristics. Eventually, decisions will have to be made regarding the use of genotypic criteria for species separation when all apparent phenotypic characteristics are identical, but major decisions in this regard would be premature at present.

Serotyping of bacterial strains is a widely accepted and useful technique for determining relationships between groups of bacteria. The nitrite oxidizers were the first nitrifiers to be studied with the fluorescent antibody (FA) technique. Using the FA technique, Fliermans et al. (1974) demonstrated that *Nitrobacter* strains were composed of two serotypes. And while employing the same technique, Stanley and Schmidt (1981) found that strains categorized in this genus were composed of several serotypes. Belser and Schmidt (1978a, b), who also used FA technique, demonstrated that the ammonia oxidizers were composed of several serotypes and that no intergeneric cross-reactions were found. Fliermans et al. (1974) and Bohlool and Schmidt (1980) showed that strains from widely separated geographic areas belonged to the same serotype. Möller (1983) and Harms and Koops (unpublished observations) found that organisms belonging to the same DNA/DNA homology group, with only one exception, belonged to the same serotype

group. No strong cross-reactions between strains of different homology groups were observed. In the future, serotyping of strains could help clarify interrelationships between strains of both ammonia- and nitrite-oxidizing bacteria.

Type genus: *Nitrobacter* Winogradsky 1892, 127. (Gen. Cons. Opin. 23 Jud. Comm. 1958, 169.)

Nitrite-Oxidizing Bacteria

STANLEY W. WATSON, EBERHARD BOCK, HEINZ HARMS, HANS-PETER KOOPS AND ALAN B. HOOPER

GENERAL CONSIDERATIONS

Habitat

Nitrite-oxidizing bacteria exist in most aerobic environments where organic matter is mineralized. They are widely distributed in soils, freshwater, seawater, and sewage. In nature, they are frequently found in suboptimal environments.

Morphological Characteristics

Cells are rod- (Fig. 20.2) to pear-shaped (Fig. 20.3), spherical (Fig. 20.4) and spirillar (Fig. 20.5) without endospores. Some, but not all, nitrite-oxidizing bacteria possess intracytoplasmic membranes which may occur as flattened lamellae or tubular structures. Cells are motile or nonmotile; when cells are motile, flagella are polar to lateral. In enrichment cultures and in nature, cells aggregate, forming cysts and zoogloeae.

Enrichment and Isolation Procedures

Pure cultures of nitrite-oxidizing bacteria are obtained from enrichment cultures grown in a mineral salts medium (Table 20.2) enriched with nitrite. The enrichment culture is normally serially diluted to eliminate many heterotrophic organisms and to decrease the organics present in the inoculum. In the lower dilutions, nitrite oxidation can be detected in a few days, while in the higher dilutions, detection of nitrification may take several months. For this reason, enrichment cultures should be kept in the dark 1–4 months. Pure cultures from these enrichment cultures are obtained by either serial diluting or plating techniques. Because their prolonged generation time, it may take a year or more to obtain pure cultures of nitrite-oxidizing bacteria by either method.

Maintenance Procedures of Stock Cultures

Active cultures of nitrite-oxidizing bacteria are maintained in such chemolithotrophic or mixotrophic media as are listed in Table 20.2 or in such heterotrophic media as are listed in Table 20.3. The pH of the medium should be adjusted to 7.5–8.0 and checked periodically to maintain this pH range when mixotrophic or heterotrophic media are used. Some nitrite oxidizers (i.e., *Nitrobacter* strains) can survive periods of starvation of 3 months or more (Bock, 1972, 1976). Most terrestrial, but not marine, strains can be freeze-dried; however, their survival rate is extremely low. The number of surviving freeze-dried cells increases with the addition of sucrose and histidine before freezing. Storage of cultures in liquid nitrogen is the method of choice, since they can be stored for years with survival rates of 90% or better.

Growth Characteristics

Growth rates of nitrite-oxidizing bacteria are controlled by the substrate concentration, temperature, pH, light and the oxygen concentration. Most strains of nitrite-oxidizing bacteria grow best chemoautotrophically at nitrite concentrations of 2–30 mM, at a pH of 7.5–8.0 and at temperatures of 25–30°C. The generation time varies from 8 h to several days.

Some, but not all, nitrite oxidizers will grow mixotrophically in a medium supplemented with yeast extract and peptone as nitrogen sources and with pyruvate or acetate as carbon source. When they are

grown mixotrophically, the generation time decreases and the cell yield may increase by a factor of 10. Only *Nitrobacter* species are able to grow heterotrophically. Most strains grow faster chemolithotrophically than heterotrophically. High concentrations of nitrite may inhibit growth.

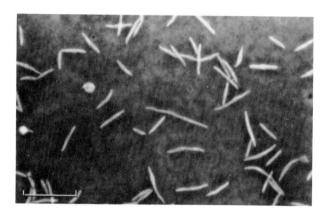

Figure 20.2. *Nitrospina gracilis.* Phase-contrast photomicrograph. *Bar,* 5 μm. (Reproduced with permission from S. W. Watson and J. B. Waterbury, Archiv für Mikrobiologie *77:* 203–230, 1971, ©Springer-Verlag, Berlin.)

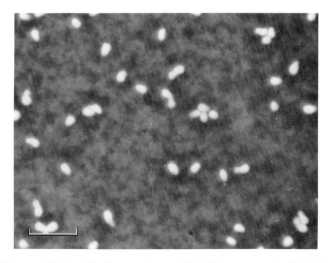

Figure 20.3. *Nitrobacter winogradskyi.* Phase-contrast photomicrograph. *Bar,* 5 μm.

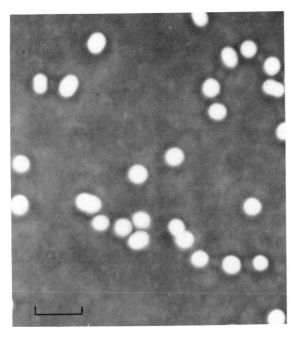

Figure 20.4. *Nitrococcus mobilis.* Phase-contrast photomicrograph. *Bar,* 5 µm. (Reproduced with permission from S. W. Watson and J. B. Waterbury, Archiv für Mikrobiologie *77:* 203–230, 1971, ©Springer-Verlag, Berlin.)

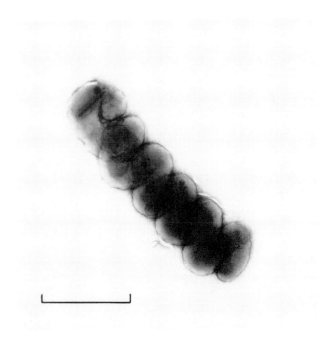

Figure 20.5. *Nitrospira marina* cell that has been negatively stained. Electron micrograph. *Bar,* 1 µm. (Reproduced with permission from S. W. Watson, E. Bock, F. W. Valois, J. B. Waterbury and U. Schlosser. Archives of Microbiology *144:* 1–7, 1986, ©Springer-Verlag, Berlin.)

Table 20.2.

Chemolithotrophic and mixotrophic media for nitrite oxidizers

	Terrestrial[a]		Marine[a]
	Aleem and Alexander (1958)	Bock, Sundermeyer-Klinger and Stackebrandt[b] (1983)	Watson and Waterbury (1971)
Distilled water (ml)	1000	1000	300
Seawater (ml)			700
$NaNO_2$ (mg)		2000	69
KNO_2 (mg)	300		
$MgSO_4 \cdot 7H_2O$ (mg)	187.5	50	100
$CaCl_2 \cdot 2H_2O$ (mg)	12.5		6.0
KH_2PO_4 (mg)	500	150	
K_2HPO_4 (mg)	500	0.750	1.74
$FeSO_4 \cdot 7H_2O$ (mg)	10	150	
$KHCO_3$ (mg)	1500		
Chelated iron (13%, Geigy Chemical) (mg)			1.0
$Na_2MoO_4 \cdot 2H_2O$ (µg)			30
$MnCl_2 \cdot 4H_2O$ (µg)			66
$CoCl_2 \cdot 6H_2O$ (µg)			0.6
$CuSO_4 \cdot 5H_2O$ (µg)			6.0
$ZnSO_4 \cdot 7H_2O$ (µg)			30
NaCl (mg)	187.5	500	
$CaCO_3$ (mg)			3
$(NH_4)_6 Mo_7O_{24} \cdot 4H_2O$ (µg)			50

[a] Amount per liter.

[b] For mixotrophic media, the following substances were added to 1 liter of autotrophic media: sodium pyruvate, 550 mg; yeast extract (Difco), 1500 mg; and peptone (Difco), 1500 mg.

Table 20.3.

Heterotrophic media for nitrite oxidizers

	Terrestrial[a]	
	Bock, Sundermeyer-Klinger and Stackebrandt (1983)	
Distilled water (ml)	1000	1000
Sodium pyruvate (mg) or	550	550
Sodium acetate (mg) or	410	
Glycerol (mg)	1400	
Yeast extract (mg) (Difco)	1500	
Peptone (mg) (Difco)	1500	
Vitamin-free casamino acids (mg) (Difco)		500

[a] Amount per liter

BIOCHEMICAL CONSIDERATIONS

Most of our knowledge on nitrite oxidation stems from investigations on strains of *Nitrobacter*. It is tacitly assumed, but not experimentally verified, that all nitrite-oxidizing bacteria will share common biochemical characteristics.

Nitrobacter strains grown chemolithotrophically oxidize nitrite to nitrate, producing ATP and NADH (Kumar and Nicholas, 1982b). NADH synthesis was shown to be an early step in energy conservation regardless of whether nitrite or organic substrates were oxidized (Sundermeyer and Bock, 1981). The source of oxygen during nitrite oxidation is H_2O (Aleem et al., 1965; Kumar et al., 1983; Hollocher, 1984).

Both *Nitrobacter* and *Nitrococcus* cells are rich in cytochromes c and a. However, members of two other genera, *Nitrospina* and *Nitrospira*, apparently lack cytochrome a. In *Nitrospira*, two cytochromes have been detected—one with an absorption peak at 558 nm and the other appearing as a shoulder at 550 nm. These peaks are interpreted as representing cytochrome b_{558} and c_{550}. Cell suspensions of *Nitrobacter* and *Nitrococcus* show characteristic (dithionite-reduced oxidized minus) absorption peaks at 420, 440, 550, 587 and 600 nm. The nitrite-oxidizing system in *Nitrobacter* is membrane-bound (Tsien et al., 1968; Aleem, 1968; O'Kelley et al., 1970). These membranes impart a brownish color which is typical of all nitrite oxidizers.

The oxidation of nitrite to nitrate is a two-electron step. The electrons are released from the enzyme-bound substrate; however, it is not known whether the actual substrate is the nitrite ion, undissociated nitrous acid or a hydrated form of one of these. Nitrite oxidoreductase of *Nitrobacter* consists of three proteins—one with a mol. wt. of 115,000, the second with a mol. wt. of 65,000, and the third with a mol. wt. of 32,000 forming an electron transport particle with a mol. wt. of 360,000. Cytochrome c, an unknown quinone, and NADH dehydrogenase are constituents of the enzyme system. The presence of molybdenum and iron as well as a high content of sulfur is typical for a molybdenum-iron-sulfur protein of the nitrate reductase type (Sundermeyer-Klinger et al., 1984).

Nitrite oxidoreductase also oxidizes nitrite to nitrate in the presence of the artificial electron acceptor, ferricyanide, and reduces nitrate to nitrite with reduced methylviologen or NADH as electron donor (Sundermeyer-Klinger et al., 1984). Nitrite oxidoreductase has been found in all *Nitrobacter* strains thus far tested but not in *Nitrospira* strains. In *Nitrospira marina,* the protein pattern of isolated membranes differed significantly (Watson et al., 1986).

Tanaka et al. (1983) suggest a somewhat simpler structure for a membrane enzyme from *Nitrobacter* which oxidizes nitrite with exogenous cytochrome c as electron acceptor. The enzyme, mol. wt. 100,000–130,000, contains subunits of 55,000, 29,000 and 19,000 and c and a hemes in the form of cytochromes c_1 and a_1. The enzyme accounts for 10% of the cell protein.

In *Nitrobacter*, the concentration of nitrite oxidoreductase varies with growth conditions. High concentrations of the enzyme are found when cells oxidize nitrite or an organic substrate in the presence of nitrate. The stimulatory substance in yeast extract and peptone (Bock, 1976) was found to be nitrate. In the absence of nitrate, nitrite oxidoreductase is repressed. The nitrite-oxidizing system is inducible. Cells grown on acetate require 9 days before they regain their ability to grow chemolithotrophically (Steinmüller and Bock, 1976). Similar studies have not yet been carried out on *Nitrococcus* and *Nitrospina*. In *Nitrospira* strains, in contrast to *Nitrobacter* strains, it appears that there is another enzyme system for nitrite oxidation (Watson et al., 1986).

In chemolithotrophic metabolism, nitrite serves the following double function: (1) as the electron donor for oxidative phosphorylation and (2) as the electron donor for NADH synthesis. According to the redox potential ($E_0' = +0.42$ V) for the NO_2^-/NO_3^- redox couple, the electrons released from the nitrite oxidoreductase penetrate the respiratory chain of *Nitrobacter* at the level of cytochrome a_1 to generate energy (Cobley 1976a, b; Bock, 1980; Aleem and Sewell, 1981).

The classical equation $NO_2^- + 0.5\ O_2 \rightarrow NO_3^- + 17$ kcal is the product of a three-step reaction:

$$NO_2^- + H_2O + 2\ \text{cytochromes}\ a_1^{3+} \rightarrow NO_3^- \\ + 2H^+ + 2\ \text{cytochromes}\ a_1^{2+} \quad \text{(a)}$$

$$2\ \text{cytochromes}\ a_1^{2+} + 2\ \text{cytochromes}\ c\ \text{oxidase}^{3+} \\ \rightarrow 2\ \text{cytochromes}\ a_1^{3+} + 2\ \text{cytochromes}\ c\ \text{oxidase}^{2+} \quad \text{(b)}$$

$$2\ \text{cytochromes}\ c\ \text{oxidase}^{2+} + 2H^+ + 0.5O_2 \\ \rightarrow 2\ \text{cytochromes}\ c\ \text{oxidase}^{3+} + H_2O \quad \text{(c)}$$

Cytochrome a_1 is assumed to be the essential electron acceptor for nitrite (Aleem, 1968; Sundermeyer and Bock, 1981; Tanaka et al., 1983). It is present in high concentrations in cells chemolithotrophically, mixotrophically and heterotrophically grown in the presence of nitrate, but it is present in low concentration in cells grown heterotrophically in the absence of nitrate (Sundermeyer and Bock, 1981). According to Reaction b, reduced cytochrome a_1 serves as the electron donor for cytochrome c and aa_3 (Tanaka et al., 1983).

Thermodynamically, the reduction of cytochrome c with nitrite as an electron donor is an energy-consuming process (Aleem, 1968). On the other hand, heterotrophic cells contain high amounts of a co-reactive b type cytochrome (Kirstein et al., 1986).

Thus it seems plausible that *Nitrobacter* species have two terminal oxidases: one for nitrite oxidation and another for heterotrophic respiration. The two terminal branches for electron transport seem to be connected via cytochrome c.

In *Nitrobacter* species, ATP is produced by oxidative phosphorylation (Aleem, 1968; Eigener, 1975). When nitrite is added to endogenous respiring cells, the ATP pool increases while the ADP pool decreases and the AMP pool remains constant. The energy charge of exponentially growing cells oxidizing nitrite is 0.37; that of endogenous respiring cells of *N. winogradskyi* is 0.5 (Eigener and Bock, 1972). At high oxygen partial pressure, when cell growth ceases and the respiration rate decreases, the ATP pool (Eigener, 1975) and the content of polyphosphates (Eigener and Bock, 1972) increase.

In *Nitrobacter*, membrane-bound nitrite oxidation is assumed to create a proton motive force, but neither washed cells nor isolated membrane vesicles show proton extrusion (Hollocher et al., 1982; Kumar and Nicholas, 1983). Isolated cytochrome c oxidase from *N. winogradskyi* does not form a pH gradient when reconstituted in liposomes (Sone et al., 1983). Although it is thought that *Nitrobacter* should be able to establish a proton motive force similar to that of other bacteria, the exact link between oxidation of nitrite and the putative proton motive force has not been established. Hooper and Dispirito (1985) suggest that all or part of the pH gradient may be generated simply by the proton-yielding oxidation of nitrite ($HNO_2 + H_2O \rightarrow HNO_3 + 2e^- + 2H^+$) in the extracytoplasmic side of the membrane, coupled to the proton-utilizing reduction of terminal electron acceptor ($2e^- + 2H^+ + 0.5O_2 \rightarrow H_2O$) on the cytoplasmic side of the membrane.

In cells oxidizing nitrite, the generation of NADH apparently requires an ATP-dependent reverse electron flow (Sewell and Aleem, 1979). After transition from a nitrogen- to oxygen-containing atmosphere, a decrease in the ATP pool and an increase in the NADH pool occur within the first second in intact *Nitrobacter* cells (Sundermeyer and Bock, 1981). NADH is generated at the expense of ATP. This energy-consuming process seems to be catalyzed by nitrite oxidoreductase. Thus the reverse electron flow system is not part of a normal respiratory chain but is possibly part of the key enzyme complex itself (Sundermeyer-Klinger et al., 1984).

The energy-consuming synthesis of NADH is presumed to be thermodynamically unfavorable. In chemolithotrophically grown cells of *Nitrobacter*, only 2–11% of the free energy generated from the oxidation of nitrite is used for cell growth; 85–115 mol of NO_2^- must be oxidized for the fixation of 1 mol of CO_2 (Bömeke, 1951). In batch culture, the maximum yield (cells produced per milligram of nitrite oxidized per milliliter) is 4×10^7 cells ml^{-1} (Bock, 1980). However, this concentration of cells can be exceeded in a mixotrophic medium. Culture filtrates of heterotrophic bacteria stimulate nitrification and cell yield of *Nitrobacter* cells. This may explain why nitrification is more rapid in contaminated cultures than in pure cultures. In mixotrophic media, some strains of *Nitrobacter* show diphasic growth; nitrite is oxidized first and then organics are oxidized. Growth rates in mixotrophic media may be used for taxonomic purposes (Steinmüller and Bock, 1976).

The nitrite-oxidizing bacteria fix carbon dioxide via the reductive pentose phosphate (RPP) cycle. In *Nitrobacter*, ribulose-1-5-bisphosphate carboxylase/oxygenase (RuBisCO) is responsible for CO_2 fixation in the RPP cycle. *N. winogradskyi* possesses mainly RuBisCO with a mol. wt. of 480,000 while "*Nitrobacter hamburgensis*" has two RuBisCO, one with a mol. wt. of 520,000 and the other with a mol. wt. of 480,000. SDS electrophoresis of both enzymes indicates a L_8S_8 quaternary structure similar to that reported for other organisms.

Polyhedral bodies called carboxysomes have been isolated from *N. winogradskyi*. The major protein component of these inclusion bodies is RuBisCO (Shively et al., 1977). Polypeptide profiles of carboxysomes correspond in molecular weight and relative abundance to the large and small subunits of RuBisCO (Biedermann and Westphal, 1979).

Carboxysomes (Fig. 20.6) occur in all *Nitrobacter* strains grown chemolithotrophically but rarely occur in heterotrophically grown cells. Numerous carboxysomes (Fig. 20.10) are also present in *Nitrococcus*

mobilis but have never been observed in *Nitrospina gracilis* (Watson and Waterbury, 1971) and in *Nitrospira marina* (Watson et al., 1986). The function of carboxysomes is not understood. It is difficult to understand why some nitrifiers have only soluble RuBisCO, while others contain both soluble and carboxysome-bound RuBisCO. The second key enzyme of the RPP cycle, phosphoribulokinase (Kiesow et al., 1977), has never been found to be associated with carboxysomes.

Neither theoretical considerations (Rittenberg, 1972) nor experimental results (Coleman, 1907/1908; Delwiche and Finstein, 1965; Ida and Alexander, 1965) indicate that *Nitrobacter* cells should be obligate chemolithotrophs. Smith and Hoare (1968) demonstrated that *Nitrobacter* would grow in a medium containing acetate and casein hydrolysate. It has also been shown that pyruvate and glycerol could serve as energy source for growth but that formate and α-ketoglutarate were less favorable substrates (Bock, 1976). Most strains of *Nitrobacter* cells grow much slower and are much less efficient when grown heterotrophically than when grown chemolithotrophically. Thus far, only strains of *Nitrobacter* have been grown heterotrophically. Why other nitrite-oxidizing bacteria fail to grow heterotrophically is not understood, but by analogy with other obligate autotrophs, this failure possibly stems from deficiencies in the tricarboxylic acid cycle enzymes, the lack of an NADH oxidase system, or a reduced permease system for organic substrates.

GENERA OF NITRITE-OXIDIZING BACTERIA

Genus I. **Nitrobacter** *Winogradsky 1892, 127*[AL] *(Nom. Cons. Opin. 23 Jud. Comm. 1958, 169)*

STANLEY W. WATSON, EBERHARD BOCK, HEINZ HARMS, HANS-PETER KOOPS AND ALAN B. HOOPER

Ni.tro.bac'ter. L.n. *nitrum* nitrate; M.L. n. *bacter* the masc. form of Gr. neut. n. *bactrum* a rod; M.L. masc. n. *Nitrobacter* nitrate rod.

Rod- or pear-shaped cells 0.5–0.8 × 1.0–2.0 μm (Fig. 20.3). Cells reproduce by budding (Fig. 20.6). **Cytomembranes occur in the form of a polar cap of flattened vesicles in the peripheral region of the cell** (Fig. 20.6). Gram-negative. **Motility may or may not occur;** if it does, it is by means of a single subterminal or lateral flagellum. **Aerobic.** The major source of energy and reducing power is from the **oxidation of nitrite to nitrate. Grows chemolithotrophically as well as chemoorganotrophically.** Occurs in aerobic environments where organic matter is being mineralized.

The mol% G + C of the DNA is 60–62 (Bd, T_m).

Type species: *Nitrobacter winogradskyi* Winslow, Broadhurst, Buchanan, Krumwiede, Rogers and Smith 1917, 552.

Further Descriptive Information

When grown chemolithotrophically, cells are pear- or rod-shaped, and buds are readily apparent (Figs. 20.3 and 20.6). Under heterotrophic conditions, cells divide by either budding or binary fission, and cell growth is often unbalanced, resulting in a large increase of poly-β-hydroxybutyrate inclusions which distort the shape and size of the cells. Cytoplasmic inclusions include carboxysomes, poly-β-hydroxybutyrate, glycogen and polyphosphates.

Cells of *Nitrobacter* have a unique cell envelope that differs from that found in other Gram-negative bacteria. The outermost cell wall layer is bipartite with an inner layer which is more electron dense than the outer layer (Figs. 20.6 and 20.7). The cytoplasmic membrane infolds into the cytoplasm, forming a polar cap of intracytoplasmic membranes (Murray and Watson, 1965) composed of 4–6 layers of paired membranes. The intracytoplasmic membranes are absent in the budding region of the cell and thus must be formed de novo in daughter cells.

Thin sections of chemolithotrophically grown cells show that the cytoplasmic side of the cytoplasmic membrane and the intracytoplasmic membrane is covered with a 10-nm electron-dense layer (Fig. 20.7). The cytoplasmic surface of these membranes, observed in freeze-

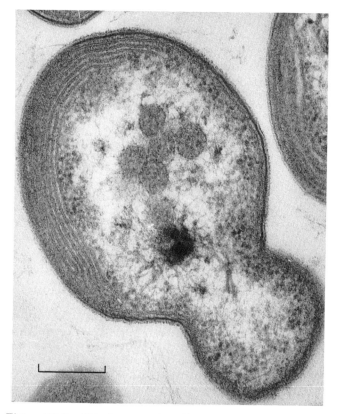

Figure 20.6. *Nitrobacter* species cell showing carboxysomes. Electron micrograph of a thin section. *Bar*, 0.25 μm.

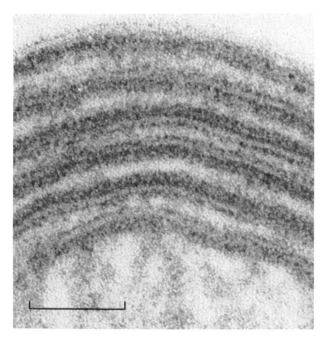

Figure 20.7. *Nitrobacter* species cell showing an electron-dense layer on cytoplasmic and intracytoplasmic membranes. Electron micrograph of a thin section. *Bar,* 50 nm. (Reproduced with permission from C. C. Remsen and S. W. Watson, International Review of Cytology *33:* 253–296, 1972, ©Academic Press, New York.)

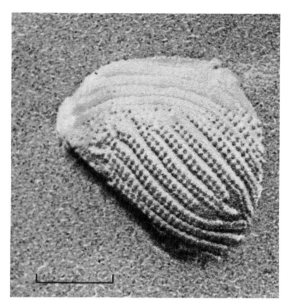

Figure 20.8. *Nitrobacter* species freeze-etched membrane showing particles arranged in rows on the membrane. Electron micrograph. *Bar,* 100 nm.

etched (Fig. 20.8) or negatively stained preparations, is studded with particles 7–9-nm in diameter which are arranged in paired rows (Remsen and Watson, 1972; Sundermeyer and Bock, 1981).

Heterotrophically grown cells often lack or have a reduced number of intracytoplasmic membranes. When present, the intracytoplasmic membranes and the cytoplasmic membranes, viewed in thin section, lack the electron-dense layer covering the cytoplasmic surface of membranes, and the 7–9-nm particles are no longer apparent in freeze-etched and negatively stained preparations (Bock and Heinrich, 1969).

Nitrobacter cells are facultative chemolithotrophs. When these organisms are grown chemolithotrophically, their energy and carbon needs are fulfilled by the oxidation of nitrite to nitrate and by the fixation of carbon dioxide. Cells grow chemolithotrophically in a basal salts medium enriched with nitrite. Most strains of *Nitrobacter* grow

faster chemolithotrophically than heterotrophically. When cells are grown heterotrophically, the generation times vary with the substrate used. Pyruvate, formate and acetate can serve as energy and carbon sources, but the highest growth yield is obtained with pyruvate (Bock, 1976). pH range for growth: 6.5–8.5. Temperature range for growth: 5–37°C.

Cells contain an unusual lipid A with 2,3-diamino-2,3-dideoxyglucose and hydroxymyristic acid in amide linkage as the only fatty acid in the one strain examined (Mayer et al., 1983). This lipid A structure is similar to that found in the budding species of *Rhodopseudomonas* (Mayer et al., 1983).

The cytoplasmic membrane and the intracytoplasmic membranes contain five major protein bands—apparent mol. wt. of 14,000, 28,000, 32,000, 65,000 and 116,000 (Sundermeyer-Klinger et al., 1984). The outer membrane fraction is characterized by the presence of 2-keto-3-deoxyoctonate and contains two major proteins with mol. wt. of 13,000 and 15,000 (Milde and Bock, 1984). The proteins associated with nitrite-oxidizing activity are associated with particles arranged in rows on the intracytoplasmic side of the membrane (Figs. 20.7 and 20.8).

Differentiation of the genus **Nitrobacter** from other genera

Table 20.1 lists characteristics differentiating *Nitrobacter* from other genera of nitrifying bacteria.

Taxonomic Comments

All organisms in the genus *Nitrobacter* have a similar shape, size and ultrastructure. Most strains are phenotypically similar to one another. Classification of strains into different species is based primarily on genotypic dissimilarities and slight differences in growth characteristics. Since the mol% G + C of the DNA ranges only from 60.1 to 61.7, this parameter cannot be employed for species differentiation. Preliminary DNA homology studies have demonstrated that genotypic differences occur between morphologically identical strains. This new information can be utilized for classification at the species level (Bock et al., 1983). With regard to the two currently recognized species in the genus, "N. hamburgensis" is only moderately related to N. winogradskyi (Engel strain) by a DNA homology value of 36%, which is indicative of separate species. Future homology studies of other strains will likely

demonstrate sufficient genotypic differences to warrant the creation of additional species.

Further Reading

Bock, E. 1976. Growth of *Nitrobacter* in the presence of organic matter. II. Chemoorganotrophic growth of *Nitrobacter agilis.* Arch. Microbiol. *108:* 305–312.

Mayer, H., E. Bock and J. Weckesser. 1983. 2,3-Diamino-2,3-dideoxyglucose containing lipid A in the *Nitrobacter* strain X$_{14}$. FEMS Microbiol. Lett. *17:* 93–96.

Milde, K. and E. Bock. 1984. Isolation and partial characterization of inner and outer membrane fractions of *Nitrobacter hamburgensis.* FEMS Microbiol. Lett. *21:* 137–141.

Murray, R.G.E. and S.W. Watson. 1965. Structure of *Nitrosocystis oceanus* and comparison with *Nitrosomonas* and *Nitrobacter.* J. Bacteriol. *89:* 1594–1609.

Remsen, C.C. and S.W. Watson. 1972. Freeze-etching of bacteria. Int. Rev. Cytol. *33:* 253–296.

Sundermeyer, H. and E. Bock. 1981. Energy metabolism of autotrophically and heterotrophically grown cells of *Nitrobacter winogradskyi.* Arch. Microbiol. *130:* 250–254.

Watson, S.W., F.W. Valois and J.B. Waterbury. 1981. The Family *Nitrobacteraceae*. *In* Starr, Stolp, Trüper, Balows and Schlegel (Editors), The Prokaryotes. A Handbook on Habitats, Isolation, and Identification of Bacteria. Springer-Verlag, Berlin, pp. 1005–1022.

Differentiation of the species of the genus **Nitrobacter**

Only two species of *Nitrobacter* are currently recognized, *N. winogradskyi* and "*N. hamburgensis.*" These species are separated primarily on genotypic differences based on DNA/DNA homology studies.

Phenotypically, "*N. hamburgensis*" differs from *N. winogradskyi* in that the former grows more rapidly heterotrophically than chemolithotrophically.

List of species of the genus **Nitrobacter**

1. **Nitrobacter winogradskyi** Winslow, Broadhurst, Krumwiede, Rogers and Smith 1917, 552, emend. mut. char. Watson 1971a, 264.[AL]

wi.no.grad'sky.i. M.L. gen. n. *winogradskyi* of Winogradsky; named after S. Winogradsky, the microbiologist who first isolated these bacteria.

Short rods, often pear-shaped, 0.6–0.8 × 1.0–2.0 μm (Fig. 20.3). Chemolithotrophically grown cells are rarely motile; when motile, the cells have a single subterminal flagellum. Other morphological characteristics are the same as those described for the genus.

Chemolithotrophs. Cells can also be grown heterotrophically in a basal salts medium enriched with pyruvate, acetate and glycerol as energy and carbon sources and with yeast extract, casamino acids, peptone, ammonia and nitrite as nitrogen sources. Chemolithotrophic and mixotrophic generation times range from 8 to 14 h, whereas chemoheterotrophic generation times range from 70 to 100 h (Bock, 1976).

The type strain was isolated from soils. Additional strains have been isolated from soils, freshwater, oceans, sewage disposal systems and compost piles and in most other aerobic environments where organic matter is being mineralized.

Many of the strains classified in this species may be found to differ genotypically but probably not phenotypically. It seems questionable that such organisms should be assigned to new species solely on the basis of genotypic differences.

The mol% G + C of the DNA in the type strain is 61.7 (Bd).
Type strain: ATCC 25391.

2. "**Nitrobacter hamburgensis**" Bock, Sundermeyer-Klinger and Stackebrandt 1983, 281.

ham'bur.gen.sis. M.L. adj. *hamburgensis* pertaining to the city of Hamburg, Federal Republic of Germany, where the organism was first isolated.

Cells are rod- to pear-shaped, 0.5–0.8 × 1.0–2.0 μm. Motile by means of a subpolar to lateral flagellum.

Cells grow chemolithotrophically, heterotrophically or mixotrophically. When grown chemolithotrophically, they are strict aerobes. Optimum growth rates are obtained in a mixotrophic medium containing nitrite, pyruvate, yeast extract and peptone. Growth is better in chemoorganic medium than in a chemolithotrophic medium.

Isolated from soils in Hamburg, Germany.

Phenotypically, this species differs from *N. winogradskyi* in that it grows better in a chemoorganic medium than in a chemolithotrophic medium.

The mol% G + C of the DNA of the type strain is 61.6 (T_m).

Type strain: #100 stored at Institut für Allgemeine Botanik, Abteilung für Mikrobiologie, University of Hamburg, Hamburg, Federal Republic of Germany.

Genus II. **Nitrospina** Watson and Waterbury 1971, 225[AL]

STANLEY W. WATSON, EBERHARD BOCK, HEINZ HARMS, HANS-PETER KOOPS AND ALAN B. HOOPER

Ni.tro.spi'na. L.n. *nitrum* nitrate; L.n. *spina* spine; M.L. masc. n. *Nitrospina* nitrate spine.

Rod-shaped cells 0.3–0.4 × 1.7–6.6 μm (Figs. 20.2 and 20.9). Spherical forms 1.35–1.45 μm in diameter are found in old cultures. Cells reproduce by binary fission. **Cells lack an extensive cytomembrane system,** but occasionally bleblike invaginations of the cytoplasmic membrane occur. Gram-negative. Nonmotile. **Aerobic.** The major source of energy and reducing power is from the **oxidation of nitrite to nitrate. Obligate chemolithotrophs;** cells will not grow mixotrophically or heterotrophically. Optimal growth requires 70–100% seawater. Cells occur in marine environments.

The mol% G + C of the DNA of the type species is 58 (Bd).

Type species: *Nitrospina gracilis* Watson and Waterbury 1971, 225.

Further Descriptive Information

Cells are straight, slender rods; spherical forms occur in senescent cultures. Cells are nonmotile and have cytochromes but no other pigments.

The organisms are obligate chemolithotrophs which oxidize nitrite to nitrate and fix carbon dioxide to fulfill their energy and carbon needs. When organisms are grown in seawater enriched with nitrite, no organic growth factors are required. Optimum growth occurs in media containing 70–100% seawater. No growth occurs in distilled water basal salts medium even if NaCl is included. The organisms are strictly aerobic.

Temperature range for growth: 20–30°C. pH range: 7.0–8.0.

Strains have been isolated from Atlantic and Pacific seawater. No terrestrial strains are known.

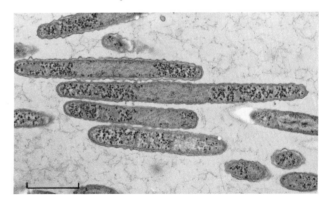

Figure 20.9. *N. gracilis* stained to demonstrate glycogen granules. Electron micrograph of a thin section. *Bar,* 1 μm. (Reproduced with permission from S. W. Watson and J. B. Waterbury, Archiv für Mikrobiologie 77: 203–230, 1971, ©Springer-Verlag, Berlin.)

Differentiation of the genus **Nitrospina** from other genera

Table 20.1 lists characteristics differentiating *Nitrospina* from other genera of nitrifying bacteria.

Taxonomic Comments

Classification of *Nitrospina* as a distinct genus of nitrifying bacteria is based presently on its unique morphological and ultrastructural characteristic differences. DNA homology studies have not yet been carried out on these organisms.

Further Reading

Watson, S.W., F.W. Valois and J.B. Waterbury. 1981. The Family *Nitrobacteraceae*. *In* Starr, Stolp, Trüper, Balows and Schlegel (Editors), The Prokaryotes. A Handbook on Habitats, Isolation, and Identification of Bacteria. Springer-Verlag, Berlin, pp. 1005–1022.

Watson, S.W. and J.B. Waterbury. 1971. Characteristics of two marine nitrite oxidizing bacteria, *Nitrospina gracilis* nov. gen. nov. sp. and *Nitrococcus mobilis* nov. gen. nov. sp. Arch. Mikrobiol. *77:* 203–230.

List of species of the genus **Nitrospina**

1. **Nitrospina gracilis** Watson and Waterbury 1971, 225.[AL]
gra′ci.lis. L. adj. *gracilis* slender.

Morphological, cultural and biochemical characteristics are the same as those described for the genus.

Figure 20.2 is a photomicrograph showing the morphology of the cells. Electron micrographs indicate that the cells are circumvallated by a well-defined cytoplasmic membrane which is surrounded by a multilayered cell wall (Fig. 20.9). Within the central region of the cells are areas which lack ribosomes and contain electron-dense strands of material resembling the nucleoplasm of other bacterial cells. Sections

treated with glycogen stains show many darkly stained bodies 30–40 nm in diameter.

No growth occurs below 14°C or above 40°C. The minimum generation time is 24 h. High concentrations of nitrite are toxic. Growth is inhibited by many organic compounds.

Only marine strains are known. The type strain was isolated from a depth of 13 m in open Atlantic Ocean waters approximately 200 miles from the mouth of the Amazon River.

The mol% G + C of the DNA of the type strain is 57.5 (Bd).
Type strain: ATCC 25379.

Genus III. **Nitrococcus** Watson and Waterbury 1971, 224[AL]

STANLEY W. WATSON, EBERHARD BOCK, HEINZ HARMS, HANS-PETER KOOPS AND ALAN B. HOOPER

Ni.tro.coc′cus. L. n. *nitrum* nitrate; Gr. n. *coccus* a grain, berry; M.L. masc. n. *Nitrococcus* nitrate sphere.

Spherical cells 1.5 μm or more in diameter (Fig. 20.4), occurring singly or in pairs. Cells reproduce by binary fission. Cells possess **tubular cytomembranes** randomly arranged throughout the cytoplasm (Fig. 20.10). Gram negative. **Motile** by means of 1 flagellum or 2 flagella. **Aerobic.** The major source of energy and reducing power is from the **oxidation of nitrite to nitrate. Obligate chemolithotrophs.** Optimal growth occurs in 70–100% seawater enriched with nitrite and other inorganic salts. No organic growth factors are required. Temperature range for growth: 15–30° C. pH range: 6.8–8.0. Organisms are isolated from marine environments.

The mol% G + C of the DNA of the type species is 61.2 (Bd).

Type species: *Nitrococcus mobilis* Watson and Waterbury 1971, 224.

Further Descriptive Information

Cells are spherical, 1.5–1.8 μm in diameter following division (Figs. 20.4 and 20.10). Just prior to division, cells are 1.8 × 3.5 μm in diameter. When swimming, cells have a turning, twisting erratic motion. The cells grow either free in media or in small clumps of a hundred or more cells embedded in a slime matrix. The cell wall is similar to that seen in most other Gram-negative bacteria.

The intracytoplasmic tubular membranes, which are randomly arranged throughout the cytoplasm (Fig. 20.10), arise by invagination of

the cytoplasmic membrane. Although numerous connections between the cytoplasmic membrane and the intracytoplasmic membranes are evident in thin sections, it is not clear whether the tubes represent a continuous cytoplasmic membrane intruding into the cytoplasm or whether this continuity is disrupted when the cell divides by binary fission. When cells are ruptured and negatively stained, the branching nature and surface structure of the membranes become apparent (Fig. 20.11). The membrane surface is covered with doughnut-shaped particles 6–8 nm in diameter.

The cytoplasm contains numerous ribosomes 13–20 nm in diameter which are dispersed between the intracytoplasmic membranes. Several kinds of inclusion bodies occur in the cells. The most prominent of these are the hexagonal bodies called carboxysomes (Fig. 20.10), which are about 100 nm in diameter. Each cell contains approximately 200 carboxysomes. Occasionally, poly-β-hydroxybutyrate granules are present. Also present are numerous electron-dense bodies believed to be glycogen storage products.

Optimal growth occurs in 70–100% seawater media; no growth has been observed in freshwater media even if NaCl is included. Optimum temperature range: 25–30°C. Optimum pH range: 7.5–8.0.

No terrestrial strains are known.

Differentiation of the genus **Nitrococcus** from other genera

Table 20.1 lists characteristics differentiating *Nitrococcus* from other genera of nitrifying bacteria.

Taxonomic Comments

Classification of *Nitrococcus* as a distinct genus of nitrifying bacteria is based presently on its unique morphological and ultrastructural characteristic differences. DNA homology studies have not yet been carried out on these organisms.

Further Reading

Watson, S.W., F.W. Valois and J.B. Waterbury. 1981. The Family *Nitrobacteraceae*. *In* Starr, Stolp, Trüper, Balows and Schlegel (Editors), The Prokaryotes. A Handbook on Habitats, Isolation, and Identification of Bacteria. Springer-Verlag, Berlin, pp. 1005–1022.

Watson, S.W. and J.B. Waterbury. 1971. Characteristics of two marine nitrite oxidizing bacteria, *Nitrospina gracilis* nov. gen. nov. sp. and *Nitrococcus mobilis* nov. gen. nov. sp. Arch. Mikrobiol. *77:* 203–230.

List of species of the genus **Nitrococcus**

1. **Nitrococcus mobilis** Watson and Waterbury 1971, 224.[AL]
mo′bi.lis. L. adj. *mobilis* movable, motile.

Morphological, cultural and biochemical characteristics are the same as those described for the genus. Figures 20.4 and 20.10 illustrate the

morphological features.

The type strain was isolated from equatorial Pacific seawater.
The mol% G + C of the DNA of the type strain is 61.3 (Bd).
Type strain: ATCC 25380.

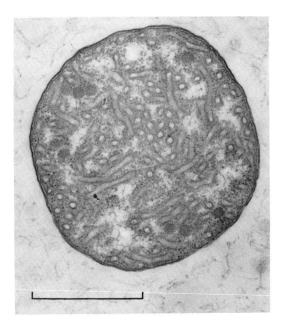

Figure 20.10. *N. mobilis* showing carboxysomes and tubular intracytoplasmic membranes. Electron micrograph of a thin section. *Bar*, 1 μm.

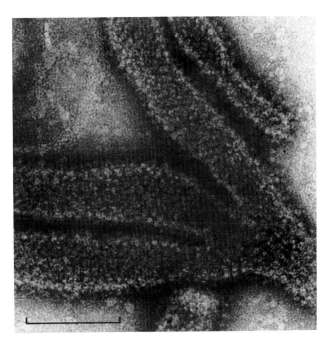

Figure 20.11. *N. mobilis* showing particles covering surface of negatively stained tubular membrane. Electron micrograph. *Bar*, 100 nm. (Reproduced with permission from S. W. Watson and J. B. Waterbury, Archiv für Mikrobiologie *77:* 203–230, 1971, ©Springer-Verlag, Berlin.)

Genus IV. **Nitrospira** *Watson, Bock, Valois, Waterbury and Schlosser 1986b, 489^{VP*} (Effective publication: Watson, Bock, Valois, Waterbury and Schlosser, 1986a, 6)*

STANLEY W. WATSON, EBERHARD BOCK, HEINZ HARMS, HANS-PETER KOOPS AND ALAN B. HOOPER

Ni.tro.spi′ra. L. n. *nitrum* nitrate; Gr. n. *spira* a coil, spiral; M.L. fem. n. *Nitrospira* nitrate spiral.

Helical to vibrioid-shaped cells having a **width of 0.3–0.4 μm** and a **spiral amplitude of 0.8–1.0 μm.** Cells reproduce by binary fission. **Cytomembranes are lacking.** Gram-negative. Usually **nonmotile. Aerobic.** The major source of energy and reducing power is from the **oxidation of nitrite to nitrate. Chemolithotrophs;** cells can grow mixotrophically. Seawater is required for growth; optimal growth occurs in a medium containing 70–100% seawater enriched with nitrite and other inorganic salts; no growth factors are required. Cells grow optimally in a mixotrophic medium. **Ubiquitous in ocean environments;** have also been isolated from soil samples.

The mol% G + C of the DNA of the type species is 50 (T_m).

Type species: *Nitrospira marina* Watson, Bock, Valois, Waterbury and Schlosser 1986b, 489.

Further Descriptive Information

Cells are curved rods which occur as tightly to loosely wound helices with 1–20 turns. When grown mixotrophically, most cells have only one turn, making them comma-shaped (Fig. 20.12). These appear spherical when viewed by phase-contrast microscopy. The true nature of the cell shapes can best be observed when the cells are negatively stained and viewed with an electron microscope (Fig. 20.5).

A general electron microscopic view of thin sections of cells is given in Figure 20.13. Like most Gram-negative bacteria, cells are surrounded by a multilayered cell wall consisting of a plasma membrane and an outer cell wall, each with a width of 6–7 nm, separated by a periplasmic space. The overall thickness of the *N. marina* cell envelope is 43–53 nm. The unique feature of this cell envelope is the width (31–41 nm) of the periplasmic space, which is approximately twice that found in

other Gram-negative bacteria. In some cells, the periplasmic space balloons out in restricted areas, forming a granular layer approximately 300–400 nm thick (Watson et al., 1986a).

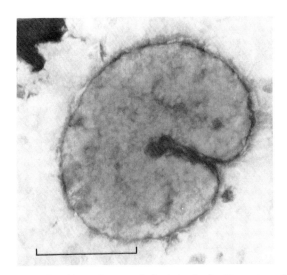

Figure 20.12. *N. marina* negatively stained cell with one turn. Electron micrograph. *Bar,* 0.5 μm. (Reproduced with permission from S. W. Watson, E. Bock, F. W. Valois, J. B. Waterbury and U. Schlosser, Archives of Microbiology *144:* 1–7, 1986, ©Springer-Verlag, Berlin.)

---

*VP denotes that this name, although not on the Approved Lists of Bacterial Names, has been validly published in the official publication, International Journal of Systematic Bacteriology.

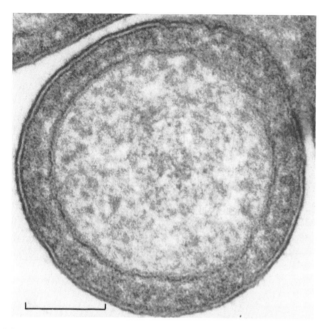

Figure 20.13. *N. marina.* Note the thickness of periplasmic space. Electron micrograph of a thin section. *Bar,* 100 nm. (Reproduced with permission from S. W. Watson, E. Bock, F. W. Valois, J. B. Waterbury and U. Schlosser. Archives of Microbiology *144:* 1–7, 1986, ©Springer-Verlag, Berlin.)

Intracytoplasmic membranes found in some other nitrite-oxidizing bacteria are lacking. Within the central region of the cells are areas which lack ribosomes and contain electron-dense strands of material resembling the nucleoplasm of other bacterial cells. Most cells contain a moderate concentration of ribosomes (10–15 nm in diameter) but lack the carboxysomes that are found in most other nitrite-oxidizing bacteria. Cells contain glycogen deposits but lack other cell inclusions.

Optimum growth occurs in 70–100% seawater enriched with 2 mM nitrite. No growth occurs in distilled water-basal salts medium even if NaCl and MgCl₂ are included. Optimum temperature range for growth: 20–30°C. Optimum pH range: 7.6–8.0. High concentrations of nitrite are toxic. The organisms grow better mixotrophically than chemolithotrophically. The minimum generation times for chemolithotrophic growth and mixotrophic growth are 90 and 23 h, respectively. Cells can be grown mixotrophically in seawater enriched with nitrite as energy source, pyruvate (55 mg/l) or glycerol (1 g/l) as carbon source, and either yeast extract or peptone (150 mg/l) as nitrogen source. High concentrations of organics are inhibitory.

Cell suspensions and cell-free extracts show characteristic (dithionite-reduced oxidized minus) absorption peaks at 416, 550 (shoulder) and 558 nm. Optimal nitrite oxidation rates are obtained in 2 mM nitrite with intact cells; no nitrite oxidation has been detected in cell homogenates. None of the five major protein bands of the nitrite-oxidizing membranes of *Nitrobacter* have been detected in *Nitrospira* membranes.

Differentiation of the genus **Nitrospira** from other genera

Table 20.1 lists characteristics differentiating *Nitrospira* from other genera of nitrifying bacteria.

Taxonomic Comments

Classification of *Nitrospira* as a distinct genus of nitrifying bacteria is based presently on its unique morphological and ultrastructural characteristic differences. DNA homology studies have not yet been carried out on these organisms.

Further Reading

Watson, S. W., E. Bock, F. W. Valois, J. B. Waterbury and U. Schlosser. 1986a. *Nitrospira marina* gen. nov., sp. nov.: a chemolithotrophic nitrite-oxidizing bacterium. Arch. Microbiol. *144:* 1–7.

Watson, S. W., F. W. Valois and J. B. Waterbury. 1981. The Family *Nitrobacteraceae. In* Starr, Stolp, Trüper, Balows and Schlegel (Editors), The Prokaryotes. A Handbook on Habitats, Isolation, and Identification of Bacteria. Springer-Verlag, Berlin, pp. 1005–1022.

List of species of the genus **Nitrospira**

1. **Nitrospira marina** Watson, Bock, Valois, Waterbury and Schlosser 1986b, 489.[VP] (Effective publication: Watson, Bock, Valois, Waterbury and Schlosser 1986a, b.)

ma.ri′na. L. fem. adj. *marina* of the sea, marine.

Morphological, cultural and biochemical characteristics are the same as those described for the genus. Figures 20.5, 20.12 and 20.13 illustrate the morphological features.

Originally isolated from Gulf of Maine water samples, this species was also the predominant nitrite oxidizer in water and sediment samples from New York Harbor and in water samples from the Black Sea. Additional strains were cultured from sediment and water samples from Woods Hole Harbor, from beach sands and salt marshes on Cape Cod, from brackish waters in the Savannah and Mississippi Rivers, and from open Atlantic Ocean waters off the coast of Angola. A cursory survey suggests that the species may be the most important nitrite-oxidizing species in marine sediments and in marine waters rich in organic matter. The habitat is apparently not restricted to the marine environment, since one strain was also cultured from soil samples collected in the Etosha Pan in Namibia.

The mol% G + C of the DNA of the type strain is 50.0 ± 0.4 (T_m).

Type strain: ATCC 43039.

Ammonia-Oxidizing Bacteria

STANLEY W. WATSON, EBERHARD BOCK, HEINZ HARMS, HANS-PETER KOOPS AND ALAN B. HOOPER

GENERAL CONSIDERATIONS

Habitat

Ammonia-oxidizing bacteria are found in most aerobic environments where organic matter is being mineralized. Species have been isolated from a great variety of soils, most oceans, brackish environments, rivers, lakes and sewage disposal systems.

Morphological Characteristics

Cells are rod-shaped (Figs. 20.14, 20.15 and 20.39), spherical (Figs. 20.16 and 20.17), spirillar (Fig. 20.18) or lobular (Fig. 20.19) without endospores. Some, but not all, species possess intracytoplasmic membranes which may occur as flattened lamellae arranged centrally, peripherally or randomly. Carboxysomes and/or polyphosphate inclusions are common in some, but not all, species. When cells are motile, flagella are polar to lateral or peritrichous. Most cells have a typical Gram-negative cell envelope; however, the marine and some other strains may have additional cell wall layers composed of repeating subunits arranged in a geometric symmetrical array. Cells occur singly, in pairs or, on occasion, in short chains. Cells often become embedded in slime-forming aggregates called zoogloeae or cysts in enrichment cultures and in nature.

Enrichment and Isolation Procedures

Enrichment cultures are grown in tubes or flasks of basal salts media enriched with ammonia (Table 20.4), and pure cultures are obtained by employing serial dilution or plating techniques. Cultures should be incubated in the dark for a period of 1–4 months. Although detection of nitrification in the lower dilutions can frequently take a few days, detection of growth in the higher dilutions may take several months.

Although organics are not added to enrichment cultures, organics present in the inoculum or those produced by the ammonia oxidizers will support the growth of heterotrophic contaminants. To minimize the organics and the growth of heterotrophic contaminants, the inoculum should be serially diluted through several orders of magnitude. Once growth is detected in the serially diluted enrichment culture, it is diluted serially again or streaked out on agar plates containing the appropriate inorganic salts. Since the ammonia oxidizers have a prolonged generation time from 8 h to several days, it may take several months to obtain pure cultures.

Maintenance Procedures of Stock Cultures

Pure cultures of ammonia-oxidizing bacteria can be maintained on agar plates and in liquid cultures in basal salts media enriched with

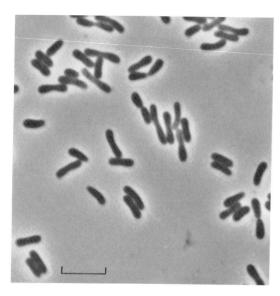

Figure 20.15. *Nitrosomonas* species terrestrial strain. Phase-contrast photomicrograph. *Bar*, 5 μm.

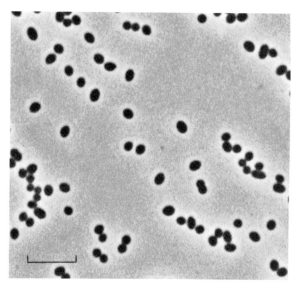

Figure 20.14. *Nitrosomonas europaea* type strain (ATCC 25978). Phase-contrast photomicrograph. *Bar*, 5 μm.

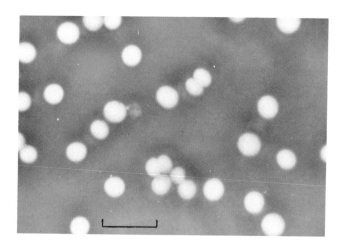

Figure 20.16. *Nitrosococcus oceanus.* Phase-contrast photomicrograph. *Bar*, 5 μm.

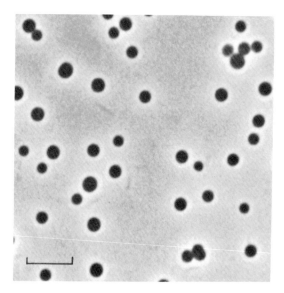

Figure 20.17. "*Nitrosococcus mobilis.*" Phase-contrast photomicrograph. *Bar*, 5 μm.

ammonia (Table 20.4). The pH of the final medium should be adjusted to 7.5–7.8. The growing cultures must be transferred every 2–4 months.

The best method for storing stock cultures is by the use of liquid nitrogen. With this technique, the survival of both the terrestrial and the marine strains is over 90%, and cultures so stored remain viable for 10 years or longer.

Most terrestrial, but not marine, strains can also be freeze-dried. The survival rate of freeze-dried cells is extremely low for all strains, and most marine strains are not viable after freeze-drying.

Growth Characteristics

Growth rates of ammonia-oxidizing bacteria in culture are primarily controlled by substrate concentration, temperature, pH, light, and oxygen tensions. Some strains have an obligate sodium requirement Watson, 1965; Koops, 1969; Koops et al., 1976; Krümmel and Harms, 1980), and all cultures should be incubated in the dark. Most species grow optimally at 25–30°C, at pH 7.5–8.0 and at substrate concentrations of 2–10 mM. As ammonia is oxidized to nitrite, the pH of the medium drops.

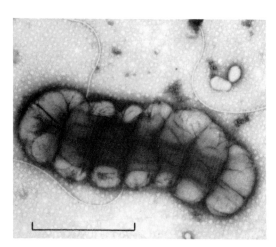

Figure 20.18. *Nitrosospira briensis* negatively stained cell. Electron micrograph. *Bar,* 1 μm. (Reproduced with permission from S. W. Watson, Archiv für Mikrobiologie *75:* 179–188, 1971, ©Springer-Verlag, Berlin.)

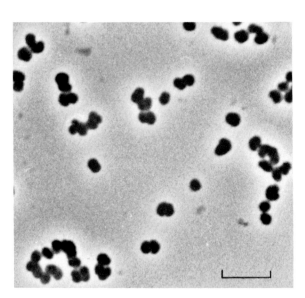

Figure 20.19. *Nitrosolobus multiformis.* Phase-contrast photomicrograph. *Bar,* 5 μm.

Table 20.4.

Growth media for ammonia oxidizers

	Terrestrial[a]		Marine[a]	Brackish[a]
	Watson et al. (1971)	Krümmel and Harms (1982)	Watson (1965)	Koops et al. (1976)
Distilled water (ml)	1000	1000		600
Seawater (ml)			1000	400
$(NH_4)_2SO_4$ (mg)	2000		1320	
NH_4Cl (mg)		535.0		500
NaCl (mg)		584.0		
$MgSO_4 \cdot 7H_2O$ (mg)	200	49.3	200	
$CaCl_2 \cdot 2H_2O$ (mg)	20	147.0	20	
KH_2PO_4 (mg)		54.4		
K_2HPO_4 (mg)	15.9		114	50
KCl (mg)		74.4		
Chelated iron (13%, Geigy Chemical) (mg)	1		1.0	
$FeSO_4 \cdot 7H_2O$ (μg)		973.1		
$Na_2MoO_4 \cdot 2H_2O$ (μg)	100		1	
$(NH_4)_6Mo_7O_{24} \cdot 4H_2O$ (μg)		37.1		
$MnCl_2 \cdot 4H_2O$ (μg)	200		2	
$MnSO_4 \cdot 4H_2O$ (μg)		44.6		
$CoCl_2 \cdot 6H_2O$ (μg)	2		2	
$CuSO_4 \cdot 5H_2O$ (μg)	20	25.0	20	
$ZnSO_4 \cdot 7H_2O$ (μg)	100	43.1	100	
H_3BO_3 (μg)		49.4		
$CaCO_3$ (mg)				5000
Phenol red (0.5%) (ml)	1			
Cresol red (0.05%) (ml)		1		1

[a] Amount per liter.

This drop in pH is a presumptive indication of ammonia oxidation, but if it is not adjusted back or is held at pH 7.5-8.0 with buffer (HEPES, 0.01 M), further oxidation is limited. The best method of pH maintenance is a pH-stat which makes continuous pH adjustments. However, adjustments can also be made manually with the aid of pH indicators such as phenol red.

The effect of various organic compounds on the growth of ammonia-oxidizing bacteria was examined by Krümmel and Harms (1982). They found that *Nitrosococcus oceanus,* compared with the other ammonia oxidizers tested, had a low tolerance to organic matter. Organic compounds scarcely affected the growth of *Nitrosomonas* strains, whereas nitrite formation by "*Nitrosococcus mobilis*" was inhibited by nearly all the substances tested. The growth of one strain of *Nitrosospira* was enhanced more than 39% by acetate and formate, but no growth was detectable in the presence of pyruvate. In contrast, another strain of *Nitrosospira* was stimulated only by pyruvate. Nitrite formation by the two strains of "*Nitrosovibrio tenuis*" was similar. The growth of both strains was enhanced considerably by formate and glucose; acetate and, to a greater extent, pyruvate inhibited these bacteria. Ammonia-oxidizing bacteria have failed to grow heterotrophically thus far, except for one strain of *Nitrosomonas europaea* grown by Pan and Umbreit (1972) in dialysis culture, but this work has received much criticism (Smith and Hoare, 1977; Matin, 1978).

Reports show that organic compounds can be assimilated in some strains of ammonia oxidizers in appreciable quantity when they are grown in the presence of inorganic energy sources (Clark and Schmidt, 1966; Kelly, 1971; Martiny and Koops, 1982). However, Williams and Watson (1968) found that resting cells of *Nitrosococcus oceanus* (*Nitrosocystis oceanus*) incubated with ^{14}C-labeled glucose and glutamate and cells grown in the presence of ^{14}C-labeled glucose, glutamate, pyruvate and methionine incorporated these compounds into cellular material but at a level too low to provide the cells major carbon and energy needs. Thus it appears that some of the ammonia-oxidizing bacteria have permeability barriers which restrict the flow of organic molecules into the cell.

In batch culture, the energy efficiency of autotrophically grown ammonia oxidizers varied from strain to strain (Belser and Schmidt, 1980). The cell yield of mixotrophically grown cultures per unit of ammonia oxidized was increased in comparison with autotrophically grown cells (Krümmel and Harms, 1982). The energy efficiency decreases with decreasing pH, starting at pH 7.4 (Terry and Hooper, 1970). Accumulation of polyphosphate occurs at pH values below 7.4.

BIOCHEMICAL CONSIDERATIONS

Most biochemical investigations of the ammonia-oxidizing bacteria have been limited to strains of *Nitrosomonas.* However, it is tacitly assumed that similar results would be obtained with other ammonia-oxidizing genera.

All species thus far studied were found to be obligate chemolithotrophs which oxidize ammonia to nitrite and fix carbon dioxide to fulfill their energy and carbon needs. The literature on mechanisms of ammonia oxidation and energy transduction has been reviewed (Drozd, 1980; Hooper, 1984). During the oxidative reaction, NH_3 rather than NH_4^+ serves as the substrate (Suzuki et al., 1974; Drozd, 1976). The oxidation of ammonia occurs in two or more steps. The first step, oxidation of ammonia to hydroxylamine or a related enzyme-bound chemical species, incorporates molecular oxygen (Hollocher et al., 1981). It is not known with certainty whether the reaction is a monooxygenase ($NH_3 + XH_2 + O_2 \rightarrow NH_2OH + X + H_2O$) or a dioxygenase ($X + NH_3 + O_2 \rightarrow NH_2OH + XO$). If a monooxygenase is involved, electrons would presumably originate from the hydroxylamine oxidation step and may be transferred via cytochrome c_{554}, as observed in extracts (Tsang and Suzuki, 1982). The cell-free oxidation of ammonia has been reconstructed with a membrane fraction, a soluble fraction containing the hydroxylamine-oxidizing enzyme and a soluble cytochrome-containing fraction (Suzuki and Kwok, 1981). Suggestive support for the monooxygenase mechanism comes from the observations of Hyman and Wood that oxidation by *Nitrosomonas* of methane (1983), ethylene (1984a) and bromocarbon compounds (1984b) requires a source of reducing power, such as hydrazine, which is oxidized to N_2 by hydroxylamine oxidoreductase (Falcone et al., 1963). The possibility that both NH_3 and the carbon compounds are oxidized by the same reaction center is supported by the observed competitive inhibition of ammonia oxidation by CO, methane and methanol (Suzuki et al., 1976) and by inhibition by ethylene (Hynes and Knowles, 1982).

The oxidation of ammonia to nitrite is sensitive to inhibition by many compounds at low concentrations, whereas the oxidation of hydroxylamine to nitrite is unaffected or much less susceptible (Lees, 1952; Hooper and Terry, 1973). Sensitivity to copper-binding agents led to the hypothesis that a copper-containing enzyme is involved (Lees, 1952). Inhibition of ammonia oxidation by 2-chloro-6-trichloromethylpyridine is used in ecological studies (Bremner and Blackmer, 1978). Acetylene, which is used in ecological studies to inhibit reduction of N_2O by dentrifying bacteria, also inhibits ammonia oxidation (and, therefore, N_2O production) by *Nitrosomonas* (Hynes and Knowles, 1978).

The second step, oxidation of hydroxylamine via NOH to nitrite, is thought to be the energy-yielding portion of the reaction. This step is catalyzed by hydroxylamine oxidoreductase (HAO). The enzyme (mol. wt. 200,000) contains 21 *c* hemes and three P-460 centers (Hooper et al., 1978). The subunit structure of the enzyme is $\alpha_3\beta_3$ with six *c* type hemes and one P-460 type heme per repeated unit (Terry and Hooper, 1981). This enzyme catalyzes the 2e$^-$ dehydrogenation of hydroxylamine to form HNO (which can spontaneously form N_2O); NO has also been detected as a product of oxidation of NH_2OH (Hooper and Terry, 1979). It is not known whether the second oxygen in nitrite is from O_2 (i.e., HNO + $0.5O_2 \rightarrow HNO_2$) or H_2O (i.e., HNO + $H_2O \rightarrow HNO_2 + 2H^+ + 2e^-$). The latter mechanism has received strong support (Andersson and Hooper, 1983).

P-460, which is easily destroyed by H_2O_2, is the CO- and NH_2OH-reactive site on the enzyme (Hooper and Terry, 1977). The hemelike P-460 has very unusual physical properties (Andersson et al., 1984). The *c* hemes of the enzyme are partially distinguishable by their electron paramagnetic resonance properties (Lipscomb and Hooper, 1982) and their optical absorption maxima and oxidation-reduction potentials which range from 295 mV to −390 mV (Prince et al., 1983). In the oxidation of NH_2OH, electrons are thought to pass through P-460 to *c* hemes of HAO (Hooper et al., 1984) and then to a terminal oxidase and cytochrome with cytochromes c_{554}, c_{552} (Yamanaka and Shinra, 1974) and c_{m553} (Dispirito et al., 1985) as possible mediators.

Cells of *Nitrosomonas* are red, reflecting the unusually high cellular content of cytochromes which are found in the periplasmic space and membrane (Hooper et al., 1972; Dispirito et al., 1985). Membranes contain ubiquinone-8 (Hooper et al., 1972). Membranes of *Nitrosococcus* and *Nitrosomonas* have predominantly 16:0 and 16:1 fatty acids, respectively (Blumer et al., 1969).

Investigations of Olson and Hooper (1983) and Dispirito et al. (1985) support the idea of a mechanism for creation of a proton gradient based on an extracytoplasmic, proton-yielding dehydrogenase coupled to a cytoplasmic proton-utilizing terminal oxidase reaction (Hooper and Dispirito, 1985). Thus uptake of the primary substrate ammonia into the cells (Drozd, 1976; Bhandari and Nicholas, 1979a, b) may be unnecessary. Oxidation of hydroxylamine to nitrite is accompanied by production of a proton gradient (Hollocher et al., 1981; Kumar and Nicholas, 1982a) in keeping with the chemiosmotic scheme proposed by Mitchell (Drozd, 1976; Olson and Hooper, 1983). Although all ammonia oxidizers oxidize hydroxylamine to nitrite, this substrate does not support growth even when added continuously at 10^{-5} M.

At reduced oxygen concentrations, oxidation of NH₃ by *Nitrosomonas* is accompanied by production of N_2O (and, to a lesser extent, NO) (Blackmer et al., 1980; Goreau et al., 1980). N_2 is apparently not a product (Ritchie and Nicholas, 1972). In cells, N_2O can be produced by reduction of nitrite (Ritchie and Nicholas, 1972). It is not known whether N_2O can also be produced in cells by direct oxidation of NH_3 or NH_2OH (without nitrite as intermediate). Extracts will catalyze producton of N_2O and NO by reduction of nitrite (Hooper, 1968; Ritchie and Nicholas, 1972, 1974) or by oxidation of hydroxylamine (Hooper and Terry, 1979).

Carbon dioxide fixed via the Calvin cycle (Campbell et al., 1966) serves as the primary carbon source. The specific activity of carbonic anhydrase of *Nitrosomonas europaea* is greater when the concentrations of CO_2 in the growth medium are low, suggesting a role for the enzyme in promoting assimilation of carbon (Jahnke et al., 1984). Although most ammonia oxidizers can grow mixotrophically on several organic compounds, such as acetate, formate, pyruvate, glucose and complex compounds (Smith and Hoare, 1977), heterotrophic growth has not been demonstrated (Krümmel and Harms, 1982). The failure of the ammonia oxidizers to grow heterotrophically may be due to deficiencies in the tricarboxylic cycle and/or the lack of a NADH oxidase system which is coupled to ATP synthesis (Hooper, 1969). This result is controversial; Williams and Watson (1968) found these activities to be present in *Nitrosococcus*.

Reduction of pyridine nucleotide in extracts of *Nitrosomonas* can be achieved in the presence of hydroxylamine and ATP (Aleem, 1966). Ammonia-nitrogen may be assimilated by an active NADPH-specific glutamate dehydrogenase (Hooper et al., 1967; Wallace and Nicholas, 1969).

Nitrosomonas is also able to oxidize ethylene (Hyman and Wood, 1984a), methane (Jones and Morita, 1983), carbon monoxide (Tsang and Suzuki, 1982) and bromocarbon compounds (Hyman and Wood, 1984b). There are some striking similarities between the hydroxylation of ammonia and methane (Hooper, 1984). Carbon from methane is incorporated into cellular components (Jones and Morita, 1983). All attempts to grow ammonia oxidizers on methane or to grow methane oxidizers on ammonia as sole energy source have failed.

The ability of cells of *Nitrosomonas* to oxidize ammonia is inactivated by ultraviolet light and by light of 410 nm (Hooper and Terry, 1974). Photoinactivation does not occur anaerobically or under conditions in which nitrite is being rapidly produced.

Taxonomic Comments

The ammonia-oxidizing bacteria are composed of two groups of organisms not phylogenetically closely related (Woese et al., 1984b). For example, *Nitrosococcus oceanus* is related to the *Chromatiaceae* branch (Woese et al., 1985), while all other species thus far studied are related to one of the *Rhodospirillaceae*. At present, the ammonia oxidizers are categorized, at both the generic and the species level, primarily by their morphological characteristics.

GENERA OF AMMONIA-OXIDIZING BACTERIA

Genus V. **Nitrosomonas** *Winogradsky 1892, 127^AL (Nom. Cons. Opin. 23 Jud. Comm. 1958, 169)*

STANLEY W. WATSON, EBERHARD BOCK, HEINZ HARMS, HANS-PETER KOOPS AND ALAN B. HOOPER

Ni.tro.so.mo′nas. M.L. adj. *nitrosus* nitrous; Gr. fem. n. *monas*, a unit, monad; M.L. fem. n. *Nitrosomonas* nitrite monad, i.e. the monad producing nitrite.

Ellipsoidal or rod-shaped cells. Cell shape and size variable between strains. Cells occur singly or, rarely, in chains and grow free in media or are embedded in a slime matrix. Cells reproduce by binary fission. **Cells have intracytoplasmic membranes arranged as flattened vesicles primarily in the peripheral region of the cytoplasm.** Gram-negative. **Motile or nonmotile. Aerobic.** Temperature range for growth: 5–30°C. pH range for growth: 5.8–8.5. The major source of energy and reducing power is from the **oxidation of ammonia to nitrite. Chemolithotrophs;** cells can grow mixotrophically but not heterotrophically. Occur in soils, most oceans of the world, lakes, rivers and sewage disposal systems.

The mol% G + C of the DNA is 45–54 (Bd, T_m).

Type species: *Nitrosomonas europaea* Winogradsky 1892, 127.

Further Descriptive Information

The size, shape and ultrastructure of various strains are illustrated in Figures 20.14, 20.15, and 20.20–20.27. Terrestrial strains (Figs. 20.24–20.26) have a typical Gram-negative type of cell wall; however, marine strains (Fig. 20.27) have an additional cell wall layer which is composed of subunits arranged in a macromolecular array (Figs. 20.28 and 20.29). Two different arrangements of the subunits have been found. In most marine strains, the sculptured outer layer is 15 nm wide and is composed of subunits that are 5 nm in diameter and have a periodicity of 12 nm (Fig. 20.28). A different arrangement of subunits has been found on one marine strain (Fig. 20.29) (Watson and Remsen, 1969).

Most strains of *Nitrosomonas* have intracytoplasmic membranes in the form of flattened vesicles located in the peripheral regions of the cytoplasm (Figs. 20.26 and 20.27). On occasion, intracytoplasmic membranes may intrude into the inner regions of the cytoplasm (Fig. 20.24). Intracytoplasmic membranes arise by an infolding of the cytoplasmic membrane. Spheroplasts do not contain internal vesicles or enzymes of the type that would be associated with such vesicles (Hooper et al., 1984). This suggests that all internal membranes of these organisms are invaginations.

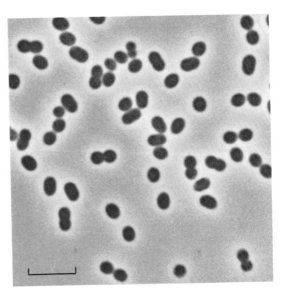

Figure 20.20. *Nitrosomonas* species terrestrial strain. Phase-contrast photomicrograph. *Bar*, 5 µm.

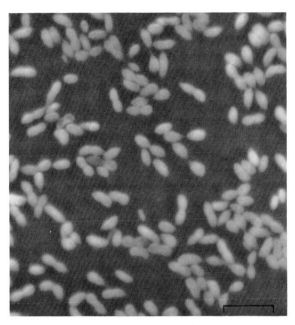

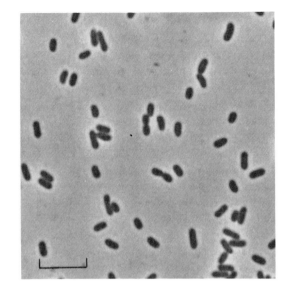

Figure 20.21. *Nitrosomonas* species sewer strain. Phase-contrast photomicrograph. *Bar,* 5 μm. (Reproduced with permission from S. W. Watson and M. Mandel, Journal of Bacteriology *107:* 563–569, 1971, ©American Society for Microbiology, Washington, D.C.)

Figure 20.22. *Nitrosomonas* species marine strain. Phase-contrast photomicrograph. *Bar,* 5 μm.

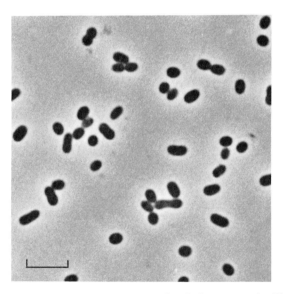

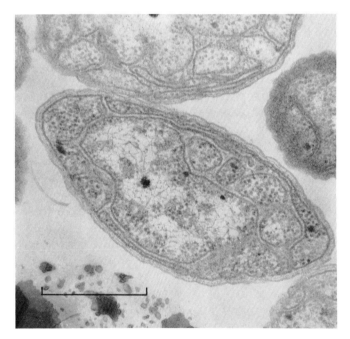

Figure 20.23. *Nitrosomonas* species brackish water strain. Phase-contrast photomicrograph. *Bar,* 5 μm.

Figure 20.24. *Nitrosomonas* species cell showing random arrangement of intracytoplasmic membranes. Electron micrograph of a thin section. *Bar,* 0.5 μm.

At the time of division the intracytoplasmic membranes are distributed nearly equally between two daughter cells. Some (Fig. 20.25), but not all, strains (Figs. 20.84 and 20.26) possess carboxysomes (Wullenweber et al., 1977) which contain RuBisCO (Harms et al., 1981). Cells are rich in cytochromes which impart a yellowish to reddish color to cell suspension. No other pigments are present.

Nitrosomonas strains grow in freshwater or seawater enriched with ammonia and inorganic salts (Table 20.4). The organisms are strictly aerobic but are capable of growing under low oxygen tensions. Many strains produce urease, which permits them to use urea as a substrate. Some strains can be grown mixotrophically in mineral salts medium (Table 20.4) supplemented with organic nutrients; however, they cannot be grown heterotrophically (Krümmel and Harms, 1982). Both high light intensities and high oxygen concentrations inhibit growth. Optimum growth occurs at 30°C at pH 7.5–8.0.

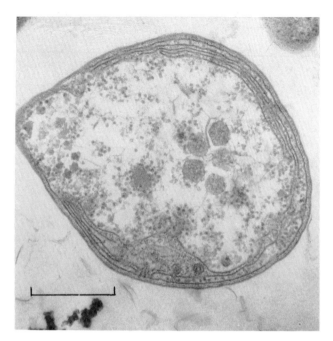

Figure 20.25. *Nitrosomonas* species cell showing carboxysomes. Electron micrograph of a thin section. *Bar,* 0.5 μm.

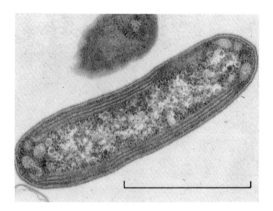

Figure 20.27. *Nitrosomonas* species marine strain. Electron micrograph of a longitudinal thin section. *Bar,* 1 μm.

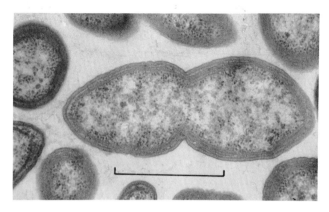

Figure 20.26. *N. europaea* type strain. Electron micrograph of a thin section. *Bar,* 1 μm.

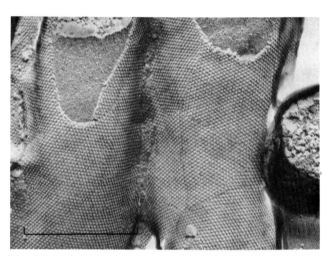

Figure 20.28. *Nitrosomonas* species freeze-etched marine cell showing additional cell wall layer. Electron micrograph. *Bar,* 0.5 μm. (Reproduced with permission from C. C. Remsen and S. W. Watson, International Review of Cytology *33:* 253–269, 1972, ©Academic Press, New York.)

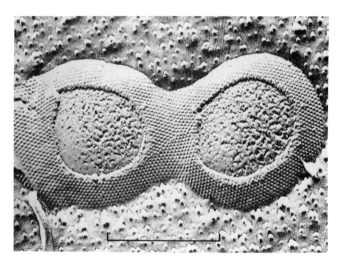

Figure 20.29. *Nitrosomonas* species freeze-etched marine cell showing additional cell wall layer. Electron micrograph. *Bar,* 0.5 μm. (Reproduced with permission from S. W. Watson and C. C. Remsen, Science *163:* 685–686, 1969, ©1968 by the American Association for the Advancement of Science.)

Differentiation of the genus **Nitrosomonas** from other genera

Table 20.1 lists characteristics differentiating *Nitrosomonas* from other genera of nitrifying bacteria.

Taxonomic Comments

At present, only a single *Nitrosomonas* species, *N. europaea*, is recognized. However, preliminary studies suggest that genotypic differences do exist between *Nitrosomonas* strains, differences which could be employed at the species level of classification. A clear-cut separation of species based on cellular morphology is impossible because of an overlap of size ranges and shapes between strains. It is likely that in the future, both genotypic and phenotypic characteristics will be employed for speciation within the genus.

Watson and Mandel (1971) showed that 13 strains of *Nitrosomonas* could be divided into three groups: the mol% G + C of the DNA of the three terrestrial strains examined was 50.7 ± 0.5 (Bd), that of the six marine strains was 47.9 ± 0.7 (Bd), and that of the four sewer strains was 48.5 ± 0.8 (Bd). Polynucleotide sequence homologies were determined for one strain of each of the three groups (Dodson et al., 1983), and the strains were readily distinguished from one another on the basis of DNA homology. Recently, Koops and Harms (1985) carried out similar studies on DNA of 44 *Nitrosomonas* strains. Results of their study suggested that the strains could be divided into six major groups having the following mol% G + C values: 45.8 ± 0.4 (T_m), 47.5 (T_m) (marine strain), 48.2 ± 0.2 (Bd, T_m) (sewer strains), 49.8 ± 0.2 (T_m), 51.0 ± 0.4 (Bd, T_m) (*N. europaea* group), and 53.9 (T_m) (Table 20.5). Based on these results, Koops and Harms (1985), using the technique described by De Ley et al. (1970), carried out DNA hybridization

studies. As shown in Table 20.5, the strains belonging to the same mol% G + C cluster, with the exception of cluster I in cross-reactions, gave relative binding percentages ranging from 63 to 100. This indicated that the strains were related at the species level (Schleifer and Stackebrandt, 1983). In cluster I, there are three subgroups with relative reassociation values between strains ranging from 56 to 100%, suggesting that this cluster should be composed of three different species. Average homologies between separate species were 36% and thus only 6% above the background value. Such studies clearly showed genotypic differences between strains of *Nitrosomonas*, which in the future may serve as a basis for creation of additional species in this genus.

Further Reading

Dodson, M.S., J. Mangan and S.W. Watson. 1983. Comparison of deoxyribonucleic acid homologies of six strains of ammonia-oxidizing bacteria. Int. J. Syst. Bacteriol. *33:* 521–524.

Koops, H.-P. and H. Harms. 1985. Deoxyribonucleic acid homologies among 96 strains of ammonia-oxidizing bacteria. Arch. Microbiol. *141:* 214–218.

Schleifer, K.H. and E. Stackebrandt. 1983. Molecular systematics of prokaryotes. Annu. Rev. Microbiol. *37:* 143–187.

Watson, S.W. and M. Mandel. 1971. Comparison of the morphology and deoxyribonucleic acid composition of 27 strains of nitrifying bacteria. J. Bacteriol. *107:* 563–569.

Watson, S.W., F.W. Valois and J.B. Waterbury. 1981. The Family *Nitrobacteraceae.* *In* Starr, Stolp, Trüper, Balows and Schlegel (Editors), The Prokaryotes. A Handbook on Habitats, Isolation, and Identification of Bacteria. Springer-Verlag, Berlin, pp. 1005–1022.

Winogradsky, S. 1892. Contributions a la morphologie des organismes de la nitrification. Arch. Sci. Biol. (St. Petersb.) *1:* 86–137.

Differentiation of the species of the genus **Nitrosomonas**

Only one species of *Nitrosomonas* is currently recognized: *N. europaea*.

List of species of the genus **Nitrosomonas**

1. **Nitrosomonas europaea** Winogradsky 1892, 127, emend. mut. char. Watson 1971a, 266.[AL]

eu.ro.pae'a. Gr. adj. *europaeus* of Europe, European.

The species description is based on characteristics of the type strain and genetically closely related strains.

Cells are rod-shaped, 0.8–0.9 × 1.0–2.0 μm, occurring either singly or, rarely, in chains, with rounded or pointed ends (Figs. 20.22 and 20.23). When motile, cells possess 1–2 subpolar flagella which are 3–4 times the length of the rod. Strains have a typical Gram-negative type of cell wall (Figs. 20.24 and 20.26). Intracytoplasmic membranes are arranged as flattened vesicles primarily in the peripheral region of the

cytoplasm (Fig. 20.26). Carboxysomes have not been detected in the type strain but are present in other strains (Fig. 20.25).

Cells grow chemolithotrophically in mineral salts medium containing ammonia or urea or mixotrophically in the medium supplemented with organic nutrients. Optimum growth temperature range: 25–30°C. Optimum pH: 7.5–8.0. Cells are obligate aerobes. Under low oxygen tensions, N_2O or NO is produced.

N. europaea strains can be distinguished from other *Nitrosomonas* species by the mol% G + C of their DNA, which is 51.0 ± 0.4 (Bd, T_m) (Table 20.6).

Type strain: ATCC 25978.

Table 20.5.
Distribution of the G + C of the DNA among strains of the genus **Nitrosomonas**[a]

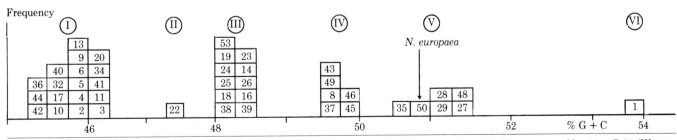

[a] Isolates are represented by their strain numbers inside the collets. The type strain *N. europaea* is marked by an arrow. Nm 50 = C-31 (Watson strain), ATCC 25978.

Table 20.6.

Relative intraspecific and interspecific reassociation of the DNA in the genus **Nitrosomonas**, *presented as % homology*

G + C group → Strain no.	(I)										(II)	(III)							(IV)					(V)		(VI)
	32	40	44	4	9	10	13	3	20	36	22	19	23	24	26	38	53	37	43	45	46	27	28	35	50[a]	1
(I) 2	80	76	62	40	44	39	31			34	39															37
44	64	83	98	33	35	34	34		38	43	38															34
5	37	33	38	84	92	85	64		42	41								36								
6	43	39	41	64	71	71	63	40	33	36																
42	33	44	40	82	94	92	65	42																		
11	41	43	40	36	41	32	31	56	60	59	30															43
17	33		42		42	34	30	97	103	75	32															
36	38		42		34		27	76	84	101	27															43
(II) 22		40		31				29	28		96	35	36	39	34	35	31			32						36
(III) 14	39										35	102	79	73	78	94	93	34		39	43					44
23								43			36	71	101	98	104	75	74			41						
39											35	104	75	73	68	101	95		25	40	38					
57[b]											40	83	71	79	69	89	82									
(IV) 8	32						34	36			38	43	37	41	38	43	36	69	70	63	96					31
37	32						34	36				40					38	97	56	65	75					
49																	39	83	73	66	78					
(V) 27			33		41													37	23	42	40	99	96	84	84	31
35					41			39					43					39		37	40	84	92	100	103	44
48																		31				98	97	82	81	
(VI) 1	44						35	39		36	37							31		43		31	44	44		103

[a] Nm 50 = C-31 (Watson strain), ATCC 25978.   [b] Nm 57 = C-91 (Watson strain).

Genus VI. **Nitrosococcus** Winogradsky 1892, 127[AL] (Nom. Cons. Opin. 23 Jud. Comm. 1958, 169)

STANLEY W. WATSON, EBERHARD BOCK, HEINZ HARMS, HANS-PETER KOOPS AND ALAN B. HOOPER

Ni.tro.so.coc′cus. M.L. adj. *nitrosus* nitrous; Gr. n. *coccus* a grain, berry; M.L. masc. n. *Nitrosococcus* nitrous sphere.

Spherical cells occurring singly, in pairs and as tetrads and often becoming embedded in slime, forming aggregates. Cells reproduce by binary fission. **Cells have intracytoplasmic membranes arranged centrally, peripherally or randomly in the cytoplasm.** Gram-negative. **Motile** by means of a tuft of flagella or a single flagellum. **Aerobic.** The major source of energy and reducing power is from the **oxidation of ammonia to nitrite. Chemolithotrophs;** cells can grow mixotrophically but not heterotrophically. Occur in soils, open oceans, salt lakes, brackish waters and industrial sewage disposal systems.

The mol% G + C of the DNA ranges from 48 to 51 (Bd, T_m).

Type species: *Nitrosococcus nitrosus* (Migula 1900) Buchanan 1925, 402.

Further Descriptive Information

This genus is reserved for spherical cells (Figs. 20.16, 20.17 and 20.30–20.32). Only two species, *N. oceanus* and "*N. mobilis*" are currently in laboratory culture. Little information is available on the type species *N. nitrosus*. The size, shape and ultrastructure of the two species in culture are shown in Figures 20.30 and 20.32. Both of these species have a typical Gram-negative cell envelope; however, they have one or more additional cell wall layers composed of repeating subunits arranged in a molecular array (Figs. 20.33 and 20.34).

Both *N. oceanus* and "*N. mobilis*" have intracytoplasmic membranes in the form of flattened vesicles which are divided nearly equally between daughter cells at the time of division. Such intracytoplasmic membranes arise by the infolding of the plasma membrane. Glycogen inclusion bodies have been observed in some, but not all, strains; other inclusion bodies have not been observed. Cells are rich in cytochromes imparting a yellowish to reddish color to cell suspensions. No other pigments have been observed.

Nitrosococcus cells are obligate chemolithotrophs, but mixotrophic growth has been demonstrated. Their energy and carbon needs are

fulfilled by the oxidation of ammonia to nitrite and by the fixation of carbon dioxide. Some strains have a urease which permits them to use urea. *Nitrosococcus* strains grow in freshwater, diluted seawater and seawater enriched with inorganic salts (Table 20.4). pH range for growth: 6.0-8.0. Temperature range for growth: 5-30°C; optimum growth temperature: 25°C. Both high light intensities, and high oxygen concentrations inhibit growth. Optimum growth occurs at 30°C and at pH 7.5–8.0.

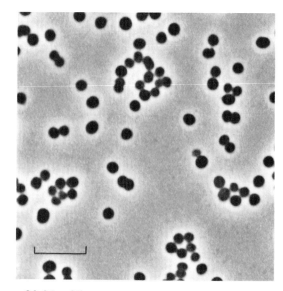

Figure 20.31. *Nitrosococcus* strain tentatively identified as *N. nitrosus.* Phase-contrast photomicrograph. *Bar,* 5 μm.

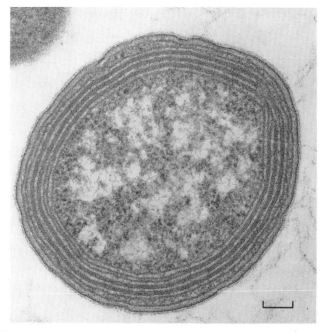

Figure 20.30. "*N. mobilis.*" Electron micrograph of a thin section. *Bar,* 100 nm.

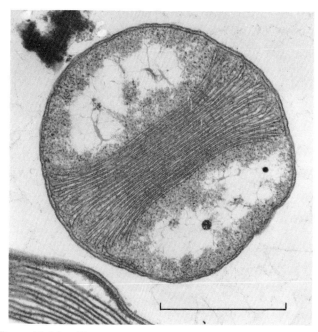

Figure 20.32. *N. oceanus.* Electron micrograph of a thin section. *Bar,* 1 μm.

Differentiation of the genus **Nitrosococcus** *from other genera*

Table 20.1 lists characteristics differentiating *Nitrosococcus* from other genera of nitrifying bacteria.

Taxonomic Comments

Strains of *Nitrosococcus* originally described by Winogradsky (1892, 1904) varied in size. The smallest strain, isolated from Buitenzorg (Java), was 0.5–0.6 μm in diameter. Other isolates were about 1.0 μm (Leningrad, U.S.S.R.), 1.5–1.7 μm (Quito, Ecuador) and 2.0 μm (Campinas, Brazil) in diameter. Migula (1900) named the strain from Quito, *N. nitrosus*. Later, this organism was accepted as the type species. Unfortunately, strains of *N. nitrosus* from Winogradsky were not preserved in laboratory culture, nor were their phenotypic characteristics clearly described; thus the taxonomy of the organisms studied by Winogradsky is questionable. In addition, information regarding their genotypic characteristics is not available.

At present, two well-characterized species of spherical ammonia oxidizers, *N. oceanus* (Fig. 20.16) and "*N. mobilis*" (Fig. 20.17), are in culture. They were isolated from marine and brackish waters, respectively. Although categorized presently in the same genus, these two species are not closely related, as revealed by recent studies (Woese et al., 1984b) and probably should not be categorized in the same genus. This genus needs to be reorganized, but this is difficult, as the type species strain is no longer available.

Recently, Koops and Harms (1985) showed that ten strains of spherical ammonia oxidizers could be divided, based on their DNA base ratios, into three major groups (Table 20.7). The clusters II and III contain strains of "*N. mobilis*" and *N. oceanus*, respectively. The strains of Group I were isolated from soil and from a sewage disposal system, respectively, and are similar in shape and size (Fig. 20.31) to the type *N. nitrosus*. If observations of these two isolates are verified, it should be possible to describe a neotype strain of *N. nitrosus* which will help facilitate the reorganization of this genus. Dodson et al. (1983) showed that there was <3% homology between the type strain of *N. oceanus* and members of the other genera of ammonia oxidizers. More recently, Woese et al. (1985) have demonstrated that *N. oceanus* is not phylogenetically related to any other species of nitrifying bacteria. Probably not more than six strains of *N. oceanus* have been isolated, and all appear phenotypically similar or identical. However, when the relative reassociation of DNA was compared (Koops and Harms, 1985), it became apparent that these strains could be divided into two subgroups (Table 20.8). Strains of "*N. mobilis*" are not phylogenetically closely related to either *N. oceanus* or any of the ammonia oxidizers thus far studied (Woese et al., 1984b).

The mol% G + C of the DNA in this genus ranges from 48.0 to 51.0 (Bd, T_m) (Watson and Mandel, 1971; Koops and Harms, 1985).

Further Reading

Koops, H.-P. and H. Harms. 1985. Deoxyribonucleic acid homologies among 96 strains of ammonia-oxidizing bacteria. Arch. Microbiol. *141:* 214–218.

Watson, S.W. 1965. Characteristics of a marine nitrifying bacterium, *Nitrosocystis oceanus* sp. n. Limnol. Ocean. (Suppl.) *10:* R274–R289.

Watson, S.W. 1971a. Taxonomic considerations of the family *Nitrobacteraceae* Buchanan. Requests for opinions. Int. J. Syst. Bacteriol. *21:* 254–270.

Table 20.7.

Distribution of the G + C of the DNA among strains of the genus **Nitrosococcus**[a]

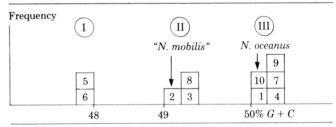

[a] Isolates are represented by their strain numbers inside the collets. The type strains of *N. oceanus* and "*N. mobilis*" are marked by arrows. Nc 1 = Gundersen strain; Nc 9 = C-27 (Watson strain); and Nc 10 = C-107 (Watson strain), ATCC 19707.

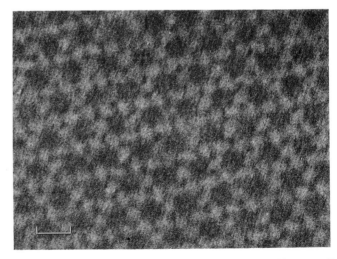

Figure 20.33. *N. oceanus* cell showing tripartite nature of intracytoplasmic membranes. Electron micrograph of a thin section. *Bar*, 10 nm.

Figure 20.34. *N. oceanus* freeze-etched cell showing additional cell wall layers. Electron micrograph. *Bar*, 100 nm. (Reproduced with permission from S. W. Watson and C. C. Remsen, Journal of Ultrastructure Research *33:* 148–160, 1970, ©Academic Press, New York.)

Table 20.8.

Relative intraspecific and interspecific reassociation of the DNA in the genus **Nitrosococcus,** *presented as % homology*

G + C group Strain no.	I 5	6	II 2	3	8	III 1	9[a]	10[b]	4	7
I 5	97	91	37	39	39	30	31	29		35
II 2	37	38	103	100	92			25	31	
III 1[c]				27		102	101	101	52	51
4			31		32	52	49	48	100	93

[a]Nc 9 = C-27 (Watson strain).
[b]Nc 10 = C-107 (Watson strain), ATCC 19707, type strain.
[c]Nc 1 = Gundersen strain.

Watson, S.W., F.W. Valois and J.B. Waterbury. 1981. The Family *Nitrobacteraceae*. *In* Starr, Stolp, Trüper, Balows and Schlegel (Editors), The Prokaryotes. A Handbook on Habitats, Isolation, and Identification of Bacteria. Springer-Verlag, Berlin, pp. 1005–1022.

Woese, C.R., W.G. Weisburg, C.M. Hahn, B.J. Paster, L.B. Zablen, B.J. Lewis,

T.J. Macke, W. Lundwig and E. Stackebrandt. 1985. The phylogeny of purple bacteria: the gamma subdivision. Syst. Appl. Microbiol. *6:* 25–33.

Woese, C.R., W.G. Weisburg, B.J. Paster, C.M. Hahn, R.S. Tanner, N.R. Krieg, H.-P. Koops, H. Harms and E. Stackebrandt. 1984b. The phylogeny of purple bacteria: the beta subdivision. Syst. Appl. Microbiol. *5:* 327–336.

Differentiation of the species of the genus **Nitrosococcus**

Table 20.9 lists differential characteristics of the three species.

List of species of the genus **Nitrosococcus**

1. **Nitrosococcus nitrosus** (Migula) Buchanan 1925, 402.[AL] (Nom. Cons. Opin. 23 Jud. Comm. 1958, 169.) (*Micrococcus nitrosus* Migula 1900, 194.)

ni.tro′sus. M.L. adj. *nitrosus* nitrous.

Cells are large spheres 1.5–1.7 μm in diameter. Motility of cells has not been observed. No information is available on ultrastructure. Knowledge of this species is based on the original description, as laboratory cultures were not preserved.

Type strain: no longer in culture.

2. **Nitrosococcus oceanus** (Watson) Watson 1971a, 267.[AL] (*Nitrosocystis oceanus* Watson 1965, R279.)

Cells spherical to ellipsoidal, 1.8–2.2 μm in diameter (Fig. 20.16), occurring singly, in pairs and, occasionally, as tetrads growing free in a liquid medium or as aggregates suspended in the medium or attached to vessel wall. When motile, cells possess 1–20 flagella. Cells divide by binary fission. Cells have a typical Gram-negative multilayered cell wall; however, they have two additional cell wall layers composed of subunits arranged in rectilinear and hexagonal arrays (Figs. 20.33 and 20.34). Cells of this species are distinguished by a centrally located membranous organelle composed of a stack of parallel, flattened vesicles that traverse the cell (Fig. 20.32) (Murray and Watson, 1965; Watson, 1965; Watson and Remsen, 1970). The triplet structure represents two closely joined unit membranes of adjacent vesicles (Fig. 20.35). The major source of energy and reducing power is from the oxidation of ammonia to nitrite. Cells contain glycogen deposits. Optimum growth temperature: 25–30°C. Optimum growth pH: 7.5–8.0. Average generation time under optimum conditions is 8–12 h, and energy efficiency is 10% (Koops, 1969).

Occurs in oceanic environments. Cells are obligate chemoautotrophs and have an obligate salt requirement similar to the salt content in seawater.

The mol% G + C of the DNA in the type strain is 50.8 (Bd).

Type strain: ATCC 19707.

3. **"Nitrosococcus mobilis"** Koops, Harms, and Wehrmann 1976, 281.

mo′bi.lis. L. adj. *mobilis* movable.

Table 20.9.

Differential characteristics of the three species of the genus **Nitrosococcus**

Species	Diameter (μm)	Habitat	Cytomembranes	G + C (mol%)
N. nitrosus	1.5–1.7	Soil	Not known	Not known
N. oceanus	1.8–2.2	Seawater	Centrally located	50.8 ± 0.4
"*N. mobilis*"	1.5–1.7 in artificial seawater 1.2–1.9 in natural seawater	Brackish water	Peripherally located	49.3 ± 0.2

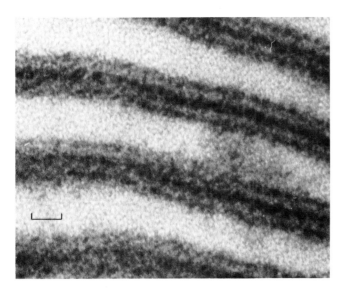

Figure 20.35. *N. oceanus* negatively stained cell showing hexagonal outer cell wall layer. Electron micrograph. *Bar*, 10 nm. (Reproduced with permission from S. W. Watson and C. C. Remsen, Journal of Ultrastructure Research *33:* 148–160, 1970, ©Academic Press, New York.)

Cells are always spherical and are 1.5–1.7 μm in diameter when grown in artificial seawater (Fig. 20.17) and slightly smaller when grown in natural seawater. Cells divide by binary fission. In liquid media, cells grow free and occur singly, in pairs and, occasionally, as short chains. When motile, cells have a tuft of 1–22 flagella which is about 12 nm wide and 3–5 μm long. Cells possess an extensive intracytoplasmic membrane system composed of flattened vesicles located peripherally (Fig. 20.30).

Cells grow chemolithotrophically and have an optimum salt requirement. Optimum growth occurs in diluted seawater enriched with inorganic salts, but growth also occurs in enriched distilled water containing 1% NaCl. Cells oxidize ammonia as energy source and fix carbon dioxide for primary carbon source. Growth is enhanced when pyruvate or glucose is added to the mineral salts medium. Growth is inhibited by many other organics.

Optimum growth occurs between 25 and 30°C; no growth occurs below 5°C or above 35°C. Optimal pH range for growth: 7.5–7.8. Under optimal growth conditions, the generation time is 12–13 h.

Found in brackish waters.

The mol% G + C of the DNA of the type strain is 49.3 (T_m).

Type strain: NC-2 is stored in stock culture in Institut für Allgemeine Botanik, Abteilung Mikrobiologie, Hamburg, Federal Republic of Germany.

Genus VII. **Nitrosospira** *Winogradsky and Winogradsky 1933, 406*[AL]

STANLEY W. WATSON, EBERHARD BOCK, HEINZ HARMS, HANS-PETER KOOPS AND ALAN B. HOOPER

Ni.tro.so.spi′ra. M.L. adj. *nitrosus* nitrous; Gr. n. *spira* a coil, spiral; M.L. fem. n. *Nitrosospira* nitrous spiral

Cells are spiral, 0.3–0.4 μm in width, with 3–20 turns; the average number of turns is 3–8, and the amplitude of the turns is 0.8–1.0 μm. **Usually tightly coiled,** spherical forms are seen in cultures. Cells reproduce by binary fission. **Cells lack cytomembrane system.** Gram-negative. **Motile or nonmotile. Aerobic.** The major source of energy and reducing power is from the **oxidation of ammonia to nitrite. Obligate chemolithotrophs.** Occur in terrestrial and freshwater environments.

The mol% G + C of the DNA in strains of this genus ranges from 52.2 to 55.4 (Bd, T_m) (Watson and Mandel, 1971; Koops and Harms, 1985).

Type species: *Nitrosospira briensis* Winogradsky and Winogradsky, 1933, 407.

Further Descriptive Information

Although cells are spiral, they usually appear as short rods when viewed with a phase-contrast microscope (Fig. 20.36); the actual shape of the cells is apparent when they are negatively stained and viewed with an electron microscope (Fig. 20.18). Cells lack intracytoplasmic membranes found in many other nitrifying bacteria, carboxysomes and other inclusions not observed (Fig. 20.37). When motile, cells are propelled by 1–6 peritrichous flagella 3–5 μm in length. Cells have cytochromes but no other pigments.

The organisms are obligate chemolithotrophs which oxidize ammonia to nitrite and fix carbon dioxide to fulfill their energy and carbon needs. Cells have urease which permits them to use urea as growth substrate. Cells grow in freshwater enriched with inorganic salts. Heterotrophic or mixotrophic growth has not been observed. Strains have been isolated from acidic (pH 4.0–4.5) soils (Walker and Wickramasinghe, 1979).

Temperature range for growth: 20–35°C. pH ranges: 7.0–8.0. High concentration of oxygen and light intensities inhibit growth. The average generation time under optimal conditions is 24 h.

Differentiation of the genus **Nitrosospira** *from other genera*

Table 20.1 lists characteristics differentiating *Nitrosospira* from other genera of nitrifying bacteria.

Taxonomic Comments

The Winogradskys (1933) described two species, *N. briensis* and *N. antarctica*, but their original laboratory cultures were never preserved. Since the two species were indistinguishable from the original descriptions, only one species, *N. briensis*, was recognized in the eighth edition of the *Manual* (Watson, 1974).

Koops and Harms (1985) showed that the isolated strains could be subdivided, based on the mol% G + C of their DNA, into two groups (Table 20.10). However, based on DNA homologies, these strains could be categorized into five species (Table 20.11). Dodson et al. (1983) showed that a strain of *Nitrosospira* had a 6.7–10.5% homology to a strain of *Nitrosolobus* and nearly no homology to strains of *Nitrosomonas* and *Nitrosococcus*. These findings were confirmed by Woese et al. (1984b) in sequence analysis of the 16S rRNA of ammonia oxidizers.

Table 20.10.

Distribution of the G + C of the DNA among strains of the genus **Nitrosospira**[a]

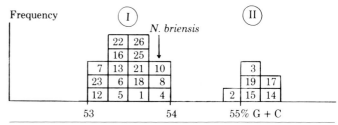

[a] Isolates are represented by their strain numbers inside the collets. The neotype strain of *N. briensis* is marked by an arrow. Nsp 4 = C-128 (Watson strain); and Nsp 10 = C-76 (Watson strain), ATCC 25961.

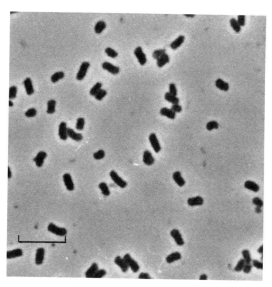

Figure 20.36. *N. briensis.* Phase-contrast micrograph. *Bar,* 5 μm.

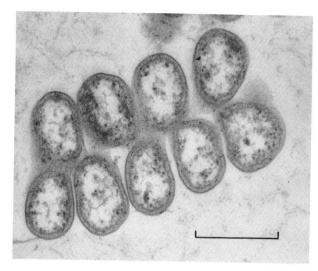

Figure 20.37. *N. briensis* cell. Electron micrograph of a thin longitudinal section. *Bar,* 0.5 μm. (Reproduced with permission from S. W. Watson, Archiv für Mikrobiologie 75: 179–188, 1971, ©Springer-Verlag, Berlin.)

Their studies revealed that *Nitrosospira* was more closely related to *Nitrosolobus* and *Nitrosovibrio* than to members of the other two genera.

Further Reading

Watson, S.W. 1971a. Taxonomic considerations of the family *Nitrobacteraceae* Buchanan. Requests for opinions. Int. J. Syst. Bacteriol. *21:* 254–270.
Watson, S.W. 1971b. Reisolation of *Nitrosospira briensis* S. Winogradsky and H. Winogradsky 1933. Arch. Mikrobiol. *75:* 179–188.

Watson, S.W., F.W. Valois and J.B. Waterbury. 1981. The Family *Nitrobacteraceae. In* Starr, Stolp, Trüper, Balows and Schlegel (Editors), The Prokaryotes. A Handbook on Habitats, Isolation, and Identification of Bacteria. Springer-Verlag, Berlin, pp. 1005–1022.
Winogradsky, S. and H. Winogradsky. 1933. Études sur la microbiologie du sol. VII Nouvelles recherches sur les organismes de la nitrification. Ann. Inst. Pasteur *50:* 350–432.

Differentiation of the species of the genus **Nitrosospira**

Only one species of *Nitrosospira* is currently recognized: *N. briensis.*

List of species of the genus **Nitrosospira**

1. **Nitrosospira briensis** Winogradsky and Winogradsky 1933, 407.[AL]

bri.en'sis. N.L. adj. *briensis* of Brie, a French place name.

Morphological, cultural and biochemical characteristics are the same as those described for the genus. Figures 20.18, 20.36 and 20.37 illustrate the morphological features.

The type strain was isolated from the soils of Crete.
The mol% G + C of the DNA of the type strain is 54.1 (Bd).
Neotype strain: ATCC 25971.

Table 20.11.

Relative intraspecific and interspecific reassociation of the DNA in the genus **Nitrosospira,** *presented as % homology* [a]

G + C group / Strain no.	1	4[a]	16	21	25	26	10	5	12	23	2	19	14	17
I 1	98	84	59	71	76	74	41	38	40	42				31
7	78	82	69	75	87	59	41		41		35			31
18	65	59	92	94	67	62	43	37	44	44				
22	76	74	70	61	89	74	34							
8	27	44		37	45	28	81	32	35	31				
10[b]	41	40				36	102	39	34	37				
6	37	41	46		49	37	45	102	78	84	39			39
13		30			45		35	84	75	101	33	34	40	36
II 15			44				38	40	40	45	99	83	48	44
19								42	41	39	78	98	52	43
3	35							38	33	34	46	48	77	70
14							37				48	52	102	63

[a] Nsp 4 = C-128 (Watson strain).
[b] Nsp 10 = C-76 (Watson strain), ATCC 25961.

Genus VIII. **Nitrosolobus** *Watson, Graham, Remsen and Valois 1971, 200[AL]*

Stanley W. Watson, Eberhard Bock, Heinz Harms, Hans-Peter Koops and Alan B. Hooper

Ni.tro.so.lob'us. M.L. *nitrosus* nitrous; M.L. n. *lobus* a lobe; M.L. fem. n. *Nitrosolobus* nitrous lobe, i.e. a lobe producing nitrite.

Pleomorphic, lobate cells with cytomembranes that partially compartmentalize the cell. Division by constriction. Gram-negative. When **motile,** cells are propelled by 1–20 peritrichous flagella. **Aerobic.** The major source of energy and reducing power is from the oxidation of ammonia to nitrite. Cells are **chemolithotrophs** but can grow mixotrophically. Cells isolated from terrestrial environments. Optimal growth occurs in a mineral salts medium. Optimum temperature: 25–30°C. Optimum pH: 7.5.

The mol% G + C of the DNA is 53–56.3 (Bd, T_m).

Type species: *Nitrosolobus mutiformis* Watson, Graham, Remsen and Valois 1971, 200.

Further Descriptive Information

Cells are pleomorphic and lobate, 1.0–1.5 μm wide and 1.0–2.5 μm long (see Fig. 20.19), and divide by constriction. Cells are motile and have a typical Gram-negative cell envelope. Electron microscopic sections reveal that the cells are partially compartmentalized by the invagination of the plasma membrane into the cytoplasm (Fig. 20.38). In cross-sections, cells never appear spherical but, occasionally, are almost triangular or rectangular. In thin section, cells appear to be composed of two or more segments. Each cell has 1–4 central compartments surrounded by 5–20 membrane-bound peripheral compartments (Fig. 20.38). Because both central and peripheral compartments contain DNA, it is obvious that complete compartmentalization of cells does not occur and that openings between compartments must exist even if they are not evident in thin sections. In addition to morphological compartmentalization of the cell, there appears to be physiological compartmentalization. When sections are stained with glycogen stain, glycogen inclusions are located primarily in the peripheral compartments. Carboxysomes and other cellular inclusions in cells have not been observed.

Although cells are strictly aerobic, low oxygen tensions can support growth. Cells require no organic growth factors but can grow mixotrophically in a medium containing formate, pyruvate and acetate. Cell yield is increased in a mixotrophic medium, but growth rates are not

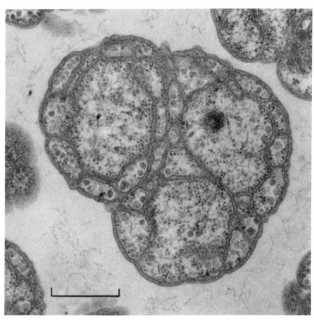

Figure 20.38.   *N. multiformis.* Electron micrograph of a thin section. *Bar,* 0.5 μm. (Reproduced with permission from S. W. Watson, L. B. Graham, C. C. Remsen and F. W. Valois, Archiv für Mikrobiologie *76:* 183–203, 1971, ©Springer-Verlag, Berlin.)

increased. Nitrite becomes toxic in concentrations of >100 mM. Urea rather than ammonia can be used as a growth substrate. Cells can oxidize hydroxylamine but cannot use it as growth substrate. About 7% of the energy derived from ammonia oxidation is used for CO_2 fixation.

Differentiation of the genus **Nitrosolobus** *from other genera*

Table 20.1 lists characteristics differentiating *Nitrosolobus* from other genera of nitrifying bacteria.

Taxonomic Comments

Although several strains have been isolated, no phenotypic differences have been established. However, based on the mol% G + C of the DNA, two groups of *Nitrosolobus* can be identified (Table 20.12). Koops and Harms (1985) found that members of this genus could be subdivided into two species (Table 20.13).

Further Reading

Watson, S.W., L.B. Graham, C.C. Remsen and F.W. Valois. 1971. A lobular, ammonia-oxidizing bacterium, *Nitrosolobus multiformis* nov. gen. nov. sp. Arch. Mikrobiol. *76:* 183–203.

Watson, S.W., F.W. Valois and J.B. Waterbury. 1981. The Family *Nitrobacteraceae. In* Starr, Stolp, Trüper, Balows and Schlegel (Editors), The Prokaryotes. A Handbook on Habitats, Isolation, and Identification of bacteria. Springer-Verlag, Berlin, pp. 1005–1022.

Table 20.12.
Distribution of the G + C of the DNA among strains of the genus **Nitrosolobus**[a]

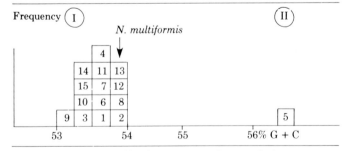

[a]Isolates are represented by their strain numbers inside the collets. The type strain of *N. multiformis* is marked by an arrow. Nl13 = C-71 (Watson strain), ATCC 25196, type strain.

Differentiation of the species of the genus **Nitrosolobus**

Only one species of *Nitrosolobus* is currently recognized: *N. multiformis.*

Table 20.13.

Relative intraspecific and interspecific reassociation of the DNA in the genus **Nitrosolobus,** *presented as %* homology

G + C group Strain no.	1	2	3	6	7	9	11	12	14	15	II 5
4	70	71	75	84	70	73	73	59	69	69	36
7	62	76	68	61	95	59	68	82	59	59	33
8	76	85	70	72	60	88	73	91	84	77	32
10	69	82	71	60	62	94	77	87	79	78	42
13[a]	68	61	71	90	75	61	59	73	67	59	37
II 5	39	39	35	40	33	35	38	39	41	39	98

[a]Nl13 = C-71 (Watson strain), ATCC 25196, type strain.

List of species of the genus **Nitrosolobus**

1. **Nitrosolobus multiformis** Watson, Graham, Remsen and Valois 1971, 200.[AL]

mul.ti.for′mis. L. adj. *multus* many; L. n. *forma* shape; M.L. adj. *multiformis* many shapes.

Morphological, cultural and biochemical characteristics are the same as those described for the genus. Figures 20.19 and 20.38 illustrate the morphological features.

The type strain was isolated from soil collected in Paramaribo, Surinam.

The mol% G + C of the DNA of the type strain is 54.6 (Bd).

Type strain: ATCC 25196.

Genus IX. **"Nitrosovibrio"** *Harms, Koops and Wehrmann 1976, 105*

STANLEY W. WATSON, EBERHARD BOCK, HEINZ HARMS, HANS-PETER KOOPS AND ALAN B. HOOPER

Ni.tro.so.vib′rio. M.L. adj. *nitrosus* nitrous; L. v. *vibrio* to move rapidly to and from, to vibrate; M.L. masc. n. *Nitrosovibrio* nitrous vibrio, i.e. a vibrio producing nitrite.

Slender curved rods, 0.3–0.4 × 1.1–3.0 μm. Spherical forms 1.0–1.2 μm in diameter present in the early stationary phase of growth. Cells reproduce by binary fission. **Extensive cytomembranes lacking.** Gram-negative. **Motile or nonmotile.** When motile, cells possess 1–4 subpolar to lateral flagella. **Aerobic.** Major source of energy and reducing power is from the **oxidation of ammonia** to nitrite. Carboxysomes and other inclusion bodies not evident. **Chemolithotrophs;** cells can grow mixotrophically but not heterotrophically.

Further Descriptive Information

Cells are curved rods (Figs. 20.39 and 20.40) occurring singly. When motile, cells possess 1–4 subpolar to lateral flagella, each about 18 nm wide and 4.2–7.5 μm long.

A general electron microscopic view of a thin section is given in Figure 20.40. The cell envelope is similar to that found in most other Gram-negative bacteria.

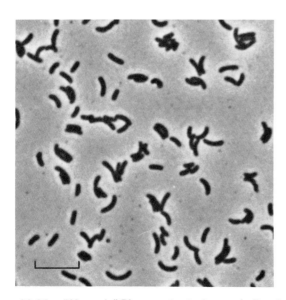

Figure 20.39. *"N. tenuis."* Phase-contrast micrograph. *Bar,* 5 μm.

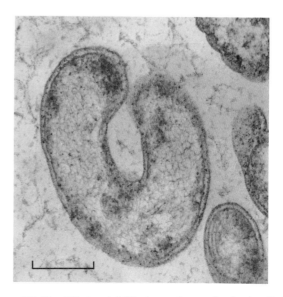

Figure 20.40. *"N. tenuis."* Electron micrograph of a longitudinal thin section. *Bar,* 0.25 μm.

Extensive intracytoplasmic membranes found in most other ammonia-oxidizing bacteria are lacking. Within the central region of the cells are areas which lack ribosomes and contain electron-dense strands of material resembling the nucleoplasm of other bacterial cells. Cells lack carboxysomes found in many other nitrifying bacteria.

Cells grow in freshwater enriched with ammonia and other inorganic salts. No organic growth factors are required. Cells can grow mixotrophically on many organic compounds. Cells are strict aerobes. Optimum growth temperature: 25–30°C. Optimum pH for growth: 7.5–7.8.

The mol% G + C of the DNA in this genus is 53.9 (T_m).

Type species: "*Nitrosovibrio tenuis*" Harms, Koops and Wehrmann 1976, 108.

Differentiation of the genus "Nitrosovibrio" from other genera

Table 20.1 lists characteristics differentiating "*Nitrosovibrio*" from other genera of nitrifying bacteria.

Taxonomic Comments

Based on DNA homologies carried out by Koops and Harms (1985), strains of "*Nitrosovibrio*" can be subdivided into two species (Table 20.14). This genus is more closely related to *Nitrosospira* and *Nitrosolobus* than to the other genera of nitrifying bacteria (Woese et al., 1984b).

Table 20.14.
Relative intraspecific and interspecific reassociation of the DNA in the genus "Nitrosovibrio," presented as % homology

Strain no.	2	13	12	6
1	83	92	42	41
2	101	91	47	41
6	41	42	98	98

Differentiation of the species of the genus "Nitrosovibrio"

Only one species of "*Nitrosovibrio*" is currently recognized: "*N. tenuis.*"

List of species of the genus "Nitrosovibrio"

1. **"Nitrosovibrio tenuis"** Harms, Koops and Wehrmann 1976, 108. te′nu.is. L. adj. *tenuis* slender.

Morphological and cultural characteristics are the same as those described for the genus. Figures 20.39 and 20.40 illustrate the morphological features.

Type strain was isolated from the soils of Hawaii (U.S.A.), but morphologically and genetically similar strains appear ubiquitous in soils throughout the world.

The mol% G + C of the DNA of the type strain is 53.9 ± 0.3 (T_m).

Type strain: Type strain (Nv-1) is stored in stock culture in the Institut für Allgemeine Botanik, Abteilung Mikrobiologie, Hamburg, Federal Republic of Germany.

Acknowledgments

This research was supported by grant BSR-8407924 from the National Science Foundation (S. W. W.) and grants from the Deutsche Forschungsgemeinschaft (E. B., H. P. K. and H. H.).

B. COLORLESS SULFUR BACTERIA

J. Gijs Kuenen

The genera of "bacteria able to oxidize reduced, or partially reduced, inorganic sulfur compounds" often have no taxonomic relationship. They have been brought together in this section for a purely practical reason, i.e. to facilitate their identification until their affiliations have been properly assigned. A number of other genera of sulfur-oxidizing bacteria have already been assigned to other groups and thus are not described in this section. For those workers not familiar with the field, this must create a very confusing situation when they attempt to identify or classify a bacterium by its sulfur-oxidizing capability. Therefore, in this introduction and in the key to the genera of sulfur-oxidizing bacteria, reference will also be made to relevant genera not covered in this section.

In many textbooks and reviews (Kuenen, 1975; Kelly and Kuenen, 1984), the bacteria able to oxidize reduced inorganic sulfur compounds are called "colorless sulfur bacteria." This not only includes the genera described in this chapter but also genera of the *Beggiatoaceae* and the genus *Achromatium*. Recently, *Sulfolobus* and *Thiodendron* have also been included in this group, as is shown in Table 20.15. The name "colorless sulfur bacteria" was originally used by Winogradsky (1890) for procaryotes that could grow autotrophically under aerobic conditions in the dark if inorganic oxidizable sulfur compounds are used as energy source. This term distinguishes this group from the colored, phototrophic sulfur bacteria which can oxidize reduced sulfur compounds under anaerobic conditions in the light (Trüper and Fischer, 1982; Pfennig and Trüper, this volume). We now know that the colorless sulfur bacteria comprise a vast range of taxonomically unrelated genera of procaryotes which have in common only their ability to oxidize reduced sulfur compounds. It is now clear that this ability is not necessarily linked to the ability to grow autotrophically and that some of the sulfur-oxidizing bacteria are essentially heterotrophs. Consequently, it is necessary to discuss sulfur and carbon metabolism separately.

All sulfur-oxidizing bacteria classified as such are able either to generate metabolically useful energy from this oxidation in the respiratory chain or to benefit metabolically from it in other ways. In the

Table 20.15.
Genera of bacteria that oxidize reduced or partially reduced inorganic sulfur compounds with oxygen or nitrate as terminal acceptor and are generally known as the "colorless sulfur bacteria" [a]

Thiobacterium	*Beggiatoa*	*Thiodendron*
Macromonas	*Thiospirillopsis*	
Thiovulum	*Thioploca*	*Sulfolobus*
Thiospira	*Thiothrix*	*Acidianus*
Thiobacillus		*Thermothrix*
Thiomicrospira	*Achromatium*	
Thiosphaera		

[a] Adapted from Kuenen, 1975. This list is not restrictive.

former, bacteria can be identified when a growth yield increase (as shown by an increase in carbon, dry weight and protein) is observed or when, after addition of a reduced sulfur compound to the culture, an increase in ATP can be demonstrated. A well-known example of a benefit other than energy generation is the detoxification by sulfide of hydrogen peroxide produced in substrate quantities during heterotrophic growth in a number of *Beggiatoa* species and *Macromonas* species and in a *Thiospira* species (Dubinina and Grabovich, 1983). The detoxification may also result in higher yields. As long as no further detailed knowledge on the role of sulfide and other reduced sulfur compounds in the metabolism of the bacteria in the second group is available, both groups will be considered as chemolithotrophs. Two genera included in this chapter, namely *Thiovulum* and *Thiobacterium*, have not yet been grown in pure culture but are thought to generate energy from reduced sulfur compounds, since they are known to thrive in habitats with co-existing sulfide and oxygen and to be able to accumulate intracellular elemental sulfur which is visible under the light microscope.

The carbon metabolism of the sulfur-oxidizing bacteria may range from complete autotrophy to heterotrophy. The more recent physiological studies, for example, on the genera *Thiobacillus* and *Beggiatoa* have shown that many genera of the colorless sulfur bacteria harbor not only typical obligate (chemolitho)autotrophs but also a complete physiological spectrum of organisms, as illustrated in Table 20.16, groups A–C. The facultative (chemolitho)autotrophs can grow autotrophically, (chemoorgano)heterotrophically, and mixotrophically, i.e. under conditions in which these two modes of growth are intermingled. Under such conditions, either the sulfur compounds may serve as additional energy source for growth on an organic compound, or an organic compound may serve as an additional carbon source during autotrophic growth. The chemolithoheterotrophs derive metabolically useful energy from the oxidation of sulfur compounds but cannot grow autotrophically. Lastly, there are heterotrophs (also included in group C, Table 20.16) that benefit in other ways from the oxidation of sulfur compounds (particularly sulfide), e.g. by detoxification of hydrogen peroxide as already mentioned. Group D of Table 20.16 refers to hetero-

trophic bacteria that can oxidize sulfur compounds but do not benefit from this oxidation.

All colorless sulfur bacteria are able to oxidize reduced inorganic sulfur compounds in the dark, but not all organisms able to carry out this oxidation fall under this name. For example, a number of the phototrophic sulfur bacteria, such as *Chromatium* species, can grow chemolithoautotrophically under aerobic conditions in the dark (Kämpf and Pfennig, 1980). Also, many heterotrophic bacteria which are able to oxidize inorganic reduced sulfur compounds are not listed as colorless sulfur bacteria. Table 20.17 gives some examples. The eucaryotes known to be able to oxidize sulfur compounds have not been included but have been reviewed recently (Wainwright, 1984). Most of the organisms in Table 20.17 belong to group D of Table 20.16 and thus do not generate energy from the oxidation or benefit from it by other means. They are, therefore, not colorless sulfur bacteria. As a matter of fact, it has been established unequivocally that only very few of the procaryotic heterotrophs can obtain useful energy from the oxidation process and thus can be identified as true chemolithoheterotrophs (Kelly and Kuenen, 1984). The primary example of a chemolithoheterotroph used to be *Thiobacillus perometabolis*, but it has recently been found to be able to grow autotrophically (Harrison, 1983; Katayama-Fujimura and Kuraishi, 1983). Therefore, at the moment there is no recognized, named species representative of this metabolic type. However, it should be realized that pure cultures of unnamed organisms from this group are available. An example of a heterotroph which can oxidize sulfur compounds but does not benefit from it is *Acidiphilium cryptum* (Harrison, 1983). This acidophile became known initially as a contaminant of *Thiobacillus ferrooxidans* cultures. As long as the affiliation of the genus *Acidiphilium* is unclear, it will be included in the key to the sulfur-oxidizing bacteria, although it obviously belongs among the organisms listed in Table 20.17.

A question that has frequently been asked is whether the ability to oxidize sulfur compounds is a sufficiently important criterion for the classification of organisms of similar morphology into one genus. The most obvious example relevant to this question is the genus *Thiobacillus*, which is by no means taxonomically homogeneous (Kelly and

Table 20.16.

Physiological types among the nonphototrophic bacteria[a] able to oxidize reduced inorganic sulfur compounds[b]

		Energy source (electron donor)		Carbon source	
Physiological type[c]	Synonyms or alternative name commonly used	Inorganic sulfur compound oxidation	Organic compound oxidation	CO$_2$	Organic compound
A. Obligate chemolithoautotroph	Obligate chemolithotroph Obligate autotroph Obligate chemoautotroph Obligate lithotroph	+	−	+	−
B. Facultative chemolithoautotroph	Facultative chemolithotroph Facultative autotroph Facultative chemoautotroph Facultative lithotroph Mixotroph	+	+	+	+
C. Chemolithoheterotroph	Heterotroph able to obtain energy from oxidation of an inorganic sulfur compound[d]	+	+	−	+
D. Chemoorganoheterotroph	Heterotroph able to oxidize sulfur compounds but unable to obtain energy	−	+	−	+

[a] By definition, the colorless sulfur bacteria belong to the first three groups.

[b] After Kelly and Kuenen, 1984.

[c] *Chemo-* indicates metabolic energy obtained from chemical oxidation rather than from photosynthesis; *litho-* indicates inorganic rather than organic (organo-) sources of energy; *auto-* indicates carbon dioxide used as the carbon source (in contrast to heterotrophic use of organic carbon sources).

[d] For taxonomic purposes, organisms which benefit from the oxidation in ways other than energy generation are provisionally included in this group.

Table 20.17.

Examples of heterotrophic bacteria reported to be able to oxidize thiosulfate, sulfur or sulfide

Organism	Reference
Streptomyces sp.	Wainwright, 1984
Pseudomonas aeruginosa	Schook and Berk, 1978
Marine *Pseudomonas*	Tuttle et al., 1974
spp.	Tuttle and Jannasch, 1972
Arthrobacter aurescens	Vitolins and Swaby, 1969
Arthrobacter simplex	Vitolins and Swaby, 1969
Arthrobacter sp.	Vitolins and Swaby, 1969
Bacillus licheniformis	Vitolins and Swaby, 1969
Bacillus brevis	Vitolins and Swaby, 1969
Flavobacterium sp.	Vitolins and Swaby, 1969
Micrococcus sp.	Vitolins and Swaby, 1969
Brevibacterium sp.	Vitolins and Swaby, 1969
Achromobacter sp.	Vitolins and Swaby, 1969
Mycobacterium sp.	Vitolins and Swaby, 1969
Pseudomonas sp.	Vitolins and Swaby, 1969
Pseudomonas fluorescens	Gleen and Quastel, 1953
Pseudomonas aromatica	Sijderius, 1946
Pseudomonas pyocyanea	Sijderius, 1946
Pseudomonas putida	Sijderius, 1946
Pseudomonas aeruginosa	Starkey, 1934
Achromobacter stutzeri	Starkey, 1934
Escherichia coli	Starkey, 1934

Harrison, this section). It seems likely that within this genus the common physiology together with rod-shaped morphology is the result of evolutionary convergence rather than the result of taxonomic relationship. In this context it should also be recalled that the genus "*Hydrogenomonas*" was abolished because the physiological grouping interfered with proper taxonomic classification (Davis et al., 1969). In an analogous way, the same might be said of the colorless sulfur oxidizers. Already there is one facultatively autotrophic sulfur oxidizer, *Paracoccus denitrificans*, which happened to be classified before it was discovered that it can grow lithoautotrophically on thiosulfate (Friedrich and Mitrenga, 1981). Had it been enriched for originally on thiosulfate, it would undoubtedly have been placed within *Thiobacillus*. It is not known how many more sulfur oxidizers exist under other generic names for lack of screening. Although it might be concluded from these examples that sulfur oxidation is insufficient as a major taxonomic criterion, it is the opinion of the author and many other workers in this field of research (see also Kelly and Harrison, this volume) that the ability to generate energy (or to benefit metabolically in other ways) from the oxidation of reduced inorganic sulfur compounds is a physiologically more elaborate and much more complex property than is the ability to oxidize molecular hydrogen. Furthermore, as has been argued above, this classification also has an ecological rationale. Therefore, the classification as an "organism metabolizing reduced inorganic sulfur compounds" or as a "colorless sulfur bacterium" is preferred and retained for purely practical purposes.

For these reasons, the key to the identification of the colorless sulfur bacteria is a necessarily practical and empirical guide. Once it has been established that an organism is a procaryote which can oxidize a reduced sulfur compound and possesses no photosynthetic pigments

(see Pfennig and Trüper, this volume), the morphology of the organism is the most important key. Thus far, the practice has been that any organism that stores microscopically visible sulfur is a candidate for the colorless sulfur bacteria. If they do not belong to the easily recognizable group of the *Beggiatoaceae* and *Achromatium* (see pages 2089 and 2131), they should belong to the genera *Thiobacterium*, *Macromonas*, *Thiovulum* or *Thiospira*. One magnetotactic species, "*Bilophococcus*" (see page 1888), also contains internal sulfur. These genera can easily be identified provisionally by morphological characteristics. Subsequently, the organism, if available in pure culture, must undergo physiological tests. For sulfur oxidizers which do not store intracellular sulfur, physiological criteria must be considered before any other keys are used, and it must be established unequivocally that they can derive energy from this oxidation or benefit from it in other ways, as already discussed. The test for the ability to derive energy from the oxidation of sulfur compounds may be easy for a number of the facultative and obligate autotrophs, since this test can be carried out in mineral medium (supplemented, if necessary, with vitamins) containing sulfide or thiosulfate and with carbon dioxide being obtained from the air supply (or bicarbonate in the case of denitrifying species). However, experience has shown that, for example, with the *Beggiatoa* species the conditions for autotrophic growth may be difficult to create in the laboratory (Nelson and Jannasch, 1983). Also, the test is extremely difficult for the few known chemolithoheterotrophs. When these organisms are grown in batch culture in organic media supplemented with a reduced inorganic sulfur compound, they may oxidize the sulfur compound but not show a cell yield increase or any other beneficial effect from this oxidation. The cell yield increase may only be revealed when the cells are grown under carbon and energy limitation in the chemostat (Kelly and Kuenen, 1984; Gommers, 1987).

If the organism can derive energy from the oxidation, its morphology is the next criterion. All rods that grow below a temperature of 55°C are classified as *Thiobacillus*. Rod-shaped organisms able to form filaments and growing at higher temperatures are classified as *Thermothrix*. Vibrioid-shaped and spiral cells are classified as *Thiomicrospira*, while typical coccoid or spherical cells are named *Thiosphaera*. Cocci which grow above 55°C belong in the genus *Sulfolobus*.

Further Reading

Bos, P. and J.G. Kuenen. 1983. Microbiology of sulphur-oxidizing bacteria. *In* Mercer, Tiller and Wilson (Editors), Microbial Corrosion. The Metals Society, London, pp. 18–27.

Dispirito, A.A. and O.H. Tuovinen. 1984. Oxidations of nonferrous metals by *Thiobacilli*. *In* Strohl and Tuovinen (Editors), Microbial Chemoautotrophy. Ohio State University Press, Columbus, Ohio, pp. 12–29.

Harrison, A.P. 1984. The acidophilic *Thiobacilli* and other acidophilic bacteria that share their habitat. Annu. Rev. Microbiol. *38:* 265–292.

Kelly, D.P. 1985. Physiology of the thiobacilli: elucidating the sulphur oxidation pathway. Microbiol. Sci. *2:* 105–109.

Kuenen, J.G., L.A. Robertson and H. van Gemerden. 1985. Microbial interactions among aerobic and anaerobic sulfur-oxidizing bacteria. Adv. Microb. Ecol. *8:* 1–59.

Larkin, J.M. and W.R. Strohl. 1983. *Beggiatoa*, *Thiothrix* and *Thioploca*. Annu. Rev. Microbiol. *37:* 341–367.

Matin, A. 1984. Mixotrophy in facultative *Thiobacilli*. *In* Strohl and Tuovinen (Editors), Microbial Chemoautotrophy. Ohio State University Press, Columbus, Ohio, pp. 57–77.

Postgate, J.R. and D.P. Kelly (Editors). 1982. Sulphur Bacteria. The Royal Society, London.

van Gemerden, H. 1983. Physiological ecology of purple and green bacteria. Ann. Microbiol. (Inst. Pasteur) *134B:* 73–92.

Key to the Organisms Metabolizing Reduced Inorganic Sulfur Compounds *and to the genera of* Organisms Metabolizing Reduced or Partially Reduced Inorganic Sulfur Compounds

All organisms are procaryotes that can oxidize one or more of the following compounds: hydrogen sulfide, **sulfides, polysulfide, elemental sulfur, thiosulfate, (poly)thionates** (e.g. tetrathionate, trithionate) and **sulfite**. The major metabolic products are sulfur and sulfate, but other oxidation products, such as polysulfide, thiosulfate, polythionates or sulfite, can also be formed.

Organisms use oxygen or nitrate as terminal electron acceptor during the oxidation of the sulfur compounds. No photosynthetic pigments have been observed. Since many of the genera are of uncertain affiliation, for convenience, reference is also made to the *Beggiatoaceae, Achromatium, Sulfolobus, Acidianus* and *Thiodendron.*

A. After incubation in liquid containing O_2 and sulfide, **cells contain intracellular** (elemental) **sulfur particles** which are visible with the light microscope (under phase contrast, the sulfur appears as yellow particles of round or irregular shape or, when the microscope is out of focus, as reddish particles).

   I. Typical "colorless cyanobacteria."

   a. Filaments or gonidia move by gliding.

   Family Beggiatoaceae, p. 2089

   II. Very large (diameter minimally 5 μm, usually 20 μm), spherical to ovoid or cylindrical cells that may contain sulfur droplets and large spherules of calcium carbonate. This organism has not been isolated in pure culture.

   Genus *Achromatium*, p. 2131

   III. Cells which have rods and are embedded in gelatinous mass are not motile. This organism has not been cultivated in pure culture.

   Genus *Thiobacterium*, p. 1838

   IV. Cells not embedded in gelatinous mass are motile.

   a. Cylindrical to bean-shaped cells; flagella polar. Organism may not be able to generate energy from sulfur oxidation but benefits from the oxidation of sulfide by detoxification of peroxide.

   Genus *Macromonas*, p. 1838

   b. Spiral cells; flagella polar. Organism may not be able to generate energy from the oxidation of sulfur compounds but benefits from the oxidation of sulfide by detoxification of peroxide.

   Genus *Thiospira*, p. 1840

   c. Round to ovoid cells; flagella peritrichous.

   Genus *Thiovulum*, p. 1841

   V. Cells magnetotactic.

   Genus *"Bilophococcus,"* p. 1888

B. **No intracellular sulfur visible under light microscope,** not even after incubation in liquid containing O_2 and sulfide.

   I. Temperature for growth: below 55°C. Organism can be grown chemolithoautotrophically (may require vitamins).

   a. Rod-shaped, motile or nonmotile.

   Genus *Thiobacillus*, p. 1842

   b. Spiral or vibrioid-shaped, motile or nonmotile, no stalks.

   Genus *Thiomicrospira*, p. 1858

   c. Vibrioid-shaped, both ends tapered, stalks (0.15–0.25 μm) on either or both poles.

   Genus *Thiodendron*, p. 1990

   d. Spherical cells, sometimes in chains.

   Genus *Thiosphaera*, p. 1861

   (See also *Paracoccus denitrificans* (Volume 1, page 399) which can, although it is not mentioned in the description, grow on thiosulfate aerobically.)

   II. a. Temperature for growth: below 55°C. Organism cannot be grown chemolithoautotrophically on sulfur compounds but does grow **chemolithoheterotrophically.** No named species are available. Known, unnamed species may fall into the genus *Thiobacillus* (Gottschal and Kuenen, 1980). At least one strain of *Hyphomicrobium* falls into this category (Suylen and Kuenen, 1986), but it is readily differentiated from the colorless sulfur bacteria by its morphology (see page 0000).

   b. **Chemoorganoheterotroph** that cannot obtain metabolically useful energy from the oxidation of inorganic sulfur compounds (check Table 20.17). If they are acidophilic, check:

   Genus *Acidiphilium*, p. 1863

   III. **Temperature optimum: above 55°C. Organism can be grown chemolithoautotrophically.**

   a. Cells rod-shaped, may form filaments.

   Genus *Thermothrix*, p. 1868

   b. Cells spherical with lobes, oxidize H_2S and S but do not reduce it.

   Genus *Sulfolobus*, p. 2250

   c. Cells spherical with lobes, oxidize H_2S and S and can also reduce it in the presence of H_2.

   Genus *Acidianus*, p. 2251

Genus **Thiobacterium** *(ex Janke 1924) Nom Rev.*

J. W. M. LA RIVIÈRE AND J. G. KUENEN

Thi.o.bac.te′ri.um. Gr. n. *thios* sulfur; Gr. dim. n. *bakterion* a small rod; M.L. neut. n. *Thiobacterium* small sulfur rod.

Rod-shaped cells, each containing one or more **sulfur globules.** Cells embedded in **gelatinous masses** which are **spherical** when free-floating or are **dendroid** when attached to a solid substrate. **Nonmotile.** No resting stages known.

Has not been grown in pure culture.

Type species: *Thiobacterium bovista* (Molisch) Janke 1924, 68.

Further Descriptive Information

Rod-shaped cells 0.4–1.5 × 2.5–9 μm with up to nine sulfur inclusions. When these are present, cell masses are white in reflected light and are black or bluish in transmitted light. Gram-negative (Scheminzky et al., 1972).

In the spherical colonies, the cells are embedded in the gelatinous walls of a bladderlike structure filled with water and up to 4 mm in diameter. Such colonies occur near the water surface and have the appearance of groups of puff balls of different sizes. Dendroid colonies show extensive branching and may reach 2–3 mm.

The only species in this genus, *T. bovista*, has been found in marine, brackish water and freshwater environments containing hydrogen sulfide and, at temperatures of up to 45°C, in thermal springs.

Enrichment and Maintenance Procedures

Molisch (1912) reported enrichment of the spherical colony type at the surface of Winogradsky columns prepared with decaying algae, mud and seawater from the Gulf of Trieste where the organism had been found. The dendroid form could not be enriched for but, after being taken from nature, could be kept alive for 3 months in the laboratory in jars with water from the original habitat kept at 20°C (Lackey and Lackey, 1961). Some further details are given by la Rivière and Schmidt (1981). For micrographs, see articles by Lackey and Lackey (1961) and Scheminzky et al. (1972). No pure cultures are known.

Taxonomic Comments

Although this genus and its type species do not appear in the Approved Lists of Bacterial Names, maintaining their descriptions in the present edition of the *Manual* and reviving the name appears justified because recent reports of *Thiobacterium* have been published (Scheminzky et al., 1972; Caldwell and Caldwell, 1974) since the eighth edition of the *Manual.*

Further Reading

Caldwell, D.E. and S.J. Caldwell. 1974. The response of littoral communities of bacteria to variations in sulfide and thiosulfate. Abstr. Annu. Meet. Am. Soc. Microbiol. *74:* 59.

la Rivière, J.W.M. and K. Schmidt. 1981. Morphologically conspicuous sulfur-oxidizing bacteria. *In* Starr, Stolp, Trüper, Balows and Schlegel (Editors), The Prokaryotes. A Handbook on Habitats, Isolation, and Identification of Bacteria. Springer-Verlag, Berlin, pp. 1037–1048.

Molisch, H. 1912. Neue farblose Schwefelbakterien. Zentralbl. Bakteriol. Parasitenkd. Infektionskr. Hyg. Abt. 2 *33:* 55–62.

Scheminzky, F., Z. Klas and C. Job. 1972. Über das Vorkommen von *Thiobacterium bovista* in Thermalwässern. Int. Rev. Gesamten Hydrobiol. *57:* 801–813.

List of species of the genus **Thiobacterium**

1. **Thiobacterium bovista** (ex Janke 1924) nom. rev. bo.vis′ta. M.L. fem. n. *bovista* puff ball.
For a description, see that of the genus.

Type *strain:* no culture available. Description is found in Janke 1924, 68.

Genus **Macromonas** *Utermöhl and Koppe in Koppe 1924, 632*[AL]

J. W. M. LA RIVIÈRE AND G. A. DUBININA

Mac.ro.mo′nas. Gr. adj. *makros* large; Gr. n. *monas* a unit, monad; M.L. fem. n. *Macromonas* large monad.

Cylindrical to bean-shaped cells, **motile by one polar flagellum, consisting of a tuft of flagella. Several large inclusions,** possibly of calcium carbonate, sometimes accompanied by sulfur globules. Multiplication by constriction, followed by fission. No resting stages known. The genus comprises two species; the type species has not been grown in pure culture.

Type species: **Macromonas mobilis** (Lauterborn, 1915) Utermöhl and Koppe in Koppe 1924, 632.

Further Descriptive Information

Cells are 3–14 μm wide and 10–30 μm long. Sluggish motility at a rate of 600–800 μm/min, probably as a result of the high specific gravity of the cells. One to four large optically dense inclusions may almost fill the cell.

The polar tuft of flagella ranges in length from 10 to 40 μm and can sometimes be seen in the light microscope.

Aerobic, aerotactic. Strains of *M. bipunctata* so far isolated are all heterotrophic but are capable of oxidizing sulfide to sulfur by means of hydrogen peroxide.

Found in freshwater environments with low oxygen concentrations, e.g. hypolimnia and upper layers of bottom muds and of sediments in sewage treatment plants. Has also been reported in acid bog waters (Schulz and Hirsch, 1973).

No methods are known for isolation and for maintenance of cultures of the type species *M. mobilis.* For *M. bipunctata,* such methods are given below.

Taxonomic Comments

The two species listed in the eighth edition of the *Manual* could only be characterized by morphological properties, as no pure cultures existed. This is still the case for the type species *M. mobilis,* which appears on the Approved Lists of Bacterial Names.

Recently, Dubinina and Grabovich isolated several strains of *M. bipunctata* and validly published a detailed description (1984).

At this time, however, we do not propose to select *M. bipunctata* as the type species in place of *M. mobilis.* We now believe that isolation of *M. mobilis* may take place in the near future and thus complete the taxonomy of the genus with a minimum of alterations.

The interest in the genus *Macromonas* may be further stimulated by the work being carried out on the populations of sulfide oxidizers encountered at the deep-sea bottom around H_2S-emitting hydrothermal vents (Jannasch, 1984).

Further Reading

Dubinina, G.A. and M.Y. Grabovich. 1984. Isolation, cultivation and characteristics of *Macromonas bipunctata.* Mikrobiologiya *53:* 748–755 (in Russian).

Jannasch, H.W. 1984. Microbial processes at deep sea hydrothermal vents. *In* Rona, Bostrom, Laubier and Smith (Editors), Hydrothermal Processes at Seafloor Spreading Centers. Plenum Publishing, New York, pp. 667–709.

la Rivière, J.W.M. and K. Schmidt. 1981. Morphologically conspicuous sulfur-oxidizing bacteria. *In* Starr, Stolp, Trüper, Balows and Schlegel (Editors), The

Prokaryotes. A Handbook on Habitats, Isolation, and Identification of Bacteria. Springer-Verlag, Berlin, pp. 1037–1048.

Schulz, E. and P. Hirsch. 1973. Morphologically unusual bacteria in acid bog water habitats. Abstr. Annu. Meet. Am. Soc. Microbiol. *73:* 60.

List of species of the genus **Macromonas**

1. **Macromonas mobilis** (Lauterborn, 1915) Utermöhl and Koppe in Koppe 1924, 632.[AL]

mo'bi.lis. L. fem. adj. *mobilis* motile.

The main, presently known feature by which this species is distinguished from *M. bipunctata* is its large cell size, which is usually 9 × 20 µm but is sometimes 6–14 × 10–30 µm (Table 20.18). Its polar tuft of flagella is 20–40 µm long.

This organism has not been grown in pure culture. For a further description, see that of the genus.

2. **Macromonas bipunctata** (ex Utermöhl and Koppe in Koppe 1924) Dubinina and Grabovich 1984, 754.

bi.punc.ta'ta. L. *bis* twice; L. part. adj. *punctatus* punctate, dotted; M.L. fem. adj. *bipunctata* twice punctate.

Cells are single or in pairs, pear-shaped, cylindrical or curved, 2.2–4 × 3.3–6.5 µm, and motile by a polar tuft of flagella (Figs. 20.41 and 20.42). Colonies are nonpigmented, slightly opalescent and flat on the surface of the agar medium and measure 0.5–4 mm.

Gram-negative. Catalase-positive. Strictly aerobic. Optimum temperature: 28°C. Optimum pH: 7.5–8.2.

Chemoorganotrophic. Acetate, succinate, malate, fumarate, benzoate and salts of other organic acids are good substrates, but sugars, alcohols and amino acids are not used. Ammonium salts and organic nitrogen compounds can serve as nitrogen source. Vitamins are required for growth. In media containing sulfides, inclusions of sulfur are formed through oxidation by hydrogen peroxide.

Isolation was performed by inoculating a semisolid medium with some material of the white deposit found on the surface of sediments in an aeration tank of a sewage treatment plant. The medium contained (per liter) of distilled water: sodium acetate, 1 g; CaCl₂, 0.1 g; casein

Table 20.18.
Differentiation between **M. mobilis** *and* **M. bipunctata**

	M. mobilis	M. bipunctata
Cell size (µm)	6–14 × 10–30	2.2–4 × 3.3–6.5

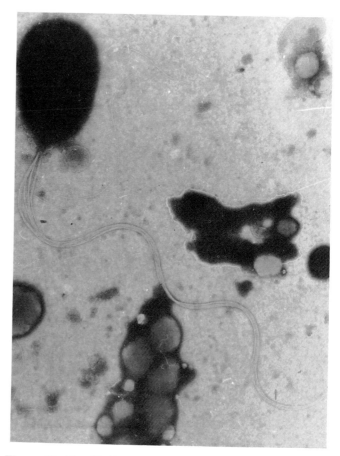

Figure 20.42. *M. bipunctata* cell showing tuft of polar flagella. Electron micrograph (× 10,000). (Reproduced with permission from G. A. Dubinina and M. Y. Grabovich, Mikrobiologiya *53:* 748–755, 1984.)

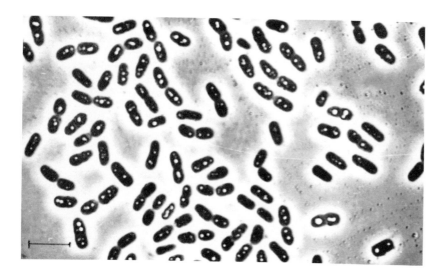

Figure 20.41. *M. bipunctata* cells grown on acetate medium. *Bar*, 10 µm. (Reproduced with permission from G. A. Dubinina and M. Y. Grabovich, Mikrobiologiya *53:* 748–755, 1984.)

hydrolysate, 0.1 g; yeast extract, 0.1 g; and agar, 1 g. After sterilization, vitamins and trace elements as well as 200 mg freshly precipitated FeS (pH 7.2–7.4) were added. Cell material growing on the surface of this medium could be purified by streaking on a solid medium of the same composition, with 10 g of agar per liter added.

The mol% G + C of the DNA is 67.6.

Type strain: VKM 1366.

This description is extracted from the paper by Dubinina and Grabovich (1984) which presents further details on the morphology and physiology of *M. bipunctata.*

Genus **Thiospira** *Visloukh 1914, 48*[AL]

J. W. M. LA RIVIÈRE AND J. G. KUENEN

Thi.o.spi′ra. Gr. *thios* sulfur; Gr. *spira* a coil; M.L. fem. *Thiospira* sulfur coil or spiral.

Spirilla, usually with pointed ends, with **sulfur inclusions. Motile** by monotrichous or polytrichous **polar flagella.** No resting stages known. Has not been cultivated in pure culture.

Type species: *Thiospira winogradskyi* (Omelianski) Visloukh 1914, 48.

Further Descriptive Information

Colorless spirilla, pointed at the ends and containing sulfur globules. Polar flagella in some cases united in a tuft, visible in the light microscope. *T. winogradskyi* is 2–2.5 µm wide and up to 50 µm long (Fig. 20.43). "*T. bipunctata*" is 1.7–2.4 µm wide and 6.6–14 µm long.

Microaerophilic and vigorously chemotactic with respect to oxygen and, possibly, H₂S.

Found in sulfurous marine and freshwater environments.

Enrichment and Maintenance Procedures

T. winogradskyi was enriched by Omelianski (1905) in Winogradsky columns kept for some months at room temperature in the dark. The cell mass appeared in the form of "bacterial plates," i.e. discrete dense layers of bacteria, and could be kept alive in the laboratory for 2 years.

Molisch (1912) enriched "*T. bipunctata*" from Black Sea mud which, when mixed with decaying algae, was used as an H₂S-generating sediment in a seawater-filled cylinder 20–30 cm high.

No pure cultures are known.

Taxonomic Comments

Although one of the species ("*T. bipunctata*") does not appear on the Approved Lists, it is retained in the present description of the genus in view of its marked differences from the type species. It should be recalled that Bavendamm (1924) recognized five species.

In 1983, Dubinina and Grabovich described the isolation of heterotrophic spirilla morphologically similar to *Thiospira* and capable of forming internal sulfur granules in sulfide-containing media. Experiments indicated that the sulfur was formed through oxidation of sulfide by hydrogen peroxide.

Since other heterotrophs capable of forming sulfur inclusions in sulfide-containing media have also been found (Skerman et al., 1957), there is a distinct possibility that on further examination the spirilla isolated by Dubinina and Grabovich may turn out to be classifiable within the existing species of the genus *Spirillum.* Also, study of the behavior of pure cultures of *Spirillum* species in sulfide-containing media would help elucidate this matter. Pending such studies, we propose to maintain the present genus *Thiospira* as described.

In spite of its present uncertain taxonomic position, the importance of the genus may prove to be considerable when further studies have been made of the population of sulfide oxidizers encountered at the deep-sea bottom around H₂S-emitting hydrothermal vents (Jannasch, 1984).

Further Reading

Bavendamm, W. 1924. Die farblosen und roten Schwefelbakterien des Süss- und Salz-wassers. *In* Kolkwitz (Editor), Pflanzenforschung. Gustav Fischer Velag, Jena, pp. 7–156.

Dubinina, G.A. and M.Y. Grabovich. 1983. Isolation of pure *Thiospira* cultures and investigation of their sulfur metabolism. Mikrobiologiya *52:* 5–12.

Jannasch, H.W. 1984. Microbial processes at deep sea hydrothermal vents. *In* Rona, Bostrom, Laubier and Smith (Editors), Hydrothermal Processes at Seafloor Spreading Centers. Plenum Publishing, New York, pp. 667–709.

la Rivière, J.W.M. and K. Schmidt. 1981. Morphologically conspicuous sulfur-oxidizing bacteria. *In* Starr, Stolp, Trüper, Balows and Schlegel (Editors), The Prokaryotes. A Handbook on Habitats, Isolation, and Identification of Bacteria. Springer-Verlag, Berlin, pp. 1037–1048.

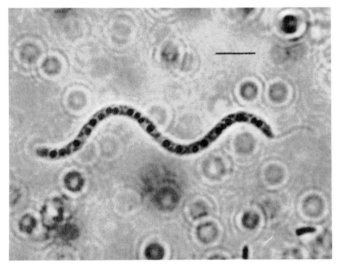

Figure 20.43. *Thiospira* species dividing cell with tuft of flagella. *Bar,* 5 µm. (Photographed by J. Klein, Delft, The Netherlands. Reproduced with permission from J. W. M. la Rivière and K. Schmidt. 1981. Morphologically conspicuous sulfur-oxidizing bacteria. *In* Starr, Stolp, Trüper, Balows and Schlegel (Editors), The Prokaryotes. A Handbook on Habitats, Isolation, and Identification of Bacteria. Springer-Verlag, Berlin, chap. 82.)

List of species of the genus **Thiospira**

1. **Thiospira winogradskyi** (Omelianski) Visloukh 1914, 48.[AL]
wi.no.grad.'sky.i. M.L. gen. n. *winogradskyi* of Winogradsky; named for S. N. Winogradsky, a Russian microbiologist.

Found in freshwater and marine environments overlaying sulfurous muds. See Table 20.19 for differentiation of *T. winogradskyi* and "*T. bipunctata.*"

2. "**Thiospira bipunctata**" (Molisch) Visloukh 1914, 48.
bi.punc.ta'ta. L. *bis* twice; L. part. adj. *punctatus* punctate, dotted; M.L. fem. adj. *bipunctata* twice punctate.

Found in sulfurous marine and brackish waters (see Table 20.19).

Table 20.19.
Differentiation of the species of the genus **Thiospira**

	T. winogradskyi	"*T. bipunctata*"
Size	2–2.5 × up to 50 µm	1.7–2.4 × 6.6–14 µm
No. of sulfur inclusions	Numerous	Few
Volutin granules at both ends	−	+

Genus **Thiovulum** Hinze 1913, 195[AL]

J. W. M. LA RIVIÈRE AND J. G. KUENEN

Thi.o'vu.lum. Gr. n. *thios* sulfur; L. n. *ovum* egg; M.L. neut. dim. n. *Thiovulum* small sulfur egg.

Cells are round to ovoid, 5–25 µm in diameter. Cytoplasm is often concentrated at one end of the cell, with the remaining space being occupied by a large vacuole. Cytoplasm normally contains **orthorhombic sulfur inclusions,** sometimes concentrated at one end and sometimes filling cells almost completely. Cell are **strongly motile by peritrichous flagella;** forward movement is accompanied by rotation around the long axis. Cells are characterized by the presence of one polar fibrillar organelle, visible in thin sections by electron microscopy; its function is not known. No resting stages are known.

Multiplication by constriction followed by fission. Gram-negative. Microaerophilic. Catalase-negative. No pure cultures are available.

Types species: *Thiovulum majus* Hinze 1913, 195.

Further Descriptive Information

Strongly chemotactic with respect to O_2 and H_2S. Cells concentrate in sharply defined, characteristic white veils or webs consisting of separate, individually moving cells held together to some extent by a loose slime matrix (Figs. 20.44–20.46). These cell masses are found in the O_2/H_2S boundary layers where both substrates occur at low concentrations (0–10 μM^{-1}) but are constantly replenished by diffusion (Jørgensen and Revsbech, 1983). Cells are killed by both anaerobic conditions and O_2 concentrations near air saturation values. The amount of sulfur present in the cells varies with the H_2S supply, and cells may be temporarily fully devoid of sulfur inclusions.

Experiments on crude laboratory cultures provide strong evidence for the chemolithotrophic and even the autotrophic nature of *Thiovulum* (Wirsen and Jannasch, 1978).

Organisms are found in freshwater and marine environments where

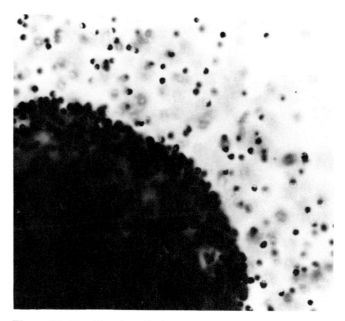

Figure 20.45. *T. majus* cells showing the periphery of a veil (× 250).

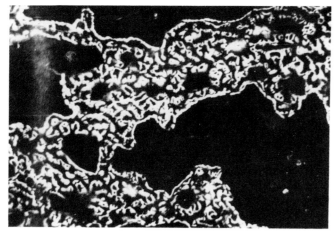

Figure 20.44. *T. majus* swarming cells showing a characteristic veil (× 3).

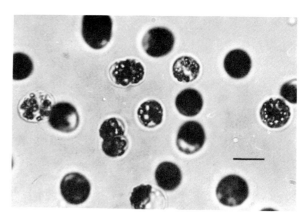

Figure 20.46. *T. majus* swarming cells showing sulfur inclusions. Note the pair of dividing cells. *Bar,* 10 µm.

sulfide-containing water or mud layers are in contact with overlaying oxygen-containing water.

Enrichment and Maintenance Procedures

There are various methods for enrichment and maintenance of *Thiovulum* from seawater, all of which are based upon the provision of a H_2S-generating system coupled to a continuous and controlled supply of dissolved oxygen (Wirsen and Jannasch, 1978; la Rivière and Schmidt, 1981). In order to exclude photosynthetic sulfur bacteria, enrichment cultures must be kept in the dark; low temperatures (<15°C) appear to be favorable.

A good example is a system consisting of a 1–10-liter jar with a layer of decaying *Ulva* on the bottom and with a continuous flow-through of seawater entering near the bottom. The sediment provides H_2S through reduction of sulfate supplied by the seawater, which is also a continuous O_2 source. The *Thiovulum* cells maintain themselves at the optimal location in the gradient thus created and, in contrast to the nonchemotactic contaminants, are not flushed out. Instead of decaying *Ulva*, several other H_2S sources can be employed, such as a pure culture of sulfate-reducing bacteria fed independently and kept separate from the *Thiovulum* culture by a membrane.

Vigorously growing laboratory cultures can be maintained by such methods for many months and can provide ample material for morphological and physiological study. So far, however, no pure cultures have become available.

Taxonomic Comments

Although there are no pure cultures, considerable progress has been made in the study of the physiology of *Thiovulum* by means of crude laboratory cultures (Wirsen and Jannasch, 1978; Jørgensen and Revsbech, 1983). The genus may gain in importance when further studies have been made of the populations of sulfide oxidizers encountered at the deep-sea bottom around H_2S-emitting hydrothermal vents (Jannasch, 1984). Furthermore, the biogeochemical sulfur cycle in which colorless sulfur bacteria play an important role is receiving increased attention (Kuenen, 1975; Ivanov and Freney, 1983).

List of species of the genus **Thiovulum**

1. **Thiovulum majus** Hinze 1913, 195.[AL]
ma′jus. L. comp. adj. *major* larger.
For a description, see that of the genus.

Further Reading

Jannasch, H.W. 1984. Microbial processes at deep sea hydrothermal vents. *In* Rona, Bostrom, Laubier and Smith (Editors), Hydrothermal Processes at Seafloor Spreading Centers. Plenum Publishing, New York, pp. 677–709.

Jørgensen, B.B. and N.P. Revsbech. 1983. Colorless sulfur bacteria, *Beggiatoa* spp. and *Thiovulum* spp., in O_2 and H_2S microgradients. Appl. Environ. Microbiol. *45:* 1261–1270.
la Rivière, J.W.M. and K. Schmidt. 1981. Morphologically conspicuous sulfur-oxidizing bacteria. *In* Starr, Stolp, Trüper, Balows and Schleger (Editors), The Prokaryotes. A Handbook on Habitats, Isolation, and Identification of Bacteria. Springer-Verlag, Berlin, pp. 1037–1048.
Wirsen, C.O. and H.W. Jannasch. 1978. Physiological and morphological observations on *Thiovulum* sp. J. Bacteriol. *136:* 765–774.

Genus **Thiobacillus** Beijerinck 1904b, 597[AL]

D. P. KELLY AND A. P. HARRISON

Thi.o.ba.cil′lus. Gr. n. *thios* sulfur; L. n. *bacillus* a small rod; M.L. masc. n. *Thiobacillus* sulfur rodlet.

Small, **Gram-negative, rod-shaped cells** (~$0.5 \times 1.0–4.0 \mu m$) with **some** species **motile by** means of **polar flagella.** No resting stages known. **Energy** is derived **from the oxidation of** one or more **reduced sulfur compounds,** including sulfides, sulfur, thiosulfate, polythionates and thiocyanate. **Sulfate is the end product** of sulfur compound oxidation, but sulfur, sulfite or polythionates may be accumulated, sometimes transiently, by most species. One species also derives energy from oxidizing ferrous iron to ferric iron. **All species can fix carbon dioxide by means of the Benson-Calvin cycle and are capable of autotrophic growth**; some species are obligately **chemolithotrophic,** while **others** are **also** able to **grow chemoorganotrophically.** The genus includes **obligate aerobes and facultative denitrifying types,** and its species exhibit pH optima of 2–8 with temperature optima of 20–43°C. Different species exhibit mol% G + C of the DNA of 50–68%. Distribution is seemingly ubiquitous in marine, freshwater and soil environments, especially where oxidizable sulfur is abundant (e.g. sulfur springs, sulfide minerals, sulfur deposits, sewage treatment areas and sources of sulfur gases, such as H_2S from sediments or anaerobic soils).

Type species: *Thiobacillus thioparus* Beijerinck 1904b, 597.

Taxonomic validity and case for retention of the genus **Thiobacillus**

As is detailed later, the range of physical growth conditions, mol% G + C of the DNA, diversity of DNA homology, range of ubiquinone and fatty acid content, and the existence of species able to grow either only chemolithoautotrophically or also heterotrophically among the "thiobacilli" is indicative of an extremely heterogeneous group, judged in terms of genetic and physiological similarity. Indeed, the only criterion for concentrating all the species into one genus is that all are rod-shaped eubacteria that obtain energy for autotrophic growth from oxidizing inorganic sulfur substrates. Physiologically, some of them bear strong similarities to other morphologically distinct species dealt with elsewhere, such as *Thiomicrospira* and "*Leprospirillum.*" Knowledge that some photosynthetic bacteria and some hydrogen-oxidizing *Alcaligenes* species can grow autotrophically in the dark with thiosulfate oxidation as their sole source of energy (Kondratieva et al., 1976; Kämpf and Pfennig, 1980; Friedrich and Mitrenga, 1981) makes validity of the genus grouping even more questionable. In our view, there is still greatest benefit in retaining the *Thiobacillus* genus for those organisms capable of dark autotrophic growth on inorganic sulfur substrates, but not of photosynthetic growth or growth on hydrogen oxidation, and in habitats where this property may be of prime importance in their metabolism. It is a physiologically and ecologically more useful category that would be lost for the purposes of intercomparison of species if some of the thiobacilli were relegated, for example, to the *Pseudomonas* genus. It could be argued that the genus name *Thiobacillus* should be retained only for the obligately chemolithotrophic strains such as the type species *T. thioparus*. This would currently serve no useful purpose, as the genetic diversity of those species is probably at least as great as that between them and the facultative species or within the latter.

Biochemical criteria for classification of the species of the genus **Thiobacillus**

Since the eighth edition of the *Manual*, a very considerable amount of information on ubiquinone and fatty acid content, DNA base composition and interspecific DNA homology has been obtained on the thiobacilli. This has enabled division of the species into distinct groups on the basis of physiology and biochemical characteristics (Harrison, 1982, 1983; Katayama-Fujimura et al., 1982, 1983a). It has also complicated consolidation of species, as DNA homology studies in some cases have shown considerable diversity among strains regarded as members of the same species, while also showing very close similarity between putatively different species.

Primary separation of most of the species of *Thiobacillus* is relatively easy to achieve by virtue of differences in gross physiological characteristics such as pH (and temperature) requirements for growth, ability or lack of ability to grow heterotrophically as well as chemolithotrophically, and differences in ability to grow anaerobically with denitrification or to use elemental sulfur. A comprehensive numerical taxonomy survey by Hutchinson et al. (1969) led to a diagnostic system and the classification of the then-known species that are of considerable interest and have been surprisingly neglected. Figure 20.47 and Table 20.20 demonstrate the major species groupings of this system. The combination of morphological, physiological and biochemical characteristics now available enable the keying out of the *Thiobacillus* species sufficiently effectively to present the data for a diagnostic table in the form of a key.

Most species of *Thiobacillus* may precipitate elemental sulfur externally to their cells during growth on sulfide, thiosulfate and, in some cases, trithionate or tetrathionate. One of the exceptions is *T. versutus*. Sulfur precipitation is not a highly distinctive diagnostic characteristic, as it is a variable property influenced by growth conditions such as oxygen availability or perturbation of steady state in chemostat culture. The precipitation of sulfur *external* to the cells is superficially comparable to the extracellular precipitation observed with the green sulfur bacteria (e.g. *Chlorobium*) and contrasts with the *intra*cellular accumulation of sulfur by *Chromatiaceae* such as *Chromatium*. It is likely, however, that some species deposit sulfur internally, subsequently oxidizing it to sulfate. Thus, *T. albertis* grown on thiosulfate is believed to contain a sulfur granule bounded by a membrane (Bryant et al., 1983) whose appearance was correlated with the production of a large amount of elemental sulfur extracellularly at the end of the growth phase. Morphologically, these inclusions resemble the sulfur found in the purple sulfur bacteria, *Beggiatoa* and *Thiothrix*. These granules did not appear during midlog growth (Bryant et al., 1983) and were not seen in earlier ultrastructural surveys of other thiobacilli (Mahoney and Edwards, 1966; Shively et al., 1970), although they may have been present in "*T. kabobis*" (Reynolds et al., 1981). This "species" is here regarded as synonymous with *T. thiooxidans*. The possibility of both extracellular depositions and intracellular accumulation of elemental sulfur in some thiobacilli is somewhat of a physiological anomaly, possibly indicative of differing mechanisms or locations of sulfur compound oxidation. Extracellular sulfur precipitation is best explained as a consequence of the conversion of sulfide or the sulfane groups of thiosulfate (or polythionates) to sulfur at the surface of the cell, presumably in the periplasmic space and catalyzed by enzyme systems located in or external to the bounding membrane of the cell. This would seem more likely than intracellular generation of sulfur and its excretion to the outside (as has indeed been suggested). The nature of the sulfur on formation is unknown, and of course, the cell wall would be likely to be a barrier to the excretion of large granules from inside the cell or even their generation from the periplasmic space. The production of intracellular sulfur from a soluble substrate (thiosulfate) implies intracellular oxidation of the substrate with the consequent implications of its transport across the membrane and the need for elucidating a mechanism for the membrane-associated electron transport systems involved in sulfur compound oxidation to sulfate. Clearly, at the present stage of our knowledge of the mechanisms for the transport of sulfur and its compounds and of the biochemistry of their conversion to

sulfate, characteristics such as intracellular sulfur accumulation cannot be employed as reliable taxonomic features.

Further Descriptive Information

Cells are usually rod-shaped and 0.5×1.0–4.0 μm, occurring singly, in pairs or in short chains. Some are motile by means of a single flagellum or multiple polar flagella. Some possess pili and other specialized surface features. All can obtain energy from the oxidation of reduced inorganic sulfur compounds and, in most cases, elemental sulfur. Some species are obligately chemolithotrophic and autotrophic, others are facultatively heterotrophic, and in some strains, best development occurs mixotrophically. Both electron transport-dependent and substrate level phosphorylations occur during sulfur compound oxidation, and reduction of NAD(P) requires an energy-dependent flow of

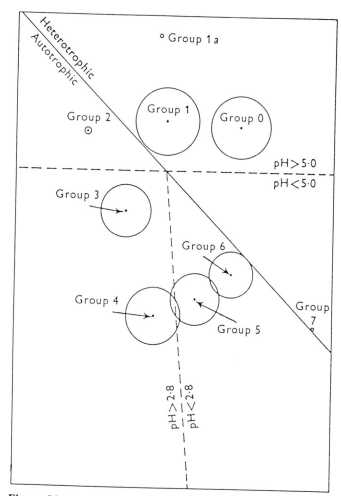

Figure 20.47. Numerical taxonomy relationships of the groups of the genus *Thiobacillus* as deduced by Hutchinson et al. (1969). Plan of the relationships of the groups of thiobacilli shows planes which separate the groups according to specific characters. Relative distance of the groups is based on the relationship $\log_2 I/S$ for the centrotype of each group. The area of the *circles* is proportional to the range of S values within the group according to the expression: $r = 2\sqrt{(d^2 n)}$, where d is the distance in terms of difference in S value between each strain and the centrotype of the group, and n is the number of strains within the group. (Reproduced by permission of the Society for General Microbiology and with permission from M. Hutchinson, K. I. Johnstone and D. White, Journal of General Microbiology 57: 397–410, 1969, ©Society for General Microbiology, Reading.)

Table 20.20.
Useful diagnostic tests for the thiobacilli as derived by Hutchinson et al. (1969) from a numerical taxonomy study of **Thiobacillus** *species*[a]

Medium	Criterion	A 0	B 1a	C 1	D 2	E 3	F 4	G 5	H 6	I 7
S6/S5	Final pH	>6.6	6.5–5.0	6.6–5.0	6.6–5.0	6.6–3.5	3.5–2.8	<2.0	<2.0	>2.0–<2.8
S6/S5	% thiosulfate oxidation	<90	<50	<30	<90	>90	>90	>90	>90	>90
S⁰ + 6% thiosulfate	% thiosulfate	<10	<10	<10	<10	<10	>10	>10	<10	<10
S6/S5 + 4% phosphate	Inhibition	±	+	+	+	+	−	−	+	+
S6/S5 + 5% NaCl	Inhibition	+	+	+	+	+	−	±	+	+
Sulfur	Final pH	ng	6.1–6.25	ng	5.15	4.6–4.1	3.2–2.8	<2.0	<2.0	>2.0–<2.8
S8	Growth	+	+	−	+	±	−	−	−	−
Anaerobic conditions	Gas formation	−	−	−	+	−	−	−	−	−
S7	Thiocyanate oxidation	−	−	−	+	+	−	−	−	−
S⁰ + 0.5% dithionate	pH change	−	−	−	−	±	−	+	−	−
Iron	Iron oxidation	−	−	−	−	−	−	−	+	−
Nutrient agar plate	Growth	+	+	+	−	−	−	−	−	+
Kosers citrate	Growth	+	−	−	−	−	−	−	−	+
Thiosulfate agar	Sulfur deposition	−	−	+	+	+	+	+	−	+

[a]Reproduced by permission of the Society for General Microbiology and with permission from M. Hutchinson, K. I. Johnstone and D. White, Journal of General Microbiology 57: 397–410, 1969, ©Society for General Microbiology, Reading.)
[b]Species A are now regarded as members of different genera. Species B are probably strains of *T. versutus*. Key to species: A, "trautweinii" types; B, group la; C, *T. novellus*, D, *T. denitrificans*; E, *T. thioparus*; F, *T. neapolitanus*; G, *T. thiooxidans*; H, *T. ferrooxidans*; I, *T. intermedius*; and ng, no growth. Symbols: +, 90% or more of strains are positive; −, 90% or more of strains are negative.

electrons from cytochrome *c* (or *b*). Autotrophic fixation of carbon dioxide occurs mainly by means of the Benson-Calvin cycle, with some fixation occurring through pyruvate or phosphoenolpyruvate carboxylation. The obligately autotrophic species possess an incomplete tricarboxylic acid cycle (lacking α-oxoglutarate dehydrogenase) used as a biosynthetic "horseshoe" pathway via oxaloacetate or succinate and α-oxoglutarate down each arm of the "horseshoe." The facultative species show diverse mechanisms for oxidation of glucose, including the simultaneous operation of the Embden-Meyerhof, Entner-Doudoroff and oxidative pentose phosphate pathways in *T. versutus* and the operation of a phosphoketolase pathway in *T. novellus*. Some species contain plasmids and have been shown to be susceptible to introduction of *Pseudomonas* plasmids into them. Little work on their genetics is available, but it is known that autotrophic and drug-resistant mutants can be obtained and that mutations that decrease autotrophic efficiency can be induced. No species is known to be pathogenic. As a genus, their distribution is ubiquitous, with the facultative species also occurring in soils and freshwater and marine environments as heterotrophs or mixotrophs. Sulfur compound-oxidizing species have been isolated from arctic, temperate and tropical waters, soil, salt marshes, freshwater lakes, rivers and canals, hot springs and sulfur-rich mine or acid mine wastewaters and other environments where oxidizable sulfur compounds occur naturally or anthropogenically. (A diagnostic key to separate the species is provided under "Differentiation of the Species of the Genus *Thiobacillus*." Table 20.21 summarizes a range of descriptive features, and Tables 20.20 and 20.22–20.26 give detailed diagnostic and physiological data.)

Enrichment, Isolation and Maintenance Procedures

Most of the species can be isolated from natural habitats by the use of mineral media containing elemental sulfur or thiosulfate as energy substrate. Use of media of different pH will assist differential selection of the neutrophilic and acidophilic species, use of acid ferrous sulfate medium will frequently select for *T. ferrooxidans*, and use of anaerobic thiosulfate medium (pH 7) supplemented with nitrate will be electively successful in selection for *T. denitrificans*. A procedure has been de-scribed for the enrichment of facultatively autotrophic, mixotrophic strains, using a continuous flow chemostat provided with both organic and inorganic substrates (Gottschal and Kuenen, 1980). This provides a means of avoiding the predomination of heterotrophs in standard batch enrichment media containing supplements such as thiosulfate and glucose or acetate. In the latter, a mixture of obligately chemolithotrophic thiobacilli and chemoorganotrophs normally develops. *T. acidophilus* was originally isolated as a commensal of *T. ferrooxidans*, although "*T. organoparus*" (now regarded as *T. acidophilus*) was enriched directly from an acid mine water environment. Media suitable for the different species are given in many places; the following bibliographic entries serve as guides to media suitable for most species: Baalsrud and Baalsrud, 1954; Barton and Shively, 1968; Bounds and Colmer, 1972; Guay and Silver, 1975; Harrison, 1982; Hutchinson et al., 1969; Jones and Kelly, 1983; Justin and Kelly, 1978; Katayama-Fujimura and Kuraishi, 1980; London and Rittenberg, 1967; Manning, 1975; Matin et al., 1980; Parker and Prisk, 1953; Silverman and Lundgren, 1959; Taylor and Hoare, 1969; Tuovinen and Kelly, 1973, 1974; Vishniac and Santer, 1957; Waksman, 1922; Wood and Kelly, 1977.

Most, if not all, strains are able to produce colonial growth on appropriate media solidified with agar. Some strains, especially those of *T. ferrooxidans*, grow poorly on agar media. In some cases, this difficulty is due to the toxicity of agar hydrolysis products and has been overcome in a number of ways (e.g. Tuovinen and Kelly, 1973). It is generally avoided by the use of a minimal concentration of agar, screening of suitable brands of purified agars, use of agarose and, in the case of *T. ferrooxidans*, a combination of low agar concentration with pH 2.2–2.5 and ferrous sulfate at only about 20 mM. The use of silica gel media is probably not normally a necessary alternative.

After cultivation on suitable media, most species survive storage at 5°C for periods of weeks to months, especially if the media for neutrophiles have not become too acid before storage. *T. ferrooxidans* survives in culture on pyrite for very long periods when stored at 5–15°C. Many strains have been successfully freeze-dried or have survived storage at liquid nitrogen temperature or in glycerol suspension at −20°C.

Table 20.21.
Descriptive characteristics of the **Thiobacillus** *species*[a]

Characteristic	1. T. thioparus	2. T. neapolitanus	3. T. tepidarius	4. T. denitrificans	5. T. novellus	6. T. versutus	7. T. intermedius	8. T. perometabolis	9. T. delicatus	10. T. ferrooxidans	11. T. thiooxidans	12. T. albertis	13. T. acidophilus
Growth at													
pH 3.0	−	−	−	−	−	−	(+)	−	−	+	+	+	+
pH 5.0	(+)	(+)	−	−	−	−	+	+	+	+	+	+	+
pH 8.0	+	+	+	+	+	+	−	−	−	−	−	−	−
30°C	+	+	+	+	+	+	+	+	+	+	+	+	+
50°C	−	−	+	−	−	−	−	−	−	−	−	−	−
Optimum pH													
2–4										+	+	+	+
5–7							+	+	+				
6–8	+	+	+	+	+	+							
Optimum temperature													
25–30°C	+	+		+	+						+	+	+
30–35°C						+	+	+	+	+			
40–45°C			+										
Motility	+	+	+	+	−	+	+	+	−	+	+	+	+
Single polar flagellum	+	+	+		−		+	+	−	+	+		
Tuft of polar flagella					−	+				−		+	
Pili (fimbriae) present						+					+	−	−
Contain carboxysomes	+	+	−	−	−		+				+	+	
May contain membrane-enclosed sulfur granules												+	
Ribulosebisphosphate carboxylase repressed by organic substrates	−	−		−	+	+	+				−		
Possess α-oxoglutarate dehydrogenase	−	−		−	+	+	(−)	(−)			−		−
Contains													
Ubiquinone-8 (Q-8)	+	+	+	+	−	−	+	−	+	+	+		−
Ubiquinone-10 (Q-10)	−	−	−	−	+	+	−	+	−	−	−		+
Fatty acid profile (see Table 20.23)													
Mol% G + C of DNA (see Tables 20.24-20.26)													
Biotin requirement for growth	−	−	−	−	+	−	−	−	−	−			−
Obligate chemolithoautotroph	+	+	+	+	−	−	−	−	−	+	+	+	−
Facultative autotroph	−	−	−	−	+	+	+	+	+	−	−		+
Optimum growth mixotrophically	−	−	−	−	−		+	+	+	−	−		
Autotrophic growth with													
Sulfur	+	+	+	+	−	−	+	+	+	+	+	+	+
Sulfide (soluble)	+	+	+	+	−	+							
Sulfide minerals (e.g. CuS, ZnS, NiS)	−	−	−	−	−	−	−	−	−	+	−	−	−
Pyrite (FeS₂)	−	−	−	−	−	−	−	−	−	+	−	−	−
Ferrous iron	−	−	−	−	−	−	−	−	−	+	−	−	−
Thiosulfate	+	+	+	+	+	+	+	+	+	+	+	+	+
Tetrathionate	+	+	+	+	+	−	+	+	+	+	+		+
Trithionate	+	+	+			−							+
Thiocyanate	(+)	−	−	−			−			−	−		−
Formate	−	−	−	−	+	+					−	−	
Methanol	−	−	−	−	(+)	(+)					−	−	
Methylamine	−	−	−	−	+	+					−	−	
Formaldehyde	−	−	−	−	+	+							
Methyl formate						+							

Table 20.21.—*continued*

Characteristic	1. *T. thioparus*	2. *T. neapolitanus*	3. *T. tepidarius*	4. *T. denitrificans*	5. *T. novellus*	6. *T. versutus*	7. *T. intermedius*	8. *T. perometabolis*	9. *T. delicatus*	10. *T. ferrooxidans*	11. *T. thiooxidans*	12. *T. albertis*	13. *T. acidophilus*
Nutritional requirement for a reduced inorganic sulfur compound							+	+	+	−			
May produce sulfur and/or polythionates from thiosulfate	+	+	+	+	+	−	+	+	+	+	+	+	−
Denitrification													
Reduce nitrate to nitrite	(+)	−	+	−	+	+	−	−	+	−	−	−	−
Reduce nitrate, nitrite or N$_2$O to nitrogen gas	−	−	−	−	+	+	−	−	−	−	−		
Anaerobic growth and denitrification with													
Thiosulfate	−	−	−	+	−	−			+		−	−	
Trithionate							−						
Tetrathionate			−	+		−			+				
Sulfide				+									
Formate				−		+							
Thiosulfate plus malate						+			+				
Glucose						+							
Sucrose						+							
Succinate						+							
Methylamine						−							
Methanol						−							
Plasmids													
5-50 Md		−			−	+	+			+			+
50-300+ Md		−			−	+	−			−			−
Drug-resistance plasmids from heterotrophs transferred and expressed		+			+								
Plasmid transfer from *E. coli* via *T. novellus*		+					+	+					+
Plasmid transfer to *E. coli*		+			+		+	+					
Growth inhibitors													
Fluoroacetate		+				+							
Fluoropyruvate		+											
2-Fluoropropionate		+											
Ampicillin					+		+						
Carbenicillin		+					+						
Chloramphenicol		+			+		+						
Gentamicin					+								
Kanamycin		+					+	+					+
Nalidixic acid					−								
Penicillin						+							
Rifampin					+			+					
Streptomycin					+		+	+					
Sulfadiazine					+								
Tetracycline		+			+		+	+					+
Trimethoprim					−								
Mercury	+	+					+			+	+		+
Tellurite							+	+					
Pyruvate							−			+	+		
Asparagine		+									+		
L-Cysteine	+	+									+		
L-Glutamate	+	(+)					−			−	(+)		
L-Histidine	−	(+)								+	(+)		
L-Methionine	−	(+)								+	+		
D-Phenylalanine		−								−			

Table 20.21.—*continued*

Characteristic	1. T. thioparus	2. T. neapolitanus	3. T. tepidarius	4. T. denitrificans	5. T. novellus	6. T. versutus	7. T. intermedius	8. T. perometabolis	9. T. delicatus	10. T. ferrooxidans	11. T. thiooxidans	12. T. albertis	13. T. acidophilus
L-Phenylalanine	+	+											
L-Serine	−	−								+	+		
L-Threonine	(+)	(+)								+	+		
L-Tyrosine	+	−								+	−		
L-Valine	−	−								(+)	−		
L-Azetidine-2-carboxylate		+								−			
DL-Thienylalanine		+								+			
Canavanine										−			
Resistance exhibited or developed against													
Fluoroacetate		+											
L-Phenylalanine		+											
Heavy metals													
Nickel										+			
3-o-Methylglucose						+				+			+
2-Deoxyglucose						+							
Gentamicin					+								
Kanamycin					+								
Nalidixic acid					+		+						
Rifampin					+								
Streptomycin					+		+	+					
Trimethoprim					+			+					
Tellurite													+
Chemoorganotrophic growth on													
Acetate	−	−	−	−	+	+				−	−		−
Adipate	−	−		−	−	+		−					
L-Alanine	−	−		−	(+)	+		+[b]					
L-Arabinose	−	−		−	+	+							
D-Arabinose	−	−		−	+	+							+
Ascorbate	−											−	+
Aspartate	−	−	−	−	−	+		+	(+)	−	−		+
Benzoate	−	−		−	−	+	.	−					−
p-Aminobenzoate	−	−		−	−	+		−					−
o-Hydroxybenzoate	−	−		−	−	−		−					
m-Hydroxybenzoate	−	−		−	−	+							
p-Hydroxybenzoate	−	−		−	−	+		−					
n-Butanol	−	−		−	(+)	+							
Butyrate	−	−		−	−	+							
Cellobiose	−	−	−	−	−	−							
Cinnamate	−	−											−
Citrate	−	−	−	−	±	±		+					−
Cyclohexane carboxylate	−	−		−	−	+							+
Cyclohexanol	−	−		−	−	−							
Cysteine	−	−		−	−	−							
2-Deoxyglucose	−	−		−	−	−							
Ethanol	−	−		−	+	+							
Ethyl acetate	−	−		−		+							
Fructose	−	−	−	−	+	+				−	−	−	+
Fumarate	−	−		−		+							
Galactose	−	−	−	−	+	+							+
Gentiobiose	−	−		−		−							+
Gluconate	−	−		−	+	+							
Glucose	−	−	−	−	+	+	(+)[c]			−	−	−	+
Glucuronate	−	−		−		−							+
Glutamate	−	−		−	(+)	+		+	(+)		−		+
Glutarate	−	−		−	(−)	+		−			−		+

Table 20.21.—*continued*

Characteristic	1. T. thioparus	2. T. neapolitanus	3. T. tepidarius	4. T. denitrificans	5. T. novellus	6. T. versutus	7. T. intermedius	8. T. perometabolis	9. T. delicatus	10. T. ferrooxidans	11. T. thiooxidans	12. T. albertis	13. T. acidophilus
Glycerol	−	−		−	+	+							
Glycollate	−	−	−	−		+							
Glyoxylate	−	−		−									−
L-Histidine	−	−		−	+	+							
L-Isoleucine	−	−		−	−	+							
Isomaltose	−	−		−		+							
Lactose	−	−		−	−	−							−
Lactate	−	−		−	+	+							−
Leucine	−	−		−	−	+							
Malate	−	−	−	−	(+)	+		+				−	+
Maltose	−	−	−	−	(+)	+							+
Mannitol	−	−		−	+	+							−
Mannose	−	−		−	−	−			−				−
Mandelate	−	−		−	−	−							
Melezitose	−	−		−		+							
Melibiose	−	−		−		−							−
Methyl α-glucoside	−	−		−		+							
Methyl acetate	−	−		−		+							
2-Oxoglutarate	−	−		−	(+)	+	−						
Oxalate	−	−		−	+	−	−						
Palatinose	−	−		−		+							
Phenol	−	−		−									−
Phenylacetate	−	−		−									
Phenylalanine	−	−		−	(+)	+							−
Pimelate	−	−		−	−	−	−						
L-Proline	−	−		−	+	+							
n-Propanol	−	−		−	+	+							
Propionate	−	−		−	(+)	+							
Pyruvate	−	−	−	−	+	+			(+)	−	−		−
Raffinose	−	−		−		−							−
Rhamnose	−	−		−									−
Ribose	−	−	−	−	+	+						−	+
Salicylate	−	−		−	−	+							−
L-Serine	−	−		−	(+)	+							
Sorbose	−	−		−		(+)							−
Succinate	−	−	−	−	(+)	+		+					+
Sucrose	−	−	−	−	(+)	+					−	−	+
Trehalose	−	−		−		+							−
Tryptophan	−	−		−	−	−							−
Tyrosine	−	−		−									
Xylose	−	−		−		+						−	+
Mixotrophic growth with thiosulfate and													
Alanine							+	+	+				
Aspartate							+	+	+				
Glutamate							+	+	+				
Malate							+	+	+				
Succinate							(+)	+	+				
Citrate							(+)	+	+				
2-Oxoglutarate							+	+	+				
Histidine							(+)	(+)	(+)				
Serine							−	+	+				
Glucose					+	+	+	(+)	(+)				
Gluconate							(−)	(+)	(+)				
Yeast extract							+	+					
Casein hydrolysate								+					
Arabinose							−	+					

Table 20.21.—*continued*

Characteristic	1. T. thioparus	2. T. neapolitanus	3. T. tepidarius	4. T. denitrificans	5. T. novellus	6. T. versutus	7. T. intermedius	8. T. perometabolis	9. T. delicatus	10. T. ferrooxidans	11. T. thiooxidans	12. T. albertis	13. T. acidophilus
Fructose							+	(+)	(+)				
Ribose								+					
Xylose								+					
Sucrose							+						
Maltose							+						
Incorporate organic substrates only if provided with an oxidizable sulfur compound	+	+		+						+[d]	+		

[a] Symbols: −, 90% or more of strains are negative; (+), indicates weakly positive characteristic or one about which there is doubt in the literature; +, 90% or more of strains are positive; (−), indicates extremely low values; ±, indicates that there are positive and negative reports for growth on citrate. Citrate may be a toxic substrate to both species, but good growth occurs under appropriate conditions (Wood and Kelly, 1983; Katayama-Fujimura and Kuraishi, 1980).

[b] Growth on these organic substrates by *T. perometabolis* occurred only after prolonged lags (Katayama-Fujimura et al., 1984).

[c] *T. intermedius* grows very poorly, if at all, in mineral media with single organic compounds. Growth on glucose or glutamate is greatly stimulated by a small amount of yeast extract. Best growth occurs mixotrophically.

[d] Reports of *T. ferrooxidans* growing heterotrophically are unsubstantiated. No facultative strain has been proved, and observed chemoorganotrophic growth can be attributed to *T. acidophilus* or *Acidiphilium cryptum* as commensals in the *T. ferrooxidans* cultures.

Table 20.22.

Generation of low pH during growth on thiosulfate or sulfur as a diagnostic characteristic for **Thiobacillus**

Species	Substrate	Lowest pH produced aerobically in optimum growth medium
T. thioparus	Thiosulfate	3.5–4.0
T. neapolitanus	Thiosulfate	2.8–3.5
T. tepidarius	Thiosulfate or tetrathionate	4.5
T. denitrificans[a]	Thiosulfate or sulfur	5.0–5.5
T. novellus	Thiosulfate (plus biotin)	5.0–5.5
T. versutus	Thiosulfate	5.8–6.5
T. intermedius	Thiosulfate	1.9–2.5
T. perometabolis	Thiosulfate or sulfur (plus yeast extract)	2.8
T. delicatus	Thiosulfate or sulfur (plus yeast extract)	2.5–3.3
T. ferrooxidans	Sulfur	1.0
T. thiooxidans	Sulfur	0.6
T. albertis	Sulfur or thiosulfate	1.8–2.0
T. acidophilus	Sulfur	1.5

[a] pH change in *anaerobically* grown culture was not as large as that in culture grown aerobically; consequently, this is not a useful criterion.

Table 20.23.

Application of ubiquinone and fatty acid content to the taxonomy of **Thiobacillus**

Group[a]	Species[b]	Type of chemolithotrophy[c]	Ubiquinone content	Major β-hydroxy acid(s) present[d]	Major nonhydroxylated fatty acids[e]	Corresponding groups in other taxonomic systems Hutchinson et al. (1969)	Key in this chapter
I-1	*T. novellus*	F	Q-10	None	*cis*-Vaccenic acid (18:1) and C_{19}-cyclopropane acid (19cyc)	1	IB1(a)
	T. versutus	F	Q-10	3-OH 10:0		1a	IB1(b)
I-2	*T. acidophilus* ("*T. organoparus*")	F	Q-10	3-OH 14:0		—	IIB
II	*T. intermedius*	F	Q-8	3-OH 10:0 and 3-OH 12:0	16:0, 16:1, 18:1, 17cyc, 19cyc	7	IB2(a)
	T. perometabolis	F	Q-8	3-OH 10:0		—	IB2(b)
	T. delicatus	F	Q-8			—	IB2(c)
III-1	*T. thioparus*	O	Q-8	3-OH 10:0 and 3-OH 12:0	16:0, 16:1, 17cyc	3	IA1(a)(i)
	T. denitrificans	O	Q-8			2	IA2
III-2	*T. neapolitanus*	O	Q-8	3-OH 12:0	16:0, 16:1, 18:1, 17cyc, 19cyc	4	IA1(a)(ii)
III-3	*T. ferrooxidans*	O	Q-8[f]	3-OH 14:0	18:1 + 19cyc (16:0, 16:1, 17cyc also significant)	6	IIA1
	T. thiooxidans	O	Q-8			5	IIA2(a)

[a] Based on Katayama-Fujimura et al. (1982). (Other data are from Katayama-Fujimura and Kuraishi, 1980, 1983; Levin 1971; Cook and Umbreit, 1963; and DiSpirito et al., 1983.)

[b] *T. tepidarius* and *T. albertis* have yet to be examined for this scheme.

[c] F, facultative; O, obligate.

[d] 3-OH 10:0, 3-hydroxydecanoic acid; 3-OH 12:0, 3-hydroxydodecanoic acid; 3-OH 14:0, 3-hydroxytetradecanoic acid.

[e] First number indicates the length of the carbon chain; second number indicates the number of double bonds; cyc indicates a cyclopropane fatty acid.

[f] ATCC 19859 also contains a small amount of Q-9.

Taxonomic Comments

1. Taxonomic Position of the Facultatively Autotrophic Species of Thiobacillus

The only factor unifying the species of *Thiobacillus* into one genus is the ability to grow (usually wholly autotrophically) by using energy from inorganic sulfur oxidation reactions. The genus was originally established on the basis of the discovery of the obligately chemolithotrophic *T. thioparus* and *T. denitrificans* (Beijerinck, 1904a) and later *T. thiooxidans* (Waksman and Joffe, 1922). The facultatively autotrophic neutrophilic species *T. novellus* (Starkey, 1935) and *T. versutus* (Taylor and Hoare, 1969) and the acidophilic species were all obtained by using elective media designed to enrich for organisms exhibiting this "classic" *Thiobacillus* physiology. Similarly, the obligately lithotrophic *T. ferrooxidans* is classified on the basis of its autotrophic sulfur-metabolizing capacities rather than on its ability to obtain energy from the iron (II) to iron (III) oxidation (Temple and Colmer, 1951; Kelly and Tuovinen, 1972). The *Thiobacillus* species can be clearly separated into either obligate or facultative autotrophs, with the obligate species that do not oxidize iron being *T. thioparus*, *T. denitrificans*, *T. thiooxidans*, *T. albertis*, *T. neapolitanus* and *T. tepidarius*. The facultative species are all capable of heterotrophic growth and, in some cases (e.g. *T. versutus*), exhibit immense versatility in the range of organic substrates supporting growth. Such species are indistinguishable from some of those bacteria grouped as *Pseudomonas*, except for the capacity for chemolithotrophic growth with reduced sulfur compounds. Earlier, it was deemed invalid to retain the genus "*Hydrogenomonas*," as all its species were facultative autotrophs and hydrogen oxidizers and could be accommodated into other genera. Hydrogen oxidation was, moreover, not the unique preserve of these bacteria. On this basis, the facultative *Thiobacillus* species could be reassigned to chemoorganotrophic genera on the basis of their reactions in diagnostic tests for heterotrophs and by using the logic that some non-thiobacilli can also grow autotrophically with reduced sulfur compounds (Friedrich and Mitrenga, 1981). Possible strength for this argument comes from the likelihood that there are different mechanisms of sulfur compound oxidation in the facultative species, such as *T. versutus* (Lu and Kelly, 1984a–c), than in the obligate species, such as *T. neapolitanus* or *T. tepidarius*, and that the sulfur-oxidizing abilities of the extant species could have arisen by convergent evolution from different ancient ancestors. At the least, the level of variation of DNA homology and the differences among some *Thiobacillus* species demonstrated by 5S RNA sequences (D. J. Lane, personal communications) indicate a major divergence if these species have a common ancient ancestry.

2. Problem of Iron-Oxidizing Rod- and Vibrioid-Shaped Eubacteria

On the basis of the chemolithotrophic physiology, capacity to oxidize sulfur compounds, morphology and DNA base composition, *T. ferrooxidans* (type strain) is a "classic" obligately chemolithotrophic *Thiobacillus*. There is an apparent problem, however, in that by using growth conditions elective for the characteristic *T. ferrooxidans* physiology, numerous strains can be isolated that are morphologically as well as genomically diverse. Thus seven different DNA homology groups were identified by Harrison (1982, 1984) within *T. ferrooxidans* (Table 20.26). A number of new isolates regarded as strains of *T. ferrooxidans* have been reported as having either polar or peritrichous flagella, with some also having pili, whereas some other isolates and culture collection strains appeared to lack flagella (DiSpirito et al. 1982). Morphologically, this species is thus disquietingly inhomogeneous. A distinct genus of iron-oxidizing vibrios ("*Leptospirillum ferrooxidans*") was isolated by Balashova et al. (1974) and subsequently found to be widespread as well as probably encompassing a variety of physiological strains (Nor-

Table 20.24.

Compilation of mol% G + C of the DNA for **Thiobacillus** *species*

Species	Strain analyzed[a]	Mol% G + C of DNA	Reference[b]
T. thioparus	ATCC8158 (T)	63, 62	1, 2
	ATCC23646	65	1
	TK21	61	3
	NCIB8349	66	4
	NCIB8370	62	4
	NCIB8085	63.3	5
	WW Umbreit	63.3	5
	(NCIB5177)[c]	63	4
T. neapolitanus	NCIB8539 (T)		
	"Strain X" (Trudinger)	56	4
	2 strains (J. London)	55.1, 54.6	5
	"Strain C" (Kelly)	57, 55.1	6, 5
	ATCC23640	52.3	2
T. tepidarius	DSM3134	66.6	7
T. denitrificans	NCIB8327	63	8
	P. A. Trudinger	64	4
	B. F. Taylor	67.9	5
	ATCC23642	63.3	2
T. novellus	ATCC8093 (T)	67.3, 68, 68.4	2, 9, 5
	NCIB8093	66	4
	NCIB9113	68	4
T. versutus	ATCC25364 (T)	67, 67.8	2
	ATCC25364 (T)	65, 66, 68	9
	ATCC25364 (T)	67.1, 67.3	5
	ATCC25364 (T)	65, 68, 69.5	7
	ATCC25364 (T)	68	1
T. intermedius	ATCC15466 (T)	64.8, 64.9, 67	5, 2, 1
T. perometabolis	ATCC23370 (T)	65, 66, 67.9	2, 1, 5
T. delicatus	IAM12624	66, 67	2, 10
T. ferrooxidans (see Table 20.27)	ATCC23270 (T)	58–59	20
	"Leathen strain"	57.8, 58.3, 58.8	11
	"Leathen strain"	56.6	5
	Diverse isolates (30)	53–65	5, 12, 13
T. thiooxidans	ATCC19377 (T)	52	12
	(NCIB8345)[d]	51–52	4
	DSM504	53	12
	DSM622	53	12
	NCIB8085	52	4
	NCIB9112	52	4
	Other strains (3)	52–53	5, 12
	DSM612[e]	62	12
	"Umbreit strain"[f]	57.9	5
	("*T. kabobis*")[g]	51.7	14, 15
T. albertis	New isolate	61.5	14
T. acidophilus	ATCC27807 (T)	62.9–63.2	16
	ATCC27807 (T)	63, 63.9, 64	17
	ATCC27807 (T)	63.5, 63–64	2, 1
	("*T. organoparus*")[h]	60.8, 60.9	8
	('*T. organoparus*')[h]	62.6	18

[a] (T) indicates type or neotype strain.

[b] 1, Harrison, 1983; 2, Katayama-Fujimura et al., 1983a; 3, Katayama and Kuraishi, 1978; 4, Jackson et al., 1968; 5, B. F. Taylor, personal communication; 6, Kelly, 1969; 7, A. P. Wood, D. P. Kelly and C. S. Dow, unpublished observations; 8, D. P. Kelly and C. S. Dow, unpublished observations; 9, Taylor and Hoare, 1969; 10, Mizoguchi et al., 1976; 11, D. P. Kelly, unpublished observations; 12, Harrison, 1982; 13, Vanyushin et al., 1964; 14, Bryant et al., 1983; 15, Reynolds et al., 1981; 16, Guay and Silver, 1975; 17, Tuovinen et al., 1978; 18, Katayama-Fujimura et al., 1982; 19, Markosyan, 1973; and 20, Harrison, 1984.

[c] Deposited as "*T. thiocyanoxidans*."

[d] Deposited as *T. concretivorus*.

[e] This strain may prove to be similar to *T. albertis*.

[f] This value is identical to *T. ferrooxidans* (Leathen strain) grown on sulfur, reduced sulfur compounds or ferrous iron.

[g] "*T. kabobis*" was published as a new species, but in our view it is not yet sufficiently well characterized to be distinguished from *T. thiooxidans*.

[h] "*T. organoparus*" was reported as a new species (see Ref. 19), but results of physiological and DNA homology studies (Table 20.25) suggest a very close relationship to *T. acidophilus*.

Table 20.25.

DNA base composition and DNA/DNA homologies among **Thiobacillus** *species*

Unlabelled DNA from test strains	Mol% G +C of DNA	% Homology[a] with ³H-labeled DNA from strain												
		1	2	3	4	5	6	7	8	9	10	11	12	13
1. *T. thioparus*	62–68	100			22	0–12	8–12	0–9	0–15		0			0
2. *T. neapolitanus*	62–68	0			0	0								0
3. *T. tepidarius*	66–67													
4. *T. denitrificans*	66–67	29			100									
5. *T. novellus*	67–68				0	100	0–14	8	0		8			0–16
6. *T. versutus*	67–68	12			0	0–7	100	0–7	0–14	9	0			0
7. *T. intermedius*	65–68	17			0	0–12	0–12	100	31–56	28	0			0
8. *T. perometabolis*	65–66	10				0	6–11	35–78	100	7	0			0
9. *T. delicatus*	66–67				6	7	6–15	25	7	100				
10. *T. ferrooxidans*[b]	56–59	0			0	0	0	10	0		100	0		0
11. *T. thiooxidans*	50–52										0	100		
12. *T. albertis*	61–62													
13. *T. acidophilus*	62–64					0–8	0–7	0	0		0			100
(13a. "*T. organoparus*")	62–63					8	7							70

[a] Values of 5% homology or less are indicated as 0.

[b] See Table 20.26.

Table 20.26.

DNA homology groups within the species designated **T. ferrooxidans**

Homology group no.	No. of strains tested	Mol% G + C of DNA	Range (%) of DNA/DNA homology of strains in one group to selected strains in each of the other groups					
			1	2	3a	3b	4	7
1[a]	4	55–56[b]	87–100	0–14	0–16	0–11	0	0–9
2	8	56–57	0	64–100	23–46	18–42	14–32	0
3a[c]		58–59	0	19–46	84–100	40–72	0–38	0–9
3b	4	57–58	0	17–47	58–73	56[d]–100	13–23	0–9
4	2	59	0	20–35	16–30	10–24	98–100	0
5	1	59	0	34–55	60–61	57–65	8	0
6	1	62	10	28–52	13–24	9–21	0	0
7[e]	1	65, 65.3	8	0–20	0–19	6–10	6	100

[a] These strains have not yet proved capable of growth on sulfur and have recently been indicated to be strains of "*Leptospirillum ferrooxidans*" (Balashova et al., 1974; Harrison and Norris, 1985; H. Hippe, personal communication).

[b] One strain assayed by three different procedures gave mol% G + C values of 53, 55.6 and 57.1. The data are means of results from DNA melting point measurements and from reverse-phase high pressure liquid chromatography following enzymatic hydrolysis.

[c] This group contains the type strain ATCC 23270.

[d] The strain showing only 56% homology with one test strain gave 75% homology with another test strain in this group.

[e] This is strain m-1 (Harrison, 1982) which is apparently unable to grow on sulfur and may be a genus distinct from the *Thiobacillus* group.

ris, 1984). Moreover, a number of iron- and sulfide-mineral-oxidizing moderate (and extreme) thermophiles have also been described in recent years. These do not conform to the criteria for inclusion in the genus *Thiobacillus* and, in one case at least ("*Sulfobacillus*"), are reported as being Gram-positive. Although it was decided some years ago (Davis et al., 1969) to reject the criterion of growth by which hydrogen oxidation as a source of energy was used as diagnostic of a discrete genus of "hydrogen bacteria" and to assign those bacteria to diverse other genera on the basis of other biochemical features, we do not believe that this is feasible for the iron-oxidizing organisms. Although evidently only some of the iron-oxidizing eubacteria can be regarded as thiobacilli, we are of the view that the criterion of ability to obtain energy for growth from the oxidation of ferrous iron should be used to create a "physiological group" of iron bacteria until such time as all the members of the group can be assigned to one or more other genera. In this way, knowledge of these organisms will not be lost through the default of their not being recognized because they have no valid nomenclatural tag. The following key illustrates the physiological and morphological similarities and differences of those iron bacteria found in common habitats such as acid mine waters, pyritic coal spoil and leach mine operations.

Key to the Nonfilamentous, Acidophilic Iron-Oxidizing Bacteria

I. Strict acidophiles: can grow in media at or below pH 3.0, with oxidation of ferrous iron used as source of energy.

    A. Optimum growth in the range of 65–85°C; may require organic supplements or enhanced CO_2 supply for growth. Also grow on sulfur or sulfide minerals.

1. Genus *Sulfolobus*

B. Optimum growth in the range of 25–35°C; obligate chemolithoautotrophs.

    1. Grow autotrophically on ferrous iron, pyrite and other sulfide minerals, sulfur and soluble reduced sulfur compounds. Rod-shaped cells; cannot grow at 45°C.

        2. *Thiobacillus ferrooxidans*

    This species is a "grouping of convenience," i.e. it contains at least five subgroups on the basis of their DNA homology; the mol% G + C of the DNA is 56–62 and is usually 56–59.

        3. Unnamed phenotypes, nonmotile; the mol% G + C of the DNA is 65.

    2. Grow autotrophically on iron but not on sulfur; some strains may grow on pyrite; cells vibrioid-shaped, forming chains of 3–12 cells giving false *Spirillum-* like morphology; some strains grow at 42°C; it cannot grow at 50°C; the mol% G + C of the DNA is 51–56 and is probably 55–56.

        4. "*Leptospirillum ferrooxidans*" representative strain DSM 2391

    This group may be as diverse as group 2 but is tentatively allocated to DNA homology group 1 (Table 20.26).

C. Optimum growth at 45–50°C; can grow at 30°C; autotrophic only when grown with increased concentration of CO_2; best growth occurs mixotrophically with ferrous iron or pyrite and yeast extract or single organic supplements (sugars, citrate); may show requirement for small amounts of reduced sulfur; variable ability to use sulfur for growth; the mol% G + C of the DNA is 48.

    5. Several rod-shaped bacteria, such as those described by Brierley (1978), Golovacheva and Karavaiko (1978), Marsh and Norris (1983) and Wood and Kelly (1984). Their DNA homology and the mol% G + C of the DNA, to date, have not been adequately studied.

3. Conclusion

We reaffirm our introductory comment that the genus should be retained with its here-named species at least until such time as the chemolithotrophic biochemistry and genomic constitutions are better understood. It may one day be desirable to reduce the number of genera of the *Thiobacillus* to only the obligate sulfur- and sulfur compound-oxidizing, iron-nonoxidizing species, to remove the facultative species into other more appropriate chemoorganotrophic genera, and to remove *T. ferrooxidans* as a separate genus (perhaps to reinstate "*Ferrobacillus*"), possibly into a family of iron-oxidizing bacteria that could include the iron-oxidizing mixotrophic thermophiles and the "*Leptospirillum*" strains (perhaps renamed more accurately as "*Ferrovibrio*").

Further Reading

Harrison, A.P. 1983. Genomic and physiological comparisons between heterotrophic thiobacilli and *Acidophilium cryptum*, *Thiobacillus versutus*, sp. nov., and *Thiobacillus acidophilus* nom. rev. Int. J. Syst. Bacteriol. *33:* 211–217.

Harrison, A.P. 1984. The acidophilic thiobacilli and other acidophilic bacteria that share their habitat. Annu. Rev. Microbiol. *38:* 265–292.

Hutchinson, M., K.I. Johnstone and D. White. 1969. Taxonomy of the genus *Thiobacillus*: the outcome of numerical taxonomy applied to the group as a whole. J. Gen. Microbiol. *57:* 397–410.

Katayama-Fijimura, Y., N. Tsuzaki and H. Kuraishi. 1982. Ubiquinone, fatty acid and DNA base composition determination as a guide to the taxonomy of the genus *Thiobacillus*. J. Gen. Microbiol. *128:* 1599–1611.

Katayama-Fujimura, Y., Y. Enokizono, T. Kaneko, and H. Kuraishi. 1983. Deoxyribonucleic acid homologies among species of the genus *Thiobacillus*. J. Gen. Appl. Microbiol. *29:* 287–295.

Kuenen, J.G. and O.H. Tuovinen. 1981. The genera *Thiobacillus* and *Thiomicrospira*. In Starr, Stolp, Trüper, Balows and Schlegel (Editors), The Prokaryotes. A Handbook on Habitats, Isolation, and Identification of Bacteria. Springer-Verlag, Berlin, pp. 1023–1036.

Lu, W.-P. and D.P. Kelly. 1984. Oxidation of inorganic sulfur compounds by thiobacilli. In Crawford and Hanson (Editors), Microbial Growth on C1 Compounds. American Society for Microbiology, Washington, D.C., pp. 34–41.

Shively, J.M., G.L. Decker and J.W. Greenawalt. 1970. Comparative ultrastructure of the thiobacilli. J. Bacteriol. *101:* 618–627.

Vishniac, W. and M. Santer. 1957. The Thiobacilli. Bacteriol. Rev. *21:* 195–213.

Differentiation of the species of the genus **Thiobacillus**

The principal differential features of the thirteen species here regarded as valid are provided in the following key and in Tables 20.21 and 20.22–20.24.

Key to the species of the genus **Thiobacillus**

I. Neutrophilic: can grow in media initially at pH 6–8 but cannot initiate growth at pH 3.0.

  A. Strictly chemolithotrophic and autotrophic: can grow in mineral media with thiosulfate as sole source of energy; cannot use glucose as source of energy for growth; contain ubiquinone Q-8.

    1. Strictly aerobic.

      a. Optimum temperature: 28–30°C

        i. Final pH 3.5–4.5 in liquid thiosulfate medium; contain 3-hydroxydecanoic and 3-hydroxydodecanoic acids; oxidize thiocyanate; the mol% G + C of the DNA is 62–68; no DNA homology has been observed for Species 2.

          1. *T. thioparus*

        ii. Produce pH >3.0 in liquid thiosulfate medium; contain 3-hydroxydodecanoic acid; do not oxidize thiocyanate; the mol% G + C of the DNA is 52–57; no DNA homology has been observed for Species 1.

          2. *T. neapolitanus*

      b. Optimum temperature: 43°C

        i. Produce pH 4.5–5.0 in thiosulfate medium; convert thiosulfate to tetrathionate before growth occurs on the latter; the mol% G + C of the DNA is 66–67.

          3. *T. tepidarius*

    2. Facultatively anaerobic: produce nitrogen from nitrate, nitrite or nitrous oxide in the absence of oxygen; the mol% G + C of the DNA is 63–68.

4. *T. denitrificans*

B. Facultatively chemolithotrophic or mixotrophic: can grow in mineral media with thiosulfate as sole source of energy; some also grow with glucose in lieu of thiosulfate.

    1. Efficient growth either chemolithotrophically or chemoorganotrophically; contain ubiquinone Q-10 but not Q-8; capable of autotrophic growth on formate.

        a. Obligate aerobes; colonies on thiosulfate agar become white with sulfur; capable of growth on tetrathionate as sole source of energy; type strain requires trace amounts of biotin; lacks hydroxy fatty acids; nonmotile; the mol% G + C of the DNA is 67–68.

5. *T. novellus*

        b. Facultative anaerobes; growth and nitrogen production from nitrate, nitrite or nitrous oxide with formate or glucose but not from thiosulfate; do not grow on tetrathionate or produce polythionates or sulfur from thiosulfate; growth on a wide range of single carbohydrates, carboxylic acids, amino acids and aromatic compounds; contain 3-hydroxydecanoic acid; motile by means of a tuft of polar flagella; the mol% G + C of the DNA is 67–69.

6. *T. versutus*

    2. Slow and poor growth on thiosulfate as chemolithotrophs; growth considerably stimulated by organic substrates; grow best as mixotrophs; negligible or poor growth with single organic substrates (may grow on these after lags of up to 2 weeks) unless thiosulfate is also present; contain ubiquinone Q-8 but not Q-10.

        a. Motile by single polar flagellum; can lower thiosulfate medium to pH 1.9–2.2; autotrophic growth markedly stimulated by glucose but not by pentoses; the mol% G + C of the DNA is 65–68.

7. *T. intermedius*

        b. Motile by single polar flagellum; can lower thiosulfate medium supplemented with yeast extract or fructose to pH 2.8; autotrophic growth stimulated by pentoses; the mol% G + C of the DNA is 65–66.

8. *T. perometabolis*

        c. Nonmotile; cannot grow on media with single carbon substrates unless supplemented with thiosulfate; lack 3-hydroxydodecanoic acid (which is present in species 7 and 8); large-scale transitory formation of tetrathionate occurs during growth on thiosulfate with yeast extract; the mol% G + C of the DNA is 66–67; show low DNA homology with species 7 (25%) and 8 (7%).

9. *T. delicatus*

II. Acidophiles: can grow in media at or below pH 3.0; cannot grow at pH 7.0; capable of good growth on elemental sulfur; strictly aerobic; contain 3-hydroxytetradecanoic acid.

    A. Strictly chemolithotrophic and autotrophic; can use sulfur, thiosulfate or tetrathionate; cannot use glucose as source of energy for growth; contain ubiquinone Q-8 but not Q-10.

        1. Can grow in minimal media at pH 1.5–3.0 by using oxidation of ferrous iron as sole source of energy for autotrophic growth; nonmotile or weakly motile; the mol% G + C of the DNA is 56–59.

10. *T. ferrooxidans*

        2. Do not oxidize ferrous iron.

            a. May produce pH ≤1.0 during growth on sulfur; motile with a single polar flagellum; the mol% G + C of the DNA is 50–52.

11. *T. thiooxidans*

            b. Can decrease medium to about pH 2.0 during growth on sulfur; motile with tuft of polar flagella; possess a glycocalyx possibly involved in adhesion to surfaces; the mol% G + C of the DNA is 61–62.

12. *T. albertis*

B. Facultatively chemolithotrophic; use sulfur and tetrathionate but not ferrous iron; can use glucose as sole source of energy; contain ubiquinone Q-10 but not Q-8; the mol% G + C of the DNA is 62–64.

13. *T. acidophilus*

List of species of the genus **Thiobacillus**

1. Thiobacillus thioparus Beijerinck 1904a, 153; 1904b, 597.[AL]

thi.o′par.us. Gk. n. *thios* sulfur; L. v. *paro* produce; M.L. adj. *thioparus* sulfur-producing.

See Tables 20.21, 20.23 and 20.24 and the generic description for many features.

Rods, averaging 0.5×1.7 μm. Motile with a polar flagellum. Gram-negative. Colonies grown on thiosulfate agar (1–2 mm in diameter) are circular and are whitish yellow due to precipitated sulfur, turning pink, then brown, especially in the center of old colonies. In static culture in liquid thiosulfate medium, sulfur is precipitated, and the medium becomes turbid with a pellicle of sulfur and cells. Sulfur granules and tetrathionate and/or trithionate may accumulate. pH drops to 4.5. In well-aerated or chemostat culture, sulfur precipitation need not occur, and quantitative oxidation of thiosulfate to sulfate takes place. Some strains oxidize thiocyanate (as well as thiosulfate, trithionate, tetrathionate, sulfur and sulfide). Obligately chemolithotrophic and auto-

trophic. Ammonium salts and nitrates are used as nitrogen source. Aerobic. Optimum temperature: 28°C. Optimum pH: 6.6–7.2, with growth occurring between pH 4.5 and pH 7.8. Some strains are claimed to initiate growth at pH 10.0. This organism is found in mud, soil, canal water and other freshwater sources. Presumably widely distributed.

The mol% G + C of the DNA is 62–63 (Bd, T_m).

Type strain: ATCC 8158.

2. Thiobacillus neapolitanus Parker 1957, 86.[AL]

ne.a.po.li.ta′nus. L. adj. *neapolitanus* Neapolitan; pertaining to the seawater at Naples from which this species was probably first isolated by Nathansohn in 1902.

See Tables 20.21, 20.23 and 20.24 and the generic description for many features.

Small rods, 0.3–0.5×1.0–1.5 μm. Motile by means of a polar flagellum. Colonies grown on thiosulfate agar are small (1–2 mm), circular, convex, glistening, and whitish yellow due to precipitated sulfur. The center of old colonies becomes pink. In static culture in liquid thiosulfate medium, sulfur and polythionates may accumulate, and the medium becomes uniformly turbid with a sulfur pellicle. Aerated cultures may show transitory accumulation of tetrathionate and trithionate. pH drops to 2.8–3.3. Chemostat cultures do not accumulate intermediates and convert thiosulfate quantitatively to sulfate. This organism oxidizes sulfur, sulfide, thiosulfate, tetrathionate and trithionate but not thiocyanate and uses ammonium salts or nitrates as nitrogen source. Obligately chemolithotrophic and autotrophic. Strict aerobe. Optimum temperature: 28–32°C; growth range: 8–39°C. Optimum pH: 6.5–6.9; growth range pH: 4.5–8.5. Isolated from seawater, canal water and corroding concrete. Frequently, this organism found in marine mud and in seawater. Presumably widely distributed in freshwater, soil and marine environments.

The mol% G + C of the DNA is 56 (Bd).

Type strain: NCIB 8539.

3. Thiobacillus tepidarius Wood and Kelly 1985, 436.^{VP}

tep.i.dar′ius. L. n. *tepidarium* a warm bath fed by natural thermal water; M.L. adj. *tepidarius* warm-bathing (*Thiobacillus*).

See Tables 20.21, 20.23 and 20.24 and the generic description for many features.

A new species isolated from the Great Roman Bath at the Temple of Sulis Minerva, Bath, Avon, England. Small rods, 0.5 × 1.0–2.0 μm. Motile by a single polar flagellum (5–10 μm). Gram-negative, nonsporeforming. Colonies grown on thiosulfate agar at 43°C are small (1–2 mm), circular, convex and smooth and become white or yellow with precipitated sulfur. In liquid batch culture on thiosulfate, quantitative production of tetrathionate takes place before growth continues, to effect complete oxidation to sulfate. Sulfur may be precipitated. pH drops to 4.5–5.0. Chemostat cultures do not accumulate intermediates during growth on sulfide, thiosulfate, tetrathionate or trithionate. This organism oxidizes sulfide, thiosulfate, trithionate, tetrathionate and sulfite but not thiocyanate. Obligately chemolithotrophic and autotrophic. Uses ammonium salts as nitrogen source. Aerobic. Optimum temperature: 43–45°C; growth ranges: 20–52°C (no growth at 15 or 55°C). Optimum pH: 6.8–7.5; growth range pH: 5.2–8.0. Distribution unknown.

The mol% G + C of the DNA is 66.6 (Bd).

Type strain: DSM 3134, ATCC 43215.

4. Thiobacillus denitrificans (ex Beijerinck 1904) nom. rev.

de.ni.tri′fi.cans. M.L. v. *denitrifico* denitrify; M.L. part. adj. *denitrificans* denitrifying.

See Tables 20.21, 20.23 and 20.24 and the generic description for many features.

Short rods, 0.5 × 1.0–3.0 μm. May be motile by means of a polar flagellum. Clear or weakly opalescent colonies are grown anaerobically on thiosulfate-nitrate agar, which on aging may become white with sulfur. Growth in anaerobic stab or roll culture results in agar splitting due to production of nitrogen gas. Facultatively anaerobic. This organism grows autotrophically aerobically on thiosulfate or tetrathionate, on which it produces growth yields approximately double those of *T. thioparus* or *T. neapolitanus*. Grows anaerobically on thiosulfate, tetrathionate or sulfide by using nitrate, nitrite or nitrous oxide as terminal respiratory oxidant. Oxidizes sulfur, sulfide, thiosulfate, tetrathionate and, probably, sulfite but not thiocyanate. Batch cultures can be grown in completely filled bottles which produce vigorous nitrogen evolution. Chemostat culture can be switched easily and repeatedly between aerobic and anaerobic growth modes, with adaptation involving derepression of nitrate and nitrite reductase synthesis. Ammonium salts and, in some strains at least, nitrate are used as nitrogen source.

Obligately chemolithotrophic and autotrophic. Optimum temperature: 28–32°C. Optimum pH: 6.8–7.4. Found in soil, mud, freshwater and marine sediments, especially under anoxic conditions. Probably very widely distributed.

The mol% G + C of the DNA is 63 (Bd, T_m).

Type strain: NCIB 8327 (newly designated).

Further comments. T. denitrificans is not on the Approved Lists and has not yet been validly published. The original isolation by Beijerinck (1904a) was unlikely to have been into pure culture (Vishniac and Santer, 1957). Later work demonstrated unambiguously that the designation is of a valid species exhibiting stable physiological characteristics (Lieske, 1912; Baalsrud and Baalsrud, 1954; Taylor et al., 1971; Justin and Kelly, 1978; Katayama-Fujimura et al., 1982). Earlier claims that its capacity to denitrify was lost on aerobic subculture and that it was facultatively heterotrophic were erroneous. The name is therefore revived with the suggested neotype or reference strain, since the early isolates are no longer extant.

5. Thiobacillus novellus Starkey 1934, 365.^{AL}

no.vel′lus. L. dim. adj. *novellus* new.

Short rods, coccoidal or ellipsoidal cells 0.4–0.8 × 0.8–2.0 μm, occurring singly and, occasionally, in pairs. Nonmotile. Colonies grown on thiosulfate agar (with biotin) are small, smooth, circular, round and opalescent, becoming white with sulfur. Thiosulfate liquid medium (lacking biotin) becomes turbid and sulfur precipitates during static incubation: thiosulfate is incompletely used; and the pH falls from 7.8 to 5.8. This poor development is due to the requirement for biotin exhibited by the type strain. The organism is facultatively chemolithoautotrophic, but best autotrophic development requires biotin, and best heterotrophic growth probably requires biotin and a small amount of a reduced sulfur source. This organism is strictly aerobic both autotrophically and heterotrophically. Oxidizes and grows on thiosulfate and tetrathionate but not on sulfur or thiocyanate. Ammonium salts, nitrates, urea and glutamate are used as nitrogen source. Optimum temperature: 25–30°C; growth range: 10–37°C (no growth at 5 or 42°C). Optimum pH: 7.0; growth range pH: 5.7–9.0. Isolated from soil. Presumably widely distributed.

The mol% G + C of the DNA is 67.3–68.4 (Bd, T_m).

Type strain: ATCC 8093.

6. Thiobacillus versutus Harrison 1983, 216.^{VP} (*Thiobacillus rapidicrescens* Katayama-Fujimura, Kawashima, Tsuzaki and Kuraishi, 1983b, 536.)

ver.su′tus. L. adj. *versutus* versatile.

See Tables 20.21, 20.23 and 20.24 and the generic description for many features.

Rods, with distinctly rounded ends, 0.4–0.6 × 1.1–1.8 μm, occurring singly or in pairs. Motile by means of a tuft of polar flagella. Colonies grown on thiosulfate agar, initially at pH 8.5, are small and clear at first but after 3–7 days develop a central opacity surrounded by a clear, spreading and flatter region ("fried egg" appearance). Colonies do not precipitate sulfur. Morphology is similar for colonies grown on formate agar and, with heavier growth, on nutrient agar or agar media containing methylamine, glucose, sucrose, citrate or succinate. This organism does not require biotin or any growth supplements for autotrophic growth or heterotrophic growth on single carbon substrates. Has been shown to oxidize glucose by a combination of Embden-Meyerhof, Entner-Doudoroff and pentose phosphate pathways and the tricarboxylic acid cycle. Grows autotrophically on thiosulfate but not on polythionates or thiocyanate. Never produces sulfur or polythionates during growth on thiosulfate. Oxidizes sulfur slowly. Uses ammonium salts or nitrates, but not urea, as nitrogen source, and uses glutamate or aspartate as nitrogen and carbon sources. Cultures in liquid autotrophic or heterotrophic media or on agar media with organic substrates have a characteristic "boiled milk" odor.

Facultatively chemolithotrophic and autotrophic, growing more rapidly on thiosulfate or numerous organic substrates than do other mixotrophic thiobacilli. Grows facultatively anaerobically (denitrification) on organic media or with formate but cannot grow anaerobically with thiosulfate. Reduces nitrate, nitrite or nitrous oxide to nitrogen gas. Optimum temperature: 30–35°C; growth range: 17–40°C (no growth at

10 or 42°C). Optimum pH: 7.5–7.9; growth range pH: 6.0–9.5. Found in soil and salt marshes and is probably widespread in occurrence.

The mol% G + C of the DNA is 67–68 (T_m, Bd).

Type strain: ATCC 25364.

7. Thiobacillus intermedius London 1963, 335.[AL]

in.ter.me'di.us L. prep. *inter* between, among; L. adj. *medius* middle; M.L. adj. *intermedius* in between, intermediate.

See Tables 20.21, 20.23 and 20.24 and the generic description for many features.

Thin, short rods, 0.6–0.8 × 1.0–1.4 μm. Motile by means of a polar flagellum. On thiosulfate agar, small colonies (up to 1 mm) with raised centers develop that are yellowish opaque with precipitated sulfur and surrounded by veillike fringes. This organism is facultatively mixotrophic. Capable of chemolithotrophic autotrophic growth on sulfur, thiosulfate or tetrathionate but not on thiocyanate. Also oxidizes sulfide. Aerobic; unable to denitrify. Unable to grow in heterotrophic media such as nutrient broth or with single organic substrates in the absence of thiosulfate. Gives very poor growth on yeast extract alone but produces substantial growth (after lags of 1–10 days) on yeast extract supplemented with glucose, fructose, sucrose, maltose, aspartate or glutamate. It is possible that a reduced sulfur compound stimulates growth under these conditions. Best growth is with mixotrophic media containing thiosulfate and yeast extract, alanine, malate, succinate, citrate, 2-oxoglutarate, serine, lactate or the supplements listed for heterotrophic growth. This organism can use ammonium salts, nitrate, urea, glutamate or aspartate as nitrogen source. Optimum temperature: 30–35°C; growth range: 15–37°C. Optimum pH: 5.5–6.0; growth range pH: 5.0–7.5, although for mixotrophic media the pH may be lowered to about 2.8. Isolated from freshwater mud; presumably widely distributed.

The mol% G + C of the DNA is 65–67 (T_m).

Type strain: ATCC 15466.

8. Thiobacillus perometabolis London and Rittenberg 1967, 218,[AL] emend. Katayama-Fujimura and Kuraishi, 1983, 650.

pe.ro.me.ta'bo.lis. Gr. adj. *peros* maimed, crippled; Gr. v. *metabole* alter, change; M.L. part. adj. *perometabolis* with a maimed metabolism.

See Tables 20.21, 20.23 and 20.24 and the generic description for many features.

Thin, short rods with rounded ends, 0.4–0.5 × 1.1–1.7 μm. Motile by means of a polar flagellum. Colonies grown on yeast extract-thiosulfate agar (1–3 mm after 1 week) are circular, entire, convex, smooth, creamy white and opaque; the center of old colonies becomes pink-orange. Colonies grown on thiosulfate agar (0.5 mm after 10 days) are circular, entire, convex, smooth, creamy white and opaque, developing with age a brown center. The original isolate of *T. perometabolis* was unable to be cultured as chemolithotrophically autotrophic or heterotrophic on single-carbon substrates (London and Rittenberg, 1967), and its "maimed metabolism" was described as "obligately mixotrophic" (Vishniac, 1974). Further study led to an emended description (Katayama-Fujimura and Kuraishi, 1983; Katayama-Fujimura et al., 1984) on which this entry is based.

Facultative chemolithoautotroph. Chemolithotrophic autotrophic growth occurs on thiosulfate, tetrathionate or sulfur but not on thiocyanate. Little or no tetrathionate or trithionate accumulates during growth on thiosulfate. This organism exhibits diauxic growth on a mixture of thiosulfate and glutamate, with preferential use of the thiosulfate. Grows slowly after lags of about 2 weeks in heterotrophic media containing one of the following: alanine, glutamate, aspartate, malate, citrate or succinate. Lags are shortened by the presence of thiosulfate. Best growth occurs in mixotrophic media with thiosulfate and organic supplements such as yeast extract, casein hydrolysate, 2-oxoglutarate, some sugars or some amino acids. Probably has a nutritional requirement for a reduced inorganic sulfur compound for heterotrophic growth. Obligate aerobe. Ammonium salts, nitrate and urea are used as nitrogen source, and glutamate and aspartate are used as both carbon and nitrogen sources. Optimum temperature: 35–37°C;

growth range: 15–42°C. Optimum pH: 5.5–6.0; growth range pH: 5.0–7.0, although for mixotrophic media the pH is lowered to about 2.8. Isolated from soil. Distribution unknown.

The mol% G + C of the DNA is 65–66 (T_m).

Type strain: ATCC 23370.

Further comments. It is clear from the emended description that there is considerable similarity between *T. perometabolis* and *T. intermedius.* There is reported to be DNA/DNA homology with the type strain (Table 20.25), but the degree of homology is in doubt, as work in two separate laboratories has separately indicated homologies of 56–78% and 31–35% (Harrison, 1983; Katayama-Fujimura et al., 1983a). These are sufficiently divergent to justify continued separation of the two species, especially as there clearly are major differences in ability for both autotrophic and heterotrophic growth, as well as minor biochemical differences, such as the apparent absence of 3-hydroxy-8-methylnonanoic acid from *T. intermedius* but its presence in *T. perometabolis.*

9. Thiobacillus delicatus (ex Mizoguchi, Sato and Okabe 1976) Katayama-Fujimura, Kawashima, Tsuzaki and Kuraishi, 1984, 142.[VP]

del.i.cat'us. L. masc. adj. *delicatus* delicate.

See Tables 20.21, 20.23 and 20.24 and the generic description for many features.

Rods, usually single, rarely in pairs, 0.4–0.6 × 0.7–1.6 μm. Nonmotile. Colonies grown on yeast extract-thiosulfate agar (1 mm in diameter) are smooth and circular and change from transparent to whitish-yellow with sulfur. Facultative chemolithotroph and mixotroph. Grows autotrophically with sulfur, thiosulfate or tetrathionate but not with thiocyanate; accumulates tetrathionate and trithionate transitorily during growth on thiosulfate. Incapable of heterotrophic growth on single-carbon compounds. Grows mixotrophically in thiosulfate media supplemented with tricarboxylic acid cycle intermediates or amino acids. Closely related biosynthetically to Species 8. Optimum growth requires both organic substances and thiosulfate or sulfur. Facultative anaerobe; reduces nitrate and produces nitrite in mixotrophic and autotrophic media with thiosulfate or tetrathionate. Ammonium salts, nitrate, urea, glutamate or aspartate can be used as nitrogen source.

Optimum temperature: 30–35°C; growth range: 15–42°C (no growth at 10 or 45°C). Optimum pH: 5.5–6.0; growth range: pH 5.0–7.0. Isolated from mine water. Distribution unknown.

The mol% G + C of the DNA is 66–67 (T_m, chem. anal.).

Type strain: IAM 12624.

10. Thiobacillus ferrooxidans Temple and Colmer, 1951, 605.[AL]

fer.ro.ox'i.dans. L. n. *ferrum* iron; M.L. v. *oxido* oxidize, make acid; M.L. part. adj. *ferrooxidans* iron-oxidizing.

See Tables 20.21, 20.22, 20.24 and 20.26 and the generic description for many features.

Rods, usually single or in pairs, 0.5 × 1.0 μm. Motile; the type strain is motile by a single polar flagellum. Small colonies (0.5–1 mm) grown on thiosulfate or tetrathionate agar are round, sometimes with irregular margins, and white with sulfur. On solid media (agar or agarose) with ferrous sulfate, microscopic colonies are formed with low iron concentrations, resulting in the appearance of an amber zone in the medium around them. With higher iron concentrations, round colonies (1 mm) are produced that become red, brown and hard with deposited ferric salts. Liquid medium with ferrous sulfate at pH 1.6 changes from a clear pale green to an amber to a red-brown with ferric sulfate. At pH 1.9 and above, considerable precipitation and encrustation with basic ferric sulfates (jarosites) take place.

Obligate chemolithotroph and autotroph. Oxidizes and grows on ferrous iron, pyrite, numerous sulfide minerals, sulfur, thiosulfate or tetrathionate. Strictly aerobic. Ammonium salts and, probably, nitrate can be used as nitrogen source; reported to be able to fix dinitrogen.

Optimum temperature: 30–35°C; growth range: 10–37°C (no growth at 42°C). Optimum pH: about 2.5; growth range pH: 1.3–4.5. Isolated in many locations worldwide where oxidizable iron, sulfide minerals and sulfur are exposed; particularly prevalent in acid drainage waters of mines for sulfide minerals, mineral leach dumps and drainage waters from coal mines and coal or spoil heaps.

The mol% G + C of the DNA of the type strain is 58–59 (T_m).

Type strain: ATCC 23270.

Further comments. The taxonomic status of *T. ferrooxidans* is discussed further under "Taxonomic Comments" and in Table 20.26. As described, the type strain is a typical obligately chemolithotrophic *Thiobacillus* with the added attribute of deriving energy from the oxidation of iron (II) to iron (III). It may also obtain energy from oxidizing Cu (I) to Cu (II) and Se (II) to Se (0) and from the oxidation of antimony compounds. Claims to have "adapted" strains of *T. ferrooxidans* to heterotrophic growth have not been substantiated (see Table 20.21, Footnote *d*); to date, no strain having the described attributes of *T. ferrooxidans* has been found that can unequivocally be described as either mixotrophic or facultatively heterotrophic.

11. **Thiobacillus thiooxidans** Waksman and Joffe 1922, 239.[AL] ("*Thiobacillus kabobis*" Reynolds, Laishley and Costerton 1981, 153.)

thio.ox′i.dans. Gr. n. *thios* sulfur; M.L. v. *oxido* make acid, oxidize; M.L. part adj. *thiooxidans* oxidizing sulfur.

See Tables 20.21, 20.23 and 20.24 and the generic description for many features.

Short rods, single, paired or in short chains, 0.5×1.0–2.0 μm. Motile by means of a polar flagellum (Doetsch et al., 1967). Minute colonies (0.5–1.0 mm) grown on thiosulfate agar appear transparent or whitish yellow which clears on prolonged incubation; edges appear complete. This organism grows in liquid medium on elemental sulfur, thiosulfate or tetrathionate. Tetrathionate and sulfur may be produced transiently during growth on thiosulfate. This organism cannot oxidize iron or pyrite but has been shown to grow on sulfur from pyrite in co-culture with "*Leptospirillum ferrooxidans*," an iron-oxidizing, sulfur-nonoxidizing vibrio. Reduces pH of sulfur media to values of 0.5–0.8.

Obligate chemolithotroph and autotroph; remarkable ability to oxidize elemental sulfur rapidly. Strictly aerobic. Ammonium sulfate used as nitrogen source. Optimum temperature: 28–30°C; growth range: 10–37°C. Optimum pH: 2.0–3.0; growth range pH: 0.5–5.5. Isolated from soil, sulfur springs, acid mine drainage waters and corroding concrete and steel environments. Likely to be widely distributed in acidic habitats with elemental sulfur or soluble reduced sulfur compounds.

The mol% G + C of the DNA is 52 (T_m, Bd).

Type strain: ATCC 19377.

Further comments. A number of isolates of extremely acidophilic and obligately chemolithotrophic sulfur-oxidizing bacteria have been designated as new species of *Thiobacillus*. Of these, only *T. albertis* is believed to be valid. *T. concretivorus* is on the Approved Lists but has no features that distinguish it from *T. thiooxidans* and should continue (as indicated in the eighth edition of the *Manual* to be regarded as synonymous with *T. thiooxidans*. The most recent "new species" is "*T. kabobis*" (Reynolds et al., 1981), distinguished on the basis of some ultrastructural features and the claim that tetrathionate accumulated during growth on thiosulfate could not be further metabolized. These criteria are not sufficient to justify a new species designation. Insufficient detailed ultrastructural information on *T. thiooxidans* is available for proper comparison, and except for *T. versutus* which cannot produce or metabolize polythionates, production and metabolism of polythionates are known to be notoriously variable characteristics influenced greatly by culture conditions (eighth edition of the *Manual*).

12. **Thiobacillus albertis** Bryant, McGroarty, Costerton and Laishley 1988, 221.[VP] (Effective publication: Bryant, McGroarty, Costerton and Laishley 1983, 1160.)

al.ber′tis. Eng. n. *Alberta* Canadian province of Alberta; M.L. adj. *albertis* Albertan (*Thiobacillus*).

See Tables 20.21, 20.23 and 20.24 and the generic description for many features.

Rods, 0.45×1.2–1.5 μm. Motile by means of a tuft of polar flagella.

Condensed glycocalyx present, extending outwards from outer membrane, apparently involved in cell adhesion to surfaces such as sulfur. This organism grows on sulfur, thiosulfate or tetrathionate; tetrathionate is accumulated transitorily during growth on thiosulfate but not on sulfur. Intracellular sulfur granules have been observed in stationary phase cells.

Obligate chemolithotroph and autotroph. Aerobic. Ammonium sulfate is used as nitrogen source. Optimum temperature: 28–30°C. Optimum pH: 3.5–4.0; growth range pH: 2.0–4.5. Isolated from extremely acidic soil adjacent to a sulfur stockpile. Probably occurs in other similar environments.

The mol% G + C of the DNA is 61.5 (UV spectrum).

Type strain: ATCC 35403.

Further comments. A comparison of the mol% G + C of the DNA from a number of *T. thiooxidans* strains (Table 20.24) and estimations of DNA homology among strains (Harrison, 1982) has indicated that most strains are very similar and the DNA composition was very different from that of *T. albertis* (mol% G + C of the DNA of 52–53 compared with 61.5). In this respect it is of interest that DSM 612, currently named *T. thiooxidans*, showed a mol% G + C of the DNA of 62 and showed little DNA homology with the original Waksman and Joffe strain of *T. thiooxidans* (ATCC 8085; Harrison, 1982). This suggests that the *T. albertis* type may be widely distributed and that physiologically similar but genomically distinct species of extremely acidophilic sulfur-oxidizing *Thiobacillus* both show wide geographical distribution.

13. **Thiobacillus acidophilus** (ex Guay and Silver 1975) Harrison 1983, 217.[VP] ("*T. organoparus*" Markosyan 1973, 1208.)

a.ci.do′phi.lus. L. adj. *acidus* sour; M.L. neut. n. *acidum* acid; Gr. adj. *philus* loving; M.L. adj. *acidophilus* acid-loving.

See Tables 20.21, 20.23 and 20.24 and the generic description for many features.

Short rods, occurring singly, mainly in pairs and rarely in chains, 0.5–0.8×1.0–1.5 μm. Motile by means of one flagellum or two subterminal flagella (Markosyan, 1973), but motility has not been seen with all strains. Colonies (1–2 mm after 6 or 7 days) grown on glucose agar are round, regular, convex, slightly translucent and cream-colored; they become rose-colored on continued incubation. This organism is a facultative chemolithoautotroph. Grows autotrophically on elemental sulfur or tetrathionate. Reportedly unable to oxidize sulfide, thiosulfate, metal sulfides or ferrous iron. Grows well on glucose in mineral medium and on a number of other sugars and organic acids. Can be transferred at will between growth on glucose and growth on sulfur. Shows no growth factor requirements. Aerobic. Ammonium salts or urea, but apparently not nitrates, can be used as nitrogen source. Optimum temperature: 27–30°C; growth range: <25–37°C. Optimum pH: 2.5–3.0; growth range pH: 1.5–5.5; the pH may fall to 1.1 on sulfur.

Type strain was isolated as a contaminant of a culture of *T. ferrooxidans* (Guay and Silver, 1975), but the extremely similar "*T. organoparus*" (Markosyan, 1973) was obtained from mine water in Armenia, so the species exhibits wide geographical distribution in habitats also suitable for *T. ferrooxidans*.

The mol% G + C of the DNA is 63–64 (T_m, Bd, UV ratios).

Type strain: ATCC 27807.

Further comments. This description is based primarily on Guay and Silver (1975) and Harrison (1982) but incorporates some original observations and details from the published description of "*T. organoparus*" (Markosyan, 1973). The latter appears identical with *T. acidophilus* in physiological properties, even to the duplication of the unusual radiorespirometric pattern of glucose oxidation exhibited by the two strains (Wood and Kelly, 1978). The mol% G + C of the DNA for the authentic "*T. organoparus*" strain (Table 20.24) is identical within errors of estimation to those reported for *T. acidophilus* (Table 20.24; and Guay and Silver, 1975). The two isolates also exhibit very high DNA/DNA homology (Table 20.25) consistent with their being strains of the same species.

Other species of the genus **Thiobacillus**

The thirteen species described (and *T. aquaesulis* described below) are currently the maximum number that can be justified on the basis of published descriptions, cultures available in culture collections, and cultures currently held in laboratory culture. Others have been inadequately reported in the literature or have been reported but are no longer available in pure culture for evaluation. Among the physiological types that have been reported but for which no new species description has been validly published are "thermophilic strains of *T. thiooxidans*" such as have been reported to occur in sulfur hot springs in several countries. Older examples of these are "*Sulfomonas (Thiobacterium)* No. 1" (Czurda, 1935, 1937) and "*Thiobacillus (Sulfomonas) thermitanus*" (Emoto, 1933). Another isolate lacking a valid name is the facultatively autotrophic neutrophilic, thermophilic *Thiobacillus* isolated from Yellowstone National Park (U.S.A.) (Williams and Hoare, 1972). This organism exhibited an optimum temperature of 50°C (grew in the range of 35–55°C but not at 60°C) and an optimum pH of 5.6 (grew in the pH range of 4.8–8.0 but not at pH 3.8). It oxidized thiosulfate and tetrathionate, and sulfur only slowly, but it did not oxidize thiocyanate. It was capable of autotrophic growth but developed better mixotrophically with acetate, malate, aspartate, glutamate or yeast extract. It could not grow heterotrophically on single organic substrates but could grow on nutrient broth. It used ammonium chloride, nitrate, urea, aspartate or glutamate as nitrogen source. It has a mol% G + C of the DNA of 66.2 (Bd). This strain sounds like a thermophilic equivalent of *T. intermedius* and would merit further study. Moderately halophilic and marine strains of thiobacilli have been reported intermittently for the past 60 years (e.g. Vishniac, 1974), but no new *Thiobacillus* species has been designated. A sporeforming, extremely thermophilic isolate was named "*T. thermophilica*" by Egorova and Deryugina (1963), but it was "probably [a] different genus" (Hutchinson et al., 1969) and seems not to have been studied further.

Metabolic types that might also await discovery among the present *Thiobacillus* genus include a facultatively heterotrophic and a thermophilic *T. ferrooxidans*, an acidophilic equivalent of *T. versutus* and an acidophilic as well as a facultatively heterotrophic equivalent of *T. deni-trificans*. The older literature indicates that at least some such strains may exist (e.g. Tyulpanova-Mosevich, 1930).

Note added in proof

Since completion of this Chapter, as additional species has been characterized. This is *T. aquaesulis*, a moderately thermophilic, facultatively autotrophic neutrophile, which would fit into the key (see above) as section I.B.3. It was isolated from the source overflow of the thermal spring at Bath, Avon, England (cf. *T. tepidarius*) by A. P. Wood (Wood and Kelly, manuscript submitted for publication). Its formal description is as follows:

Thiobacillus aquaesulis Wood and Kelly sp. nov.

a.quae.su′lis. L. n. *aquae* waters; L. n. *Sulis* pertaining to the Temple of Sulis Minerva (Minerva, the Roman goddess of wisdom); M.L. adj. *aquaesulis* from the waters of Sulis Minerva.

A new species isolated from the thermal springs at Bath, Avon, England. Short rods, 0.3×0.9 μm, containing some polyphosphate inclusions. Motile, Gram-negative, non-sporeforming. Colonies on thiosulfate agar at 43°C are small (1–2 mm), circular, convex and smooth, becoming white or yellow with precipitated sulfur. In liquid batch culture sulfur precipitation and a drop in pH without tetrathionate accumulation occur. Initiates growth at pH 7–9 (30–55°C), dropping the pH to 6–7. No growth at pH 6.4 or 9.4 or at 26 or 58°C. Chemostat cultures do not accumulate sulfur or other intermediates during growth on thiosulfate, trithionate or tetrathionate at pH 7.6 and 43°C. Facultatively heterotrophic on complex media (yeast extract or nutrient broth) but unable to grow on common sugars, organic acids, formate or methylamine as single substrates. Uses ammonium salts as nitrogen source. Inefficiently facultatively anaerobic in batch culture, producing nitrite and sulfur from thiosulfate and nitrate. Optimum temperature: 40–50°C. Optimum pH: 7.6–8.2.

Contains ubiquinone-8.

The mol% G + C of the DNA is 65.7 (UV ratios).

Type strain: to be catalogued by DSM and ATCC.

Genus **Thiomicrospira** *Kuenen and Veldkamp 1972, 253*[AL]

J. G. KUENEN AND L. A. ROBERTSON

Thi.o.mi.cro.spi′ra. Gr. n. *thios* sulfur; Gr. adj. *micros* small, little; Gr. n. *spira* spiral; M.L. fem. n. *Thiomicrospira* small sulfur spiral.

Small **spiral-shaped cells** forming long screws or portions of a turn. Dimensions: 0.2–0.3 μm in diameter, between 1 and 2 μm long, sometimes seen in spirals of individual cells up to 30 μm long. Gram-negative. Motile by means of a polar flagellum (Fig. 20.48) or nonmotile. No resting stages are known. **Metabolism respiratory. Energy derived from** the **oxidation of** one or more reduced or partially **reduced inorganic sulfur compounds** including sulfide, elemental sulfur and thiosulfate. The final oxidation product is sulfate, but elemental sulfur may accumulate in the medium. **Chemolithotrophs** able to use carbon dioxide as their major or only carbon source. At least one strain requires vitamin B$_{12}$. Metabolic properties are very similar to those of the genus *Thiobacillus*.

The mol% G + C of the DNA varies from 36 to 44 (T_m).

Type species: *Thiomicrospira pelophila* Kuenen and Veldkamp 1972, 253.

Further Descriptive Information

Members of the genus *Thiomicrospira* require an external electron acceptor for respiration. *T. pelophila* and *T. crunogena* are obligate aerobes requiring oxygen, but they grow best when low dissolved oxygen concentrations are used. *T. denitrificans* can only use oxygen under extreme microaerophilic conditions and grows best when supplied with nitrate or nitrite under anaerobic conditions. Although *T. pelophila* is an obligate chemolithotroph and thus, by definition, must use carbon dioxide as its main carbon source, it can assimilate small amounts of organic substrates such as acetate, while growing autotrophically under thiosulfate limitation. This can lead to an increase in biomass of up to 20%. However, this species does not have functional citric acid or glyoxylate cycles. The citric acid cycle of *T. denitrificans* also does not appear to be active, and the enzymes serve for biosynthetic purposes only.

All named species of *Thiomicrospira* were isolated from estuarine mud or seawater rich in sulfide. However, one strain, *T. denitrificans*, does not have a requirement for NaCl, and the genus should not be regarded as exclusively marine. Equally important is the fact that although the known species in this genus are all obligate chemolithotrophs, the inclusion of facultative chemolithotrophs, as in the genus *Thiobacillus*, cannot be excluded.

Enrichment and Isolation Procedures

Procedures for the enrichment and isolation of these organisms have been published (Kuenen and Tuovinen, 1982; Ruby et al., 1981). The best source of inoculum for *T. pelophila* is estuarine or marine mud rich in sulfide. This should be passed slowly through a membrane filter of pore size 0.22 μm to exclude members of the genus *Thiobacillus*. The resulting filtrate can be directly mixed with soft (1%, w/v) thiosulfate

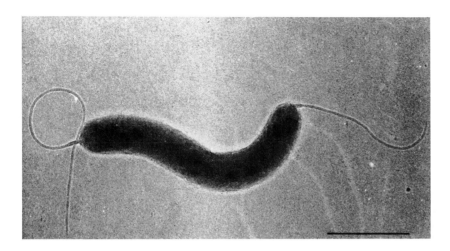

Figure 20.48. *T. pelophila* cell platinum-shadowed to show shape and flagellation. Electron micrograph. *Bar*, 0.5 μ.

agar to promote the formation of the distinctive colony type. The filtrate can also be used as an inoculum for various enrichment procedures such as sulfide gradients or continuous culture. A mineral salts medium which includes NaCl and, for *T. denitrificans*, nitrate should be used. For the cultivation of the aerobes, thiosulfate is a more convenient energy source than sulfide, as this avoids the complications of chemical oxidation. However, aerobic growth on sulfide is possible in a sulfide-limited chemostat, as has been described for *Thiobacillus* species (Beudeker et al, 1982). For the enrichment of *T. denitrificans*, the use of oxygen-free nitrogen and oxygen-proof tubing and equipment is essential, as this species is easily outcompeted by other organisms if the redox of the medium is not sufficiently low. *T. denitrificans* was isolated from a rigorously anaerobic chemostat inoculated with unfil-

tered mud and maintained under sulfide limitation. For growth on agar, anaerobic techniques are advisable, and plastic Petri dishes should not be used, as the plastic contains oxygen which is given off during incubation.

Maintenance Procedure

Members of this genus are best maintained in liquid nitrogen. They can be subcultured on mineral salts medium with sulfide or thiosulfate, but *T. denitrificans* must be kept anaerobically.

Thiomicrospira species can be differentiated from the related genus, *Thiobacillus*, by their spiral cell form and lower mol% G + C.

For additional information, the reader should consult Kuenen and Tuovinen (1982).

Differentiation of the species of the genus **Thiomicrospira**

Characteristics useful for the differentiation of the species of the genus *Thiomicrospira* are given in Tables 20.27 and 20.28.

List of species of the genus **Thiomicrospira**

1. **Thiomicrospira pelophila** Kuenen and Veldkamp 1972, 253.[AL]

pe.lo′phi.la Gr. n. *pelos* mud; Gr. adj. *phila* loving; N.L. adj. *pelophila* mud-loving.

Tables 20.27 and 20.28 summarize the important characteristics of this species.

Colonies on thiosulfate agar are small and white and are often surrounded by a halo of sulfur. On soft thiosulfate agar, colonies may be up to 1 cm in diameter and grow down into the agar as large disks (Fig. 20.49). These disks are white from precipitated sulfur and only sparsely populated with bacteria. In media containing more than 0.2–0.3 mM thiosulfate, sulfur is formed. Liquid cultures should be maintained at neutral pH with carbonate, as acid formation might easily result in the irreversible inhibition of growth.

Cells are motile by means of a single, polar flagellum or nonmotile.

Chemolithotrophic, obtaining energy from the oxidation of molecular sulfur and reduced sulfur compounds such as sulfide, thiosulfate or tetrathionate. Sulfide tolerance is high in this species compared with *Thiobacillus* species. CO_2, fixed via the Calvin cycle, is the primary source of carbon, although small amounts of organic compounds may serve as a secondary source.

Ammonium salts serve as nitrogen source.

This species is strictly aerobic.

Requires 1.5–3.0% NaCl for growth. Some strains require vitamin B_{12}.

Found in marine mud flats in which sulfide is produced and in the vicinity of hydrothermal vents.

Type strain: ATCC 27801 (DSM 1534, LMD 80.69).

2. **Thiomicrospira denitrificans** Timmer ten Hoor 1975, 344.[AL]

de.ni.tri′fi.cans. L. prep. *de* away from; L. n. *nitrum* soda; M.L. n. *nitrum* nitrate; M.L. v. *denitrifico* denitrify; M.L. part. adj. *denitrificans* denitrifying.

Tables 20.27 and 20.28 summarize the important characteristics of this species.

Colonies are brown, 1–2 mm in diameter. Sulfur is not deposited.

Chemolithotrophic, obtaining energy from the oxidation of reduced sulfur compounds such as sulfide and thiosulfate. CO_2, fixed via the Calvin cycle, is the primary source of carbon.

Ammonium salts serve as nitrogen source.

This species is microaerophilic, only able to use oxygen as an electron acceptor when pO_2 is <0.5%. In practice, aerobic growth has only been attained in an oxygen-limited chemostat. Nitrate or nitrite can serve as electron acceptors, being reduced to molecular nitrogen. The dissimilatory nitrate reductase is constitutive.

Although isolated from marine samples, this species does not have a requirement for NaCl.

Found in the mud of marine tidal flats where sulfide is produced.

Type strain: DSM 1251 (LMD 81.3).

3. **Thiomicrospira crunogena** Jannasch, Wirsen, Nelson and Robertson 1985, 422.[VP]

cru.no.ge′na. Gr. n. *crunos* spring; Gr. v. *genomai* to be generated; Gr. part. adj. *crunogena* spring-born.

Tables 20.27 and 20.28 summarize the important characteristics of *T. crunogena* and its differentiation from the other two species.

Table 20.27

Differential characteristics among the species of the genus **Thiomicrospira**[a]

Species	Motility	Mol% G + C of DNA (T_m)	μ_{max} (h^{-1})[b]	Fully aerobic growth	Denitrification	Diameter (µm)
T. pelophila	+	44[c]	0.3	+	−	0.2-0.3
T. denitrificans	−	36	0.1	−	+	0.3
T. crunogena	+	42-43	0.8	+	−	0.5

[a]Symbols: +, 90% or more of strains are positive; −, 90% ormore of strains are negative.
[b]$S_2O_3^{2-}$ as energy source.
[c]Correction of original 48% (Kuenen and Veldkamp, 1972) to 44% (Kuenen and Tuovinen, 1982; Jannasch et al., 1985).

Table 20.28.

Main characteristics of the species comprising the genus **Thiomicrospira**[a]

Characteristic	1. *T. pelophila*	2. *T. denitrificans*	3. *T. crunogena*
Cells vibrioid-shaped or spiral	+	+	+
Diameter (µm)	0.2–0.3	0.3	0.5
Length (µm)	1–2	var	1.5
Motility	+	−	+
Optimum temperature (°C)	28–30	22	28–32
Optimum pH	6.5–7.5	7.0	7.5–8.0
NaCl requirement	+	−	+
Mol% G + C of DNA (T_m)	44	36	42–43
Main electron acceptor			
Oxygen	+	−	+
Nitrate or nitrite	−	+	−
Microaerophilic growth	+	+	+
μ_{max} (h^{-1}), with thiosulfate as the source of energy	0.3	0.1	0.8

[a] Symbols: +, 90% or more of strains are positive; var, variable; −, 90% or more of strains are negative.

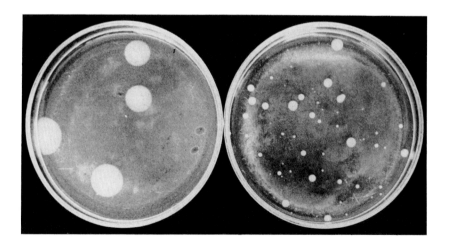

Figure 20.49. Typical colonies of *T. pelophila*, formed on soft (1%, w/v) agar.

Colonies are white, smooth, dull, entire and similar to those produced by *T. pelophia*. In soft agar, the diameter may be as much as 1 cm. Sulfur is deposited in the colony.

Cells are motile by means of a single, polar flagellum.

Chemolithotrophic, obtaining energy from the oxidation of reduced sulfur compounds including sulfide, thiosulfate and sulfur, but not sulfite or thiocyanate. *T. crunogena* can withstand relatively high concentrations of sulfide, continuing to fix CO_2 at concentrations up to 800 μM. Sulfide is toxic at 2000 μM. CO_2, fixed via the Calvin cycle, is the main source of carbon.

Ammonium salts serve as nitrogen source.

This species is strictly aerobic and does not denitrify.

Requires NaCl (at least 0.5%) for growth.

At 260 atm, the CO_2 fixation rate is 80% of that obtained at 1 atm. Growth does not occur at 400 atm or above.

Isolated from a marine hydrothermal vent system (21°N, 109°W) at a depth of 2600 m.

Type strain: ATCC 35932 (LMD 84.20).

OTHER ORGANISMS

Sulfide-oxidizing bacteria other than *T. crunogena* have been isolated from the waters and surfaces around the deep-sea volcanic vents off the Galapagos Islands (Ruby et al., 1981; Ruby and Jannasch, 1982). These bacteria appear to be among the primary producers in a complex food chain based on sulfide oxidation rather than on photosynthesis. One isolate, reported to be essentially indistinguishable from 11 other strains, has been described in detail (Ruby and Jannasch, 1982). This isolate, *Thiomicrospira* strain L-12, is very similar to *T. pelophila* in its morphology, mol% G + C and physiology, but the colonial form is slightly different. Growth occurs over a pH range of 5.0–8.5 and a temperature range of 4.0–38.5°C. Sulfide, thiosulfate and molecular sulfur can all serve as energy source for growth. The maximum growth rate in artificial seawater with thiosulfate is around 0.22 h^{-1}. *Thiomicrospira* L-12 has a requirement for NaCl.

Genus **Thiosphaera** Robertson and Kuenen 1984a, 91^{VP} (Effective publication: Robertson and Kuenen 1983, 2854)

J. G. KUENEN AND L. A. ROBERTSON

Thi.o.sphae'ra. Gr. n. *thios* sulfur; Gr. n. *sphaera* a sphere; Gr. n. *Thiosphaera* sulfur sphere.

Cells **coccoid** (but on rich media may fail to divide), **occurring singly, in pairs and as a chain.** Gram-negative. No resting stages are known. **Metabolism respiratory,** able to use oxygen and/or nitrate, nitrite or a nitrogen oxide as terminal electron acceptor. **Facultative chemolithoautotroph** able to **utilize reduced sulfur compounds as energy source** for growth. CO_2 can serve as source of carbon. Oxidase- and catalase-positive.

The mol% G + C of the DNA is 66 (T_m).

Type species: *Thiosphaera pantotropha* Robertson and Kuenen 1984a, 91.

Further Descriptive Information

The type species, *T. pantotropha,* is a very versatile facultative chemolithoautotroph which typically appears as a coccus in pairs or as a chain (Fig. 20.50). During growth on rich substrates, *T. pantotropha* becomes somewhat pleomorphic (Fig. 20.51) and can give the appearance of rods and cocci in one chain. *T. pantotropha* is capable of heterotrophic nitrification, converting ammonium to nitrite in the presence of oxygen and an organic substrate.

Like most other facultatively chemolithotrophic species, *T. pantotropha* has an advantage over specialized species such as the obligate chemolithotrophs in environments where an inorganic reduced sulfur compound and a low molecular organic compound are present in growth-limiting concentrations (Gottschal and Kuenen, 1980). The primary ecological niche of *T. pantotropha* involves denitrifying conditions, and the ability of this species to denitrify in the presence of dissolved oxygen (Robertson and Kuenen, 1984b) could confer a selective advantage in situations in which oxygen is limiting or fluctuates and nitrate or nitrite is present.

Enrichment and Isolation Procedures

Mixotrophic species such as *T. pantotropha* are most successfully enriched for by means of a chemostat with equivalent and growth-limiting amounts of sulfide or thiosulfate and an organic substrate such as acetate (Kuenen and Tuovinen, 1982). The known mixotrophic *Thiobacillus* species can be excluded by supplying nitrate to the culture and maintaining anaerobic conditions. The resulting enrichment culture should be streaked on mineral salts medium with thiosulfate and nitrate and then incubated anaerobically. *T. pantotropha* has been obtained at 37°C and pH 8.0–8.3 from enrichments inoculated from a denitrifying industrial wastewater treatment plant.

Maintenance Procedures

T. pantotropha can be maintained on mineral salts agar and a suitable substrate. It survives lyophilization well and may also be stored in liquid nitrogen.

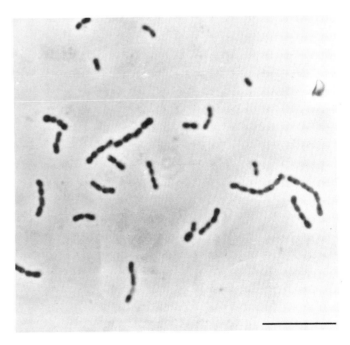

Figure 20.50. *T. pantotropha* cells grown on a rich medium to promote chain formation. Phase-contrast micrograph. *Bar,* 10 μ.

Differentiation of the genus **Thiosphaera** *from other closely related taxa*

The genus *Thiosphaera* is differentiated from its most closely related genus, *Thiobacillus*, by the coccoid shape of the cells. Under certain conditions, however, *Thiobacillus versutus* may form coccoid to oval cells. *Paracoccus denitrificans* is also of coccoid shape and grows aerobically on thiosulfate. Characteristics of use in discriminating between these three species are summarized in Table 20.29.

1. **Thiosphaera pantotropha** Robertson and Kuenen 1984a, 91.[VP] (Effective publication: Robertson and Kuenen 1983, 2854.)

pan.to'troph.a. Gr. pre. *panto* all; Gr. n. *trophos* feeder; M.L. adj. *pantotrophus* omnivorous.

T. pantotropha grows as off-white, round, entire colonies. On agar plates containing thiosulfate, sulfur deposition has not been observed, but the agar is acidified. This organism can grow autotrophically on sulfide, thiosulfate and hydrogen under both aerobic and anaerobic (denitrifying) conditions. It has a μ_{max} on thiosulfate of approximately 0.03 h^{-1} (aerobically) or 0.02 h^{-1} (anaerobically). All three substrates can be used for mixotrophic growth. *T. pantotropha* does not grow on methane, methanol or formate. On heterotrophic media, growth is much more rapid (e.g. $\mu_{max} = 0.34$ h^{-1} in mineral medium at a dissolved oxygen concentration of 80% of air saturation, with acetate and nitrate supplied). Since the growth rate is strongly affected by the degree of aeration, the dissolved oxygen concentration in cultures in which the growth rate is important should be monitored and, preferably, controlled.

Ammonium salts, nitrate, nitrite and urea can all serve as nitrogen source for growth, but methylamine cannot. The following organic substrates support aerobic and anaerobic (denitrifying) growth: glucose, fructose, acetate, lactate, malate, pyruvate, succinate, fumarate, citrate, mannose, propionate, acetone, propane-1,2-diol, isopropanol, gluconate, glutamate, isoleucine, serine, leucine, alanine, histidine, proline, yeast extract, casamino acids, propanol, acetol and propionaldehyde. Benzoate and adipate support aerobic growth but not anaerobic (denitrifying) growth. The following additional substrates do not support growth: arabinose, lactose, galactose, pimelate, methyl acetate, methyl ethyl ketone, propylene oxide, dulcitol and glycogen. *T. pantotropha* is capable of the simultaneous use of oxygen and nitrate (aerobic denitrification) and the aerobic oxidation of ammonium to nitrite if an extra source of energy is supplied (heterotrophic nitrification) (Robertson and Kuenen, 1984b and c).

Indole is not produced, gelatin is not liquified, β-galactosidase is not present, and sulfide is not produced. Oxidase and catalase are both present.

T. pantotropha can grow at a pH range of 6.5–10.5, with an optimum pH at 8.0. The temperature range permitting growth lies between 15 and 42°C, with an optimum at 37°C.

The mol% G + C of the DNA is 66 (T_m).

Type strain: ATCC 35512 (LMD 82.5).

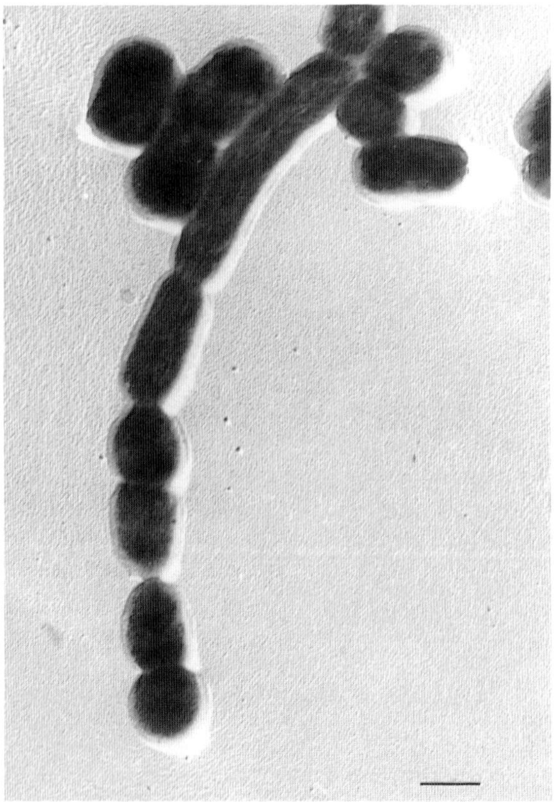

Table 20.29.

Physiological differences between **Thiosphaera pantotropha, Thiobacillus versutus**[a] *and* **Paracoccus denitrificans**[b, c]

Characteristic	*T. pantotropha*		*T. versutus*		*P. denitrificans*	
Motility	−		+		−	
Anaerobic (denitrifying) growth on reduced sulfur compounds	+		−		−	
Anaerobic growth with fumarate as electron acceptor	+		+		−	
Methylamine as nitrogen source	−		+			
Acetoin production	+		−		−	
Acid from:						
Sucrose	+		+		−	
L(+)-Arabinose	−		+		−	
Mannitol	+		+		−	
Fructose	+		+		−	
Glucose	+		+		−	
Maltose	+		+		−	
Sorbitol	+		+		−	
Growth on the following organic substrates:	aer	anaer	aer	anaer	aer	anaer
Adipate	+	−	−	−	+	+
Arabinose	−	−	−	−	+	+
Citrate	−	−	+	+	+	−
Galactose	−	−	+	+	+	+
Serine	+	+	+	+	−	−
Mannose	+	+	+	+	−	−
Dulcitol	−	−	+	+	+	+
Glycogen	−	−	+	+	+	+
Formate	−	−	+	+	+	−

[a] *Thiobacillus versutus* LMD 80.62, ATCC 25364.

[b] *Paracoccus denitrificans* LMD 22.21, ATCC 17741 (type strain).

[c] Data are taken from Robertson and Kuenen, 1983. Symbols and abbreviations: −, 90% or more of strains are negative; +, 90% or more of strains are positive; aer, aerobic growth; anaer, anaerobic (denitrifying) growth.

Figure 20.51. *T. pantotropha* platinum-shadowed to show atypical forms produced during very rapid growth. *Bar,* 0.5 μ. (Reproduced by permission of the Society for General Microbiology and with permission from L. A. Robertson and J. G. Kuenen, Journal of General Microbiology *129:* 2847–2855, 1983, ©Society for General Microbiology, Reading.)

Genus **Acidiphilium*** Harrison 1981, 211^{VP}

ARTHUR P. HARRISON, JR.

A.ci.di.phi′li.um. M.L. n. *acidum* an acid; Gr. adj. *philus* loving; M.L. neut. n. *Acidiphilium* acid lover.

Straight rods with rounded ends. Strains vary from 0.3 to 1.2 μm in diameter and from 0.6 to 4.2 μm in length. **Gram-negative.** Motile by means of a polar flagellum or by means of two lateral flagella. Some few strains are nonmotile. **Endospores are not formed.**

Aerobic. Weakly catalase-positive. **Acidophilic.** Grows in the pH range of 2.5–5.9 but not at pH 6.1. Some strains grow at pH 2.0. **Mesophilic.** Growth is slow below 20°C, is fastest between 31 and 41°C and is absent at 47°C. The cells die rapidly at 67°C.

The mol% G + C of the DNA is between 63 and 70 (T_m, Bd, Ez).

Chemoorganotrophic. Upon initial isolation, however, most strains **will not grow in concentrations of peptones and extracts customarily employed in organic media.** This organism grows in 0.01% trypticase or 0.005–0.05% yeast extract, especially if 0.1% glucose is present. Will not grow with elemental sulfur, inorganic sulfur compounds, or Fe^{2+} as source of energy. But weak oxidation of elemental sulfur may occur gratuitously in some strains as cells grow as chemoorganotrophs, and Fe^{2+} may stimulate growth. In inorganic media, growth is due to organic impurities in reagents and glassware and from the atmosphere.

In agar media with dilute organic substrates (pH 3) after 2 weeks at 30°C, surface colonies are smooth, opaque, and white, pink, or light brown and are 0.5–2 mm in diameter. In ferrous sulfate-agarose medium used to cultivate *Thiobacillus ferrooxidans*, and lacking added organic material, subsurface colonies of *Acidiphilium* are barely visible to the unaided eye and are smooth, especially when near a colony of *T. ferrooxidans* (Fig. 20.52), but surface colonies may be lobate (Fig. 20.53) and 0.3 mm or less in diameter.

Acidiphilium is common in acidic mineral environments such as pyritic mine drainage, pyritic coal refuse, and copper and uranium mine tailings. It may be isolated, unwittingly, with *Thiobacillus ferrooxidans* in Fe^{2+} enrichment cultures; thus it is a common contaminant in these cultures (Table 20.30).

Type species: *Acidiphilium cryptum* Harrison 1981, 211.^{VP}

Further Descriptive Information

Motility of the type strain ATCC 33463 is unusual. Cells grown in liquid medium (mineral salts containing 0.005% yeast extract and 0.1% glucose) swim in circles, with all cells in the field of view swimming in the same direction. When some cells reverse direction, the others do so also, as if on signal. When they collide with the underside of the coverslip, they stick to it, perhaps attaching thereto by means of their abundant pili (Fig. 20.54). These cells spin about their point of attachment, always in the same direction as the swimming cells. Stained with Leifson's stain (BBL flagella stain no. 04-104, BBL Microbiology Systems, Cockeysville, Maryland 21030), the cells appear to have solely polar flagellation, whereas when examined with the transmission elec-

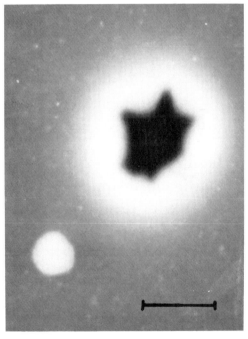

Figure 20.52. A white colony of *A. cryptum* strain ATCC 33463 near a black colony of *T. ferrooxidans* strain IFO 14245. From a mixed culture of the two species in liquid mineral salts containing 4% FeSO₄·7H₂O (Fe^{2+} as energy source for *T. ferrooxidans*) to which no organic material was overtly added. Plated on mineral salts medium containing Fe^{2+} and gelled with agarose. Incubated at 28°C for 2 weeks. Viewed with a dissecting microscope (× 20), *Bar,* 0.5 mm. (Reproduced, with permission, from the Annual Review of Microbiology *38:* 265–292, ©1984 by Annual Reviews Inc., and from A. P. Harrison, Jr.)

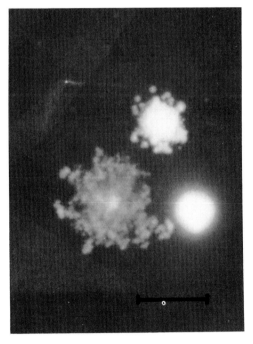

Figure 20.53. Two lobate colonies of *A. cryptum* strain ATCC 33463 on mineral salts medium lacking overtly added organic substrate. The bright spot is an air bubble in the gel. *A. cryptum* had been carried through numerous serial passages in liquid mineral salts medium before being plated on this gel. *Bar,* 0.5 mm. (Reproduced, with permission, from the Annual Review of Microbiology *38:* 265–292, ©1984 by Annual Reviews Inc., and from A. P. Harrison, Jr.)

* Although *Acidiphilium* is a chemoorganotroph, it is discussed here because of its close association with autotrophic thiobacilli in the natural habitat and in laboratory cultures.

Table 20.30.

Examples of heterotrophs in presumably pure cultures of **T. ferrooxidans**[a]

Example no.	Citation for impurity	Pedigree of mixture	Mol% G + C of DNA[b]	Intrapair DNA homology
1	Guay and Silver, 1975	*T. ferrooxidans* ATCC 13661 (TM) *T. acidophilus* ATCC 27807 (DSM 700)	56 63–64	nd[c]
2	Harrison et al., 1980, Harrison, 1981	*T. ferrooxidans* BCU-4 *Acidiphilium* sp. DSM 2390 (KG-4)	nd 68	nd
3	Harrison et al., 1980, Harrison, 1981	*T. ferrooxidans* IFO 14245 (Lp) *A. cryptum* ATCC 33463 (DSM 2389, Lhet2 or NCIB 11690)	57 69–70	0
4	Harrison et al., 1980 Harrison, 1981; Arkesteyn and de Bont, 1980[d]	*T. ferrooxidans* ATCC 13598 *A. cryptum* NCIB 11691 (13598het)	59 70	0
5	Harrison, unpublished observations	*T. ferrooxidans* AP-44 *Acidiphilium* sp. DSM 2613	57 70	nd
6	Johnson and Kelso, 1983	*T. ferrooxidans* NCIB 8455 *Acidiphilium* sp. NCIB 11822	59 nd	nd
7	Johnson and Kelso, 1983	*T. ferrooxidans* NCIB 10435 *Acidiphilium* sp. NCIB 11745, NCIB 11746	nd nd	nd
8	Lobos et al., 1986	*T. ferrooxidans* *A. organovorum* ATCC 43141	nd 64	nd

[a] Extended from Harrison, 1984, and reproduced, with permission, from the Annual Review of Microbiology *38:* 265–292, ©1984 by Annual Reviews Inc., and from A. P. Harrison, Jr.

[b] The mol% G + C of the DNA was determined by buoyant density, melting point, and enzymatic hydrolysis followed by chromatography, as designated in the citation.

[c] nd, not determined.

[d] These investigators mislabeled the heterotroph *T. acidophilus. A. cryptum* had not been described and named at the time of their study.

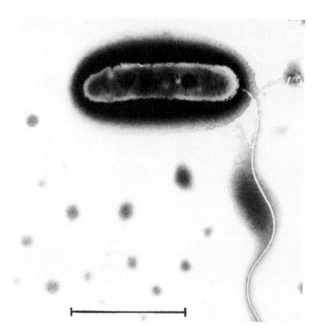

Figure 20.54. *A. cryptum* strain ATCC 33463. Electron micrograph. *Bar,* 1 μm. (Reproduced with permission from A. P. Harrison, Jr., International Journal of Systematic Bacteriology *31:* 327–332, 1981, ©American Society for Microbiology, Washington, D.C.)

tron microscope, they show both polar (Fig. 20.54) and lateral (Fig. 20.55) flagella.

Two strains of *A. cryptum*, ATCC 33463 and NCIB 11691 (13598het), produce colonial variants. After 2 weeks of culturing at 28°C, one strain is white and 2 mm in diameter, whereas the other strain is pink and 0.5 mm or less in diameter. Stock cultures prepared from the white colonies, upon streaking, give white colonies; cultures prepared from the pink colonies give both white and pink colonies.

Many organic substances are metabolized (see Table 20.31; Wichlacz and Unz, 1981; and Wichlacz et al., 1986). However, 0.01% sodium acetate is usually not attacked and may be inhibitory. Some strains are inhibited by 0.2% glucose when they are first isolated but later, after "adaptation," grow well in laboratory media. In glucose media at pH 5.7, the pH drops concomitant with growth. Shuttleworth et al. (1985) reported that glucose catabolism is by a combination of the Entner-Doudoroff and pentose phosphate pathways.

The several strains studied by Harrison et al. (1980) and Harrison (1981) were very similar in the phenotype and showed high DNA/DNA homology with type strain ATCC 33463. Different phenotypes were isolated by Wichlacz and Unz (1981) from Pennsylvania coal mine drainage (Table 20.31) and show <20% DNA/DNA homology with *A. cryptum* ATCC 33463. Wichlacz et al. (1986) further characterized these strains and established three new species: *A. angustum, A. rubrum* and *A. facilis*. Lobos et al. (1986) described another biotype which they named *A. organovorum*, which grows to high cell density in high concentrations of organic substrates. Johnson (1983) isolated acidic hetertrophs, probably *Acidiphilium*, in "acidic streamers" from a pyrite mine in Wales. Likewise, similar acidophiles were encountered, but not extensively described, by Zavarzin (1972) from a peat bog in Soviet Europe, by Belly and Brock (1974) from coal refuse, by Manning (1975) from coal mine drainage, and by DiSpirito et al. (1982) from uranium ore-leaching sites in Canada. These heterotrophic bacteria are wide-

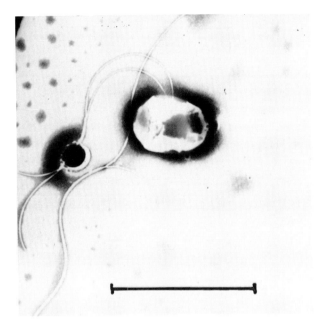

Figure 20.55. *A. cryptum* strain ATCC 33463. Electron micrograph. *Bar*, 1 µm.

Chemoorganotrophs have been isolated many times from presumably pure cultures of *T. ferrooxidans*. Table 20.30 enumerates eight well-documented instances. Strain KG-4, isolated by Shafia et al. (1972) and sometimes incorrectly designated *T. acidophilus*, was an early isolate of *Acidiphilium*. The contaminant grows with *T. ferrooxidans* in liquid mineral salts-Fe²⁺ media by consuming organic impurities in the media and substances released by the chemolithotroph (Harrison, 1984).

Isolation of single colonies of *T. ferrooxidans*, if interactions between the lithotroph and the organotroph are not appreciated, may lead to mixed cultures. The colonies on the gel (Fig. 20.57) are not clones. Selecting them guarantees impurity of the transplants. Organic impu-

Table 20.32.
Comparison of **A. cryptum** *with* **T. acidophilus** *and* **T. ferrooxidans**

Species	Mol% G + C of DNA[a]	Used as sole source of energy for growth		
		Glucose	Sulfur	Fe²⁺
A. cryptum	66–70	±[b]	−[c]	−[c]
T. acidophilus	63–64	+[d]	+[d]	−[c]
T. ferrooxidans	57–62 (usually 57–59)	−[e]	+[d]	+[d]

[a] The mol% G + C of the DNA was determined by buoyant density, melting point, and enzymatic digestion followed by chromatography.
[b] Growth is poor (<10⁸ cells/ml) unless medium is supplemented with peptone or yeast extract.
[c] Although the designated substrate is not attacked, the population may attain 10⁷ cells/ml through the use, by the cells, of traces of organic impurities in the mineral salts medium.
[d] Good growth.
[e] Although some strains of *T. ferrooxidans*, under certain circumstances, may be able to consume both Fe²⁺ and glucose concurrently (Barros et al., 1984), no strain has been isolated, to date, which can grow as a chemoorganotroph using glucose or some other organic substrate as the sole source of energy.

spread, and undoubtedly additional phenotypes will be encountered by using suitable enrichment culture techniques.

When compared with the strains of *Thiobacillus*, *A. cryptum* most closely resembles *T. acidophilus*. Table 20.32 compares the two species and *T. ferrooxidans*. Note that *T. acidophilus* can grow either as a chemoorganotroph, using glucose (or other organic substrate) as sole source of energy, or as a chemolithotroph, using elemental sulfur or inorganic sulfur compounds as sole source of energy (Guay and Silver, 1975). Figure 20.56 establishes the phylogeny among these other species.

Table 20.31.
Acidiphilic heterotrophs from coal mine drainage similar to **A. cryptum**[a–c]

Characteristic	Group 1		Group 2		Group 2ₐ		A. cryptum strain ATCC 33463
	Strain KLB	Strain OP	Strain PW1	Strain PW2	Strain AWB	Strain BBW	
Mol% G + C of DNA	67	63	65	65	65	65	69 ± 1
Size (µm) in citrate	2.4 × 0.6	2.0 × 0.6	1.9 ± 0.8	1.4 × 0.8	2.0 × 0.7	1.6 × 0.6	1.3 × 0.5
Pigmentation	+	+	−	−	−	−	±
Urea hydrolyzed	−	−	+	+	−	−	nd
H₂S from cysteine	−	−	−	−	+	+	−
Growth on citrate inhibited by acetate	+	+	−	−	−	−	+
Use as sole source of energy							
Glucose, glycerol and lactose	−	−	+	+	+	+	+
Glutamate	−	−	+	+	+	+	−
Succinate and fumarate	−	−	+	+	+		nd
Malate	−	+	+	+	+	+	nd
α-Ketoglutarate	−	+	+	+	−	−	nd
Ethanol	+	−	+	+	+	+	nd

[a] Compiled from Wichlacz and Unz (1981, 1982, and personal communication), and reproduced, with permission, from the Annual Review of Microbiology 38: 265–292, ©1984 by Annual Reviews Inc., and from A. P. Harrison, Jr.
[b] All strains utilize citrate as sole source of energy, but none use acetate. All strains grow with glucose if a trace of yeast extract is added. All strains grow at pH 2.6–6. DNA/DNA homology between *A. cryptum* strain ATCC 33463 and the other strains examined (PW2, AWB, OP and KLB) was <20%.
[c] Symbols and abbreviations: +, 90% or more of strains are positive, −, 90% or more of strains are negative; and nd, not determined.

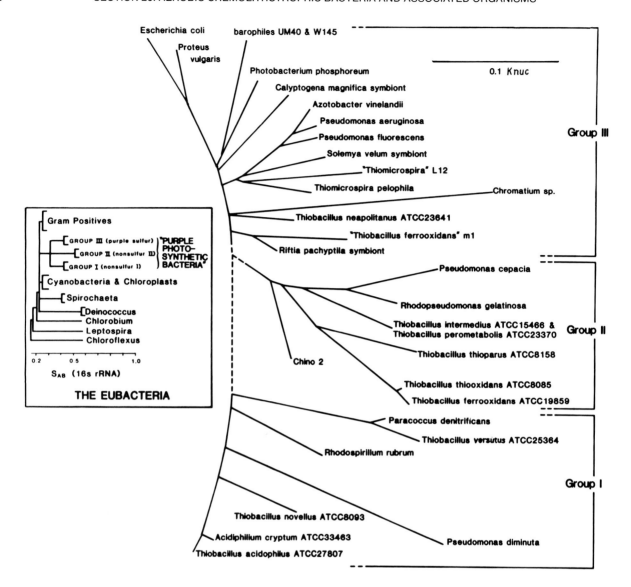

Figure 20.56. Phylogenetic relationships among various bacteria and *A. cryptum*. The length of the branches of this "tree" (described, in part, by Stahl et al. in 1984) are in proportion to "evolutionary distances," i.e. the degree of dissimilarity between species based on the number of nucleotide differences in 5S RNA. The *insert diagram* summarizes the lines of eubacteria descent so far defined by partial 16S rRNA sequence characterization (Fox et al., 1980). (Reproduced with permission from D. J. Lane, D. A. Stahl, G. J. Olsen, D. J. Heller and N. R. Pace, Journal of Bacteriology *163:* 75-81, 1985, ©American Society for Microbiology, Washington, D.C.)

rities in the gel inhibit the growth of *T. ferrooxidans* except at foci where cells of the organotroph consume these impurities or degradation products of the agar. At these foci, *T. ferrooxidans* first forms its characteristic rust-colored colonies which are mistakenly assumed to be pure and may be selected for transplants (Harrison, 1984). *A. cryptum* maintains itself indefinitely through serial transfers in liquid ferrous sulfate media lacking overtly added organic matter. The scavenging ability of heterotrophic bacteria is well-documented (Harrison, 1984). Beijerinck and van Delden (1903) appreciated the scavenging capability of nonacidophilic heterotrophs, and they suggested that these bacteria be used to purify air. In an English language reprint (van Iterson et al., 1983), A. J. Kluyver summarizes Beijerinck's conclusions.

In the natural habitat, *A. cryptum* may aid mineral leaching through the consumption of organic matter inhibitory to *T. ferrooxidans*. Moreover, *A. cryptum* may aid leaching more directly, as a result of its own metabolism. However, the role of acidophilic heterotrophs in mineral environments has yet to be established.

Isolation, Cultivation and Maintenance Procedures

A suitable general-purpose medium comprises 0.2% $(NH_4)_2SO_4$, 0.01% KCl, 0.05% K_2HPO_4, and 0.05% $MgSO_4 \cdot 7H_2O$ (pH 3), to which are added 0.1% glucose and 0.01% yeast extract (or trypticase). The organic supplements are autoclaved separately (as 10% and 1% solutions, respectively) and are then added to the autoclaved and cooled mineral salts. For isolation of *Acidiphilium* directly from mineral environments and for enrichment cultures, the medium can be adjusted to pH 2 to minimize growth of mold, but not all strains grow below pH 2.5. Colonies may be selected from the same medium (pH 3–4) solidified with 1.2% agar or 0.4% agarose. Double-strength acidic mineral salts solution is autoclaved separately from the agar-organic supplement mixture which is also double-strength. After cooling to 45°C, the two solutions are mixed. Some strains when first isolated are inhibited by customary bacteriological agar. A good gelling agent for these sensitive strains is type I, no. A-6013, 0.4% agarose (Sigma Chemical Co., St.

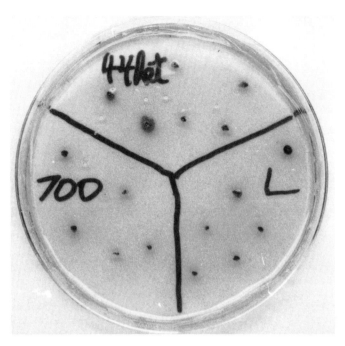

Figure 20.57. Impure colonies containing a mixture of *T. ferrooxidans* with acidophilic heterotroph. The Petri dish is 9 cm in diameter. Mineral salts medium containing 0.15% FeSO₄·7H₂O gelled with 1.5% agar (BBL Microbiology Systems, Cockeysville, Maryland 21030) was thickly seeded over its entire surface with *T. ferrooxidans* strain AP-19. After this inoculum was absorbed by the gel, heterotrophic bacteria were pricked into the gel on the tip of a pin. The autotroph, *T. ferrooxidans*, can be seen growing only at the points on the gel where the heterotrophic bacteria were deposited. The heterotrophs consume organic impurities in the agar which are inhibitory to the autotroph. (The white specks on the gel are air bubbles.) *L, A. cryptum* strain ATCC 33463; *44het,* a strain of *Acidiphilium* from an allegedly "mixotrophic" *T. ferrooxidans* (strain AP-44); *700, T. acidophilus* strain DSM 700. (Reproduced, with permission, from the Annual Review of Microbiology *38:* 265–292, ©1984 by Annual Reviews Inc., and from A. P. Harrison, Jr.)

Louis, Missouri 63178). Stock cultures may be maintained in liquid or gelled media at pH 3–4 and at 20°C and transferred monthly. Or cells may be emulsified in 8% aqueous polyvinylpyrrolidone (PVP-360, Sigma Chemical Co.) and lyophilized. The same media can be used to separate *Acidiphilium* from cultures of *T. ferrooxidans*. Purifying *T. ferrooxidans* from such mixtures, however, is more difficult, but means are available (Harrison, 1984). Johnson and Kelso (1983) isolated *Acidiphilium* contamination cultures of *T. ferrooxidans* with similar acidic mineral salts enriched with 0.1% mannitol and 0.01% tryptone soy broth (Oxoid). And Johnson (1983) used this medium to acquire similar bacteria from the "acid streamers" of pyrite mines. Wichlacz and Unz (1981) used a medium of 0.015% (NH₄)₂SO₄, 0.015% KCl, 0.015% K₂HPO₄, 0.0336% MgSO₄·7H₂O, 0.097% CaCl₂, 0.0225% Al₂(SO₄)₃·18H₂O, and 0.012% MnSO₄·H₂O (pH 3), enriched with 0.05% citric acid or other organic compounds.

Taxonomic Comments

In terms of "evolutionary distances" (Fig. 20.56), *A cryptum* is more closely related to *T. acidophilus* than to other species of the *Thiobacillus*. It diverges from *T. acidophilus* to about the same degree as *T. thiooxidans* diverges from *T. ferrooxidans* and as *Pseudomonas aeruginosa* diverges from *Azotobacter vinelandii*. The phylogenetic "tree" (Fig. 20.56) illustrates that acidophily, which is here defined as the ability of an organism to grow when inoculated into media poised at pH <3, is widely scattered among the branches. The following species on the tree share this property: *A. cryptum, T. acidophilus, T. thiooxidans, T. ferrooxidans*, and strain m-1, labeled *"Thiobacillus ferrooxidans* m-1." This last organism is an iron oxidizer similar in phenotype to *T. ferrooxidans* but unable to utilize elemental sulfur for energy (Harrison, 1984). In fact, utilization of Fe²⁺ or sulfur as sources of energy for growth are also properties widely dispersed over the tree.

List of species of the genus **Acidiphilium**

1. **Acidiphilium cryptum** Harrison 1981, 211.^VP

cryp′tum. Gr. adj. *kryptos* hidden.

Description for this species is generally the same as the genus, with rods 0.3–0.5 × 0.6–1.5 μm. It grows between pH 2.0 and 6.0 and is inhibited by acetate.

The mol% G + C of the DNA is 66 (Ez), 69 (Bd) and 68–70 (T_m).

Type strain: ATCC 33463 (Lhet2, DSM 2389, NCIB 11690).

Other species of the genus **Acidiphilium**

At this time, the following additional species of *Acidiphilium* have been named and described.

Acidiphilium rubrum Wichlacz, Unz and Langworthy 1986, 200.^VP

ru′brum. L. adj. *rubrum* red.

Distinguished by red-violet pigmentation of colonies and broth cultures. In citric acid-salts medium, the cells are 0.6 × 2.2 μm, with polar flagellation. This organism is inhibited by acetate and shows a lack of nutritional versatility, utilizing citrate, glucose, L-malate and α-ketoglutarate but not *cis*-aconitate, glycerol, lactose, fumarate, pyruvate and ethanol.

The mol% G + C of the DNA is 63 (Bd).

Type strain: ATCC 35903 (strain OP).

Acidiphilium angustum Wichlacz, Unz and Langworthy 1986, 200.^VP

an.gus′tum. L. adj. *angustum* limited with respect to nutritional versatility.

Distinguished by a pink pigmentation of colonies and brown cultures. In citric acid-salts medium, the cells are often swollen and distended, 0.8 × 2.9 μm, with polar flagellation. This organism is inhibited by acetate. Ethanol, citric acid and glycerol support growth, whereas α-ketoglutarate, *cis*-aconitate, glutamate, glucose, lactose, succinate, L-malate, pyruvate and fumarate do not.

The mol% G + C of the DNA is 67 (Bd).

Type strain: ATCC 35903 (strain KLB).

Acidiphilium facilis Wichlacz, Unz and Langworthy 1986, 200.^VP

fac′i.lis. L. adj. *facilis* ready, quick, with respect to growth.

Distinguished by white to light brown colonies. In citric acid-salts medium, the cells are 0.7 × 1.8 μm, often occurring in chains and small flocs, with polar flagellation. This organism is not inhibited by acetate.

Growth is more rapid and heavy for this species than for the other species. Urea is hydrolyzed, and glucose, citric acid, glycerol, lactose, *cis*-aconitate, glutamate, succinate, L-malate, fumarate, α-ketoglutarate and ethanol support growth.

The mol% G + C of the DNA is 65 (Bd).

Type strain: ATCC 35904 (strain PW2).

Acidiphilium organovorum Lobos, Chisolm, Bopp and Holmes 1986, 143.[VP]

or.gan′o.vor.um. N.L. n. *organum* organic compound; L. v. *voro* eat,

consume; N.L. adj. *organovorum* organisms that use organic compounds.

Colonies are white. Cells are 0.6 × 0.8–1.0 μm. Growth is inhibited by acetate and pyruvate, and no growth occurs on lactose, maltose and cellobiose. Other simple sugars support growth, as do sugar alcohols, carboxylic acids and amino acids. This organism is distinguished by heavy growth even in high concentrations of organic substrates.

The mol% G + C of the DNA is 64 (Ez).

Type strain: ATCC 43141.

Genus **Thermothrix** *Caldwell, Caldwell and Laycock 1981, 217*[VP] *(Effective publication: Caldwell, Caldwell and Laycock 1976, 1515)*

Douglas E. Caldwell

Ther′mo.thrix. Gr. adj. *thermos* hot; Gr. n. *thrix* hair; N.L. fem. n. *Thermothrix* hot hair.

Rod-shaped cells, usually 0.5–1.0 × 3–5 μm. **Filamentous cells are produced when the oxygen concentration limits the rate of growth.** Rod-shaped cells are motile by a single polar flagellum. **Facultatively anaerobic and facultatively chemolithotrophic,** using an oxidative type of metabolism. Temperature range: 40–80°C. pH range: 6.0–8.0. Inorganic sulfur compounds and organic compounds can be used as electron donor. Either oxygen or nitrate can be used as the terminal electron acceptor. **Gram-negative.** No resting stages are known. **The rod-shaped growth form is easily confused with *Thiobacillus* spp.**

Type species: *Thermothrix thiopara* Caldwell, Caldwell and Laycock 1981, 217.

Further Descriptive Information

Under highly aerated conditions in batch culture, the cells are rod-shaped and possess a single polar flagellum (Caldwell et al., 1983, 1984). Under oxygen-limited conditions in continuous culture, filamentous cells are produced (Fig. 20.58). When these are aerated, they fragment to form rod-shaped cells approximately 0.5–1.0 × 3–5 μm in size. Cell filaments, observed in thin section (Fig. 20.59), consist of a series of protoplasts separated by peptidoglycan septa (Caldwell et al., 1976). The filament is surrounded by an outer membrane which may invaginate between individual protoplasts but which does not completely separate them.

Respired substrates include glucose, sulfide and thiosulfate. When thiosulfate is oxidized to sulfate, elemental sulfur, sulfite, and poly-

thionates accumulate as transient intermediates in batch culture (Brannan and Caldwell, 1980, 1983). Elemental sulfur is often deposited extracellularly as spherical granules (Fig. 20.60).

This organism is found in situ within the sulfide-oxygen interfaces of neutral pH geothermal springs, including Mammoth Hot Springs (Yellowstone National Park, Wyoming) and Jemez Hot Springs (Jemez Springs, New Mexico) (both in the U.S.A.). Microscopic cell mats, several cells thick, form on calcite surfaces in situ (Brannan and Caldwell, 1982; Caldwell et al., 1984; Kieft and Caldwell, 1984a and b). The sulfuric acid produced during metabolism causes the dissolution of the carbonate substratum and results in cell nets suspended above one another in the aqueous phase. The mats and nets generally consist of a mixture of filamentous and rod-shaped cells. Cells growing on the reducing side of the interface form filaments (Fig. 20.61) which intertwine, forming streamers up to 10 cm or more in length, and which are visible macroscopically (Fig. 20.62). When these extend beyond the interface, they fragment to form flagellated, rod-shaped cells. When the location of the interface is shifted by applying a plastic covering, the filaments relocate within a period of 8 days or less. Streamers of *Thermothrix* species may be distinguished from those of *Beggiatoa* and *Thiothrix* species by the lack of intracellular sulfur granules and the elevated temperature requirements of *Thermothrix* species (40–80°C).

Enrichment and Isolation Procedures

Representatives of the genus are found within the sulfide-oxygen interface of hot springs (40–80°C). Under these conditions, metabolism

Figure 20.58. *T. thiopara* cell filaments produced under oxygen-limited growth conditions in nutrient broth. In well-aerated cultures, filaments are not produced. Phase-contrast micrograph. *Bar,* 10 μm.

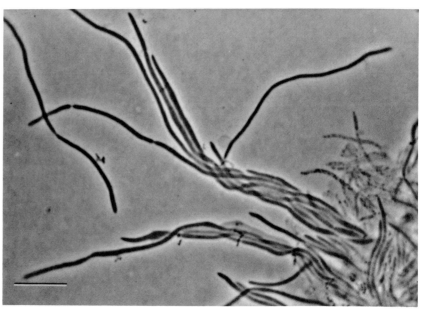

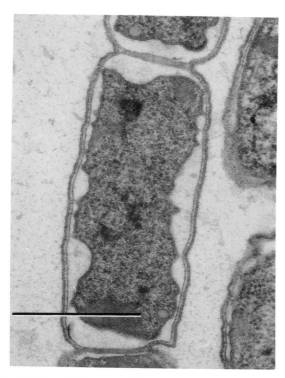

Figure 20.59. *T. thiopara* cell filament portion. The filament consists of a series of protoplasts surrounded by an outer membrane and separated by peptidoglycan septa. The outer membrane invaginates slightly between the protoplasts but does not completely separate them. This sample was collected from the sulfide-oxygen interface of a thermal spring (Jemez Springs, New Mexico). Electron micrograph of a thin section (see Fig. 20.61 for the corresponding light micrograph). *Bar*, 0.5 μm. (Reproduced by permission of the National Research Council of Canada and from D. E. Caldwell, S. J. Caldwell and J. P. Laycock, Canadian Journal of Microbiology *22:* 1509-1517, 1976.)

is autotrophic, with sulfide serving as the electron donor and oxygen as the electron acceptor. Consequently, a synthetic medium with either sulfide or thiosulfate as sole energy source is normally used for initial cultivation. The following medium has been used: $Na_2S_2O_3 \cdot 5H_2O$, 3.0 g/l; $NaHCO_3$, 2.0 g/l; NH_4Cl, 1.0 g/l; KNO_3, 2.0 g/l; $MgSO_4 \cdot 7H_2O$, 0.5 g/l; KH_2PO_4, 2.0 g/l; and $FeSO_4 \cdot 7H_2O$-EDTA chelate, 0.02 g/l; plus trace elements (pH 6.8) (Brannan and Caldwell, 1980). Care should be taken to avoid the loss of bicarbonate as carbon dioxide if the medium is autoclaved and when the medium is stored or incubated. Organic media are generally inadequate for initial cultivation, although the cells may be adapted to grow heterotrophically after the initial isolation. Either nutriet broth or nitrate broth supports heterotrophic growth. Nitrate broth is preferred, however, since it avoids the problem of aeration at high temperature. Transfer from autotrophic to heterotrophic media and vice versa is difficult, often resulting in loss of the culture. Although syntehtic media can be used for heterotrophic growth, the growth rate is very low despite the addition of reduced, organic sulfur compounds.

Streamers consisting of intertwined filaments are collected, added to the enrichment medium, and incubated at 73°C with vigorous aeration. At 73°C, the stationary phase in batch culture continues only 4 h before the death phase begins. As a result, it is important either to maintain the cells in the log phase of growth or to transfer them to the refrigerator for storage (up to 5 days). Cells maintained at 73°C without adequate nutrient are killed within 24 h. Because of the low solubility of oxygen at this temperature (approximately 3 mg/l), the organisms should be cultivated in shake flasks with a large head space to provide sufficient aeration. Although it is possible to clone the cells on agar, recovery is poor. As a result, cloning is normally by dilution in liquid media.

Maintenance Procedures

Cells may be either frozen in a 15% solution of glycerol and stored at −15°C or lyophilized and stored at 4°C. Cells are more easily recovered from frozen cultures than from lyophilized cultures. Cultures adapted to grow on nitrate broth (Difco) were more easily maintained than were autotrophically grown cells.

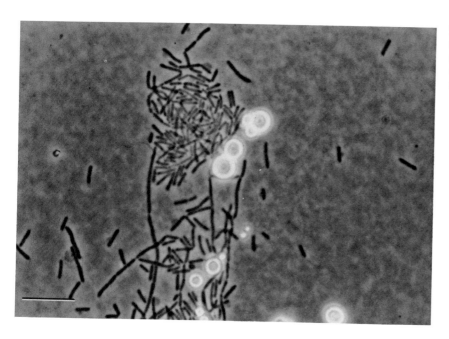

Figure 20.60. *T. thiopara* during oxidation of thiosulfate, with extracellular deposition of elemental sulfur (spherical granules) shown. The culture was highly aerated, thus producing rod-shaped cells and cell chains but no cell filaments.

Figure 20.61. *T. thiopara* filaments. The filaments form streamers which are visible macroscopically, as is shown in Figure 20.62. This sample was collected from the sulfide-oxygen interface of a thermal spring (Jemez Springs, New Mexico). Phase-contrast micrograph (see Fig. 20.59 for the electron micrograph of these filaments). *Bar,* 10 μm.

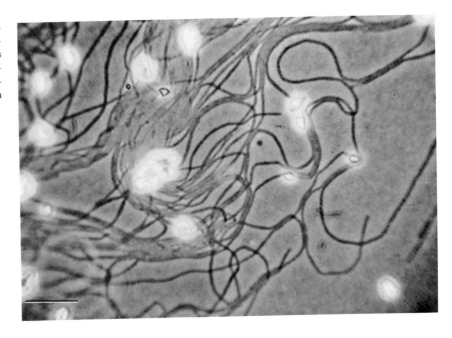

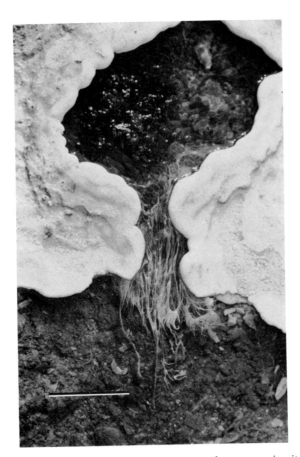

Figure 20.62. *T. thiopara* streamers as they appear in situ. The streamers consist of intertwined cell filaments. See Figures 20.59 and 20.61 for electron and phase micrographs, respectively, of streamer filaments. *Bar,* 10 cm. (Reproduced with permission from D. E. Caldwell, T. L. Kieft and D. K. Brannan, Geomicrobiology Journal *3*(3): 181–200, 1984. ©Crane, Russak & Company, Inc., New York.)

Differentiation of the genus **Thermothrix** from other closely related taxa

The primary basis for discrimination of *Thermothrix* species from thermophilic *Thiobacillus* species is the production of filaments when the concentration of the electron acceptor limits the rate of growth. Cells obtained during the initial isolation are usually motile and rod-shaped, however. Induction of the filamentous growth form requires continuous cultivation under oxygen-limited conditions. The oxygen tension should be maintained at 1 mg/l or less.

Further Reading

Brannan, D.K. and D.E. Caldwell. 1980. *Thermothrix thiopara;* growth and metabolism of a newly isolated thermophile capable of oxidizing sulfur and sulfur compounds. Appl. Environ. Microbiol. *40:* 211–216.

Brannan, D.K. and D.E. Caldwell. 1980. *Thermothrix thiopara;* growth and metabolism of a newly isolated thermophile capable of oxidizing sulfur and sulfur compounds. Appl. Environ. Microbiol. *40:* 211–216.

Brannan, D.K. and D.E. Caldwell. 1986. Ecology and metabolism of *Thermothrix thiopara.* Adv. Appl. Microbiol. *31:* 233–270.

Caldwell, D.E., T.L. Kieft and D.K. Brannan. 1984. Colonization of sulfide-oxygen interfaces on hot spring tufa by *Thermothrix thiopara.* Geomicrobiol. J. *3:* 181–200.

Mason, J., D.P. Kelly, and A.P. Wood. 1987. Chemolithotrophic growth of *Thermothrix thiopara* and some thiobacilli on thiosulfate and polythionates, and a reassessment of the growth yields of *Thx. thiopara* in chemostat culture. J. Gen. Microbiol. *133:* 1249–1256.

Differentiation of the species of the genus **Thermothrix**

The type species is the sole species in the genus.

List of species of the genus **Thermothrix**

1. **Thermothrix thiopara** Caldwell, Caldwell and Laycock 1981, 217.[VP] (Effective publication: Caldwell, Caldwell and Laycock 1976, 1515.)

thi.o′par.a. Gr. n. *thios* sulfur; L. v. *paro* produce; M.L. adj. *thiopara* sulfur-depositing.

For most features of the species, see the description of the genus.

The cardinal temperatures are 60, 73, and 80°C (minimum, optimum, and maximum) for cells grown by using either inorganic or organic media (Caldwell et al., 1976; Caldwell and Brannan, 1982). The generation time at 73°C is approximately 2 h on either medium. When this species is cultivated by using reduced sulfur compounds as electron donor, elemental sulfur is frequently deposited as extracellular granules but is not deposited intracellularly (Fig. 20.60). In batch culture,

elemental sulfur, sulfite and polythionates accumulate as transient intermediates but are subsequently oxidized completely to sulfuric acid. In continuous culture, elemental sulfur is not deposited during steady-state growth but is deposited during the transition from low to high dilution rates. During transfer from nitrate broth to autotrophic media containing thiosulfate, cell filaments often form and become encased in a coating of elemental sulfur (Fig. 20.63).

Denitrification occurs only heterotrophically (Brannan and Caldwell, 1982). During denitrification, dinitrogen is the primary end product, although small amounts of nitrous oxide are also produced. Nitrite accumulates as a transient intermediate.

Type strain: ATCC 29244.

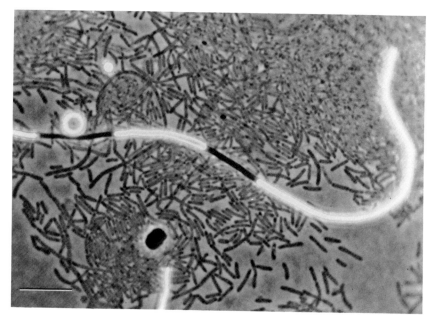

Figure 20.63. Deposition of elemental sulfur in a smooth refractile layer partially surrounding a filament of *T. thiopara* (*center*) during the transition from nitrate broth to a synthetic medium with thiosulfate as sole energy source. Phase-contrast micrograph. *Bar,* 10 μm.

C. OBLIGATELY CHEMOLITHOTROPHIC HYDROGEN BACTERIA

Genus **Hydrogenobacter** Kawasumi, Igarashi, Kodama and Minoda 1984, 9[VP]

T. KAWASUMI

Hy.dro.ge.no.bac′ter. Gr. n. *hydro* water; Gr. n. *genus* offspring; M.L. neut. n. *hydrogenum* hydrogen, that which produces water; M.L. n. *bacter* masc. form of Gr. neut. n. *bacterium* a rod; M.L. masc. n. *hydrogenobacter* hydrogen rod.

Straight rods, 0.3–0.5 × 2.0–3.0 μm, occurring singly or in pairs. **Gram-negative. Nonmotile**; cells do not possess flagella. Endospores absent. **Aerobic. Optimum temperature: 70–75°C**; maximum temperature: ~80°C. The optimum pH for growth is around neutrality. **Chemolithotrophic, using molecular hydrogen** as electron donor **and carbon dioxide** as carbon source. Chemoorganotrophic growth has not been observed. Growth factors are not required.

The mol% G + C of the DNA is 43.5–43.9 (T_m).

A straight-chain saturated $C_{18:0}$ acid and a straight-chain unsaturated $C_{20:1}$ acid are the major components of the cellular fatty acids. 2-Methylthio-3-VI,VII-tetrahydromultiprenyl[7]-1,4-naphthoquinone (methionaquinone) is the major component of the quinone system.

Type species: *Hydrogenobacter thermophilus* Kawasumi, Igarashi, Kodama and Minoda 1984, 9.

Further Descriptive Information

No filamentous bacterial form such as that of *Thermus aquaticus* (Brock and Freeze, 1969) or *Methanobacterium thermoautotrophicum* (Zeikus and Wolfe, 1973) is observed regardless of the growth temperature or phase. In Figure 20.64, an electron micrograph of an ultrathin section of *H. thermophilus* TK-6, a Gram-negative type of cell wall profile can be seen. Organelles, like mesosomes, are present. Intracytoplasmic membrane structures such as those present in methylotrophs and nitrifying bacteria cannot be seen.

All members of the genus can be easily cultivated on basal inorganic medium in an atmosphere consisting of H_2, O_2 and CO_2 (75:15:10). Liquid cultivation is routinely used because after prolonged cultivation, no bacterial colonies grew on agar media under either autotrophic or heterotrophic conditions. The specific growth rate under autotrophic conditions at the optimum temperature is 0.33–0.42 (h^{-1}). Ammonium and nitrate ions are utilized as nitrogen source, but urea and gaseous nitrogen are not. Nitrite inhibits growth. Assimilatory nitrate reduction and peroxidase are positive. Urease is negative.

None of the following organic compounds (0.1%) or media are used as sole sources of energy and carbon: glucose, fructose, galactose, maltose, sucrose, xylose, raffinose, L-rhamnose, D-mannose, D-trehalose, mannitol, starch, formate, acetate, propionate, pyruvate, succinate, malate, citrate, fumarate, maleate, glycolate, gluconate, DL-lactate, α-ketoglutarate, p-hydroxybenzoate, DL-β-hydroxybutyrate, betaine, methanol, ethanol, methylamine, dimethylamine, trimethylamine, glycine. L-glutamate, L-aspartate, L-serine, L-leucine, L-valine, L-tryptophan, L-histidine, L-alanine, L-lysine, L-proline, L-arginine, nutrient broth, yeast extract-malt extract medium and brain-heart infusion. Under an atmosphere containing 90% CO, 5% CO_2 and 5% O_2, no growth in the strains has been observed.

No oxygen uptake by intact cells of strain TK-6 has been detected with use of the following organic compounds (1 mM): glucose, fructose, acetate, pyruvate, citrate, α-ketoglutarate, succinate, fumarate, malate, oxalacetate and glutamate. In the case of cell-free extracts, oxygen uptake is observed clearly only with use of malate and is scarcely detected or is not detected at all with use of the other organic substrates. The rate of oxygen uptake is significantly higher in the presence of NADH and hydrogen than in the presence of malate. These organic compounds have different effects on the autotrophic growth of strain TK-6. Succinate, α-ketoglutarate, citrate and formate inhibit autotrophic growth, while fumarate and glucose have no effect on growth. Fructose stimulates autotrophic growth slightly at relatively low concentrations (5–10 mM) but strongly inhibits growth at concentrations higher than 50 mM. Acetate, pyruvate and malate markedly stimulate autotrophic growth at low concentrations (2–3 mM) and inhibit it at concentrations higher than 100, 10 and 10 mM, respectively.

Strain TK-6 has deficient carbohydrate metabolic pathways and an incomplete tricarboxylic acid cycle (Shiba et al., 1982). Several enzymes of the Embden-Meyerhof pathway and key enzymes of the pentose phosphate pathway are present in cell-free extracts, but their activities are low. Phophofructokinase, aldolase, pyruvate kinase, lactate dehydrogenase and two enzymes of the Entner-Doudoroff pathway (6-phosphogluconate dehydrase and KDPG aldolase) have not been detected. Activities of all enzymes of the tricarboxylic acid cycle except

Figure 20.64. *H. thermophilus* strain TK-6. Electron micrograph of ultrathin section. *Bar*, 1 μm.

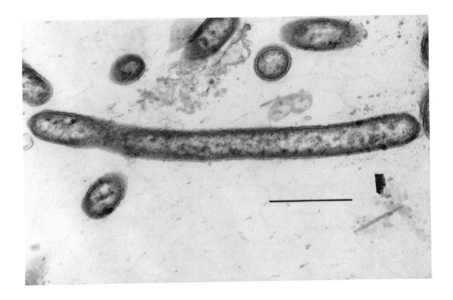

α-ketoglutarate dehydrogenase are present, though pyruvate dehydrogenase activity has not been detected. Enzyme activities of the glyoxylic acid cycle are also lacking.

Membrane-bound hydrogenase activity has been observed in cell-free extracts of strain TK-6, but NAD-dependent soluble hydrogenase activity has not.

Type b and c cytochromes have been found in cell-free extracts of all the strains of the genus.

The electrophoretic patterns of the total soluble proteins are essentially the same among all strains of the genus, though there are differences in the relative mobilities of several proteins.

Hydrogenobacter strains so far described were all isolated from hot (>45°C) water-containing soils from various hot springs in Japan.

Enrichment and Isolation Procedures

H. thermophilus can be enriched with inorganic agar medium in the atmosphere containing H_2, O_2 and CO_2 (85:5:10) at 65°C. Colonies which are developed on plates are inoculated into the same liquid medium and gas mixture. After repeated liquid cultivation, *H. thermophilus* can be isolated in pure culture by the dilution method (Kawasumi et al., 1980). Once purified, none of the strains could grow as colony on agar medium. This can be explained by the fact that the organism is sensitive to agar or only grows as a colony in mixed culture. To clarify this, further investigations are required.

Maintenance Procedures

Hydrogenobacter strains can be preserved for about 1 year by L-drying. As the suspending medium, 0.1 M phosphate buffer (pH 7.0) containing 3% sodium glutamate is used.

Taxonomic Comments

Studies on DNA or RNA homology and an analysis of the oligonucleotide catalogs from 16S rRNA may prove useful for investigating the phylogenic relationships of *Hydrogenobacter* to other genera or higher taxa. "*Calderobacterium hydrogenophilum*" seems to be closely related to *H. thermophilus* in its morphology, growth characteristics, obligate autotrophy and mol% G + C of the DNA (Kryukov et al., 1983). However, determination of the taxonomical relationships will depend on future studies on chemotaxonomy or DNA homology.

List of species of the genus **Hydrogenobacter**

1. **Hydrogenobacter thermophilus** Kawasumi, Igarashi, Kodama and Minoda 1984, 9.[VP]

ther.mo'phi.lus. Gr. n. *therme* heat; Gr. adj. *philus* loving; M.L. masc. adj. *thermophilus* heat-loving.

The description of this species is the same as that of the genus. *Type strain:* TK-6; IAM 12695.

D. IRON- AND MANGANESE-OXIDIZING AND/OR DEPOSITING BACTERIA

The iron and manganese bacteria are a diverse group of bacteria that are able to oxidize and/or deposit iron or manganese oxides extracellularly or, sometimes, intracellularly. Many of these bacteria are classified elsewhere in the *Manual*. For example, the genus of stalked iron bacteria, *Gallionella,* is classified in Section 21 with the "Budding and/or Appendaged Bacteria." Another species, *Thiobacillus ferrooxidans,* is classified in Section 20 with the "Colorless Sulfur Bacteria." Both of these iron bacteria are chemolithotrophs deriving energy from the oxidation of ferrous iron (Fe (II)) with the formation of ferric hydroxide (Fe (III)). Likewise, both of these groups are able to fix carbon dioxide by the ribulose pentose phosphate cycle. However, many other taxa treated here and elsewhere in the *Manual* are capable of iron or manganese oxidation and/or deposition and are not known to derive energy from the process. Nonetheless, these organisms are also important in the biogeochemical cycling of these metals.

One of the reasons the iron and manganese bacteria are considered as a special group of bacteria is that their deposition of ferric and manganese oxides makes them very conspicuous when viewed under the light microscope. Thus, when material from iron springs or natural waters is examined microscopically, these bacteria are a recognizable and, often, a directly identifiable component of the microbial community.

In addition to those iron and manganese bacteria that form microscopically obvious deposits of metal oxides about their cells, there are many bacteria, cultivated from a variety of aquatic habitats, soils, and rock varnishes (i.e. desert varnish), that are able to oxidize Mn (II) to Mn (IV). Most of these bacteria are identifiable to well-known heterotrophic taxa such as the genera *Bacillus* (van Veen, 1973; Nealson and Ford, 1980; Gregory and Staley, 1982; Palmer et al., 1985), *Micrococcus* (Ehrlich, 1966; Palmer et al., 1985), *Pseudomonas* (Zavarzin, 1962; van Veen, 1973; Nealson, 1978; Gregory and Staley, 1985), *Cytophaga* (Gregory and Staley, 1982), *Flavobacterium* (Nealson, 1978), *Chromobacterium* (Gregory and Staley, 1982), *Oceanospirillum* (Ehrlich, 1978), *Caulobacter* (Gregory and Staley, 1982), *Arthrobacter* (Ehrlich, 1966; Bromfield, 1974; Palmer et al., 1985), *Nocardia* (Schweisfurth, 1968), and *Streptomyces* (Bromfield, 1979). This particular group of genera is not included in the key below, although they are probably also important in the geochemical cycling of these metals.

Bacteria that are involved in the reduction of oxidized iron and manganese are not treated specifically in the *Manual*. These are a diverse group of bacteria, including many of the well-known heterotrophic taxa, that are undoubtedly also very important in the geochemical cycling of these elements. For more information on these organisms, the reader is referred to Nealson (1983a, b).

Key to the identification of **Iron- and Manganese-Oxidizing and/or Depositing Bacteria**

I. Bacteria which deposit iron or manganese oxides externally to the cell
  a. Unicellular bacteria
    i. Cells with appendages
      aa. Prosthecate bacteria (Section 21):
          Genus *Pedomicrobium,* p. 1910
          Genus *Hyphomicrobium,* p. 1895
          Genus "*Caulococcus*," p. 1986

FAMILY "SIDEROCAPSACEAE" PRIBRAM 1929, 377

O. H. TUOVINEN, P. HIRSCH AND G. A. ZAVARZIN

Si.de.ro.cap.sa′ce.ae. M.L. fem. n. *Siderocapsa* type genus of the family; M.L. fem. pl. n. *Siderocapsaceae* the *Siderocapsa* family.

Cells display much variation in morphology and capsulation. Spherical, ellipsoidal and rod-shaped cells have been described which are typically encrusted with oxides of iron (III) and manganese (IV).

The taxonomic validity of *"Siderocapsaceae"* is questionable due to the lack of physiological and biochemical characterization of the members of this family, most of which have not been obtained in pure culture. Pure culture studies are scarce and have not been verified. Thus the taxonomic status of nearly all species of this family is based on sketchy morphological description of either environmental or enriched samples.

Genera incertae sedis are *"Ferribacterium"* (*"Sideroderma"*), *"Siderobacter," "Sideromonas," "Sideronema," "Siderosphaera"* and *"Siderocystis."* The most recent diagnostic key to these genera was published by Švorcová (1979), but due to the lack of pure culture data, it cannot presently be validated.

The remaining four genera, *"Siderocapsa," "Naumanniella," "Ochrobium"* and *"Siderococcus,"* are presently viewed as poorly described morphovars of some resemblance to better characterized genera in other families. The description of these four genera has emerged from environmental observations supported by morphological data from enrichment cultures or, in a very few cases, pure cultures. The taxonomic existence of *"Siderocapsaceae"* is retained here primarily for reason of reference in order to conserve its identity until new evidence becomes available to substantiate the status of this family.

These bacteria are found in environments which may be characterized by elevated concentrations of iron and/or manganese. There appears to be an association between members of *"Siderocapsaceae"* and the presence of iron and manganese; the cells become nuclei of metal precipitation, resulting in **the formation of insoluble metal oxides** which **may completely encrust and envelop the cell. Capsular material characteristically serves as** **the core of iron and manganese oxide deposition.** There is no evidence to suggest that the oxidation and subsequent precipitation of iron or manganese are biologically favorable reactions. These bacteria have not been cultured chemolithotrophically (with Fe^{2+} or Mn^{2+} as electron donor), nor has the autotrophic mode of metabolism been documented. Hence members of *"Siderocapsaceae"* should not be referred to as iron- or manganese-oxidizing bacteria but should be regarded as a part of the group of "iron- and/or manganese-precipitating bacteria." This terminology has no taxonomic significance but indicates the practical consequences associated with the occurrence of such bacteria in various environments.

Previous descriptions of *"Siderocapsaceae"* indicate that **these bacteria are aerobic or microaerophilic**, although **facultative or obligate anaerobicity has been reported for *"Ochrobium"*** (Jones, 1981). **In aquatic environments**, these bacteria are found as **either planktonic or attached to algae, plants or other submerged surfaces.** Oxic-anoxic interfaces appear to be abundant sources for enrichment of many of these bacteria; however, some members of the *"Siderocapsaceae"* have been found in large numbers in the aerobic epilimnion or in the anaerobic hypolimnion of lakes. **Under microscopic examination, *"Siderocapsaceae"* appear rust-brown due to iron encrustation and, sometimes, dark brown or olive-green to black due to the presence of manganese dioxide.** The discoloration and metal precipitation, although possibly abiotic, are prime diagnostic characteristics in microscopic examination (it is possible, however, that iron oxidation in some cases may have occurred only after sampling and transportation to the laboratory, i.e. by subsequent oxygenation (Jones, 1981)).

Various members of *"Siderocapsaceae"* have also been diagnosed from well-water samples, groundwater, field drainage tiles and effluents as well as from soil samples. Most of the published information stems from a limited number of studies in European countries.

Key to the genera of the family "Siderocapsaceae"

I. Iron or manganese oxides deposited.
  A. Oxides deposited in (on) capsular material which surrounds groups of spherical or ovoid cells; deposition often ring-shaped:
      Genus I. *"Siderocapsa"*

B. Oxides deposited as a sheath enveloping the cell's margin; cells usually rod-shaped and single, although aggregates of cells occur where each cell has the deposit.
    1. Sheath of deposits completely envelops the cell in a very regular fashion; multiplication may be by budding:
        Genus II. *"Naumanniella"*
    2. Sheath not continuous, usually open at one end, resembling a horseshoe:
        Genus III. *"Siderococcus"*
II. Iron oxide deposited only, manganese oxides absent. Encrustations bright orange-yellow. Cells spherical; multiplication is by budding:
        Genus IV. *"Ochrobium"*

Genus I. **"Siderocapsa"** *Molisch 1909, 29*

P. HIRSCH, G. A. ZAVARZIN AND O. H. TUOVINEN

Si.de.ro.cap′sa. Gr. n. *siderus* iron; L. fem. n. *capsa* box; M.L. fem. n. *Siderocapsa* iron box.

One or several spherical to ovoid cells surrounded by a common capsule partially or completely **encrusted with oxides of iron or manganese.** Capsular material appears to precede the deposition of iron or manganese. **Deposits often ring-shaped** (and not completely spherical) **when the cells live attached to surfaces.** The more or less loose **capsular material may be rust-brown, owing to the presence of iron oxides, or greenish to olive-colored, owing to the presence of manganese oxides.**

Common in freshwater habitats on surfaces or planktonic. **Some species bear resemblance to** *Arthrobacter* **species when cultivated in the laboratory but attain the morphology described above when reintroduced into the normal aquatic habitat** (Schmidt, 1984). Accordingly, Dubinina and Zhdanov (1975) suggested that *"S. eusphaera"* be recognized as a new species of *Arthrobacter (A. sidercapsulatus),* but this revision needs to be substantiated by further work with pure cultures.

The differentiation of *"Siderocapsa"* species is presently based on morphological characteristics as outlined by Skuja (1974). Cell morphology is often obscured due to iron or manganese encrustation which can be removed by sample pretreatment with dilute solutions of either oxalic acid, hydrochloric acid or EDTA.

Successful enrichment cultures were based on amending the sample with $FeCO_3$ or $MnCO_3$ (1 mg/l each) or on using liquid or solid media which additionally contained a low concentration of complex organic carbon substrates such as yeast extract, beef extract or peptone (Hanert, 1981).

"Siderocapsa" coenobia may be visualized under the electron microscope on film-covered electron microscopic grids exposed in the natural environment (Hirsch and Pankratz, 1970).

Type species: *"Siderocapsa treubii"* Molisch 1909, 29.

Further Descriptive Information

Caldwell and Hirsch (D. E. Caldwell and P. Hirsch, unpublished observations, 1975) observed bacteria resembling *"Siderocapsa"* species from a sample collected at a 2-m depth from a small meromictic lake (Knaack Lake) in Wisconsin (U.S.A.). These organisms had olive-colored, loose, thick capsules, and the cells contained gas vesicles (Fig. 20.65).

Differentiation and characteristics of the species of the genus **"Siderocapsa"**

The differential characteristics of the species of the genus *"Siderocapsa"* are provided in Table 20.33.

Further Reading

Schmidt, W.D. 1984. Die Eisenbakterien des Pluβsees. II. Morphologie und

Feinstruktur von *Siderocapsa geminata* (Skuja 1954/57). Z. Allg. Mikrobiol. *24:* 391–396.

Švorcová, L. 1975. Iron bacteria of the genus *Siderocapsa* in mineral waters. Z. Allg. Mikrobiol. *15:* 553–557.

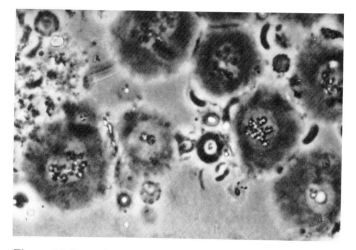

Figure 20.65. *"S. eusphaera"* (?) from the metalimnion of Knaack Lake (Wisconsin) at a 2-m depth. This sample was collected May 14. The cells shown in Figure 20.68 carry gas vesicles.

Table 20.33.

Characteristics differentiating the species of the genus "Siderocapsa"[a]

Characteristic	1. "S. treubii"	2. "S. major"	3. "S. monoica"	4. "S. anulata"	5. "S. geminata"	6. "S. coronata"	7. "S. arlbergensis"	8. "S. eusphaera"	9. "S. hexagonata"	10. "S. quadrata"
Cell form	Cocci	Cocci	Cocci	Cocci	Ovoid	Cocci	Cocci to rods	Cocci to rods	Cocci to ovoid cells	Cocci to ovoid cells
Diameter (μm)	0.4–0.6	0.7–1.8	0.5–0.8	0.2–0.5	0.5–0.6		0.4–1.0	1–2	0.6–0.8	0.5–1.0
Growth attached to surfaces	+	+	+	−		−	−	−	−	−
Free-floating cells	−	−	−	+		+	+	+	+	+
No. of cells/capsule	Several	Several	1	1	(1)–2	Several	1–4	Up to 60	Several	1?
Capsule size and structure	Large	Large; loose	Small	Small	Large radially structured or granular and layered		Granular	Stratified: 2–3 concentric layers	Hexagonal (cross-section lenticular)	Square (cross-section lenticular)
Neustonic	−	−	−	−	−	+	−	−	−	−
Aggregating capsules	−	−	−	−	−	+	(+)	−	−	−
Remarks	Type species				May be an Arthrobacter sp.			Arthrobacter siderocapsulatus	An obligate autotroph?	

[a]Symbols: +, 90% or more of strains are positive; −, 90% or more of strains are negative; and (+), rarely positive.

Key to the species of the genus "Siderocapsa"

I. Grow attached to aquatic plants or other surfaces.
  A. Multiple cells occur, surrounded by a large, common capsule.
    1. Cocci, 0.4–0.6 μm in diameter:
        1. "Siderocapsa treubii"
    2. Cocci, 0.7–1.8 μm in diameter:
        2. "S. major"
  B. Single cocci, each surrounded by a thin capsule; 0.5–0.8 μm in diameter:
        3. "S. monoica"
II. Cells planktonic or mostly free-floating.
  A. Single cocci, each surrounded by a thin capsule of homogeneous appearance; 0.2–0.5 μm in diameter:
        4. "S. anulata"
  B. Capsular layer is thick and round, often with a distinct radial or granular appearance.
    1. Cells ovoid, 0.5–0.6 μm in diameter and 0.8 μm in length, usually 1 pair/capsule:
        5. "S. geminata"
    2. Multiple spherical cells in each capsule.
      a. Neustonic forms in large aggregates cemented together with a network of capsular material:
        6. "S. coronata"
      b. Planktonic forms, no distinct aggregation.
        aa. Cells 0.4–1.0 μm in diameter, 1–4/capsule:
        7. S. arlbergensis"
        bb. Cells 1–2 μm in diameter, up to 60/capsule:
        8. "S. eusphaera"
  C. Capsule hexagonal or square, lenticular in cross-section.
    1. Cells 0.6–0.8 μm in diameter; capsule hexagonal; possibly autotrophic:
        9. "S. hexagonata"
    2. Cells 0.5–1.0 μm in diameter; capsule square:
        10. "S. quadrata"

Species Incertae Sedis (Švorcová, 1979)

"S. lanceolata," "S. rectangulata," "S. conglomerata," "S. monoeca" and "S. solitaria."

List of species of the genus "Siderocapsa"

1. **"Siderocapsa treubii"** Molisch 1909, 29.

treu' bi.i. M.L. gen. n. *treubii* of Treub; named for Professor Treub, an early director of the tropical garden in Buitenzorg, Java.

Capsules encrusted with iron oxide. This species is found widely distributed on surfaces in aquatic environments. Capsular material may also appear dark brown to black due to precipitation of manganese oxide.

2. **"Siderocapsa major"** Molisch 1910, 13.

ma'jor. L. comp. adj. *major* larger.

Similar to *S. treubii*, but cells are larger (0.7–1.8 µm in diameter), and the capsule is less defined. Often, there are 2–4 cells/capsule, and the cells may be ovoid to short rod-shaped (Fig. 20.66). Widely distributed on surfaces in aquatic environments.

Comment. Intermediate forms occur which would be ascribed to either *S. treubii* or *S. major*.

3. **"Siderocapsa monoica"** Naumann 1921, 49.

mon.o'ica. Gr. adj. *monos* single; Gr. n. *oicus* house; M.L. fem. adj. *monoica* solitary dwelling.

A single coccoid cell/capsule. Capsular layer is typically thin but, owing to the precipitation of iron and manganese oxides, develops a dark color and encrustation. Cells 0.5–0.8 µm in diameter, attached to submerged aquatic plants.

4. **"Siderocapsa anulata"** Kalbe, Keil and Thiele 1965, 35.

a.nu.la'ta. L. fem. adj. *anulata* with a ring.

Cells are single cocci, 0.2–0.5 µm in diameter. Capsular layer is thin, appearing granular or radially organized; outer diameter: 1.2–1.9 µm; inner diameter: 0.7–1.9 µm. Capsule is thick and rust-brown when encrusted with iron oxides. Often, nonencrusted inner capsules surround each of several small cells which are jointly encased by the densely iron-stained outer capsule (Fig. 20.67).

5. **"Siderocapsa geminata"** Skuja 1956, 19.

gem.in.a'ta. L. v. *gemino* to double; M.L. fem. part. adj. *geminata* doubled, paired.

Cells are ovoid to short rod-shaped, 0.5–0.6 × 0.6–1.6 µm and in pairs, although single cells are often seen after division to daughter cells. Capsular layer is characteristically round and 7–11 µm in diameter. Iron encrustation initiates at the outermost part of the capsule and proceeds concentrically, resulting in a stratified appearance. This species is found in the hypolimnion of Swedish lakes and also in the epilimnion during vernal or autumnal circulation. Also found in slow-flowing iron springs in Northern Germany (P. Hirsch, unpublished observations) (Fig. 20.68). Schmidt (1984) described the morphology and fine structure of this organism. Additional information on the life cycle and ecology of this species was published by Schmidt (1984).

6. **"Siderocapsa coronata"** Redinger 1931, 413.

co.ro.na'ta. L. fem. part. adj. *coronata* crowned.

Two to eight cells in an irregularly spherical capsule of up to 24 µm in diameter, with the characteristic discoloration due to iron or manganese encrustation. This species is found in the neuston of alpine or subalpine lakes and pools. Occurs also under microaerophilic conditions.

7. **"Siderocapsa arlbergensis"** Wawrik 1956, 21.

arl.berg.en'sis. L. adj. suff. *-ensis* belonging to; M.L. adj. *arlbergensis* from Arlberg, a town in Tyrol, Austria.

Capsule is irregularly spherical, 6–15 µm in diameter and typically granular. Capsular aggregation is rare. Cells 0.4–1.0 µm in diameter, with 1–4/capsule. This species was originally found in alpine pools in Austria.

8. **"Siderocapsa eusphaera"** Skuja 1948, 13.

eu.sphae'ra. Gr. prep. *eu* true, nice, beautiful; Gr. n. *sphaera* ball, sphere; M.L. n. *eusphaera* beautiful sphere.

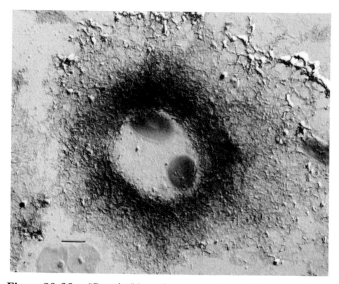

Figure 20.66. *"S. major"* from the neuston of a small forest pond near Westensee (Kiel, Holstein, Federal Republic of Germany), growing attached to an electron microscopic grid which had been coated with formvar and was exposed for 4 days. *Bar,* 10 µm. (Micrograph by W. C. Ghiorse, Ithaca, New York.)

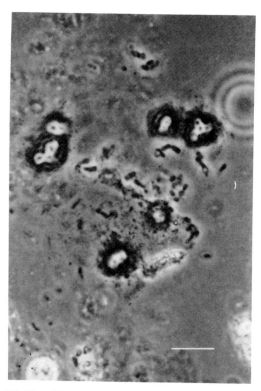

Figure 20.67. *"S. anulata"* from an iron spring at Reselithberg (Waaken, Holstein, Federal Republic of Germany). This sample was collected July 2. *Bar,* 10 µm.

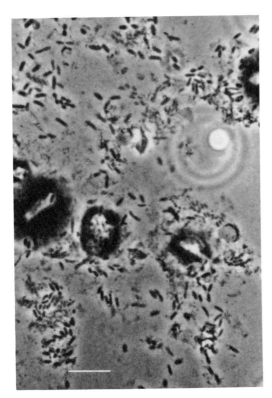

Figure 20.68. *"S. geminata"* from an iron spring at Reselithberg (Waaken, Holstein, Federal Republic of Germany). This sample was collected July 2. *Bar, 10 μm.*

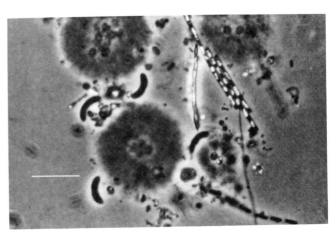

Figure 20.69. *"S. eusphaera"* (?) from the metalimnion of Knaack Lake (Wisconsin) at a 2-m depth. This sample was collected May 14. The cells shown in Figure 20.68 carry gas vesicles. *Bar, 10 μm.*

Capsules are regularly spherical, 10–50 μm in diameter and usually give a stratified appearance with two or three concentric layers of iron encrustation. According to Dubinina and Zhdanov (1975), cells display, depending on the culture age and condition, both coccoidal and rod-shaped morphology. Encapsulated cells are typically planktonic. This species was originally found in hypolimnion and epilimnion layers of lakes. Older cells may have central gas vesicles (compare Fig. 20.69 with Fig. 20.65).

Comment. Dubinina and Zhdanov (1975) proposed that *"S. eusphaera"* is appropriately placed in the genus *Arthrobacter* as *A. siderocapsulatus*; further work has not been reported to substantiate this proposal.

9. **"Siderocapsa hexagonata"** Švorcová 1975, 555.

hex.a.go.na′ta. M.L. fem. adj. *hexagonata* hexagonal.

Cells spherical to ellipsoidal, 0.6–0.8 μm in diameter and surrounded by a regularly hexagonal capsule which is lenticular in cross-section. The lightly rust-colored to dark brown capsule is surrounded by a less encrusted envelope. This organism may be a strict autotroph, as it was cultured in mineral water without addition of organic compounds.

10. **"Siderocapsa quadrata"** Švorcová 1975, 556.

qua.dra′ta. M.L. fem. adj. *quadrata* square.

Cells spherical to ellipsoidal, 0.5–1.0 μm in diameter, with a square capsule 2.2–2.5 μm large. The capsule is lightly rust-colored to dark brown. This species has been found in mineral water from Karlovy Vary.

Acknowledgments

We gratefully acknowledge obtaining information and/or micrographs from W. M. Gorlenko and G. Dubinina (Moscow, U.S.S.R.), R. Schweisfurth (Homburg, Federal Republic of Germany), G. Jones (Ambleside, England) and D. R. Gabe (Leningrad, U.S.S.R.). One of us (P. H.) had extended discussions with H. Skuja (Uppsala, Sweden).

Genus II. **"Naumanniella"** Dorff 1934, 19

P. Hirsch, G. A. Zavarzin and O. H. Tuovinen

Nau.man.ni.el′la. M.L. dim. ending *-ella;* M.L. fem. n. *Naumanniella* named for Einar Naumann, a Swedish limnologist.

Cells most often **rod-shaped,** sometimes **ellipsoidal or almost coccoid,** with each cell **surrounded by a delicate, regular capsule which becomes encrusted with iron oxide** (yellow or rust-brown) **or manganese oxide** (dark brown to black). **Capsular encrustation** emphasizes the cell margin and **gives the appearance of a chain link.** Readily enriched from iron- and/or manganese-bearing waters; presumably able to decompose complex organic compounds of iron and manganese.

Multiplication by fission, but a budding mechanism has been claimed for two species. Some cells may show a morphology reminiscent of branching (Y shapes), but this may be due to the budding process. Not obtained in pure culture.

Type species: *"Naumanniella neustonica"* Dorff 1934, 20.

Further Descriptive Information

"Naumanniella" species have been found in cold iron springs and deep wells (Beger, 1949; Hanert, 1981; P. Hirsch, unpublished observations) or in brown forest soils and iron-manganese crusts of podzols; in all cases, conditions were aerobic or microaerophilic.

Motility of the buds has been observed in one case (*"N. polymorpha"* (Ten, 1969)). Isolation and enrichment procedures have been described by Hanert (1981) and Ten (1969).

Differentiation of the genus "**Naumanniella**" from other closely related taxa

The morphology is so characteristic that it can be used for identification: the relatively sharp margin and shape of a chain link make the "*Naumanniella*" cells appear like minute diatoms. Budding and rod-shaped forms sometimes appear to resemble "*Blastobacter*" species. Iron and/or manganese deposition by "*Blastobacter*" species has not been studied so far, although "*B. henricii*" was originally found in iron-containing water.

Taxonomic Comments

The differences in morphology suggest that the species of this genus may be quite unrelated to each other.

Differentiation of the species of the genus "**Naumanniella**"

Characteristics differentiating the species of the genus "*Naumanniella*" are listed in Table 20.34. As most species have never been cultured, differentiation is by morphology only.

List of species of the genus "**Naumanniella**"

1. "**Naumanniella neustonica**" Dorff 1934, 20.
neus.to′ni.ca. Gr. adj. *neustus* swimming, floating; M.L. adj. *neustonica* of the neuston or surface film.

Cells rod-shaped and straight. Cell size with capsule: 1.8–3.3 × 4.9–10.0 μm. Cells occur singly and may be constricted. Multiplication is by binary fission.

Growth in ferrous citrate solutions produces a golden-brown surface film and voluminous deposits of iron hydroxide. Growth in other media has not been reported.

Comment. Sometimes the cells may adhere to each other and thus become surrounded by a common capsule (Fig. 20.70). Also, branching forms have been observed by one of us (P. H.); these could be interpreted as budding cells.

2. "**Naumanniella minor**" Dorff 1934, 21.
mi′nor. L. comp. adj. *minor* smaller.

Cells are frequently curved or spiral and occur singly. Cell size with capsule: 1.2–1.5 × 3.1–3.6 μm.

3. "**Naumanniella catenata**" Beger 1943, 321.
ca.te.na′ta. L. part. adj. *catenatus* in chains.

Cells are slightly curved rods and occur mostly in short chains. Cell size with capsule: 1.0–1.2 × 4.9–5.5 μm. The rods may be very short at times (Fig. 20.71).

4. "**Naumanniella pygmaea**" Beger 1949, 65.
pyg·mae′a. Gr. adj. *pygmaea* dwarfish.

Table 20.34.

Characteristics differentiating the species of the genus "Naumanniella"

Characteristic	1. "N. neustonica"	2. "N. minor"	3. "N. catenata"	4. "N. pygmaea"	5. "N. elliptica"	6. "N. polymorpha"
Cell shape	Straight rods	Curved or spiral	Rods, slightly curved	Straight rods with rounded ends	Ellipsoidal	Ellipsoidal to coccoid
Cell size (with capsule) (μm)	1.8–3.3 × 4.9–10.0	1.2–1.5 × 3.1–3.6	1.0–1.2 × 4.9–5.5	1.0 × 2.0	2.0 × 2.5–3.0	0.7–1.0 × 1.0–2.0[a]
Cell aggregation	Single	Single	In chains	Single	Single	Single
Multiplication	Binary fission	Binary fission	Binary fission?	Budding?		Budding
Habitat	Neuston	Sediment from an iron well				
Growth conditions	Ferrous citrate solution			Soil extract agar (Ten, 1967)		Growth in manganese carbonate agar or manganese acetate agar; no growth in ordinary organic media
Remarks	Type species psychrophilic[b]	Psychrophilic[b]	Psychrophilic[b]	Psychrophilic[b]		Buds motile; oxidizes only manganese

[a] Measurements without capsule.
[b] Hanert, 1981.

Figure 20.70. *"N. neustonica"* from an acid bog iron spring in Michigan (U.S.A.). A clean glass slide was exposed in October for 5 days. Some of the cells show lateral branching or exhibit a Y shape, while others share a joint capsule. The encrustations are yellowish olive. *Bar*, 10 μm.

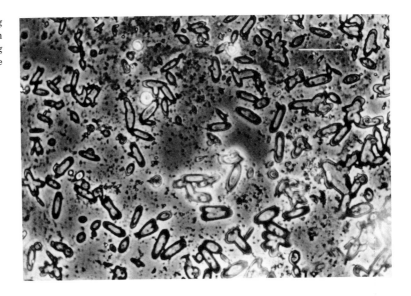

Figure 20.71. *"N. catenata"* (?) from a Lake Konstanz surface water sample collected in November. Cells are in short chains and, sometimes, slightly bent. The encrustations are yellowish brown. *Bar,* 10 μm.

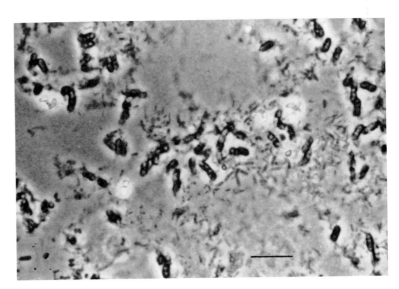

Cells are straight rods with rounded ends and occur singly. Cell size with capsule: 1.0×2.0 μm. Multiplication by budding has been claimed. This organism grows slowly on soil extract agar, producing minute brownish colonies (Ten, 1967).

5. **"Naumanniella elliptica"** Beger 1949, 66.

el·lip′ti·ca. Gr. adj. *elliptica* elliptical.

Cells ellipsoidal with pronounced capsule. Cell size with capsule: 2.0×2.5–3.0 μm.

6. **"Naumanniella polymorpha"** Ten 1969, 698.

po·ly·mor′pha. Gr. adj. *poly* many; Gr. n. *morphus* form, shape; M.L. adj. *polymorpha* of many shapes.

Cells ellipsoidal or, sometimes, coccoid, 0.7–1.0×1.0–2.0 μm. Multiplication is by budding; the bud is motile and free from metal oxides.

Colonies on manganese carbonate or manganese acetate agar are dark brown, minute and swarm on the surface. No growth in ordinary organic media has been observed. This organism oxidizes manganous but not ferrous compounds. Originally isolated from soils of Sachalin with high manganese content.

Acknowledgments

Some of the observations on *Naumanniella* occurrence were made by Jan W. Krul (Wageningen) during a research period in the laboratory of one of us (P. H.) in Michigan.

Genus III. **"Siderococcus"** *Dorff 1934, 9*

P. HIRSCH, G. A. ZAVARZIN AND O. H. TUOVINEN

Si.de.ro.coc′cus. Gr. n. *siderus* iron; Gr. n. *coccus* a berry, sphere; M.L. masc. n. *Siderococcus* iron sphere.

Cells are spherical and small, 0.2–0.5 μm in diameter and occur **singly or in small aggregates** which may sometimes resemble an ear of corn (*Zea mays*) and sometimes are just irregular. Zavarzin (1974) claimed these were motile, but the type of flagellation was unknown. Other authors do not mention motility.

Cells were originally described as carrying filamentous appendages

(Dorff, 1934; Kutuzova, 1974). The latter author observed very fine branching filaments, especially when the cells were kept under reducing conditions. Dorff (1934) was unable to find capsules, but **Kutuzova (1974) stresses that electron microscopic studies definitely showed capsules to be present and that the iron oxides were precipitated into (onto) these.**

Multiplication is by budding; the cells may then become slightly pear shaped. Often, young buds occur again, thus **giving rise to budding cell chains or even nets** (Kutuzova, 1974; P. Hirsch, unpublished observations).

The organisms usually develop as large accretions. Iron oxidation and deposition around the cells may be considerable; the **deposits are bright yellowish orange** and may be seen as distinctly colored horizons on stratified sediments or sediment-water interfaces. **The deposits contain only ferric hydroxide.** *"Siderococcus"* microzones are especially common in mud horizons with low concentrations of oxygen and at neutral pH (Perfil'ev and Gabe, 1964), such as in groundwater iron springs in which the cold water oozes out horizontally, and are widely distributed in freshwater bottom deposits. These organisms have not been obtained in pure culture.

Type species: *"Siderococcus limoniticus"* Dorff 1934, 9.

Ecological Observations and Attempted Enrichments

"Siderococcus" were found in lakes in Russia and Sweden, as well as in tropical freshwater habitats (Dorff, 1934). Growth in slit peloscopes that were exposed in mud for 15 days to 2 months resulted in the formation of minute cocci that arose by budding from still young mother cells (Kutuzova et al., 1972; Kutuzova, 1974). Dorff (1934) obtained growth of *"Siderococcus"* in test tube water samples containing some mud after incubation for 3–4 days. Under these conditions, large amounts of iron oxide were precipitated. The original type location was a spring horizon (Quellhorizont) at Teufelsee near Freienwalde (Mark, Germany) with 4.5 mg Fe per liter. One of us (P. H.) found bright yellowish-orange *"Siderococcus"* iron deposits for 12 consecutive years in an iron spring horizon near Itzehoe (Holstein, Germany). Good in situ growth was indicated by the presence of many buds of different size. Some environmental parameters were measured; the observed ranges were: 9–12°C; pH 6.2–7.0; and 1–15 mg Fe^{2+} per liter. Of several adjacent springs, only those that had these properties carried *"Siderococcus"* cells. In all of these cases the concentration of oxygen was between 2 and 4 mg/l.

Differentiation of the genus **"Siderococcus"** from other genera

The small size, the spherical shape, the budding process (Fig. 20.72) and the bright yellowish-orange iron deposition allow an easy separation from other bacteria. *"Planctomyces condensatus"* (Skuja, 1964) with a similar morphology also aggregates, but it never produces the bright yellowish-orange iron oxide deposits on the cell surface. Other *Planctomyces* species normally have stalks that consist of excreted fibers, bands or tubes (Schmidt and Starr, 1978). *Pirella* species (Schlesner and Hirsch, 1984) are normally pear- or drop-shaped and do not deposit iron oxides on their cell surfaces.

Taxonomic Comments

Although the genus *"Siderococcus"* clearly multiplies by a budding process, closer relationships to other budding bacteria do not appear to exist. Phylogenetic relationships, of course, can only be studied when pure cultures become available.

List of species of the genus **"Siderococcus"**

1. **"Siderococcus limoniticus"** Dorff 1934, 9.

li.mo.ni′ti.cus. M.L. n. *limonitum* limonite, a mineral, ferrous oxide; M.L. adj. *limoniticus* of limonite.

The description of the species is the same as that for the genus.

Comment. Dorff (1934) suspected that the organism might be a chemoautotroph because of the large amounts of iron that were oxidized.

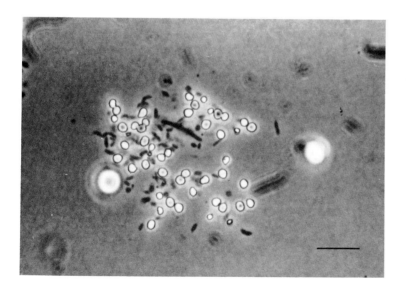

Figure 20.72. *S. limoniticus* from the hypolimnion of Knaack Lake (Wisconsin). This sample was drawn from a 10-m depth in May. The original micrograph shows bright yellowish-orange iron deposits on the cell surfaces. Note budding cells. *Bar*, 10 μm.

Genus IV. "Ochrobium" Perfil'ev in Visloukh 1921, 88

P. HIRSCH, G. A. ZAVARZIN AND O. H. TUOVINEN

O.chro'bi.um. Gr. n. *ochra* yellow-ochre; Gr. n. *bios* life; M.L. neut. n. *Ochrobium* yellow life, referring to color imparted by iron oxides.

Cells ellipsoidal to rod-shaped, 0.5–0.7 × 0.7–1.5 µm, and **partially surrounded by a marginal thickening (capsule) that may be impregnated with iron oxides to a varying degree. The whole organism with capsule may measure 1–3 × 1.5–5 µm. The capsule leaves one end open; through this end the flagellum emerges. This results in a horseshoe appearance. Cells may unite to form aggregates of 2, 4** or, rarely, 8 cells. According to Dubinina and Kusnetzov (1976), "*Ochrobium*" cells may be gas-vacuolated.

This organism is widely distributed in iron-bearing freshwater. **May be capable of anaerobic growth** (Jones, 1981). Not obtained in pure culture.

Type species: "*Ochrobium tectum*" Perfil'ev in Visloukh 1921, 88.

Enrichment Procedures and Comments on the Organism's Ecology

Apparently, "*Ochrobium*" cells are widely distributed in freshwater of low oxygen content. Skuja (1948) found "*O. tectum*" at the end of August in lakes at a 7-m depth, associated with "*Siderocapsa*" species, *Cryptomonas* species and *Macromonas bipunctata*. Skuja (1956) observed this organism in bog waters collected at a 10–17-m depth from Lapland; here it was associated with "*Peloploca pulchra*," "*Pelosigma cohnii*," etc., bacteria considered to be anaerobes. Under these conditions, the "*Ochrobium*" aggregates were "quite vividly motile, rotating evenly." More detailed observations were reported by Jones (1981). "*Ochrobium*"-like bacteria did not have an open capsule and they were never motile. However, all organisms with open capsules had either a discrete nucleus under fluorescence microscope or were motile and showed chlorophyll fluorescence. Such properties are consistent with those of a eucaryote flagellate. "*Ochrobium*"-like bacteria with closed capsules appeared to occupy the redox niche between the NO_3^-/NH_4^+ and the SO_4^{2-}/S^{2-} couples. They did not develop in the presence of NO_3^- or S^{2-}. Furthermore, "*Ochrobium*"-like bacteria wintered over in the sediments of Esthwaite Water, a eutrophic lake in the English Lake District. At the onset of summer, with the water column becoming anoxic, "*Ochrobium*" cells migrated into the free water. Direct counts made on 0.45-µm Millipore membrane filters reached 1.5×10^4 cells ml^{-1}. "*Ochrobium*" cells also grew on agar-coated slides (prepared with 2% water agar) when these were inserted into the upper sediment layer of core samples. After incubation at 8°C for 24 h, cell densities of up to 4.7×10^5 cells/cm^2 were obtained. Jones calculated an apparent in situ generation time of 29 h. Anaerobic growth in the laboratory was obtained.

Differentiation of the genus "Ochrobium" from other closely related taxa

"*Ochrobium*" differs from other bacterial forms with morphological similarity mainly in that it has one open end (horseshoe shape) and, under normal conditions, is motile. This excludes "*Siderocapsa*" and "*Naumanniella*" species.

Dorff (1934) suggested that "*Ochrobium tectum*" might be a flagellate similar to the genus *Pteromonas*. This was denied by Skuja (1956) who pointed out that "*Ochrobium*" cells were smaller than the minimum size known for algae. According to Jones (1981), "*Ochrobium*" development in samples was inhibited by chloramphenicol but was not affected by Acti-Dione, an indication for its procaryotic nature.

Further Comments

The variable degree of deposition of iron oxides onto (into) the "*Ochrobium*" capsule (Skuja, 1948, 1956; Jones, 1981) makes it quite unlikely that this organism is a chemoautotroph gaining energy from the oxidation of ferrous iron. Jones (1981) suggested that iron impregnation of the capsule might only occur after the removal from the (anoxic) natural habitat by contact with oxygen during the microscopic examination.

List of species of the genus "Ochrobium"

1. **"Ochrobium tectum"** Perfil'ev in Visloukh 1921, 88.
tec'tum. L. neut. past part. *tectum* of L. v. *tego* covered.
Its morphology is the same as that described for the genus.

Originally found in the region around Leningrad (U.S.S.R.); later found independently in Sweden by Naumann (1929) and in wells near Berlin by Beger (1949).

E. MAGNETOTACTIC BACTERIA

R. P. BLAKEMORE, N. A. BLAKEMORE, D. A. BAZYLINSKI AND T. T. MOENCH

The magnetotactic bacteria (Blakemore, 1975, 1982) are cells whose swimming direction is influenced by the direction of the local (geo)magnetic field. This phenetic assemblage includes morphologically diverse procaryotes inhabiting marine, brackish water and freshwater environments. Whereas large numbers of these microorganisms can be obtained from natural environments by taking advantage of their magnetic properties (Moench and Konetzka, 1978), only two isolates, both of which are spirilla, exist in axenic culture. Consequently, phylogenetic information based upon measurements of genetic relatedness must await the isolation and taxonomic characterization of additional strains.

The magnetotactic bacteria examined to date share certain characteristics in addition to magnetism. They all appear to be Gram-negative, motile by means of flagella, and microaerophilic. It is possible that nonmotile and, consequently, nonmagnetotactic forms of magnetic bacteria exist or that soil or host-associated forms may eventually be found. However, the magnetic methods which have been used to recover these unusual microorganisms (Blakemore, 1975; Moench and Konetzka, 1978) have selected for aquatic and magnetotactic cells.

Magnetotactic bacteria are morphologically and metabolically diverse. The diversity of magnetotactic cell types is illustrated in Figures 20.73–20.76. We interpret this variability to indicate widespread phylogenetic distribution of the trait. Only one species, *Aquaspirillum magnetotacticum* (Fig. 20.73*d*), has been isolated, grown axenically and taxonomically characterized (Blakemore et al., 1979; Maratea and Blakemore, 1981). Cells of this species are denitrifying (Escalante-Semerena et al., 1980; Bazylinski and Blakemore, 1983a), nitrogen-fixing (Bazylinski and Blakemore, 1983b), obligately microaerophilic, chemoheterotrophic spirilla. A coccoid magnetotactic bacterium containing sulfur (Fig. 20.74*c*) has been proposed as a new species, "*Bilo-*

phococcus magnetotacticus" (T. T. Moench, *Antonie van Leeuwenhoek Journal of Microbiology* in press). Still other forms appear similar to "*Ochrobium*" and other species of "iron bacteria."

An especially fascinating magnetotactic "organism" has been recovered from sediments in Brazil (Farina et al., 1983) and in salt marshes in New England (U.S.A.) (our unpublished results). Each is a highly motile, spherical cell aggregate or microcolony up to approximately 13 μm in diameter (Fig. 20.76, a–c). A smaller type, 3–5 μm in diameter, has also been observed. An aggregate has the appearance of a morula, consisting of a uniform cluster or ball of from 7 to approximately 20, or so, ovoid, magnetic, procaryotic cells, each 0.8–1.4 μm long $\times$ 0.6–0.8 μm wide. Each cell bears numerous flagella along one side and contains numerous (average of 30) magnetosomes somewhat irregular in shape and distribution. Each cell assemblage is extremely motile and swims in a coordinated spinning fashion. It is magnetotactic and swims at speeds of up to 100 μm/s in a unidirectional fashion even when in a homogeneous magnetic field such as the geomagnetic field (e.g., like other magnetotactic bacteria, it is not "pulled" by the field). Upon heating or drying, cell aggregates quickly disintegrate into loose groups of nonmotile, single cells which appear morphologically identical. Thus, the assemblage appears not to be a consortium of more than one microbial species. Both large and small forms have been found in brackish environments containing free H_2S. The "organism" has not been grown in axenic culture but is distinct from any known genus of microorganism.

The permanent magnetic character of magnetotactic bacteria results from a striking and consistent cell structural feature which characterizes the group—the "magnetosome" (Balkwill et al., 1980). In forms in which they have been studied, magnetosomes are enveloped single crystals of the iron oxide magnetite (Frankel et al., 1983; Towe and Moench, 1981; Matsuda et al., 1983; Mann et al., 1984a). Each is a single magnetic domain with a crystal size approximately 400–1000 Å, depending upon the species. Consequently, individual magnetosomes are not evident within cells observed with the light microscope. Their high iron content, however, renders them quite impenetrable by electrons, and even in unstained cells they are easily visualized by means of electron microscopy. The structure and composition of the magnetosome envelope has not been studied. A second iron biomineral, ferrihydrite (5 $Fe_2O_3 \cdot 9H_2O$), is abundant in cells of the magnetotactic spirillum, in a nonmagnetotactic mutant strain of this organism, and in wild type cells physiologically blocked in magnetite formation.

Magnetosomes within a given strain or cell type are homogeneous in grain size and are uniform in shape and arrangement within the cell. The maximum size of the magnetosome within a given bacterial species is limited by an unknown mechanism. The number of magnetosomes per cell, however, can vary in response to culture conditions, including iron supply and dissolved oxygen. For instance, the average number of magnetosomes within cells of a magnetic spirillum varied from 0 to 17 in response to culture pO_2, and optimal numbers were produced under microaerobic conditions (Blakemore et al., 1984).

Within a given sample of magnetotactic bacteria separated from sediments, different cell types may have magnetosomes of different morphology. However, only one morphological type of magnetosome is found in a given cell type, suggesting genetic control of crystal morphology. The known magnetosome types are illustrated in the selection of cell types appearing in Figures 20.73–20.76. Again, it is important to note that the illustrated cells, with the exception of those of *A. magnetotacticum*, have not been grown axenically but have been magnetically separated from natural environments and enrichments and prepared for transmission electron microscopy. Magnetosomes within *A. magnetotacticum* are truncated octahedral prisms (Mann et al., 1984a). Viewed in the horizontal plane, they give various projections similar to those within other types of cells, as is illustrated in Figure 20.73, a–d. Magnetosomes within coccoid cells studied by Mann et al. (1984b) as well as those within an unidentified cell from a pond in Japan (Matsuda et al., 1983) were truncated hexagonal prisms. The lateral projections of these shapes are rectangular with beveled corners, as is illustrated in Figure 20.74, a–d. The prismatic crystals of either the hexagonal or

the octahedral type were oriented with their easy axes of magnetization (the axis lying perpendicular to [111] planes) along the chain axis. The crystal structure and morphology of teardrop or bullet-shaped magnetosomes illustrated by Figure 20.75, a–d, are completely unknown.

In some cell types, the magnetosomes occur in clusters predominantly at one side of the cell. In other species or types, the magnetosomes occur as a string or chain of particles arranged along the motility axis of the cell. The magnetosomes situated at ends of such chains are often smaller (Figs. 20.73 and 20.74). This suggests that magnetosome chains "grow" bidirectionally along their long axis as iron newly transported into the cell is transformed into magnetite. At cell division, magnetosomes, whether in chains or not, normally appear to be partitioned between each daughter cell, although, infrequently, dividing cells have been observed in which one daughter cell has no apparent magnetosomes.

Because they contain magnetosomes, cells of magnetotactic bacteria each have a permanent magnetic moment. The cell magnetic moment interacts with the local geomagnetic field, tending to passively align the cell in the field (Frankel and Blakemore, 1980). Inasmuch as cell orientation and not absolute cell velocity is directly affected by the magnetic field, the observed behavior is a true taxis and not a klinokinesis. The geomagnetic field over most of the earth is inclined from the horizontal (i.e. it has an angle of dip). The vertical component of the local geomagnetic field exerts strong selective pressure on natural populations for cells with a direction of magnetization, tending to direct them downward along the inclined field lines (Blakemore et al., 1980; Frankel and Blakemore, 1980; Blakemore and Frankel, 1981; Frankel et al., 1981). This was first evident with monopolarly flagellated forms which consistently swam forward and in the direction of the magnetic field (i.e. the direction indicated by the north-seeking end of a compass needle); it was further substantiated by field observations which revealed that cells in Southern Hemisphere natural populations were of opposite magnetic polarity to those in the Northern Hemisphere. Consequently, magnetotaxis tends to direct unidirectionally swimming cells downward in each hemisphere. Interestingly, this also applies to the colonial form of magnetotactic bacterium; the aggregates found in Brazil (Farina et al., 1983) swim south and down, whereas those from New England (our unpublished results) swim north and down. Some magnetotactic bacteria are bipolarly flagellated and swim principally along the inclined geomagnetic field lines but in either direction. The direction actually taken at any instant depends not only upon magnetism but also upon other "taxes." Aerotaxis, for instance, has been shown to override magnetotaxis in bipolarly flagellated magnetotactic spirilla (Spormann and Wolfe, 1984). The observed effect of Earth's magnetic field in orienting cells so that they may swim preferentially downward is consistent with their observed natural distribution. These organisms are found in sediments and in the sediment-water interface, not in surface films or the surface microlayer. Because strong selection pressure is exerted upon natural populations for cells of appropriate magnetic polarity, care must be taken in examining sediments for these microorganisms that the appropriate magnetic field direction is used.

As mentioned, magnetosome production appears to be a genetically stable character, i.e. a given cell type produces magnetosomes of a particular morphology and arrangement within the cell. Cultured in the laboratory, nonmagnetic mutants of magnetic spirilla survive many passages without producing magnetosomes. Since this trait can be lost, often abruptly, but with no obvious detrimental effect on cells, and since diverse species or morphological types of bacteria in natural environments possess magnetosomes, it would not be surprising if genes encoding magnetosome formation were clustered and carried on plasmids or insertion elements. Extensive efforts in several laboratories to detect plasmids within magnetotactic spirilla have met with negative results, however.

Several types of magnetotactic bacteria have been studied in sufficient detail to conclude that they are of separate genera. These are, notably, the magnetic spirilla, magnetic coccoid forms and the colonial aggregates of magnetic cells.

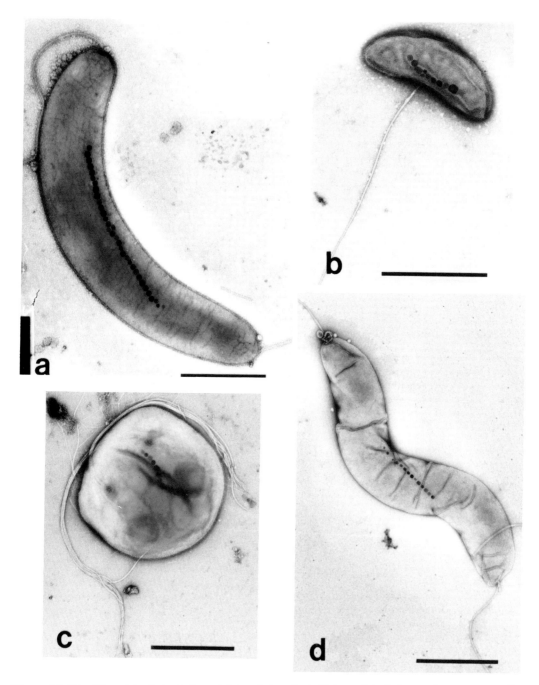

Figure 20.73.   Magnetotactic bacteria containing chains of cuboidal or octahedral magnetosomes, *a–c,* cells are of undescribed species magnetically separated from sediments collected from a Durham, New Hampshire, water treatment plant (*a*), a river in Exeter, New Hampshire (*b*), and Cedar Swamp, Woods Hole, Massachusetts (*c*). *d, A. magnetotacticum* strain MS-1 ATCC 31632. Transmission electron micrographs of negatively stained cells. *Bars,* each 1 μm. (*c* is reproduced with permission from R. P. Blakemore and R. B. Frankel, Scientific American *245:* 58–65, 1981; and *d* is reproduced with permission from D. Maratea and R. P. Blakemore, International Journal of Systematic Bacteriology *31:* 425–455, 1981, ©American Society for Microbiology, Washington, D.C.)

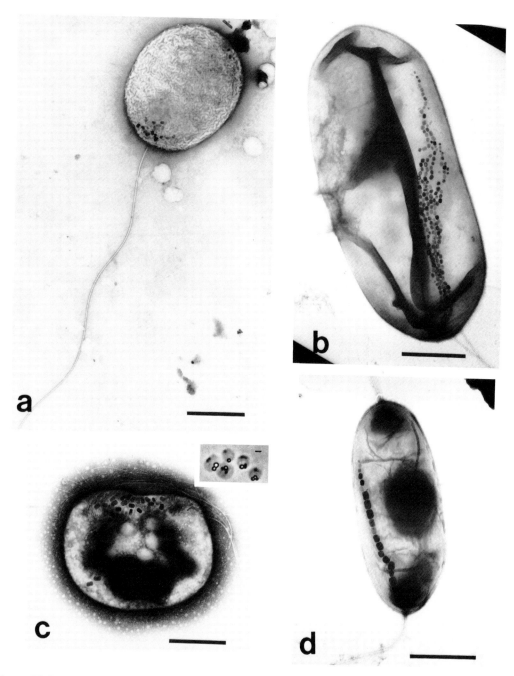

Figure 20.74. Magnetotactic bacteria containing magnetosomes which appear rectangular in the horizontally projected plane. Cells were magnetically separated from sediments collected at a bog in Amherst, New Hampshire (*a* and *b*), a sewage oxidation pond in Bloomington, Indiana *c*), and a river in Exeter, New Hampshire (*d*). Transmission electron micrographs of negatively stained cells. *Bars,* each 1 μm. (*a* is reproduced, with permission, from *Annual Review of Microbiology 36:* 217–238, ©1982 by Annual Reviews Inc. and from R. P. Blakemore; and *c* is reproduced with permission from K. M. Towe and T. T. Moench, *Earth Planet Science Letter 52:* 213–220, 1981.)

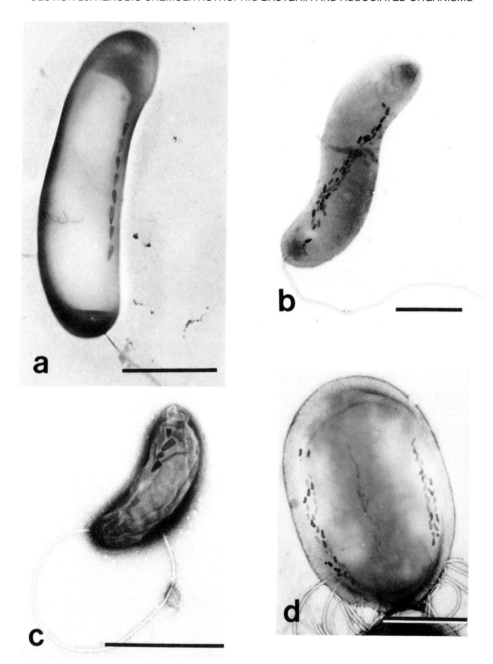

Figure 20.75. Magnetotactic bacteria containing teardrop or bullet-shaped magnetosomes. Cells are of undescribed species collected with magnets from sediments of the Little Styx River, Christchurch, New Zealand (*a*), a river in Exeter, New Hampshire (*b* and *c*), and a bog in Amherst, New Hampshire (*d*). Transmission electron micrographs of negatively stained cells. *Bars,* each 1 μm. (*c* is reproduced with permission from R. P. Blakemore, R. B. Frankel and A. J. Kalmijn, Nature *286:* 384–385, 1980; and *d* is reproduced, with permission, from Annual Review of Microbiology *36:* 217–238, ©1982 by Annual Reviews Inc., and from R. P. Blakemore.)

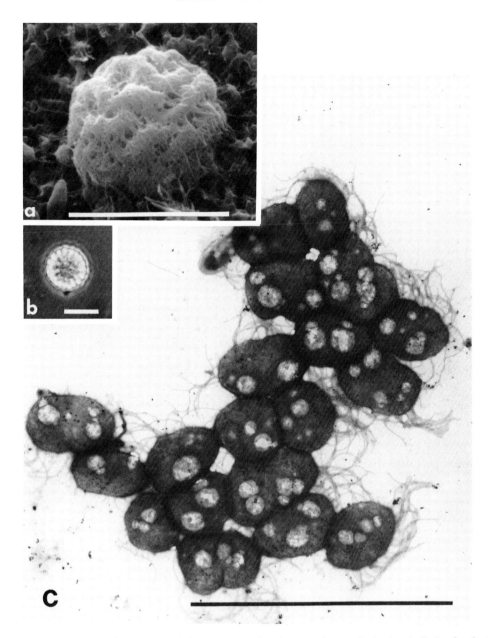

Figure 20.76. A colonial magnetotactic form. *a*, a scanning electron micrograph of a chemically fixed and critical point-dried cell aggregate showing numerous flagella. *b*, a phase-contrast light micrograph showing the overall morphology of this organism which looks like a morula. *c*, a transmission electron micrograph of negatively stained cells of an unfixed aggregate which has disintegrated. Each cell is multiflagellate and contains numerous magnetosomes. *Bars*, each 10 μm. (Reproduced with permission from D. Maratea and D. Bazylinski, unpublished data.)

Key to the identification of the **Magnetotactic Bacteria**

I. Helical cells

Species Aquaspirillum magnetotacticum

II. Coccoid unicells

Genus *"Bilophococcus"*

Genus **Aquaspirillum** *Hylemon, Wells, Krieg and Jannasch 1973, 361**

NOEL R. KRIEG

Aq.ua.spi.ril′lum. L. *aqua* water; Gr. n. *spira* a spiral; M.L. dim. neut. n. *spirillum* a small spiral; *Aquaspirillum* small water spiral.

Rigid, generally helical cells, 0.2-1.4 μm in diameter; however, one species is vibrioid, another consists of straight rods. A **polar membrane** underlies the cytoplasmic membrane at the cell poles in all species so far examined for this characteristic by electron microscopy. Intracellular **poly-β-hydroxybutyrate** is usually formed. Some species form thin-walled **coccoid bodies** which predominate in old cultures. **Motile by polar flagella**, generally **bipolar tufts**; one species is monotrichous, others have a single flagellum at each pole. **Aerobic** to microaerophilic, having a respiratory type of metabolism with oxygen as the terminal electron acceptor; a few species can grow anaerobically with nitrate. The optimum temperature for most species if 30-32°C. Chemoorganotrophic; however, one species is a facultative hydrogen autotroph. **Oxidase-positive.** Usually catalase- and phosphatase-positive. Indole- and sulfatase-negative. Casein, starch and hippurate are not hydrolyzed. **No growth occurs in the presence of 3% NaCl.** A few species can denitrify. Nitrogenase activity occurs in some species, but only under microaerobic conditions. **Carbohydrates are not usually catabolized,** but a few species can attack a limited variety. Amino acids or the salts of organic acids serve as carbon sources. Vitamins are not usually required. Usually occur in **stagnant, freshwater environments**.

The mol% G + C of the DNA ranges from 49 to 66 (T_m).

Type species: *Aquaspirillum serpens* (Müller 1786) Hylemon, Wells, Krieg and Jannasch 1973, 366.

Partial list of species of the genus **Aquaspirillum**

R. P. BLAKEMORE

18. **Aquaspirillum magnetotacticum** Maratea and Blakemore 1981, 454.[VP]

mag.ne.to.tac′ti.cum. Gr. n. *magnes* magnet, comb. form magneto-; Gr. adj. *taktikos* showing orientation or movement directed by a force or agent; *magnetotacticum* capable of orientation with respect to a magnet.

Helical (clockwise) spirilla, 0.2–0.4 × 4.0–6.0 μm, with a tendency to form long chains and coccoid bodies in older cultures; the wavelength is 1–2 μm. Gram-negative. Motile by means of a single flagellum at each pole. Magnetotaxis is displayed by cells cultured at low (~1 kPa) O_2. Each magnetotactic cell contains enveloped magnetite (Fe_3O_4) particles arranged in a chain within the cytoplasm; each enveloped particle (magnetosome) is approximately 40–50 nm on a side. Magnetosomes are of the truncated octahedral prismatic type. Intracytoplasmic granules presumed to be poly-β-hydroxybutyrate are present. Optimal growth occurs at 30°C. This organism is chemoheterotrophic. Microaerophilic. Growth in the presence of KCN is inhibited. This organism denitrifies (see below) but cannot grow anaerobically with nitrate. Does not hydrolyze casein, starch, hippurate, esculin or gelatin. Selenite is not reduced. Hydrogen sulfide is not produced from cysteine. Catalase, oxidase, urease, sulfatase and indole are negative. Oxidase test is faintly positive with toluene-treated cells. Phosphatase is positive. There is no alkaline reaction in litmus milk. This organism grows in the presence of 1% glycine, but growth is inhibited by 1% bile or 1% NaCl. No pigment is produced from aromatic amino acids. A water-soluble fluorescent pigment is not produced. Nitrate is reduced to dinitrogen with transient accumulation of nitrous oxide but without nitrite accumulation. Under nitrogen limitation, dinitrogen is fixed (acetylene is reduced). Ammonia is formed during growth in nitrate-containing medium. A variety of tricarboxylic acid cycle intermediates are used as sole carbon source. Carbohydrates are not used as sole carbon source. Nitrate or ammonium ions are utilized as sole nitrogen source.

The mol% G + C of the DNA is 65 (Bd, T_m).

Isolated by myself at the University of Illinois from sediments collected in Cedar Swamp, Woods Hole, Massachusetts (U.S.A.).

Type strain: strain MS-1 (ATCC 31632). The description for the type strain is the same as that for the species.

A magnetotactic, chemoheterotrophic, microaerophilic, spirillum designated strain MS-2 has been isolated by N. A. Blakemore (personal communication) from the water treatment plant in Durham, New Hampshire (U.S.A.). Cells of this incompletely characterized organism are similar to those of strain MS-1 with respect to their overall nutrition, physiology and morphology and in the characteristics of their magnetosomes. They also have an identical cell outer membrane protein profile (L. C. Paoletti, unpublished observations).

The mol% G + C of the DNA is 63, which is very similar to that of strain MS-1.

Genus **"Bilophococcus"**

T. T. MOENCH

Bi.lo.pho.coc′cus. L. adv. *bis* twice; Gr. n. *lophos* a tuft; Gr. n. *coccus* a berry; N.L. masc. n. *bilophococcus* doubly tufted spherical bacterium.

Spherical cells approximately 1.6 μm in diameter. **Gram-negative. Actively motile** by means of **two adjacent flagellar tufts** of 10–15 flagella each. Forward motion is **continuous** with a **wobbly** characteristic. In the region of the flagellar tufts, a **polar membrane** underlies the cytoplasmic membrane. Iron is precipitated intracellularly as magnetite inclusions (**magnetosomes**). **Magnetotaxis** is exhibited.

---

* **Editorial note:** The description of the genus has been reprinted from Volume I of the *Manual.*

The cytoplasm **contains sulfur. Catalase-negative.** Habitat: microaerobic aquatic sediments. This organism has not been grown in axenic culture.

The mol% G + C of the DNA is 61–62 (Bd).

Type species (monotype): "*Bilophococcus magnetotacticus.*"

Further Descriptive Information

"*B. magnetotacticus*" was originally designated "the magnetococcus" (Moench, 1978; Moench and Konetzka, 1978). It is most commonly observed in microaerophilic freshwater sediments, being found most prevalently in association with sulfurous muds. Cells are coccoid (1.6 ± 0.2 μm) and easily recognized microscopically by the presence of 1–3 refractile bodies (cell anterior), a darkened area (cell posterior), and a distinctive wobbling forward motion and magnetic orientation (Fig. 20.74c).

The refractile bodies are sulfur inclusions which constitute 1.8–9.9% cellular dry weight. Thin sections reveal that the sulfur is enclosed by invaginations of the cytoplasmic membrane (T. T. Moench, *Antonie van Leeuwenhoek Journal of Microbiology* in press; Moench and Konetzka, 1978.)

The darkened area at the posterior portion of the cell corresponds to the accumulated magetite inclusions or magnetosomes which constitute the greatest part of the 3.8 ± 0.3% cellular iron by dry weight. In whole-cell and thin-section transmission electron micrographs, the magnetosomes appear as electron-dense inclusions. Each magnetosome has a hexagonal prism habit (i.e. is a parallelepiped) measuring 99.3 ± 8.7 × 62.3 ± 6.1 nm. These dimensions fall within the theoretical considerations for single-domain magnets (Butler and Banerjee, 1975; Towe and Moench, 1981) and account for the stability of the magnetic dipole moment. Generally, the magnetosomes are localized along the posterior cell membrane in the region between the flagellar tufts. They are enclosed by a triple-layer membrane. It is proposed that the biogenesis of the magnetite crystal occurs at the surface of this membrane at a single nucleation site (Mann et al., 1984).

"*B. magnetotacticus*" is actively motile with a mean velocity of 69 ± 16 μm s^{-1} (Moench and Konetzka, 1978). The positioning of two flagellar tufts near one another results in translational movement with a characteristic wobble. The presence of a stable magnetic dipole moment results in unidirected magnetotaxis in a magnetic field. During such magnetic behavior, the wobble of the cell is most pronounced. The anterior portion of the cell follows a line along the cell axis, while the posterior portion of the cell shifts from side to side about the cell axis.

Forward motion appears continuous and lacks tumbling and random walk pattern motility.

Cell division is proposed to occur longitudinally, resulting in a partitioning of the sulfur bodies, the magnetosomes and one flagellar tuft to each daughter cell (Blakemore, 1982; T. T. Moench, *Antonie van Leeuwenhoek Journal of Microbiology* in press). The only species in this genus, "*B. magnetotacticus*," is ubiquitously found in marine and freshwater sediments.

Enrichment, Isolation and Maintenance Procedures

The procedure for the enrichment and maintenance of "*B. magnetotacticus* consists of overlaying sewage aeration basin sulfurous muds with secondarily treated wastewater and then incubating them at room temperature until an ecological succession occurs (Moench and Konetzka, 1978). After 4–5 weeks, "*Bilophococcus*" was found to be present in the water column in numbers isolatable by using a magnetic collection technique.

An example of this procedure of enrichment is to layer 5 cm of black, sulfurous, aeration basin mud in the bottom of a 2-liter beaker. One liter of secondary effluent is added, and the jar is wrapped with an opaque material to minimize the growth of photosynthetic bacteria in the mud layer. The jar is covered with plastic wrap to prevent evaporation. "*Bilophococcus*" appears to be quite aerotolerant, as it becomes enriched in the water column where H_2S and oxygen levels are apparently optimal. Cultures such as these can be maintained up to a year.

Isolation of the bacterium is accomplished by attaching a bar magnet to the outside of an enrichment vessel with the south pole positioned 5–8 cm above the sediment surface. Cells migrate and accumulate at the magnetic pole and can be removed and studied. The cells enriched and isolated in this manner are 99% "*B. magnetotacticus*" (Moench and Konetzka, 1978). Thus far, no axenic cultures of "*Bilophococcus*" have been obtained.

Taxonomic Comments

"*B. magnetotacticus*" is easily differentiated from both the colorless sulfur-oxidizing genera and other magnetic bacteria because of its unique morphology and motility pattern. Within the colorless sulfur group, only *Thiovulum* species bears any resemblance whatsoever to "*B. magnetotacticus*," but *Thiovulum* exhibits no response to an imposed magnetic field and has both a different distribution of sulfur globules and a translational motility pattern (my own unpublished results).

List of species of the genus "Bilophococcus"

1. "**Bilophococcus magnetotacticus.**"
mag.ne.to.tac′ti.cus. Gr. n. *magnes* magnet; comb. form magneto-; Gr. n. *tacticus* showing orientation or movement directed by an agent or force; N.L. masc. adj. *magnetotacticus* showing oriented movement with respect to a magnet.

The characteristics of the species are the same as those described for the genus.

SECTION 21

Budding and/or Appendaged Bacteria

James T. Staley and John A. Fuerst

The budding and/or appendaged bacteria are a diverse group of morphologically distinctive procaryotes. Many have unusual shapes, have complex life cycles, and divide by budding. Most but not all of these bacteria are unicellular, and many have appendages which are sufficiently prominent that they can be detected by phase-contrast light microscopy.

The appendage may either be *cellular* (i.e. contain cytoplasm), in which case it is termed a **prostheca** (pl. -ae) (Staley, 1968), or it may be *acellular*. An example of a prosthecate bacterium, *Ancalomicrobium adetum,* which has several prosthecae per cell, is shown in Figure 21.1. Thin sections of this bacterium clearly demonstrate that the appendages of the organism contain cytoplasm and are bound by the cell wall (Fig. 21.2). *Caulobacter* and *Asticcacaulis* produce distinctive cross-bands in their prosthecae, a feature that is of deterministic value for this group (Fig. 21.3).

There are two major types of acellular appendages. One type is referred to as a **stalk** (Henrici and Johnson, 1935) because it mediates attachment in such organisms as *Planctomyces* and *Gallionella.* A specimen of *Planctomyces maris* shows a typical fibrillar stalk that is characteristic for this group (Fig. 21.4). Another type of acellular appendage is termed a **spina** (pl. -ae) (Easterbrook and Coombs, 1976) for a select group of as yet unnamed planktonic heterotrophs. This appendage is analogous to a large fimbria, but it is sufficiently wide that when it is stained, it can be

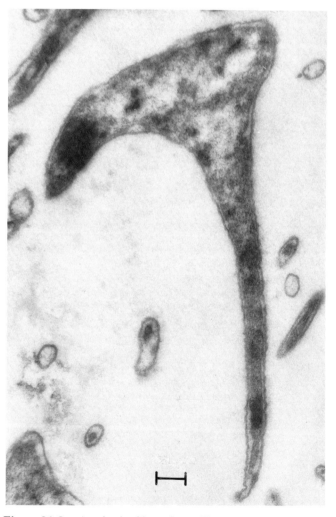

Figure 21.2. *Ancalomicrobium adetum.* Thin section showing a prostheca. Note that the cell envelope extends around the appendage and that the appendage contains cytoplasmic constituents. *Bar,* 0.2 μm. (Reproduced with permission from J. T. Staley, Journal of Bacteriology *95:* 1921-1942, 1968, ©American Society for Microbiology, Washington, D.C.)

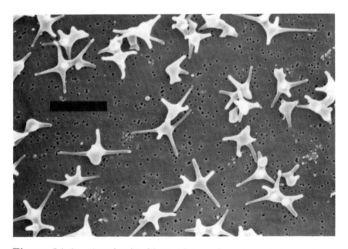

Figure 21.1. *Ancalomicrobium adetum.* Scanning electron micrograph showing the appearance of prosthecae. *Bar,* 5 μm. (Courtesy of A. R. W. van Neerven.)

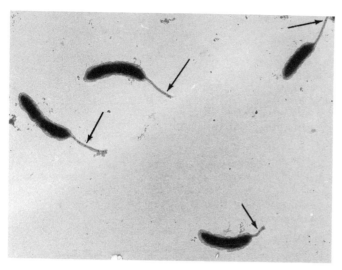

Figure 21.3. *Caulobacter* species. An electron micrograph showing stalked cells with cross-bands (*arrows*). Also see Figure 21.28 in the genus description.

observed by light microscopy. Spinae have characteristic cross-striations when viewed by electron microscopy (see Fig. 21.84).

Still other terms have been used to describe appendages, but these have more restricted definitions that refer to the appendage type of a specific genus or limited group of genera. Thus, the hypha (pl. -ae) is the prostheca of *Hyphomicrobium*, *Hyphomonas*, and *Pedomicrobium*, and a fascicle refers to the multifibrillar bundle of some *Planctomyces* spp. in which an attachment function for a stalk has not been demonstrated.

Attachment is never due to an appendage per se but to a **holdfast** structure (Poindexter, 1964) which is often borne at the tip of an appendage. Many of the bacteria in this section can attach to inanimate substrata, detritus, or other organisms (particularly sheathed bacteria and cyanobacteria) via their holdfast.

A number of bacteria in this group divide by a process termed **budding** rather than by binary transverse fission. Several definitions have been proposed for budding (cf. Staley, 1973a; Hirsch, 1974a; Whittenbury and Dow, 1977; Staley et al., 1981). It is a process of asymmetric polar growth which culminates in cell division. In its most highly developed form, budding results in the de novo synthesis of wall material of the newly formed daughter cell or bud (Fig. 21.5). Labeling studies have been performed for a more thorough understanding of this process in some of these bacteria, such as *Planctomyces* (Tekniepe et al., 1982) and *Seliberia* (Schmidt and Starr, 1984b). Characteristically, a bud develops as a small protuberance at a particular location (i.e. the reproductive pole) on the mother cell and

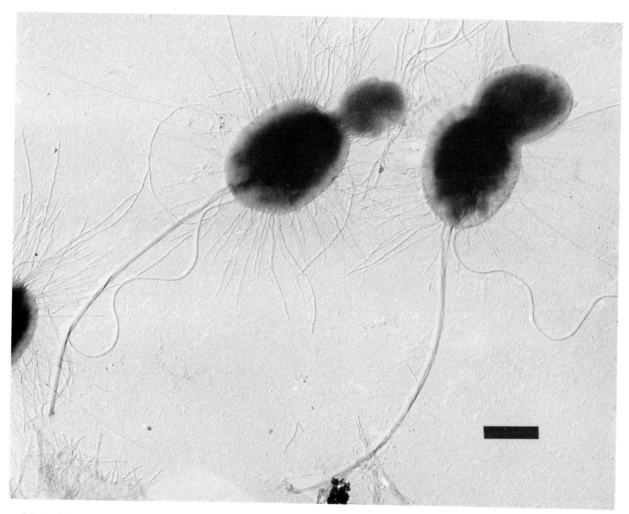

Figure 21.4. *Planctomyces maris.* An electron micrograph showing whole cells. Note that the two cells are producing buds at their non-stalked reproductive poles. Note also the fibrillar nature of the stalks, the numerous fimbriae of the cells, and the subpolar flagellum on each of the mother cells. *Bar,* 0.5 μm.

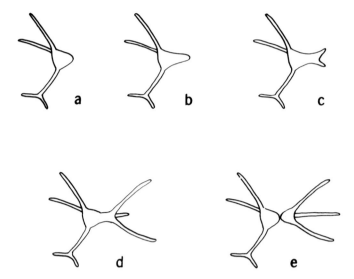

Figure 21.5. A diagram of *Ancalomicrobium adetum,* illustrating the life cycle of this budding bacterium. The mother cell has three appendages, one of which is bifurcated (*a*). Bud formation occurs at the apex of the conical cell (*b*). The bud begins to differentiate (*c* and *d*) and ultimately separates from the mother cell (*e*). Following division, the mother cell, whose appearance after reproduction remains essentially identical with its initial appearance in *a*, will produce another daughter cell from the same location. This process will be repeated again and again as long as conditions are favorable for growth. (Reproduced with permission from J. T. Staley, Journal of Bacteriology *95:* 1921–1942, 1968, ©American Society for Microbiology, Washington, D.C.)

enlarges before separation from the mother cell. The bud becomes the daughter cell, and the mother cell continues to produce additional daughter cells generation after generation, typically at the same location on its surface. Thus, each clone develops a genealogy, and often the oldest cell can be identified because of its unique morphology even after many generations.

Budding and prostheca formation are independent characteristics. Thus, budding occurs in some nonprosthecate bacteria as well as in some prosthecate bacteria. Buds may be formed directly on the cell surface or at the tip of a prostheca, depending upon the genus. Several bacteria in this group have dimorphic life cycles consisting of a motile, undifferentiated daughter cell and an immotile, prosthecate or stalked mother cell.

It is increasingly clear that this section contains an artificial collection of organisms representing at least two and probably several phylogenetically separate groups. For example, research using 16S rRNA oligonucleotide cataloguing procedures indicates that the *Planctomyces* group, which lacks peptidoglycan (König et al., 1984), is a distinct and perhaps either relatively ancient (Stackebrandt et al., 1984) or a rapidly evolving group of the eubacteria (Woese, 1987). Recently, a new order, *Planctomycetales,* and family, *Planctomycetaceae,* have been proposed in recognition of this information (Schlesner and Stackebrandt, 1986). In addition to the genus *Planctomyces,* the genera *Pirella* and *Isosphaera* are members of this new order.

In contrast, the hyphomicrobia belong to the alpha group of the purple photosynthetic bacteria (Moore, 1977; Fox et al., 1980; Stackebrandt, 1985), a result which is consistent with the phenotypic similarities between these organisms and certain budding and, in some cases, prosthecate members of the purple nonsulfur bacterial genera *Rhodomicrobium* and *Rhodopseudomonas.* Interestingly, the genus *Prosthecomicrobium* has also been reported to be a member of this same group of purple bacteria (Stackebrandt, 1985) despite its strong morphological resemblance to *Prosthecochloris* and *Ancalochloris,* two genera of green sulfur bacteria. Further work on informational macromolecules of the bacteria in

Table 21.1.

Characteristics of heterotrophic budding and/or appendaged bacteria that have been grown in pure culture and named[a]

Characteristic	*Hyphomicrobium*	*Hyphomonas*	*Pedomicrobium*	*Ancalomicrobium*	*Prosthecomicrobium*	*Labrys*	*Stella*	*Caulobacter*	*Asticcacaulis*
Prosthecae	+	+	+	+	+	+	+	+	+
Polar or subpolar	+	+	−	−	−	−	−	+	+
Multiple, radiating	−	−	+	+	+	−	−	−	−
Multiple, one plane	−	−	−	−	−	+	+	−	−
Bud formation	+	+	+	+	+	+	+	−	−
Tip of prostheca	+	+	+	−	−	−	−	−	−
Cell surface	−	−	−	+	+	+	+	−	−
Flagella	+	+	+	−	D	−	+	+	+
Gas vacuoles	−	−	−	+	D	−	D	−	−
Stalks (acellular)	−	−	−	−	−	−	−	−	−
Crateriform structures	−	−	−	−	−	−	−	−	−
Peptidoglycan	+	+	?	?	+	?	?	+	?
Obligate aerobes or microaerophiles	−	+	+	−	+	+	+	+	+
Denitrifiers	+	−	−	−	−	−	−	−	−
Facultative anaerobes (fermentative)	−	−	−	+	−	−	−	−[b]	−
Obligate anaerobes	−	−	−	−	−	−	−	−	−
Methanol utilizers	+	−	−	−	D	−	−	−	−
Mol% G + C of DNA	59–65	57–62	62–67	70–71	64–70	68	69–74	62–67	55–61

[a]Symbols: +, 90% or more of strains are positive; −, 90% or more of strains are negative; D, varies from one species to another; and ?, unknown.
[b]See the comment in genus description.

this section is needed to assess more fully their relatedness to one another and to other bacteria.

Some of the bacteria in this group are involved in iron and manganese oxidation and deposition and on that basis could be placed with bacteria in other sections. However, until further information about their true phylogenetic relatedness is available, any changes would be premature and speculative. Indeed, some metal-oxidizing members of the section, such as *Pedomicrobium*, bear such a strong phenotypic resemblance to the hyphomicrobia that it seems likely that they are appropriately classified with them. Furthermore, iron and manganese oxidation and deposition are properties that are widespread among the bacteria and hence do not seem to be significant phylogenetic features beyond the level of the species or genus.

Finally, it is important to realize that budding and/or appendaged bacteria have been placed in other groups because of their nutritional and physiological similarities to nonbudding, nonappendaged bacteria. Thus, the chemolithotrophic bacterium *Nitrobacter winogradskyi* has been classified in Section 20 with the nitrifying bacteria. Likewise, "*Methylosinus*" is a budding bacterium that has been classified with the methanotrophs. Also, several genera of photosynthetic bacteria are prosthecate bacteria and are treated in Section 18. These include the green sulfur bacteria in the genera *Ancalochloris* and *Prosthecochloris,* the purple nonsulfur bacteria in the genus *Rhodomicrobium,* and some members of the genus *Rhodopseudomonas.*

The genera of this section that have been isolated in pure culture are included in Table 21.1 which contains morphological and physiological properties that may assist in their identification. In addition, the following key is used to differentiate all the genera included in this group.

Key to the differentiation of **Budding and/or Appendaged Bacteria**

I. Prosthecate Bacteria
　A. Divide by budding
　　1. Buds produced at tip of prostheca
　　　a. Nonphotosynthetic
　　　　i. Bud lengthens parallel to long axis of prostheca
　　　　　aa. Methylotrophic
　　　　　　　Genus *Hyphomicrobium*, p. 1895
　　　　　bb. Not methylotrophic
　　　　　　　Genus *Hyphomonas*, p. 1904
　　　　ii. Bud lengthens perpendicular to long axis of prostheca
　　　　　　　Genus *Pedomicrobium*, p. 1910
　　　b. Photosynthetic
　　　　　　Genus *Rhodomicrobium* (see Section 18)
　　2. Buds produced on cell surface
　　　a. Nonphotosynthetic
　　　　i. Facultative anaerobic
　　　　　　Genus *Ancalomicrobium*, p. 1914

Table 21.1.—*continued*

Characteristic	*Prosthecobacter*	*Planctomyces*	"*Isosphaera*"	*Ensifer*	*Blastobacter*	*Angulomicrobium*	*Gemmiger*	*Gallionella*	*Seliberia*
Prosthecae	+	−	−	−	−	−	−	−	−
Polar or subpolar	+	−	−	−	−	−	−	−	−
Multiple, radiating	−	−	−	−	−	−	−	−	−
Multiple, one plane	−	−	−	−	−	−	−	−	−
Bud formation	−	+	+	+	+	+	+	−	+
Tip of prostheca	−	−	−	−	−	−	−	−	−
Cell surface	−	+	+	+	+	+	+	−	+
Flagella	−	+	−	+	D	−	−	+	+
Gas vacuoles	−	−	+	−	−	−	−	+	+
Stalks (acellular)	−	+	−	−	−	−	−	+	−
Crateriform structures	−	+	+	+	−	−	−	−	−
Peptidoglycan	?	−	−	−	?	?	?	?	?
Obligate aerobes or microaerophiles	+	+	+	+	+	+	−	+	?
Denitrifiers	−	−	+	?	?	+	−	+	+
Facultative anaerobes (fermentative)	−	−	−	−	+	+	−	−	D
Obligate anaerobes	−	−	−	−	−	−	+	−	−[b]
Methanol utilizers	−	−	−	−	−	+	−	−	+
Mol% G + C of DNA	54–60	50–59	62	63–67	59–69	64–69	59	55	63–66

[a]Symbols: +, 90% or more of strains are positive; −, 90% or more of strains are negative; D, varies from one species to another; and ?, unknown.
[b]See the comment in genus description.

I. PROSTHECATE BACTERIA

A. BUDDING BACTERIA

1. BUDS PRODUCED AT TIP OF PROSTHECA

Genus **Hyphomicrobium** Stutzer and Hartleb 1898, 76[AL*]

P. HIRSCH

Hy.pho.mi.cro'bi.um. Gr. *hyphe* thread; Gr. adj. *micros* small; Gr. masc. n. *bios* life; M.L. neut. n. *Hyphomicrobium* thread-producing microbe.

Cells 0.3–1.2 × 1–3 μm; rod-shaped with pointed ends, or **oval, egg-** or **bean-shaped;** produce **monopolar** or **bipolar filamentous outgrowths** (hyphae or prosthecae) of varying length and 0.2–0.3 μm in diameter, when stained. The hyphae are not septate, but hyphal cytoplasmic membranes show conspicuous constrictions. **Hyphae** may be **truly branched;** secondary branches are rare. Cells stain with carbol fuchsin but stain only feebly with aqueous aniline dyes. Gram-negative and non-acid-fast. Do not form spores.

Multiplication: **daughter cell formation by** a **budding** process at one hyphal tip at a time (Fig. 21.6); mature buds become **motile** as **swarmers,** break off, and may attach themselves to surfaces or other cells to form clumps or **rosettes.** Motility is lost soon after swarmer cell liberation and/or attachment. Older cultures nearly lack motile swarmer cells. **Poly-β-hydroxybutyrate** is stored by most cells, **usually at a** distinct **cell pole.**

Colonies on solid media are **small,** even after prolonged incubation; they are brownish in transmitted light and **bright beige or colorless** in reflected light. Colony surface is shiny or granular, folded or smooth. Older colonies often display concentric rings and change color to darker brown or bright yellow-orange.

Chemoorganotrophic, aerobic. Carbon dioxide is required for growth. **Oligocarbophilic,** i.e. growth can occur on mineral salts media without added carbon sources. Growth may be stimulated by soil extract if the pH remains near neutral. **Good growth with** 0.1–0.2% (w/v) of **one-carbon compounds** such as **methanol** or **methylamine.** NH_4^+ is a good nitrogen source, but organic nitrogen compounds (amino acids) may also be utilized. Do not nitrify.

Mesophilic. Optimum pH: above 7.0, except for one species with a lower optimum.

The mol %G + C of the DNA ranges from **59 to 65** (T_m). Widely distributed in soils and aquatic habitats.

Type species: *Hyphomicrobium vulgare* Stutzer and Hartleb 1898, 76. A viable type culture does not exist.

Further Descriptive Information

The cell morphology may vary with the growth conditions. In media with low nutrient concentrations the hyphae may elongate up to a length of 300 μm. Also, the degree of branching depends on the concentration and type of carbon source present. Some strains have helically twisted hyphae. Stirring laboratory cultures may result in an increased intercalary bud formation in the hyphae.

The number and attachment site of flagella are variable among the nine species described. Most hyphomicrobia that utilize C_1 compounds have one to three subpolar flagella which are easily shed. Cell walls of one strain (B-522) have been analyzed and found to contain α,ε-diaminopimelic acid as well as the other normal components of most Gram-

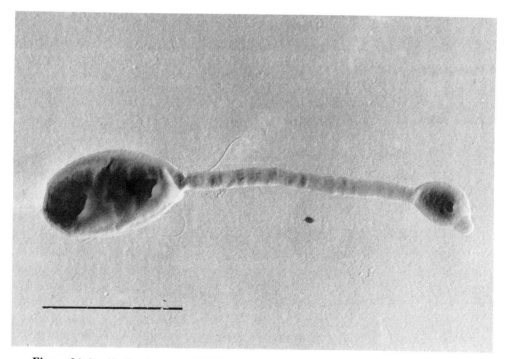

Figure 21.6. *Hyphomicrobium facilis* B-522. Mother cell with hypha and young bud. *Bar,* 1 μm.

---

*AL denotes inclusion of this name on the Approved Lists of Bacterial Names (1980).

melic acid as well as the other normal components of most Gram-negative walls (Jones and Hirsch, 1968). Fine structural studies of a few isolates have shown intracytoplasmic membrane systems which develop under certain growth conditions (Conti and Hirsch, 1965).

Liquid media may become turbid or remain clear upon growth of hyphomicrobia, depending on the strain. In the latter case, growth occurs as a surface pellicle or ring on the glass walls near the medium surface. Attachment to glass walls may be inhibited by light in some strains. Surface pellicles, when shaken, will fall to the bottom of the vessel, especially in older cultures.

Colonies on solid media remain quite small, even after long incubation. Some pellicle-forming strains have colonies of different sizes.

The life cycle of *Hyphomicrobium* species is complicated and has been studied, with special emphasis placed on the budding process (Kingma-Boltjes, 1936; Mevius, 1953) or on bud nucleation and the possibility of obtaining synchronous swarmer cells (Moore and Hirsch, 1973; Matzen and Hirsch, 1982b). As several consecutive buds can be formed on one hyphal tip, the size of the swarmer cells produced increases with mother cell age. Synchronous swarmer cells of nearly identical size were produced by Matzen and Hirsch (1982b) from chemostat cultures that had been transferred to a glass wool-packed column which was then washed with fresh medium for several hours.

All species described so far are methylotrophs; highest growth yields are obtained with methanol and/or methylamine as the carbon and energy source. Most strains are also stimulated by a variety of other carbon sources, but in that case the growth rates and yield are usually substantially lower than with the C_1 compounds (Matzen and Hirsch, 1982a).

Nitrate is reduced anaerobically by some strains; for these organisms a special enrichment technique using KNO_3 and methanol has been described by Attwood and Harder (1972). Vitamin B_{12} stimulates growth of some species (Matzen and Hirsch, 1982a), but there is no absolute vitamin requirement. Most strains grow in the presence of 2.5% NaCl, but they also develop at total salt concentrations of or approaching distilled water. Milk is coagulated by one strain. H_2S evolution and gelatin liquefaction have also been observed in this organism. Some isolates of *Hyphomicrobium* grow at 4–6°C; others can still multiply at 45°C (Hirsch, unpublished observations).

Bacteriophages have been isolated for several strains of *Hyphomicrobium* (Voelz and Gerencser, 1971; Gliesche et al., 1988; Preissner et al., 1988). Mutants with amino acid auxotrophy or resistance against antibiotics have been obtained (Wieczorek and Hirsch, unpublished observations). Serological relationships among some hyphomicrobial isolates have been studied by Powell et al. (1980).

Twelve strains were tested for pathogenicity against mice or guinea pigs; all were avirulent (Famurewa et al., 1983). Genome sizes of three species ranged from 2.13 to 2.62×10^9 mol. wt. (Kölbel-Boelke et al., 1985; Moore and Hirsch, 1973).

Hyphomicrobium species have been isolated from all soil samples tested so far; they were present in nearly all water samples as well (Hirsch and Conti, 1964a; Hirsch and Rheinheimer, 1968). In freshwater habitats they are especially prevalent in the neuston layer, on submerged surfaces and in the upper layer of the sediment, even when this is anaerobic. *Hyphomicrobium* strains were found to grow in temporary puddles, in sewage treatment plants and on the surface of indoor flower pots (Hirsch, 1974a).

Enrichment and Isolation Procedures

A variety of enrichment techniques has been proposed. In all cases, growth of hyphomicrobia is slow; they may be overgrown especially in the presence of other heterotrophic bacteria. Most enrichment cultures for nitrifying bacteria contain hyphomicrobia in large numbers (Stutzer and Hartleb, 1898; Hirsch and Rheinheimer, 1968; Hirsch, 1970). Under oligotrophic conditions and after prolonged incubation the hyphomicrobia usually outcompete other organisms. A slow but successful method consists of allowing a natural water sample to stand at room temperature in the dark for several weeks or months. Eventually, hyphomicrobia become part of the dominant microflora, even in the presence of amoeba. Another method prescribes the addition, to a natural water sample or soil suspension, of methylamine hydrochloride at 3.38 g/l and/or incubation in an atmosphere of methanol. Such an enrichment culture should be monitored frequently in order to determine the optimal time for subculturing. Inoculation of a natural sample into mineral salts medium "337" containing 0.1–0.2% (w/v) of a C_1 compound and dark incubation at 20–25°C for a few weeks usually yields hyphomicrobia in large numbers (Hirsch and Conti, 1965). Improvements of medium "337"[†] resulting in faster growth and higher yields have been reported by Matzen and Hirsch (1982a).

Isolation of rosette-forming and denitrifying *Hyphomicrobium* strains, especially from aquatic sediments, can be achieved by inoculating the sediment sample into a mineral salts medium containing KNO_3 at 5 g/l and up to 0.5% (v/v) of methanol; incubation is anaerobic at room temperature (Attwood and Harder, 1972). It must be stressed, however, that each of these methods will yield different *Hyphomicrobium* species The application of an oligotrophic medium containing low concentrations of peptone, yeast extract and glucose ("PYG") (Staley, 1968) has often yielded *Hyphomicrobium*-like bacteria. But such isolates usually do not grow on C_1 compounds and may be pigmented; they comprise a different group of possibly generic rank.

Once hyphomicrobia occur or predominate in liquid enrichments, they can be isolated and purified by repeatedly streaking these on mineral salts medium "337" and incubating the plates in the dark at 20–25°C. To avoid excessive drying of the plates, they should be placed in plastic bags, or thicker layers of agar should be used. Concerning the purification procedure, it should be remembered that some pellicle-forming strains normally grow with colonies of different size (e.g. NQ-521Gr). Subculturing small or large colonies will again result in both types.

Hyphomicrobium colonies are often tough and coherent; these should be ground properly before being spread on plates. Typical colonies of hyphomicrobia appear dark brown in transmitted light, often with folds and concentric rings. Under reflected light the colonies are shiny and bright beige or even colorless.

Maintenance Procedures

Most hyphomicrobia growing on slants can be kept well at 4–5°C. Subculturing every 5–6 months is sufficient. Lyophilization in skim milk is the optimal method for maintenance of cultures. Suspension in phosphate buffer and sterile glycerol, followed by immediate vortexing and cooling down to −25°C, is another technique; such preparations may be kept for several years in the freezing compartment of a refrigerator. For subculturing, the glycerol suspension is streaked directly onto agar plates. Warming up of the glycerol suspension should be avoided, since rapid death of the cells results.

Procedures for Testing Special Characters

Cell Shape and Morphogenesis

An agar slide culture is prepared with medium "337" and 1.8% Bacto Noble agar. The agar medium is spread thinly over sterile glass slides and allowed to solidify. With the use of sterile coverslips, agar is then cut off to leave two agar squares side by side and separated only by a small ditch. One of the squares is inoculated with a thin *Hyphomicrobium* suspension, the other square receives a small droplet of 0.5% methanol. Both squares are covered with one large coverslip, and the edges can be sealed with vaspar. Spreading of methanol over to the inoculated square should be avoided, since direct contact at this concentration is toxic for the bacteria. Growth and morphogenesis can then be followed over a period of up to 48 h or more.

[†]Composition of medium "337": KH_2PO_4, 1.36 g; Na_2HPO_4, 2.13 g; $MgSO_4 \cdot 7H_2O$, 0.3 g; $(NH_4)_2SO_4$, 0.5 g; $CaCl_2 \cdot 2H_2O$, 1.99 mg; $FeSO_4 \cdot 7H_2O$, 1.0 mg; $MnSO_4 \cdot H_2O$, 0.35 mg; $Na_2MoO_4 \cdot 2H_2O$, 0.5 mg; vitamin B_{12} (if needed), 2.5 µg; distilled water, to 1000 ml; pH, 7.2.

Cell Size Measurements

Only living cells, preferentially those from agar slide cultures, are used for size measurements. Phase-contrast light micrographs are prepared and enlarged 10 times; sizes are measured on these enlargements from at least 50-100 cells, since considerable size variation exists in an asynchronous *Hyphomicrobium* culture.

Growth on Carbon Sources

Medium "337" is used as a base, and sterile-filtered carbon sources are added at 0.1-0.2% (w/v). Most hyphomicrobia are oligocarbophilic; i.e. they may grow (although slowly) on the expense of laboratory contaminations of the air. It is mandatory, therefore, to have control plates inoculated which do not contain the carbon source to be tested; the growth on these controls has to be considered. Growth on plates can be scored after 1, 2 and 4 weeks. Furthermore, oligotrophic growth makes it necessary to subculture, at least two additional times, with the same carbon source to ensure that the growth observed is due to the substrate offered and not to substrate carried over from the inoculum. Liquid carbon utilization tests can be scored by measuring optical density at 650 nm (OD_{650}). However, dramatic changes of cell size and morphology may result from some carbon sources, and light microscopy has to ascertain that this is not the case. Protein determination has been applied widely as a better method for growth estimation (Matzen and Hirsch, 1982a). In all such experiments it is crucial to have a really homogeneous suspension in the initial inoculation procedure.

Growth Stimulation by Vitamins

Growth of some hyphomicrobia is markedly stimulated by vitamin B_{12}, especially in chemostat cultures where the population consists mainly of younger cells. Thus, obviously, nutrient requirements may change with cell age. Static cultures, being asynchronous, contain a large number of older mother cells and do not require B_{12} addition for growth. It was found that application of a vitamin mixture (vitamin solution no. 6) (Van Ert and Staley, 1971) led to less stimulation than the application of B_{12} alone (Matzen and Hirsch, 1982a).

Growth Inhibition by Visible Light

Hyphomicrobia which form surface pellicles rather than growing as turbidity are markedly inhibited by light (Hirsch and Conti, 1964b). Experiments to determine the influence of light on *Hyphomicrobium* growth can be carried out by illuminating (with sunlight) agar plates or liquid cultures. Care must be taken to ensure temperature constancy and avoid water condensation and/or drying out of the plates. In the case of liquid cultures, the light inhibition can be detected by the failure of the bacteria to attach to the glass walls on the illuminated side.

DNA Extraction for the Determination of Base Ratios

Disintegration of hyphomicrobia is often difficult; a variety of techniques have been described for DNA extraction (Gebers et al., 1985). For the "cell mill A" method, 1-2 g of bacterial wet weight are suspended in 20 ml of saline-EDTA supplemented with 1 mg proteinase K. Then 50-g glass beads (0.1 mm diameter) are added, and the precooled mixture is shaken for 5-10 s in an MSK cell homogenizer (Braun, Melsungen, Germany). Cell lysis is completed by adding 20 mg sodium dodecyl sulfate per ml to the suspension. For DNA extraction, $NaClO_4$ and chloroform-isoamyl alcohol are added, and the suspension is shaken for 15 min at 100 rpm. Centrifugation at $1350 \times g$ for 20 min results in a separation of the emulsion into two layers, from which the nucleic acids can be precipitated. This is followed by a 45-min ribonuclease treatment and by a 2-h treatment with proteinase K (200 µg/ml) at 37°C. We then add 1 volume of phenol saturated with $1 \times SSC$ (0.15 M NaCl plus 0.015 M Na_3-citrate, pH 7) and 0.1 volume of chloroform-isoamyl alcohol and agitate the preparation for 10 min at 100 rpm. Centrifugation at $27,000 \times g$ for 20 min results in the separation of the emulsion into three layers, the upper one of which is used for the precipitation of DNA by ethanol (Gebers et al., 1986).

In some cases, a similar method described by Gebers et al. (1981) and called the "enzyme A" method may yield better results.

Differentiation of the genus **Hyphomicrobium** from other closely related taxa

All *Hyphomicrobium* species described so far will grow with C_1 compounds, especially methanol, although this was not mentioned in the first description of the type species, *H. vulgare,* which grew well on formate. C_1 compounds do not support growth of any of the other genera listed in Table 21.2. Cell shape, arrangement of the bud on the hyphal tip, and the tapering of prosthecae are the best differential characters for the group of hyphal, budding bacteria. It should be pointed out, however, that the cell shape can vary with the carbon source, growth temperature, nutrient concentration, etc.

Natural samples may contain other organisms which superficially resemble *Hyphomicrobium* species. *Achromatium oxaliferum* from acid bog lakes undergoes constrictive division, and its umbilical cord which holds the two daughter cells together may be mistaken for a thin hypha (Hirsch, 1974a). Fell (1966) described the *Sterigmatomyces* species, a true fungus which has a surprising resemblance to hyphomicrobia, except that the cells are much larger and usually carry true vacuoles.

Taxonomic Comments

The genus *Hyphomicrobium*—considered monospecific until recently—has been defined mainly by morphological characters and the conspicuous life cycle. Consequently, many authors named their isolates *H. vulgare* because they saw mother cells, hyphae and motile swarmer cells (Kingma-Boltjes, 1936; Mevius, 1953; Zavarzin, 1961a; Hirsch and Conti, 1964a; Shishkina and Trotsenko, 1974; Lebedinskii, 1981). Several authors have already noted substantial morphological differences among their isolates (Hirsch and Conti, 1964a; Lebedinskii, 1981), and it became increasingly clear that "*H. vulgare*" apparently was composed of several different species. A detailed study has been carried out on the taxonomy of some 80 hyphomicrobia with the ability for C_1 utilization (Hirsch, manuscript in preparation). A computer analysis of these

strains carried out by R. Colwell revealed the presence within the strain matrix of 8 different groups separated by similarity values of 50-65% S (Colwell and Hirsch, manuscript in preparation). This may, indeed, be an indication of the need for separation on a higher level than that of species. A confirmation of these results came from DNA/DNA hybridization data obtained with 19 *Hyphomicrobium* strains (see Table 21.6) (Gebers et al., 1986). Those strains which fell within the computer-selected groups showed high homology (86-100%); homology between members of different groups was in most cases below 10%. Differences among the species of *Hyphomicrobium* shown in Tables 21.3-21.5 concern morphological, physiological and ecological characteristics.

In culture collections a large number of *Hyphomicrobium*-like bacteria exist which form hyphae and buds from mother cells and which cannot usually grow with C_1 compounds. These require at least low concentrations of peptone, yeast extract, etc. In some cases such organisms have been called "*Hyphomonas*," but much information is still lacking on the properties of such strains. Base ratios of these "organic hyphomicrobia" may be lower than those of the C_1 hyphomicrobia (Gebers et al., 1985).

Hyphomicrobium neptunium Leifson 1964, 249 was isolated from seawater and does not resemble C_1 hyphomicrobia other than by its morphology. Recently, this organism has been compared with *Hyphomonas* species (Moore and Hirsch, 1972; Hirsch, 1974a, b; and Weiner et al., 1985), and Moore et al. (1984) transferred *Hyphomicrobium neptunium* to the genus *Hyphomonas*.

A bacterium isolated from seawater by Weisrock and Johnson (1966) and supposedly resembling hyphomicrobia was described as *Hyphomicrobium indicum*. It has already been pointed out by Hirsch (1974a, b) that there were substantial differences between this facultatively anaerobic organism and the type species, *Hyphomicrobium vulgare*. The organism forms acid from sugars, is indole-, nitrate-, and H_2S-positive, and

Table 21.2.

Differentiation of the genus **Hyphomicrobium** *from other closely related genera[a]*

Characteristic	Hyphomicrobium	Hyphomonas	Pedomicrobium	Bacterium T[b]	Bacterium D[c]	Ancalomicrobium	Prosthecomicrobium
Cells ovoid, pear- or bean-shaped	+	+	+	+	−	−	+
Cells nearly spherical	−	+	−	−	−	−	−
Cells nearly tetrahedral	−	−	−	−	+	+	−
Hyphae formed regularly	+	+	+	+	+	−	−
Prosthecae normally tapering	−	−	−	−	−	+	+
Bud elongates with long axis of hypha	+	+	−	+	+	−	−
Bud elongates perpendicularly to hyphal long axis	−	−	+	−	−	−	−
C₁ compounds support growth	+	−	−	−	−	−	−
Moderately thermophilic and halophilic	−	−	−	−	+	−	−
Fe and/or Mn are oxidized	v	−	+	−	−	−	−
May possess gas vesicles	−	−	−	−	−	+	+

[a]Symbols: +, 90% or more of strains are positive; −, 90% or more of strains are negative; and v, variable, depending on growth conditions.
[b]Data are from Eckhardt et al. (1979).
[c]Data are from Hirsch (1980).

Table 21.3.

Characteristics differentiating the species of the genus **Hyphomicrobium**[a]

Characteristic	1. H. vulgare[b]	2. H. vulgare IFAM MC-750	3. H. aestuarii IFAM NQ-521Gr	4. H. hollandicum IFAM KB-677	5. H. facilis IFAM H-526	5a. H. facilis subsp. tolerans IFAM I-551	5b. H. facilis subsp. ureaphilum IFAM CO-582	6. H. zavarzinii IFAM ZV-622	7. H. coagulans 10-2	8. H. methylovorum KM-146
Mother cells bean-shaped	−	−	+	−	−	−	−	−	−	−
Mother cells oval or pear-shaped	+	+	−	+	+	+	+	+	+	+
Rosette formation	−	−	−	−	−	−	−	+	−	−
Pellicles formed on liquids	v	−	+	v	−	−	−	v	+	−
Optimum pH:>7.0	−	−	−	−	−	−	−	−	+	−
Growth with peptones	−	−	+	−	−	+	−	+	+	NT
Growth with acetate	+	+	+	−	(+)	−	−	(+)	−	−
Gelatin liquefied, milk coagulated	−	−	−	−	−	+	+	−	+	+
Origin: soil	+	+	−	−	+	+	+	+	+	+
Mol% G + C of DNA (T_m)	NT	61	64	62	59	59	60	65	NT	61

[a]Symbols: −, 90% or more of strains are negative; +, 90% or more of strains are positive; v, variable, depending on growth conditions; NT, not tested; and (+), growth stimulation weak but significant.
[b]Data are from Stutzer and Hartleb (1898).

Table 21.4.
Morphological characteristics of the species of the genus **Hyphomicrobium**[a]

Characteristic	1. *H. vulgare*[b]	2. *H. vulgare* IFAM MC-750	3. *H. aestuarii* IFAM NQ-521Gr	4. *H. hollandicum* IFAM KB-677	5. *H. facilis* IFAM H-526	5a. *H. facilis* subsp. *tolerans* IFAM I-551	5b. *H. facilis* subsp. *ureaphilum* IFAM CO-582	6. *H. zavarzinii* IFAM ZV-622	7. *H. coagulans* 10-2	8. *H. methylovorum* KM-146
Mother cells oval, pear- or drop-shaped	+	+	−	+	+	+	+	+	+	+
Mother cells bean-shaped	−	−	+	−	−	−	−	−	−	−
Mother cell width 0.5–1.2 µm	+	+	+	+	+	+	+	+	+	−
Mother cell width 0.3–0.65 µm	−	−	−	−	−	−	−	−	−	+
Mother cell length (average in µm)	1–3[b]	2.00	1.64	1.66	2.00	1.93	1.90	1.78	1.2–2.0	0.5–1.2
Flagella polar	NT	−	−	−	−	−	−	−	+	−
Flagella lateral	NT	−	−	−	−	−	−	−	−	+
Flagella (1–3) subpolar	NT[c]	+	+	+	+	+	+	+	−	−
Mother cells with polar holdfast	−	−	−	−	−	−	−	+	−	−
Rosette formation or cell clumping	C	C	C	C	−	−	−	R	C	−
Growth as turbidity or pellicle	v	T	P	v	T	T	T	v	P	T
Older cells yellow	−	−	−	−	−	−	−	−	+	+
Isolated from soil, water or sewage	S	S	W	Sw	S	S	S	S	S	S

[a]Symbols: +, 90% or more of strains are positive; −, 90% or more of stains are negative; NT, not tested; C, cell clumping; R, rosette formation; v, variable, depending on growth conditions and culture age; T, turbidity; P, pellicle; S, soil; W, water; and Sw, sewage.
[b]Data are from Stutzer and Hartleb (1898), from stained preparations.
[c]Motility was observed.

deaminates phenylalanine. It is psychrotrophic, requires 50–100% seawater, and lacks true budding and hyphal branching.

The mol% G + C of the DNA is 40 for "*Hyphomicrobium indicum*," which is also in contrast to all other, true hyphomicrobia, where the range is 59–65. This bacterium can no longer be included in the genus *Hyphomicrobium*.

A budding bacterium labeled "*Hyphomicrobium variabile*" is available from culture collections; evidently it is a patented strain, and information on its properties is lacking.

The definition of the genus *Hyphomicrobium* has been hampered seriously by the lack of a type culture; *H. vulgare* as described by Stutzer and Hartleb (1898) no longer exists. A search for a neotype culture has been difficult, since the tests described in the 1898 publication can only partly be used or checked at the present time. Within the matrix of some 80 C_1 hyphomicrobia a strain was found with properties essentially identical with those of *H. vulgare* (IFAM MC-750). This strain also showed a high similarity to the hypothetical median organism of these hyphomicrobia (Colwell and Hirsch, manuscript in preparation). It is proposed, therefore, to accept this strain as the neotype culture for the genus *Hyphomicrobium* (Hirsch, manuscript in preparation). DNA/DNA hybridization studies of 19 hyphomicrobia indicated at least weak relationships between IFAM (Institut für Allgemeine Mikrobiologie, Kiel, Germany) MC-750 and *H. aestuarii* (18–24% homology), *H. zavarzinii* (14%), *H. hollandicum* (11–12%), and *H. facilis* (4–11%) (Gebers et al., 1986; and Table 21.6).

Further Comments

Hyphomicrobium species have been investigated for phospholipids (Goldfine and Hagen, 1968), hopanoids (Rohmer et al., 1984), ubiquinones (Köhler and Schwartz, 1981), cytochromes (Hirsch, unpublished observations) and poly-β-hydroxybutyrate (Jacobsen, G., M.S. thesis, University of Kiel, 1975).

Acknowledgments

Donation of cultures by M. Feil, C. Gliesche, W. Harder, T. Y. Kingma-Boltjes, E. Leifson, M. Macpherson-Kraviec, G. T. Sperl, B. Speralski, Y. Trotsenko, R. Weiner, G. A. Zavarzin and many others are gratefully acknowledged. Critical discussions with R. Colwell, C. Dow, R. Gebers, W. Harder, T. Roggentin and R. Weiner helped in organizing this material. This work would not have been possible without the able technical assistance of G. Maisch, A. Graeter, B. Hoffmann, M. Beese and K. Lutter-Mohr.

Further Reading

Harder, W., and M.M. Attwood. 1978. Biology, physiology and biochemistry of hyphomicrobia. Adv. Microb. Physiol. *17*: 303–359.
Moore, R.L. 1981. The biology of *Hyphomicrobium* and other prosthecate, budding bacteria. Annu.Rev. Microbiol. *35*: 567–594.
Moore, R.L. 1981. The genera *Hyphomicrobium*, *Pedomicrobium*, and *Hyphomonas*. *In* Starr, Stolp, Trüper, Balows and Schlegel (Editors), The Prokaryotes. A Handbook on Habitats, Isolation, and Identification of Bacteria. Springer-Verlag, Berlin, pp. 480–487.

Table 21.5.

Physiological properties of species of the genus **Hyphomicrobium**[a]

Property	1. H. vulgare[b]	2. H. vulgare IFAM MC-750	3. H. aestuarii IFAM NQ-521Gr	4. H. hollandicum IFAM KB-677	5. H. facilis IFAM H-526	5a. H. facilis subsp. tolerans IFAM I-551	5b. H. facilis subsp. ureaphilum IFAM CO-582	6. H. zavarzinii IFAM ZV-622	7. H. coagulans 10-2	8. H. methylovorum KM-146
Carbon sources										
Formate	+	+	+	+	(+)	+	+	+	+	(+)
Acetate	+	+	+	−	(+)	−	−	(+)	−	−
n-Butyrate	NT	+	(+)	−	−	+	+	+	NT	NT
Lactate	+	−	+	+	+	−	−	−	−	−
Succinate	+	+	+	+	−	−	−	−	NT	−
Ethanol	NT	−	+	−	(+)	−	(+)	+	+	−
Glycerol	+	+	+	+	+	+	+	+	NT	−
Amygdalin	NT	+	−	+	(+)	−	−	(+)	NT	NT
Peptones	−	−	+	−	−	+	−	+	+	NT
N-Acetylglucosamine	NT	+	(+)	+	+	+	(+)	−	NT	NT
Formamide	NT	−	+	−	−	−	−	−	NT	+
Aspartate	NT	−	−	+	−	−	−	+	+	+
Asparagine	+	(+)	(+)	−	−	−	−	−	NT	NT
Oligocarbophilic	+	+	+	+	+	+	+	+	NT	−
Nitrate reduction	+[c]	+	+	−	−	−	−	+	−	−
Growth in presence of 2.5% NaCl	+	+	+	−	+	+	+	+	NT	NT
Growth at 5°C	NT	−	−	−	+	−	−	−	NT	−
Growth at 15°C	+	+	+	−	+	+	+	+	NT	+
Growth at 37°C	NT	+	+	+	+	+	+	+	NT	−
Growth at 45°C	NT	−	+	−	−	+	+	−	NT	−
Optimum pH:>7.0	NT	+	+	+	+	+	+	+	−	+
Optimum pH:~6.0	NT	−	−	−	−	−	−	−	+	−
Inhibition by visible light	NT	−	+	+	−	−	−	+	NT	NT
Growth stimulation by vitamin B_{12}	NT	−	−	−	+	−	−	−	NT	+
Gelatin liquefaction	−	−	−	−	−	−	−	−	+	−
Milk coagulation	NT	−	−	−	−	−	−	−	+	NT
H_2S evolution	NT	−	−	−	−	−	−	−	+	−
α-Hemolysis of sheep blood	NT	+	−	−	−	−	+	+	NT	NT
Genome size mol. wt. ($\times 10^9$)[d]	NT	2.13	2.62	2.43	NT	NT	NT	NT	NT	NT
Mol% G + C of DNA (T_m)	NT	61	64	62	59	59	60	65	NT	61

[a]Symbols: +, 90% or more of strains are positive; (+), growth stimulation weak but significant; −, 90% or more of strains are negative; and NT, not tested.

[b]Data are from Stutzer and Hartleb (1898).

[c]There was anaerobic growth with KNO_3, but nitrate reduction was considered to be negative.

[d]Data are from Kölbel-Boelke et al. (1985).

Table 21.6.
Levels of DNA/DNA homologies of **Hyphomicrobium** *species[a]*

Species	IFAM no.	ATCC no.	Mol% G + C of DNA[b]	% homology with labeled DNA from				
				Mc-750	NQ-521Gr	EA-617[c]	B-522	ZV-622
H. vulgare[T] (neotype)	MC-750	27500	61.38	100	4		2	3
H. aestuarii[T]	NQ-521Gr	27483	64.11	18	100	101	5	9
H. aestuarri	EA-617		63.46	20	110	100	2	
H. aestuarii	MEV-533Gr	27488	64.68	24	103	70	4	
H. aestuarri	WH-563		63.09	19	92	102	4	
H. facilis[T]	H-526	27485	59.53	5		3	88	
H. facilis	B-522	27484	59.34	4	0	3	100	2
H. facilis	F-550		59.91	5			106	
H. facilis subsp. *tolerans*[T]	I-551	27489	59.40	5	1		86	1
H. facilis subsp. *tolerans*	CO-558	27491	59.78	7			91	
H. facilis subsp. *ureaphilum*[T]	CO-582	27492	60.54	11	1		87	2
H. zavarzinii[T]	ZV-622		64.8[d]		8			100
H. zavarzinii	ZV-580		61.77	14		11	5	91
H. hollandicum[T]	KB-677	27498	62.41	12	3	10	4	4
H. hollandicum	MC-651	27497	62.91	11				

[a]Data are from Gebers et al. (1986).
[b]Data are from T_m determinations (Gebers et al., 1985).
[c]Data are from Moore and Hirsch (1972).
[d]Data are from Bd determinations (Mandel et al., 1972).

Differentiation of the species of the genus **Hyphomicrobium**

The differential characteristics of the species of *Hyphomicrobium* are indicated in Table 21.3, morphological characteristics of the species are listed in Table 21.4, and physiological properties are listed in Table 21.5.

List of species of the genus **Hyphomicrobium**

1. **Hyphomicrobium vulgare** Stutzer and Hartleb 1898, 76.[AL]

vul.ga´re. L. neut. adj. *vulgare* common.

Mother cells oval, pear-, or drop-shaped, 0.5–1.2 × 1–3 µm, with hyphae of varying lengths and a diameter of 0.2–0.3 µm (up to 0.4 µm when stained). In liquids, cells do not form rosettes; growth may occur as turbidity or (rarely) as pellicle and turbidity. Swarmer cells with one to three subpolar flagella. Colonies remain small even after long incubation, colorless or beige, in transmitted light brownish. Colony surface shiny but granular, the edge is wavy.

Chemoorganotrophic, aerobic, oligocarbophilic. Grow well with methanol, methylamine·HCl, formate, acetate, *n*-butyrate, isovalerate, propionate, lactate (except for MC-750), isobutanol, glycerol, L-arabinose, D-mannose, D-melibiose, raffinose, dextrin, amygdalin, aesculin, D-glucosamine, *N*-acetylglucosamine, dilute human urine, succinate and asparagine. Growth is slow but stimulated by pyruvate, α-oxoglutarate, β-hydroxybutyrate, oxalate, galacturonate, chitin, lactose and D-maltose. Most amino acids are inhibitory. The type strain grew well with propionate, isobutyrate, valerate and mannitol. It did not grow with fructose or sucrose.

Nitrogen sources utilized (in the order of growth stimulation) are: NH_4^+, NO_3^-, NO_2^- and ureate. Do not use urea or fix N_2, although slow oligonitrophilic growth has been observed. Do not nitrify. Anaerobic growth occurs in the presence of NO_3^-, but NO_2^- has not been detected. There is slow growth on sheep blood agar.

Strain MC-750 is inhibited by 30-µg disks each of kanamycin, neomycin and novobiocin and 10 µg of streptomycin. It tolerates 5.5% NaCl, but growth is retarded at this concentration. The pH optimum is between 6.5 and 7.5, the temperature range for growth is 15–37°C. MC-750 is catalase- and cytochrome oxidase-positive, sheep blood is hemolyzed (α-hemolysis), and most cells form poly-β-hydroxybutyrate as a storage product. MC-750 is not pathogenic for mice and guinea pigs.

Habitat: soil. The neotype strain came from construction soil.

The mol% G + C of the DNA is 61.4 (IFAM MC-750; T_m).

Genome size: 2.13×10^9 (Kölbel-Boelke et al., 1985).

Type strain: the original type strain no longer exists; a neotype culture is being proposed: IFAM MC-750 (ATCC 27500).

2. **Hyphomicrobium vulgare** (neotype strain IFAM MC-750; ATCC 27500).

3. **Hyphomicrobium aestuarii** sp. nov.

ae.stu.a´ri.i. L. n. *aestuarium* estuary; M.L. gen. n. *aestuarii* of the estuary.

Mother cells bean-shaped, often with short hyphae; the bud is also bean-shaped but bent at a 90° angle from the mother cell. Cell sizes: mother cells 0.6 (0.5–1.0) µm wide and 1.6 (0.6–5.0) µm long. Older hyphae branched. Swarmers with one to three subpolar flagella. Cells do not form rosettes but clump easily and grow as surface pellicles in liquids.

Shaking precipitates the pellicle. In liquids, growth occurs also on the glass surface near the top of the vessel. Attachment of swarmer cells to the glass walls is inhibited by light. Colonies on solid media brownish, strongly folded irregularly and often with concentric rings, very cohesive.

Chemoorganotrophic, aerobic, oligocarbophilic. Grow well with methanol, methylamine·HCl, formate, formamide, dilute human urine, acetate, pyruvate, malate, ethanol and acetamide. Growth is stimulated but slow with n-butyrate, isovalerate, lactate, α-oxoglutarate, succinate, crotonate, β-hydroxybutyrate, oxalate, glucuronate, ethanol, n-propanol, isobutanol, formaldehyde, glycerol, chitin and Bacto peptone. Also stimulatory (as C sources) are: d,l-aspartate, l-asparagine and N-acetylglucosamine.

Nitrogen sources utilized for growth: NH_4^+, NO_3^- and urea; the organisms are oligonitrophilic. There is slow growth on Bacto peptone with methylamine·HCl added and on sheep blood agar, but there is no hemolysis.

Inhibited by 30 µg each of kanamycin, neomycin, tetracycline and erythromycin and 10 µg of streptomycin (all administered as disks). Grow well in the presence of 3.5% NaCl and faintly in the presence of 5.5% NaCl. Temperature range: 5–45°C. Optimum pH: 6.5–7.5. Inhibited by visible light. With methanol and KNO_3 there is anaerobic growth and gas formation; grow anaerobically with methylamine in the presence of thioglycolate. Cytochrome oxidase- and catalase-positive, gelatin is not liquefied. Not pathogenic for mice or guinea pigs.

Habitat: Isolated from brackish water of the Elbe River estuary near Cuxhaven, West Germany (Mevius, 1953) and from harbor water of Woods Hole, Massachussetts (Hirsch and Rheinheimer, 1968). Originally present in enrichments of nitrifiers.

The mol% G + C of the DNA is 64.1 (strain IFAM NQ-521Gr).

Genome size: 2.62×10^9 (Kölbel-Boelke et al., 1985).

Type strain: IFAM NQ-521Gr (ATCC 27483).

Additional strains: IFAM MEV-533, MEV-533Gr (ATCC 27488), IFAM WH-563, IFAM EA-617, IFAM EN-616, IFAM NQ-521 and IFAM NQ-528.

Further comments: With the exception of strain IFAM WH-563, all of these strains are descendants of the strain "B" which was originally isolated by Mevius (1953).

4. Hyphomicrobium hollandicum sp. nov.

hol.lan'di.cum. M.L. neut. adj. *hollandicum* pertaining to the Netherlands.

Mother cells oval or pear-shaped, 0.70 (0.6–0.8) µm wide and 1.66 (1.5–3.5) µm long. Older hyphae branched. Swarmer cells subpolarly flagellated. Growth in liquid media as pellicle or turbidity; cells may tend to clump. Colonies on solid media are brownish in transparent light and beige in reflected light with entire edges and shiny.

Chemoorganotrophic, aerobic, oligocarbophilic. Grow well with methanol, methylamine·HCl, formate, glycerol, cellobiose, raffinose, dextrin, amygdalin, esculin, N-acetylglucosamine, and ureate. Growth is stimulated with isovalerate, pyruvate, lactate, succinate, oxalate, isobutanol, formaldehyde, L-sorbose, D-maltose, chitin, d,l-aspartate, D-glucosamine, and dilute urine.

Nitrogen sources utilized are: NH_4^+, NO_2^-, NO_3^-. The organisms grow slowly without added nitrogen source, i.e. oligonitrophilically. Strain IFAM KB-677 is inhibited by 30 µg each of kanamycin, neomycin and tetracycline. There is no growth in the presence of 2.5% NaCl. Temperature range: 25–37°C. Optimum pH: >7.5. Strain KB-677 is slightly inhibited by visible light. Catalase- and cytochrome oxidase-positive, gelatin liquefaction and hemolysis-negative. Poly-β-hydroxybutyric acid is formed as a storage product. Not pathogenic for mice or guinea pigs.

Habitat: Strain IFAM KB-677 was obtained from T. Y. Kingma-Boltjes, who isolated it from sewage.

The mol% G + C of the DNA is 62.4 (T_m; strain KB-677).

Genome size: 2.43×10^9 (Kölbel-Boelke et al., 1985).

Type strain: IFAM KB-677 (ATCC 27498).

Further comments: Strain IFAM MC-651 (ATTC 27 497) is related and was isolated from soil by M. Macpherson-Kraviec.

5. Hyphomicrobium facilis sp. nov.

fa'ci.lis. L. adj. *facilis* ready, quick.

Mother cells pear- or drop-shaped, 0.95 (0.6–1.5) µm wide and 2.00 (0.9–6.0) µm long; on some media, hyphae are richly branched and often bipolar. Swarmer cells with one to three subpolar flagella. Growth in liquid media as turbidity; on solid media, colonies are light brownish to beige with a smooth and shiny surface and entire edges. Vigorous stirring of liquid cultures may result in intercalary bud formation in hyphae. Chemoorganotrophic, aerobic.

Grow well with methanol, methylamine·HCl, N-acetylglucosamine and gelatin (strain IFAM B-522). Growth is significantly stimulated by formate, acetate, lactate, α-oxoglutarate, succinate, β-hydroxybutyrate, oxalate, glucuronate, ethanol, glycerol, amygdalin, chitin, and poly-β-hydroxybutyrate (*Bacillus megaterium*). Oligocarbophilic. Growth is also stimulated significantly by d,l-leucine, d,l-lysine and d,l-phenylalanine. There is no growth in dilute human urine.

Nitrogen sources utilized: NH_4^+, NO_3^-, urea and (slow) Bacto peptone. Slow growth oligonitrophilically. There is faint growth on sheep blood agar but no hemolysis. Inhibited by 30 µg each of kanamycin, neomycin, tetracycline and erythromycin and 10 µg streptomycin. There is slow growth in the presence of 3.5% NaCl. Temperature range: 5–37°C. Optimum pH: 6.5–7.0. Light does not inhibit growth. Grow anaerobically with methylamine·HCl and thioglycolate; denitrification-negative; catalase- and cytochrome oxidase-positive. Gelatin is not liquefied and poly-β-hydroxybutyrate is formed as a storage product. Lysine decarboxylase-negative.

Not pathogenic for mice or guinea pigs.

Habitat: soil.

The mol% G + C of the DNA is 59.5 for strain IFAM H-526 and 59.3 for strain IFAM B-522.

Genome size: 2.35×10^9 (strain IFAM B-522).

Type strain: IFAM H-526 (ATCC 27485).

Additional strains: IFAM D-524, E-525, G-527, K-529, L-530 and B-522 (ATCC 27484).

5a. Hyphomicrobium facilis subsp. tolerans subsp. nov.

to'le.rans. L. part. adj. *tolerans* tolerating; pertaining to the tolerance of high CO concentrations.

Morphology and cell sizes as in *H. facilis.*

Colonies on solid media are light brown to beige, smooth and shiny, with entire edges. Grow in liquids as turbidity.

Chemoorganotrophic, aerobic, oligocarbophilic. Good growth on methanol, methylamine·HCl, formate, n-butyrate, isovalerate, glycerol, N-acetylglucosamine. Slow growth, but significant stimulation by pyruvate, crotonate, β-hydroxybutyrate, isobutanol, formaldehyde, Bacto Peptone and ureate. Nitrogen source utilized: NH_4^+. Slow growth on sheep blood agar but no hemolysis. Inhibited by 30 µg each of kanamycin, neomycin, tetracycline and erythromycin and 10 µg of streptomycin. Growth in the presence of 2.5% NaCl has been observed; growth is faint in the presence of 5.5% NaCl. Temperature range: 15–45°C. Optimum pH: 6.5–7.5. Not inhibited by visible light. Do not denitrify, but growth occurs with methylamine·HCl anaerobically with thioglycolate. Catalase- and cytochrome oxidase-positive. Tolerate up to 90% (v/v) of CO in the atmosphere. Gelatin is not liquefied; poly-β-hydroxybutyrate is formed. Not pathogenic for mice or guinea pigs.

Habitat: soil.

The mol% G + C of the DNA is 59.4 (strain IFAM I-551; T_m).

Type strain: IFAM I-551 (ATCC 27489).

Additional strains: IFAM 0-545, P-546, Q-547, R-549, M-552, CO-553, CO-557 and CO-558 (ATCC 27491).

5b. Hyphomicrobium facilis subsp. ureaphilum subsp. nov.

u.re.a.phi'lum. Gr. n. *urum* urine; Gr. adj. *philus* loving, M.L. adj. *ureaphilum* loving urea.

Cell sizes and morphology are very similar to IFAM I-551 (Fig. 21.7). Mother cell width 1.10 (1.0–1.25) µm. Grow as turbidity in liquid media. Colonies on solid media are brownish to beige, smooth, shiny with entire edges. Physiological properties as for *H. facilis* subsp. *tolerans* IFAM

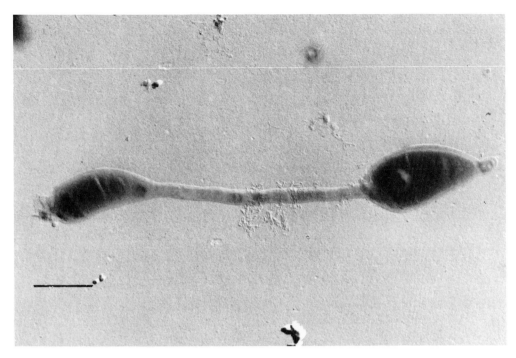

Figure 21.7. *H. facilis* subsp. *ureaphilum.* Mother cell, hypha and mature bud. The mother cell contains a storage granule (poly-β-hydroxybutyrate?). Shadow-cast. *Bar,* 1 μm.

I-551, except for the following: growth is stimulated significantly by α-oxoglutarate but not crotonate, by ethanol but not by Bacto peptone, by urea and ureate as carbon sources. Urea as a nitrogen source is also utilized in the presence of methanol. Temperature range: 25–37°C; there is weak growth at 15° and 45°C. There is weak growth and α-hemolysis on sheep blood agar. Poly-β-hydroxybutyrate may be formed.

Habitat: soil.

The mol% G + C of the DNA is 60.5 (strain CO-582).

Type strain: IFAM CO-582 (ATCC 27492)

Additional strains: IFAM CO-573, CO-574, CO-587, CO-611, CO-613, CO-614, CO-610 and CO-645.

6. Hyphomicrobium zavarzinii sp. nov.

za.var.zin′i.i. M.L. gen. n. *zavarzinii* of Zavarzin; named for G. A. Zavarzin, the Russian microbiologist who isolated these bacteria.

Mother cells drop- or pear-shaped, somewhat slender, with hyphae which rarely branch (Fig. 21.8). Mother cells 0.63 (0.5–0.9) μm wide and 1.78 (0.7–2.5) μm long. Swarmer cells with one to three subpolar flagella. In liquid media under most growth conditions, rosettes are formed, since mother cells produce a polar holdfast. Growth in liquids initially as turbidity and later also as a pellicle and precipitation on the bottom. Colonies on solid media are lightly brownish to colorless beige, smooth and shiny, with entire edges.

Chemoorganotrophic, aerobic, oligophilic. Good growth with the following carbon sources: methanol, methylamine·HCl, formate, *n*-butyrate, isovalerate, crotonate, β-hydroxybutyrate, ethanol, *n*-propanol, isobutanol and glycerol. Growth is stimulated significantly by acetate, *n*-valerate, α-oxoglutarate, galacturonate, formaldehyde, D-glucose, D-mannose, D-melibiose, amygdalin, esculin, chitin, Bacto peptone, *d,l*-lysine, *d,l*-aspartate and dilute human urine. Nitrogen sources utilized are: NH₄⁺, NO₂⁻, NO₃⁻ and (poorly) Bacto peptone. There is slow growth in the absence of added nitrogen sources. Poor growth on sheep blood agar with α-hemolysis. The following antibiotics at 30 μg each inhibit growth: kanamycin, neomycin and tetracycline. Streptomycin at 10 μg is also inhibitory. There is growth in the presence of 3.5% NaCl. Temperature range: 15–37°C. Optimum pH: 6.5–7.5. Visible light inhibits slightly.

There is anaerobic growth with nitrate and gas formation (methanol as carbon source). With methylamine·HCl and thioglycolate there is little growth. Catalase and cytochrome oxidase are positive; gelatin liquefaction is negative. Poly-β-hydroxybutyrate is a storage product.

Not pathogenic for mice or guinea pigs.

Habitat: peaty and moist soil near Moscow, Russia.

The mol% G + C of the DNA is 64.8 (Bd) for strain ZV-622 and 61.8 (T_m) for strain ZV-580.

Genome size: 2.73×10^9 (strain ZV-580; Kölbel-Boelke et al., 1985).

Type strain: IFAM ZV-622.

Additional strains: IFAM ZV-580, ZV-620, MY-619, MC-625, MC-629, MC-630 and MC-627.

7. Hyphomicrobium coagulans (ex Takada 1975) nom. rev.

co.a′gu.lans. L. part. adj. *coagulans* curdling, coagulating.

Mother cells ovoid or pear-shaped, 0.6–1.2 × 1.2–2.0 μm. Hyphae polar or bipolar, branched in older cultures. Swarmer cells motile with one to three polar flagella. In liquid media, growth occurs as turbidity or pellicle. Growth on solid media may become yellow.

Chemoorganotrophic, aerobic. Good growth on methanol, methylamine and ethanol. Other carbon sources utilized are: *n*-propanol, *n*-butanol, isobutanol, benzyl alcohol, furfuryl alcohol, trimethylene glycol, formate and citrate. Carbon sources not utilized: acetate, lactate, formaldehyde and glycerate. Growth is stimulated by glucose, sucrose and lactose.

Acid but no gas is formed from: glucose, lactose, glycerol, methyl-α-glucoside, sucrose, maltose, salicin, arabinose, galactose mannitol, inulin, xylose and soluble starch.

Gelatin is liquefied, peptone is utilized, and milk is slowly coagulated but not peptonized. Casein is not hydrolyzed, indole is not produced. H₂S-positive; methyl red test and Voges-Proskauer tests are positive. Nitrate reduction-negative.

Optimum pH: about 6.0; pH range: 5.7–8.0. Temperature optimum: 35°C.

Nitrogen sources utilized are: casamino acids, polypeptone, aspartate, KNO₃ and NH₄⁺.

Methane is utilized as a carbon source.

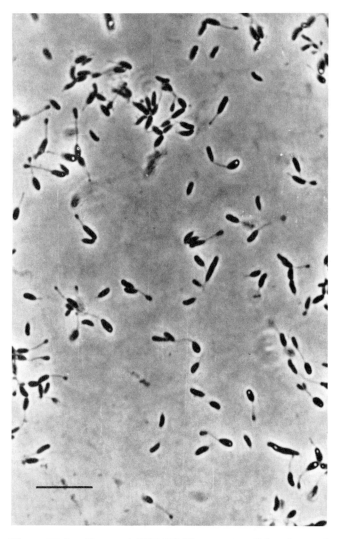

Figure 21.8. *H. zavarzinii* ZV-580. Phase-contrast light micrograph of young growing culture showing all stages of development as well as rosettes. Some of the mother cells carry large granules of poly-β-hydroxybutyric acid (bright granules). *Bar*, 10 µm.

Habitat: rice field soil of Hirakata, Osaka, Japan.

The mol% G + C of the DNA has not been reported.

Type strain: Takada 10-2.

8. **Hyphomicrobium methylovorum** Izumi, Takizawa, Tani and Yamada 1983, 439. ^{VP‡} (Effective publication: Izumi et al. 1982, 373.)

me.thy.lo.vo′rum. M.L. n. *methyl* the methyl radical; L. v. *voro* devour; M.L. n. *methylovorum* methyl devourer.

Mother cells oval, 0.3–0.65 × 0.5–2.0 µm, with monopolar or bipolar hyphae. Swarmer cells motile with a single lateral flagellum. On solid media, colonies white to faintly yellow, circular, convex, smooth and glistening.

Chemoorganotrophic, aerobic, aminopeptidase-positive. Carbon sources utilized for growth: methanol, methylamine, dimethylamine and trimethylamine. Poor growth on formate and formamide. Compounds not utilized are: methane, formaldehyde, ethanol, *n*-propanol, glycerol, D-glucose, D-fructose, D-lactose, D-arabinose, sucrose, trehalose, melibiose, cellobiose, mannitol, inositol, dextrin, starch, acetate, pyruvate, lactate, succinate, oxalate, glycolate, glyoxylate, citrate, fumarate, malate, tartrate, glycine and serine.

Nitrogen sources utilized: NH_4^+ and *l*-glutamine; poor growth on peptone, casamino acids, *l*-cysteine and *l*-aspartate. Nitrogen compounds not utilized: nitrate, urea, yeast extract, meat extract, glycine and *l*-serine.

Nitrate reduction, Voges-Proskauer, indole, H_2S, starch hydrolysis, citrate and urease were negative.

Catalase-positive. Temperature range for growth: 14–33°C. Optimum temperature: around 28°C. Optimum pH: around 7.0. Vitamins are not required.

Habitat: soil.

The mol% G + C of the DNA is 60.6 (T_m).

Type strain: KM-146 (Institute for Fermentation, Osaka, Japan, IFO 1480).

Genus **Hyphomonas** *(ex Pongratz 1957) Moore, Weiner and Gebers 1984, 71*^{VP}

R. L. MOORE AND R. M. WEINER

Hy.pho.mo′nas. Gr. n. *hyphos* filament; Gr. n. *monas* a unit, monad; M.L. fem. n. *Hyphomonas* hypha-bearing unit.

The main cell body of the **rod-shaped to oval mature cells** measures 0.5–1.0 µm × 1.0–3.0 µm and may become larger and rounder just prior to bud formation. **Buds are produced at tips of polar hyphae** (prosthecae) which measure 0.2–0.3 µm in diameter and are 1–5 times the length of the cell body. Hyphae are nonseptate and rarely branch under normal growth conditions. **Pleomorphic. Young daughter cells** (i.e. newly formed **buds**) **are oval** to pear-shaped, **lack hyphae,** and are smaller than the mother cell. Motile by means of a **single polar to lateral flagellum located on** developing **buds** or young daughter cells. Gram-negative. Not acid-fast. Aerobic. Non-sporeforming. **Chemoorganotrophic.** All strains investigated thus far are catalase-positive, oxidase-positive, nonproteolytic, nonsaccharolytic and nonpathogenic. **Amino acids are required** for growth. Optimum temperature for growth ranges from 22 to 37°C. Prefer slightly alkaline conditions for growth. The majority of available strains were isolated from marine sources.

The mol% G + C of the DNA is 57–62 (Bd, T_m).

Type species: *Hyphomonas polymorpha* Moore, Weiner and Gebers 1984, 71.

Further Descriptive Information

Normal-appearing cells of the type strain of *Hyphomonas polymorpha* (ATCC 33881, IFAM PS 728) are shown in Figure 21.9. Some strains also possess obvious capsules. Old cultures or poor growth conditions produce a large number of aberrant cell forms. These include giant cells, spindle-shaped or triangular cells, cells with unusually long or branched

---

‡*VP denotes that this name, although not on the Approved Lists of Bacterial Names, has been validly published in the official publication, *International Journal of Systematic Bacteriology*.

hyphae, cells with intercalary buds and cells with hyphae originating from locations other than the poles. Daughter cells may be half their normal dimensions. Polyphosphate and poly-β-hydroxybutyrate granules which are normally present (Weiner et al., 1985) may become especially pronounced under poor growth conditions.

The appearance of the cell wall in thin sections is typical of other Gram-negative bacteria. The cytoplasmic membrane is continuous with the cell wall, and no organized membrane structures are observed. The composition of the cell wall of *Hyphomonas neptunium* was found to be much more similar to that of *Escherichia coli* than to a strain of *Hypho-microbium* (Jones and Hirsch, 1968). The cells are sensitive to detergents (see Table 21.9) and are readily lysed in a solution of ethylenedia-minetetraacetate with 1% sodium lauryl sulfate. Cells stain well with aniline dyes. The use of Lugol's iodine as a mordant facilitates the staining of the narrow hyphae. Best results are obtained with silver impregnation.

The life cycle of these organisms is generally similar to those of other prosthecate, budding bacteria (Hirsch, 1974a) and has been investigated in some detail (Wali et al., 1980; Moore, 1981b). At 36°C, *Hyphomonas neptunium* requires about 265 min to complete a full cycle. During the first 85 min, the cell exists as a motile swarmer cell. The flagellum becomes detached, and the cell produces a hypha at one, usually the narrower, of the cell poles. This hyphal growth stage requires approximately 95 min of the total cycle. At the end of this stage, the size of the main cell body may increase by up to 2–4 times. The bud development stage occupies the remaining 85 min of the life cycle. The bud is produced at the very tip of the hypha and, at an as yet undetermined time, produces a single flagellum. The mother cell is pushed through the medium by the motile bud, in contrast to *Hyphomicrobium* species, which are pulled by the motile bud (Moore, 1981b). Whether this constitutes a serious diagnostic feature, however, is uncertain. The mature bud eventually separates from the mother cell by fission of the hyphal tip. After a short period of hyphal growth, further daughter cells may be produced by the mother cell. Altering the temperature of growth not only influences the time course of the life cycle but also results in a shift in the relative proportion of the vari-

ous cell types present in a given culture. DNA synthesis is discontinuous and occurs just prior to bud formation.

Good growth occurs on casamino acids, blood agar and other rich media. The addition of sea salts is required by some strains and is stimulatory to others (Havenner et al., 1979). Growth in a defined medium supplemented with a mixture of glutamic acid, aspartic acid, methionine and serine as substrates has been reported for *Hyphomonas neptunium* (Havenner et al., 1979). *H. hirschiana* and *H. polymorpha* have the same requirements as *H. neptunium; H. jannaschiana* requires biotin but not methionine; *H. oceanitis* requires the four amino acids plus biotin, folic acid, pyridoxine, riboflavin and *p*-aminobenzoic acid (Devine and Weiner, manuscript in preparation). No growth on mineral salts media with $CaCO_3$, acetate, propionate, lactate, ethanol, glycerol, glycine or C_1 compounds as the sole source of carbon. Growth is not influenced by light. Some strains may produce a dark brown, acid-insoluble, base-soluble pigment under certain conditions (see Table 21.9).

Carbon dioxide is the primary end product of metabolism, and the medium becomes alkaline, probably due to the evolution of ammonia (Leifson, 1964; Havenner et al., 1979). Deamination and tricarboxylic acid cycle oxidation of amino acids is the major catabolic pathway (Havenner et al., 1979).

Enrichment and Isolation Procedures

Most of the currently available isolates have been obtained by direct plating of samples onto commonly used media such as blood agar, medium 383 (casitone, 2 g/l; yeast extract, 1 g/l; $MgCl_2$, 1 g/l; Leifson, 1964) and, for marine strains, marine agar (Difco 2216; Zobell, 1941). However, a simple procedure has been reported for their isolation from water samples (Moore, 1981a). The sample is brought to 0.005% (w/v) peptone and 0.005% (w/v) yeast extract. The cultures are incubated aerobically and after times ranging from about 1 day to a week or more, are plated onto solid medium. The colonies which arise are screened microscopically for cells with the typical morphology of *Hyphomonas* species and are replated for purification and identification. Two of the nine species have been isolated from shellfish beds of the warm water hydrothermal vents

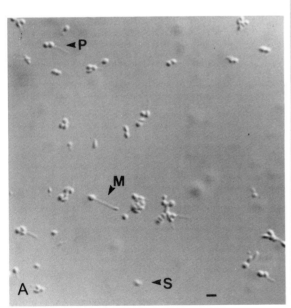

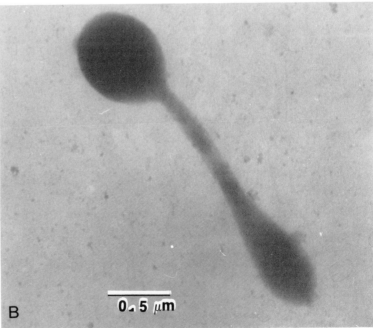

Figure 21.9. *H. polymorpha,* type species. *A,* type strain S (ATCC 33881; IFAM PS 728). Nomarski photomicrograph showing budding mother cell (*M*), cell with prostheca (*P*) and swarmer cells (*S*). Flagella are not visible. *Bar,* 1 μm. *B,* strain R (ATCC 33880; IFAM PR 727). Scanning electron micrograph of mother cell showing bud formation. (Reproduced with permission from P. A. Sorando and R. M. Weiner, *Electron Microscopy Newsletter 10:* 15, 1982, ©University of Maryland EM Central Facility.)

near the Galapagos Islands, at a depth of 2600 m (Jannasch and Wirsen, 1981).

Maintenance Procedures

The members of this genus are generally quite hardy and will survive up to several months in liquid or solid growth medium at 4°C. They are easily revived from lyophilized cultures and can be stored at −20°C over a period of several years in a solution of 60% glycerol in 0.05 M KH$_2$PO$_4$ at pH 7.

Differentiation of the genus **Hyphomonas** from other taxa

Table 21.7 lists the major features which differentiate *Hyphomonas* from other genera of prosthecate, budding bacteria. Support for the separation of this genus is also indicated by the low level of intergeneric cross-reactions seen in serological studies (Powell et al., 1980), DNA/DNA homology studies (Moore and Hirsch, 1972; Moore and Staley, 1976; Gebers et al., 1984), rRNA/DNA studies (Moore, 1977), and comparisons of membrane protein profiles (Dagasan and Weiner, 1986).

Acknowledgments

The authors thank J. Poindexter, R. Gebers and H. Jannasch for providing isolates and helpful discussion and B. Devine, L. Dagasan and D. Powell for their contributions to the manuscript.

A portion of this material is based upon work supported by National Science Foundation under grant no. PCM 8316178.

Further Reading

Hirsch, P. 1974. Budding bacteria. Annu. Rev. Microbiol. *28*: 391–444.
Moore, R.L. 1981. The genera *Hyphomicrobium*, *Pedomicrobium*, and *Hyphomonas*. *In* Starr, Stolp, Trüper, Balows and Schlegel (Editors), The Prokaryotes. A Handbook on Habitats, Isolation, and Identification of Bacteria. Springer-Verlag, Berlin, pp. 480–487.
Moore, R.L. 1981. The biology of *Hyphomicrobium* and other prosthecate, budding bacteria. Annu. Rev. Microbiol. *35*: 567–594.
Moore, R.L., R.M. Weiner and R. Gebers. 1984. Genus *Hyphomonas* Pongratz 1957 nom. rev. emend., *Hyphomonas polymorpha* Pongratz 1957 nom. rev. emend., and *Hyphomonas neptunium* (Leifson 1964) comb. nov. emend. (*Hyphomicrobium neptunium*). Int. J. Syst. Bacteriol. *34*: 71–73.
Weiner, R.M., R.A. Devine, D.M. Powell, L. Dagasan and R.L. Moore. 1985. *Hyphomonas oceanitis* sp. nov., *Hyphomonas hirschiana* sp. nov., and *Hyphomonas jannaschiana* sp. nov. Int. J. Syst. Bacteriol. *35*: 237–243.

Differentiation of the species of the genus **Hyphomonas**

The major diagnostic features are listed in Table 21.8. The two species also differ slightly in their resistance to mechanical disruption, penicillin and streptomycin (Table 21.9). DNA homology studies (filter method; Moore and Hirsch, 1972) have shown relatedness values of 40% and 28% between *H. neptunium* and *H. polymorpha* strains PR 727 and PS 728, respectively. No serological relationships between the two species have been observed (Powell et al., 1980; Weiner et al., 1985; and Table 21.10), and *H. polymorpha* has been reported to have a greater tendency for producing new buds prior to the separation of existing buds than does *H. neptunium* (Weiner et al., 1985). Membrane protein profiles (Jones and Krieg, 1984) support the species placements in Table 21.9 (Dagasan and Weiner, 1986).

List of species of the genus **Hyphomonas**

1. **Hyphomonas polymorpha** (ex Pongratz 1957) Moore, Weiner and Gebers 1984, 71.[VP]

po.ly.mor'pha. Gr. adj. *poly* many; Gr. n. *morphe* shape, body; M.L. adj. *polymorpha* many shapes.

Pongratz (1957) reported that upon isolation on solid media, colonies appear as smooth or rough types. The smooth colonies are round, convex, watery and translucent and can be emulsified easily. A capsule covers the main body of the cell. Rough colonies are rare. They are smaller and dry and form a central crater after several days. The colonies are not readily emulsified, and suspensions remain granular. They lack capsules.

No growth on inulin, dextrin, glycogen, esculin, glycerol, erythritol, mannitol, sorbitol or urea. Reduces neutral red, methylene blue and Janus green. Produces H$_2$S. Other characteristics are given in Table 21.9.

Contrary to the original description (Pongratz, 1957), NO$_3^-$ and NO$_2^-$ are not reduced, indole is not formed from tryptophan, and the rough

Table 21.7.
Differential characteristics of the genera of bacteria which reproduce by budding from the tip of hyphae[a]

Characteristic	Hyphomonas	Hyphomicrobium	Pedomicrobium	Rhodomicrobium
Photosynthetic	−	−	−	+
Able to use C$_1$ compounds as the sole source of carbon	−	+	D	−
Requires amino acids as a source of carbon	+	−	−	−
Able to use a variety of organic acids and alcohols as a source of carbon	−	−	+	+
Produces spores or cysts	−	−	−	+
Capable of depositing a heavy layer of iron or manganese salts on the cell surface	−	−	+	−
Main cell body of mother cell retains size and shape during cell cycle	−	+	−	+
Number of hyphae	1 (occasionally 2), polar	1 (occasionally 2), polar	1–5	2, polar

[a]Symbols: −, 90% or more of strains are negative; +, 90% or more of strains are positive; and D, differs, depending upon species of genus. Reproduced with permission from R. L. Moore, R. M. Weiner and R. Gebers, International Journal of Systematic Bacteriology *34*: 71–73, 1984, ©International Union of Microbiological Societies.

Table 21.8.
Differential characteristics of species of the genus **Hyphomonas**[a]

Characteristic	*H. polymorpha* PS 728 and PR 727	*H. neptunium* LE670[T] and H13	*H. oceanitis* SCH1325[T]	*H. jannaschiana* VP1, VP2[T], VP3 and VP4	*H. hirschiana* VP5[T]
Nutritional requirements					
NaCl (%)	0.5–5.0	1.0–7.5	1.0–7.5	2.0–15.0	2.0–15.0
Methionine	+	+	+	−	+
Biotin	−	−	+	+	−
Biochemical properties					
Nitrate reduction	−	+	+	+	+
Hemolysis	α/γ	α	γ	α	γ
Brown pigment (31–37°C)	−	−	−	+	−
Growth at 37°C	+	+	−	+	−
Susceptibility to					
Mechanical lysis (min)[b]	2–5	<2	6–8	≥9	≥9
Tween 80 (0.01–1%)	R	R	S	R	R
Novobiocin (30 μg)	S	S	R	S	S
Penicillin (10 IU)	S	S	R	S	I
Ampicillin (10 μg)	S	S	R	S	S
Streptomycin (10 μg)	I	S	R	S	I
Level of DNA homology (%) with[c]					
H. polymorpha PS728[T]	100 & 111	23 &25	6	29, 8, 36, 10	0
H. neptunium LE670[T]	21 & 20	100 & 110	3	15, 0, 0, 0	0

[a]Symbols: +, 90% or more of strains are positive; −, 90% or more of strains are negative; R, resistant; S, sensitive; and I, intermediate. Data are reproduced with permission from R. M. Weiner, R. A. Devine, D. M. Powell, L. Dagasan and R. L. Moore, International Journal of Systematic Bacteriology 35: 237–243, 1985, ©International Union of Microbiological Societies.

[b]Time required for lysis by a sonicator.

[c]Data are from a study by Gebers et al., 1984.

strain, PR 727, is motile. It is not known whether these differences are due to the continuous subculturing of these strains.

Not virulent for mice (5 ml), rats (1 ml), guinea pigs (1 ml) or rabbits (1 ml) if a suspension which contains 5×10^9 cells/ml is injected subcutaneously or intraperitoneally. The organisms cannot be recovered from treated animals.

Isolated only once from a patient with infectious sinusitis.

Type strain: smooth (ATCC 33881; IFAM PS 728).

The mol% G + C of the DNA is 60 (Bd) (Mandel et al., 1972). The mol% G + C of the DNA of the rough strain (IFAM PR 727; ATCC 33880) is 61 (Bd) (Mandel et al., 1972).

2. **Hyphomonas neptunium** (Leifson 1964) Moore, Weiner and Gebers 1984, 71.[VP] (*Hyphomicrobium neptunium* Leifson 1964, 249.)

nep.tu′ni.um. L. n. *neptunus* god of the sea (probably should be L. gen. n. *neptuni*).

See Tables 21.8–21.10 for characteristics. Relatedness of *H. neptunium* by DNA/DNA homology to *H. polymorpha* strains PR 727 and PS 728 is 40% and 28%, respectively (filter method; Moore and Hirsch,

1972) or 20% and 21%, respectively (in solution nuclease S_1 method; Gebers et al., 1984).

Isolated from a sample of stored seawater originally obtained from the harbor at Barcelona, Spain.

The mol% G + C of the DNA is 61.7 (Bd) (Mandel et al., 1972).

Type strain: LE 670 (IFAM LE 670; ATCC 15444).

3. **Hyphomonas jannaschiana** Weiner, Devine, Powell, Dagasan and Moore 1985, 240.[VP]

jan′nasch.i.an.a. L. fem. adj. *jannaschiana* pertaining to Jannasch; named for H. Jannasch for his contributions to marine microbiology.

Mature mother cells are 0.5–0.8 × 1.0–3.0 μm, and the main body of the cell tends to be elongated and bullet- or spindle-shaped. Young swarmer cells are motile and pear-shaped and resemble those of other members of the genus. On blood agar, colonies are small, dull gray, dry, and circular to irregular with dimpled elevations and lobate margins (strains VP1 and VP3) or gray, circular, convex, entire, glistening, and mucoid (strains VP2[T] and VP4), resembling *H. neptunium* colonies, which have similar shape and are white. In broth, growth appears granu-

Table 21.9.
Characteristics of species of the genus **Hyphomonas**[a]

Characteristic	1. H. polymorpha PS 728/PR 727[T]	2. H. neptunium LE617[T]/H13	3. H. jannaschiana VP1/VP3	H. jannaschiana VP2[T]/VP4	4. H. hirschiana VP5[T]	5. H. oceanitis SCH 1325[T]
Type of growth in broth	Turbid	Turbid	Granular	Ropy	Pellicle	Turbid
Optimal temperature (°C)	30–37	30–37	37	37	25–31	20–30
%NaCl for maximum growth	0.5–3.5	2.0–5.0	3.5–7.5	3.5–7.5	3.5–7.5	2.0–5.0
%NaCl for growth	0.5–5.0	1.0–7.5	2.0–15.0	2.0–15.0	2.0–15.0	1.0–7.5
Optimum pH	7.0–7.4	8.0	7.6	7.6	7.6	7.6
Microacrophotic growth	−	−	Slight	Slight	−	Slight
Requires methionine	+/−s	+	−	−	+	+
Requires biotin	−	−	+	+	−	+
Film formation on growth vessel	− or slight	Slight	+	Slight	Slight	−
Rosette formation	−	−	+	−	−	−
Brown pigment at 31–41°C	−	−	+	+	−	−
Resistance to mechanical lysis[b]	2–5	2	9	9	9	6–8
Hemolysis on sheep blood agar						
Growth on TSI agar	−	−	−	−	−	−
Growth on MacConkey agar	−	−	−	−	−	−
Mannitol fermentation	−	−	−	−	−	−
Acid from glucose, lactose	−	−	−	−	−	−
Gelatin hydrolysis	−	−	−	−	−	−
Starch hydrolysis	−	−	−	−	−	−
Indole from tryptophan	−	−	−	−	−	−
$NO_3^- \rightarrow NO_2^-$	−	+	+	+	+	+
$NO_2^- \rightarrow N_2, NH_3$	−	−	−	−	−	−
DNAse	−	−	−	−	−	−
Ornithine decarboxylase	−	−	−	−	−	−
Lysine decarboxylase	−	−	−	−	−	−
Coagulase	−	−	−	−	−	−
Sensitivity to						
Tellurite (0.5%)	S	S	S	S	S	S
Ox bile (10%)	I	I	I	I	I	I
Crystal violet (0.2%)	S	S	S	S	S	S
Neutral red (0.4%)	R	R	R	R	R	R
Brilliant green (0.2%)	S	S	S	S	S	S
Methylene blue (10%)	S	S	S	S	S	S
Sodium lauryl sulfate (1%)	S	S	S	S	S	S
Teepol 610 (80%)	S	S	S	S	S	S
Methyl violet (0.04%)	R	R	R	R	R	R
Pyronin (0.4%)	S	S	S	S	S	S
NP-40 (0.01%)	I	S	S	S	S	S
Tween 80 (0.01–1.0%)	R	R	R	R	R	S
Erythromycin (15 µg)	S	S	S	S	S	S
Rifampin (5 µg)	S	S	S	S	S	S
Cephalothin (30 µg)	S	S	S	S	S	S
Novobiocin (30 µg)	S	S	S	S	S	R
Kanamycin (30 µg)	S	S	S	S	S	S
Chloramphenicol (30 µg)	S	S	S	S	S	S
Penicillin (10 IU)	S[c]	I	S	S	I	R
Ampicillin (10 µg)	S	S	S	S	S	R
Streptomycin (10 µg)	I	S	S	S	S	I
Mol% G + C of DNA	60, 61	62, 60	60	60	57	59

[a]Symbols: −, 90% or more of strains are negative; +, 90% or more of strains are positive; −s, negative but stimulatory; S, sensitive; I, intermediate; and R, resistant. Data are reproduced with permission from R. M. Weiner, R. A. Devine, D. M. Powell, L. Dagasan and R. L. Moore, International Journal of Systematic Bacteriology *35:* 237–243, 1985, ©International Union of Microbiological Societies.

[b]Minutes required for 99% lysis by Brownwill Biosonik IV sonicator; low probe at full power

[c]Sensitivities were assessed on 50% concentrations of marine broth (Zobell, 1941). Sensitivity on other medium may be different (Hirsch, 1974a)

Table 21.10

Serological relationships of the strains of the genus **Hyphomonas**[a]

Antiserum to strain:	*H. polymorpha* strains		*H. Neptunium* strains		*H. jannaschiana* strains				*H. hirschiana* VP5^T	*H. oceanitis* SCH 1325
	PS 728^T	PR 727	LE670^T	H13	VP1	VP3	VP2^T	VP4		
PS 728^T	1280	1280	—	20	—	—	—	—	20	40
PR 727	1280	1280	—	320	—	—	—	—	—	—
LE670^T	—	—	320	1280	—	—	—	—	40	40
VP1	—	—	—	—	160	320	320	320	160	—
VP2^T	—	—	—	—	320	320	320	640	80	—
VP3	—	—	—	—	80	160	320	160	—	40
VP4	—	—	—	—	160	160	320	320	80	—
VP5^T	—	—	—	—	20	20	40	20	320	20
SCH1325	—	—	—	—	—	—	—	—	40	1280

[a]The titers listed are reproduced with permission from R. M. Weiner, R. A. Devine, D. M. Powell, L. Dagasan and R. L. Moore, International Journal of Systematic Bacteriology *35*: 237–243, 1985, ©International Union of Microbiological Societies.

lar, and a film of tan cells covers the sides and bottom of the culture vessel (strains VP1 and VP3), or growth may appear ropy and produce only a slight film (strains VP2^T and VP4). Strains VP1 and VP3 tend to form rosettelike cell aggregates.

A brown pigment with chemical properties characteristic of melanins is produced in type 2216 marine broth at 31–37°C. A mixture containing glutamic acid, aspartic acid and serine as substrates and the cofactor biotin is required for chemoorganotrophic growth. The temperature for optimum growth is 37°C. The NaCl concentration for optimum growth is 3.5–7.5%. Optimum pH: 7.6.

Nitrate is reduced. Produces α-hemolysis on Zobell marine medium supplemented with 5% sheep blood. Susceptible to NP-40 (0.01%), novobiocin, penicillin, ampicillin and streptomycin. Resistant to Tween 80 (1.0%). Very resistant to breakage by sonication.

Possesses some surface antigens in common with *H. hirschiana* but none in common with *H. oceanitis*, *H. polymorpha* or *H. neptunium* (Table 21.10).

Four strains, strains ATCC 33882 (VP1), ATCC 33883^T (VP2^T), ATCC 33884 (VP3) and ATCC 33885 (VP4) of *H. jannaschiana*, were isolated in 1979 from shellfish beds near hydrothermal vents on the floor of the mid-Pacific Ocean.

The appearance is typical of Gram-negative bacteria. The only notable difference among the strains is the consistent presence of large dark granules in strains VP1 and VP3. The occurrence of these granules is independent of the medium used for culturing.

The mol% G + C of the DNA of strains VP1, VP2^T, VP3 and VP4 is 60.

Low levels of DNA homology occur between all four isolates and *H. polymorpha* PS 728^T (Gebers et al., 1984).

Strains cannot be differentiated on the basis of morphological, serological, nutritional or biochemical tests.

Type strain: VP2 (ATCC 33883).

4. Hyphomonas hirschiana Weiner, Devine, Powell, Dagasan and Moore 1985, 242.^VP

hir′schi.an.a. L. fem. adj. *hirschiana* pertaining to Hirsch; named for P. Hirsch for his contributions to the study of prosthecate, budding bacteria.

Cellular morphology is like that of *H. polymorpha*. Colonies are small (1.0 mm in diameter after 48 h), dull gray, dry, and circular to irregular, with dimpled elevations and lobate margins. Growth in broth produces a pellicle at the surface and a light film of growth on the sides and bottom of the culture vessel.

A mixture of L-glutamic acid, L-aspartic acid, L-serine and L-methionine is required for growth. The temperature range for optimum growth is 25–31°C. The NaCl concentration for growth is 2.0–15.0%. Optimum pH: 7.6.

Nitrate is reduced. Sheep erythrocytes are not hemolyzed. Pigment is not formed. Susceptible to 0.01% NP-40, novobiocin and ampicillin. Resistant to 1.0% Tween 80. Intermediate susceptibility to penicillin and streptomycin. Treatment for 9 min or more with a Brownwill Biosonik IV sonicator (low probe at full power) is required to produce 99% lysis of cells.

H. hirschiana possesses some surface antigens in common with other *Hyphomonas* species but no DNA homology to *H. polymorpha* or *H. neptunium* in solution with endonuclease treatment (Gebers et al., 1984).

The type strain was isolated in 1979 from shellfish beds near hydrothermal vents on the floor of the mid-Pacific Ocean by H. Jannasch.

The mol% G + C of the DNA is 57.

Type strain: VP5 (ATCC 33886).

5. Hyphomonas oceanitis Weiner, Devine, Powell, Dagasan and Moore 1985, 240.^VP

o.cean.i′tis. N.L. fem. n. *oceanitis* daughter of the ocean.

Cells are round to oval and ~0.9 μm in diameter and usually have one hypha which is up to 3 times the length of the mother cell. Under favorable growth conditions, a small proportion of cells produce two hyphae, one at each of the poles. Both hyphae are capable of producing buds concurrently. Buds (daughter cells) are pear-shaped and become larger and rounder when they are mature (mother cells) and producing buds. Intercalary buds (i.e. two or more daughter cells remaining attached to the distal pole(s) of the stalk(s) of the mother cell) are common. Buds are motile until the hyphae form.

Gram-negative. Not acid-fast. No endospores. Aerobic or microaerophilic.

On agar, the colonies are colorless, raised, semitranslucent or opaque and, after 3 days, up to 1.5 mm in diameter.

In liquid media, growth produces uniform turbidity without a pellicle or sediment. The best growth occurs in media containing sea salts. Does not grow on the mineral salts medium used for *Hyphomicrobium vulgare*. A mixture of L-glutamic acid, L-aspartic acid, L-serine and L-methionine is required for growth. Requires biotin.

The temperature range for optimum growth is 20–30°C. The NaCl concentration for optimum growth is 1.0–7.5%. Optimum pH: 7.6. Nitrate is reduced. Sheep erythrocytes are not hemolyzed. Under optimal conditions in marine broth, growth is slower than the growth of other species of *Hyphomonas*.

Susceptible to NP-40 (0.01%) and Tween 80 (0.1 to 1.0%). Resistant to novobiocin, penicillin, ampicillin and streptomycin. Requires 6–8 min of treatment with a Brownwill Biosonik IV sonicator (low probe at full power) to produce 99% lysis of cells.

Hyphomonas oceanitis has marginal antigenic relatedness to *H. polymorpha*, *H. neptunium*, *H. hirschiana* and *H. jannaschiana*. The levels of genetic relatedness to *H. polymorpha* and *H. neptunium*, as determined by DNA homology studies (in solution with endonuclease treatment) (R. Gebers, personal communication), are 6% and 3%, respectively.

Isolated from the Baltic Sea in 1979 by H. Schlesner.

The mol% G + C of the DNA is 59.

Type strain: SCH 1325 (IFAM 1325; ATCC 33879).

Genus **Pedomicrobium** Aristovskaya 1961, 957,[AL] emend. Gebers 1981, 313

R. GEBERS

Pe.do.mi.cro′bi.um. Gr. n. *pedon* soil; Gr. adj. *micros* small; Gr. masc. n. *bios* life; M.L. neut. n. *Pedomicrobium* soil microbe.

Oval or spherical cells, 0.4–2.0 × 0.4–2.5 µm. **Up to five or more hyphae** (i.e. cellular outgrowths or prosthecae of constant diameter with reproductive function) are formed per cell body. Hyphae are 0.15–0.3 µm in diameter. **At least one hypha originates laterally;** others may appear at the cell poles. Multiplication is by **budding at the hyphal tips** (Figs. 21.10 and 21.11); mature buds either separate from the hyphae as uniflagellated swarmers or remain attached. Extracellular polymers can be stained with ruthenium red and sometimes are visible in India ink mounts as thick capsules around mother cells. **Oxidized iron or manganese compounds or both are deposited on mother cells and also on hyphae.** Resting stages are not known. **Gram-negative,** older cells variable. Swarmer cells are motile by a single sub-polar flagellum (Fig. 21.12). Other stages of the cell cycle (Fig. 21.13) are nonmotile. Colonies are yellowish brown to dark brown, due to accumulated iron and manganese oxides. **Aerobic.** Catalase-positive (for catalase, test in absence of MnO₂ and at neutral pH). **Chemoorganotrophic.** Acetate, caproate or pyruvate are utilized as carbon sources. Protein digests such as yeast extract, peptone, casamino acids or soytone serve as nitrogen sources.

Inorganic nitrogen compounds allow only poor growth of some strains. **Slow and poor growth occurs on agar media with 0.1–1% fulvic acid iron sesquioxide complexes as sole carbon and nitrogen sources.** Vitamin mixtures stimulate growth; lack of vitamins results in pleomorphic cells which produce large granules of poly-β-hydroxybutyric acid.

The mol% G + C of the DNA is 62–67 (T_m, Bd).

Type species: *Pedomicrobium ferrugineum* Aristovskaya 1961, 957.

Further Descriptive Information

Cells are sometimes tetrahedral, pear- or bean-shaped. Hyphae vary in length with cultural conditions; true branching occurs. Buds may arise in an intercalary fashion by localized hyphal swelling. Occasionally, direct budding of mother cells or division of single mother cells has been observed (Aristovskaya, 1961). Deposition of iron and manganese oxides has occurred with all strains studied so far (Aristovskaya, 1961; Khakmun, 1967; Hirsch, 1968; Gebers and Hirsch, 1978; Ghiorse and Hirsch, 1979).

Intracytoplasmic membranes have been observed. Up to three granules of poly-β-hydroxybutyric acid are stored per cell. Small, dense granules stainable with Loeffler methylene blue are suggestive of storage of polyphosphates.

On solid media, two types of colonies may develop. Type 1 colonies are round or convex and have even or radially frayed edges; sometimes they exhibit concentric rings. These colonies have a soft consistency. Type 2 colonies are round, flat and even; they may be crateriform (due to growth into the agar), and the edges are even or radially frayed. The cells in the center of these colonies are often lysed, giving them a granular appearance. Type 2 colonies have a cartilaginous consistency and may be removed from the agar intact. Upon spreading on solid media, type 1 and 2 colonies give rise to both types of colonies. In the course of cultivation with frequent transfers to fresh medium, large colonies tend to predominate over small ones.

Generally, organic acids appear to be the most appropriate carbon sources for *Pedomicrobium* species. Alcohols and carbohydrates are uti-

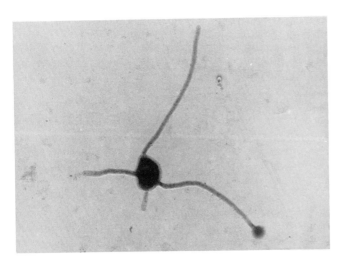

Figure 21.10. *P. manganicum* E-1129. Transmission electron micrograph showing mother cell with hyphae and young bud. Platinum/carbon (Pt/C)-shadowed. *Bar,* 2.5 µm.

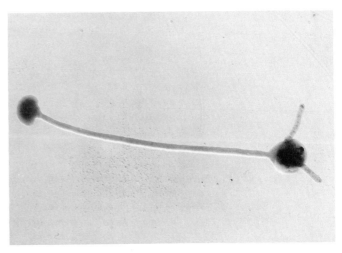

Figure 21.11. *P. manganicum* E-1129. Transmission electron micrograph showing mother cell with hyphae and almost mature daughter cell. Pt/C-shadowed. *Bar,* 1 µm.

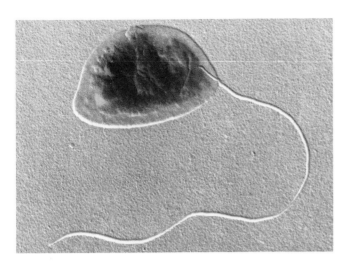

Figure 21.12. *P. ferrugineum* S-1290. Transmission electron micrograph showing swarmer cell with subpolarly inserted flagellum. Pt/C-shadowed. *Bar,* 1 µm.

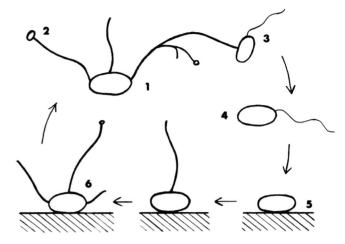

Figure 21.13. Life cycle of *Pedomicrobium* species: *1,* mother cell with hyphae and buds; *2,* young bud; *3,* mature bud with flagellum; *4,* swarmer cell; *5,* young mother cell attached to solid surface; and *6,* mature mother cell with hyphae and beginning bud formation.

lized only in some cases. All strains grow at 20 and 30°C and in the pH range of 7–9.

P. ferrugineum S-1290 and *P. manganicum* E-1129 are not pathogenic for guinea pigs after intraperitoneal injection of 10^8 cells and are not hemolytic.

Pedomicrobium species are widely distributed in podzolic and other soils, in freshwater lakes and ponds, in iron springs and in seawater; they are ubiquitous.

Enrichment and Isolation Procedures

Isolation of *P. ferrugineum* and *P. manganicum* from soil, especially from podzolic soil, is achieved by Aristovskaya's procedure (1961) as described by Gebers and Hirsch (1978): Soil samples are suspended by repeatedly shaking in 0.85% (w/v) saline solution and streaked onto humic gel agar.* Since fulvic acids serve as sole carbon and nitrogen sources, this medium is rather selective but allows only slow growth of *Pedomicrobium* species. After 3–12 weeks incubation at 20 or 30°C in the dark, *Pedomicrobium*-containing parts of the enrichment may be recognized by their yellowish brown to dark brown color due to accumulation of iron and/or manganese oxides. Identification of iron-depositing colonies by the Prussian blue reaction is difficult because humic gel usually contains Fe (III) and thus stains intensely. Screening for manganese-depositing colonies, however, is facilitated by flooding the enrichment plate with leuko-berbelin blue I. Since *Pedomicrobium*-containing colonies are strongly coherent, spreading onto agar plates is enhanced by sterile grinding of the inoculum in a drop of saline solution.

For final purification streaks, humic gel agar is supplemented with a vitamin solution.† This is because *Pedomicrobium* cells in pure colonies have an irregular, pleomorphic appearance when they are grown without vitamins.

Pedomicrobium standard medium (PSM)‡ supplemented with 0.015% (w/v) Acti-Dione (Roth, Darmstadt, Germany) and 1.8% agar may serve as an alternative medium for enrichment and isolation of aquatic or soil pedomicrobia. Acti-Dione inhibits many fungi, but this medium allows growth of many contaminating bacteria; therefore, the selectivity for *Pedomicrobium* species is low.

Aquatic strains of *Pedomicrobium* spp. not classified as yet can be enriched by a procedure of Staley et al. (1980): Freshwater samples are diluted in a series of test tubes with dilute peptone medium (DPM)§ up to the 10^{-9} dilution. Inoculated tubes are incubated at 20–30°C until surface pellicles develop in the highest dilution tubes. For isolation of *Pedomicrobium* species, the pellicles are streaked onto DPM solidified with 1.8% agar.

Maintenance Procedures

Pedomicrobium species grown on PSM agar slants survive for more than 2 years in tightly sealed screw-capped tubes at 20 or 30°C. For longer periods of preservation, 1 part of an exponentially growing liquid culture is mixed with 1 part of sterilized milk (fat content, 0.3% of dry weight) and freeze-dried at −55°C; addition of milk may be omitted. PSM, either autoclaved or sterile-filtered, is recommended for revival of lyophilized cultures and subculturing.

Procedures for Testing Special Characters

Testing for iron and manganese oxide accumulation from fulvic acid sesquioxide complexes is impractical, because these humic substances

---

***Humic gel agar:* Humic gel (fulvic acids complexed with metal sesquioxides) is prepared by hydrochloric acid extraction from (podzolic) humus soil (Ponomareva, 1964; Gebers and Hirsch, 1978). Five g (wet weight) humic gel and 18 g agar (Difco) are suspended in 1 l distilled water and autoclaved, and the mixture is poured as thick layers into Petri plates; the final pH will be 5–6.

†Vitamin solution (Staley, 1968) consists of: 2 mg biotin, 2 mg folic acid, 5 mg thiamine·HCl, 5 mg calcium pantothenate, 0.1 mg cyanocobalamin, 5 mg riboflavine, 5 mg nicotinamide, 5 mg *p*-aminobenzoic acid, 10 mg pyridoxin·HCl, and 1000 ml distilled water.

‡PSM consists of 10 mM sodium acetate, 0.5 g yeast extract (Difco), 1 ml "metals 44" (see below), 10 ml vitamin solution (see Footnote †), and distilled water to 1000 ml. Adjust the pH to 9.0; final pH after autoclaving: 7.0. "Metals 44" (Cohen-Bazire et al., 1957) consists of: 125 mg EDTA, 547.5 mg $ZnSO_4·7H_2O$, 250 mg $FeSO_4·7H_2O$, 77 mg $MnSO_4·H_2O$, 19.6 mg $CuSO_4·5H_2O$, 12.4 mg $Co(NO_3)_2·6H_2O$, 8.85 mg $Na_2B_4O_7·10H_2O$, and 50 ml distilled water. Adjust pH to 6.8.

§DPM consists of: 0.1 g peptone (Difco), 20 ml Hutner's modified salts solution (see below), 10 ml vitamin solution (see Footnote †), and distilled water to 1000 ml. Hutner's modified salts solution (Cohen-Bazire et al., 1957) (amount per liter) consists of: 10 g nitrilotriacetic acid, 29.7 g $MgSO_4·7H_2O$, 3.3 g $CaCl_2·2H_2O$, 12.7 mg $NaMoO_4·2H_2O$, 99.0 mg $FeSO_4·H_2O$, and 50 ml "metals 44" (see Footnote ‡). Distilled water is added to the volume after pH adjustment. The nitrilotriacetic acid is first neutralized with potassium hydroxide. Then the remaining ingredients are added before the pH is adjusted to 7.2 with KOH and H_2SO_4. Distilled water is added to make 1 liter of solution.

are solely available from podzolic soils, which only occur in certain regions on earth. Therefore, it is recommended that instead of fulvic acid complexes, elemental iron or FeS and $MnSO_4$, respectively, embedded in agar media be employed. The specificity of the test is reduced, however, since autoxidation of elemental iron and pyrite occurs at physiological pH and various bacteria are capable of accumulating the oxidized products.

Presence of ferric iron is indicated by a blue color around cells or colonies when a solution of 2% $K_4[(Fe(CN)_6]$ acidified with HCl has been added (Prussian blue reaction). Manganese (IV) is demonstrated by a blue color reaction with a 0.4% (w/v) solution of leuko-berbelin blue I (Krumbein and Altmann, 1973) or with Feigl's reagent: 1% (w/v) benzidiniumhydrochloride in a 7% (v/v) acetic acid solution. In contrast to Feigl's reagent, berbelin blue I does not inhibit viability of the cells.

Differentiation of the genus **Pedomicrobium** from other genera

Table 21.11 provides the primary characteristics that can be used to differentiate the genus *Pedomicrobium* from morphologically similar taxa.

Taxonomic Comments

Originally, three species of *Pedomicrobium* were described: *P. ferrugineum*, *P. manganicum* (Aristovskaya, 1961), and "*P. podsolicum*" (Aristovskaya, 1963). None of the *Pedomicrobium*-like isolates known to us fit the description of "*P. podsolicum*." Therefore, this species was omitted from the Approved Lists of Bacterial Names.

Since *Pedomicrobium* species reveal neither prominent biochemical capabilities nor distinct morphological differences, DNA/DNA homologies are valuable tools for subdividing the genus. DNA/DNA hybridizations between pedomicrobia and other hyphal, budding bacteria resulted in homologies of 7% and below (see Table 21.14).

Acknowledgments

I gratefully acknowledge provision of *Pedomicrobium*-like strains by J. A. Babinchak and P. Hirsch, E. Dale and W. C. Ghiorse, and J. T. Staley.

Further Reading

Gebers, R. 1981. Enrichment, isolation, and emended description of *Pedomicrobium ferrugineum* Aristovskaya and *Pedomicrobium manganicum* Aristovskaya. Int. J. Syst. Bacteriol. *31:* 302–316.
Gebers, R., and M. Beese. 1988. *Pedomicrobium americanum* sp. nov. and *Pedomicrobium australicum* sp. nov. from aquatic habitats, *Pedomicrobium* gen. emend., and *Pedomicrobium ferrugineum* sp. emend. Int. J. Syst. Bacteriol. *38:* 303–345. (Describes two new species)
Hirsch, P. 1974. Budding bacteria. Annu. Rev. Microbiol. *28:* 391–444.
Moore, R. L. 1981. The biology of *Hyphomicrobium* and other prosthecate, budding bacteria. Annu. Rev. Microbiol. *35:* 567–594.
Moore, R. L. 1981. The genera *Hyphomicrobium, Pedomicrobium,* and *Hyphomonas. In* Starr, Stolp, Trüper, Balows and Schlegel (Editors), The Prokaryotes. A Handbook on Habitats, Isolation, and Identification of Bacteria. Springer-Verlag, Berlin, pp. 480–487.

Differentiation of the species of the genus **Pedomicrobium**

The differential characteristics of the species of *Pedomicrobium* are listed in Table 21.12. Other descriptive characteristics are summarized in Table 21.13. Table 21.14 presents DNA/DNA homologies of *Pedomicrobium* strains.

Table 21.11.

Differential characteristics of the genus **Pedomicrobium** *and other morphologically similar taxa[a]*

Characteristic	*Pedomicrobium*	*Hyphomicrobium*	*Hyphomonas neptunium*	*Hyphomonas polymorpha*	*Rhodomicrobium*
Number of hyphae per mother cell	1–5 (or more)	1 (or 2)	1 (or more)	1	1 or 2
Origin of hyphae:					
Lateral	+	−	−	−	−
Polar	+	+	+	+	+
Septation of hyphae	−	−	−	−	+
Accumulation of heavy metal oxides	+	−	−	−	−
Photosynthetic pigments	−	−	−	−	+
Carbon source utilization					
Formate	D	+		−	
Acetate	+	+		−	
Nitrogen source utilization					
4% (w/v) $NaNO_2$	−	+			
9% (w/v) $NaNO_3$	−	+			
Growth in the presence of 5% (w/v) NaCl	−	+			
Mol% G + C of DNA	62.8–67.3	59.2–66.8	61.7	60.2–61.2	61.8–63.8

[a]Symbols: numbers in parentheses are based on rare observations; +, 90% or more of strains are positive; −, 90% or more of strains are negative; and D, differs among species.

Table 21.12.

Characteristics differentiating the species of the genus **Pedomicrobium**[a]

Characteristic	1. *P. ferrugineum*	2. *P. manganicum*
Deposition of oxidized iron compounds on cell surfaces	+	−[b]
Deposition of oxidized manganese compounds on cell surfaces	−	+
Reduction of ferric iron in fulvic acid sesquioxide complexes	−[b]	+[b]
Sensitivity to		
Ampicillin	+	−
Cephalothin	+	−
Bacitracin	−	+
Polymyxin B	−	+
Rifampin	+	−
Tetracycline	+	−
Chloramphenicol	+	−
Nitrofurazon	+	−

[a]Data are from Gebers (1981), p. 309. Symbols: +, 90% or more of strains are positive; and −, 90% or more of strains are negative.
[b]Tested on humic gel agar.

Table 21.14.

DNA homology of **Pedomicrobium** *and* **Hyphomicrobium** *strains with* **P. ferrugineum** *S-1290 reference DNA*[a]

Species	Strain	% homology to S-1290 DNA
P. ferrugineum	S-1290	100
	P-1196	98
	Q-1197	99
	R-1198	101
	T-1130	97
	F-1225	104
P. manganicum	E-1129	13
Pedomicrobium sp.	WD-1355	17
	ST-1306	18
	868	18
	869	22
Hyphomicrobium sp.	MC-750	7
	H-526	7
	B-522	4
Hyphomonas polymorpha	PS-728	3
Rhodomicrobium vannielii	1178	0

[a]Data are from Gebers et al. (1981), p. 285, and from unpublished data.

Table 21.13.

Other characteristics of species of the genus **Pedomicrobium**[a]

Characteristic	1. *P. ferrugineum*	2. *P. manganicum*
Shape of mature cell		
Oval	+	+
Spherical	−	+
Tetrahedral	+	+
Pear-shaped	+	−
Bean-shaped	+	+
Size of mature cells up to	$1.7 \times 2.5\ \mu m$	$0.9 \times 1.5\ \mu m$
Number of hyphae per cell up to	3	5
Outgrowth of hyphae		
Laterally	+	+
Polarly	+	+
Pili or fimbriae	−	−
Storage granules of		
Poly-β-hydroxybutyric acid	+	+
Polyphosphate	+	+
Growth on		
Ribose	−	+
Glucose	d	+
Lactose	−	
Formate	d	+
Acetate	+	+
Caproate	+	+
Pyruvate	+	+
Lactate	d	+
Succinate	+	
Fumarate	+	
Malate	+	
Sensitivity to		
Cycloserine	−	−
Nalidixic acid	−	−
Gentamycin	+	+
Neomycin	+	+
Sulfanilamide	−	−

[a]Data are from Gebers (1981), p. 302. Symbols: +, 90% or more of strains are positive; −, 90% or more of strains are negative; and d, 11–89% of strains are positive.

List of species of the genus **Pedomicrobium**

1. **Pedomicrobium ferrugineum** Aristovskaya 1961, 957,[AL] emend. Gebers 1981, 314.

fer.ru.gi′ne.um. M.L. neut. adj. *ferrugineum* of iron color.

The morphology of cells and colonies are as given for the genus. Further characteristics of morphology and physiology are listed in Tables 21.12 and 21.13.

The temperature for optimum growth is 30°C, and the temperature range is 10–40°C. The pH for optimum growth is 9.0; the pH range is 3.5–10.0. Growth occurs in the presence of up to 0.1% (w/v) NaCl; no growth, but survival, has been observed in the presence of 1–5% NaCl. Higher concentrations of NaCl are bacteriocidal.

Isolated from podzolic soils.

The mol% G + C of the DNA is 64.5–66.8 (T_m, Bd).

Type strain: ATCC 33119.

2. **Pedomicrobium manganicum** Aristovskaya 1961, 957,[AL] emend. Gebers 1981, 315.

man.ga′ni.cum. M.L. neut. adj. *manganicum* of manganese.

The cell morphology and the colonial morphology are as given for the genus. Further characteristics of morphology and physiology are listed in Tables 21.12 and 21.13.

Isolated from a quartzite rock pool.

The mol% G + C of the DNA is 65 (T_m) to 67.3 (Bd).

Type strain: ATCC 33121.

Further Comments

Budding bacteria which resemble pedomicrobia have been isolated from manganese deposits of hydroelectric pipelines (Tyler and Marshall, 1967) and from seawater (Hirsch, 1968). The organisms accumulate iron and manganese oxides and show multiple formation of hyphae from all over the cell surface under particular culture conditions.

Pedomicrobium-like organisms have been observed in soils containing fulvic acid iron/manganese complexes (Khakmun, 1967) and in ooze containing iron and manganese (Kutuzova, 1972).

Morphological characteristics of *Pedomicrobium*-like budding bacteria, strains 868 and 869, have been investigated by Ghiorse and Hirsch (1979). Both strains accumulated iron as well as manganese oxides. They were isolated from a temporary pond.

Strains 868 and 869, as well as strains ST-1306, WD-1355, and G-1381, recently isolated from freshwater habitats, are presently under investigation. They reveal DNA/DNA homologies of 17–22% to *P. ferrugineum* S-1290 (Table 21.14).

The mol% G + C of the DNA is 62.8–65.0 (T_m) (Gebers et al., 1985).

2. BUDS PRODUCED ON CELL SURFACE

Genus **Ancalomicrobium** Staley 1968, 1940[AL]

J. T. STALEY

An.ca′lo.mi.cro′bi.um. Gr. masc. n. *ancalos* arm; Gr. adj. *micros* small; Gr. masc. n. *bios* life; M.L. neut. n. *Ancalomicrobium* arm (-producing) microbe.

Unicellular bacterium with conical cells, about 1.0 µm in diameter. Cells produce from **two to eight or more prosthecae.** Prosthecae are cylindrical without cross-bands and taper gradually from the cell to a distal diameter of about 0.2 µm and a length of 2–4 µm when fully differentiated. Prosthecae may be bifurcated. **Budding bacterium.** Buds are formed directly from mother cell, never from tips of prosthecae. Cells occur singly or in pairs prior to division; rarely form aggregates.

Gram-negative. Flagella and holdfasts are not produced. **Gas vacuoles** are produced by type strain.

Facultative anaerobic. Chemoorganotrophic. Use sugars anaerobically and aerobically. Ferments sugars by mixed acid fermentation. Some organic acids are utilized aerobically but are not fermented. Ammonium can be used as sole source of nitrogen. Vitamins required for growth. Oxidase- and catalase-positive. Temperature range for type strain: 9–39°C. Optimum pH: 7.0; pH range: from <6.3 to >7.5. Found in natural waters and pulp mill oxidation ponds.

The mol% G + C of the DNA (type strain) is 70.4 (Bd).

Type species: *Ancalomicrobium adetum* Staley 1968, 1940.

Further Descriptive Information

The most distinctive features of the genus *Ancalomicrobium* are the size, shape and location of the prosthecae that extend from the base of the conical cells (Fig. 21.14). When fully developed, the prosthecae attain a length of 2–3 µm and are occasionally bifurcated (Fig. 21.15). Shorter prosthecae, as are found in the genus *Prosthecomicrobium*, are not produced under normal conditions for growth.

Buds begin as small protuberances from the apex of the cell cone. As they enlarge, they differentiate to produce the multiple appendages of the newly forming daughter cell. The daughter cell is a pseudo-mirror image of the mother cell at the time of cell separation. The mother cell retains its original prosthecae, and each bud is produced at the same location on the mother cell. The daughter bud is synthesized largely de novo during the budding process (Staley, 1973; Staley et al., 1981) as illustrated in Figure 21.5.

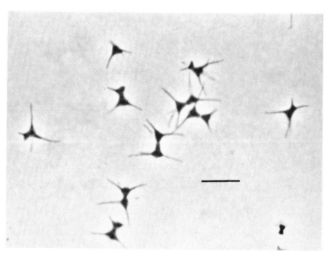

Figure 21.14. *A. adetum.* Phase photomicrograph showing several cells. *Bar,* 5.0 µm. (Reproduced with permission from J. T. Staley, Journal of Bacteriology *95:* 1929, 1968, ©American Society for Microbiology, Washington, D.C.)

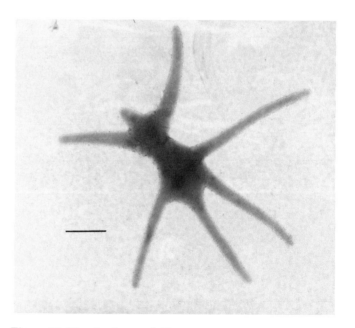

Figure 21.15. *A. adetum* cell. Electron micrograph. *Bar,* 1.0 µm. (Reproduced with permission from J. T. Staley, Journal of Bacteriology *95:* 1929, 1968, ©American Society for Microbiology, Washington, D.C.)

Flagella are not produced by *Ancalomicrobium*. The type of strain produces gas vacuoles. Gas vacuoles are not formed aerobically during active growth on sugars; some are occasionally found during stationary phase under these conditions. They are produced anaerobically on sugars at low temperatures (i.e. <18°C) (A. van Neerven and J. Staley, unpublished observations). Gas vacuoles are also produced during microaerophilic growth on organic acids including acetic, pyruvic and succinic acids (R. Irgens and J. Staley, unpublished observations).

The minimal temperature for growth of the type strain is between 6 and 9°C, whereas the maximum lies between 39 and 43°C. The optimum pH for growth was between 6.9 and 7.3, and the range extended throughout all tested values from 6.3 to 7.5.

Sugars are fermented by a mixed acid fermentation (van Neerven and Staley, 1988). Glucose is fermented to form acetic acid, ethanol, lactic acid, formic acid, succinic acid, hydrogen gas and carbon dioxide. The same products are produced by *Escherichia coli* growing under the same conditions.

Colonies of *A. adetum* are nonpigmented and may be translucent to white in appearance. Colonies are circular in form, have an entire margin, and have convex elevation.

A variety of sugars including monosaccharide hexoses, pentoses, sugar alcohols and some disaccharides as well as organic acids can be used as carbon sources for aerobic growth. These include arabinose, ribose, glucose, fructose, mannose, galactose, lyxose, maltose, cellobiose, lactose, trehalose, fucose, rhamnose, inositol, glycerol, glucosamine, acetate, pyruvate and malate. Some carbon sources can also be used anaerobically by fermentation, including some sugars and sugar alcohols. Agar is digested slowly. Ammonium salts are utilized as a sole source of nitrogen. Pantothenic acid is required for growth by the type strain, and biotin, thiamine, folic acid, and nicotinamide are stimulatory for growth.

The type strain of *A. adetum* grows on a defined medium* containing glucose, ammonium salts, phosphate, a modified Hutner's organic salts solution, and vitamins. Better growth is obtained in complex media such as modified medium B (MMB)† which contains yeast extract in addition to the constituents provided in the defined medium. Highest yields have been obtained on a richer complex medium‡ (R. Irgens, personal communication).

Ancalomicrobium strains are not known to be pathogenic to humans.

A. adetum occurs in freshwater habitats including mesotrophic lakes and eutrophic habitats such as ponds, rivers and pulp mill oxidation lagoons (Staley, 1971; Stanley et al., 1979; Staley et al., 1980).

Enrichment and Isolation Procedures

The type strain was isolated from a eutrophic stream from enrichment cultures containing 0.01% peptone (10 mg peptone in 100 ml of natural water sample). Initial isolation was obtained by passing portions of the positive enrichment through a column of glass beads to absorb attaching forms and permit the free passage of planktonic forms such as *Ancalomicrobium* and *Prosthecomicrobium* which lack holdfasts and do not preferentially attach to glass (Staley, 1968). However, now that more is known about the nutrition of this group it is often possible to obtain pure cultures by direct streaking from positive enrichment cultures onto media such as dilute peptone§ or MMB media (Staley, 1981a). The procedure is described below.

Enrichments of 100 ml are normally used. Graduated 150-ml beakers containing 10 mg of peptones are covered with aluminum foil and autoclaved. Natural water samples are collected aseptically, and 100 ml are added to the beaker. Enrichment cultures are incubated at room temperature without shaking. Cultures should be examined periodically for the appearance of multiple appendaged prosthecate bacteria by preparing wet mounts for phase microscopic observation from the time the cultures become turbid (usually 4–7 days) until 2–3 weeks have elapsed. Whereas *Caulobacter* species are frequently observed attached to debris in the surface film of the enrichment, these planktonic multiple appendaged forms are rarely encountered there. They are usually found moving with the currents in the wet mount and are most likely seen in areas where free-floating forms have accumulated near debris or air bubbles. When multiple appendaged forms comprise a significant portion of the enrichment culture (~1%), attempts should be made to isolate them by streaking onto MMB plates. Alternatively, 10^{-3}–10^{-5} dilutions of the enrichment culture can be plated by spread-plating onto MMB. Plates should be incubated at room temperature for 1–2 weeks before examination. Individual colonies are selected for examination by wet mount. When positive colonies are found, they are restreaked for purification.

Maintenance Procedures

A. adetum can be maintained for at least 1 month on MMB slants that have been refrigerated. Long term preservation is effected by lyophilization of cultures grown on complex media.

Differentiation of the genus **Ancalomicrobium** from other genera

The striking overall morphology of the genus *Ancalomicrobium* permits it to be readily distinguished from nonappendaged bacteria and from most of the other prosthecate bacteria. However, some of the multiple appendaged bacteria may appear similar. The genus *Stella* can clearly be distinguished from *A. adetum* because its appendages lie in one plane. The most morphologically similar genus is *Prosthecomicrobium*. Some

---

*Defined medium contains (amount/l): ammonium sulfate, 0.25 g; disodium phosphate, 0.0005 M; glucose, 0.25 g; Hutner's modified salts solution (see below), 20 ml; vitamin solution (see below), 10 ml; and distilled water added to volume (for solid medium, 1.5% agar should be added). The Hutner's modified salts solution contains (amount/l): nitrilotriacetic acid, 10.0 g; MgSO₄·7H₂O, 29.7 g; CaCl₂·2H₂O, 3.3 g; NaMoO₄·2H₂O, 12.7 mg; FeSO₄·7H₂O, 99.0 mg; "metals 44" (see below), 50 ml; and distilled water added to volume after pH adjustment (see below).

The nitrilotriacetic acid is first neutralized with potassium hydroxide. The remaining ingredients are added before the pH is adjusted to 7.0 with KOH and H₂SO₄. Distilled water is added to make 1 liter of solution. "Metals 44" contains (amount/100 ml): EDTA, 250 mg; ZnSO₄·7H₂O, 1095 mg; FeSO₄·7H₂O, 500 mg; MnSO₄·H₂O, 154 mg; CuSO₄·5H₂O, 39.2 mg; CoCl₂·6H₂O, 20.3 mg; and Na₂B₄O₇·10H₂O, 17.7 mg. A few drops of sulfuric acid are added to prevent precipitation before making to volume with distilled water.

The vitamin solution contains (amount/l): B₁₂, 0.1 mg; biotin, 2 mg; calcium pantothenate, 5 mg; folic acid, 2 mg; nicotinamide, 5 mg; pyridoxine·HCl, 10 mg; riboflavin, 5 mg; thiamine·HCl, 5 mg; and distilled water added to volume.

†MMB agar contains (amount/l): peptone, 0.15 g; yeast extract, 0.15 g; glucose, 1.0 g; ammonium sulfate; 0.25 g; Hutner's modified salts solution, 20 ml; vitamin solution (see Footnote *), 10 ml; agar, 15 g; and distilled water added to volume (pH should be adjusted to 7.0–7.5 prior to autoclaving).

‡Irgens super MMB contains (amount/l): peptone, 0.2 g; yeast extract, 1.0 g; NH₄Cl, 0.2 g; CaCl₂·2H₂O, 0.01 g; NaCl, 0.2 g; MgSO₄·7H₂O, 0.2 g; Fe-citrate, 0.005 g; modified Pfennig's SL-6 trace elements solutions (see below), 1.0 ml; vitamin solution (see Footnote *), 20.0 ml; KH₂PO₄, 5.0 g; and distilled water to 1 l (pH should be adjusted to 7.0 before autoclaving).

After autoclaving, glucose is added to 0.3%. The medium is nearly colorless with no precipitate. Less KH₂PO₄ may be used with nonfermentable substrates.

Pfennig's modified SL-6 trace elements solution (Irgens, 1977) contains (amount/l distilled water): ZnSO₄·7H₂O, 0.10 g; MnCl·4H₂O, 0.03 g; H₃BO₃, 0.3 g; CaCl₂·6H₂O, 0.2 g; CuCl₂·2H₂O, 0.01 g; NiCl₂·6H₂O, 0.02 g; and Na₂MoO₄·2H₂O, 0.03 g (pH should be adjusted to 3–4 with HCl).

§Dilute peptone agar contains (amount/l): peptone, 0.1 g; Hutner's modified salts solution, 20 ml; vitamin solution, 10 ml; agar, 15 g; and distilled water added to volume.

cells of *P. hirschii*, in particular, appear identical to *A. adetum*, although short appendaged cells are also produced by *P. hirschii*. Also, all *P. hirschii* strains are motile, whereas *A. adetum* is nonflagellated. Furthermore, *P. hirschii* strains do not produce gas vacuoles, whereas the type strain of *A. adetum* does. More significantly, these two groups are physiologically distinct. All species of *Prosthecomicrobium* are obligately aerobic, whereas *Ancalomicrobium* is a fermentative facultative anaerobe. Table 21.15 summarizes the important differential characteristics to distinguish these two genera. One other organism, reported from aquatic habitats and as yet not named or isolated, resembles *A. adetum*, but buds are produced at the tip of a prostheca emanating from the apex of the conical cell (Staley, 1968; Hirsch, 1974a).

Taxonomic Comments

DNA/DNA hybridization studies have shown that *Ancalomicrobium* bears no strong relatedness to any of the strains of *Prosthecomicrobium* with which it was compared (Moore and Staley, 1976). This finding is consistent with the current taxonomy of these two genera.

Although further taxonomic work on this genus is desirable, the difficulty encountered in obtaining isolates has hindered taxonomic investigations of the genus. However, since the initial isolation of the type strain, a number of strains have been isolated from pulp oxidation lagoons. DNA phages have also been obtained from the same source (Stanley, 1976).

It is noteworthy that *A. adetum* is currently the only fermentative heterotrophic budding and prosthecate bacterium in pure culture. Further studies are warranted to assess the evolutionary relatedness of this organism to other nonprosthecate fermenters as well as other budding and prosthecate bacteria. Of special note in this regard is the discovery that *A. adetum* is a mixed acid fermenter. Furthermore, the phosphoenolpyruvate: sugar phosphotransferase system of this organism has been compared to that of certain enteric bacteria (Saier and Staley, 1977). The most interesting discovery from this investigation was that enzymatic cross-reactivity was detected between the membrane-

Table 21.15.

Characteristics differentiating **Ancalomicrobium** *from* **Prosthecomicrobium**[a]

Characteristic	Ancalomicrobium	Prosthecomicrobium spp.
Long prosthecae (i.e. 2–4 μm when fully developed)	+	D[b]
Short prosthecae (i.e. <2 μm when fully developed)	−	+
Flagella	−	D
Gas vacuoles	+	D[c]
Hugh-Leifson (acid from glucose fermentatively)	+	−
Mol% G + C of DNA	70–71	65–70

[a]Symbols: +, 90% or more of strains are positive; D, differs, depending on species; −, 90% or more of strains are negative.
[b]*Prosthecomicrobium* species all produce short appendages (i.e. <2 μm in length). For example, *P. hirschii* produces some cells with long appendages that resemble *A. adetum;* however, short-appendaged cells are also produced during active growth; other species, such as *P. pneumaticum*, occasionally produce cells with one or two longer prosthecae.
[c]*P. pneumaticum* produces gas vacuoles.

associated enzyme II complexes of *A. adetum* and the soluble enzyme I components of the enteric bacterium *Salmonella typhimurium*. These results suggest this bacterium may be related to the enteric bacteria.

The morphological similarities between *Ancalomicrobium adetum* and the green sulfur genera *Ancalochloris* and *Prosthecochloris* is also suggestive of an evolutionary relationship between these two groups.

List of species of the genus **Ancalomicrobium**

1. **Ancalomicrobium adetum** Staley 1968, 1940.[AL]
   a'de.tum. M.L. adj. *adetum* arm or appendage.
   The characteristics are as described for the genus.
   Occur in freshwater.
   Type strain: ATCC 23632.

Further Reading

Hirsch, P. 1974. Budding bacteria. Annu. Rev. Microbiol. *28:* 371–444.

Staley, J.T. 1981. The genera *Prosthecomicrobium* and *Ancalomicrobium*. In Starr, Stolp, Trüper, Balows and Schlegel (Editors), The Prokaryotes. A Handbook on Habitats, Isolation, and Identification of Bacteria. Springer-Verlag, Berlin, pp. 456–460.
Staley, J.T., P. Hirsch and J.M. Schmidt. 1981. Introduction to the budding and/or appendaged bacteria. In Starr, Stolp, Trüper, Balows and Schlegel (Editors), The Prokaryotes. A Handbook on Habitats, Isolation, and Identification of Bacteria. Springer-Verlag, Berlin, pp. 456–460.

Genus **Prosthecomicrobium** Staley 1968, 1940,[AL] emend. Staley 1984, 304

J. T. STALEY

Pros.the 'co.mi.cro.bi.um. Gr. fem. n. *prosthece* appendage; Gr. adj. *micros* small; Gr. masc. n. *bios* life; M.L. neut. n. *Prosthecomicrobium* appendage (-bearing) microbe.

Unicellular bacterium with coccobacillary to rod-shaped cells ranging in diameter from 0.8 to 1.2 μm and **containing numerous prosthecae** extending from all locations on the cell surface. **Prosthecae** which may number from 10 to more than 30/cell **are typically short** (i.e. <1.0 μm in length); some species, however, also produce longer prosthecae (>2.0 μm).

Cells divide by **budding.** Buds are produced directly from the mother cell, never from tips of prosthecae.

Gram-negative. Motile and nonmotile species exist. **Motile organisms produce single polar to subpolar flagella;** one species forms gas vacuoles but not flagella.

Obligately aerobic, nonfermentative, **heterotrophic.** A variety of sugars and organic acids are used as energy sources for growth. All strains tested require one or more B vitamins for growth. **Oxidase- and catalase-positive.** Found in soils and fresh and marine waters.

The mol% G + C of the DNA ranges from 64 to 70 (Bd).
Type species: *Prosthecomicrobium pneumaticum* Staley 1968, 1940.

Further Descriptive Information

The genus *Prosthecomicrobium* comprises a diverse collection of multiply-appended prosthecate bacteria. All produce short prosthecae, i.e. prosthecae that are typically <1.0 μm in length. The shortest prosthecae appear as small bumps on the surface of the cell and cannot be readily discerned by light microscopic examination of cells. The "corn cob" organism (now named "*P. polyspheroidum*") was so named because of the numerous short stubby prosthecae that were regularly arranged on the surface of the cell. Somewhat longer prosthecae are conical in shape and are typical for many species. These range in length from <0.25 μm to >1.0 μm, depending upon the species and the growth medium (longer prosthecae may be produced when phosphate is limiting growth). Even longer prosthecae are produced by some strains. For example, *P. pneumaticum* occasionally produces prosthecae >2.0 µm long. This, however, occurs rarely (Staley, 1968). Some strains of the marine species *P. litoralum* also produce longer appendages. One species, *P. hirschii*, produces both short-appendaged as well as long-appendaged cells. The long-appendaged cells closely resemble those of *Ancalomicrobium adetum* and could be confused with them if morphology is used as the sole criterion for identification of organisms from natural samples.

Buds are produced as outgrowths at or near one pole of the cell (Vasilyeva, 1972; Staley, 1984). These typically appear as a forked protuberance from the dividing pole. The bud enlarges and differentiates to produce a mirror image of the mother cell. As in *Ancalmocrobium*, buds appear to be synthesized de novo (Staley, 1973a; Staley et al., 1981).

Some species of *Prosthecomicrobium* produce flagella. Flagella are always single and may be found in a polar or subpolar position on the cell. One species, *P. pneumaticum*, does not produce flagella but produces gas vacuoles. Some species are immotile and do not produce either flagella or gas vacuoles.

All species are obligately aerobic chemoorganotrophs that use a variety of sugars, organic acids, and sugar alcohols for growth. All species can grow on a simple, defined medium (see *Ancalomicrobium*). All species require one or more water-soluble vitamins for growth.

Prosthecomicrobium species are not known to be pathogenic to humans.

Prosthecomicrobium species are found in soils, freshwater habitats of all trophic states (Staley et al., 1980), as well as in the marine habitat (Bauld et al., 1983). They have been reported as important components of biofilms in sewage treatment processes and in pulp mill aeration lagoons (Stanley et al., 1979). Bacteria which resemble these forms have also been reported in the intestinal tracts of insects and other animals (Cruden and Markovetz, 1981); however, it is uncertain whether they have been concentrated from the foodstuff or are truly indigenous to this environment.

Enrichment and Isolation Procedures

The same procedures described for *Ancalomicrobium* isolation can be used for isolation of *Prosthecomicrobium*. The dilute peptone enrichment procedure has been used successfully for the isolation of most strains. Recognition of short-appendaged species in the enrichment culture is difficult because they are not as noticeable as the longer appendaged species. Nonetheless, even with the phase-contrast microscope, they can be detected because of their slightly irregular surface (Fig. 21.16). However, it may be desirable to observe preparations from wet mounts with the transmission electron microscope to confirm their presence in the enrichments. When their numbers have reached significant proportions of the total numbers of bacteria (i.e. 1–5%), then attempts at isolation should be made. Dilute peptone agar plates should be streaked and incubated at room temperature for 2 weeks or more. Colonies are typically small. Wet mounts of each colony type should be prepared and examined by phase-contrast microscopy for identification. The morphology of the resulting pure culture should be confirmed by examination of whole cells with the transmission electron microscope. Additional information on isolation has been published elsewhere (Staley, 1981a).

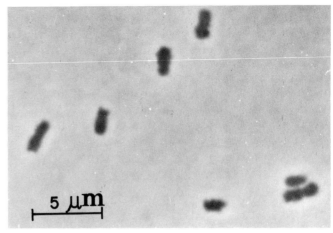

Figure 21.16. *P. enhydrum.* Phase photomicrograph showing several cells. Note the irregular surface of the cells due to the presence of numerous short prosthecae. *Bar,* 5 µm.

Maintenance Procedures

Strains can be maintained on slants in the refrigerator for at least 1 month. MMB agar (cf. *Ancalomicrobium*) with glucose as a carbon source provides a favorable growth medium. Lyophilization can be used for long term preservation.

Differentiation of the genus **Prosthecomicrobium** from other genera

Only one other genus poses major problems for differentiation. This is the genus *Ancalomicrobium*. Differentiation from that genus is discussed in detail in the section on *Ancalomicrobium*. Morphologically, that genus can be distinguished from *Prosthecomicrobium* because of its conical cells and lack of short-appendaged cells. Furthermore, *Ancalomicrobium* is a genus of facultative anaerobes that ferments selected sugars. Thus, the Hugh-Leifson test can be used to distinguish between these two groups (cf. Table 21.15, *Ancalomicrobium*).

Taxonomic Comments

When these bacteria were first described, they were regarded as dividing by binary transverse fission (Staley, 1968; Vasilyeva, 1969). However, they are now known to be budding bacteria (Vasilyeva, 1972; Staley, 1984). The initial difficulty in determining the mode of reproduction of these bacteria was due to the small size of their cells. Unlike *Ancalomicrobium*, the short appendages formed by most species of *Prosthecomicrobium* during development of the bud cannot be readily distinguished in slide culture. Thus, it is more difficult to identify the process of cell division as budding.

Morphologically, *Prosthecomicrobium* comprises a diverse collection of bacteria. There are differences in appendage length, motility, gas vacuole formation, habitat, and carbon source utilization among the species so far described.

The mol% G + C of the DNA within the genus ranges from 64 to 70 (Staley and Mandel, 1973). Results of DNA/DNA hybridization studies (Moore and Staley, 1976) suggest that additional species exist that have not yet been fully described. Several unnamed strains have been deposited in the ATCC (ATCC nos. 27825, 27826 and 27833). *Ancalomicrobium adetum* shows only low levels of homology with *Prosthecomicrobium* species that have been tested.

Other relevant taxonomic comments are included in the discussion of *Ancalomicrobium*.

Differentiation of the species of the genus **Prosthecomicrobium**

The characteristics differentiating among the species of the genus *Prosthecomicrobium* are listed in Table 21.16.

List of species of the genus **Prosthecomicrobium**

1. **Prosthecomicrobium enhydrum** Staley 1968, 1940.[AL]

en.hy′drum. N.L. adj. *enhydrum* living in water, aquatic.

Prosthecae are always short, i.e. <0.5 µm, giving the cell an irregular surface when observed by phase-contrast microscopy (Fig. 21.16). Cells are motile by a polar to subpolar flagellum (Fig. 21.17). Gas vacuoles are not produced. Ammonium but not nitrate can be used as a sole source of nitrogen in media containing an appropriate carbon source and vitamins. Pentoses and hexoses are commonly used by the type strain. Some disaccharides and organic acids are also used as carbon sources (Table 21.16). Thiamine is required for growth.

The temperature range for growth of the type strain is 9–37°C. The pH optimum for growth is 7.0.

Colonies may be white (type strain) or pigmented yellow or red.

The mol% G + C of the DNA of the type strain is 65.8 (Bd).

Type strain: ATCC 23634.

2. **"Prosthecomicrobium polyspheroidum"** (Nikitin and Vasilyeva 1968) Vasilyeva and Lafitskaya 1976, 768. (*Agrobacterium polyspheroidum* Nikitin and Vasilyeva 1968, 444.)

po.ly.spher.oi′dum. N.L. adj. *polyspheroidum* many spheroids, i.e. having numerous bumps.

Cells have many (up to 230/cell) short prosthecae (i.e. <0.1 µm in length). They are distributed in slightly spiral rows along the length of the rod-shaped cells, giving the appearance of a corn cob (Fig. 21.18). Cells, which measure about 0.5 µm in diameter and up to 5.1 µm in length, are motile by a polar flagellum. Lateral buds may be formed under

some conditions of growth. Prosthecae may not be evident in cultures containing more than 0.1% organic nutrients. Monosaccharides and disaccharides are metabolized by pentose phosphate and the Entner-Duodoroff pathway, with the formation of alcohols, organic acids, and

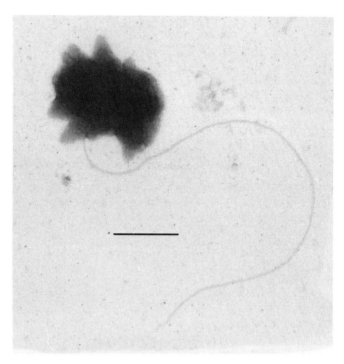

Figure 21.17. *P. enhydrum.* Electron micrograph. Note the subpolar location of the single flagellum. *Bar,* 1.0 µm.

Table 21.16.

Characteristics differentiating the species of the genus **Prosthecomicrobium**[a]

Characteristic	1. *P. enhydrum*	2. *"P. polyspheroidum"*	3. *P. pneumaticum*	4. *P. litoralum*	5. *P. hirschii*
Short prosthecae (<1.0 µm) on MMB	+	+	+	+	+
Long prosthecae (>2.0 µm) on MMB	−	−	−[b]	−[b]	+
Lateral buds	−	+[c]	−	−	−
Flagella	+	+	−	−	+
Gas vacuoles	−	−	+	−	−
Sodium ion requirement; optimum salinity of 25 ⁰/₀₀	−	−	−	+	−
Carbon source utilization					
Maltose, cellobiose, lactose	+	+	+	+	−
Melibiose	−	?	+	+	−
Rhamnose	+	−	+	+	−
Sorbitol	−	±	+	+	−
Pyruvate	+	−	−	+	+
Propionate	−	±	−	−	+
Agar digestion	−	−	−	+	?
Mol% G + C of DNA	66	64–67	69–70	66–67	68–70

[a]Symbols: +, 90% or more of strains are positive; −, 90% or more of strains are negative; ?, not determined; and ±, indefinite.

[b]Strains of both species rarely produce long appendages.

[c]These are formed rarely.

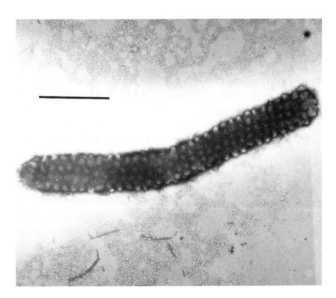

Figure 21.18. *"P. polyspheroidum."* Electron micrograph. Note the arrangement of the numerous short prosthecae in rows. *Bar,* 2.0 µm. (Courtesy of Dr. L. V. Vasilyeva.)

aromatics (cf. Lafitskaya et al., 1976). Thiamine and riboflavin are required for growth. Nitrate reduced to nitrite. Voges-Proskauer and methyl red tests are negative.

Colonies are punctiform after 2–3 days of growth and attain a diameter of about 1 mm after 10 days. They are raised with entire margins, opaque, cream colored and slimy. Optimum temperature: 28–30°C; optimum pH: 6.5–7.1.

The mol% G + C of the DNA ranges from 64 to 67 (Bd).

Type strain: AUCM B-1313.

3. **Prosthecomicrobium pneumaticum** Staley 1968, 1940.[AL]

pneu.ma′ti.cum. N.L. adj. *pneumaticum* inflated, containing gas vacuoles.

Most prosthecae are short (i.e. <1.0 µm in length); however, long prosthecae are occasionally produced (Fig. 21.19). Gas vacuoles are formed by the type strain. Flagella are not produced.

Ammonium, but not nitrate, can be used as a sole nitrogen source for growth. A variety of sugars, both hexoses and pentoses, monosaccharides and disaccharides, can be used as carbon sources for growth (Table 21.16). Sugar alcohols and methyl sugars fucose and rhamnose can also be used.

Biotin, thiamine and vitamin B_{12} are required for growth.

The temperature range for the type strain is 9–42°C. Optimum pH: 6.0–6.5, although good growth also occurs at pH 7.0.

Colonies are translucent to opaque white (the chalky white color is due to the formation of gas vacuoles). Colony size is quite variable.

The mol% G + C of the DNA ranges from 69 to 70 (Bd).

Type strain: ATCC 23633.

4. **Prosthecomicrobium litoralum** Bauld, Bigford and Staley 1983, 613.[VP]

li.to.ra′lum. L. adj. *litoralis* of the seashore.

Prosthecae are mostly short (i.e. <0.5 µm in length), although occasionally long prosthecae are formed. Nonmotile. Neither flagella nor gas vacuoles are produced.

Ammonium can be used as a sole source of nitrogen. A variety of pentoses and hexoses can be used for growth as well as some sugar alcohols and organic acids (Table 21.16). Agar digestion occurs on prolonged incubation. Sodium ions are required for growth.

The minimum salinity at which growth occurs is 5 ⁰/₀₀; the optimum, 25 ⁰/₀₀ (Table 21.16). These bacteria are psychrotrophic. Their minimum temperature for growth is 1–5°C, depending upon the strain, and their optimum is between 27 and 34°C.

Colonies are white and raised initially and, after prolonged incubation, become cream-colored and umbonate. Agar digestion is noticeable around colonies on plates incubated at least 30 days at room temperature.

The mol% G + C of the DNA is 66–67 (Bd).

Type strain: ATCC 35022.

5. **Prosthecomicrobium hirschii** Staley 1984, 304.[VP]

hirsch′i.i. N.L. gen. *hirschii* of Hirsch; named in honor of P. Hirsch, an authority on budding bacteria.

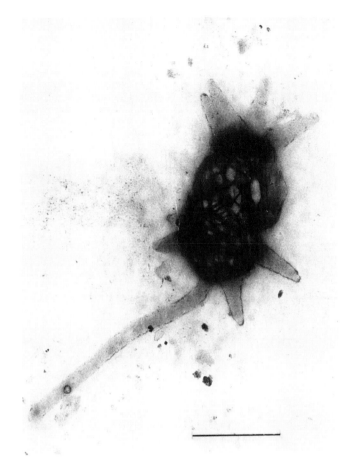

Figure 21.19. *P. pneumaticum* as observed by electron microscopy. Note the gas vesicles within the cell and the single long prostheca. *Bar,* 1.0 µm.

Prosthecae may be short (i.e. <1.0 µm in length) or long (>2.0 µm in length), depending on the cell. Both short- and long-appendaged cells occur simultaneously in culture (Fig. 21.20). Cells may be motile by single polar or subpolar flagella. Gas vacuoles are not formed.

Sugars and organic acids are commonly used as carbon sources. Long chain organic acids such as valerate and caproate are used. Methanol and ethanol can also be used as carbon sources. Biotin, nicotinic acid, pantothenate and thiamine are required for growth.

Colonies are circular in form and umbonate in elevation. They have an entire margin and are pink in color.

The mol% G + C of the DNA of strains ranges from 67.9 to 69.9 (Bd).

Type strain: ATCC 27832.

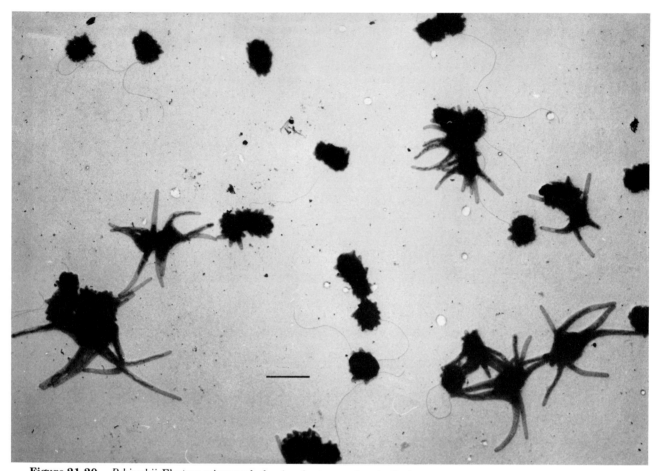

Figure 21.20.   *P. hirschii.* Electron micrograph showing short-appendaged cells, long-appendaged cells, and flagella. *Bar,* 2.0 μm.

Genus **Labrys** *Vasilyeva and Semenov 1985, 375[VP] (Effective Publication:
Vasilyeva and Semenov 1984, 92)*

L. V. VASILYEVA

Lab′rys. Gr. n. *Labrys* double-headed ax, an organism resembling Minoan ax by the shape of the cell.

Unicellular flat bacterium; cells possess **triangular radial symmetry.** Dimensions are 1.1–1.3 × 1.3–1.5 μm. **Two to three tapering short prosthecae** (<0.6 μm) protrude from two corners of the triangle; the third remains free and is associated with multiplication.

Cells divide by budding. Buds are produced directly from the mother cell at the tip of the triangle lacking prosthecae. In this stage, cells resemble a double-headed ax or labrys.

Gram-negative, nonmotile, and do not possess fimbriae.

Obligately aerobic, nonfermentative, **chemoorganotrophic.** Utilize carbohydrates and some organic acids as sole carbon and energy source. Type strain requires B vitamins for growth. Oxidase- and catalase-positive. Found in freshwater lakes.

The mol% G + C of the DNA is 67.9 (T_m).

Monotypic.

Type species: *Labrys monachus* Vasilyeva and Semenov 1985, 375.

Enrichment and Isolation Procedures

Strain was isolated from the silt samples from Lake Mustijärv (Esto-

nian S.S.R.). The medium was horse manure extract obtained by heating dry manure in 100 parts of water. The sediment was left to settle, and a liquid medium was prepared from the supernatant; 2% agar was added for solidification and colony isolation. Incubation was at 28°C for 10–14 days.

Minute colonies were isolated and examined under a phase-contrast microscope for the presence of bacteria with unusual morphology. Repeated subculturing of individual colonies produced a pure culture.

Maintenance Procedures

Potato agar provides a favorable growth medium. Growth occurs on MMB agar (see *Ancalomicrobium*) with glucose, only if supplemented by yeast extract of up to 0.25% (Vasilyeva and Semenov, 1984). The type strain is maintained on slants in the refrigerator for at least 3 months. Lyophilization can be used for long term preservation.

Differentiation of the genus **Labrys** *from other genera*

Labrys combines morphological features typical for budding bacteria with prosthecae such as *Prosthecomicrobium* and *Ancalomicrobium* and for flat bacteria with radial symmetry such as *Angulomicrobium* and *Stella* (Vasilyeva, 1980).

Physiological differences among these organisms are minimal.

Labrys, unlike *Angulomicrobium,* possesses prosthecae, which makes differentiation easy in spite of the resemblance in cell shape and budding. Unlike *Ancalomicrobium,* it has flat cells.

Taxonomic Comments

Labrys combines features of a number of genera and inclusion of these organisms into other genera would necessarily change their diagnoses. Only a single strain has so far been isolated. DNA/DNA hybridization studies revealed no homology with *Stella* (Lysenko et al., 1984). Further work is needed to reveal a phylogenetic interrelation among budding prosthecobacteria.

List of species of the genus **Labrys**

1. **Labrys monachus** Vasilyeva and Semenov 1985, 375.[VP] (Effective publication: Vasilyeva and Semenov 1984, 92.)

mon.ach′us. N.L. adj. from ancient Gr. *monachos* meaning the only, unique, single.

The description is as for the genus.

Unicellular flat triangular budding prosthecobacterium. Dimensions 1.1–1.5 µm. Prosthecae are short, <0.6 µm, tapering and protruding from two corners of triangle (Fig. 21.21). Cells nonmotile. Gas vacuoles are not produced.

Gram-negative. On the outer cell surface is an irregular visible capsular microlayer (Fig. 21.22). No laminated membranous structures in the cells.

Division is by budding on the corner free from prosthecae. Daughter cell separates when it approaches mother cell size and shape (Fig. 21.23).

Utilizes the following carbohydrates as a single source of carbon and energy: D-erythrose, D-ribose, L-arabinose, D-xylose, D-lyxose, D-glucose,

L-sorbose, L-rhamnose, D-fructose, D-talose, L-fucose, D-mannose, D-galactose, D-tagatose, trehalose, glycerol, mannitol, L-arabitol, adonitol, L-dulcitol and D-sorbitol. Not utilized: D-lactose, D-cellobiose, D-melibiose, sucrose, D-raffinose, melezitose, starch, inulin, pectin, glycogen, dextrin and inositol. The medium is acidified during growth on carbohydrates in all instances. Morphology is altered when luxurious growth occurs. Utilization of amino acids, organic acids and alcohols is limited. Yeast extract above 0.25% inhibits growth; B vitamins required for growth.

A considerable quantity of poly-β-hydroxybutyrate accumulates in cells immediately after inoculation on all utilized substrates.

Colonies circular about 2 mm in diameter, colorless or gray, slightly convex, flat, opaque, glistening smooth and viscous.

Optimal temperature: 28°C; the generation time: 8 h.

Type strain: All Union Collection of Microorganisms (AUCM) B-1479. Isolated from silt of Lake Mustijärv (Estonian S.S.R.) as strain 42.

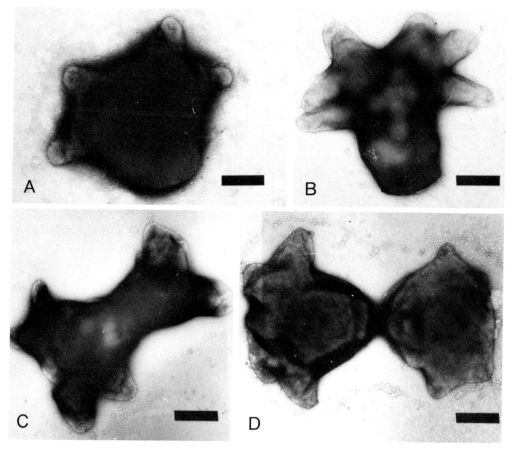

Figure 21.21.   *L. monachus. A–D,* electron microscopy showing cells in sequential stages of a multiplication. Note prosthecae protruding from two angles of the cell end, the "double ax" shape of the figure formed by the mother and daughter cells (D). Uranyl acetate-negative stain. *Bar,* 0.5 µm.

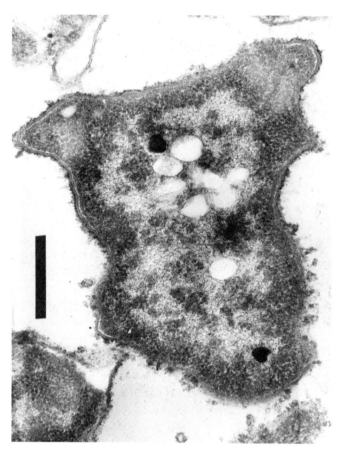

Figure 21.22. *L. monachus.* Thin section. Note cytoplasm in prosthecae, granules of poly-β-hydroxybutyrate, and an external microcapsular layer on the outer side of the typical Gram-negative cell wall. *Bar,* 0.5 μm.

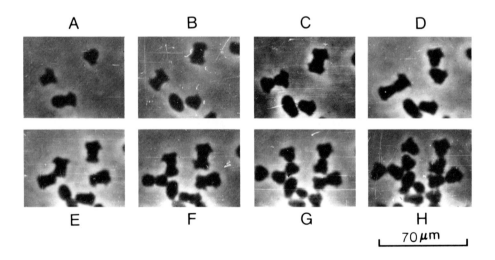

Figure 21.23. *L. monachus.* Phase-contrast micrographs. Slide microculture. Hours: *A*, 0; *B*, 4; *C*, 7.5; *D*, 8.5; *E*, 11.5; *F*, 12.5; *G*, 13; and *H*, 15.

Genus **Stella** Vasilyeva 1985, 521[VP]

L. V. VASILYEVA

Stel′la. M.L. fem. n. *Stella* star, to denote star-shaped morphology of cells.

Cells are flat, six-pronged stars, radially symmetrical, and 0.7–3.0 μm. Occur singly or in pairs. Some strains possess **gas vesicles.** Spores are not formed. **Gram-negative.** Aerobic. Reproduction is by **symmetrical cell division.**

Chemoorganotrophic, using a variety of amino acids or organic acids. Aerobic and oxidative. **Oligocarbophilic.**

Occur in soil, freshwaters, and artificial ecosystems where complete decomposition of organic matter is underway; typically representative of the microflora of dispersal systems.

The mol% G + C of the DNA ranges from 69.3 to 73.5 (T_m).

Type species: *Stella humosa* Vasilyeva 1985, 521.

Further Descriptive Information

Flat, star-shaped bacteria were first observed by Nikitin and colleagues (Nikitin et al., 1966) and shortly thereafter by Staley (Staley, 1968). Since that time, these prosthecobacteria have been discussed in a number of publications (Vasilyeva, 1970, 1972, 1980; Vasilyeva et al., 1974; Hirsch et al., 1977; Hirsch and Schlesner, 1981; Staley et al., 1981; Terekhova et al., 1981; Schlesner, 1983).

The characteristic morphology of *Stella* species is that of a flat, six-pointed star ("Star of David"). There are also intermediate forms between the flat prosthecobacteria, such as the flat triangles observed in organisms assigned to the genus *Labrys* (Vasilyeva and Semenov, 1984), and the genus *Angulomicrobium* (Vasilyeva et al., 1979).

The reproduction of star-shaped bacteria is quite similar in all strains examined so far. Cell division proceeds by cross-wall formation along a line where the cell has the smallest diameter and between opposite pairs of prongs. Both daughter cells retain three prongs each from the mother cell and then form three new additional prongs (Vasilyeva, 1972). The cell cytoplasm appears to be similar to that of other Gram-negative bacteria, and so far no obvious intracellular membrane component has been observed that might account for the prong structures that occur on the flat cells of the organism. Poly-β-hydroxybutyrate storage granules are apparent within some cells. Morphology of the star-shaped forms can vary with changes in concentration of nutrient in the broth, as well as within different strains.

Phylogenetic position of the genus *Stella* is difficult to interpret. The high S_{AB} values of 16S rRNA found between stellas and members of the α-group of purple bacteria indicate that the star-shaped organisms are nonphototrophic representatives of the purple bacteria (Fischer et al., 1985).

Strains of the genus *Stella* are able to utilize a variety of organic acids or amino acids as substrates. The majority of strains utilize: pyruvate, citrate, α-ketoglutarate, succinate, malate, acetate and glutamate. Some strains utilize: lysine, glutamine, cysteine, cystine, L-alanine, asparagine, aspartate and gluconate. Only one or a few strains utilize: fumarate, butyrate, valerate, D-alanine, arginine, proline, threonine, histidine. None of the strains utilize: propionate, benzoate, urea, ethanol, methanol, monomethylamine, leucine, isoleucine, methionine, valine, tryptophan, phenylalanine, glycine and oxyproline. Complex carbohydrate or protein polymers, cellulose, starch and gelatin are not catabolized. In addition to the compounds listed, star-shaped bacteria require 0.01% yeast extract or casamino acids in the growth medium. A mixture containing 0.1% L-glutamic acid and various B vitamins can be substituted for the yeast extract. Star-shaped bacteria are obligately aerobic, and their metabolism is oxidative (Vasilyeva et al., 1974).

The strains of *Stella* were obtained from a variety of soil, aquatic and from animal fecal materials (Hirsch and Schlesner, 1981; Vasilyeva, 1985).

From ecological observations performed with direct microscopic techniques and enrichment broth cultures, it is apparent that these organisms are found in habitats where active degradation of organic substances is occurring. Thus, these prosthecobacteria are typical representatives of the aerobic oligotrophic microflora of dispersal (Zavarzin, 1970), which are defined as an ecological group of bacteria that utilize low molecular weight compounds formed by other microorganisms during anaerobic degradation.

Enrichment and Isolation Procedures

The most successful method of recovery of *Stella* species involves the use of enrichment cultures containing prosthecobacteria growing in association with aerobic cellulose-decomposing bacteria on Hutchinson medium. The unique morphology of these star-shaped bacteria is usually obvious under phase-contrast microscopy. Colonies on agar plates are usually mixed, and a long series of subculturing and reisolation of single colonies is required for selection of pure cultures.

Pure cultures of organisms can be maintained either in dilute meat-peptone media (1:5), such as nutrient broth with beef extract and peptone added, and medium solidified with 2% (w/v) agar or in media described by Staley (see *Ancalomicrobium*). This defined medium supplemented with 0.01% yeast extract can be used for determination of carbon source utilization.

Maintenance Procedures

Strains can be maintained on slants in the refrigerator for at least 6 months. Lyophilization can be used for long term preservation.

Differentiation of the genus **Stella** from other genera

The cluster of star-shaped bacteria appears to represent a clear and distinct group within the collection of budding and/or appendaged bacteria. The mode of cell division occurring as a cross-wall separating two equal daughter cells whose profile is that of two three-pronged flat crowns provides a major means to separate organisms in the genus *Stella* from other prosthecobacteria, such as *Hyphomicrobium, Hyphomonas,* *Pedomicrobium, Rhodomicrobium, Ancalomicrobium, Ancalochloris, Prosthecomicrobium* and *Prosthecochloris.* The flat cellular morphology of *Stella* is shared with the genus *Labrys,* but the latter multiplies by budding. DNA/DNA homology between *Stella* species and *Labrys* is quite low.

Differentiation of the species of the genus **Stella**

Two species, *S. humosa* and *S. vacuolata,* in the genus *Stella* are differentiated by the presence or absence of gas vesicles which correlate with a number of other characters, such as substrate utilization and a slightly different mol% G + C content of their DNA. All vacuolate strains had DNA/DNA homologies in a range of 74–100%; however, some of nonvacuolated strains had DNA/DNA homologies in a range of 60–72%, while others had homologies as low as 3%, with this group indicating that stellas are heterogenous.

Two additional species, "*S. aquatica*" and "*S. pusilla*," were described by Schlesner (Schlesner, 1983); differentiating characters, however, remain unclear.

List of species of the genus **Stella**

1. **Stella humosa** Vasilyeva 1985, 521.[VP] (Effective publication: Vasilyeva, Lafitskaya, Aleksandrushkina and Krasil'nikova 1974, 712.) hu.mo′sa. M.L. fem. adj. *humosa* soil, earth.

Cells are flat, six-pronged stars 0.7–3.0 μm in diameter and occur singly or in pairs (Fig. 21.24). No clusters or other aggregates are formed. Gram-negative with typical three-layered cell envelope. Nonmotile. Multiplication by symmetrical cell division. Aerobic. Poly-β-hydroxybutyrate granules are formed as the reserve substance.

Colonies are grayish white, circular, compact and up to 2.5 mm in diameter after incubation for 14 days at 28°C.

Chemoorganotrophic, utilizing as sole energy source a limited number of organic acids of the tricarboxylic acid cycle and amino acids for respiration. Carbohydrates are not fermented or utilized. Yeast extract is required by all strains but may be replaced by glutamic acid and B vitamins in some strains. No hydrolytic activity. Polysaccharides and proteins not degraded. Oligocarbophilic.

Optimal temperature for growth is 28–30°C. Optimal pH is neutral for the type strain and is slightly alkaline for others. Some strains are stimulated by up to 1% NaCl. Catalase- and oxidase-positive.

Sensitive to neomycin (0.5–1.0 μg/ml); moderately sensitive to penicillin (8 μg/ml for type strain) and monomycin (2–10 μg/ml) as well to most other antibacterial antibiotics (Terekhova et al., 1981).

The mol% G + C of the DNA ranges from 69.3 to 72.9 (T_m). Plasmids have so far not been detected.

Type strain: AUCM B-1137.

2. **Stella vacuolata** Vasilyeva 1985, 521.[VP]

va′cu.o.la.ta. L. adj. *vacuus* empty, void; L. adj. *latus* broad, wide; M.L. *vacuolata* large areas in cytoplasm that appear empty due to gas vesicle formation.

Cells are flat, six-pronged stars 1.9–2.5 μm in diameter. Occur singly or in pairs. Clusters or aggregates are not formed. Gram-negative, nonmotile. Multiplication by symmetrical division into two three-pronged daughter cells. Distinctive morphological feature is presence of **gas vesicles** throughout cell cytoplasm (Fig. 21.25). Cells exhibit considerable buoyancy.

Colonies on agar prepared with dilute meat-peptone media (1:5) are **milky white,** circular and viscous and may reach 2.5 mm in diameter.

Growth in liquid broth: A pellicle is formed and sediment occurs on the bottom of tube. Growth is inhibited by shaking cultures and by 1% NaCl.

Chemoorganotrophic, aerobic. Selected amino acids and organic acids of the tricarboxylic acid cycle are utilized as energy sources. Yeast extract is required for growth, although casamino acids or L-glutamic acid and a B vitamin mixture can substitute for yeast extract. Carbohydrates are not utilized but do not inhibit growth. Do not possess the ability to utilize polymers.

Optimal temperature: 28°C. Optimal pH: neutral or slightly alkaline.

The mol% G + C of the DNA ranges from 70 to 73.5 (T_m). Plasmids were not detected.

Habitat: isolated from horse manure and sewage sludge from a piggery.

Type strain: AUCM B-1552.

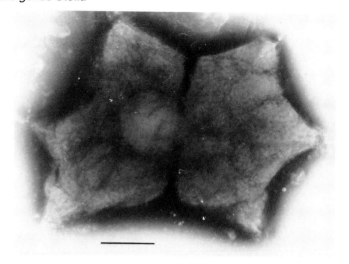

Figure 21.24. *S. humosa* type strain AUCMB-1337. Phosphotungstic acid-negative stain. *Bar,* 0.5 μm. (Reproduced with permission from E. N. Mischustin, Izvestiya Akademii Nauk S.S.S.R. Seriya Biologicheskaya *5:* 730, fig. 3, 1980.)

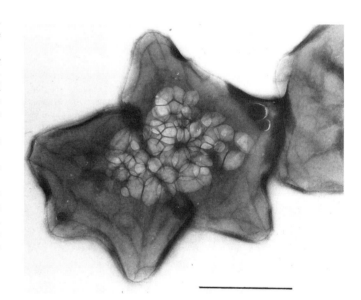

Figure 21.25. *S. vacuolata.* Bright areas in cytoplasm are gas vesicles. Uranylacetate-negative stain. *Bar,* 1.0 μm.

B. BACTERIA THAT DIVIDE BY BINARY TRANSVERSE FISSION

Genus **Caulobacter** *Henrici and Johnson 1935, 83*[AL]

JEANNE S. POINDEXTER

Cau′lo.bac′ter. L. n. *caulis* stalk; M.L. *bacter* masc. form of Gr. neut. n. *bactrum* rod; M.L. masc. n. *Caulobacter* stalk(ed) rod.

Cells **rod- or vibrioid-shaped** or **fusiform,** 0.4–0.6 × 1–2 μm; rarely larger. Morphology of the dividing cell is unique among unicellular procaryotes: The younger pole of the cell bears a **single flagellum,** and the older pole bears a prostheca (the **stalk**) derived from the cell envelope. The stalk includes outer membrane, peptidoglycan, cell membrane, and a core sometimes observed to be occupied in part by membranes but not in any case by any other discernible cytoplasmic components. Stalk diameter is constant along its length, varying from 0.11 to 0.18 μm among isolates. At the base of the flagellum and at the outer tip of the stalk is a small mass of adhesive material, the **holdfast,** which confers adhesiveness on each of the progeny. Binary fission is **constrictive** and is completed without formation of a septum. The stalk-bearing progeny cell grows and eventually repeats the **asymmetric cell division.** The flagellum-bearing progeny cell, after a period of motility, releases the flagellum and develops its stalk at the previously flagellated site as it grows and proceeds to its **asymmetric cell division.**

Gram-negative. Polar, single flagellum in motile stage. Strictly **respiratory** and **aerobic***; only O_2 serves as terminal electron acceptor for growth, although nitrate may be reduced to nitrite. Colonies are circular, convex and glistening, with smooth margin; are butyrous or (rarely) glutinous in texture; and may be colorless or any of several shades of pink, yellow or orange due to production of carotenoid pigments or, upon aging, may be light brown. In unagitated liquid cultures, cells accumulate as a **surface film** or heavier **pellicle** and develop as a ring of growth on the vessel wall at or just below the air-liquid interface. Growth in agitated liquid cultures is evenly dispersed.

Chemoorganotrophic and **oligotrophic;** grow readily in media such as peptone-yeast extract below 0.1% (w/v) organic material but not in standard nutrient broth with 0.8% (w/v) organic solutes. During growth, do not produce acid or gas from sugars. Optimal temperature for growth: 20-25°C; tolerated range for growth: 10-35°C. Optimal pH near neutrality: pH 6-9 tolerated. Maximum specific rates of exponential growth: 0.12-0.46 h⁻¹. Typically require organic growth factors: B vitamins, amino acids or other unidentified substances. Glucose and glutamic acid are the most widely utilized carbon sources.

The mol% G + C of the DNA is 62-67 (Bd).

Type species: *Caulobacter vibrioides* Henrici and Johnson 1935, 84.

Further Descriptive Information

Cell morphology is a major characteristic in classification within this genus, in that morphology is uniform within a species among cells grown in a standard, dilute peptone-yeast extract medium. However, cell shape varies among populations of a given clone according to medium composition (Figs. 21.27, 21.28, 21.31 and 21.32). Cells may be short and fusiform in complex medium but may be long, slender and rod-shaped (not tapered) in defined medium. Cells described as "subvibrioid" are tapered and gently curved, and some cells in the population may not exhibit any curvature of the long axis. Isolates that are vibrioid have this shape in all media, but mean cell length prior to constriction may vary from <1 to 3 μm, depending on medium composition. Rod-shaped isolates exhibit the least variability with medium composition but may vary in mean cell length.

Stalk length varies greatly among isolates. For any isolate, mean stalk length decreases with increasing concentration of nutrients in peptone-yeast extract media and with increasing phosphate concentration in both complex and defined media (Schmidt and Stanier, 1966; Haars and Schmidt, 1974; Poindexter, 1984). Growth of the majority of freshwater isolates is inhibited by phosphate concentrations in excess of 5 mM; marine isolates grow, but also die, faster in media containing 1 mM or more of phosphate.

Stalk bands occur in all known isolates except one. Each band is a set of concentric rings that are more electron opaque and structurally more rigid than the remainder of the stalk (Jones and Schmidt, 1973). The function of the bands is unknown; there is evidence that one band is added to the growing stalk during each cell cycle completed by the mature stalked cell (Staley and Jordan, 1973). Bands may be regarded as indicative of a *Caulobacter* or *Asticcacaulis* (q.v.) prostheca.

All isolates examined possess a thin peptidoglycan sacculus that extends continuously through the cell pole into the stalk. In most species, whole-cell peptidoglycan exhibits a 50% excess of muramic acid over

glucosamine (Poindexter and Hagenzieker, 1982). Stalk peptidoglycan has been assayed separately only for *C. crescentus;* the relative proportions of the two sugars appears reversed, implying that stalk outgrowth involves a modification of the peptidoglycan or of its synthesis. The composition of the peptide side chains of the peptidoglycan appears to vary with medium composition; in some media, glycine appears to be a component (Markiewicz et al., 1983), but glycine is not invariably detected in the peptidoglycan.

The membrane proteins of *Caulobacter* species also seem distinctive, particularly the outer membrane. Although medium composition has some influence on the variety of proteins assembled in the outer membrane of *C. crescentus,* its composition under all conditions differs from that of other genera by the greater number and sizes (majority, >70,000 daltons) of the polypeptides present (Agabian and Unger, 1978). These characteristics extend also to other vibrioid species and to fusiform and rod-shaped isolates (Poindexter, unpublished observations). Major membrane proteins unique to the stalk have not been discerned.

The flagellum of most species comprises two flagellins of slightly different mobilities in denaturing electrophoretic gels (Lagenaur and Agabian, 1977). The flagellum is microstructurally simple, not decorated; the two component proteins appear to be present in each flagellar filament. In *C. crescentus,* the larger protein predominates in the proximal region of the filament, and the smaller predominates in the distal regions (Koyasu et al., 1981; Weissborn et al., 1982).

Because cell division is typically asymmetric, any exponentially growing population comprises three types of cells: nonstalked, flagellated "swarmer" cells; unconstricted stalked cells; and constricted stalked cells that bear a flagellum at the nonstalked pole before the constriction is completed. In wild type isolates of species other than *C. leidyi* and *C. variabilis,* growing under optimal conditions, constrictions are only rarely seen in cells prior to initiation of stalk development, and stalk development is not initiated at the cell's younger pole until after cell separation. The latter type of development, however, does occur at a significant frequency in slowly growing populations and is frequently seen in caulobacters in natural materials. In the two exceptional species, nonstalked constricted cells are frequent during exponential growth, especially in phosphate-excess media (see Fig. 21.31); such cells have not been seen to bear more than one flagellum.

The majority of isolates have not been cultivated in defined media. This seems attributable principally to lack of identification of required growth factors, since all isolates can be cultivated on a variety of organic compounds as principal carbon source, with ammonium as nitrogen source, in basal media containing concentrations of peptone and yeast extract sufficient only as sources of growth factors. A major consequence of their undefined nutrition has been a concentration of *Caulobacter* research on a single, somewhat atypical species, *C. crescentus,* which grows more rapidly than the other isolates, is nutritionally independent of organic growth factors, is less sensitive to elevated nutrient concentrations, and is rarely encountered in enrichment and isolation procedures. Nevertheless, since the principal interest of research with this genus is its unique developmental sequence from swarmer to stalked cell to asymmetric fission, and that sequence is nearly universal among isolates, *C. crescentus* is an adequate representative for developmental studies.

As far as tested, *Caulobacter* species employ the Entner-Doudoroff pathway for hexose catabolism. Enzymes for catabolism of some carbohydrates are induced by exposure to substrate, but induced levels are not significantly greater than 10-fold higher than uninduced levels (reviewed in Poindexter, 1981). Ammonium assimilation has been examined only in *C. crescentus,* which lacks glutamic dehydrogenase and employs the glutamine synthetase-glutamic synthase system only (Ely et al., 1978).

Genetic studies, like developmental research, have focused on *C. crescentus.* A linear map of the *C. crescentus* genome has been constructed on the basis of linkage and complementation studies among mutations in biosynthetic processes, drug resistance, phage sensitivity, and

---

* Several isolates have been observed which are capable of forming colonies on peptone-yeast extract plates incubated under conditions sufficiently anaerobic to allow development of colonies of *Clostridium sporogenes* (J. Smit, personal communication).

motility (Barrett et al., 1982a, b). Stable, unconditionally stalkless mutants have not been reported; defective stalk development as a result of pleiotropic mutations is known (reviewed in Poindexter, 1981), but a direct selection for developmental mutations has not been devised. Both conjugation and transduction can be used to transfer genetic markers between substrains of *C. crescentus* strain CB15. *C. crescentus* isolates lack native plasmids but can propagate promiscuous plasmids originally isolated from other genera (Ely, 1979). Plasmids have been detected in other *Caulobacter* species, even after years of maintenance of the strains on laboratory media; these plasmids are cryptic and have been detected only by physical methods (Schoenlein and Ely, 1983). One unstable plasmid has been reported whose loss was coincidental with loss of capacity for manganese oxidation (see Gregory and Staley, 1982; E. Gregory, personal communication). Bacteriocins are produced by some species; they are active only against other *Caulobacter* isolates and may be produced by strains lacking detectable plasmids (Schoenlein and Ely, 1983).

A variety of bacteriophages has been isolated for *Caulobacter* species; in a few instances, the source of phage was a *Caulobacter* culture (reviewed in Poindexter, 1981). The majority of phages have large (50–65 × 170–260 nm), prolate cylindrical heads with long (200–320 nm), flexible noncontractile tails. These phages exhibit wide host ranges among *Caulobacter* species. Six other morphological types of phages have been described, including small RNA phages. None of the phages tested is lytic for any other genus, and phages lytic for other genera are not lytic for *Caulobacter* species, with one exception: Two phages isolated on *Asticcacaulis excentricus*, another prosthecate species, are lytic for a few *Caulobacter* isolates (see Table 21.19). Generally, *Caulobacter* appears isolated from other genera with respect to phage propagation. Within the genus, most phages are lytic either for vibrioid isolates or for rod-shaped and fusiform isolates, but some are lytic for both subgroups. Phage typing has not proved useful in *Caulobacter* taxonomy.

Because of their unique morphology, *Caulobacter* cells can be recognized in natural materials by phase-contrast and electron microscopy. Generally, they are most readily observed in samples of water of low nutrient content and among the bacteria attached to the surfaces of algal thalli. They are commonly found among bacterial contaminants of unialgal cultures and may influence the course of development in the algae (Klaveness, 1982). They are also frequently detected in moist soils, either attached to diatoms or among members of rhizosphere communities, and in activated sludge. However, only in waters (not soils) of very low nutrient concentrations—open ocean samples or stored distilled water, for examples—do they occur as numerically prominent members of bacterial populations. They have not been encountered as plant or animal parasites, although they may occur as epibionts of fungi in arthropod intestines. Their distinctive distribution is in oligotrophic habitats. Their role is presumed to be that of scavengers of soluble nutrients from low concentrations. Their adhesiveness presumably contributes to their efficiency in this role by allowing them to persist on wetted surfaces where sorption of organic materials would occur. Similarly, the production of a motile cell at each reproductive event would allow continual dispersal of the population within the nutrient-poor environment, thereby reducing intraclonal competition for sparse resources. Whether the extended cell surface represented by the stalk also serves to improve the efficiency of nutrient capture by *Caulobacter* cells remains to be demonstrated experimentally.

Enrichment and Isolation Procedures

The lack of identification of any physiologic peculiarity within this group has prevented the development of a strong selective enrichment procedure. Enrichment depends on a mechanical process: the accumulation of stalked cells in the air-water interface of a water sample or soil extract carefully protected during incubation and examination against turbulence that would disturb the air-water interface. The most dependable, although tedious, procedure for enrichment and isolation of *Caulobacter* species. has not changed in 30 years (Houwink, 1955). A sample of clean water (fresh, brackish, or sea) or a water extract of soil is enriched with at most 0.01% (w/v) peptone and allowed to stand at room tempera-

ture. Within a few days, a sample of the surface film, taken with a bacteriological loop or a coverslip (Schmidt, 1981a), is examined by phase-contrast microscopy for the presence of stalked cells. Some cells may possess a stalk at each pole and so be indistinguishable from *Prosthecobacter* (q.v.); distinguishing these two genera is dependable only after clones have been isolated and examined for motility (characteristic of *Caulobacter*). When such cells account for 10–50% of the population (see Fig. 21.26), a sample (again, taken with a loop, not a pipette) is streaked on a dilute (0.05%, maximum 0.1%, w/v) peptone or peptone-yeast extract medium prepared with 1.0% or 1.5% agar. By the third or fourth day of incubation of the plates, small, hyaline or crystalline noniridescent colonies of caulobacters begin to appear. It is helpful to remove these colonies while they are very small, by using sterile toothpicks, to small sites ("patches") on secondary plates, for two reasons. First, samples of oligotrophic populations often include bacteria that swarm as a continuous film on the agar surface. Second, preparation of a wet mount to screen the initial, small colony may consume the entire colony. It is preferable to begin microscopic screening only after the patches of growth on the secondary plate have developed.

Identification requires phase-contrast microscopy (see Figs. 21.27, *A* and *B*; 21.29*A*; 21.30*A*; and 21.33*A*) because of the small diameter of the stalk (<0.2 μm), which is below the resolution afforded by ordinary light microscopy. The addition of a stain to the wet mount or the use of a mordanted stain such as is designed for flagella may be helpful. The mordant alone applied to dried smears clearly reveals stalks by phase-contrast microscopy (see Figs. 21.27*C*; 21.31*A*; 21.32, *A* and *B*; and 21.33*B*). However, examination of wet mounts of living cells is necessary because motility is characteristic of *Caulobacter* species, and its detection aids particularly in distinguishing *Caulobacter* from *Prosthecobacter*. In the dense populations developed on an agar surface, *Caulobacter* cells will adhere to each other's holdfasts, and the characteristic rosettes, with cells peripheral to the stalks united in a common holdfast, are often the most dependable way to detect the presence of stalks. In enrichment samples and in pure populations, stalked cells become trapped within air bubbles in wet mounts, and stalks not clearly discernible in the suspended population are more obvious in such regions (see Fig. 21.27*B*).

Typical caulobacters do not multiply so rapidly as do bacteria such as *Pseudomonas* and *Flavobacterium* species that are often present in the same samples. It has been suggested that serial dilutions of the sample would allow the caulobacters to develop without becoming outnumbered by such other types. However, this procedure is suitable only when the caulobacters are initially predominant *and* not attached to other cells, two conditions not commonly met.

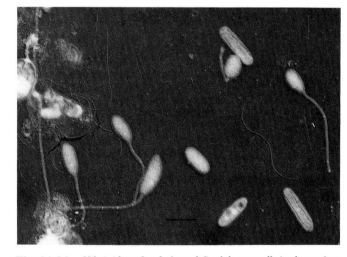

Fig. 21.26. Vibrioid- and rod-shaped *Caulobacter* cells in the surface film of an enrichment culture. Electron microscopy, shadowed specimen, negative image. *Bar*, 1 μm.

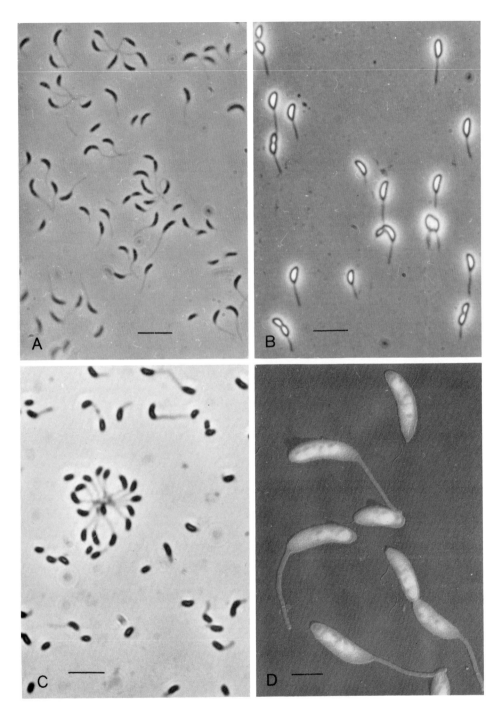

Figure 21.27. *C. crescentus* strain CB2 grown in peptone-yeast extract (*A–C*) and in glucose-glutamate mini-mal medium (*D*). *A*, phase-contrast microscopy, wet mount. *B*, phase-contrast micrograph of cells trapped under an air bubble within a wet mount. *C*, phase-contrast micrograph of dried smear to which a droplet of Gray's flagella stain mordant (only) and coverslip were added. *D*, electron microscopy, shadowed specimen, negative image. *Bars*, 5 μm for *A–C*; 1 μm for *D*.

It is also possible to enrich a water sample in situ by "baiting" the caulobacters with coverslips, to which they will attach. The submerged coverslip can be removed, rinsed well with sterile water, then used as inoculum for a stationary culture as described above. *Caulobacter* attachment is tenacious; the cells cannot be efficiently scraped from the coverslip but should be allowed to release swarmers by cell division. Some success with thin plastic foil carefully laid on the surface of quiet water has also been reported.

In any of these procedures, the overriding factor important to successful isolation is that the sample be low in nutrient content. Caulobacters are not necessarily absent from richer samples, but their proportion is invariably too low, and their reproductive rate is not competitive in nutrient-rich cultures. Until a physiologic enrichment procedure is developed, the caulobacters of habitats such as the rhizosphere and activated sludge may continue to elude isolation.

Maintenance Procedures

Once isolated, *Caulobacter* species can be dependably maintained in at least four ways. First, vegetative stocks should be maintained on 1% agar slants of dilute (0.05–0.3% organic material) complex medium or defined medium (if possible, with a given isolate) that contains at least 100 mg organic carbon/mg phosphate-phosphorus. Such a medium promotes the storage of carbon reserves and prolongs the viability of the population during storage. Freshwater, soil and marine isolates should be transferred every 8 or 9 weeks, incubated 2 or 3 days at 20–25°C (higher incubation temperatures reduce stability during storage), then refrigerated. Second, cells grown in dilute complex medium can be stored in small volumes frozen at −70°C without cryoprotectant. Survival varies among isolates, ranging from 10 to 50%. Such frozen cultures can be thawed at room temperature and transferred to growth medium to resume vegetative cultivation. This is the most dependable method of maintenance of freshwater and soil caulobacters; it has not been used for marine isolates. Third, washed cells diluted to 10^3–10^4 cells/ml of sterile water and sealed in ampuls can be stored at room temperature for 2–3 years. This procedure is more dependable than lyophilization but requires periodic recultivation. It has not been attempted with marine isolates. Fourth, lyophilization is the least dependable means of maintenance but is suitable for many freshwater and soil isolates. Marine isolates, in particular, are difficult to revive. If a protectant such as milk solids is used, the rehydrated specimen should be diluted immediately in order to avoid the inhibitory effect of the solids. Lyophilization on strips of sterile filter paper, without any additive, has proved the most dependable environment for lyophilization.

Procedures for Testing for Special Characteristics

The genus *Caulobacter* is distinguished by the morphology of the dividing cell—specifically, by the asymmetry of its appendages. Both appendages are best characterized by electron microscopy. Shadowed specimens provide the clearest image (see Figs. 21.26; 21.27D; 21.28; 21.29, B and C; 21.30, B and C; 21.31, B–D; 21.32D; 21.33, C–E; and 21.34), but negatively stained specimens need not be washed and so preserve a higher proportion of attached flagella. The holdfast is best detected by its function, adhesiveness, although it, too, is discernible by electron microscopy.

Differentiation of the genus **Caulobacter** from other closely related taxa

Four other groups of bacteria produce long cellular appendages of the envelope that are of constant diameter; these bacteria also tend to occur in habitats with caulobacters. They are distinguishable from *Caulobacter*, and from each other, by the morphology of their reproductive stages. These groups are described in Table 21.17.

Taxonomic Comments

The genus *Caulobacter* was created by Henrici and Johnson (1935) on the basis of their observations of bacterial populations attached to slides submerged in a freshwater lake. They did not obtain isolates or study pure cultures. Nevertheless, they correctly inferred the developmental sequence and recognized that this type of bacterium was unique. Subsequent study has justified the recognition of this group as a genus, seemingly long isolated—genetically—from other Gram-negative bacteria including other prosthecate groups except *Asticcacaulis*, a more recently created genus. In addition to their unique developmental sequence, the caulobacters have also been found unusual with respect to cell envelope and flagellum composition, isolated with respect to bacteriophage propagation, and (most recently) possibly different in significant ways with respect to the sequence structure of regulatory (Winkler et al., 1984) and ribosome-function genes (Filer and Furano, 1980, 1981; Stringfellow et al., 1980). Much less is as yet known about the only closely related genus, *Asticcacaulis*, which is also far less commonly encountered in nature. The more widely distributed genus, *Caulobacter*, is indeed distinctive, presumably of some antiquity, and consequently difficult to position taxonomically among bacterial genera. On the bases of carbohydrate catabolism, mode of flagellation, and certain aspects of molecular biology, the genus can be provisionally accepted as prosthecate relatives of the aerobic pseudomonads.

The initial system for subgeneric classification (Poindexter, 1964) and the key to species in the previous edition of the *Manual* employed cell morphology as the principal subdividing criterion. Because morphology is flexible and must be described for exponentially growing populations under standard conditions, this may seem an unwise choice of characteristics. Nevertheless, the practice is continued in the subgeneric classi-

Table 21.17.

Differential morphology of reproductive stages among genera that produce cylindrical prosthecae[a]

	Caulobacter	*Asticcacaulis*	*Prosthecobacter*	*Ancalomicrobium*	*Hyphomicrobium*
Reproductive mechanism					
Constriction	+	−	+	−	−
Septation	−	+	−	−	−
Budding from cell surface	−	−	−	+	−
Budding from prostheca	−	−	−	−	+
Prostheca					
Number/dividing cell					
1	+	+	−	−	+
2	−	+	+	−	−
>2	−	−	−	+	−
Site					
Polar	+	−	+	−	+
Subpolar	+	+	−	−	−
Lateral	−	+	−	+[b]	−
Associated structures					
Bands	+	+	−	−	−
Holdfast	+	−	+	−	−
Flagellum					
Polar	+	−	−	−	+
Subpolar	+	+	−	−	+

[a]Symbols: +, 90% or more of strains are positive; and −, 90% or more of strains are negative.

[b]Cells are multiply prosthecate; the identity of the "pole" is not distinctive.

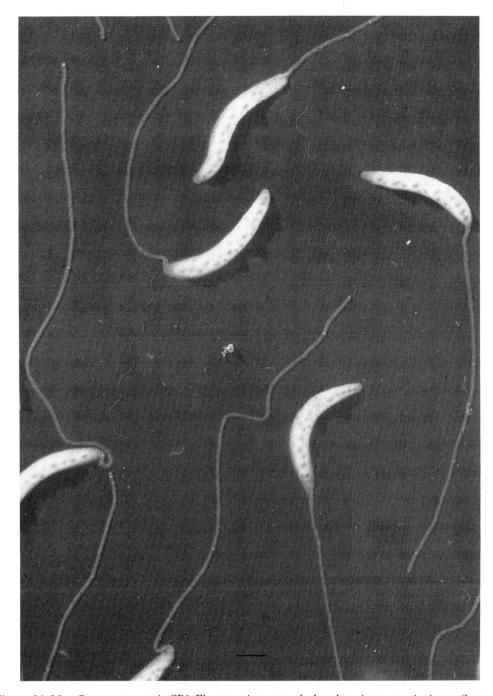

Figure 21.28. *C. crescentus* strain CB2. Electron microscopy, shadowed specimen, negative image. Swarmer cells were suspended in glucose-glutamate minimal medium without phosphate and incubated 23 h to allow stalk development. *Bar*, 1 μm.

fication here, for four reasons. First, it is consistent with a genus designation based exclusively on morphology and life cycle. Second, although flexible, morphology under standard conditions does not seem mutable (as are, for examples, catabolic, biosynthetic, motility, drug resistance, and bacteriophage propagation properties), presumably be-

cause the pattern of construction of the sacculus is under the direction of a complex of genetic properties, each of whose expression is essential to the physical integrity of the cell under a given set of conditions. Similarly, the shape of the cell pole reflects to a significant extent the mechanics of fission, the essentially normal occurrence of which is (by definition, with

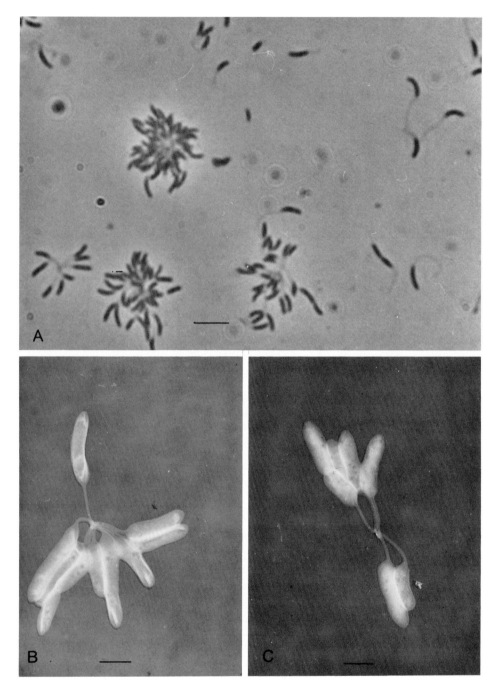

Figure 21.29. *C. subvibrioides* grown in peptone-yeast extract medium. *A,* strain 18 (VKM v-1187). Phase-contrast microscopy, wet mount. *Bar,* 5 μm. *B* and *C,* strain 20 (VKM v-1489). Electron microscopy, shadowed specimen, negative image. *Bars,* 1 μm for each.

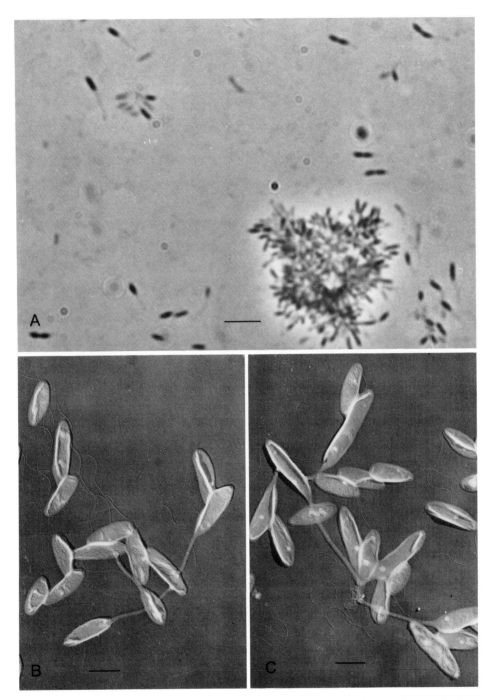

Figure 21.30. *C. fusiformis* strain CB27 grown in peptone-yeast extract medium. *A*, phase-contrast micros-copy, wet mount. *Bar*, 5 µm. *B* and *C*, electron microscopy, shadowed specimen, negative image. *Bars*, 1 µm.

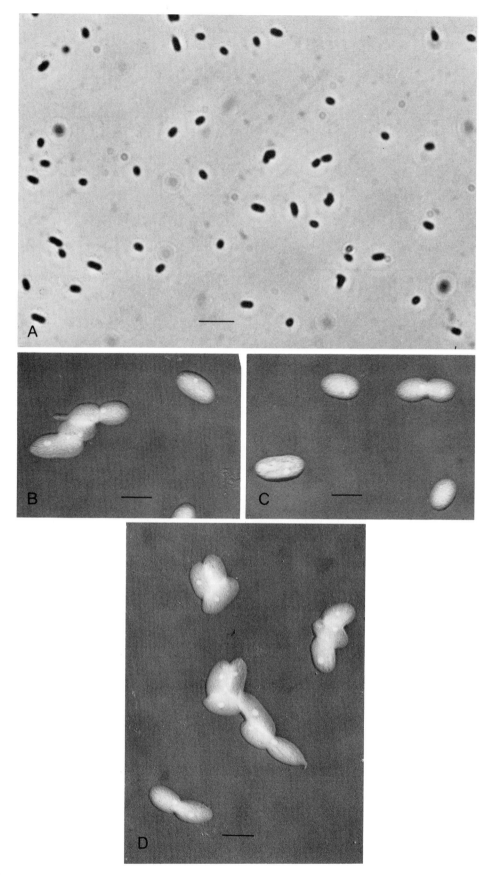

Figure 21.31. *C. leidyi* strain CB37 grown in peptone-yeast extract medium. *A*, phase-contrast micrograph of dried smear mounted in Gray's flagella stain mordant. *Bar*, 5 μm. *B–D*, electron microscopy, shadowed specimen, negative image. *Bars*, 1 μm for each.

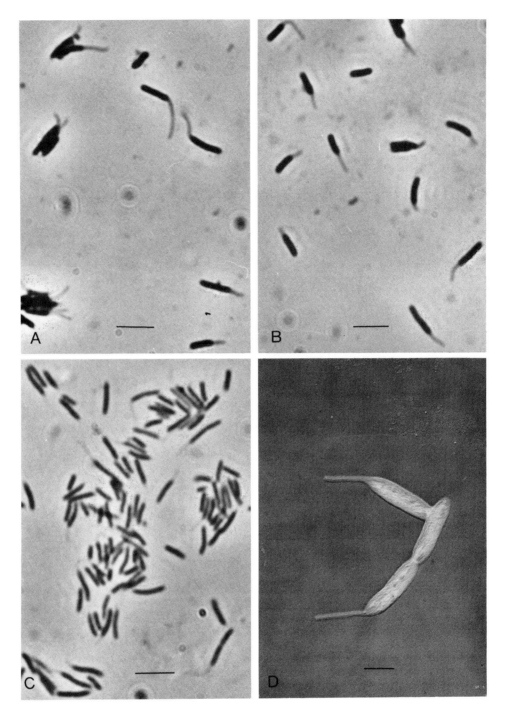

Fig. 21.32. *C. leidyi* strain CB37 grown in glucose-glutamate minimal medium containing phosphate as the yield-limiting nutrient. *A* and *B*, phase-contrast micrographs of dried smear mounted in Gray's flagella stain mordant. *Bars*, 5 μm. *C*, phase-contrast microscopy, wet mount. *Bar*, 5 μm. *D*, electron microscopy, shadowed specimen, negative image. *Bar*, 1 μm.

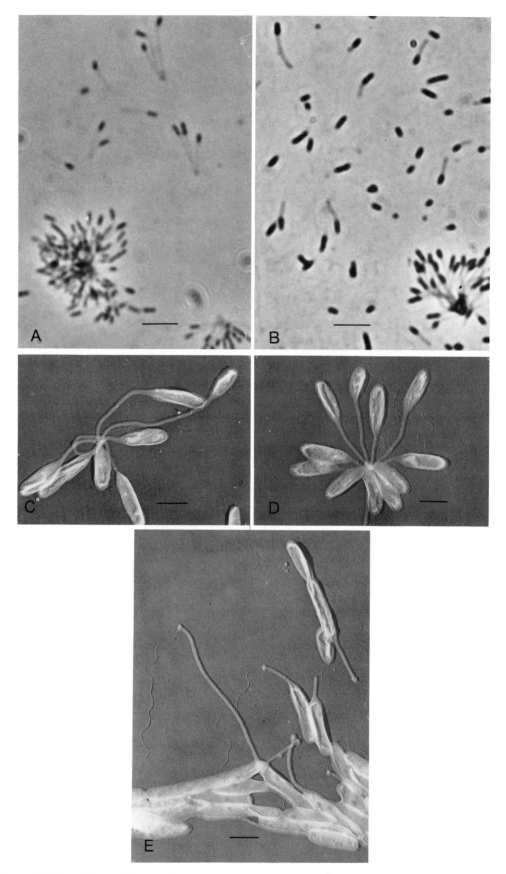

Figure 21.33. *C. bacteroides* grown in peptone-yeast extract medium. *A, B,* and *E,* strain 25 (VKM v-1183). *C* and *D,* strain CB11a (ATCC 19090). For *A,* phase-contrast microscopy, wet mount. *Bar,* 5 μm. For *B,* phase-contrast micrograph of dried smear mounted in Gray's flagella stain mordant. *Bar,* 5 μm. For *C–E,* electron microscopy, shadowed specimens, negative image. *Bars,* 1 μm for each.

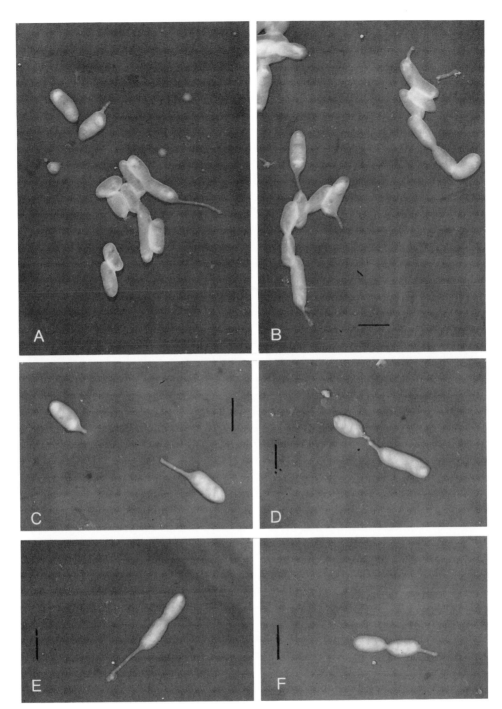

Figure 21.34. *C. variabilis* strain 5 (VKM v-1192) grown in peptone-yeast extract medium. *A–D*, clone *t*. *E* and *F*, clone *l*. Electron microscopy, shadowed specimens, negative image. *Bars*, 1 µm.

unicellular organisms) essential for viability. Third, there is too little comparative information available regarding other types of characteristics within this genus. The physiologic characteristics that are available serve classification better within than between morphological groups. DNA/DNA homology is difficult to detect between isolates of different morphological groups (Moore et al., 1978) and so is not yet available as a test of the validity of the species groups. Finally, this group seems so isolated from other superficially similar groups, such as the pseudomonads, that their morphology must have been determined long ago as important to their survival; accordingly, it can be expected that it is an expression of conserved properties within this group.

If Table 21.18 were arranged as a dichotomous key, the first and second levels of subdivision would be seen to be morphological. The order used in the previous edition of the *Manual* is reversed here, placing cell curvature above the shape of the poles; the reversal reflects the opinion of Krasil'nikov and Belyaev (1970) that cell curvature distinguishes two principal subgroups within this genus. Results of several studies, particularly of nutritional requirements and bacteriophage sensitivities, also imply that cell curvature is a characteristic significantly correlated with other types of properties.

It must be emphasized that the 13 species listed here are not adequate to accommodate all the known varieties of *Caulobacter* isolates. Several subspecies have been proposed that are not listed here. Species are described broadly enough to accommodate subspecific groups, and formal use of subspecies is not advisable within a group where the characters available cannot yet be evaluated for their phylogenetic significance. It is hoped that future studies, perhaps at the level of nucleic acid fine structure or expression, will provide the insight needed to recognize historical relationships among *Caulobacter* varieties and allow a phylogenetic classification within the genus.

Acknowledgments

The author is grateful to the U.S.S.R. Academy of Sciences for providing 24 representative strains of the *Caulobacter* collection of Krasil'nikov and Belyaev to allow their comparison with the author's isolates, to C. G. Poindexter for technical assistance in the comparative studies, to J. T. Staley, E. Gregory and D. Klaveness for providing isolates over the years, and especially to J. M. Schmidt, whose laboratory was the safe haven for the author's collection for 9 years.

Further Reading

Babinchak, J.A. and V.F. Gerencser, 1976. Bacteriophage typing of the "*Caulobacter* group." Int. J. Syst. Bacteriol. *26:* 82–84.
Henrici, A.T. and D.E. Johnson. 1935. Studies on freshwater bacteria. II. Stalked bacteria, a new order of schizomycetes. J. Bacteriol. *30:* 61–93.
Krasil'nikov, N.A. and S.S. Belyaev. 1973. Taxonomy and classification of the genus *Caulobacter*. Izv. Akad. Nauk S.S.S.R. Ser. Biol. *3:* 313–323.
Moore, R.L., J. Schmidt, J. Poindexter and J.T. Staley. 1978. Deoxyribonucleic acid homology among the caulobacters. Int. J. Syst. Bacteriol. *28:* 349–353.
Poindexter, J.S. 1964. Biological properties and classification of the *Caulobacter* group. Bacteriol. Rev. *28:* 231–295.
Poindexter, J.S. 1981. The caulobacters: ubiquitous unusual bacteria. Microbiol. Rev. *45:* 123–179.
Poindexter, J.S. and R.F. Lewis. 1966. Recommendations for revision of the taxonomic treatment of stalked bacteria. Int. J. Syst. Bacteriol. *16:* 377–382.
Schmidt, J.M. 1981. The genera *Caulobacter* and *Asticcacaulis*. *In* Starr, Stolp, Trüper, Balows and Schlegel (Editors), The Prokaryotes. A Handbook on Habitats, Isolation, and Identification of Bacteria. Springer-Verlag, Berlin, pp. 466–476.
Schmidt, J.M. and R.Y. Stanier. 1965. Isolation and characterization of bacteriophages active against stalked bacteria. J. Gen. Microbiol. *39:* 95–107.
Staley, J.T. 1973. Budding and prosthecate bacteria. *In* Laskin and Lechevalier (Editors), CRC Handbook of Microbiology, vol. 1, Organismic Microbiology. CRC Press, Cleveland, OH, pp. 29–49.
Staley, J.T., P. Hirsch and J.M. Schmidt. 1981. Introduction to the budding and/or appendaged bacteria. *In* Starr, Stolp, Trüper, Balows and Schlegel (Editors), The Prokaryotes. A Handbook on Habitats, Isolation, and Identification of Bacteria. Springer-Verlag, Berlin, pp. 451–455.

Table 21.18.
Differential characteristics of the species of the genus **Caulobacter**[a]

Characteristic	1. C. vibrioides	2. C. intermedius	3. C. henricii	4. C. crescentus	5. C. subvibrioides	6. C. fusiformis	7. "C. kusnezovii"	8. C. leidyi	9. C. maris	10. C. halobacteroides	11. C. bacteroides	12. "C. glutinosus"	13. C. variabilis
Morphology[b]													
Long axis of cell curved	+	+	+	+	±	−	−	−	−	−	−	−	−
Nonstalked pole tapered	+	+	+	+	±	+	+	+	−	−	−	−	−
Stalk invariably central	+	+	+	+	+	+	+	+	+	+	+	+	−
NaCl													
≥0.05% required for growth	−	−	−	−	−	−	−	−	+	+	−	−	−
4% tolerated	−	−	−	−	−	−	−	−	−	+	−	−	−
Carbon sources generally used													
Carbohydrates	+	+	+	+	+	−	+	+	+	+	+	+	+
Amino acids	d	+	+	+	+	+	+	+	−	+	d	+	+
Other organic acids	d	+	d	+	d	−	d	d	−	+	+	−	d
Primary alcohols	−	−	−	+	−	−	−	−	−	−	−	−	−
Organic growth factors needed													
Vitamin B$_2$	+	−	−	−	−	−	−	−	−	−	−	−	−
Biotin	−	+	−	−	−	−	−	−	−	−	−	d	−
Vitamin B$_{12}$	d	−	d	−	−	−	−	−	−	−	−	−	−
Amino acids	−	−	d	−	−	−	+	−	−	−	d	+	−
Other, unidentified	+	+	−	−	+	+	+	−	−	−	+	+	+
Colonies distinctly pigmented at all ages	d	−	+	−	d	+	+	−	−	−	d	−	d

[a]Symbols: +, 90% or more of strains are positive; ±, varies among cells within a clone; −, 90% or more of strains are negative; and d, 11–89% of the strains are positive.
[b]Morphology as observed during growth in 0.1% (w/v) peptone, 0.05% (w/v) yeast extract, 0.01% (w/v) MgSO$_4$·7H$_2$O broth prepared in tap water or, for marine strains, in 0.05% (w/v) peptone, 0.05% (w/v) casamino acids prepared in 80% seawater; agitated cultures, 30°C. Cell shape and stalk position are illustrated in Figures 21.27–21.34.

Table 21.19.

Other characteristics of the species of the genus **Caulobacter**[a]

Characteristic	1. C. vibrioides	2. C. intermedius	3. C. henricii	4. C. crescentus	5. C. subvibrioides	6. C. fusiformis	7. "C. kusnezovii"	8. C. leidyi	9. C. maris	10. C. halobacteroides	11. C. bacteroides	12. "C. glutinosus"	13. C. variabilis
Maximum specific rate of exponential growth >0.35 h^{-1}	−	+	−	+	−	−	−	+	−	−	−	−	−
Sugar utilization													
Arabinose	+	+	d	d	−	−	−	−	−	+	+	+	−
Ribose	+	−	d	−	−	−	−	−	−	+	+	+	−
Xylose	+	+	+	+	+	−	d	d	+	+	+	+	d
Glucose	+	+	+	+	+	−	d	+	+	+	+	+	+
Galactose	+	+	+	+	+	−	d	d	−	+	+	+	+
Mannose	+	+	d	+	−	−	−	+	−	+	+	+	−
Fructose	+	−	d	−	−	−	−	+	−	+	+	+	−
Lactose	+	+	d	+	−	−	−	−	−	+	d	+	−
Maltose	+	+	+	+	+	−	d	d	+	+	d	+	+
Sucrose	+	+	+	+	+	−	d	d	+	+	+	+	d
Starch hydrolysis	+	+	+	d	+	−	−	−	−	+	+	+	d
Amino acid utilization													
Alanine	+	+	+	+	+	−	d	+	−	−	d	+	d
Aspartate	+	+	+	+	+	−	−	+	−	−	d	+	−
Glutamate	+	+	+	+	+	+	+	+	−	−	d	+	+
Proline	+	+	+	+	d	−	d	+	−	+	d	+	+
Tyrosine	d	−	d	+	−	−	−	−	−	−	−	−	−
Utilization of other acids													
Acetate	−	+	+	+	+	d	d	d	−	+	+	−	d
Butyrate	d	+	+	+	d	−	−	−	−	+	d	−	+
Pimelate		+	+	+	−	−	−	+			−	−	−
Pyruvate	d	+	+	d	+	−	−	−	−	+	+	+	+
Malate	d	+	+	d	d	−	−	+	−	−	d	−	−
Fumarate	+	+	+	d	+	−	−	+	−	−	+	−	+
Succinate	+	+	+	−	+	−	−	+	−	−	+	−	+
Utilization of primary alcohols													
Methanol	−	−	−	+	−	−	−	−	−	−	−	−	−
Ethanol	−	d	d	+	−	−	−	−	−	−	d	−	−
Propanol	−	−	−	+	−	−	−	−	−	−	−	−	−
Butanol	+	+	+	+	−	−	−	−	−	−	−	−	d
Pentanol	−	−	−	+	−	−	−	−	−	−	−	−	−
Nitrate reduction to nitrite	d	−	−	d	−	−	−	−	+	−	d	−	−
Sensitivity to[b]													
Penicillin G	d	+	+	−	+	+	+	−		+	+	+	+
Ampicillin			−	−		+		−					
Streptomycin	+	+	+	+	+	+	+	−		+	+	+	+
Rifampin			+	+		+		−					
Chloramphenicol			+	+		+		+					
Kanamycin			+	+		+		+					
Tetracycline			+	+		+		+					
Sensitivity to bacteriophages[b]													
I (I)[c]	−		−	+	−		+	−			+	+	
I (II)	+		−	+	+		+	−			+	+	
I (III)	+		+	+	−						−	−	
III	+		+	−									
VII (IV)	−		−	−							+	−	
VII (V)	+		−	+	−		−				−	−	
VII (Va)	+		−	+	−		−				−	−	
VII (VI)	−		−	−	−		+	−			−	−	
AC phages[d]	−		+	−	+	+					+	+	
Plasmid(s) detected[b]			+			+		+			+		
Number of known isolates[e]	46	2	11	6	35	2	13	11	3	7	62	10	3
		28			4		5				18		

[a]Symbols: −, 90% or more of strains are negative; +, 90% or more of strains are positive; and d, 11–89% of strains are positive.

[b]Tested for selected representative strains only. The plasmid-containing (E. Gregory, personal communication), orange-pigmented isolate of Gregory and Staley (1982) has been identified as *C. bacteroides* (Poindexter, unpublished observation).

[c]Roman numerals refer to phage groups of Poindexter (1981); numerals in parentheses refer to phage groups of Schmidt and Stanier (1965).

[d]Phages isolated on strains of *Asticcacaulis* species.

[e]Numbers in the lower row represent the isolates reported by Babinchak and Gerencser (1976), for which only cell morphology and phage sensitivities have been reported.

List of species of the genus **Caulobacter**

1. **Caulobacter vibrioides** Henrici and Johnson 1935, 84.[AL]

vib.ri.oi′des. M.L. n. *vibrio* name of genus; Gr. n. *eidus* form, shape; M.L. adj. *vibrioides* resembling a vibrio.

Vibrioid cells slender or nearly ovoid. Colonies colorless or pale yellow. Vitamin B₂ essential for growth, but additional unidentified growth factors available in peptone-yeast extract also required by most strains.

The mol% G + C of the DNA is 64–65 (Bd, determined for two isolates). Isolates reported from water and from soil.

Neotype strain: CB51 (Poindexter and Lewis, 1966).

Krasil'nikov and Belyaev (1973) reported 20 isolates of *C. vibrioides.* Babinchak and Gerencser (1976) reported 28 vibrioid isolates; however, characteristics other than morphology and phage sensitivities have not been described for their isolates.

2. **Caulobacter intermedius** Poindexter 1964, 288.[AL]

in.ter.med′i.us. L. adj. *intermedius* in the middle degree, between extremes.

Vibrioid cells short. Colonies colorless. Biotin stimulates growth, but additional unidentified growth factors available in peptone-yeast extract also required.

Type strain: CB63 (ATCC 15262).

3. **Caulobacter henricii** Poindexter 1964, 288.[AL]

hen.ric′i.i. M.L. gen. n. *henricii* of Henrici; named for A. T. Henrici, who observed stalked bacteria on slides that had been submerged in freshwater.

Vibrioid cells slender; cells of some strains unusually small (<0.5 μm × <1 μm.) Colonies yellow or golden-red. Vitamin B₁₂ and/or a complex of amino acids required as growth factors.

The mol% of the DNA is 62–65 (Bd, determined for two isolates).

Type strain: CB4 (ATCC 15253).

Krasil'nikov and Belyaev's (1973) strain 44 (VKM v-1190), designated "*C. rutilus*" sp. nov. is not distinguishable from *C. henricii.* As described here, *C. henricii* accommodates all known *Caulobacter* isolates of brightly pigmented vibrioid types.

4. **Caulobacter crescentus** Poindexter 1964, 288.[AL]

cres′cen.tus. L. adj. *crescentus* of the moon in its first quarter, crescent.

Vibrioid cells slender. Colonies colorless, with centers becoming dark pink on aging. Lack of growth factor requirements is unique among vibrioid *Caulobacter* types.

The mol% G + C of the DNA is 62–67 (Bd, determined for one isolate; T_m, determined for three isolates; paper electrophoresis of hydrolysate, determined for one isolate). (Illustrated in Figures 21.27 and 21.28.)

Type strain: CB2 (ATCC 15252).

5. **Caulobacter subvibrioides** Poindexter 1964, 289.[AL]

sub.vib.ri.oi′des. L. pref. *sub* almost, somewhat, near; M.L. n. *vibrio* name of a genus; Gr. n. *eidus* resembling; M.L. adj. *subvibrioides* somewhat like a vibrio.

Cell morphology variable within a clone: some poles distinctly tapered, others rounded; long axis gently curved or not curved. Colonies orange, golden or colorless. Organic growth factor requirements not satisfied by mixtures of B vitamins, amino acids, and purine and pyrimidine bases.

The mol% G + C of the DNA is 67 (Bd, determined for one isolate). Isolates reported from water and from soil. (Illustrated in Figure 21.29.)

Type strain: CB81 (ATCC 15264).

Krasil'nikov and Belyaev's (1973) strain 23 (VKM v-1188), designated "*C. robiginosus*" sp. nov., and strains 18 (VKM v-1187) and 20 (VKM v-1489), designated "*C. metschnikovii*" sp. nov., are not distinguishable from *C. subvibrioides.* As described here, *C. subvibrioides* accommodates all known subvibrioid isolates of *Caulobacter* able to utilize sugars for growth. Subvibrioid isolates that grow poorly, if at all, at the expense of sugars remain unassigned to any species. Known isolates of this type are colorless or very pale golden and include Krasil'nikov and Belyaev's (1973) strain 10 (VKM v-1180), designated "*C. bacteroides modicus*"

subsp. nov., and CB66, designated type I (Poindexter, 1964). Babinchak and Gerencser (1976) reported four subvibrioid isolates; however, characteristics other than morphology and phage sensitivities have not been reported for their isolates.

6. **Caulobacter fusiformis** Poindexter 1964, 289.[AL]

fus.i.form′is. L. n. *fusus* spindle; L. n. *forma* shape, form; M.L. adj. *fusiformis* spindle-shaped.

Fusiform cells slender. Colonies bright yellow. Sugars not utilized as sources of carbon. Organic growth factor requirements not satisfied by mixtures of B vitamins, amino acids, and purine and pyrimidine bases. (Illustrated in Figure 21.30.)

Type strain: CB27 (ATCC 15257).

Krasil'nikov and Belyaev's (1973) strain 25 (VKM v-1183) was assigned by them to this species. However, on the basis of its morphology (Fig. 21.33, *A–C*), pigmentation and ability to utilize a variety of sugars, it is assignable to *C. bacteroides.* Another fusiform isolate, strain 1 (VKM v-1189), designated "*C. rossii*" sp. nov. by Krasil'nikov and Belyaev (1973), is not assignable to *C. fusiformis;* because only one such isolate is known and its physiological characteristics are predominantly inabilities and appear variable, "*C. rossii*" is not included in this list. Babinchak and Gerencser (1976) reported five fusiform isolates; however, characteristics other than morphology and phage sensitivities have not been described for their isolates.

7. "**Caulobacter kusnezovii**" Krasil'nikov and Belyaev 1973, 320.

kus.ne.zov′i.i. M.L. gen. n. *kusnezovii* of Kusnetsov; named for S. I. Kusnetsov.

Fusiform cells slender. Colonies dark golden or dark orange. Growth is stimulated by amino acid mixtures, but additional growth factors available in peptone-yeast extract are also required. Most isolates are able to utilize at least one sugar.

Type strain: CB26 (ATCC 15256).

This species, as described by Krasil'nikov and Belyaev (1973), appears indistinguishable from type II (Poindexter, 1964).

8. **Caulobacter leidyi** Poindexter 1964, 289.[AL]

leid′y.i. M.L. gen. n. *leidyi* of Leidy; named for J. Leidy, who observed tufts of (bacterial) growth on fungi in insect guts in 1853.

Cell morphology in dilute peptone-yeast extract medium predominantly short, uncurved, slightly tapered, sometimes nearly ovoid, with short stalks. In phosphate-deficient media, morphology predominantly uncurved, cylindrical, with poles more rounded than tapered, and stalks distinctly longer. Colonies colorless. Organic growth factors not required.

The mol% G + C of the DNA is 67 (Bd, determined for one isolate). Isolates known from water, millipede hindgut, and soil. (Illustrated in Figures 21.31 and 21.32.)

Type strain: CB37 (ATCC 15260).

Krasil'nikov and Belyaev's (1973) strain 15 (VKM v-1486), designated "*C. bacteroides modicus*" subsp. nov., is distinguishable from the type strain of *C. leidyi* only by the presence of bands in its stalks; strain CB37 is the only known isolate of *Caulobacter* to lack stalk bands. As described here, *C. leidyi* should provisionally accommodate growth factor-independent uncurved *Caulobacter* isolates. Additional characterization of such isolates with respect to plasmids, bacteriocin production, antibiotic sensitivities, and number of flagellins is needed to clarify the limits of this species. To date, only strain CB37 has been characterized and is unusual among *Caulobacter* isolates with respect to each of these properties. It is resistant to several antibiotics, resistant to mercury, carries a large (cryptic) plasmid, and produces a bacteriocin active against most *Caulobacter* isolates, but not against any other of several genera tested.

9. **Caulobacter maris** Poindexter 1964, 289.[AL]

mar′is. L. gen. n. *maris* of the sea.

Rod-shaped cells slender. Colonies colorless. Organic growth factor requirements not satisfied by mixtures of B vitamins and amino acids. Growth requires NaCl (1–4%, w/v). Known isolates utilize few sugars and do not utilize individual amino acids as carbon sources but grow on peptone-casamino acids media.

Type strain: CM11 (ATCC 15268).

One of two marine species included in this list. Vibrioid marine and estuarine isolates, also dependent on NaCl supplementation for growth in complex organic media, are known; their characteristics have not been reported. Whether cell morphology will serve as a suitable subgeneric criterion among marine *Caulobacter* types has yet to be determined.

10. **Caulobacter halobacteroides** Poindexter 1964, 289.[AL]

hal.o.bac.ter.oi'des. Gr. n. *hals* salt; M.L. *bacter* masc. form of Gr. neut. n. *bactrum* rod; Gr. n. *eidus* form, shape; M.L. adj. *halobacteroides* salt (-needing) and rod-shaped.

Rod-shaped cells slender. Colonies colorless. Organic growth factor requirements not satisfied by mixtures of B vitamins and amino acids. Most sugars but few amino acids can be utilized as sole sources of carbon for growth. Growth requires NaCl (0.5–3%, w/v).

Type strain: CM13 (ATCC 15269).

See comments under *C. maris* regarding diversity among marine *Caulobacter* isolates.

11. **Caulobacter bacteroides** Poindexter 1964, 289.[AL]

bac.ter.oi'des. M.L. *bacter* masc. form of Gr. neut. n. *bactrum* rod; Gr. n. *eidus* form, shape; M.L. adj. *bacteroides* rod-shaped.

Rod-shaped cells slender. Stalk typically with a bulbous distal tip (Fig. 21.33*E*). Colonies colorless or brightly pigmented yellow or orange. Organic growth factor requirements not satisfied by mixtures of B vitamins, amino acids, and purine and pyrimidine bases. Individual sugars and organic acids are generally utilized as sources of carbon, but utilization of amino acids is limited.

The mol% G + C of the DNA is 66 (Bd, determined for one isolate). Isolates reported from water and from soil. (Illustrated in Figure 21.33.)

Type strain: CB7 (ATCC 15254).

Krasil'nikov and Belyaev (1973) assigned 60 isolates to this species, for which they proposed three new subspecies. As described, the strains they assigned to *C. bacteroides* and to "*C. bacteroides creteus*" subsp. nov. are accommodated by this species. However, at least two isolates designated "*C. bacteroides modicus*" subsp. nov. cannot be accommodated; one

(strain 10, VKM v-1180) is recognized here as subvibrioid (see comments under *C. subvibrioides*), and another (strain 15, VKM v-1486) is recognized here as *C. leidyi* (see comments under *C. leidyi*). Their description of "*C. bacteroides podsolicum*" subsp. nov. is recognized here as closer to that of "*C. glutinosus*" (see comments under "*C. glutinosus*"). Bacteroid types IV and V of Poindexter (1964) are still not assignable.

12. "**Caulobacter glutinosus**" Krasil'nikov and Belyaev 1973, 319.

glu.ti.no'sus. L. masc. adj. *glutinosus* glutinous, gluey.

Rod-shaped cells slender. Colonies colorless; viscous or gummy consistency in most isolates is unique among *Caulobacter* types. Unidentified growth factors available in peptone-yeast extract required; biotin stimulates growth of some isolates. Sugars and amino acids widely utilized as individual sources of carbon, but other organic acids not generally utilized.

Type strain: KA5 (ATCC 15267).

This species as described by Krasil'nikov and Belyaev (1973) appears indistinguishable from type III (Poindexter, 1964). On the basis of morphology, growth factor requirements, and inability to utilize organic acids, Krasil'nikov and Belyaev's proposed "*C. fulvus*" sp. nov. can also be accommodated here. On the basis of morphology, growth factor requirements, and gummy consistency of colonies, their proposed "*C. flexibilis*" sp. nov. can also be accommodated; their strain 3 (VKM v-1487), reported as unable to utilize carbohydrates, does so but grows slowly.

13. **Caulobacter variabilis** (ex Poindexter 1964, 292) nom. rev.

var.i.a'bil.is. M.L. adj. *variabilis* variable.

Rod-shaped cells short and thick; position of the stalk variable, arising from the center of the cell pole or from a subpolar (excentral) site. Colonies red-orange or colorless. Organic growth factor requirements not satisfied by mixtures of B vitamins, amino acids, and purine and pyrimidine bases. Utilization of carbon sources diverse but limited for any individual isolate. Isolates reported from water and from soil. (Illustrated in Figure 21.34.)

Type strain: CB17 (ATCC 15255).

Besides stalk position, the shape of cell poles can vary from blunt through rounded to gently tapered. These variations occur within individual clones in any growing population so far examined; morphologically constant subclones have not been isolable.

Genus *Asticcacaulis* Poindexter 1964, 282[AL]

JEANNE S. POINDEXTER

A'stic.ca.cau'lis. Gr. *alpha* privative without; Anglo-Saxon n. *sticca* stick; L. n. *caulis* stalk; L. masc. n. *Asticcacaulis* stalk that does not stick.

Cells **rod-shaped**, 0.5–0.7 × 1–3 μm; poles blunt or gently rounded. Some cells in any growing population with one subpolar or one or two lateral **prosthecae.** Each prostheca includes outer membrane, peptidoglycan, cell membrane, and a core sometimes observed to be occupied in part by membranes, but through most of its length, other cytoplasmic components cannot be discerned. Beyond the cell-prostheca juncture, prostheca diameter is constant, 0.10–0.15 μm. Other cells in the same population bear a **single, subpolar flagellum.** Each type of cell bears a small mass of adhesive material, the **holdfast,** at one pole; the holdfast site is not coincident with the site of the flagellum or of the prostheca(e). Binary fission occurs by **septation,** typically resulting in the production of a longer, prosthecate cell and a shorter, flagellated cell. Fission may occur in cells lacking prosthecae. In both instances, **cell division is unequal.**

Gram-negative. Subpolar, single flagellum in motile stage. Strictly **respiratory** and **aerobic** but may be somewhat O₂ sensitive; only O₂ serves as terminal electron acceptor for growth, although nitrate may be reduced to nitrite. Colonies circular, convex, glistening, with smooth margin, butyrous in texture, and colorless. In unagitated liquid cultures, cells accumulate as a **surface film** or a heavier **pellicle** and develop as a ring of growth on the vessel wall at or just below the air-liquid interface.

Growth in agitated liquid cultures is evenly dispersed.

Chemoorganotrophic and **oligotrophic;** grow readily in media such as peptone-yeast extract below 0.1% (w/v) organic material and may not grow in standard nutrient broth with 0.8% (w/v) organic solutes. During growth, may produce acid from sugars but do not produce gas. Optimal temperature for growth: 20–25°C; tolerated range for growth: 15–35°C. Optimal pH near neutrality: 6–9 tolerated. Maximum specific rates of exponential growth: 0.23–0.57 h⁻¹. All isolates require biotin as the only organic micronutrient. Each of glucose, fructose, maltose and lactose is utilized by all isolates as the sole carbon source.

The mol% G + C of the DNA is 55–61 (Bd, T_m).

Type species: *Asticcacaulis excentricus* Poindexter 1964, 292.

Further Descriptive Information

The prosthecae of all isolates are banded. Each band is a set of concentric rings that are more electron opaque and structurally more rigid than the remainder of the prostheca (Schmidt and Swafford, 1975). The function of the bands is unknown. They do not occur in prosthecae of most genera; their presence may be regarded as indicative of an *Asticcacaulis* or *Caulobacter* (q.v.) prostheca.

The pattern of prostheca development in *Asticcacaulis* species as it relates to the cell cycle appears to vary among isolates and, in a given isolate, with composition of the growth medium (Pate et al., 1973; Larson and Pate, 1975). In some cultures, development occurs only toward the end of exponential growth; in others, practically all dividing cells are prosthecate in all growth phases of the culture. So far as is known, only one progeny cell of each reproductive event is flagellated, whether or not the other progeny cell bears a prostheca. Prosthecae that arise laterally are usually inherited by the nonmotile progeny cell but may also be inherited by the motile cell. However, the capacity for development is not lost by a clone arising from a nonmotile, nonprosthecate cell; prosthecaless clones have not been encountered as frequent variants. Like that of isolates of *Caulobacter* (q.v.), the prostheca length of *Asticcacaulis* is greatly increased in dilute media; in defined media, prostheca length is promoted especially when phosphate concentration is growth limiting (Schmidt and Stanier, 1966) but also when the available carbon source is only slowly utilized (Larson and Pate, 1975).

The outer membrane proteins of strains examined so far are numerous and predominantly >70,000 daltons in molecular size. Major proteins unique to the prostheca have not been detected. The thin peptidoglycan layer of the cell body continues without interruption into the prostheca. Peptidoglycan of both known species is similar with respect to the glycan, in which muramic acid is present in a 50% excess over glucosamine (Poindexter and Hagenzieker, 1982). The species differ in peptide composition. *A. biprosthecum* contains a significantly higher proportion of glutamic acid than is found in *A. excentricus* and other Gram-negative bacteria. Prostheca peptidoglycan has not been separately assayed in either species.

Intermediary metabolism has been examined in only a preliminary fashion. The Entner-Doudoroff pathway is present for carbohydrate dissimilation; the glycolytic pathway has not been detected. Enzymes for catabolism of some carbohydrates are induced by exposure to substrate, but induced levels are only 1.5- to 10-fold higher than uninduced levels.

Three morphological types of bacteriophages lytic for *Asticcacaulis* species have been reported (reviewed in Poindexter, 1981). All are two-stranded DNA phages with long, flexible, noncontractile tails. Heads may be icosahedral, prolate cylindrical, or elongated polyhedral. Of more than 40 phage isolates known, only two (of the prolate cylindrical type) are lytic for a few *Caulobacter* isolates; all others are lytic only for *Asticcacaulis* isolates, and no phages lytic for any other genus are lytic for *Asticcacaulis* isolates. Generally, this genus appears isolated from other genera with respect to phage propagation. The genetics of this genus has not been investigated.

Asticcacaulis has been isolated only from freshwater ponds. Although its phages can be isolated from sewage, the distribution of the bacteria appears to be limited to oligotrophic freshwaters. However, it is not frequently observed in natural samples, and isolation of representatives of this genus has been reported by only three laboratories.

Enrichment and Isolation Procedures

Isolation of *Asticcacaulis* species has been achieved by the same procedure as described for *Caulobacter* (q.v.). A sample of clean water is enriched with at most 0.01% (w/v) peptone and allowed to stand at room temperature. Within a few days, a sample of the surface film, taken with a bacteriological loop or a coverslip (Schmidt, 1981a), is examined by phase-contrast microscopy for the presence of prosthecate cells or for rosettes of rod-shaped cells. When such cells account for 10–50% of the population, a sample (again, taken with a loop, not a pipette) is streaked on a dilute (0.05%; maximum: 0.1%, w/v) peptone or peptone-yeast extract medium prepared with 1.0 or 1.5% agar. By the third or fourth day of incubation of the plates, small, hyaline or crystalline, noniridescent colonies of prosthecate bacteria begin to appear. Such colonies, or patches of growth inoculated from such colonies, are then screened by phase-contrast microscopy. Clones of *Asticcacaulis* are often difficult to recognize during the microscopic screening. However, any clone that includes frequent rosettes should be purified, cultivated in dilute (0.1% peptone, 0.05% yeast extract) broth, and examined by electron microscopy for prosthecate and flagellated cells in whole-cell mounts such as shadowed or negatively stained specimens.

A. biprosthecum has been isolated only once, by a modification of this procedure in which a loopful of the enrichment culture was streaked on a dilute medium containing 0.02% beef extract, 0.05% tryptone, 0.05% yeast extract and 0.02% sodium acetate, prepared with 1.5% agar. After several days incubation of the plates at 30°C, very small colonies were transferred to the same medium prepared with 0.4% agar as deep cultures. *A. biprosthecum* was detected by microscopic examination of the submerged colonies (Pate et al., 1973).

Maintenance Procedures

Once isolated, *Asticcacaulis* species can be maintained as vegetative, frozen or lyophilized populations. Vegetative stocks should be maintained on 1% agar slants of dilute (0.05–0.3% organic material) complex medium, transferred every 8 or 9 weeks, incubated 2 or 3 days at 20–25°C, then refrigerated. Cells grown in dilute complex medium can be stored in small volumes frozen at −70°C without cryoprotectant. Such frozen cultures can be thawed at room temperature and transferred to growth medium to resume vegetative growth. Lyophilization is a dependable means for maintenance, either in milk solids or on strips of filter paper.

Procedures for Testing for Special Characteristics

This genus is distinguished by the number, position and substructure of its appendages, particularly the prosthecae. The appendages are best examined by electron microscopy. Shadowed specimens provide the clearest image (see Figs. 21.35 and 21.36*C*), but negatively stained specimens need not be washed and so preserve a higher proportion of attached flagella. The holdfast is best detected by its function, i.e. adhesiveness, although it, too, is discernible by electron microscopy.

Differentiation of the genus **Asticcacaulis** from other closely related taxa

See Table 21.17 under *Caulobacter*.

Taxonomic Comments

The genus *Asticcacaulis* was created by Poindexter (1964) to accommodate isolates originally regarded as *Caulobacter* species but whose prosthecae were not adhesive and therefore not entirely analogous to *Caulobacter* stalks. Subsequent investigations of a greater variety of prosthecate bacteria have revealed that only the *Caulobacter* and *Asticcacaulis* appendages lack cytoplasm along most or all of their length, and only in these two genera are the bandlike substructures found. Accordingly, the appendages appear structurally very similar in these two genera, and they may well be homologous. Nevertheless, the ranges of mol% G + C of the DNA of the two genera do not overlap, only 2 of well over 100 phage isolates are lytic for both genera, and DNA/DNA homology cannot be detected between them (Moore et al., 1978). Thus, the two genera may be more closely related to each other than either is to any other genus, but their divergence from each other appears to be significant. On the bases of mode of flagellation and carbohydrate catabolism, *Asticcacaulis* seems most closely (although still distantly) related to pseudomonads, among nonprosthecate bacteria.

Two species are recognized (Tables 21.20 and 21.21), distinguished by number and position of the prosthecae. Two (icosahedral) phages are lytic for representatives of both species, but only intraspecies DNA/DNA homology has been detected (Moore et al., 1978).

Acknowledgment

The author is grateful to J. Pate for providing isolates of both species of *Asticcacaulis* for comparison with the author's isolates of *A. excentricus*.

Further Reading

Moore, R.L., J. Schmidt, J. Poindexter and J.T. Staley. 1978. Deoxyribonucleic acid homology among the caulobacters. Int. J. Syst. Bacteriol. *28:* 349–353.
Pate, J.L., J.S. Porter and T.L. Jordan. 1973. *Asticcacaulis biprosthecum* sp. nov.

Table 21.20.

Differential characteristics of the species of the genus **Asticcacaulis**[a]

Characteristic	A. excentricus	A. biprosthecum
Number of prosthecae		
1	+	−
2	−	+
Position of prostheca		
Subpolar	+	−
Lateral	−	+

[a]Symbols: +, 90% or more of strains are positive; and −, 90% or more of strains are negative.

Life cycle, morphology and cultural characteristics. Antonie van Leeuwenhoek J. Microbiol. Serol. *39:* 569–583.

Poindexter, J.S. 1964. Biological properties and classification of the *Caulobacter* group. Bacteriol. Rev. *28:* 231–295.

Poindexter, J.S. 1981. The caulobacters: ubiquitous unusual bacteria. Microbiol. Rev. *45:* 123–179.

Schmidt, J.M. 1981. The genera *Caulobacter* and *Asticcacaulis. In* Starr, Stolp, Trüper, Balows and Schlegel (Editors), The Prokaryotes. A Handbook on Habitats, Isolation, and Identification of Bacteria. Springer-Verlag, Berlin, pp. 466–476.

Staley, J.T., P. Hirsch and J.M. Schmidt. 1981. Introduction to the budding and/or appendaged bacteria. *In* Starr, Stolp, Trüper, Balows and Schlegel (Editors), The Prokaryotes. A Handbook on Habitats, Isolation, and Identification of Bacteria. Springer-Verlag, Berlin, pp. 451–455.

Table 21.21.

Other characteristics of the species of the genus **Asticcacaulis**[a]

Characteristic	A. excentricus	A. biprosthecum
Maximum specific rate of exponential growth >0.35 h⁻¹	+	−
Sugar utilization		
Arabinose	d	−
Ribose	−	
Xylose	+	+
Glucose	+	+
Galactose	+	+
Mannose	+	−
Fructose	+	+
Lactose	+	+
Maltose	+	+
Sucrose	+	−
Starch hydrolysis	+	+
Amino acid utilization		
Alanine	+	+
Aspartate	+	+
Glutamate	+	+
Proline	+	+
Tyrosine	d	−
Utilization of other acids		
Acetate	+	−
Pyruvate	+	+
Malate	+	−
Fumarate	+	−
Succinate	+	−
Utilization of primary alcohols		
Methanol	d	−
Ethanol	+	+
Propanol	d	−
Butanol	d	−
Pentanol	d	−
Nitrate reduction to nitrite	d	−
Sensitivity to bacteriophages		
I–IX[b]	+	−
X–XII[b]	−	+
VII[c]	+	+
Number of known isolates	19	1

[a]Symbols: +, 90% or more of strains are positive; −, 90% or more of strains are negative; and d, 11–89% of strains are positive.

[b]Phage groups of Middleton and Pate (1976).

[c]Phage group of Schmidt and Stanier (1966).

List of species of the genus **Asticcacaulis**

1. **Asticcacaulis excentricus** Poindexter 1964, 292.[AL]

ex.cen′tri.cus. L. pref. *ex* out, beyond; Gr. n. *centron* center of circle; M.L. adj. *excentricus* out from the center.

Rod-shaped cells thick. A single prostheca arises from a subpolar site previously occupied by a single flagellum. Colonies colorless. Biotin the only growth factor required in glucose-ammonium-salts medium.

The mol% G + C of the DNA is 55–60 (Bd, determined for one isolate; T_m, determined for one isolate). (Illustrated in Figure 21.35.)

Type strain: AC48 (ATCC 15261).

2. **Asticcacaulis biprosthecum** Pate, Porter and Jordan 1973, 582.[AL]

bi.pros.thec′um. L. pref. *bi, bis* twice; Gr. fem. n. *prosthece* appendage; M.L. adj. *biprosthecum* twice-appendage(d).

Rod-shaped cells thick. One or, more often, two prosthecae arise near the equator of the cell at roughly diametrically opposite positions from each other; neither site is coincidental with the site occupied by the single, subpolar flagellum. Colonies colorless. Biotin the only growth factor required in glucose-ammonium-salts medium, but growth is markedly

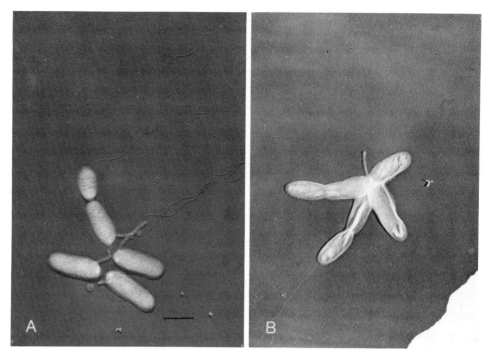

Figures 21.35. *A. excentricus* strain S-3 grown in peptone-yeast extract medium. Electron microscopy, shadowed specimen, negative image. *Bar,* 1 μm.

stimulated by mixtures of amino acids. Somewhat sensitive to dissolved O_2, growing faster and more efficiently (as yield) when allowed to reduce medium prior to aeration. Pili as well as holdfast material participate in adhesion.

The mol% G + C of the DNA is 61 (T_m, determined for one isolate). (Illustrated in Figure 21.36.)

Type strain: C-19 (ATCC 27554).

There is a single known isolate of this species; strain C-19 was the original strain designation, but this isolate also appears in the literature as AC-2. This is the only prosthecate species in which enzyme activities and nutrient uptake properties of isolated, cell-free prosthecae have been reported.

Genus **Prosthecobacter** *Staley, de Bont and de Jonge 1976, 341*[VP] *(Validated in Staley, de Bont and de Jonge 1980, 595)*

JEANNE S. POINDEXTER AND JAMES T. STALEY

Pros.the′co.bac′ter. Gr. fem. n. *prosthece* appendage; M. L. *bacter* masc. form of Gr. neut. n. *bactrum* rod; N.L. masc. n. *Prosthecobacter* appendage(d) rod.

Cells **fusiform** or **vibrio-shaped,** 0.5–0.9 × 2–5 μm, exclusive of appendages. Each cell bears at least **one polar prostheca** of a type unique to this genus. Prosthecal diameter is 0.1–0.2 μm, tapering gently away from the cell pole but typically with a bulbous distal tip, which is **adhesive.** Interior of the prostheca is a continuation of the protoplast, including cytoplasmic membrane and ribosomes. Binary fission is **constrictive** and is completed without formation of a septum. Prostheca development occurs at the younger pole as the cell grows; at the time of fission, each progeny cell bears a single polar prostheca, so that cell division is morphologically **symmetrical.**

Gram-negative. Nonmotile. Strictly **aerobic.** Colonies circular, convex, glistening, with smooth margin; butyrous in texture; may be colorless or pale yellow. Growth in agitated liquid cultures is evenly dispersed. Catalase-positive, oxidase-negative.

Chemoorganotrophic and **oligotrophic,** grow readily in complex media containing <0.1% (w/v) organic material. Optimal temperature for growth: 20–30°C; tolerated range for any isolate is wide, with lows ranging from 1–10°C and with highs ranging from 35–40°C. Optimal pH: near neutrality; range tolerated: 6.6–8.2 for the type strain. Exogenous organic micronutrients not required. Sugars are the only generally utilized carbon sources.

The mol% G + C of the DNA is 54–60 (Bd).

Type species: *Prosthecobacter fusiformis* Staley, de Bont and de Jonge 1976, 341.

Further Descriptive Information

Cell morphology is constant for a given isolate. The cells of all known isolates are distinctly tapered, but the long axis may be straight or curved (Fig. 21.37). Prostheca length is not reported to vary significantly with cultivation conditions, generally reaching a maximum approximately equal to cell body length. The prosthecae are not banded, as in *Caulobacter* (q.v.) and *Asticcacaulis* (q.v.), and do not produce buds, as in, for example, *Hyphomicrobium* (q.v.). Fimbriae are produced by all strains. They extend from all surfaces of the cell except from the distal end of the prostheca (Fig. 21.38). They are most evident when cultures are incubated without agitation.

Neither intermediary metabolism nor any aspect of the genetics of this genus has been studied. Bacteriophages have been sought but have not been obtained; isolates are not lysed by any phages lytic for *Caulobacter* or *Asticcacaulis* that have been tested.

Prosthecobacter cells were first described by Henrici and Johnson (1935) among bacteria attached to slides that had been submerged in a freshwater lake. They are commonly seen in freshwater and estuarine samples, typically attached to inanimate particles, cyanobacteria, or

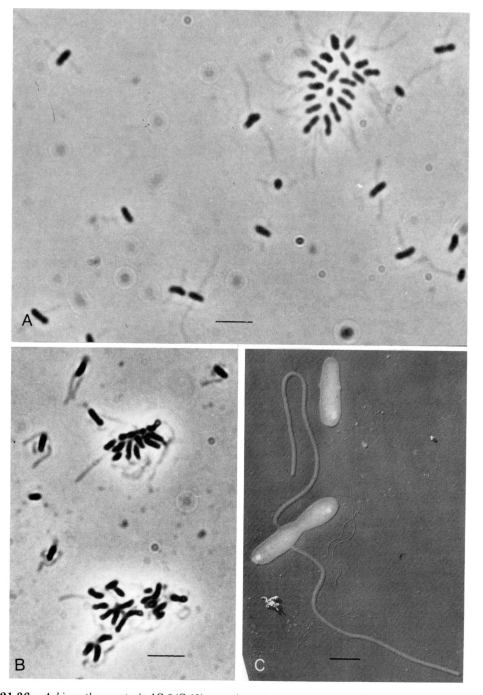

Fig. 21.36. *A. biprosthecum* strain AC-2 (C-19) grown in peptone-yeast extract medium. *A*, phase-contrast microscopy, wet mount. *Bar*, 5 μm. *B*, phase-contrast micrograph of dried smear to which droplet of Gray's flagella stain mordant (only) and coverslip were added. *Bar*, 5 μm. *C*, electron microscopy, shadowed specimen, negative image. *Bar*, 1 μm.

algal thalli. Isolates have been obtained from freshwater and sewage; marine isolates have not been reported. In natural materials, they may be difficult to distinguish from fusiform or vibrio-shaped *Caulobacter* cells that produce stalks at the unattached pole prior to cell division. In pure cultures, however, *Prosthecobacter* cells usually initiate prostheca development prior to cell division and do not produce motile cells, whereas *Caulobacter* cells typically produce nonprosthecate, flagellated cells.

Because *Prosthecobacter* isolates grow well on dilute media and occur in habitats common to *Caulobacter*, *Prosthecobacter* may be regarded as

oligotrophic. However, sensitivity of *Prosthecobacter* to elevated nutrient concentrations has not been systematically explored.

Enrichment and Isolation Procedures

Enrichment of *Prosthecobacter* depends on their ability to multiply in dilute organic environments. A water or sewage sample is enriched to not more than 0.01% (w/v) peptone, then incubated at room temperature in a beaker or bottle; the sample volume should be about two thirds of the capacity of the vessel. In order for prosthecae to be visualized, samples of

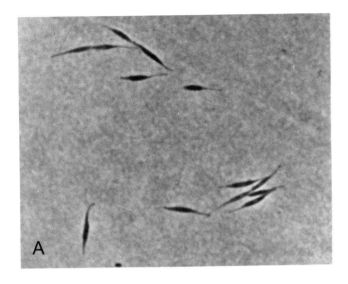

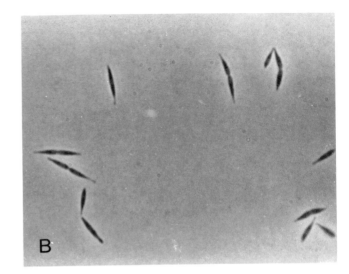

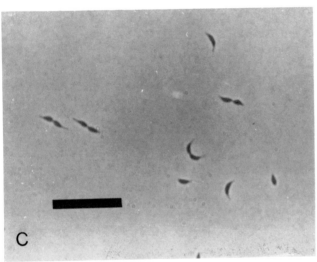

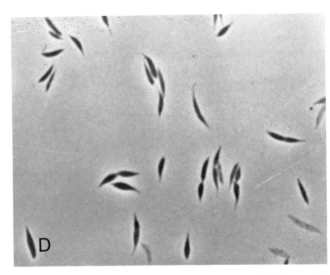

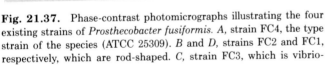

Fig. 21.37. Phase-contrast photomicrographs illustrating the four existing strains of *Prosthecobacter fusiformis. A,* strain FC4, the type strain of the species (ATCC 25309). *B* and *D,* strains FC2 and FC1, respectively, which are rod-shaped. *C,* strain FC3, which is vibrio-shaped. *Bar,* 10 μm. (Reproduced with permission from J. T. Staley, J. A. M. de Bont and K. de Jonge, Antonie van Leeuwenhoek Journal of Microbiology and Serology *42:* 333–342, 1976, ©H. Veenman en Zonen, Wageningen, The Netherlands.)

the enrichment population must be examined by phase-contrast microscopy or with the aid of mordanted stains such as those used for flagella. Within 1–2 weeks of incubation, *Prosthecobacter* cells should appear in the enrichment culture. Fusiform or slender vibrio-shaped cells of *Prosthecobacter* can be distinguished from *Caulobacter* cells by any of several traits of *Prosthecobacter:* Cells are typically quite slender, they taper into the prostheca, so that a distinct site cannot be recognized as the cell-prostheca juncture, and the prostheca is relatively wide. Typically, dividing *Caulobacter* cells will bear only one prostheca, and the nonprosthecate incipient offspring will bear an active flagellum that vibrates the attached cell. *Prosthecobacter* cells will be nonvibrating and bear a prostheca at each pole. However, *Caulobacter* cells—particularly in dilute environments such as these enrichment cultures—often initiate stalk development prior to fission; so this last criterion is not dependable until isolated clones can be examined.

When significant numbers of probable *Prosthecobacter* cells have accumulated, samples of the enrichment culture should be streaked on plates of dilute (0.01%, w/v) peptone agar prepared with Hutner's mineral base (see *Ancalomicrobium*), and the plates should be incubated 1–2

weeks at room temperature. Samples of small, circular, convex, colorless or pale yellow colonies should be examined by phase-contrast microscopy in wet mounts. *Prosthecobacter* colonies will contain polarly prosthecate cells dividing symmetrically and will lack motile cells; rosettes will be small and infrequent. Isolates are purified by repeated restreaking on the dilute peptone agar or on "MMB" (0.015% peptone, 0.015% yeast extract, 0.1% glucose, and 0.025% ammonium sulfate, prepared in modified Hutner's mineral base).

Maintenance Procedures

Prosthecobacter isolates can be maintained on slants of MMB, transferred at monthly intervals, and stored refrigerated. Lyophilization is suitable for long term maintenance, but lyophilized populations require lengthy incubation (about 2 weeks at room temperature) after rehydration prior to resumption of vegetative growth.

Procedures for Testing Special Characteristics

This genus is distinguished by the morphology of the dividing cell, specifically, by the symmetry of its polar appendages. The appendages are best characterized by electron microscopy, to determine tapering, diameter, presence of the bulbous tip, and absence of bands. The holdfast is best detected by its function, i.e. adhesiveness, although it, too, is discernible by electron microscopy.

Differentiation of the genus **Prosthecobacter** *from other closely related taxa*

See Table 21.17 under *Caulobacter*.

Taxonomic Comments

The genus *Prosthecobacter* was created by Staley, de Bont and de Jonge (1976) to accommodate organisms superficially similar to *Caulobacter* (de Bont et al., 1970) but which, upon isolation, proved different in several ways. Nutritionally, *Prosthecobacter* isolates are independent of organic micronutrients, in contrast to the majority of *Caulobacter* (and all *Asticcacaulis*) isolates. In defined media, they are unable to utilize compounds such as amino acids, alcohols, and nonnitrogenous organic acids as sole sources of carbon for growth; such compounds are commonly utilized by other genera of caulobacters (i.e. *Caulobacter* and *Asticcacaulis*). The base composition ranges of *Prosthecobacter* and *Asticcacaulis* are similar but do not overlap with that of *Caulobacter*. Intergeneric DNA/DNA homology is not detectable (Moore et al., 1978); indeed, no significant DNA/DNA homology was detected even among the four known extant strains of *Prosthecobacter* that were included in that study. Finally, the fine structure of the *Prosthecobacter* appendage is sufficiently different from that of *Caulobacter* and *Asticcacaulis* to imply a lack of structural homology. These traits, in addition to the lack of a motile stage in *Prosthecobacter*, imply that the niche of *Prosthecobacter*, as well as its natural history, is distinct from that of the other caulobacters.

There is a single species. Two strains have been deposited in the ATCC: the type strain and ATCC 27091.

Further Reading

de Bont, J.A.M., J.T. Staley and H.S. Pankratz. 1970. Isolation and description of a non-motile, fusiform, stalked bacterium, a representative of a new genus. Antonie van Leeuwenhoek J. Microbiol. Serol. *36*: 397–407.

Henrici, A.T. and D.E. Johnson. 1935. Studies on freshwater bacteria. II. Stalked bacteria, a new order of schizomycetes. J. Bacteriol. *30*: 61–93.

Moore, R.L., J. Schmidt, J. Poindexter and J.T. Staley. 1978. Deoxyribonucleic acid homology among the caulobacters. Int. J. Syst. Bacteriol. *28*: 349–353.

Staley, J.T. 1981. The genus *Prosthecobacter. In* Starr, Stolp, Trüper, Balows and Schlegel (Editors), The Prokaryotes. A Handbook on Habitats, Isolation, and Identification of Bacteria. Springer-Verlag, Berlin, pp. 477–479.

Staley, J.T., J.A.M. de Bont and K. de Jonge. 1976. *Prosthecobacter fusiformis* nov. gen. et sp., the fusiform caulobacter. Antonie van Leeuwenhoek J. Microbiol. Serol. *42*: 333–342.

List of species of the genus **Prosthecobacter**

1. **Prosthecobacter fusiformis** Staley, de Bont and de Jonge 1976, 341.[VP] (Validated in Staley, de Bont and de Jonge 1980, 595.)

fus.i.form′is. L. n. *fusus* spindle; L. n. *forma* shape, form; N.L. adj. *fusiformis* spindle-shaped.

Tapered cells uncurved (fusiform) or curved (vibrio-shaped). Colonies colorless or pale yellow. Sugars the only utilizable carbon sources known.

The mol% G + C of the DNA is 55–60 (Bd, determined for four isolates). Isolates reported from water and from sewage.

Type strain: FC4 (ATCC 25309).

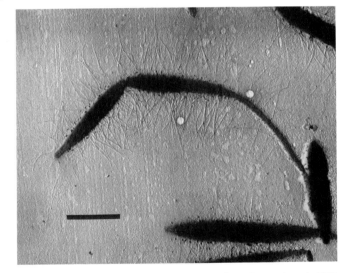

Fig. 21.38. Electron micrograph, shadowed specimen of strain FC2. Numerous fimbriae cover the surface of the cell except for the distal end of the prostheca. *Bar,* 2.0 μm. (Reproduced with permission from J. T. Staley, J. A. M. de Bont and K. de Jonge, Antonie van Leeuwenhoek Journal of Microbiology and Serology *42*: 333–342, 1976, ©H. Veenman en Zonen, Wageningen, The Netherlands.)

II. NONPROSTHECATE BACTERIA

A. BUDDING BACTERIA

1. LACK PEPTIDOGLYCAN

Genus **Planctomyces** *Gimesi 1924, 4*[AL]

MORTIMER P. STARR AND JEAN M. SCHMIDT

(*Blastocaulis* Henrici and Johnson 1935, 84; the *Blastocaulis-Planctomyces* group of budding and nonprosthecately appendaged bacteria, Schmidt and Starr 1978, 1981)

Planc.to.my′ces. Gr. adj. *planktos* wandering, floating; Gr. n. *mykes* fungus; M.L. masc. n. *Planctomyces* floating fungus.

Gram-negative bacteria. **Divide by budding.** Often relatively **large** (ignoring appendages and aggregations, individual vegetative cells range up to 3.5 µm in greatest dimension; immature buds smaller). **Cells are spherical, ovoid, ellipsoidal, teardrop-shaped or bulbiform.** Have at least one **major multifibrillar (nonprosthecate) appendage** (called a **spike, spire, fascicle, bristle, or stalk**) which does not always have the true stalk function of connecting the cell to a substratum. A **holdfast**—which is not always an easily visualized, discrete structure—is often present at the distal end of an appendage or at one end of the cell. Often form **homologous aggregations, rosettes or bouquets,** by joinings at the holdfasts. Some species have a **dimorphic life cycle:** a **sessile mother cell** buds; the bud develops into a **swarmer** that is **motile** by means of a **flagellum** (often **ensheathed**); after maturation, the swarmer loses its flagellum and becomes a sessile, budding mother cell. Typical Gram-negative **ultrastructure,** except for the **rather thin cell envelope** and **lack of a visible peptidoglycan layer.** Generally **resistant to β-lactam antibiotics.** Produce **crateriform surface structures** (surface pits 12 nm in diameter, circumscribed by a grommet with a 30-36-nm outside diameter) and **pili** in characteristic patterns. Occur worldwide in both eutrophic and oligotrophic freshwaters, as well as in estuarine and marine habitats. Sometimes become **encrusted with iron and manganese oxides.** Often **associated** in nature with **algae** and **cyanobacteria.** A **heterogeneous** assemblage, the classification of which is presently best treated—in a taxonomically noncommittal manner—as several **morphotypes** of the **Blastocaulis-Planctomyces** group. Although several species have now been **isolated in pure culture,** the type species and various others have **not been cultivated axenically.**

Type species: *Planctomyces bekefii* Gimesi 1924, 4.

Taxonomic Comments

The genus *Planctomyces* Gimesi 1924 was originally established to accommodate the peculiar aquatic "fungus" observed by Gimesi (1924) in a pond (Lake Lágymányos) in Budapest, Hungary. Gimesi's organism, named by him *Planctomyces bekefii,* has been reported many times from all over the world (Teiling, 1942; Wawrik, 1952; Fott and Komárek, 1960; Heynig, 1961; Zavarzin, 1961b; Hortobágyi, 1965, 1968; Kristiansen, 1971; Parra, 1972; Oláh and Hajdú, 1973; Tell, 1975; Schmidt and Starr, 1978). The notion that this organism was a fungus persisted during the next half century; in fact, several additional species were assigned to this "fungal" genus *Planctomyces* (Wawrik, 1952; Skuja, 1964; Hortobágyi, 1965). This situation was not altered until Hirsch (1972) reported that a freshwater bacterium, described under the name "*Blastocaulis sphaerica*" (Henrici and Johnson, 1935), was identical with *Planctomyces bekefii.* Examination of material from the type localities of both organisms (Schmidt and Starr, 1980a) has provided conclusive evidence that the two organisms are indeed indistinguishable and that both are bacterial rather than fungal. Thus, a bacterial genus ("*Blastocaulis*" Henrici and Johnson 1935) has the dubious distinction of being an exact later synonym of a group which had, for some 50 years, been considered to be a "fungal" genus (*Planctomyces* Gimesi 1924).

Neither the type species (*P. bekefii*) nor several other species have ever been cultivated axenically, making it difficult to establish the limits of the genus *Planctomyces* solely on the basis of the cultivated members. To avoid premature taxonomic commitment, this rather heterogeneous assemblage in its entirety has been treated as morphotypes of the *Blastocaulis-Planctomyces* group (Schmidt and Starr, 1978, 1981). Descriptions of each morphotype and a diagnostic key are given in Table 21.22; the major distinguishing features of each morphotype are provided in Table 21.23. Present indications make it appear likely that some organisms comprising the *Blastocaulis-Planctomyces* group do not fit within the boundaries of a single well-conceived bacterial genus. However, the paucity and fragmentary nature of existing knowledge about these bacteria, including unavailability of axenic cultures of the type species of the genus *Planctomyces* (as well as of other key organisms), presently precludes precise delineation of alternative genera. Hence, as an interim measure, all validly published members of this group are formally classified here as species of the genus *Planctomyces,* within a framework of the vernacular morphotype designations. Where later synonyms have been published, they are referenced here, albeit definitive comparative studies are often lacking.

Enrichment and Isolation Procedures

Of the five morphotypes of the *Blastocaulis-Planctomyces* group, representatives only of morphotypes III and IV have been isolated in axenic culture. Although they have not yet been isolated axenically, morphotypes I, II and V have been substantially enriched in the laboratory.

Enrichment and Axenic Isolation of Morphotypes III and IV

Morphotypes III and IV can be enriched (Schmidt, 1978; Schmidt and Starr, 1978, 1981) by adding a small amount of peptone (0.001-0.005%) to freshwater samples placed in beakers covered with clear plastic wrap and held for several days or weeks at room temperatures (24-28°C). These budding and appendaged bacteria occur in the surface film, often closely associated with green algae and cyanobacteria. Exposure of the enrichment beakers to ambient light is usually accompanied by development of algae and cyanobacteria. Enrichment of morphotypes III and IV is improved by the presence of these phototrophs and, consequently, by incubation of the samples in the light rather than in the dark. Microscopic examination of the samples is done on a weekly basis by brief contact of a small coverslip with the surface film in the beaker; these preparations are then observed by phase-contrast microscopy, looking for ellipsoidal, ovoid, or spherical budding bacteria possessing a very thin, nonprosthecate major appendage. The appendage may be difficult to visualize by light microscopy, and it may be desirable to touch electron microscope grids to promising surface films and, after negative staining, examine these in the transmission electron microscope. Enrichment cultures containing such organisms in their surface films are suitable candidates for streaking on solid media as described below.

The water agar-coverslip technique (Hirsch et al., 1977) is another useful method for enrichment and isolation of morphotypes III and IV. Relatively nutrient-poor water samples are solidified with 1.8-2.0% agar without any additions ("water agar"); a layer 0.5-0.75 cm deep is placed in the bottom of a Petri dish 20 cm in diameter. In addition, coverslips are coated with the same water agar. Several such coated coverslips, as well as several uncoated ones, are inserted perpendicularly into the solidified layer of agar in the Petri dish. The water sample providing the inoculum is then added in a volume that almost fills the Petri dish, leaving only the

Table 21.22.

A descriptive key to the morphotypes of the **Blastocaulis-Planctomyces** *group of budding and nonprosthecately appendaged bacteria most frequently encountered in aquatic environments, mainly as they appear in nature or in laboratory enrichments*

Definition of the *Blastocaulis-Planctomyces* group: Identical, for the time being, with the definition of the genus *Planctomyces*, as presented herein. The invariant diagnostic features are budding cell division, at least one multifibrillar (nonprosthecate) appendage, crateriform surface structures, a relatively thin cell envelope lacking a discernible peptidoglycan layer, and resistance to β-lactam antibiotics.

I. Major appendage is a stalk, which usually looks flattened or ribbonlike but actually is tubular.
  A. Width (diameter) of the tubular stalk 0.25–0.35 μm in the absence of manganese or iron encrustations; stalk length variable. Cells spherical (mature nonbudding cells are about 1.4–1.7 μm in diameter). Several cephalotrichous spires with fibrillar substructure are distributed on the hemisphere opposite the stalk attachment site. Peritrichous pili may be present. Commonly occur in multicellular, homologous rosettes of many individuals (usually 12; sometimes as many as 30), radiating from a collective of holdfasts, one of which is assumed to be located at the end of the single, multifibrillar, major appendage (the stalk) of each cell. Assumed holdfast at distal terminus of stalk is discrete, nonfibrillar, and without scattered fibrils at its tip. Stalk lengths within a given rosette are quite uniform. Active motility not observed. Generally resistant to β-lactam antibiotics. Species occur worldwide in ponds and lakes, especially those of eutrophic character, frequently following blooms of algae and cyanobacteria.

   1. Substructure of stalk shows a regular longitudinal array of microtubles, with a center-to-center spacing of 12–13 nm, held in place by an osmophilic matrix. The uniform width of the tubular stalk over its length is a constant feature. Cells are always resistant to β-lactam antibiotics.

Morphotype Ia

   2. Substructure of stalk shows a microfibrillar bundle, not regularly arranged, with the bundle of fibrils spreading out at the end distal to the cell. Stalks are usually shorter and thicker than in morphotype Ia and often appear to taper. Resistance to β-lactam antibiotics not determined.

Morphotype Ib

  B. Narrow stalk, which is probably tubular but appears ribbonlike, is <0.2 μm wide and several times the cell width in length. Cells are not spherical but rather are ovoid, in the classical sense of the term. A multifibrillar stalk emanates from the narrower end of the ovoid cell. Holdfast (at distal end of stalk) is diffuse, fibrillar, extensive. Crateriform surface structures, scattered over most of the cell, extrude as cornicula (small hornlike processes) in preparations stained with 1.0% uranyl acetate. Several cephalotrichous flagella occur on the broader, nonstalked, budding end of the cell. Petritrichous pili may be present. Buds, ovoid mirror images of the mother cell, develop cephalotrichous flagella before release from the mother cell. Several cells are attached, by their holdfasts, to form homologous bouquets. Often occur in surface films of dilute peptone enrichments prepared from water samples from eutrophic ponds and lakes. Usually periphytic, attached to detritus or other organisms.

Morphotype II

II. Major appendage is a ropelike stalk (i.e. a fascicle of braided fibrils). Homologous rosette formation is not typical, but attachments to other organisms and debris—mediated by a fibrillar holdfast at the distal end of the stalk—are common in most forms. Cells often have a motile stage; usually with a single sheathed flagellum attached either near or opposite to the stalk origin, sometimes with several sheathed flagella arranged peritrichously. Characterized strains are obligate aerobes.
  A. Ellipsoidal or spherical cells. Ropelike, coarsely stranded stalks up to 2.5 cell widths in length and usually shorter. Crateriform surface structures distributed randomly over entire cell surface. Species occur worldwide in various aquatic (freshwater, brackish, and marine) habitats; have also been enriched from soil samples.

   1. Conventional double membrane (i.e. the "typical" Gram-negative) cell envelope profile but lacking a visible peptidoglycan layer.

     a. Pili absent or very rare.

Morphotype IIIa

     b. Cell has an extra wall (outermost) layer consisting of goblet- or shuttlecock-shaped elements.
Morphotype IIId

   2. Cell envelope has a tripartite appearance: a very narrow, faintly electron-dense, single-track (*not* the usual double-track) outer layer; a narrow, electron-transparent region; and a slightly thicker, more electron-dense inner layer.

     a. Pili absent or rare. Cytoplasm is lobed or membrane-compartmentalized. Several flagella may be present; usually arranged peritrichously.

Morphotype IIIc

     b. Numerous peritrichous pili. Single-sheathed flagellum originates at pole from which the stalk emanates.
Morphotype IIIb

  B. Cells are ellipsoidal or ovoid, tapering toward the stalk attachment site (when it is present) or having a slightly narrower hemisphere with a holdfast at the pole. The major appendage is a ropelike (braided) stalk, a fascicle, made up of fine strands; it may exceed three cell widths in length. After isolation, homologous rosettes are formed in pure culture via a very adhesive holdfast located at the narrower pole of the cell. Typical crateriform surface structures are densely distributed over the top third of the budding end of the cell, and smaller porelike craters are lo-

Table 21.22.—*continued*

cated at the opposite end of the cell (the end from which the stalk fibers may emanate). The sheathed flagellum is attached at the budding pole. Species occur worldwide in freshwater ponds, lakes, and streams. Typically periphytic or associated with neuston.
Morphotype IV

III. Relatively large bacteria. Major appendage is not a stalk (i.e. it lacks a distal holdfast and, hence, a stalk's connecting function). Mother cells and mature buds are bulbiform (i.e. shaped like an incandescent lamp, a globose sphere merging into a cylinder, or a truncated cone). Early in its development, the bud is a small sphere, which soon assumes the bulbiform shape; the mature bud is a mirror image of the mother cell; i.e. the globose ends of the bud and the mother cell are conjoined. Amorphous holdfast region occurs only at narrow end of cell, never on globose hemisphere. Crateriform surface structures occur only on the globose hemisphere. Homologous multicellular rosettes (radiating from holdfasts at the narrower ends of cells) are very common. Cells are not actively motile. Rosettes occur as planktonic forms in eutrophic ponds and lakes.

A. Bulbiform; in this case, a sphere merging into a cylinder. Major appendage is a single, relatively broad and long, gradually tapering, rigid, brittle, multifibrillar, polar or slightly subpolar, nonprosthecate spike. The spike and the globose end of the developing bud are located at the globose pole of the mother cell. Numerous fine pili (7–10 nm wide) on globose hemisphere. Cell size varies with environmental conditions; a typical mature cell is about 3.0 μm long, 1.3 μm wide through the globose hemisphere, and 0.6 μm in diameter at the narrow pole.
Morphotype Va

B. Bulbiform; in this case, a sphere merging into the broader end of a truncated cone. Major appendages are numerous multifibrillar bristles located on the globose hemisphere and often accompanied by many entrapped smaller bacteria. The bristles are 1.8–2.0 μm long and 20–25 nm wide at the base; they taper to a fine point at the distal end. Spikes are entirely absent. Size of a mature cell: 3.0–3.5 μm long, 1.5–1.7 μm in diameter through the globose hemisphere, tapering to about 1.1 μm at the narrower end.
Morphotype Vb

Table 21.23.
Some characteristics useful in distinguishing morphotypes of the **Blastocaulis-Planctomyces** *group of budding and nonprosthecately appendaged bacteria[a]*

Characteristic	Morphotype				
	I	II	III	IV	V
Appendages					
Tubular stalk	+	+?	0	0	0
Spires	+	0	0	0	0
Spike	0	0	+	+	+/0
Fascicle	0	0	0	0	0
Bristles	0	0	0	0	+/0
Cellular shape	Spherical	Ovoid	Ellipsoid	Ovoid or ellipsoid	Bulbiform
Distribution of crateriform surface structures	Uniform	Uniform[b]	Uniform	On budding hemisphere	On budding hemisphere
Flagellation[c]	0	Multiple	Single	Single	0
Multicellular aggregates	R, H, P	B, I, D	D, I, (R)	D, I, (R)	R, H, P
Axenic growth	0	0	+	+	0
Enrichment with					
Peptone	0	+	+	+	0
Phototrophs[d]	+	+	+	+	+

[a]Symbols: +, trait occurs; ?, trait is of questionable occurrence; 0, trait does not occur; R, rosettes occur; H, only homologous rosettes and not mixed rosettes; P, characteristically occur in natural samples as planktonic (floating, suspended), multicellular, homologous rosettes, seldom as individual unattached cells; B, bouquetlike arrangements, with bases of several stalks attached to detritus; I, can occur individually as well as in attached situations; D, attached to detritus or to other microbes in natural samples; and (R), rosettes sometimes occur.
[b]Except at stalked pole.
[c]Flagella are generally ensheathed.
[d]Algal and cyanobacterial cells or cell extracts.

top 2–3 mm of the coverslips not submerged. The dishes are incubated at room temperatures, under ambient light to encourage development of phototrophs, which, in turn, seem to enhance development of these budding bacteria. The coverslips that were not coated with water agar are monitored weekly, or even more often, by examining them with a phase-contrast microscope for the occurrence of attached budding bacteria.

When such bacteria are present, the agar-coated coverslips provide the inoculum for preparation of streak or dilution-spread plates. The locations at which the budding bacteria were observed microscopically to occur on the uncoated coverslips is used as a guide in selecting the regions of the agar-coated coverslips to be plated.

Isolation Media

The media used for isolation of morphotypes III and IV are typically low in nutrients. Often the natural water sample itself, with 1.5–1.8% agar added, is suitable. Staley's (1981a) MMB agar (0.15% peptone, 0.015% yeast extract, 0.1% glucose, 0.025% ammonium sulfate, 1.0% vitamin solution, 1–2% Hutner's vitamin-free mineral base, 1.5% agar, and distilled water) also is useful. A number of strains have been isolated by using Schmidt's (1978) medium I (0.02% peptone, 0.01% yeast extract, 0.1% filter-sterilized glucose, 1.0% Hutner's vitamin-free mineral base, 1.0–1.5% agar, and distilled water) and Staley's (1981b) PYG medium (0.025% peptone, 0.025% yeast extract, 0.025% glucose, 2.0% Hutner's vitamin-free mineral base, 1.0% vitamin solution, 1.5% agar, and distilled water or artificial seawater). Media with higher concentrations of organic nutrients may also be employed. Sometimes, isolations are facilitated by additions of 5 mM $MgSO_4$, 0.005 M Trizma buffer (pH 7.5–7.8) (Sigma Chemical Company), and/or NaCl or artificial seawater (the latter is particularly desirable for isolations from brackish or marine sources). Use of solidifying agents other than agar may improve the chances of securing axenic cultures.

Direct streaking and spreading of diluted material are the most effective of the various routines used for inoculating the primary isolation plates. Morphotypes III and IV grow rather slowly in culture. Plates must be incubated for 2–5 weeks at room temperature; hence, precautions must be taken to avoid dessication of the medium, such as sealing the Petri dishes with Parafilm or using plastic bags or boxes. Colonies are very small, rather inconspicuous, usually quite adherent or cohesive, and white or pigmented (pink or light brown). Patch plates, prepared with the same medium used for the primary isolation, may then be used to produce enough material for microscopic examination and restreaking.

Enrichment of Morphotype Ia

The enrichment of morphotype Ia, *P. bekefii*, the type species of the genus *Planctomyces*, has been facilitated by taking advantage of the considerable resistance of all members of this group to antibiotics which, in other bacteria, affect peptidoglycan integrity. Addition of a β-lactam antibiotic, such as ampicillin (about 250 µg/ml), to pond water samples containing detectable but low amounts (1–5 × 10^4/ml) of morphotype Ia rosettes results, within 3 days, in a 5- to 6-fold increase in the number of rosettes as determined by direct microscopic counts. This increase may have resulted from (a) release of nutrients or growth factors from other bacteria lysed by action of the antibiotic or (b) inhibition by the antibiotic of organisms antagonistic to the development or proliferation of *P. bekefii* rosettes. The success of the enrichment by β-lactam antibiotics appears to be dependent upon the types and numbers of other microbes present in the water samples. Many workers, including phycologists and limnologists, have reported that occurrence of planktonic morphotype Ia often coincides with occurrence of various algae and cyanobacteria. The dominant algae and cyanobacteria present during and immediately preceding *P. bekefii* blooms in natural aquatic environments may be useful as "helpers" to enhance growth of *P. bekefii* in co-cultivation trials in the laboratory. Albeit numerous solid media and cultivation conditions have been tried, morphological forms resembling the organisms in the natural rosettes have never been found. Axenic cultivation of *P. bekefii* (morphotype Ia), the type species of the genus *Planctomyces*, and the closely related "*P. crassus*" (morphotype Ib) remains a challenge.

Enrichment of Morphotype II

Morphotype II, an ovoid budding organism with a long multifibrillar stalk, occurs individually and in clusters ("bouquets") in pond water enrichments to which 0.001–0.005% peptone has been added. The pond waters in which this relatively uncommon organism occurs are typically eutrophic. About 1 or 2 weeks after peptone is added to pond waters of this sort, these morphotype II organisms are found in the surface films.

They have not been isolated axenically, nor have they been cultivated on any solid medium.

Attempted Enrichment of Morphotype V

P. guttaeformis (morphotype Va) and *P. stranskae* (morphotype Vb) are planktonic bacteria bulbiform in shape and characteristically occurring in multicellular rosettes in pond or lake waters where they accompany algal and/or cyanobacterial blooms. They seem not to be inhibited by addition of ampicillin (250 µg/ml); neither do they seem to be enriched by the presence of this antibiotic, as is *P. bekefii*. Additions of various organic nutrients (e.g. peptones, amino acid mixtures, individual amino acids, vitamin mixtures, and/or individual vitamins) to pond water samples containing easily detectable numbers of morphotype V have not provided any clue to specific enrichment conditions for these bacteria. Their natural aquatic habitats usually have a distinctly eutrophic character, and the number of rosettes of these bacteria often increases significantly (4- to 5-fold) in such water samples held in the collection bottle for a week or so in the laboratory without any additions (e.g. antibiotics, preservatives or possible nutrients). No representative of morphotype V has been observed to grow on any solid medium.

Maintenance Procedures

The existing axenic cultures, all belonging to morphotypes III and IV, have successfully been preserved by lyophilization of cell suspensions in skim milk. Addition of 10% (v/v) of glycerol to liquid cultures of morphotypes III and IV, followed by freezing and storage at −70°C, has satisfactorily preserved these strains for several months.

Acknowledgments

Our studies on these bacteria have been supported by research grants AI-08426 from the National Institutes of Health and U.S. Public Health Service and DEB-78-23281 from the National Science Foundation. We are grateful to Phoebe Betty Starr for bibliographic and redactional assistance.

Further Reading

Bauld, J. and J.T. Staley. 1976. *Planctomyces maris* sp. nov.: a marine isolate of the *Planctomyces-Blastocaulis* group of budding bacteria. J. Gen. Microbiol. 97: 44–55.

Gimesi, N. 1924. Hydrobiologiai Tanulmányok [Hydrobiologische Studien]. I. *Planctomyces Békefii* Gim. nov. gen. et sp. [Ein neues Glied des Phytoplanktons.] [Hungarian; partial German translation.] Kiadja a Magyar Ciszterci Rend, Budapest, pp. 1–8.

Henrici, A.T. and D.E. Johnson. 1935. Studies of freshwater bacteria. II. Stalked bacteria, a new order of Schizomycetes. J. Bacteriol. 30: 61–93.

Hirsch, P. 1972. Two identical genera of budding and stalked bacteria: *Planctomyces* Gimesi 1924 and *Blastocaulis* Henrici and Johnson 1935. Int. J. Syst. Bacteriol. 22: 107–111.

Hortobágyi, T. 1965. Uj Planctomyces fajok. [Neue Planctomyces-Arten.] [Hungarian, with German résumé.] Bot. Közl. 52: 111–115.

Schmidt, J.M. 1978. Isolation and ultrastructure of freshwater strains of *Planctomyces*. Curr. Microbiol. 1: 66–71.

Schmidt, J.M. and M.P. Starr. 1978. Morphological diversity of freshwater bacteria belonging to the *Blastocaulis-Planctomyces* group as observed in natural populations and enrichments. Curr. Microbiol. 1: 325–330.

Schmidt, J.M. and M.P. Starr. 1981. The *Blastocaulis-Planctomyces* group of budding and appendaged bacteria. *In* Starr, Stolp, Trüper, Balows and Schlegel (Editors), The Prokaryotes. A Handbook on Habitats, Isolation, and Identification of Bacteria. Springer-Verlag, Berlin, pp. 496–504.

Staley, J.T. 1973. Budding bacteria of the *Pasteuria-Blastobacter* group. Can J. Microbiol. 19: 609–614.

Starr, M.P., R.M. Sayre and J.M. Schmidt. 1983. Assignment of ATCC 27377 to *Planctomyces staleyi* sp. nov. and conservation of *Pasteuria ramosa* Metchnikoff 1888 on the basis of type descriptive material. Request for an opinion. Int. J. Syst. Bacteriol. 33: 666–671.

Starr, M.P. and J.M. Schmidt. 1984. *Planctomyces stranskae* (ex Wawrik 1952) sp. nov. nom. rev. and *Planctomyces guttaeformis* (ex Hortobágyi 1965) sp. nov. nom. rev., distinguishable members of the *Blastocaulis-Planctomyces* group of budding bacteria. Int. J. Syst. Bacteriol. 34: 470–477.

Wawrik, F. 1952. *Planctomyces*-Studien. Sydowia 6: 443–452.

Zavarzin, G.A. 1961. Budding bacteria. Mikrobiologiya 30: 952–975 (English translation: 774–791).

List of species of the genus **Planctomyces**

1. **Planctomyces bekefii** Gimesi 1924, 4.[AL] (*Blastocaulis sphaerica* Henrici and Johnson 1935, 84 (Hirsch, 1972); morphotype Ia of the *Blastocaulis-Planctomyces* group (Schmidt and Starr, 1980a, 1981.)

be.ke'fi.i. M.L. *bekefii* of Békefi; named for Remigius Békefi (1858–1924), cultural historian, university professor, and abbot of the Hungarian Cistercian Order.

Gram-negative, budding bacteria. Cellular shape is spherical. Mature cells are 1.4–1.7 µm in diameter. Each mature cell has a tubular, nonprosthecate stalk (Fig. 21.39, *A* and *B*) 0.25–0.35 µm wide and varying in length from very short (<0.2 µm) to several micrometers. The tubular stalk is comprised of a regular array (Fig. 21.39 *B*) of longitudinally aligned microtubules (12–13 nm in diameter) enmeshed in an osmophilic matrix (Fig. 21.39*C*). The distal end of each stalk is characteristically attached to several other distal stalk tips to form multicellular homologous rosettes (Fig. 21.39*A*); however, no distinctive or obvious holdfast structure can be discerned at the junction. Crateriform surface structures (Fig. 21.39*B*) are uniformly distributed over the entire cell. Numerous cephalotrichous, tapering, multifibrillar spires (Fig. 21.39, *A* and *B*) emanate from the hemisphere of the cell opposite the site of attachment of the stalk. Pili are present over the entire cell.

Nonmotile. Divide by budding from a site precisely opposite to the pole from which the stalk originates. The nonstalked and nonmotile daughter cells, after they are released from the mother cell, may associate with the center of the originating or another rosette and subsequently form a stalk, thus resulting in an increased number of stalked cells in a rosette. Stalks may be encrusted with manganese and/or iron oxides (Schmidt et al., 1982). Resistant to β-lactam antibiotics. Rosettes are planktonic, occurring in eutrophic freshwater lakes, ponds, and reservoirs, typically with waters of a slightly alkaline pH. Occurrence usually is concomitant with or subsequent to blooms of various algae and cyanobacteria, especially during the late summer in temperate climates. Mesophilic. Worldwide in distribution. Complete life cycle is unknown; however, nonstalked budding bacteria, with morphological and ultrastructural features (shape; size; occurrence and distribution of crateriform surface structures and spires; distinctive cell envelopes) identical to those of *P. bekefii*, occur in clusters in the same aquatic samples. Although the relationship of these nonstalked forms to *P. bekefii* has not yet been demonstrated conclusively, the circumstantial evidence is strong that they may be immature (i.e. nonstalked) forms of *P. bekefii*. *P. bekefii* has not been cultivated axenically; hence, archival (Gimesi, 1924) and modern (Schmidt and Starr, 1980a, 1980b) descriptive type material from the type locality, a pond in the Lágymányos district of Budapest, Hungary, must suffice in place of a type culture.

No species belonging to morphotype II has been validly published, nor has the axenic cultivation of any strain been reported, although substantial laboratory enrichment has been achieved (Schmidt and Starr, 1979b). The unmistakable arrangement into a bouquet of several stalked cells of a typical representative of morphotype II, as sketched by Henrici and Johnson (1935), is reproduced here in Figure 21.40*B*. This organism was referred to as "*Blastocaulis* sp." by these authors, with the remark that "specific names are withheld until further studies have been completed" (Henrici and Johnson, 1935). Unfortunately, no further publication about this organism by these authors seems to have appeared.

2. **Planctomyces maris** Bauld and Staley 1976, 54.[VP] (Validated in Bauld and Staley 1980, 657.) (Morphotype IIIb of the *Blastocaulis-Planctomyces* group (Schmidt and Starr, 1981). Other names are sometimes encountered for organisms belonging to morphotype III; most of these names have no taxonomic standing. Two red-pigmented strains belonging to morphotype IIIa provided the basis for the description of the species *Planctomyces limnophilus* by Hirsch and Müller (1985). A single morphotype IIIc strain is the basis of a description by Franzmann and Skerman (1984) of the genus *Gemmata* and its sole species *Gemmata obscuriglobus*. However, rigorous comparisons of these taxa with *Planctomyces maris* and/or with other presently unnamed representa-

tives of morphotype III (Schmidt and Starr, 1978, 1981) remain to be made.)

mar'is. L. gen. n. *maris* of the sea.

Gram-negative, budding bacteria. Mature cells are spherical or ellipsoidal, 1.0–1.5 µm in major dimension. Numerous crateriform surface structures and pili (5–6 nm in diameter) are distributed randomly over the entire cell (Fig. 21.41, *B* and *C*). In the budding process, the newly released daughter cells (0.4 µm in minimum diameter) are usually smaller than mature cells. Mature cells generally have a braided, multifibrillar, nonprosthecate stalk extending from a pole exactly opposite to the budding pole (Fig. 21.41, *A–C*). Individual fibrils (5 nm in diameter) of the multifibrillar stalk, emanating from separate pores at the basal structure when anchored to the cell, are joined into a bundle (a fascicle) to form the stalk, which may be up to 5 µm long. The many finer fibrils, which extend from the distal tip of the stalk, may serve as a "holdfast" device (Fig. 21.41*C*); some stalked cells, joined by the distal tips of their stalks, are depicted here in Figure 21.41*A*. The daughter cells are motile by a single, subpolar, sheathed flagellum, which is attached to the cell at or near the pole from which the stalk originates.

Of marine origin, with an absolute requirement for 1.5–4.0% (w/v) NaCl. Heterotrophic, obligately aerobic, mesophilic (optimum temperature: 30–33°C). Colonies on marine agar (Difco) are white or slightly cream-colored, 2–4 mm in diameter, slightly mucoid, and glistening. Carbon sources utilized: glucose, galactose, mannose, rhamnose, xylose, maltose, cellobiose, melibiose, furanose, trehalose, *N*-acetylglucosamine, glucuronic acid, lactic acid, pectin and aesculin. Vitamins are not required, but colonies grow more rapidly in the presence of peptone and yeast extract than in the glucose-salt medium. Growth is relatively slow, with a minimum doubling time of 13 h at 30°C.

The mol% G + C of the DNA of ATCC 29201 is 50.5 (Bauld and Staley, 1976) or 52.0 (M. Mandel, personal communication, 1979) as determined by buoyant density.

Type strain: ATCC 29201. Source: Neritic waters, Puget Sound, Washington, U.S.A.

Strains essentially identical to *P. maris* in morphological and ultrastructural features, and probably also related in other ways, have been isolated from freshwater samples originating in many parts of the world (Hirsch et al., 1977; Schmidt, 1978; Schmidt and Starr, 1978, 1981; Franzmann and Skerman, 1984; Gebers et al., 1985; Hirsch and Müller, 1985). With the exceptions of *G. obscuriglobus* Franzmann and Skerman 1984, a taxon based upon a single morphotype IIIc strain not yet compared rigorously with other members of morphotype III, and *P. limnophilus* Hirsch and Müller 1985, a taxon based solely upon two red-pigmented morphotype IIIa strains, none of these strains has as yet been validly named. They do not require 1.5% NaCl.

The mol% G + C of the DNA is 54–68 as determined by buoyant density (M. Mandel, personal communication, 1979–1980) or thermal denaturation (Gebers et al., 1985); genome sizes (renaturation kinetics) of the few strains examined ranged from 2.67 to 3.65 × 10⁹ (Kölbel-Boelke et al., 1985); to the extent examined, no peptidoglycan can be detected by chemical analysis (O. Kandler, personal communication, 1979–1980; König et al., 1984) or electron microscopy (Schmidt and Starr, 1978, 1981; König et al., 1984), thus correlating with the demonstrated resistance to β-lactam antibiotics (Schmidt et al., 1980; König et al., 1984), existence of other characteristics atypical of ordinary eubacteria (Schmidt and Starr, 1981), and their postulated evolutionary origin (Stackebrandt et al., 1984). Some of these freshwater strains form pink or red colonies, though their colonies are more typically cream-colored or white; some develop a brown (melaninlike) pigmentation after several days of growth. The single strain tested was not pathogenic to mice (Famuwera et al., 1983).

3. **Planctomyces limnophilus** Hirsch and Müller 1986, 355.[VP] (Effective publication: Hirsch and Müller 1985, 278.) (This taxon is based on two red-pigmented strains belonging to morphotype IIIa of the

Blastocaulis-Planctomyces group (Schmidt and Starr, 1981). Synonymy is unclear, since direct comparisons of *Planctomyces limnophilus* with nonpigmented morphotype IIIa strains or with the earlier published *Gemmata obscuriglobus* Franzmann and Skerman 1984, a representative of morphotype IIIc of this group, seem not to have been made.)

lim.no'phi.lus. Gr. n. *limnos* lake; Gr. adj. *philus* loving; M.L. adj. *limnophilus* lake-loving.

Gram-negative, budding bacteria. Mature cells are spherical to ellipsoidal, 1.1–1.5 μm in diameter. Numerous crateriform structures and pili occur on the cell surface. Mature cells have a braided or twisted,

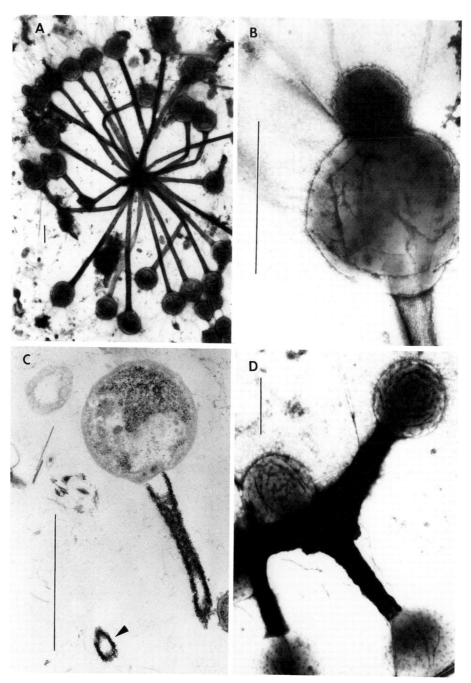

Figure 21.39.   Morphotype I of the *Blastocaulis-Planctomyces* group. *A,* morphotype Ia (*P. bekefii*) from the eutrophic man-made pond at The Lakes, Tempe, Arizona; rosette with several budding cells. 1.0% uranyl acetate; × 3,960. *B,* budding cell of morphotype Ia (*P. bekefii*) from Lake Mendota, Madison, Wisconsin. Note bud, spires, crateriform surface structures, and stalk substructure showing parallel fibrils. 1.0% uranyl acetate; × 40,135. *C,* thin section of cell of morphotype Ia (*P. bekefii*) from the pond at The Lakes, Tempe, Arizona, showing a tangential section of the tubular stalk as well as a separate transverse section (*arrow*) of another stalk. Fixed by the acrolein-glutaraldehyde procedure of Burdett and Murray (1974) (see also Schmidt and Starr (1980b)); × 36,000. *D,* rosette of morphotype Ib *"P. crassus"* in a sample from the railroad-bridge pond, Budapest, Hungary, showing heavy metallic oxide encrustation of its stalks (Schmidt et al., 1981). 1.0% uranyl acetate; × 15,000. *Bars,* 1.0 μm for *A–D.*

Figure 21.40. Morphotype II of the *Blastocaulis-Planctomyces* group. *A,* several morphotype II cells, some with buds, arranged in a typical bouquet, from a dilute peptone enrichment of water from a lake near Hesteskodam, Hillerød, Denmark. These organisms can be found in the surface film or pellicle of such enrichments. × 1,900. *B,* drawing of *"Blastocaulis* sp." (Henrici and Johnson, 1935). × 1,900. *C,* two morphotype II organisms, one with a bud and each with a long major appendage (a stalk) terminating in a holdfast (one holdfast is attached to detritus). Several cephalotrichous flagella and numerous crateriform surface structures are found on the budding (nonstalked) hemisphere. Dilute peptone enrichment of water sample from highly eutrophic pond at the sewage works in Strandfontein, Republic of South Africa. 1.0% uranyl acetate; × 11,200. *D,* a budding cell of morphotype II with crateriform surface structures everted as cornicula, as they often do when stained with 1.0% uranyl acetate (Schmidt and Starr, 1979b); pili, several flagella, and the major appendage (a stalk) are evident. Dilute peptone enrichment of water sample from an ornamental fountain, University of the Witwatersrand, Johannesburg, Republic of South Africa. 1.0% uranyl acetate; × 51,300. *Bars,* 5.0 μm for *A* and *B* and 1.0 μm for *C* and *D.*

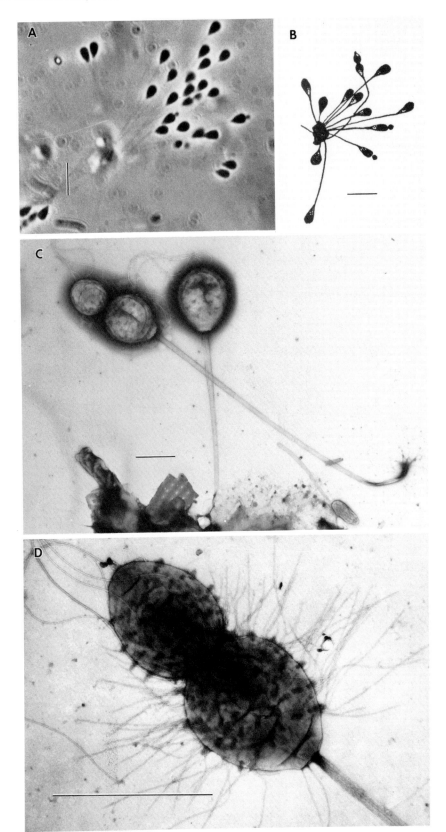

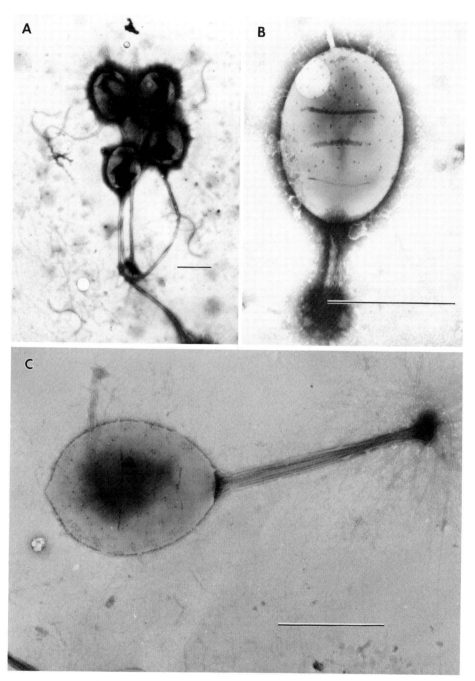

Figure 21.41. Morphotype III of the *Blastocaulis-Planctomyces* group. *A,* several cells of *P. maris,* ATCC 29201, morphotype IIIb of the *Blastocaulis-Planctomyces* group. Stained with 1.0% potassium phosphotungstate following fixation with 0.5% glutaraldehyde. A braided, multifibrillar fascicle (a stalk) extends from a pole of each cell, and the distal ends of the fascicles are attached to each other. × 8,960. *B,* cell of a morphotype III organism from a freshwater enrichment (water sample from Old Main Fountain, Arizona State University, Tempe, Arizona). The crateriform structures are scattered over most of the cell surface. Note the ellipsoidal cellular shape, and compare with morphotype IV cells (see Fig. 21.42), which are usually ovoid in shape. The prominent, braided, multifibrillar fascicle with its electron-dense (i.e. heavily stained) holdfast is typical of morphotype III. 1.0% potassium phosphotungstate; × 35,100. *C,* cell of morphotype III from an enrichment (water sample from Willow Springs Lake, northern Arizona), showing a very early stage of budding (the tiny protuberance at the pole opposite to the stalk) as well as the typical braided stalk with electron-dense holdfast. 0.5% potassium phosphotungstate; × 28,700. *Bars,* 1.0 μm for *A–C.*

multifibrillar, nonprosthecate stalk (a fascicle) extending from a pole exactly opposite the budding pole; the noncellular end of the fascicle serves as a "holdfast" device. Multiplication is by budding on the pole of the cell distal to the fascicle. Daughter cells are monotrichously and polarly or subpolarly flagellated; the flagellum is attached at or near the pole from which the stalk originates. Nonacidfast; colonies red; do not form endospores.

Temperature range: 17–39°C; optimum: 30–32°C. NaCl tolerance: <1% (w/v). pH tolerance: 6.2–8.0; pH optimum: 6.2–7.0.

The following substances are utilized as carbon sources (0.1% (w/v)): D-glucose, D-galactose, maltose, cellobiose, N-acetylglucosamine. The following substances are not utilized as carbon sources (0.1% (w/v) except where different concentrations are noted): glucuronic acid, D-fructose, D-ribose, mannitol, starch, dextrin, inulin, salicin, pyruvate, citrate, α-oxoglutarate, succinate, fumarate, malate, formamide, methylamine hydrochloride (0.136%), formate (0.136%), urea (0.09%), methane (0.5%), methanol (0.4%), ethanol (0.4%), lactate, acetate, propionate, tartrate, glutarate, caproate, phthalate, glycerol (0.186%), L-arginine, L-aspartate, DL-alanine, L-glutamate, L-glycine, L-histidine, L-leucine, DL-phenylalanine, L-proline and L-serine. No aerobic acid formation from D-glucose, saccharose, D-fructose, maltose, D-galactose or mannitol. Anaerobic acid formation from D-glucose, saccharose, maltose or galactose; no anaerobic acid formation from D-fructose or mannitol. No anaerobic gas formation in the Hugh-Leifson tests.

The following substances are utilized as nitrogen sources (0.1% (w/v) except where a different concentration is noted): $(NH_4)_2SO_4$ (0.05%), Bacto peptone, Bacto yeast extract, or casamino acids (vitamin free). The following substances are not utilized as nitrogen sources: $NaNO_2$ (0.2–0.69%), $NaNO_3$ (0.2–0.85%), methylamine hydrochloride (0.675%), and urea (0.46%).

Vitamins not required. The following reactions are positive: nitrate reduction (dissimilatory), gelatin liquefaction, H_2S formation, and tolerance to 30 vol% carbon monoxide. The following reactions are negative: decarboxylation of lysine or arginine, deamination of phenylalanine or lysine, oligocarbophilic growth, urease, nitrification, nitrate reduction (assimilatory), anaerobic gas formation with nitrate, formation of acetoin or indole, growth in or changes of litmus milk, tolerance to 50 vol% carbon monoxide, or extracellular DNase.

The mol% G + C of the DNA (T_m) is 53.24 ± 0.59 for strain 1008 and 54.4 ± 0.7 for strain 1007. Genome size (strain 1008): 2.67 ± 0.05 × 10⁹ daltons.

Isolated from surface water of the freshwater lake Pluβsee, Holstein, Federal Republic of Germany.

Type strain: IFAM 1008 (Mü 290). Practically identical with strain IFAM 1007 (Mü 279) (DSM 1115).

4. **Planctomyces staleyi** Starr, Sayre and Schmidt 1983, 667.^VP (*Pasteuria ramosa* sensu Staley (Staley, Hirsch and Schmidt, 1981). Not *Pasteuria ramosa* Metchnikoff 1888 sensu stricto (Sayre and Starr, 1985; Starr, Sayre and Schmidt, 1983; cf. genus *Pasteuria* by R. M. Sayre and M.P. Starr in Volume IV of the *Manual*); morphotype IV (in part) of the *Blastocaulis-Planctomyces* group (Schmidt and Starr, 1982; Tekniepe et al., 1981); *Pirella staleyi* Schlesner and Hirsch 1984, 494.^VP)

sta′ley.i. M.L. adj. *staleyi* of Staley; named in honor of J. T. Staley.

Gram-negative, budding bacteria. Ovoid or ellipsoidal. Mature cells are 0.5–1.0 × 1.0–1.7 μm or larger. Forms a fragile fascicle (Fig. 21.42, A and C), a bundled or braided multifibrillar appendage (Schmidt and Starr, 1982; Starr et al., 1983). Holdfast occurs, usually at narrower pole of cell. Two kinds of crateriform or porelike surface structures occur. The larger crateriform structures (12 nm in diameter; enlarging with age) are located on the reproductive (budding) pole of the cell (Fig. 21.42B), from which many short and brittle pili (5–6 nm in diameter) also extend. The smaller porelike structures (5–7 nm in diameter) are located on the nonreproductive and nonpiliated pole of the cell. In the budding process, the newly released daughter cells are usually much smaller than mature cells; the envelope of the bud (Fig. 21.42C) is synthesized de novo (Tekniepe et al., 1982). Dimorphic life cycle (Tekniepe et al., 1981): A mature bud develops a sheathed flagellum attached to the piliated pole and

becomes a motile swarmer; the swarmer loses its flagellum and becomes a sessile mother cell; the mother cell buds, and the cycle repeats. Highly resistant to β-lactam antibiotics (methicillin, ampicillin, penicillin G, cephalosporin C).

Type strain: ATCC 27377 (ICPB 4128), isolated from Lake Lansing, Michigan, U.S.A.

The mol% G + C of the DNA is 59 (Bd).

Other strains of morphotype IV—some of which may belong to *P. staleyi*—have been isolated from freshwater habitats in North America, South America, Europe and Africa. Colonies of the various strains are white, pink and (in one case) brown; all are extremely adherent to substrata (agar, glass, each other). In those morphotype IV strains thus examined, peptidoglycan cannot be found by chemical analysis (O. Kandler, personal communication, 1979–1980; König et al., 1984) and no discrete peptidoglycan layer can be visualized in thin sections by electron microscopy (Schmidt and Starr, 1981, 1982; Starr et al., 1983; König et al., 1984), thus correlating with the demonstrated resistance to β-lactam antibiotics (Schmidt et al., 1980; König et al., 1984), other characteristics atypical of ordinary eubacteria (Schmidt and Starr, 1981), and their postulated evolutionary origin (Stackebrandt et al., 1984). The single strain tested was not pathogenic to mice (Famuwera et al., 1983).

The mol% G + C of the DNA of several strains range from 56 to 63 as determined by buoyant density (M. Mandel, personal communication, 1979–1980; Schmidt and Starr, 1981) or, for a different series of strains, from 54 to 58 as determined by thermal denaturation (Gebers et al., 1985). Genome sizes of the strains thus examined range from 2.73 to 4.43 × 10⁹ (Kölbel-Bolke et al., 1985).

5. **Planctomyces guttaeformis** (ex Hortobágyi 1965) Starr and Schmidt 1984a, 473.^VP (*Planctomyces guttaeformis* Hortobágyi 1965, 111, emend. Hajdú (Hortobágyi and Hajdú, 1984); morphotype Va of the *Blastocaulis-Planctomyces* group (Schmidt and Starr, 1979a; Starr and Schmidt, 1984a).)

gutt.ae.form′is. L. gen. n. *gutta(e)* (of a) drop; L. suffix -*formis* in the form or shape of; M.L. adj. *guttaeformis* drop-shaped.

Gram-negative, budding bacteria. Mature cells are relatively large (2.9–3.0 μm in length, 1.15–1.3 μm for the diameter of the globose end, and 0.6–0.7 μm for the diameter of the cylindrical end). Bulbiform (bulb-shaped; in this case, a cylinder blending into a spherical terminal dilatation; shaped like a common screw-in incandescent lamp). A prominent multifibrillar appendage, a spike (Fig. 21.43, A–C), extends from the globose end of the cell. Division is by budding, with a mirror-image bud (Fig. 21.43C) formed at the globose end of the cell; the bud is often slightly off center with respect to the longitudinal axis of the mother cell, whereas the spike is usually exactly polar. Numerous crateriform surface structures and fine pili occur on the globose end of the cell (Fig. 21.43C). Fine structure is that of a typical bacterium, except for the rather thin cell envelope, the spike and its basal attachment site, and the crateriform surface structures. Cells are resistant to β-lactam antibiotics. Occur in rosettes (Fig. 21.43A) consisting of as many as a dozen cells attached via holdfasts located at the narrower ends of the several cells. Neither motility nor flagella have been observed. Common in eutrophic aquatic habitats, usually accompanying phototrophs (algae and cyanobacteria). Species has not been cultivated axenically, though blooms occur in laboratory enrichments. Descriptive type material in Starr and Schmidt (1984a). The type locality is a eutrophic man-made pond in a residential district (The Lakes) in Tempe, Arizona, U.S.A. Frequently confused with *P. stranskae,* from which it can readily be distinguished on the basis of the characteristic cellular sizes and shapes, the presence of a multifibrillar spike in *P. guttaeformis* and its absence in *P. stranskae,* and the presence of numerous multifibrillar bristles in *P. stranskae* and their absence in *P. guttaeformis.*

6. **Planctomyces stranskae** (ex Wawrik 1952) Starr and Schmidt 1984a, 473.^VP (*Planctomyces stranskae* Wawrik 1952, 448; morphotype Vb of the *Blastocaulis-Planctomyces* group (Starr and Schmidt, 1984a).)

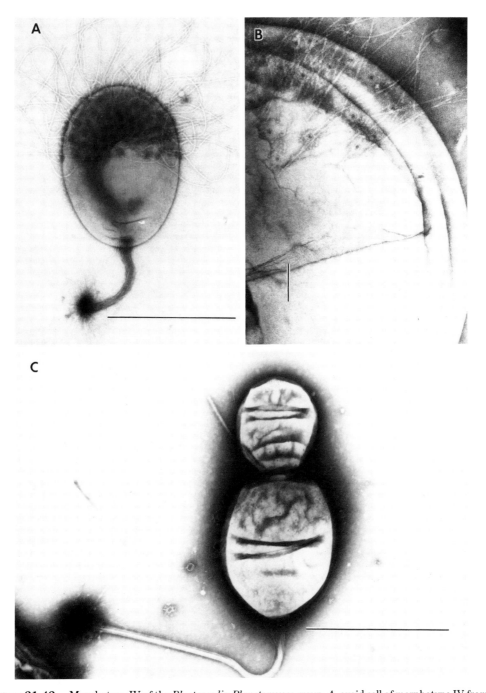

Figure 21.42. Morphotype IV of the *Blastocaulis-Planctomyces* group. *A,* ovoid cell of morphotype IV from a freshwater enrichment, showing the typical braided, multifibrillar fascicle with a presumed terminal holdfast. Note the numerous pili and crateriform surface structures on the hemisphere opposite the fascicle. 1.0% potassium phosphotungstate; × 34,400. *B, P. staleyi,* ATCC 27377; portion of a cell showing crateriform surface structures and pili on the hemisphere opposite to the pole with the fascicle. 1.0% uranyl acetate; × 100,800. *C,* budding cell of morphotype IV, with a fascicle on the mother cell; dilute peptone enrichment from water in a birdbath at the Lanzerac Hotel, Stellenbosch, Republic of South Africa. 1.0% potassium phosphotungstate; × 39,150. *Bars,* 1.0 μm for *A* and *C* or 0.1 μm for *B.*

stran′skae. M.L. gen. n. *stranskae* of Stransky; named originally by F. Wawrik in honor of her biology teacher, M. L. Stransky.

Gram-negative, budding bacteria. Mature cells are relatively large (3.0–3.5 μm in length, 1.5–1.7 μm for the diameter of the globose end, about 1.3–1.4 μm for the initial diameter of the conical end, and 1.0–1.1 μm for the diameter of the terminus of the cell). Bulbiform (i.e. bulb-shaped; in this case, a truncated cone blending into a spherical terminal dilatation; shaped like a common screw-in incandescent lamp). Numerous multifibrillar appendages, termed bristles (Fig. 21.43, *D–F*), extend from the globose end of the cell; many smaller bacteria are associated with the bristles, especially in preparations made directly from natural samples. Division is by budding, with a mirror-image bud (Fig. 21.43F)

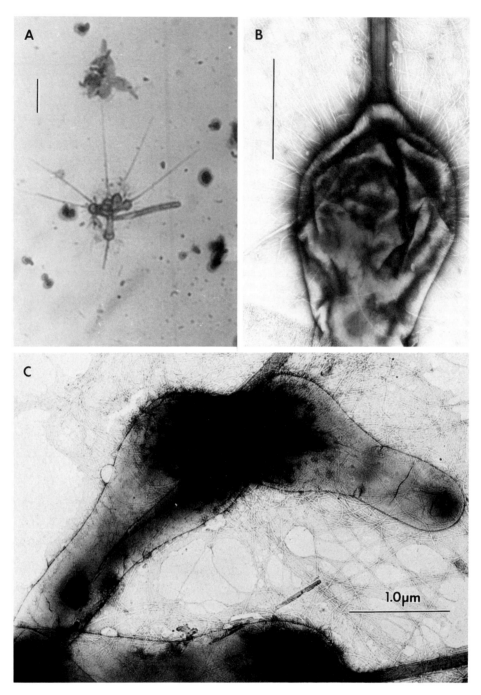

Figure 21.43. Morphotype V of the *Blastocaulis-Planctomyces* group. *A,* stained (Kodaka et al., 1982) preparation of a rosette of morphotype Va (*P. guttaeformis*), homologous as to cell type, showing the typical bulbiform cellular shape and the prominent spikes. × 1,800. *B,* bulbous end of morphotype Va (*P. guttaeformis*) cell, showing pili, crateriform surface structures, and basal portion of the spike. 1.0% uranyl acetate; × 25,200. *C,* budding cell of morphotype Va (*P. guttaeformis*) from the pond at The Lakes, Tempe, Arizona, showing pili, crateriform surface structures, and base of the spike. The bud is a mirror image of the bulbiform mother cell. 1.0% uranyl acetate; × 27,333. *D,* stained (Kodaka et al., 1982) preparation showing a rosette, homologous as to cell type, of morphotype Vb (*P. stranskae*). Note that this organism lacks the spikes typical of morphotype Va but does have a prominent halo of bristles with entrapped bacteria. × 1,800. *E,* Globose hemisphere of a morphotype Vb (*P. stranskae*) cell from the pond at The Lakes, Tempe, Arizona, showing the typical multifibrillar bristles. Neither a spike nor the "socket" from which the spike emanates in morphotype Va is present. 1.0% uranyl acetate; × 45,000. *F,* rosette of cells of morphotype Vb (*P. stranskae*) cells from the pond at The Lakes, Tempe, Arizona, one with a mirror-image bud. Note the numerous multifibrillar bristles on the globose hemispheres of each cell. 1.0% uranyl acetate; × 11,560. *Bars,* 5.0 μm for *A* and *D;* 1.0 μm for *B, C* and *F;* and 0.5 μm for *E.*

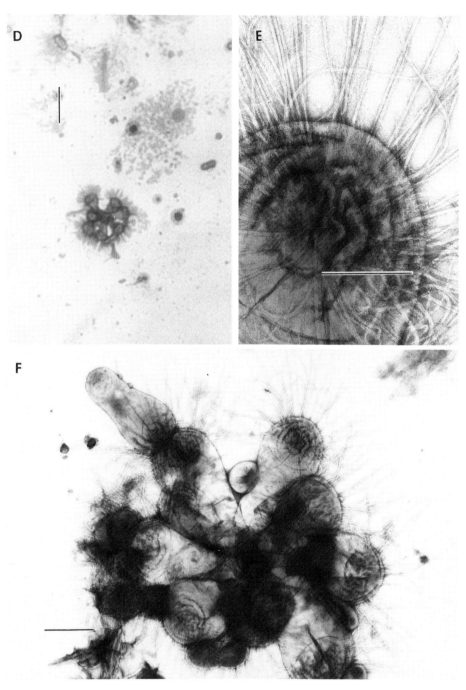

Figure 21.43*D–F.*

formed at the globose end of the cell. Numerous crateriform surface structures (Fig. 21.43*E*) occur on the globose end of the cell; presence of pili is uncertain. Fine structure is that of a typical bacterium, except for a rather thin cell envelope, the crateriform surface structures and the many multifibrillar bristles. Cells are resistant to β-lactam antibiotics. Occur in rosettes consisting of as many as a dozen cells attached via holdfasts at the narrower ends of the several cells. Neither motility nor flagella have been observed. Common in eutrophic freshwater habitats,

usually accompanying phototrophs (algae and cyanobacteria). Metallic oxide encrustations of the cells have been observed in specimens from Austria and Arizona. Species has not been cultivated axenically, though blooms occur in laboratory enrichments. Descriptive type material in Starr and Schmidt (1984a). The type locality is a eutrophic man-made pond in a residential district (The Lakes) in Tempe, Arizona, U.S.A. Frequently confused with *P. guttaeformis,* from which it can readily be distinguished on the basis of the characteristic cellular sizes and shapes, the absence of a multifibrillar spike in *P. stranskae* and its presence in *P. guttaeformis,* and the presence of numerous multifibrillar bristles in *P. stranskae* and their absence in *P. guttaeformis.*

Species Incertae Sedis

a. **"Planctomyces condensatus"** Skuja 1964, 16.

Skuja (1964) stated that this organism differs from *P. bekefii* Gimesi "durch die viel kürzeren und sich zentralwärts nicht merklich verdickten Zellstielchen, die kleineren Kolonien, durch das gewöhnlich solitäre Vorkommen von terminalen Kugelzellen sowie die verhältnissmässig mächtige und anscheinend immer auftretende zentrale Eisenhydroxykonkretion."

b. **"Planctomyces crassus"** Hortobágyi 1965, 111. (Morphotype Ib of the *Blastocaulis-Planctomyces* group (Schmidt et al., 1981).)

In the German résumé of his paper, Hortobágyi (1965), using the mycological terminology then in vogue, stated that *"P. crassus"* was distinguished from all other species of the genus *Planctomyces* "durch die Ausbildung der Sporenträger und die aus den Armen hevorschiebenden Sporen"—a view based on comparisons of the remarkably broad and tapering stalks (in the mycological terminology used by Hortobágyi, these are called "Sporenträger" or "conidiophores") of *"P. crassus"* with the rather thin and uniformly dimensioned stalks of *P. bekefii,* and of the spherical cells ("Sporen" or "conidia") of *"P. crassus"* with the bulbiform cells of *P. guttaeformis.* Our examination (Schmidt et al., 1981) of this relatively uncommon bacterial form (Fig. 21.39*D*) supports the distinctions made by Hortobágyi (1965) and adds others concerning its bacterial nature, the fine structure of the stalk, and deposition of metallic oxides.

c. **"Planctomyces crassus** subsp. **maximus"** Hortobágyi 1980.

Its author stated: "The subspecies differs from *Planctomyces crassus* Hortobágyi in its robust thallus similar to that of *Planctomyces condensatus* Skuja, but its shape is different[,] as is the development of reproductive cells."

d. **"Planctomyces ferrimorula"** Wawrik 1956, 296.

The entire description of this rare organism by Wawrik (1956) follows: "In einer zarten Gallerthülle lagern locker um eine zentrale Eisenoxyhydratausfällung von 1–8 µm diam., 1–100 und mehr farblose (?) kugelige Zellen von 0.5–1.5 µm diam. Das Endstadium der Entwicklung ist ein morulaartiges Gebilde von 12–20 µm diam., in dem sich die Zellen nach allen Richtungen des Raumes dicht an die dunkelbraune Eisen-konkretion angelagert haben. Es wurden auch zusammengesetzte Kolonien beobachtet."

e. **"Planctomyces gracilis"** Hortobágyi 1965, 112.

This unusual rosette-forming and filamentous organism (Fig. 21.44) is not a member of the *Blastocaulis-Planctomyces* group (Starr et al., 1984).

f. **"Planctomyces hajdui"** Hortobágyi 1980.

Its author stated: "The species is nearest to *Planctomyces crassus* Hortobágyi but differs from it in its broad thallus and the projecting thinner stalks."

g. **"Planctomyces kljasmensis"** (Razumov 1949) Hirsch 1972, 110.

An accessible description of this organism has been presented by Zavarzin (1961b) under the names *"Blastocaulis kljasmensis"* Razumov 1949 and *"Gallionella planctonica"* Krasil'nikov 1949. From Zavarzin's description, this organism—except for its smaller cells (reported by Zavarzin as spherical and 0.3–0.5 µm in diameter, although he stated that "sometimes larger cells are encountered")—seems to be similar to iron-encrusted *P. bekefii.*

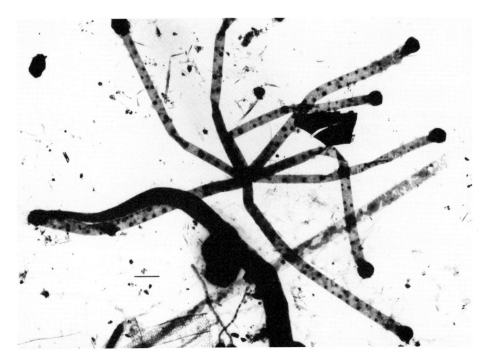

Figure 21.44.   Rosette of *"P. gracilis"* Hortobágyi 1965. Water sample from the pond at The Lakes, Tempe, Arizona. This unusual rosette-forming and filamentous bacterium, which lacks crateriform surface structures and multifibrillar appendages, does not belong to the *Blastocaulis-Planctomyces* group (Starr et al., 1984). 1.0% uranyl acetate; × 6,710. *Bar,* 1.0 µm.

Genus "**Isosphaera**" *Giovannoni, Schabtach and Castenholz 1987, 283*

S. J. GIOVANNONI AND R. W. CASTENHOLZ

(*Isocystis* Borzi 1878 (cyanobacteria))

I.so.sphaer'a. Gr. adj. *iso* equal; L. fem. n. *sphaera* ball or sphere; *Isosphaera* sphere of equal size.

Spherical cells 2.0-2.5 µm in diameter, **forming chains.** Chain length indefinite, often over 100 cells. Cell division by **budding.** Buds intercalary or at chain ends. Chain branching does not occur. Capsules are not formed. Gas vesicles are usually present, normally forming one "vacuole" per cell. Resting stages are not known. **Motile by gliding.** Pili, but not flagella, present. Gram-variable.

Strictly aerobic. Temperature range: 40-55°C. Optimal pH range: 7.8-8.8. **Chemoheterotrophic** with **respiratory** metabolism. Glucose or lactate only known carbon sources. Oligotrophic, glucose above 0.025% inhibitory. Carotenoids present. No chlorophyll or bacteriochlorophyll present.

The mol% G + C of the DNA for one strain (IS1B) is 62.2.

Type species: "*Isosphaera pallida*" (Woronichin 1927) Giovannoni, Schabtach and Castenholz 1987, 283.

Further Description Information

Cell size is variable in actively growing chains. Negatively stained specimens show no signs of capsules, although cells often appear capsulated under phase-contrast microscopy. Although no resting stages are known, some cells may appear to be more refractile. Numerous pili are observed by transmission electron microscopy (TEM). Gliding motility is slow, ~0.05 µm/s. Chains and colonies are often phototactic. Motility is known only on plates of 0.4% agarose or Gelrite. On 1.5% agar, colonies are convex with entire edges.

Ultrastructural characterization of "*I. pallida*" by TEM has demonstrated an unusual wall structure. Periodically spaced ring-shaped structures of 27 nm in diameter are observed in negatively stained cells and isolated cell walls (Fig. 21.45). Transmission electron micrographs of "*I. pallida*" thin sections show a wall consisting of two electron-dense layers separated by an electron-transparent layer (Figs. 21.46 and 21.47). Growth of "*I. pallida*" is not inhibited by penicillin G (2338 units/ml). Lipids are ester-linked.

Enrichment and Isolation Procedures

"*I. pallida*" has been isolated from numerous North American hot springs including Mammoth Hot Springs, Yellowstone National Park, Wyoming, and Kah-nee-ta Hot Springs, Oregon. It has been identified microscopically and reported from other North American hot springs and several European hot springs (Anagnostidis, 1961). "*I. pallida*" is usually found in association with cyanobacteria in the temperature range 35-55°C and is frequently a minor component of cyanobacterial mats.

"*I. pallida*" may be selectively isolated by streaking samples onto plates of IM medium (Table 21.24) and incubating in the dark at 45°C under a 5% CO_2/95% air atmosphere. Under these conditions, the bicarbonate/CO_2 buffer system maintains a pH of ~7.9. Small (1-2 mm), pink, convex colonies appear after 1-2 weeks. Colonies are firm and not viscous. "*I. pallida*" is usually a minor component of the flora in its habitat and may frequently be isolated from inocula even when microscopic examination does not readily reveal its presence. Cyanobacterial

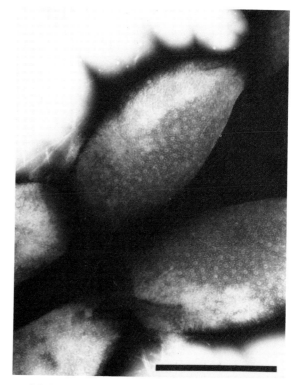

Figure 21.45. Transmission electron micrograph of negatively stained "*Isosphaera pallida*," showing "crateriform" structures. *Bar,* 1 µm. (Reproduced with permission from S. J. Giovannoni, E. Schabtach and R. W. Castenholz, Archives of Microbiology *147:* 276-284, 1987, ©Springer-Verlag.)

enrichment cultures containing "*I. pallida*" were obtained from a saline (~13 °/₀₀) hot spring in Utah, U.S.A. Attempts to obtain pure cultures failed, even when 0.2 M NaCl was added to the isolation medium. Thus, it appears that "*Isosphaera*" strains exist which cannot be readily isolated by the above methods.

Maintenance Procedures

"*Isosphaera*" cultures have been maintained by monthly transfer on slants of medium IMC (Table 21.24). Cultures are incubated at 45°C in an atmosphere of 5% CO_2/95% air. Slants may be stored at room temperature, in air, for 1 month without losing viability. It is not known whether "*I. pallida*" survives lyophilization or freezing at −196°C.

Differentiation of the genus "**Isosphaera**" *from other genera*

Size and morphology are adequate criteria for preliminary identification of "*Isosphaera.*" It is the only nonphotosynthetic, budding organism known which forms chains of spherical cells. Possible exceptions are species of *Isocystis* which at this time may still be regarded as cyanobacteria, and *Gemmiger* species, which are not free-living. "*Isosphaera pallida*" (formerly *Isocystis pallida*) is presently the only species of "*Isosphaera*" cultured and characterized by bacteriological methods. However, it is easily distinguished microscopically. The mature cells are completely spherical, although buds may appear to be ovoid (Fig. 21.48). An asymmetric clear spot (gas vacuole) is evident in most cells (Fig. 21.48). Cells

are pale pink but usually appear colorless under the light microscope. Some cyanobacteria, particularly *Nostoc* species, also consist of chains of nearly spherical cells. However, typically the red or orange autofluorescence of chlorophyll *a* or phycoerythrin, respectively, is seen with epifluorescence microscopy.

Additional Taxonomic Comments

The complete 5S rRNA sequence of "*Isosphaera pallida*" has been determined (unpublished data). When this sequence was compared with those of approximately 100 other procaryotic organisms, no homology

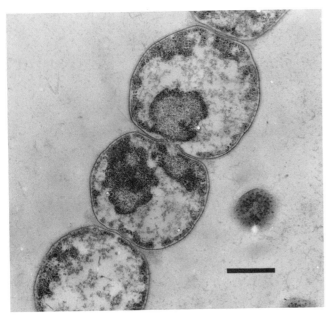

Figure 21.46. Transmission electron micrograph of a thin section of "*Isosphaera pallida*," showing a budding cell in a late stage of bud formation. *Bar,* 1 μm. (Reproduced with permission from S. J. Giovannoni, E. Schabtach and R.W. Castenholz, Archives of Microbiology *147:*276–284, 1987, ©Springer-Verlag.)

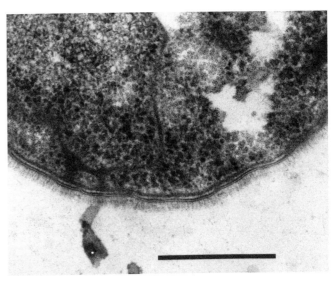

Figure 21.47. Transmission electron micrograph of a thin section of "*Isosphaera pallida*," showing wall ultrastructure in cross-section. *Bar,* 0.5 μm. (Reproduced with permission from S. J. Giovannoni, E. Schabtach and R.W. Castenholz, Archives of Microbiology *147:*276–284, 1987, ©Springer-Verlag.)

Table 21.24.
Composition of **"Isosphaera"** *medium*

	Ingredients	Amounts
Solution A[a]	CaCl₂·2H₂O	0.32 g/l
	MgSO₄·7H₂O	0.4 g/l
	KCl	0.5 g/l
	NaCl	1.0 g/l
	(NH₄)₂SO₄	0.5 g/l
	KH₂PO₄	0.3 g/l
	FeCl₃	0.292 mg/l
	Trace element solution SL-7[b]	10 ml/l
	Vitamin B₁₂	5 μg/l
Solution B[c]	NaHCO₃	42.0 g/l
Medium IM[d]	Solution A	250 ml
	H₂O	650 ml
Medium IMC	D-Glucose	0.025%
	Casamino acids	0.025%
	Vitamin solution[e]	0.5 ml/l

[a]Adjust solution to pH 7.6 with NaOH, remove precipitate by filtration through Whatman no. 1 filter paper, and store at 4°C.
[b]Pfenning and Trüper (1981).
[c]Autoclave, then bubble vigorously with CO₂ for 1 h.
[d]After autoclaving, add 100 ml sterile solution B.
[e]After autoclaving, add the vitamin solution which contains: nicotinic acid, 2 mg/ml; thiamine HCl, 1 mg/ml; *p*-aminobenzoic acid, 0.2 mg/ml; and biotin, 0.02 mg/ml.

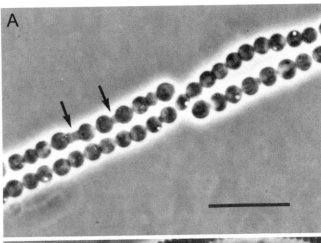

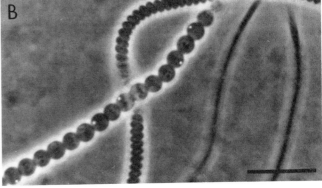

Figure 21.48. Phase-contrast photomicrographs of "*Isosphaera pallida*." *A,* exponentially growing cells of strain IS1. *Arrows* indicate pair of buds forming between adjacent cells. *B,* field specimens from Mammoth Hot Springs, Yellowstone National Park. The coiled filament is a cyanobacterium (*Spirulina* species). The light spots showing in some cells are gas vacuoles. *Bars,* 10 μm. (Reproduced with permission from S. J. Giovannoni, E. Schabtach and R.W. Castenholz, Archives of Microbiology *147:*276–284, 1987, ©Springer-Verlag.)

values of >0.75 were obtained (Hori and Osawa, 1979). The results of this analysis indicate that *"I. pallida"* belongs in a unique and deeply rooted phylogenetic division of the eubacteria. Since 5S rRNA sequences were not available for other budding bacteria, no conclusions regarding the relationship of *"I. pallida"* to these organisms could be drawn from this data at this time.

The ultrastructure of the cell wall of *"I. pallida"* is similar to that observed in the *Blastocaulis-Planctomyces* group of budding bacteria (Schmidt and Starr, 1981, 1982). *I. pallida* is also similar in terms of Gram staining reaction and penicillin resistance, suggesting that these organisms may be related. Recently, Stackebrandt et al. (1984) suggested an early evolutionary origin for budding, peptidoglycan-less bacteria including *Planctomyces* and related organisms.

The genus *Isocystis* was originally described as a Nostocacean cyanobacterium by Borzi (1878, ex Bornet and Flahault, 1888) on the basis of morphological criteria. Since then, this genus has been ignored by many authors of cyanobacterial taxonomies, with notable exceptions (e.g.

Geitler, 1932; Elenkin, 1949; Starmach, 1966). However, other members of this genus have not been cultured; other species, at least, may be cyanobacteria. The type species, *Isocystis messanenis* Borzi, was described as blue-green or olive in color.

Isocystis pallida Woronichin 1927 was described as *pale* blue-green but otherwise as characterized here. The original collection was from warm springs in the Caucasus. Because of the apparent budding nature of the cells, Geitler (1955, 1963) reclassified *Isocystis pallida* and other species of *Isocystis* as yeasts (e.g. *Torulopsidosira pallida*). Anagnostidis and Rathsack-Kunzenbach (1967), who were very familiar with *Isocystis pallida* from hot spring collections in Greece, concluded that this species was a cyanobacterium. Their extensive description and discussion indicate that *Isocystis pallida* from their collections and *"Isosphaera pallida"* from our cultures and collections are the same. However, a weak red fluorescence was seen in their collected material, a fluorescence we have been unable to confirm with North American collections.

List of species of the genus "Isosphaera"

1. **"Isosphaera pallida"** Giovannoni, Schabtach and Castenholz 1987, 283 (*Isocystis pallida* Woronichin 1927—as cyanobacterium; *Torulopsidosira pallida* (Woronichin) Geitler 1963—as a yeast.) pal'li.da. L. adj. *pallida* pale.

The characteristics are as the same as those described for the genus. Occur in hot springs (40-55°C).
Type strain: IS1B (ATCC 43644).

2. CONTAIN PEPTIDOGLYCAN

Genus **Ensifer** *Casida 1982, 339*[VP]

L. E. CASIDA, JR.

En'si.fer. L. adj. *ensifer* sword-bearing; M.L. masc. n. *Ensifer* sword bearer.

Rods 0.7-1.1 × 1.0-1.9 μm, occurring singly or in pairs. **Reproduction by budding at one pole of the cell,** with the bud then elongating to give **asymmetric polar growth** (Fig. 21.49). **Attaches endwise to vari-** **ous Gram-positive and Gram-negative host bacteria. It may cause lysis of the host bacterium. Host cells not required.** Gram-negative but may stain poorly. **Motile** by means of **a tuft of three to**

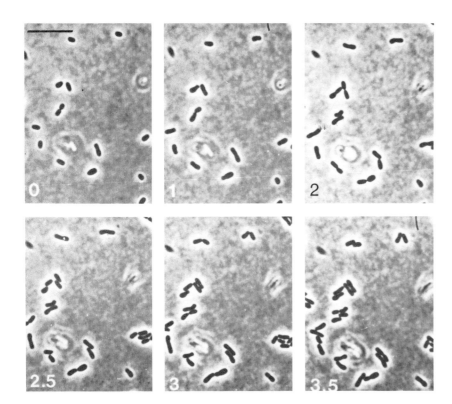

Figure 21.49. Growth of *Ensifer adhaerens* on full-strength heart infusion agar. Incubation was for 0, 1, 2, 2.5, 3 and 3.5 h. Phase-contrast microscopy of a slide culture. *Bar,* 10 μm. (Reproduced with permission from L. E. Casida, Jr., International Journal of Systematic Bacteriology 32: 339-345, 1982, ©International Union of Microbiological Societies.)

five flagella that are attached subterminally. **Aerobic;** does not grow anaerobically in the presence of light. Optimal growth occurs at 27°C; good growth at 20 and 37°C. Not heat-resistant. Weakly catalase-positive. Nitrate and nitrite are reduced. Nitrification is negative for ammonia and nitrite. The **metabolism of glucose and galactose is oxidative.** Growth is inhibited by 4% NaCl but not by 2% NaCl. Grows well on most media. Definite but slow growth on soil extract agar and 1.5% Noble agar in distilled water. Agar not hydrolyzed. Utilizes a variety of organic carbon sources.

The mol% G + C of the DNA is 67 (T_m) and 63 (Bd).

Type species (monotype): *Ensifer adhaerens* Casida 1982, 339.

Further Descriptive Information

E. adhaerens was originally designated merely as "strain A" (Casida, 1980).

Growth of *E. adhaerens* is initiated by budding at one pole of a cell, and the bud then elongates to give asymmetric polar growth. This growth usually widens to equal the diameter of the mother cell. The daughter cell eventually separates from the mother cell by binary fission. Either the mother and daughter cells are the same size, or the daughter cell is smaller.

Measurements of cell size from electron micrographs show that some of the nonattached daughter cells are 20–30% smaller (length or width or both) than the nondividing mother cells. There is no tube or filament between the mother and daughter cells at the time of binary fission. After fission, growth resumes as new buds at the newly formed poles of both the mother and daughter cells. There does not seem to be any requirement for a rest or maturation period before growth resumes. Bud formation does not always occur at the pole of the cell. In old cultures, buds formed from the side of a mother cell are sometimes observed.

The budding and division processes of *E. adhaerens* somewhat resemble those described by Eckersley and Dow (1980) for *Rhodopseudomonas blastica*. However, the latter organism is photosynthetic and grows anaerobically in the light; also, it divides only when the mother and daughter cells are of equal size. The daughter cell has to undergo an obligate period of maturation before it initiates growth.

Whole-cell preparations of *E. adhaerens* stained with uranyl acetate and observed by transmission electron microscopy often show darkly stained material as a bar along the side of the cell. This bar becomes wider near one or both poles of the cell. When cells of *E. adhaerens* are attached to host cells, such as cells of *Micrococcus luteus*, this bar often extends between the *E. adhaerens* cell and the *M. luteus* cell. The chemical and morphologic composition of this bar is not known. Also, this bar is not readily apparent in whole-cell preparations of *E. adhaerens* that are negatively stained with phosphotungstic acid instead of uranyl acetate.

When *E. adhaerens* is grown in the presence of *M. luteus* (or some other sensitive bacterium) on an agar medium, large numbers of *E. adhaerens* cells attach endwise to the *M. luteus* cells. These *E. adhaerens* cells are arranged side by side, closely packed, in a picket fence arrangement. If the prevailing nutritive and pH conditions (either in soil or on laboratory media; pH 6 is optimal) are satisfactory, this arrangement eventually results in lysis of the *M. luteus* cells. There is no specialized terminal morphological structure on the cell for attachment purposes. Rosettes are not formed.

E. adhaerens is not an obligate predator. It grows well on most media in the absence of potential host cells. In fact, except for the occurrence of tracking (Casida, 1980), the overall growth of *E. adhaerens* usually does not increase as a result of tracking or lysis of *M. luteus* cells. However, some increased growth of *E. adhaerens* does occur when both organisms are placed on Noble agar with or without 0.1% glucose. Therefore, it appears that the only benefits of this interaction to *E. adhaerens* occur on a medium of very low nutritive value. This is comparable to the presumed low-nutrient availability that occurs in soils that have not recently received organic matter. In soil, the *E. adhaerens* cells attach to host cells, so that even small amounts of lytic factor produced under these conditions can be used effectively in lysing the host cells. On agar media, this lytic factor is diffusible and can act on host cells at a distance from the *E. adhaerens* cells.

Indigenous *E. adhaerens* cells in soil attack only certain species of bacteria that are added to the soil. Based on tests using indirect phage analysis (Germida and Casida, 1983), *E. adhaerens* attacks *Agromyces ramosus*, *Myxococcus luteus*, *Myxococcus* species soil isolate, *Staphylococcus aureus*, and two *Streptomyces* species soil isolates (Zeph, 1985). It does not attack *Actinomyces humiferus*, *Agrobacterium tumefaciens*, *Arthrobacter globiformis*, *Azotobacter vinelandii*, *Bacillus stearothermophilus*, *B. subtilis*, *B. thuringiensis*, *Escherichia coli*, *Pseudomonas aeruginosa*, *Rhizobium leguminosarum*, *R. meliloti* or *Salmonella typhosa*. However, in a few instances *E. adhaerens* will attack another bacterial predator, such as the *Myxococcus* species, that is itself attacking certain of the above organisms (Germida and Casida, 1983).

After 6 days growth, colonies 10–15 mm in diameter are produced on heart infusion agar prepared at one tenth of the recommended strength (1.5% agar). The colonies are grayish white, convex, circular with undulate margins, slimy, moist and opaque; they may appear almost translucent, due to excessive slime production. Growth on agar slants is abundant, opaque, grayish white, smooth, flat, slimy and moist. Pellicle and sediment (little turbidity) are produced in a broth medium containing 0.5% peptone, 0.1% yeast extract and 0.1% glucose.

Definite but slow growth occurs during sequential transfers on 1.5% Noble agar in distilled water. Host cells are not required, and agar is not hydrolyzed. This growth is equivalent to that obtained on soil extract agar. A good synthetic medium contains 0.1% glucose, 0.1% NH_4NO_3, 0.1% KH_2PO_4, 0.1% $MgSO_4 \cdot 7H_2O$, 0.1% NaCl, 0.1% L-glutamic acid, and 1.5% agar (pH 7.0). *E. adhaerens* utilizes a variety of organic carbon sources including glucose, galactose, mannose, rhamnose, xylose, mannitol, sorbitol, glycerol, L-glutamic acid, L-alanine, L-asparagine and L-glutamine. Acetate is used only slowly and does not inhibit glucose utilization. *E. adhaerens* grows on pure gelatin without hydrolysis. Starch is not hydrolyzed. Good growth occurs on blood agar; *E. adhaerens* is nonhemolytic. Good growth also occurs on desoxycholate agar; initially the growth is whitish purple and then changes to buff.

The metabolism (Hugh and Leifson, 1953) of glucose and galactose is oxidative; no growth occurs under petrolatum; in the absence of petrolatum, gas is not produced, and only trace amounts of acid, if any, are produced.

E. adhaerens cells do not survive 30 s of heating in tap water at 71°C.

The habitat for *E. adhaerens* is soil. The numbers of *E. adhaerens* cells in soil can be estimated (Casida, 1980) by gently applying soil dilutions to the surfaces of pregrown lawns of *M. luteus* cells (heart infusion agar made up at one-tenth strength, 1.5% agar). After further incubation, *E. adhaerens* produces small, thin, transparent colonies appearing as small moist areas that can expand and coalesce. These colonies are not visible by transmitted light. The plates must be viewed from above by using light arriving at an oblique angle. The *E. adhaerens* colonies are on the surface of the *M. luteus* cell lawn. Under these conditions, they neither penetrate nor lyse the *M. luteus* cells.

E. adhaerens has been isolated from a range of soil types. However, the strains obtained from various soils do not necessarily cross-react when they are tested by phage typing (Germida and Casida, 1983). The predatory activity of *E. adhaerens* and its host range can be detected and followed in soil via the indirect phage analysis procedure of Germida and Casida (1983). Some bacteria, such as a myxobacterium and a *Streptomyces* predatory bacterium, succumb to *E. adhaerens* attack in soil but do not do so in laboratory cultures.

E. adhaerens is a component of a sequence of three predatory bacteria in soil that respond naturally when host cells, such as those of *M. luteus*, are added to the soil (Casida, 1980). A *Streptomyces* predator responds quickly with growth and attack on *M. luteus*. This is followed by multiplication of *E. adhaerens*, which attaches to and lyses both *M. luteus* and the streptomycete. Finally, a myxobacterium (*Myxococcus*) multiplies for attack on the residual *M. luteus* cells but is itself attacked by *E. adhaerens*. *E. coli* is not attacked directly by *E. adhaerens* is soil. Instead, the *E. coli* cells activate germination of the myxobacterium microcysts so that *E. coli* is destroyed, and this is followed by *E. adhaerens* attack on the myxobacterium (Germida and Casida, 1983; Liu and Casida, 1983).

E. adhaerens attaches to other bacteria in soil, but it also attaches to other bacteria (or does not become detached) during the preparation of dilutions of soil for plating for other soil organisms. Therefore, it may be in the colonies of the other soil organisms, and it may not be apparent that this is the case. *E. adhaerens* is difficult to remove from cultures of other bacteria unless the other bacteria will grow on media containing 4% NaCl. *E. adhaerens* does not grow in the presence of 4% NaCl.

Enrichment and Isolation Procedures

Variations of two procedures can be used for the enrichment and isolation of *E. adhaerens*. For the first procedure, washed *M. luteus* cells, or cells of some other host organism, are added to natural soil, followed by addition of enough water to adjust the soil water content to approximately 50–65% of the soil's moisture-holding capacity. Alternatively, the cells are mixed with soil and sand in a soil percolation apparatus (Germida and Casida, 1983), and water is percolated through the column of soil. Incubation is for 4–6 days at 25–27°C. After this time, dilutions of the soil are plated on desoxycholate agar or MacConkey agar. Alternatively, the dilutions can be carefully spread over the surfaces of pregrown lawns of *M. luteus* (one-tenth strength heart infusion agar), followed by further incubation of the *M. luteus* plates. (See the previous description for the appearance of the resulting *E. adhaerens* colonies.)

For the second procedure, washed *M. luteus* cells, or cells of some other host organism, are applied as a smear to a sterile glass slide. The cells are allowed to become just dry at room temperature. They are then immediately placed in contact with natural soil. The slides can be partially buried in soil, either outdoors or in the laboratory. They are placed vertically in the soil so that only the top approximately 2 cm protrude. Water is added to the soil at intervals to maintain a range of 40–65% of moisture-holding capacity. Alternatively, a sterile glass ring 11 mm high × 25 mm in diameter (e.g. as cut from a test tube) can be placed on the smear and filled with soil. The soil is tamped lightly to ensure contact with the smear. Moisture-holding capacity is adjusted to 65%, and incubation is at 27°C in sterile Petri plates. Additional water is added as needed. The incubation time for *M. luteus* host cells is 3–4 days. At completion of incubation of these slides, or of the above buried slides, the soil is gently removed to expose the slide surface where the *M. luteus* smear was placed. An inoculating loop that has been heated and plunged into agar while still hot is touched against this area of the slide. The loop is then streaked through a lawn of *M. luteus* cells or onto the surfaces of plates of desoxycholate or MacConkey agars without bacterial lawn.

Maintenance Procedures

E. adhaerens survives well on refrigerated slants of heart infusion agar made up at one-tenth strength (1.5% agar). It can be lyophilized by common procedures used for aerobes.

Differentiation of the genus Ensifer from other genera

The genus *Ensifer* is separated from other genera of aerobic, motile, nonphotosynthetic, Gram-negative rods by its method of multiplication. It reproduces by budding at one pole of the cell, with the bud then elongating to give asymmetric polar growth. Separation of the cells occurs by binary fission. After fission, growth resumes immediately as new buds at the newly formed poles of both the mother and daughter cells.

In addition to the above, *E. adhaerens* attaches with one of its poles to various Gram-positive and Gram-negative bacteria. If enough *E. adhaerens* cells are present, they will position themselves side by side in a picket fence arrangement around the other bacterium. *M. luteus* is a good organism for demonstrating this. Under suitable conditions of pH and background nutritional level, and depending on the species of other bacteria involved, *E. adhaerens* may proceed to kill and lyse the host bacterium.

E. adhaerens can be differentiated from, or even removed from, some other genera of bacteria by using medium containing 4% NaCl. *E. adhaerens* does not grow in the presence of 4% NaCl but does grow in the presence of 2% NaCl.

Taxonomic Comments

E. adhaerens-like bacteria have been isolated from several soils. These bacteria have the characteristics of *E. adhaerens* but do not demonstrate a cross-reaction with strains A or 7A when they are examined by phage typing. These *E. adhaerens*-like bacteria are considered to be strains of *E. adhaerens*, with the lack of cross-reaction being due to strain specificity of the particular bacteriophages that have been used.

List of species of the genus Ensifer

1. **Ensifer adhaerens** Casida 1982, 339.[VP]

ad.haer′ens. L. adj. *adhaerens* adherent.

Description as for the genus. The type strain of *E. adhaerens* is strain A, which is deposited with the American Type Culture Collection under the number ATCC 33212. The description of the type strain is the same as that for the genus and species. Two variants have been isolated from cultures of this organism. These variants produce less slime, which results in smaller colonies and a drier and slightly whiter appearance of the colonies.

A strain of this bacterium that differs from strain A somewhat in its rate of attack on *M. luteus* cells but not in most other characteristics, in-

cluding phage typing, was isolated from the same soil as strain A. However, the soil had been incubated with added *B. subtilis* spores instead of *M. luteus* cells. This strain (strain 7A) is deposited with the American Type Culture Collection under the number ATCC 33499. Strain 7A can be differentiated from strain A by its growth on desoxycholate agar; strain 7A growth remains purple throughout 10 days and then becomes whitish purple.

The habitat is soil.

The mol% G + C of the DNA is 67 (T_m) and 63 (Bd).

Type strain: ATCC 33212.

Genus Blastobacter Zavarzin 1961, 962[AL]

Y. A. Trotsenko, N. V. Doronina and P. Hirsch

Blas.to.bac′ter. Gr. n. *blastos* bud shoot; Gr. masc. n. *bactrum* rod; M.L. n. *bacter*; M.L. masc. n. *Blastobacter* budding rod.

Cells ovoid rods, wedge- or club-shaped, or pleomorphic, often slightly curved and **occasionally branching.** Cell poles rounded or slightly tapering on one pole. **Cell size range: 0.5–1.0 × 1.0–4.5 (10)** μm. New cell formation and **multiplication** occur by a budding process on the free cell pole, subpolarly or even laterally. **Young buds initially rod-shaped, ovoid, or spherical to oblong; later, these may**

be motile (three species). **Some strains produce** large amounts of **exopolymer. Grow in liquids as turbidity, pellicle or precipitate; three species form rosettes. Colonies** raised, **mostly colorless,** pale pink **or yellow.**

Gram-negative, aerobic, mesophilic and heterotrophic. Some strains may fix CO_2 reductively when grown on methanol or methylated amines. Optimum pH: between 6.8 and 7.8. Temperature range for growth: 10–46°C. **Carbon and energy sources may be alcohols, sugars, organic acids or some amino acids.** NH_4^+, NO_3^-, urea, peptones, yeast extracts or casein hydrolysates may be utilized as nitrogen source. Some strains reduce NO_3^- or NO_2^-. Nitrification activity has not been observed.

Oxidase-, catalase- and peroxidase-positive.

The mol% G + C of the DNA ranges from 58.9 to 69 (T_m). *Blastobacter* species occur in lakes, ponds, activated sludge, groundwater, or freshwater swimming pools.

Type species: *Blastobacter henricii* Zavarzin 1961, 962 (not obtained in pure culture).

Further Descriptive Information

Some strains tend to be pleomorphic and may occasionally form branches and/or lateral buds. Fine structural studies revealed the presence, in some cultures, of storage granules (polyphosphates, poly-β-hydroxybutyrate) and "vacuoles"; the latter may have been lipids removed during the embedding procedure. There were no internal membrane structures, as have been observed in nitrifying, photosynthetic or some methylotrophic bacteria (Loginova and Trotsenko, 1979).

Under adverse conditions, buds may grow out to rods which are substantially longer than the mother cell. Subpolar attachment of buds may not be detected microscopically if the bud lies over the mother cell. Rosette-forming *Blastobacter* cells may stand upright in thicker slide wet mounts and thus appear to be coccal in shape.

Organic growth factors (vitamins) are not required. Acetoin, indole or H_2S are not produced. Some strains alkalize litmus milk but do not peptonize or coagulate it; other strains do not alter milk at all. Good growth occurs with ammonium salts, nitrates, peptones or some amino acids as the nitrogen source.

Most *Blastobacter* isolates came from the surface of freshwater lakes or ponds (Hirsch et al., 1977; Hirsch and Müller, 1985, 1986). Others were isolated from activated sludge (Loginova and Trotsenko, 1979; Doronina et al., 1983) or a swimming pool (Sly, 1985). Recently, *Blastobacter* strains were isolated from the Solar Lake (Elat, Sinai; Hirsch 1980), from Antarctic rocks and from groundwater (Hirsch and Rades-Rohkohl, unpublished observation). The type species, *B. henricii,* was originally found in forest brook water rich in iron and to which shreds of filter paper had been added.

Enrichment and Isolation Procedures

The simplest procedure consists of supplementing a surface water sample with 0.005% (w/v) of Bacto peptone and incubating it aerobically in the dark at 18–23°C (Hirsch, 1981a; Hirsch and Müller, 1986). After 1–3 weeks, *Blastobacter* cells or aggregates can be observed. Care must be taken to prevent much mechanical agitation during the preparation, since the young buds (needed to recognize the cells as *Blastobacter*) detach easily. The successful enrichment is then streaked onto a low-nutrient medium containing peptone, yeast extract and glucose, such as "PYG" described by Staley (1968).

On PYG medium, growth is visible within 2–3 days. Even direct streaking of a water sample onto PYG medium may yield *Blastobacter* colonies that can be purified easily by restreaking on the same medium. *B. denitrificans* was obtained by concentrating lake surface water 40-fold via centrifugation. The concentrated sample was incubated without any further addition (5 weeks, 18–23°C, dark). It was then diluted 1:10³ and plated on PYG agar. The shiny, whitish colonies were observed 4 weeks later (M. Müller, Ph.D. thesis, Kiel, West Germany, 1977).

Inoculation of an activated sludge sample from a paper mill into 100 ml of a mineral salts medium containing 1% (w/v) methanol, resulted in the enrichment of *B. viscosus* after 7 days incubation (30°C, dark). Purification was achieved by plating on the enrichment medium supplemented with agar (Loginova and Trotsenko, 1979).

Maintenance Procedures

Blastobacter cultures have been stored for several months on PYG agar slants at 5°C. For long term preservation, *Blastobacter* strains can be lyophilized in PYG liquid medium or skim milk by using common procedures for aerobes.

Differentiation of the genus **Blastobacter** *from other morphologically similar genera*

The genus *Blastobacter* was proposed by Zavarzin (1961b) for budding bacterial rods. Although some of his original cells had one tapering cell pole, his drawings indicate bud formation, in this case, on the blunt pole. This separates *Blastobacter* species from "*Methylosinus* spp.," where the pointed cell pole produces the "exospore" (Whittenbury et al., 1970a). Also, fine structural investigation of several different *Blastobacter* strains indicated absence of intracellular membranes which are so characteristic of methanotrophic bacteria (Whittenbury et al., 1970b).

Bacteria of the genus *Pirella* (Schlesner and Hirsch, 1984) are shorter and club-shaped and always have one pointed cell pole; the young bud is usually also tapered on the distal cell pole. *Pirella* cells always show pits ("crateriform structures") on their surface; *Blastobacter* cells lack such structures.

Rhodopseudomonas (*Rhodobacter*) species (*Rhodopseudomonas palustris, Rhodopseudomonas viridis*) may superficially resemble *Blastobacter* cells, but the former are anaerobic photosynthetic bacteria which carry internal membranes and the corresponding pigments, while *Blastobacter* species lack bacteriochlorophylls. Occasionally, budding bacteria of the genus *Hyphomicrobium* may show a certain resemblance to *Blastobacter* cells. Bud formation in hyphomicrobia is always preceded by the formation of at least a short hypha (narrow cellular extension), a feature which has never been observed in *Blastobacter* species. A new budding bacterium, *Gemmata obscuriglobus,* has a life cycle with a multitrichous swarmer stage and produces a phase-dark inclusion of packed ribosomes and nuclear material (Franzmann and Skerman, 1984) as distinct from *Blastobacter* species.

Taxonomic Comments

The original enrichment culture of the type species, *Blastobacter henricii,* no longer exists. As its description was largely morphological, a true neotype culture may never be obtainable. The generic description should be emended, therefore, and an existing pure culture should be accepted as the neotype. Unfortunately, the range of morphological and physiological variation in *Blastobacter* species is larger than in other comparable genera. A future subdivision into two or more genera may become necessary.

Differentiation of the species of the genus **Blastobacter**

The differential characteristics of the species of *Blastobacter* are indicated in Table 21.25. Other characteristics of the species are presented in Table 21.26.

Acknowledgments

Helpful discussions with G. A. Zavarzin (Moscow) and the provision of information by L. I. Sly (Brisbane) are gratefully acknowledged. We also thank N. I. Govorukhina (Pushchino), A. Graeter, B. Hoffmann and K. Lutter-Mohr (Kiel) for skillful technical assistance and G. Gentzen for the preparation of manuscripts.

Table 21.25.
Differential characteristics of the species of the genus **Blastobacter**[a]

Characteristic	1. B. henricii	2. "B. viscosus"	3. "B. aminooxidans"	4. B. natatorius	5. B. aggregatus	6. B. capsulatus	7. B. denitrificans
Initial bud shape							
Rods	−	−	−	−	+	−	+
Ovoid or spherical	+	+	+	+	−	+	−
Exopolymer and capsule	−[b]	+	+[c]	−	−	+	−
Rosette formation	+	−	−	+	+	−	−
Motility	−[b]	−	−	+	+	−	+
Colony pigmentation yellow	ND	+	+	+	−	−	−
Utilization of methanol (0.5%, w/v)	ND	+	−	ND	−	−	+
Utilization of ethanol (0.4%, w/v)	ND	+	+	−	+	−	+
Acid from D(+)-glucose (aerobically)	ND	+	−	+	+	+	−
NO_3^- reduction (assimilatory)	ND	+	+	−	−	+	−

[a]Symbols: −, 90% or more of strains are negative; +, 90% or more of strains are positive; and ND, not determined.
[b]Would have been reported if positive.
[c]Fibrillar capsule

Table 21.26.
Other characteristics of the species of the genus **Blastobacter**[a]

Characteristic	1. B. henricii	2. "B. viscosus"	3. "B. aminooxidans"	4. B. natatorius	5. B. aggregatus	6. B. capsulatus	7. B. denitrificans
Utilization of carbon sources (1 or 10 g/l)							
Sucrose; cellobiose	ND	+	+	ND	+	+	−
Salicin	ND	ND	ND	ND	−	+	−
Glucuronic acid lactone; N-acetyl-glucosamine	ND	ND	ND	ND	−	−	+
Succinate; malate	ND	+	+	ND	−	−	+
Formate; formamide	ND	+	+	ND	−	−	+
Tartrate; glutarate	ND	−	ND	ND	−	−	+
L-Arginine	ND	−	−	ND	+	−	−
L-Proline	ND	−	ND	ND	+	+	−
Methanol (0.5%,v/v)	ND	+	−	−	−	−	+
Ethanol (0.4%,v/v)	ND	+	+	ND	+	−	+
Acid from D(+)-glucose (aerobically)	ND	+	−	+	+	+	−
Acid from mannitol (aerobically)	ND	ND	ND	−	−	+	−
Utilization of nitrogen sources							
Urea (4.6 g/l)	ND	−	ND	−	+	−	+
NO_3^- reduction (assimilatory)	ND	+	+	−	−	+	−
NO_3^- reduction (dissimilatory)	ND	ND	ND	−	−	+	+

[a]Symbols: ND, not determined; +, 90% or more of stains are positive; and −, 90% or more of strains are negative.

List of species of the genus **Blastobacter**

1. Blastobacter henricii Zavarzin 1961, 962.[AL]

hen.ri'ci.i. M.L. gen. n. *henricii* of Henrici; named for A. Henrici, an American microbiologist who may have been the first to see bacteria belonging to the genus *Blastobacter*.

Cells rod-, wedge-, or club-shaped, 0.6–0.8 × 1.5–2.3 μm. Cells form rosettes by attaching to each other with the (often tapering) nonreproductive pole. A glistening corpuscle (holdfast?) was seen in the center of the rosette. Single buds (spherical to oblong) are formed terminally on the blunt cell pole; they are 0.3 μm wide and nonmotile.

Originally found in a cylinder containing iron-rich forest brook water from Northern Russia and to which shreds of filter paper had been added. Growth was best in a zone of reduced iron at a pH of 6.2. A pure culture was not obtained.

Comment: Namsaraev and Zavarzin (1972) referred to this organism incorrectly as *"Methylosinus trichosporium"* because they had isolated a morphologically similar but methanol-utilizing bacterium from the same location as *B. henricii*.

2. "Blastobacter viscosus" Loginova and Trotsenko, 1979, 650.

vis.co'sus. L. adj. *viscosus* sticky.

Cells rod-shaped to pleomorphic, often bent, and occasionally branched, sometimes possessing microcapsules (Figs. 21.50–21.53). Cell size range: 0.5–0.9 × 1.0–3.2 μm. Buds are produced polarly and laterally and are ovoid and not motile. On agar plates containing peptone and glucose, they form colonies 3–4 mm in diameter, round, convex and shiny, with an even edge and a slimy consistency. Colony pigmentation yellow. In liquid medium with methanol and glucose, growth occurs as turbidity, finally with a slimy sediment. An exopolysaccharide formed consists of galactose, glucose, rhamnose, xylose and glucuronic acid. Cells do not form rosettes.

This species grows autotrophically in an atmosphere of $H_2 + O_2 + CO_2$ or with methanol. In both cases, cells assimilate CO_2 via the ribulosebisphosphate pathway and show active phosphoribulokinase (PRK) and ribulosebisphosphate carboxylase (RBPC).

In contrast to PRK, the RBPC is completely repressed in glucose-grown cells. The primary CO_2 acceptor is regenerated by transaldolase and transketolase activity.

The cells possess dehydrogenase activity, catalyzing methanol oxidation via formaldehyde and formate to CO_2. The serine and hexulose-phosphate pathways of C_1 metabolism do not operate due to the absence of hydroxypyruvate reductase, serine-glyoxylate aminotransferase, ATP malate lyase, and hexulose-phosphate synthase, respectively. Fructose-1,6-bisphosphate aldolase and glyceraldehyde-phosphate dehydrogenase (NAD) play an important role in metabolic conversions of phosphotrioses.

The cells contain all enzymes of the citric acid cycle, with lower levels in methanol-grown cells than in glucose-grown cells. C_4 compounds are resynthesized mainly by carboxylation of pyruvate and phosphoenolpyruvate. Carbon sources utilized are galactose and sucrose but not methane, alanine or glycine.

Figure 21.50. *"Blastobacter viscosus."* Cells from a culture in the exponential growth phase on a medium with 0.3% glucose. *Bar,* 10 μm.

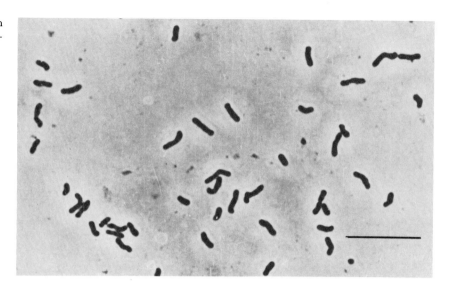

Figure 21.51. *"B. viscosus."* Cells grown with 0.5% methanol (exponential growth phase). Negative contrast. *Bar,* 1 μm.

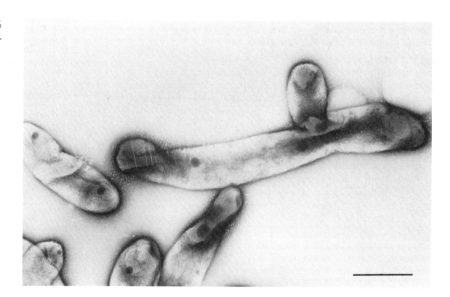

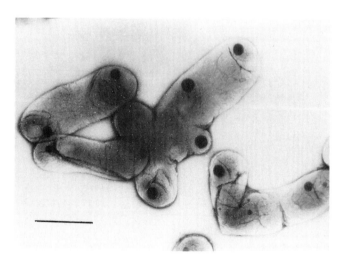

Figure 21.52. *"B. viscosus."* Methanol-grown cells (see Fig. 21.51) with polyphosphate granules and branches. *Bar,* 1 μm.

NH_4^+ is assimilated by reductive amination of pyruvate and glyoxylate as well as by the glutamate cycle. Nitrate, but not nitrite, can be used as a nitrogen source.

The organisms do not hydrolyze gelatin, starch or cellulose. They alkalinize milk but do not peptonize or coagulate it. Catalase-and oxidase-positive, strictly aerobic. *"B. viscosus"* does not form acetoin, indole or H_2S.

Resistant to penicillin, ampicillin, lincomycin, erythromycin, oleandomycin; weakly sensitive to nalidixic acid, neomycin, streptomycin, novobiocin; and inhibited by kanamycin and gentamicin. The main fatty acid of PYG agar-grown cells is: $C_{18:1}$ (76.0%).

Aerobic, mesophilic. Optimal temperature: 28–30°C. Optimal pH for growth: 6.8–7.2. Vitamins are not required.

Isolated from activated sludge of the drainage system of the Baikal paper mill, U.S.S.R.

The mol% G + C of the DNA is 66.3 ± 0.9 (T_m).

Type strain: UCM V-1439D^T, carried in the culture collection of the Institute of Microbial Biochemistry and Physiology, Academy of Sciences, Pushchino, U.S.S.R.

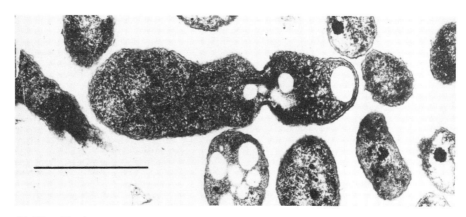

Figure 21.53. *"B. viscosus."* Ultrathin section showing cell wall structure and polar storage granules believed to be poly-β-hydroxybutyrate. *Bar*, 1 μm.

3. "Blastobacter aminooxidans" Doronina et al. 1983, 552.

a.mi.no.ox′i.dans. M.L. n. *aminum* amine; M.L. v. *oxido* make acid, oxidize; M.L. part. adj. *aminooxidans* oxidizing amines.

Cells 0.8–1.0 × 1.5–3.0 μm, rod-shaped, often pleomorphic, and apparently branching to form Y-shaped cells. Sometimes, cells possess minute tubelike appendages on one pole. Multiplication is by nonmotile, oval buds formed terminally or laterally. Colonies on agar media with trimethylamine or glucose are yellow and of about 2 mm in diameter, convex, round, glistening and opaque. These colonies have a smooth surface.

Aerobic, mesophilic. Temperature range for growth: 10–34°C. pH range: 6.5–8.0. At optimum temperature 29–32°C and optimum pH 7.2–7.8, the generation time is 5–6 h. Cells do not produce exopolymer.

Vitamins are not required. Gelatin and starch are hydrolyzed; milk is alkalinized. Organisms are positive for catalase, peroxidase and oxidase. Nitrates are reduced to NO_2^-. With glucose medium, acid and gas are not produced. Methyl red and Voges-Proskauer tests are not negative. Carbon sources utilized are: monomethylamine, dimethylamine or trimethylamine, ethanol, butanol, mannitol, xylose, glucose, raffinose, fumarate, malate and lactate. Nitrogen sources utilized are: NH_4^+, NO_3^-, peptone, methylated amines, and certain amino acids, but not NO_2^-.

Trimethylamine and methylamine are oxidized by dehydrogenases, and dimethylamine is oxidized by a monooxygenase (NADH or NADPH). Formaldehyde is oxidized via formate to CO_2 by dehydrogenases; the CO_2 is refixed into 3-phosphoglyceric acid by using the autotrophic ribulose-1,5-bisphosphate pathway. Phosphoribulokinase is also present and active. The *"B. aminooxidans"* cells may also grow autotrophically in an atmosphere of H_2, CO_2, and O_2.

The dominating fatty acid of whole cells grown on PYG agar is $C_{18:1}$ (75%).

The mol% G + C of the DNA is 69 ± 0.9 (T_m).

Habitat: Activated sludge of a sewage purification system at a pulp and paper mill.

Type strain: "Blastobacter aminooxidans" 14A. This organism is carried in the culture collection of the Institute of Microbial Biochemistry and Physiology, Academy of Sciences, U.S.S.R.

4. Blastobacter natatorius Sly 1985, 43.[VP]

na.ta.to′ri.us. M.L. masc. adj. *natatorius* of a swimming place (pool).

Cells 0.5–0.8 × 1–3 μm, rod- or wedge-shaped, with straight or only slightly curved axis. Older cells may reach 10 μm in lengths. Cells occur singly or in pairs. Buds are spherical, ovoid or rod-shaped and formed polarly. The buds become motile with a single polar flagellum. The cells do not have capsules. Colonies on peptone-yeast extract agar are yellow and round with entire edges and high convex elevations. Colony surface shiny. Growth is easily emulsified. Older colonies become rubbery in texture and may be removed intact from the agar surface. Colonies grown on PYG medium (Staley, 1968) are pink after 4 days.

Temperature range for growth: 11–39°C; optimum temperature: 25–30°C. There are no vitamin requirements. The organisms produce acid from fructose, glucose, glycerol, maltose, mannose, melezitose or sucrose. Methanol or H_2 + O_2 + CO_2 do not support growth. Gelatin and Tween 80 are hydrolyzed, but cellulose or starch are not. There is no urease activity, but catalase, oxidase and phosphatase are positive. H_2S or indole are not formed. An extracellular DNAse activity has been detected.

The mol% G + C of the DNA is 65 (T_m).

Isolated from a freshwater swimming pool.

Type strain: UQM 2507[T] (ATCC 3595, NCIB 12035, DSM 3183), deposited in the culture collection of the Department of Microbiology, University of Queensland, Brisbane, Australia.

5. Blastobacter aggregatus Hirsch and Müller, 1986, 354.[VP] (Effective publication: Hirsch and Müller 1985, 284.)

ag.gre.ga′tus. L. adj. *aggregatus* joined together, referring to the frequent formation of rosettes.

Cells 0.6–0.8 × 1.5–2.3 μm, ovoid to rod-shaped (Fig. 21.54). Multiplication by rod-shaped buds formed at the narrow and unattached cell pole. Bud cells motile and attaching to each other to form rosettes. Colonies colorless to slightly beige or brownish, round with entire edges, dull to shiny. Liquid cultures turbid. A definite capsule has not been observed. Carbon and nitrogen sources utilized are listed in Table 2.26.

Tolerance of NaCl: grow in presence of up to 36 g/l. A mixture of CO and air (80:20) is tolerated during growth. Temperature range for growth: 13–43°C; optimum temperature: 36°C. Optimum pH for growth: 6.9.

Grow well on dilute media such as PYG (Staley, 1968). Vitamins not required.

Isolated from the water surface of Lake Höftsee (Holstein, West Germany) in October.

The mol% G + C of the DNA is 60.4 ± 0.4 (T_m).

Type strain: IFAM 1003[T] (Müller 161, DSM 1111).

6. Blastobacter capsulatus Hirsch and Müller 1986, 354.[VP] (Effective publication: Hirsch and Müller 1985, 285.)

cap.su.la′tus. L. n. *capsule* a small chest, capsule; M.L. neut. adj. *capsulatus* encapsulated.

Cells 0.7–0.9 × 1.5–2.3 μm, rod-shaped to short ovoid, often bent and narrowing on one cell pole. Older cells may be Y-shaped (Fig. 21.55). Buds of ovoid shape are produced terminally on the narrow cell pole or occasionally laterally. Cells with capsules; they are not motile and do not form rosettes. Grow in liquids as turbidity or pellicle. Cultures grown at 25°C form much exopolymer. Nitrate is reduced. Tolerance of NaCl: growth occurs in the presence of up to 27 g/l. A mixture of CO and air (80:20) is not tolerated during growth. Temperature range for growth: 14–35°C; optimum temperature: 27°C. Optimum pH for growth: 7.3–7.8.

Figure 21.54. *B. aggregatus.* Actively growing culture on medium PYG, showing budding cells and rosettes. *Bar,* 10 µm.

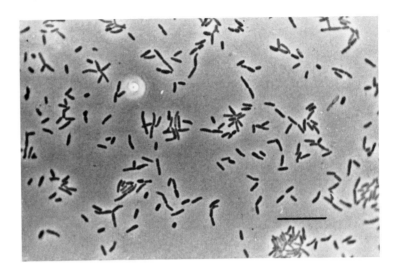

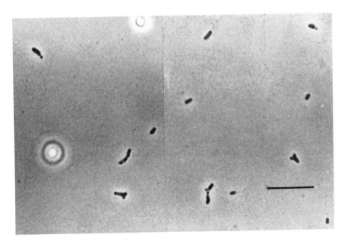

Figure 21.55. *B. capsulatus.* Young, growing culture with budding and Y-shaped cells. *Bar,* 10 µm.

Isolated from a shallow eutrophic pond near Westensee (Kiel, West Germany).

The mol% G + C of the DNA is 58.9 ± 1.3 (T_m).

Type strain: IFAM 1004[T] (Müller 216, DSM 112).

7. **Blastobacter denitrificans** Hirsch and Müller 1986, 354.[VP] (Effective publication: Hirsch and Müller 1989, 285)

de.ni.tri'fi.cans. L. prep. *de* away from; L. n. *nitrum* soda; M.L. n. *nitrum* nitrate; M.L. v. *denitrifico* denitrify; M.L. part. adj. *denitrificans* denitrifying.

Cells 0.6–0.8 × 1.5–2.3 µm, rod-shaped with rounded cell poles (Fig. 21.56). Rod-shaped buds formed subpolarly, motile with 1–3 subpolar flagella. Do not have capsules or form rosettes. Growth in liquid media is turbid. Colonies glistening, round with entire edges, initially colorless, later beige to brownish in transmitted light.

Grow well with C_1 compounds such as methanol, formate or formamide as well as autotrophically in an atmosphere of $H_2 + O_2 + CO_2$.

Nitrogen gas is formed from nitrate anaerobically. A mixture of CO and air (80:20) is tolerated during growth. Tolerance of NaCl: growth occurs in the presence of up to 27 g/l. Temperature range for growth: 13–46°C; optimum temperature: 41°C. Optimum pH for growth: 6.8–7.2.

Isolated from Lake Plußsee (Holstein, West Germany) from surface water in April.

The mol% G + C of the DNA is 64.5 ± 0.8 (T_m).

Type strain: IFAM 1005[T] (Müller 222, DSM 1113).

Figure 21.56. *B. denitrificans.* Well-grown culture on PYG with subpolar buds and free swarmer cells. *Bar,* 10 µm.

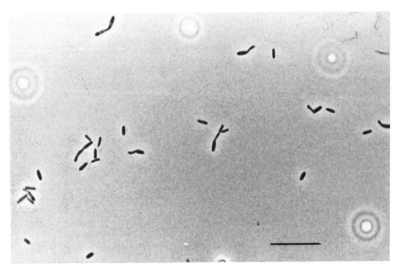

Genus **Angulomicrobium** *Vasilyeva, Lafitskaya and Namsaraev 1979, 1037^VP*

L. V. VASILYEVA

An.gu.lo.mi.cro'bi.um. M.L. fem. n. *angularis* angular; Gr. adj. *micros* small; Gr. masc. n. *bios* life; M.L. neut. n. *Angulomicrobium* angular microbe.

Unicellular bacterium, polygonal cells with radial symmetry ranging in dimensions from 1.1 to 1.5 µm. The shape of the cells is tetrahedral or mushroomlike. Flat triangular bacteria are provisionally included within the genus.

Cells divide by budding. Buds are produced on the tetrahedron directly on the conical point of elongation of the mother cell, a short tube connecting two cells. **Gram-negative. Nonmotile.** Cells lack prosthecae, or lamellated membranous structures, or gas vacuoles.

Obligately aerobic, nonfermentative, **chemoorganotrophic.** A variety of organic acids, monosaccharides and amino acids is utilized. Menthanol and formate can serve as energy sources only in the presence of yeast extract. Methane and hydrogen are not utilized. **Catalase- and oxidase-positive.**

The mol% G + C of the DNA ranges from 64.3 to 68.4.

Monotypic.

Type species: *Angulomicrobium tetraedrale* Vasilyeva, Lafitskaya and Namsaraev 1979, 1037.

Further Descriptive Information

Budding bacteria which resembled a "mushroom" during some stages of its growth cycle were isolated from aquatic environments (Whittenbury and Nicoll, 1971; Namsaraev and Zavarzin, 1972; Lafitskaya and Vasilyeva, 1976; Stanley et al., 1976). Slide cultures indicate that the bacteria reproduce by a budding process. Newly divided organisms are rounded on one side, while the area where cell separation occurs appears conical. This conical section elongates to form a tube, and at this stage the cell outline resembles a mushroom. The growing tube then enlarges. Just before cell division, the mother and daughter cells are of equal size. The region between the mother and daughter cells constricts, and the two cells separate. Both mother and daughter cells synchronously produce lateral buds at the point of separation (see Fig. 21.59).

The same cycle is observed for the flat triangular bacterium. After separation, growth begins by an elongation of the apex of the triangle at the point of division, and new buds are formed synchronously by the mother and daughter cells (Vasilyeva et al., 1979).

The cell wall structure is typical for Gram-negative bacteria, but the flat triangular form, in contrast to the form of the type strains, has no visible rigid layer in its cell wall. No membranous structures were observed except for the small loops of membranes close to the cell wall (Fig. 21.60).

All strains are capable of growth in the mineral medium with glucose or a variety of carbohydrates as the sole source of energy and organic carbon. None of the strains grew anaerobically with or without nitrate or sulfate.

Sugars are used via the hexose-monophosphate and Entner-Doudoroff pathways.

Strain Z-2821 could grow with methanol or formate as a sole energy source, but in this case a limited amount of yeast extract should be added (Namsaraev and Zavarzin, 1974). Acetate enhances methylotrophic growth. Hydrolytic activity is absent (Lafitskaya and Vasilyeva, 1976).

DNA homology reassociation showed no relation of the mushroom-shaped bacteria to *Hyphomicrobium, Rhodopseudomonas, Ancalomicrobium* or *Prosthecomicrobium* (Stanley et al., 1976).

The flat triangular strain 1109 differs from the type strains and might be representative of another taxon. Particularly, the shape of its flat cells makes it closer to the prosthecobacteria *Stella* and *Labrys.* However, it is premature to establish a new species until additional isolates have been characterized.

Enrichment and Isolation Procedures

No elective procedure for enrichment is known. Strains were isolated as colonies on the mineral base medium supplemented by low concentrations of organic substances, e.g. glucose. Numerous colonies were examined in wet mounts by phase-contrast microscopy, and those containing cells with unusual morphology were isolated. The type strain was isolated as a satellite in the methane-oxidizing community from a swamp (Namsaraev and Zavarzin, 1972). Another strain was isolated from freshwater (Whittenbury and Nicoll, 1971). A pulp mill aeration lagoon contained up to 10^6 cells/ml (Stanley et al., 1976). The flat triangle was isolated from the peat bog in the Moscow River valley (Lafitskaya and Vasilyeva, 1976).

Maintenance Procedures

Strains can be maintained on slants in the refrigerator for at least 6 months. Potato infusion agar or mineral base medium (e.g. MMB agar, cf. *Ancalomicrobium*) with glucose or other sugars is a favorable growth medium. Lyophilization can be used for long term preservation.

Differentiation of the genus **Angulomicrobium** from other genera

Angulomicrobium is differentiated from other genera of budding bacteria by its characteristic morphology. It differs from *Labrys* by the absence of prosthecae, and it differs from *Nitrobacter* and similar budding bacteria by the absence of lamellated membranous structures. The flat triangular strain 1109 might be compared with the flat dividing bacteria with the radial symmetry of the genus *Stella*.

Taxonomic Comments*

Angulomicrobium represents a distinct morphological type in the oligocarbophilic "microflora of dispersal" (Zavarzin, 1970). It utilizes either carbohydrates in low concentrations or methanol produced by incomplete oxidation of methane in methane-utilizing communities. It is not related to other genera of budding bacteria by DNA/DNA homology studies. On the basis of DNA base composition (mol% G + C of the DNA of 68) the strains of *Angulomicrobium* cannot be closely related to other budding bacteria, such as *Gemmiger formicilis* (mol% G + C of the DNA of 59, *Nitrobacter* (mol% G + C of the DNA of 61–62) or *Hyphomicrobium* (mol% G + C of the DNA of 59–61); they are close to *Rhodopseudomonas palustris* (mol% G + C of the DNA of 65–66), but they do not possess intracytoplasmic membranous structures (Stanley et al., 1976). DNA/DNA homology studies indicated a relatedness among all four strains of *Angulomicrobium* in the range of 40–85% (Stanley et al., 1976). Substrate utilization is similar for all strains except the flat triangular strain.

---

*Editorial note: Sequencing 16S rRNA studies indicate that *Angulomicrobium tetraedrale* (strain WAL-4, Stanley et al., 1976) belongs to the alpha group of the purple photosynthetic bacteria and is most closely related to *Rhodopseudomonas acidophilus* and *R. palustris* (S. Giovannoni, personal communication).

Differentiation of the species of the genus **Angulomicrobium**

1. **Angulomicrobium tetraedrale** Vasilyeva, Lafitskaya and Namsaraev 1979, 1037.[VP] ("Mushroom-shaped bacterium" Whittenbury and Nicoll 1971, 123; Stanley, Moore and Staley 1976, 522; "tetrahedron" Namsaraev and Zavarzin 1972, 999.)

tet′ra.ed′ra.le. Gr. pref. *tetra-* four; Gr. n. *edra* seat, face; Gr. adj. *tetraedralis* tetrahedral.

Unicellular budding bacterium. The cells have radial symmetry; cells of the type strain have a tetrahedral form, 1.1–1.5 µm (Fig. 21.57); cells of other strains (1109) have a flat form, 0.95–1.2 µm (Fig. 21.58). Single or in pairs. Gram-negative. Nonmotile.

Multiplication is by budding from the top of the tetrahedron (Fig. 21.59) or from the top of the triangle. Mother and daughter cells are similar in form and size. Ultrastructure typical to Gram-negatives with no complex membranous system (Fig. 21.60).

Colonies are white, round and mucous with a pearly shine.

Aerobic. Catalase- and oxidase-positive.

Chemoorganotroph. Carbohydrates, amino acids, organic acids, and alcohols are utilized as sole sources of carbon and energy. All strains utilize: arabinose, glucose, L-histidine, L-proline, acetate and mannitol. Some strains utilize: mannose, ribose, xylose, propionate, citrate, ethanol, methanol and methylamine; but they do not utilize lactose, raffinose, pectin, glycogen, gelatin, L-tryptophan, L-arginine, L-leucine, DL-methionine and Tween 80.

Only flat strain 1109 utilizes sucrose, cellobiose and melibiose, but this strain does not utilize methanol, organic acids and glycerol. Organic acids are not produced from carbohydrates.

Sugars are used via the hexose-monophosphate and Entner-Doudoroff pathways. Type strain has enzymes of the Embden-Meyerhof pathway (Lafitskaya and Vasilyeva, 1976).

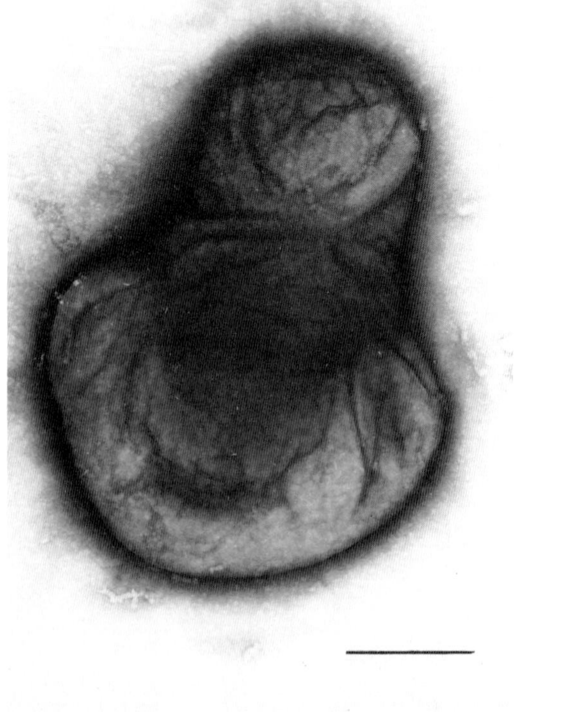

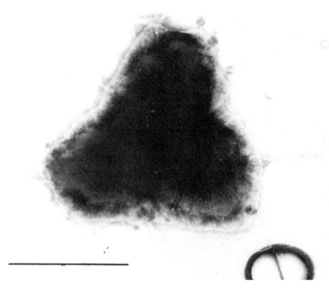

Figure 21.57. Cell of type strain AUCM B-1335. Phosphotungstic acid. *Bar*, 0.5 µm. (Reproduced with permission from E. N. Michustin, Izvestiya Akademii Nauk S.S.S.R. Seriya Biologicheskaya 5: 732, 1980.)

Figure 21.58. Cell strain AUCM B-1336. Phosphotungstic acid. *Bar*, 0.5 µm. (Reproduced with permission from E. N. Michustin, Izvestiya Akademii Nauk S.S.S.R. Seriya Biologicheskaya 5: 732, 1980.)

Figure 21.59. *A. tetraedrale.* Sequential series of phase photomicrographs illustrating the growth cycle of the type strain. Time in hours: *A,*0; *B,* 0.5; *C,* 1; *D,* 2; *E,* 2.5; *F,* 3.5; *G,* 4; and *H,* 4.5. *Bar*, 5 µm. (Reproduced with permission from L. V. Vasilyava, T. N. Lafitskaya and B. B. Namsaraev, Microbiologiya 48: 1033–1039, 1979.)

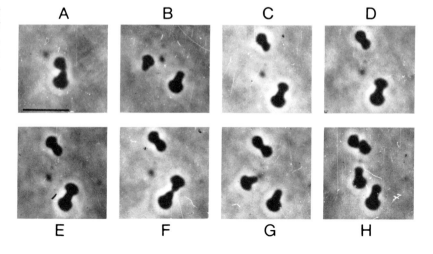

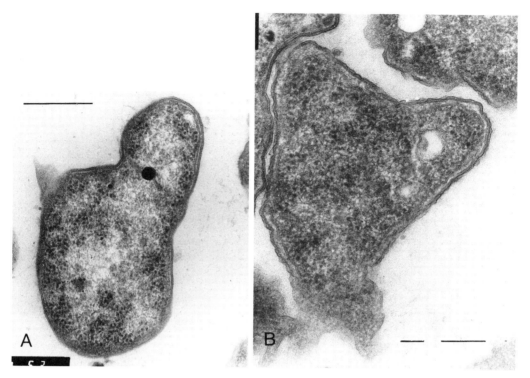

Figure 21.60. Thin section of *Angulomicrobium. A*, type strain AUCM B1335. *Bar*, 0.5 μm. *B*, flat triangular AUCM B-1336. *Bar*, 0.5 μm.

Organic growth factors are not required, but they stimulate growth. Strain 1109 requires yeast extract.

Temperature range: 15–35°C; optimum temperature: 28–30°C. Optimum pH for growth: near neutrality (6.8–7.0).

Sensitivity towards antibiotics (μg/ml) for type strain and 1109: penicillin G, 30 and 100; chloramphenicol, 100 and 0.5; erythromycin, 10 and 30; actinomycin D, 5.0 and 8.0; and polymyxin M, 50 and 10.

The mol% G + C of the DNA is 64.3 (1109) and, for the type strain, 64.5 (T_m) (68.2 according to Stanley et al., 1976, p. 525).

Habitat: type strain isolated from swamp near Moscow. Other related strains isolated from freshwater and pulp mill aeration lagoon.

Type strain: Z-2821 (AUCM B-1335).

Genus **Gemmiger** Gossling and Moore 1975, 206[AL]

JENNIFER GOSSLING

Gem′mi.ger. L. n. *gemma* a bud; L. v. *gero* to bear: M.L. masc. n. *Gemmiger* bud bearer.

Ovoid to hourglass-shaped bacteria, 0.9–2.5 μm long and up to 1.0 μm wide, that apparently divide at a constriction, giving the **appearance of budding.** Rapidly growing organisms may form chains. Gram-variable to Gram-negative. Non-sporeforming, **nonmotile** and with no external structures.

Obligately **anaerobic chemoorganotrophs using carbohydrate** as the only or major energy source. Growth on glucose or other sugars **produces butyrate,** usually lactate and formate, and sometimes small amounts of other compounds. Catalase-negative.

The mol% G + C of the DNA is 59 (T_m) as determined for one strain.

Type species: *Gemmiger formicilis* Gossling and Moore 1975, 206.

Further Descriptive Information

The cells most commonly have a bowling pin shape and are 0.9–2.5 μm long; the diameter of the larger end is 0.5–1.0 μm, that of the smaller end is 0.2–0.8 μm, and that of the constriction is 0.2–0.5 μm (Figs. 21.61 and 21.62). The constriction may not be resolved under the light microscope, and the organism is seen as a pair of cocci, usually with one smaller than the other, resembling a budding yeast. Where the constriction is relatively long, secondary constrictions may be seen by electron microscopy. The bacteria are often seen in pairs, especially in logarithmic phase cultures; the two bacteria are attached to each other by the smaller ends (Figs. 21.62 and 21.63). Long chains are also formed, including pairs with

the smaller ends together. At low concentrations of penicillin, sufficient to inhibit division but not growth, long filaments are formed (Salanitro et al., 1976).

There is a multilayered cell wall (Fig. 21.63) (Gossling and Moore, 1975; Salanitro et al., 1976). Intracellular granules of a glycogenlike substance may be found (Salanitro et al., 1976).

Colonies are 1–2 mm in diameter after 48 h of growth. They are usually circular, entire, smooth and low convex. They may be clear, translucent or opaque cream or white, depending on the medium. Broth cultures may become turbid initially, but the growth usually settles to form a ropy sediment.

Strict anaerobes, they have been cultured by using the roll tube, glove box and steel wool (Mitsuoka, 1980) techniques but cannot be cultured on agar medium which has been exposed to air and is incubated in a conventional anaerobic jar (Gossling and Moore, 1975; Croucher and Barnes, 1983). Carbon dioxide is normally added to the gas phase for incubation and appears necessary for good growth.

Carbohydrates or related compounds are required for growth. Most strains use glucose; fresh isolates—from humans—which do not use glucose will use maltose (Holdeman et al., 1976; Mitsuoka, 1980). For strains from chickens, NH_4^+ has been shown to be the preferred nitrogen source (Salanitro et al., 1976). Various unidentified factors present in ruminal, fecal, liver or yeast extracts are necessary for growth. Growth of strains

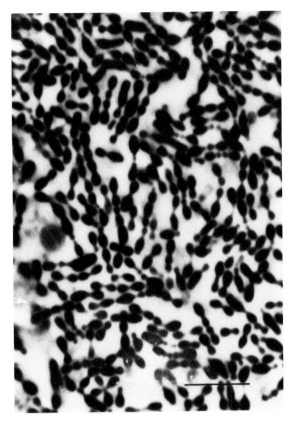

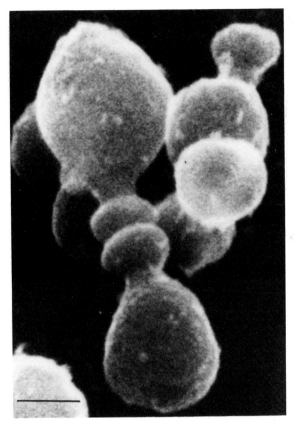

Figure 21.61. *G. formicilis* strain SC3/5. Phase-contrast photomicrograph of broth culture. *Bar,* 5 µm. (Reproduced with permission from S. C. Croucher and E. M. Barnes, Revue de l'Institut Pasteur de Lyon *14:* 95–102, 1981, ©Institut Pasteur de Lyon.)

Figure 21.62. *G. formicilis* strain L61. Scanning electron micrograph. *Bar,* 0.5 µm. (Reproduced with permission from J. Gossling and W. E. C. Moore, International Journal of Systematic Bacteriology *25:* 202–207, 1975, ©International Union of Microbiological Societies.)

from chickens is stimulated by thiamine, riboflavin, pantothenate and straight chain volatile fatty acids (Salanitro et al., 1976). Growth of some strains from humans is stimulated by Tween 80 (0.01–0.10%), but this is inhibitory to other strains (Gossling and Moore, 1975; Salanitro et al., 1976).

Glucose is fermented with the production of butyrate and usually formate and lactate; other products may include acetate, pyruvate, succinate and malonate. All strains use and ferment a range of the following substances: amygdalin, arabinose, arabinoxylan, cellobiose, dextrin, esculin, fructose, galactose, glucose, glycogen, inulin, lactose, maltose, mannose, melibiose, raffinose, salicin, starch, sucrose, trehalose and xylose. Lactate and nitrogenous compounds are not fermented.

The few strains that have been tested grow in the presence of tetracycline (10 µg/ml), doxycycline (10 µg/ml), streptomycin (10 µg/ml), neomycin (100 µg/ml), kanamycin (100 µg/ml), gentamicin (10 µg/ml), colistin (10 µg/ml) or nalidixic acid (100 µg/ml). They do not grow in the presence of penicillin (10 units/ml), erythromycin (10 µg/ml), lincomycin (2 µg/ml), clindamycin (1 µg/ml), vancomycin (5 µg/ml), or bacitracin (10 µg/ml) (Croucher and Barnes, 1983).

Gemmiger isolates have been obtained from chickens and humans. In chickens up to 6 weeks of age, these bacteria live in the lumen of the large intestine and the ceca, forming a significant proportion—often >10%—of the flora (Salanitro et al., 1976; Croucher and Barnes, 1983). In adult humans they comprise about 1–2% of the fecal bacteria (Moore and Holdeman, 1974; Gossling and Moore, 1975; Holdeman et al., 1976).

Enrichment and Isolation Procedures

Via the roll tube technique, *Gemmiger* strains are isolated on media enriched with ruminal fluid, fecal extract or liver extract and containing carbohydrates (glucose, maltose and/or cellobiose, soluble starch). No successful selection or enrichment techniques have been reported. Samples are diluted under strictly anaerobic conditions and streaked out on agar media for isolated colonies. After incubation for 3–7 days, large samples of colonies are picked for identification. *Gemmiger* can be distinguished microscopically by using phase contrast (Fig. 21.61) or Gram stain (Mitsuoka, 1980).

Maintenance Procedures

Gemmiger strains are maintained by lyophilization, via methods suitable for strict anaerobes.

Differentiation of the genus **Gemmiger** from other genera

The key feature which distinguishes *Gemmiger* from aberrant minicell-producing bacilli, budding cocci or streptococci is the appearance of two small forms between two large ones (Fig. 21.61). Metabolically, *Gemmiger* can be distinguished from most other intestinal anaerobes by their requirement for carbohydrates together with the production of butyrate and no gas.

Taxonomic Comments

Gemmiger does not fit into any described higher taxon. Metabolically, these bacteria have been compared with other anaerobic intestinal bacilli, such as *Eubacterium* and the *Bacteroidaceae* (Moore and Holdeman, 1974; Salanitro et al., 1976), but *Gemmiger* has a higher mol%

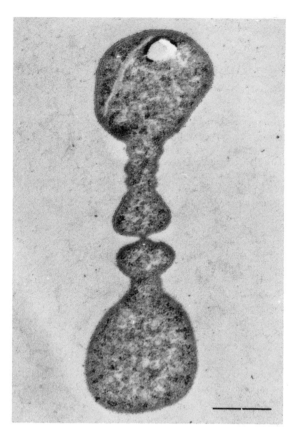

Figure 21.63. *G. formicilis* strain L61. Transmission electron micrograph of a thin section. *Bar,* 0.5 μm. (Reproduced with permission from J. Gossling and W. E. C. Moore, International Journal of Systematic Bacteriology 25: 202–207, 1975, ©International Union of Microbiological Societies.)

G + C of the DNA than do any of these. The mode of division may be similar to that of the facultative, prosthecate, freshwater bacterium *Ancalomicrobium* (Staley, 1968), but this bacterium has a higher mol% G + C of the DNA than does *Gemmiger*. Other bacteria which may have a similar mode of division are even more different metabolically (Whittenbury and Nicoll, 1971; Hirsch, 1974a).

Gemmiger have been grouped with the anaerobic cocci (Moore and Holdeman, 1974; Mitsuoka, 1980), but the formation of filaments in sublethal concentrations of penicillin (Salanitro et al., 1976) does not indicate a typical coccal morphology.

Further Reading

Croucher, S.C. and E.M. Barnes. 1983. The occurrence and properties of *Gemmiger formicilis* and related anaerobic budding bacteria in the avium caecum. J. Appl. Bacteriol. *54:* 7–22.
Gossling, J. and W.E.C. Moore. 1975. *Gemmiger formicilis* n. gen., n. sp., an anaerobic budding bacterium from intestines. Int. J. Syst. Bacteriol. *25:* 202–207.
Salanitro, J.P., P.A. Muirhead and J.R. Goodman. 1976. Morphological and physiological characteristics of *Gemmiger formicilis* isolated from chicken ceca. Appl. Environ. Microbiol. *32:* 623–632.

List of species of the genus **Gemmiger**

1. **Gemmiger formicilis** Gossling and Moore 1975, 206.[AL]

for.mi′ci.lis. M.L. adj. *formicilis* pertaining to formic acid.

Strictly anaerobic, mesophilic bacteria conforming to the generic description. Require glucose, fructose, maltose or other carbohydratelike substances (see generic description) for growth. Produce butyrate and usually formate and lactate and no gas from glucose and other sugars. The predominant product varies with the strain and the sugar used. The terminal pH in weakly buffered media is 4.8–6.0. Erythritol, inositol, mannitol, melezitose, rhamnose and ribose are not fermented. Indole, lecithinase, lipase, acetylmethylcarbinol, hydrogen sulfide and urease are not produced. Nitrate is not reduced. Hippurate is not hydrolyzed. Casein and meat are not digested; there may be a weak action on gelatin (Gossling and Moore, 1975).

Study of poultry strains indicates that most of them belong to one of two groups on the basis of the fermentation products and carbon sources used (Table 21.27) (Salanitro et al., 1976; Croucher and Barnes, 1983). Human strains may be divided similarly on the basis of fermentation products, but the groups obtained do not correspond with the poultry groups on the basis of carbon sources used.

All poultry strains use raffinose and salicin; most human strains do not. However, the type strain is a human strain which uses salicin (Gossling and Moore, 1975).

It has been suggested that the human strains, which grow poorly in culture, do not use glucose on initial isolation, and do not produce formate, belong to a separate species (Holdeman et al., 1976); however, strains which normally produce formate may not do so when not growing well (Gossling and Moore, 1975).

The mol% G + C of the DNA is 59 (T_m).
Type strain: ATCC 27749.

Table 21.27.
Differential characteristics of the groups of **G. formicilis** *from poultry[a]*

Characteristic	Group	
	1	2
Major fermentation product from glucose		
Butyrate or formate	−	+
Lactate	+	−
Growth on		
Cellobiose	+	−
Mannose	+	−
Sucrose	+	−
Trehalose	+	−

[a]Symbols: −, 90% or more of strains are negative; and +, 90% or more of strains are positive.

B. NONBUDDING, STALKED BACTERIA

Genus **Gallionella** Ehrenberg 1838, 166[AL]

HANS H. HANERT

Gal.li.o.nel'la. M.L. dim. ending *-ella;* M.L. fem. n. *Gallionella;* named for B. Gaillon, a receiver of customs and zoologist (1782–1839) in Dieppe, France.

Cells (fully developed) kidney-shaped, 0.5–0.7 μm in diameter and 0.8–1.8 μm in length; daughter cells rounded immediately after fission. Cells grown in ferrous iron-containing natural waters or mineral media **secrete colloidal ferric hydroxide** from the concave side without any organic matrix, **forming twisted** (periphytic community) or **nontwisted** (pelagic community) **inorganic stalks** 0.3–0.5 μm in width (primary stalks) and up to 400 μm in length. **Stalks consist of a bundle of numerous fibers** each ~2 nm in thickness at the point of excretion by the cell. Stalk fibers and **stalks dissolve completely in reducing agents** and weak acids (therefore there is no similarity to flagella tufts of *Selenomonas* species). **Cells always lie apically at the tip of the stalk,** with the long axis of the cell perpendicular to the long axis of the stalk. **Multiplication by transverse binary fission,** and continuous stalk production during cell fission results in **dichotomous branching of the stalks. Rotary motion of the apical cell** causes stalk twisting. Capsules not formed. Endospores not formed. Gram-negative. **Cells motile by means of a single polar flagellum** when dislodged from a stalk (naturally liberated as swarmer cells or artificially liberated by dissolving the stalks in reducing agents). **Intracytoplasmic membranes** from membrane vesicles and long **vesicotubular** channels into the central region of the cell, predominantly starting from an invagination of the cytoplasmic membrane of the concave cell side. **All membranes are exceptionally thin** (only 4–5 nm thick) but show typical structures of Gram-negative bacteria, i.e. two dense layers separated by an electron-transparent region; **cell envelope totally developed with inner and outer membrane and peptidoglycan** (i.e. not like mycoplasmas). **Poly-β-hydroxybutyrate (PHB)** and **glycogenlike granules** are formed as storage inclusions.

Strictly aerobic (microaerobic). Only ferrous iron ions as electron donor and CO₂ as carbon source in almost **neutral mineral medium** are required for growth. Organisms **do not oxidize manganous ions. Cultural characteristics** (low redox potential with an E_h ranging from +200 to +320 mV, low O_2 content of about 1%, low temperature of about 17°C, Fe (II) of 5–25 mg/l and CO_2 of about 150 or more mg/l are optimum batch culture conditions. Depend on the stability conditions of bivalent ionic iron at a pH near 6. **Chemolithotrophic and chemoautotrophic. CO₂ fixation via the enzymes of the Calvin cycle,** i.e. D-ribulose-1,5-bisphosphate carboxylase **(RuBPCase), present in the cytosol** (carboxysomes do not occur), and D-ribulose-5-phosphate kinase. Under lithoautotrophic conditions, batch culture growth yield (dry weight) (Y_{Fe}) per g atom Fe (II) oxidized was found to be 0.36 g × g atom⁻¹, indicating the **same energy metabolism as known for *Thiobacillus ferrooxidans* with a consumption of about 150 g ferrous iron per g dry weight.** Organisms occur most abundantly in oligotrophic ferrous iron-bearing waters (freshwater or marine habitats); have also been found in the metalimnion of a eutrophic lake.

The mol% G + C of the DNA is 54.6 (Bd, *Gallionella ferruginea* strain BD).

Type species: *Gallionella ferruginea* Ehrenberg 1838, 166.

Further Descriptive Information

The information given above on the ultrastructure, physiology and biochemistry of *Gallionella* may clarify the uncertainties and earlier confusion about the fundamental metabolism and bacterial development in this genus. The axenic culture of *Gallionella ferruginea*, which served as the basis for the described features, has been maintained in our laboratory since 1970 and is named "*Gallionella ferruginea* strain BD" (B for

Braunschweig and D for drain pipe, the place and the habitat from which this strain was isolated). Because other pure cultures of *Gallioniella* do not presently exist, the ultrastructural, physiological and biochemical characteristics of strain BD have been used for generic definition.

As may be concluded from the description of the genus, the pure culture of *G. ferruginea* strain BD does not contain the following structures described in literature as evidence for a complex cycle of development in this genus: (a) sporangia in the form of membrane sacs on the stalks (van Iterson, 1958; Zavarzin, 1965); (b) side bacterial cells on the stalks (van Iterson, 1958; Zavarzin, 1965); (c) budding cells of submicroscopic size on the filaments of the stalk (Perfil'ev, 1926; van Iterson, 1958; Aristovskaya, 1965; Zavarzin, 1965; Balashova, 1967); and (d) zoogloea-type of growth (Perfil'ev, 1926; Aristovskaya, 1965; Balashova, 1967). These structures must have been contaminants in the observed material collected from natural habitats or enrichment cultures. Furthermore, there are no "mycoplasma" forms in either the cell or the stalk, as proposed by Zavarzin (1965), Balashova (1968, 1969), and Balashova and Cherni (1970). The only structures in strain BD are (a) the apical cells (always placed at the end of the stalk, provided special observation techniques, such as direct microscopy of developing cells in microculture or submerged glass slides or electron microscope grids, are used for proving mode of development in natural environments as well as pure culture (Hanert, 1970, 1974, 1981)) and (b) the stalks. The stalks do not represent and do not contain living elements; they absorb UV, but they do not contain protein and DNA as hypothesized (Hanert, 1968); the UV absorption is only due to the ferric iron content of the fibers. Fibers as well as all "buds" of submicroscopic size are only inorganic ferric iron hydroxide structures. Convincing proof of this is the complete solubility of these structures in reducing or chelating or acid agents. Because of the importance of this feature, we have carefully investigated the solubility of the stalks. One of the results is that 0.12% (w/v, final concentration) sodium thioglycolate added to the cultures at the end of incubation dissolves all structures except cells, resulting in pure cell suspensions without any stalk material but with maintenance of the motion of cells, indicating their viability (more details in Gebauer, 1985). Furthermore, protein was not detected in a chemical analysis of protein in the stalks, which may be seen in the result of the analysis of at least 10¹¹ μm of stalk material (Hanert, 1975). Therefore, "confirmations" of the supposed living nature of *Gallionella* stalks and their relationship to mycoplasmas may be a thing of the past. This may also be concluded from the lack of phosphorus in stalks, established by Heldal and Tumyr (1983) using x-ray energy-dispersive microanalysis for cells and stalks from natural environments. *Gallionella* cells also do not contain any mycoplasma forms within the cytoplasm and do not consist of a mycoplasma cell body deficient in the usual peptidoglycan component as described by Balashova (1969) and Balashova and Cherni (1970). As shown in Figure 21.64C, the ultrathin sections of *Gallionella* cells of strain BD reveal a clear appearance of the ultrastructure expected for Gram-negative bacteria. As members of this group, they have two cell envelope membranes, the outer membrane and the cytoplasmic membrane (CM) separated by a visible peptidoglycan layer. Additionally, the cells contain an extensive system of intracytoplasmic membranes (ICMs) which are shown to be connected with the CM. The presence of ICMs also implies that *Gallionella* is a metabolic specialist related to the chemolithoautotrophic bacteria. (The following procedure for ultrathin sectioning is recommended: Chemolithoautotrophically grown cells of strain BD from 10 l of culture medium were harvested by centrifugation after the stalks were dissolved with sodium thioglycolate. Cells (their viability indicated by motility)

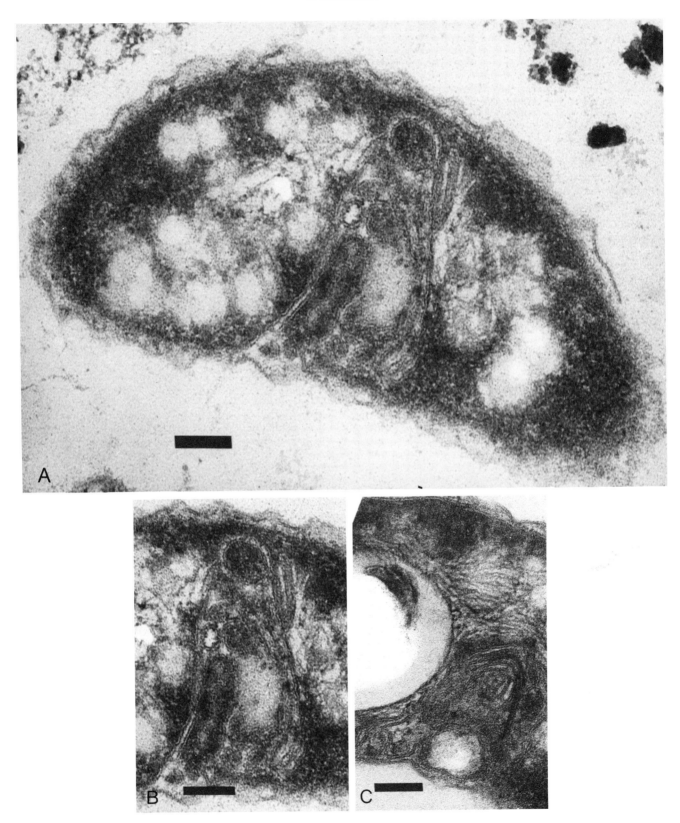

Figure 21.64. Ultrathin section of *G. ferruginea* strain BD at the end of exponential growth phase. *A,* ICMs with invaginations of CM from the concave side of the cell, small electron-transparent regions, which represent glycogenlike material (Walther-Mauruschat et al., 1977), and ribosomes. *Bar,* 0.1 μm. *B,* long vesicotubular ICMs continuous with the CM (at higher magnification). *Bar,* 0.1 μm. *C,* Gram-negative cell envelope with outer membrane, peptidoglycan layer and CM (the *large white area* is indicative of PHB) (Cohen-Bazire and Kunisawa, 1963; Kran et al., 1963), further ICM, nucleoplasm ribosomes and glycogenlike material visible. *Bar,* 0.1 μm. For preparation and abbreviations, see the text.

were prefixed in glutaraldehyde, fixed in OsO_4, enrobed in agar (Merck), dehydrated by transfer through a graded series of ethyl alcohol, embedded in Epon 812 (Mollenhauer, 1964), sectioned with a diamond knife (essential) and stained with uranyl acetate and lead citrate (more details in Lütters, 1985).)

Rigorous proof of chemolithotrophic metabolism of *G. ferruginea* strain BD by analyzing the ferric iron content of *Gallionella* stalks in statu nascendi has been described formerly (Hanert, 1975). A microscopic method was developed to differentiate freshly produced stalks ("primary stalks") from elder ones ("secondary stalks") and intermediate stages of higher iron level caused by subsequent chemical iron oxidation on the surface of the primary *Gallionella* ferric iron stalks. Via this method, it was possible to say that the primary stalks shown in Figure 21.65A contain 4×10^{-8} µg ferric iron per 1 µm stalk length and that those shown in Figure 21.65B contain 25×10^{-8} µg ferric iron per 1 µm stalk length. By estimating stalk production, cell number and protein content per culture, growth yields (dry weight) ($Y_{Fe\,(II)}$) of *G. ferruginea* strain BD were measured to be 0.37 (± 0.05) g × g atom^{-1} (8 determinations) when cell carbon is supplied from CO_2 as sole source. This value is in the same range of chemolithotrophically grown *Thiobacillus ferrooxidans* (Y'_{Fe}, 0.35–0.39), indicating the same fundamental metabolism of both microorganisms (Kelly and Jones, 1978).

Recently, the chemoautotrophy of *Gallionella* via Calvin cycle has also been proven by using a micromethod for estimating in vivo activity of RuBPCase and phosphoribulokinase. This work has been performed in our laboratory (in collaboration with A. Gebauer) and in close cooperation with B. Bowien (Institute of Microbiology, University of Göttingen, Federal Republic of Germany), who developed the microassay. We reported on the results in an abstract (Gebauer et al., 1984) and in two oral presentations (82nd Annual Meeting of the American Sociology for Microbiology, Atlanta, Georgia, U.S.A., 1982 and XIIIth International Congress of Microbiology, Boston, Massachusetts, U.S.A., 1982) by this author. Because evidence for *Gallionella* autotrophy has not yet been published (cf. Ghiorse, 1984), the curves of RuBPCase activity of *G. ferruginea* in Figure 21.66, *A* and *B*, are presented. The procedure used is as follows: Chemolithoautotrophically grown cells of strain BD from 30–40 Fernbach culture vessels (1.8-l size; cell concentration of 2×10^6 cells/ml) were harvested by continuous flow centrifugation at $48,000 \times g$ after the stalks were dissolved by sodium thioglycolate and were twice washed and resuspended in 220 µl of buffer (0.02 Tris-HCl (pH 7.8), 1 mM EDTA, 0.01 M $MgCl_2$, 0.05 M $NaHCO_3$, and 1 mM dithioerythritol). Ten assays (at pH optimum curve) were carried out (20 µl cell suspension per assay + 20 µl for protein determination (Bio-Rad protein assay)). Viability of cells was checked by observing cell motion. The reaction mixture (final volume, 350 µl) contained 20 µl cell suspension (163 µg cell protein optimum pH curve, 230 µg temperature curve), 50 µl 0.5 M assay buffer (see legends), 10 µl 0.25 M $MgCl_2$, 50 µl 0.25 M $NaH^{14}CO_3$ (4.2 µCi), 63.6 µl distilled weeks and 6.4 µl 0.5% CTAB (cetyl-trimethyl-ammonium bromide) for cell permeabilization (3 min). The reaction was started by addition of 50 µl 7.5 mM ribulosebisphosphate (RuBP) and allowed to proceed for 3 min, after which it was stopped by the addition of 100 µl 43% H_3PO_4. To remove unfixed CO_2, the mixture was shaken for 1 h. Samples of 100 µl were measured in the scintillation counter against controls without RuBP. Radioactive counts were converted to disintegrations and, subsequently, to moles of CO_2 via conventional procedures. Controls containing no RuBP gave disintegrations of about 150 dpm (see Gebauer, 1985).

The results obtained illustrate *Gallionella* to be a true chemoautotroph possessing high RuBPCase activity with an optimum pH of about 6.5 and an optimum temperature of about 35°C under test conditions. Ribulose-5-phosphate kinase in vivo activity (optimum pH: 7.5) has also been shown by using corresponding procedures. (3-Phosphoglycerate was found radiochromatographically to be the primary CO_2 fixation product.) The established specific RuBPCase activity of 0.055 µmol CO_2 per min and mg cell protein is sufficient for synthesizing total cell carbon from carbon dioxide (Gebauer et al., 1984; see details in Gebauer, 1985).

Genetics, antigenetic structure, antibiotic sensitivity and pathogenicity of *Gallionella* are not known.

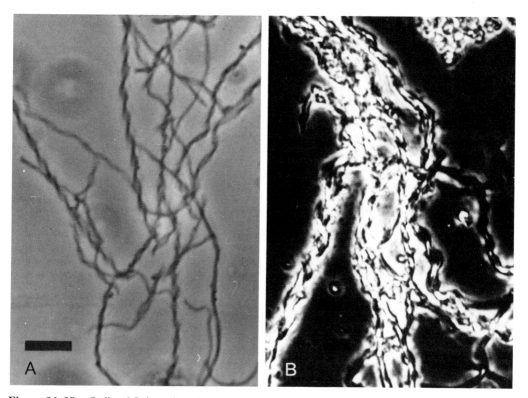

Figure 21.65. Stalks of *G. ferruginea* showing *"primary stalks"* (*A*, Fe (III) content of 4×10^{-8} µg Fe (III) per µm stalk length (*bar*, 10 µm)) and *"secondary stalks"* (*B*, Fe (III) content of 25×10^{-8} µg Fe (III) per µm stalk length).

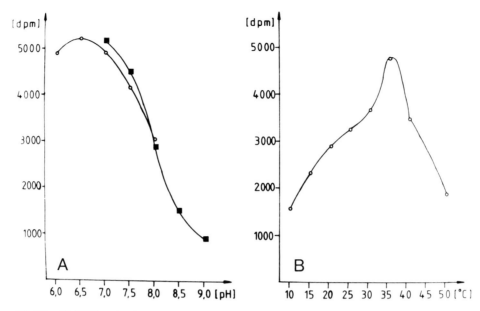

Figure 21.66. RuBPCase in vivo activity of *G. ferruginea* strain BD. *A*, optimum pH curve (*circles*, 0.1 M imidazole-HCl buffer; *squares*, 0.1 M Tris-HCl buffer, dpm per 47 µg cell protein). *B*, optimum temperature curve (0.1 M imidazole-HCl buffer (pH 6.5), dpm per 66 µg cell protein). See text for explanation.

The mol% G + C of the DNA of *G. ferruginea* strain BD is 51.0. It was calculated from its buoyant density and by using a micromethod with novel collimating optics described by Flossdorf (1983) (*E.coli* B was used as a reference; the DNA base composition was calculated according to Schildkraut et al., 1962).

Enrichment and Isolation Procedures

Until now, all of the successful *Gallionella* cultures were able to develop only in mineral media with iron (II) as energy source. The excellent culturing procedures of Kucera and Wolfe (1957) that use ferrous sulfide as a source of reduced iron have proven useful. To obtain the mentioned optimum culture conditions, the following procedure for enrichments in test tubes is suitable: Cotton-plugged test tubes are filled (9 ml) with modified mineral Wolfe's medium (1 g NH_4Cl, 0.2 g $MgSO_4 \cdot H_2O$, 0.1 g $CaCl_2 \cdot 2H_2O$ and only 0.05 g $K_2HPO_4 \cdot 3H_2O$ (one-tenth original concentration per liter distilled water); then, 22.8 cm³ CO_2 are bubbled through each tube by using a 1-ml pipette (length of bubbling, ~5 s; the pH of the medium is now 4.5–4.8); 1 ml FeS precipitate is then slowly added with a pipette; to prepare ferrous sulfide precipitate, 78 g ferrous ammonium sulfate are reacted with 44 g sodium sulfide (50°C) (ferrous salt is added in solid form while the mixture is being stirred), the resulting FeS precipitate must be washed with extraordinary care with deionized water (decanting of the supernatant and its replacement with deionized water at 50°C), removing Na^+, NH_4^+ and, above all, S^{2-} ions until the precipitate reacts neutrally (pH measurement in FeS, not in the supernatant); 6 h after the addition of FeS, and subsequent to dissolving 5–10 ppm bicarbonatic Fe (II) in the medium, and the inoculation follows; meanwhile, the tubes are stored in jars at 17°C under an atmosphere of 94% N_2 + 5% CO_2 + 1% O_2; the cultures are then incubated in preserving jars at 17°C in an atmosphere of the same gas mixture; this gas mixture can also be used for bubbling through the cultures (135 cm³ for each test tube).) *Gallionella* growth is macroscopically visible after 3–5 days (see Hanert, 1981).

Two isolation procedures have been described in detail (Hanert, 1968, 1975, 1981; Nunley and Krieg, 1968); in both, Wolfe's FeS medium is used as a selective isolation medium for *Gallionella*, in which neither sheathed nor capsulated iron bacteria will grow. The procedure of Nunley and Krieg is based on an assumed resistance of *Gallionella* to 0.5% formalin, requires much less time, and, according to the authors, results in a pure culture in 7 of 10 cases. Because we were not able to reproduce this quick

procedure (our *Gallionella* pure cultures as well as material from habitats do not grow after formalin treatment), the other procedure, i.e. isolation by dilution and serial transfer, has successfully been applied twice in our laboratory (this isolation technique is demonstrated in Fig. 21.67). The same enrichment culture procedure is used aseptically: An enrichment

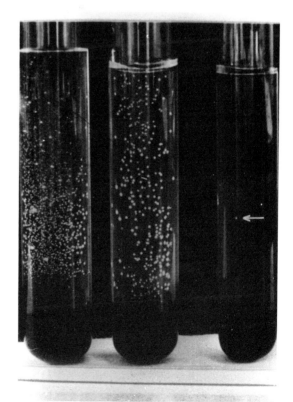

Figure 21.67. Isolation procedure for *G. ferruginea* (*arrow*, one-colony culture). (Reproduced with permission from H. H. Hanert, Archives of Microbiology *60:* 348–376, 1968, ©Springer-Verlag, Berlin.)

test tube culture with colonies which are attached to the wall of the test tube is carefully rinsed, by using a pipette, with approximately 200 ml of fresh, sterile medium without FeS, after initial disposal of the FeS sediment and the 9 ml of mineral medium. Then one colony is transferred 5 times into test tubes containing 10 ml of sterile medium (without FeS) and washed with gentle shaking to rid the colony of clinging contaminants. The washed colony is then suspended in sterile medium (10 ml) and again inoculated into test tubes containing the FeS culture medium at dilutions of maximally 10^{-6} (30–50 parallel cultures starting with a 10^{-4} dilution). Five to ten serial transfers, each starting from one colony, are necessary to achieve pure cultures in this manner. This procedure requires up to 10 weeks but is a very certain method of continually reducing the number of contaminants and obtaining a pure culture. Purity is checked microscopically and by use of a variety of heterotrophic and autotrophic test media; i.e. yeast extract bouillon, nutrient agar, *Nitrosomonas* medium and *Thiobacillus ferrooxidans* medium (length of observation up to 4 weeks).

Maintenance Procedures

Preservation of *Gallionella* culture material in viable form for at least 13 weeks by freezing has been reported by Nunley and Krieg (1968). Culture material was centrifuged at $3000 \times g$ for 3 min, resuspended in the fluid portion of fresh Wolfe's medium containing 15% glycerol, and stored in 1-ml quantities in a low-temperature cabinet at $-80°C$. Survival was shown.

Maintaining pure stock cultures of *Gallionella* strain BD over the past 14 years was performed by using the described culture conditions with transfers every 4 weeks.

Differentiation of the genus **Gallionella** from other genera

The genus *Gallionella* is separated from all other genera of aerobic, curved, motile Gram-negative nonsporing rods by its unique stalks and physiological characteristics. The characteristic, spirally twisted or nontwisted, stalk structure consisting of a bundle of numerous fibers makes *Gallionella* very easy to identify. There are no other bacteria which secrete colloidal ferric hydroxide stalks. The special physiological feature of the genus is its capacity to grow on ferrous iron as energy source and to assimilate carbon dioxide as sole carbon source in neutral mineral media, both of which distinguish this genus from *Thiobacillus ferrooxidans* growing in acid media and so-called "classic iron bacteria" genera, i.e. *Leptothrix, Siderocapsa* (see family "*Siderocapsaceae*" and the group "Sheathed Bacteria") unable to grow in pure mineral media without addition of organic substances. The morphology of the cells of *Gallionella* closely resembles that of *Desulfovibrio vulgaris* NCIB 8303 (Fig. 7.4 of the *Manual*, Vol. 1).

Taxonomic Comments

The phylogenetic relationships of *Gallionella* to other genera or higher taxa are not known, and precise knowledge will depend on nucleic acid studies, such as DNA/rRNA hybridization or rRNA oligonucleotide cataloging, requiring cell amounts in the Gram range which are not presently available.

The ultrastructure of the cells, especially the cell envelope with two membranes, peptidoglycan layer and periplasmic space, and the physiological properties, i.e. chemolithoautotrophic metabolism, indicate that the genus *Gallionella* is not related to "*Metallogenium*" and *Mycoplasma*. There are no mycoplasmoid forms, in either the cell or the stalk. Classification of *Gallionella* based upon its physiology, biochemistry and ultrastructure results in a close taxonomic position of this organism to the Gram-negative chemolithotrophic bacteria which may be divided in organisms oxidizing ammonia or nitrite (family *Nitrobacteraceae*), those metabolizing sulfur (*Thiobacillus*) and those metabolizing and/or depositing iron or manganese oxides. In the latter group, two families could be proposed: family I, "*Gallionellaceae*" (metabolizing ferrous iron chemolithoautotrophically), and family II, "*Siderocapsaceae*" (depositing iron or manganese oxides without any chemolithoautotrophic metabolism). Such a classification would be consistent with the characteristics of *Gallionella*, viz. (a) a relationship to *Thiobacillus ferrooxidans* based upon common physiology and biochemistry with ferrous iron used for chemolithoautotrophic growth and (b) a relationship to members of the *Nitrobacteraceae*, also based upon common fundamental chemolithoautotrophy. The occurrence of intracytoplasmic membranes in *Gallionella* supports relationships to the "lithoautotrophs" and to *Nitrobacteraceae*. The arrangement of *Gallionella* intracytoplasmic membranes closely resembles the extensive tubular cytomembrane system with invaginated cytoplasmic membrane of the marine obligate chemoautotrophic *Nitrococcus mobilis* (Watson and Waterbury, 1971) and the photosynthetic *Thiocapsa pfennigii* (Eimhjellen, 1970). In connection with recent results showing a close phylogenetic relation between *Rhodopseudomonas palustris* and members of the genus *Nitrobacter* (Seewaldt et al., 1982), the existence of an intracytoplasmic membrane system may indicate relationships of *Gallionella* not only to chemosynthetic bacteria but also to photosynthetic organisms.

The recent findings about *Gallionella* confirm Winogradsky's hypothesis on the chemolithoautotrophic life of iron bacteria (Winogradsky, 1888, 1922). They also support Cholodny's ideas (1924) on the life cycle of *Gallionella* and the nature of its stalks. However, it has taken a long time and necessitated numerous experimental steps to prove these ideas.

Acknowledgments

I wish to thank Professor Dr. E. Bock and Miss E. Manshard, University of Hamburg, for their help in ultrathin sectioning. This work was supported by grants from the Deutsche Forschungsgemeinschaft to the author.

Differentiation of the species of the genus **Gallionella**

The taxonomy of the species of the genus *Gallionella* has been based on the different form of the stalk. However, light and electron microscopic investigations have revealed extreme pleomorphism of stalks, both in nature and in pure cultures, obviously caused by additional iron encrustation on the surface of the secreted primary stalks which become more and more thick. Many workers have observed these phenomena and doubt the existence of all species of *Gallionella* which have been described, except *Gallionella ferruginea* (Perfil'ev, 1926; Pringsheim, 1949; Cholodny, 1953; van Iterson, 1958; Zavarzin, 1961b; Poindexter and Lewis, 1966; Hanert, 1975, 1981). Moreover, the descriptions have been carried out on natural populations from ecological systems differing in physicochemical conditions which also give rise to various stalk forms; furthermore, strains of the dubious "species" either are not available or have not been obtained in pure culture. Because of the uncertainties regarding these other species, we are recognizing only a single species, *G. ferruginea*, at this time. All other described species are regarded as ecological or physiochemical growth forms of it.

List of species of the genus **Gallionella**

1. **Gallionella ferruginea** Ehrenberg 1838, 166.[AL]

fer.ru.gin′e.a. L. fem. adj. *ferruginea* rust-colored.

Morphology, flagellar arrangement and ultrastructure are the same as those of the genus. See Figures 21.64, *A–C* (ultrastructure), 21.68 (cell morphology and flagellar arrangement in cell suspensions after dissolving the stalks) and 21.69 (apical cell on the end of stalk) for these features.

The cells secrete colloidal ferric hydroxide from the concave side of the

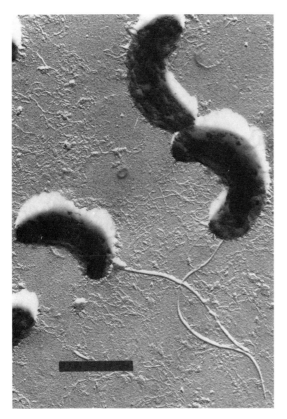

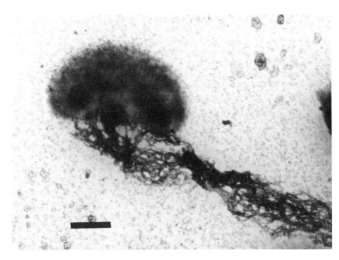

Figure 21.69. Apical cell, region of stalk secretion, and ultrastructure of the stalk of ongrowing *G. ferruginea* from the drain pipe from which strain BD was isolated. Four electron-dense regions indicate PHB granules. (Reproduced with permission from H. H. Hanert, Archives of Microbiology *60:* 348–376, 1968, ©Springer-Verlag, Berlin.)

Figure 21.68. *G. ferruginea* strain BD cell morphology and flagellar arrangement in cell suspension after the stalks were dissolved in sodium thioglycolate. *Bar,* 0.1 μm.

cell, forming bandlike "primary stalks" (Fig. 21.65*A*) which consist of a bundle of up to 90 fibers. Additional chemical iron encrustation of these primary stalks results in "secondary stalks" of various shapes, becoming more and more thick (cause for description of various genera and species).

Cultural, physiological and biochemical characteristics are the same as those for the genus. Chemolithoautotrophic metabolism with vesicotubular intracytoplasmic membranes which are continuous with the cytoplasmic membrane. Cells oxidize the ferrous iron ion for energy production and assimilate carbon dioxide as their sole carbon source in neutral mineral media.

Widely distributed in ferrous iron-bearing waters. Most common environmental conditions are: pH 6.0–7.6 (no growth in acid habitats), E_h ranging from +200 to +320 mV (very good example of a gradient organism), O_2 of 0.1–1 mg/l (microaerobic, but occurrence at higher oxygen contents is possible), temperature of 8–16°C (but also under snow and in thermal springs at 47°C), CO_2 of 20 or more mg/l, very slight content of organic material (not above 12 mg/l) and, above all, ferrous iron of 5–25 mg/l (most important factor for occurrence, stability of bivalent iron, is the only essential condition; Fe (II) range larger than common values presented). Freshwater and marine habitats. Most frequently found in ferruginous mineral springs, wells, drain pipes and storage basins in waterworks. Swamp ditches and lakes are unusual habitats, but a major population in the metalimnion of an eutrophic lake has recently been reported. Growth causes problems in pipe lines but is of high usefulness for quantitative removal of iron in rapid sand filters of waterworks.

The mol% G + C of the DNA is 54.6 (Bd)

Type strain: original type strain does not exist in pure culture; description is based upon strain BD (Institute of Microbiology, University of Braunschweig strain collection).

Genus **Nevskia** *Famintzin 1892, 484*[AL]

H.-D. BABENZIEN

Nev′ski.a. M.L. fem. n. *Nevskia* from the Neva, a river in Leningrad.

Cells elongated rod-shaped, usually slightly bent with **acellular hyaline stalks.** The **stalks branch dichotomously** as a result of binary fission of mature cells and the preference for laterally excreted slime material (Fig. 21.70). Undisturbed and slowly growing cells form **bushlike microcolonies** (Fig. 21.71) up to 80 μm in size **on the surface of freshwater.** Faster growth results in the formation of a thin surface pellicle without distinct stalks (Fig. 21.72*A*) and with polymer all around the cells. Cells filled with numerous globules (Fig. 21.72*B*) which consist mainly of poly-β-hydroxybutyrate. Resting stages are not known. **Gram-negative.** In young cultures, cells **motile by** means of **polar flagella;** they are set free from the stalks and can start new colonies. **Aerobic.** Originally found in aquarium water. Occur on the surface of freshwater (neuston community).

The original strain described by Famintzin (1892) as the type strain was not isolated in pure culture.

Type species: *Nevskia ramosa* Famintzin 1892, 484.

Further Descriptive Information

The type species was described by Famintzin (1892) as being 2–6 × 12 μm in size, but he also mentioned organisms identical with *N. ramosa* of "much smaller dimensions." Henrici and Johnson (1935) described an organism practically identical with *N. ramosa* in morphology but of smaller dimensions, i.e. 1 × 3–4 μm, Babenzien (1965, 1967) isolated some strains from the surface of swamp ditches and ponds. The average size was 0.7 × 2.4–2.7 μm. Hirsch (1981b) reported on some other findings of *Nevskia*-like organisms also in this size range.

The globular bodies were thought to be composed of "etheral oils" and could be dissolved with 70% ethanol (Famintzin, 1892), whereas it was assumed by Henrici and Johnson (1935) that vacuoles contained sulfur. According to Babenzien (1974), globules contain chiefly poly-β-hydroxybutyrate.

In the enrichment cultures of Henrici and Johnson (1935), the bac-

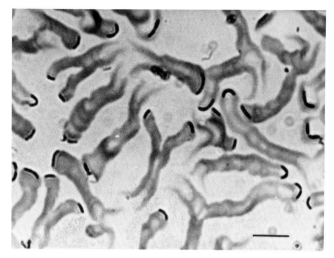

Figure 21.70. Enrichment culture of *Nevskia ramosa,* showing the cells at the tip of slime stalks. Formalin-toluidine blue. *Bar,* 10 μm.

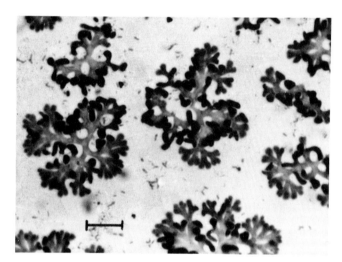

Figure 21.71. Habitat form of *N. ramosa.* Formalin-carbol-fuchsin. *Bar,* 20 μm.

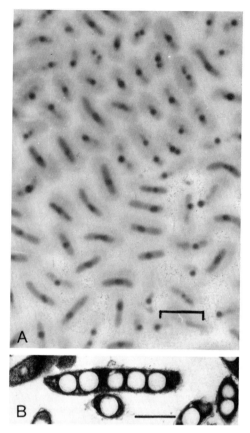

Figure 21.72. *N. ramosa* strain IMET 10965. *A,* without distinct stalks in this growth phase. Phase-contrast micrograph. *Bar,* 10 μm. *B,* ultrastructure of organism grown with Na-lactate. Cells filled with poly-β-hydroxybutyrate granules (*white areas*). *Bar,* 1 μm.

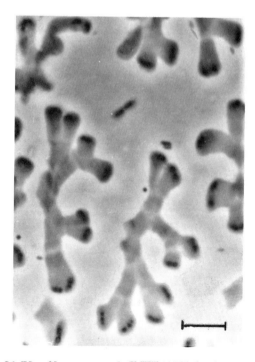

Figure 21.73. *N. ramosa* strain IMET 10965 showing typical morphology. Phase-contrast micrograph. *Bar,* 10 μm.

teria were distinctly favored by the addition of sulfide, which made it presumptive that *Nevskia* was either a sulfur bacterium or a microaerophile. As reported by Babenzien (1965) and Hirsch (1981b), enrichment cultures were definitely favored by addition of 0.1% sodium lactate or acetate, respectively. Hirsch (1981b) summarized various other recent unpublished observations of *Nevskia*-like organisms from brackish water and anaerobic habitats. In some cases, the short rods contained gas vesicles. Typical morphological features were compiled by Babenzien and Hirsch (1974).

Enrichment and Isolation Procedures

Surface films of swamp ditches, greenhouse pools, ponds, etc., are collected with sterile glass slides, paper strips or foils. This material has to be transferred to Petri dishes with sterile water from the same sites. Under microscopic control, suspect bacterial colonies from the surface are picked up with a loop and transferred repeatedly into sterile Erlenmeyer flasks with sterile water from the habitat supplemented with 0.05–0.1% Na-lactate. Incubation in the dark at room temperature (18–22°C) yields *Nevskia* microcolonies on the surface within 10 days (Babenzien, 1965). Similar procedures were recommended by Hirsch (1981b): Surface water samples are poured into Erlenmeyer flasks and supplemented with either peptone or yeast extract (0.005%, Difco), and with 1 ml vitamin solution no. 6 (Van Ert and Staley, 1971) in 500 ml. *Nevskia* microcolonies will occur on the surface within 30–40 days in the dark at room temperature.

Pure cultures are obtained by repeated application of dilution series in test tubes with the same medium. Babenzien (1967) also used the micromanipulator technique for this purpose. *Nevskia* does not grow in nutrient broth (control tube). Streaking these prepurified organisms onto the same medium solidified with agar (1.6%, Difco) yielded colorless to yellow cultures of slime-producing bacteria. However, such organisms produce polymers all around the cells rather than just laterally. Hirsch (1981b) has confirmed this. The bushlike colonies obviously emerge only under the specific physicochemical conditions at the water-air interface and with nutrient conditions in the culture media resembling the natural condition most closely.

Maintenance Procedures

Stock cultures can be maintained in Erlenmeyer flasks with liquid medium (pond water + Na-lactate, 0.1%), covered with cotton plugs, at 12°C, with transfers every 3 months.

Taxonomic Comments

The phylogenetic relationships of *Nevskia* to other taxa are not known, and its discussion in view of our sparse knowledge would be only speculative. In all probability, the two morphological/cytological properties, lateral slime stalks and intracellular granules, are not sufficiently distinctive, and thus different bacteria may have to be recognized as *Nevskia.*

However, in his reisolation studies, Babenzien (1965, 1967) documented all typical features of the organisms studied by Famintzin (1892). A new culture and a neotype strain (IMET 10965) not yet validly published show these morphological and structural peculiarities only when grown as a surface film on dilute media (Fig. 21.73). The cell wall exhibits the multilayered structure common to Gram-negative bacteria but is also surrounded by a thick layer of hyaline slime.

The mol% G + C of the DNA is 60.4 (T_m).

Further Reading

Hirsch, P. 1981. The genus *Nevskia. In* Starr, Stolp, Trüper, Balows and Schlegel (Editors), The Prokaryotes. A Handbook on Habitats, Isolation, and Identification of Bacteria. Springer-Verlag, Berlin, pp. 520–523.

List of species of the genus **Nevskia**

1. **Nevskia ramosa** Famintzin 1892, 484.[AL]
ra.mo′sa. L. adj. *ramosus* branched.

Morphology and description are the same as those of the genus. Organisms occur in freshwater habitats, especially in the surface communities (neuston); prefer slightly acidic conditions. Strictly aerobic, chemoorganotrophic, Gram-negative. Further taxonomic comments must be delayed until a neotype strain becomes available and is effectively published.

C. OTHER BACTERIA

1. NONSPINATE BACTERIA

Genus **Seliberia** Aristovskaya and Parinkina 1963, 56[AL]

JEAN M. SCHMIDT AND MORTIMER P. STARR

Se.li.be′ri.a. M.L. fem. n. *Seliberia* of Seliber; named for the Russian microbiologist, Professor G. L. Seliber.

Rods, 0.5–0.8 µm in diameter and 1–12 µm in length, with a **helically sculptured** or **furrowed** topography. The ends of the cell may be either blunt or rounded. **Stellate aggregates (rosettes)** of **sessile rods** joined at one pole; and individual, shorter **motile rods (swarmers)** occur in the same culture. An adhesive **holdfast**, secreted at one cell pole, mediates attachment in rosettes. Growth on appropriate soil extract media may permit formation of round to ovoid **"generative" cells.** Capsules are not produced. Resting stages are not known. Gramnegative. Following **unidirectional polar cell growth,** a shorter motile cell (a **swarmer**) and a longer sessile cell are produced by **asymmetric transverse fission.** A single **subpolar ensheathed flagellum** is characteristically present on the swarmer; **several lateral flagella, not ensheathed,** may also be present. **Strictly aerobic.** Optimum temperature: 25–30°C; maximum: ~37°C; minimum: 15–20°C. Chemoorganotrophic, having an **oxidative type of metabolism.** Catalase- and oxidase-positive. These organisms occur in soil and freshwater environments as autochthonous microflora, often where oligotrophic conditions prevail.

The mol% G + C of the DNA is 63–66 (Bd).

Type species: *Seliberia stellata* Aristovskaya and Parinkina 1963, 55.

Further Descriptive Information

The typical cells are helically sculptured rods of varying length (Figs. 21.74, 21.77 and 21.78). In a growing culture, the shorter cells are motile swarmers; the longer cells are sessile and include the predivisional cells. The rods become very long (10 µm or more in length) when grown on fulvic acid medium (Aristovskaya, 1974); in aquatic environments with very dilute organic nutrient conditions, seliberias also occur as very long helically sculptured rods. In media containing ulmic acid complexes (Aristovskaya, 1974; Schmidt and Swafford, 1979) or when a plentiful supply of organic nutrients are available (Schmidt and Swafford, 1979), the cells are shorter, and the longest cells seldom exceed 5 µm in length. Growth of some strains of *S. stellata* on soil extract media (Aristovskaya and Parinkina, 1963; Aristovskaya, 1964; Aristovskaya, 1974) may give rise to round to ovoid "generative cells"; production of the round to ovoid generative cells with the type strain of *S. stellata* (ICPB 4130) has not been verified (Schmidt and Starr, 1984).

Cell wall composition has not been examined in detail. The cell walls are damaged by treatment with lysozyme in the presence of ethylenediaminetetraacetate (Schmidt and Swafford, 1981), resulting in blurring of the helical ridges and in cell lysis. Ultrastructural features of *S. stellata* are shown in Figure 21.75.

Cell growth occurs unidirectionally, at the pole of the rod opposite to the pole with the secreted holdfast. The end of the predivisional rod that consists of the newly made surface components eventually becomes a motile swarmer as a result of an asymmetric division. The remaining (longer) portion of the predivisional cell retains the surface components of the parent without redistributing them into the zone of new growth. The subpolar flagellum of the new swarmer is found at the apical end of the predivisional cell, shortly before its division. The asymmetry perpendicular to the division plane results in unequal division products (Schmidt and Starr, 1984). Swarmer cell production by unidirectional polar growth in the genus *Seliberia* meets two of the major criteria (de novo synthesis of the bud surface and transverse asymmetry of division) of accepted definitions of budding (Staley, 1973a; Staley et al., 1981); however, a third feature typical of most budding bacteria, an increasing diameter of the bud during its development (Hirsch, 1974a), is not found in *Seliberia:* The developing daughter cell (swarmer) (a) is not initially narrower than the parent and (b) does not increase in diameter (width) during growth (Schmidt and Starr, 1984).

Figure 21.74. Scanning electron micrograph of *S. stellata* strain Z/A fixed with 2.0% glutaraldehyde, critical-point dried and gold-coated, showing the helically sculptured topography of the bacteria. *Bar*, 1 μm. (Courtesy of J. R. Swafford.)

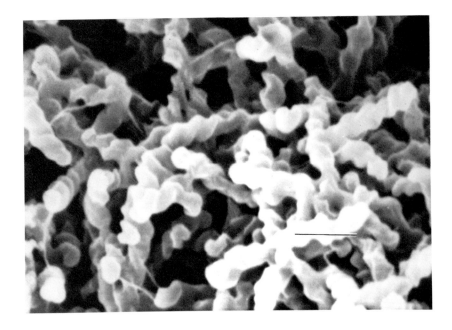

Figure 21.75. Thin section of *S. stellata* strain Z/A, prepared with a modification of the Ryter-Kellenberger fixation method (Kellenberger et al., 1958), 1.0% osmic acid in 0.1-strength buffer for 2 h, and embedded in Spurr resin. The thin cell envelope and wavy outline are characteristic of seliberias. *Bar*, 0.1 μm. (Courtesy of J. R. Swafford.)

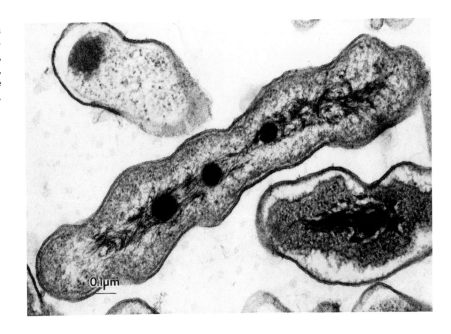

The proportion of cells in stellate aggregates (rosettes) varies in *Seliberia* cultures, but rosettes are readily detectable microscopically under most cultural conditions (Fig. 21.76). The stellate aggregates are formed by association of a swarmer, which has produced an adhesive holdfast at one pole, with sessile cells—often with those stationary rods located in the immediate vicinity of the predivisional cell that produced the swarmer. Also, at high cell densities in liquid cultures, polar aggregation of swarmer cells occurs (Schmidt and Starr, 1984), akin to the manner of formation of *Caulobacter* rosettes (Poindexter, 1964, 1981).

Growth of *Seliberia* occurs on dilute organic media, such as yeast extract plus peptone or casamino acids (Difco), soil extract agar, or pond water agar; media containing organomineral complexes of either fulvic or ulmic acid with sesquioxides have been used (Aristovskaya and Parinkina, 1963; Aristovskaya, 1974; Schmidt and Swafford, 1981). With these media, aerobic incubation at 25°C gives satisfactory growth.

Although the genus *Seliberia* has been previously described as "facultatively anaerobic" (Aristovskaya, 1974), the available strain (Z/A = ICPB 4130) of the type species, *S. stellata*, and all of the several *Seliberia*-like aquatic strains are strictly oxidative; all lack the capacity to carry out anaerobic fermentations. *S. stellata* strain Z/A is a strong nitrate reducer and can grow anaerobically in the presence of 0.1% $NaNO_3$, indicating a nitrate/nitrite respiration. Most of the aquatic *Seliberia*-like strains are not able to reduce nitrate anaerobically (Schmidt and Swafford, 1979, 1981).

Seliberias are quite resistant to low concentrations (10 μg) of most of the common antibiotics; most *Seliberia* and *Seliberia*-like strains are inhibited by ampicillin, penicillin G, vancomycin, chlortetracycline, streptomycin and rifampin at concentrations of 100 μg/ml.

The habitats of *Seliberia* include soil and freshwater environments. Although they appear to be widely distributed, they have not received much attention from bacteriologists. Seliberias are well-suited to conditions of limited nutritional resources and are considered to be oligotrophic (Aristovskaya and Parinkina, 1963).

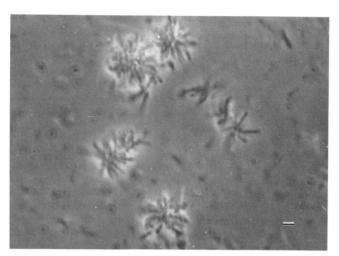

Figure 21.76. Phase-contrast light micrograph of *S. stellata* rosettes. *Bar,* 1 μm. (Courtesy of J. R. Swafford.)

Enrichment and Isolation Procedures

Specific enrichment procedures for podzol-inhabiting seliberias have not been described, although it has been noted (Aristovskaya and Parinkina, 1963) that these bacteria occur frequently in pedoscopes. Seliberias of both aquatic and soil origin can be enriched, nonspecifically, by oligotrophic conditions (Schmidt and Swafford, 1979, 1981). Glass beakers, to which water samples (e.g. 200–800 ml of pond, lake, or even tap water) are added, with or without addition of 0.001–0.005% peptone (Difco), are covered with plastic film to prevent evaporation and incubated for several days to several weeks or months at 24–26°C. To adapt the aquatic enrichment technique to soil inocula, suspensions of 1 g (or less) of soil are made in 500 ml of filtered pond or tap water, to which either no nutrients or very low concentrations of peptone are added.

The seliberias usually occur at the air-water interface of the enrichment (in the surface pellicle, if heavy growth has occurred). They will be easier to isolate, subsequently, if heavy growth of other, more rapidly growing bacteria has not occurred in the enrichment beaker; hence, the use of several beakers with varying concentrations of added nutrients may facilitate the enrichment procedure. Observation of the bacteria at the surfaces of the enrichments, by using transmission electron microscopy and negative stains (Schmidt and Starr, 1981), is useful for determining whether significant numbers of seliberias are present.

To obtain pure cultures of seliberias, several types of solid culture media have been employed. To isolate seliberias from soil samples, agar media containing dilute organomineral complexes (ulmic or humic acids or fulvic acid) obtained from soil humus (Aristovskaya and Parinkina, 1961, 1963) have been used successfully. Soil samples thought to contain seliberias are streaked on the ulmic or fulvic acid agar media; after 4–7 days, the slow-growing colonies that show some browning (due to accumulation of iron oxide) are examined for characteristic morphological features. The accumulation of ferric hydroxide by seliberias of soil origin is characteristic of their behavior in mixed culture; in pure culture, an atmosphere of about 1% CO_2 stimulates deposition of iron oxide (Aristovskaya and Parinkina, 1963).

Seliberia-like bacteria of aquatic or soil origin may be isolated (from enrichment cultures) by streaking from the liquid enrichment surface onto a dilute organic medium, such as the PYE medium or dilute medium I.* After 2–3 weeks of incubation at 25°C, the plates are examined with a dissecting microscope for minute (0.5–1.0 mm in diameter) white colonies. Colonies of *Seliberia*-like bacteria of aquatic origin usually adhere very strongly to the agar. The selected colonies are transferred onto patch plates and, after additional incubation for several days, are observed by phase-contrast light microscopy to screen for rosette-forming, asymmetrically dividing, rod-shaped bacteria which have a motile stage. Transmission electron microscopy, with negative stains used, should be done to check for the helically sculptured topography of the rods, a characteristic of the seliberias (Schmidt and Swafford, 1981).

Maintenance Procedures

Stock cultures grown aerobically on slants of PYE medium in screw-capped test tubes remain viable for several weeks at room temperatures (24–26°C). The slant cultures survive several weeks longer at 4°C. Suspensions of cells scraped (with some difficulty) from agar surfaces and suspended in sterile distilled water also survive well for several weeks at room temperature. For longer term preservation (several years), lyophilization is a satisfactory method.

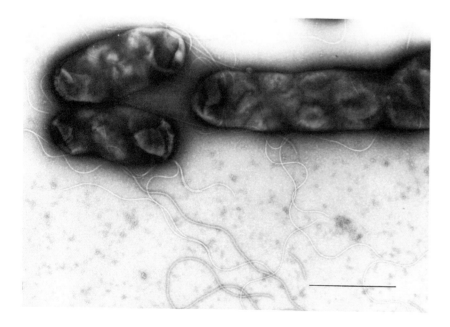

Figure 21.77. Two types of flagella—ensheathed and thinner, ordinary (i.e. not ensheathed)—of *S. stellata* strain Z/A grown on PYE agar. Negative contrast, 0.5% potassium phosphotungstate. *Bar,* 1 μm. (Courtesy of J. R. Swafford.)

*PYE medium: 0.2% peptone (Difco), 0.1% yeast extract, 1.0% Hutner's vitamin-free mineral base (Cohen-Bazire et al., 1957), 1.2 or 1.5% Bacto agar (Difco), and distilled water. *Dilute medium I:* 0.02% peptone, 0.01% yeast extract, 1.0% Hutner's mineral base, 1.2 or 1.5% agar (Difco), and distilled water (the addition of 0.1% (filter-sterilized) glucose is optional) (Schmidt and Swafford, 1981).

Figure 21.78. *Seliberia*-like aquatic strain ICPB 4133 from a liquid PYE culture, illustrating furrowed topography and an asymmetric plane of division. Negative contrast, 0.5% potassium phosphotungstate. *Bar*, 1 μm. (Courtesy of J. R. Swafford.)

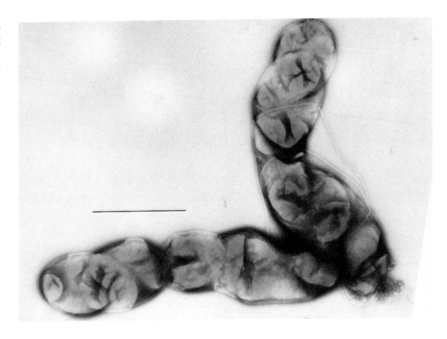

Differentiation of the genus **Seliberia** *from other genera*

The most obvious features of the genus *Seliberia* are a collection of morphological, developmental and ultrastructural characteristics. However, in making use of the more readily observable of these characteristics at the resolution achievable with the light microscope, seliberias can be confused with various other rosette-forming bacteria including certain members of the genera *Agrobacterium, Pseudomonas* and caulobacters (*Caulobacter* or *Asticcacaulis*) (Table 21.28). In addition to formation of multicellular rosettes (starlike aggregates of several to many cells), other features these various bacteria may have in common include: their occurrence in the same types of natural habitats and preference for aerobic environments, similarities in cell size and apparent rodlike shape, and presence of shorter motile and longer sessile rods. It should be noted that the seliberias (at least those which have been characterized, to date) are not prosthecate, whereas the mature *Caulobacter* and *Asticcacaulis* cells ordinarily have at least one prostheca or cellular stalk (Poindexter, 1964, 1981).

To approach confirmation that an isolate belongs to the genus *Seliberia*, it is usually necessary to make some ultrastructural observations in order to discern the presence of the furrowed screwlike cell surface of the seliberias and the thick, sheathed subpolar flagellum of *Seliberia* swarmers. Transmission electron microscopic preparative techniques (such as negative contrast, with 0.5–1.0% sodium or potassium phosphotungstate used, or shadowing with a heavy metal) provide sufficient contrast and resolution to distinguish between seliberias and other bacteria, such as caulobacters. A critical-point drying technique to prepare bacterial specimens has also been used, in conjunction with either scanning or transmission electron microscopy, to demonstrate the screwlike furrowing of the surface of seliberias (Schmidt and Swafford, 1979; Swafford, 1980). The screwlike cell topography should be present in the majority of bacteria in the population if the strain is representative of this genus.

Use of morphological characteristics as the sole guide to generic assignment is not a desirable situation. Information on the physiology, relationship to oxygen, mol% G + C of DNA, and mode of growth and division are necessary to confirm membership in the genus *Seliberia*. Since the seliberias characteristically exhibit unidirectional polar growth and their swarmers are generated at the end of the dividing cell (Schmidt and Starr, 1984), this unusual mode of cell division may be particularly useful in defining members of the genus.

Taxonomic Comments

To determine the phylogenetic relationships of the genus *Seliberia* to other genera or higher taxa, future studies on its nucleic acids (such as rRNA oligonucleotide sequencing) are desirable. At the species level, it will be necessary to provide information on nucleic acid homologies among the type species, *S. stellata,* and the available *Seliberia*-like aquatic and soil strains (see "Other Organisms") to determine whether establishment of any additional species might be warranted. It will be of interest to include *Pseudomonas* (formerly *Seliberia*) *carboxydohydrogena* (Meyer et al., 1980) in such comparative studies of the nucleic acids, along with selected members of other genera, such as *Pseudomonas, Caulobacter, Agrobacterium* and *Rhizobium,* since the nearest taxonomic neighbors of the genus *Seliberia* have not yet been located.

Table 21.28.

Differential morphological and developmental characteristics of the genus **Seliberia**[a] *and other biochemically and morphologically similar taxa*[b]

Characteristic	*Seliberia*	*Caulobacter*	*Pseudomonas*	*Agrobacterium*
Unidirectional polar cell growth	+	−	−	−
Asymmetric division products	+	+	−	−
Ensheathed polar or subpolar flagellum	+	−	D	−
Prostheca production	−	+	−	−
Helically sculptured cell surface	+	−	−[c]	−
Stellate aggregate (rosette) formation	+	+	D	D
Mol% G + C of DNA	63–66	62–67[d]	58–70[e]	58–62

[a] *S. stellata* and the aquatic and soil *Seliberia*-like strains.

[b] Symbols: +, 90% or more of strains are positive; −, 90% or more of strains are negative; and D, different reactions occur in different species.

[c] Data are from Meyer et al., 1980.

[d] Data are from Poindexter, 1981.

[e] Data are from Bergan, 1981.

Acknowledgments

We thank George A. Zavarzin, Institute of Microbiology, Academy of Sciences of the U.S.S.R., Moscow, for the culture of *S. stellata* Aristovskaya strain Z/A (ICPB 4130) (culture history: Aristovskaya → Nikitin → Zavarzin → Starr → Schmidt). DNA base compositions were determined by Manley Mandel. Micrographs were kindly supplied by James R. Swafford. Some of the data on the characterization of the aquatic *Seliberia*-like strains was obtained in collaboration with Suzanne V. Kelly.

Further Reading

Aristovskaya, T.V. 1974. Genus *Seliberia* Aristovskaya and Parinkina. *In* Buchanan and Gibbons (Editors), Bergey's Manual of Determinative Bacteriology, 8th ed. The Williams and Wilkins Co., Baltimore, p. 160.

Aristovskaya, T.V. and V.V. Parinkina. 1963. New soil microorganism *Seliberia stellata* n. gen. n. sp. Izv. Akad. Nauk S.S.S.R. Ser. Biol. *28:* 49–56.

Schmidt, J.M. and J.R. Swafford. 1979. Isolation and morphology of helically sculptured, rosette-forming, freshwater bacteria resembling *Seliberia.* Curr. Microbiol. *3:* 65–70.

Schmidt, J.M. and J.R. Swafford. 1981. The genus *Seliberia. In* Starr, Stolp, Trüper, Balows and Schlegel (Editors), The Prokaryotes. A Handbook on Habitats, Isolation, and Identification of Bacteria. Springer-Verlag, Berlin, pp. 516–519.

List of species of the genus Seliberia

There is presently only one validly published species.

1. **Seliberia stellata** Aristovskaya and Parinkina 1963, 55.[AL]

stel.la′ta. L. adj. *stellata* starred.

Colonies on peptone-yeast extract agar (PYE medium, see "Enrichment and Isolation Procedures" and "Maintenance Procedures") are smooth, convex and white. The diameter is 0.5–1.5 mm, with a regular border. On ulmic acid agar, a soil extract medium (Aristovskaya and Parinkina 1961, 1963), growth is sparse, and colonies are <1.0 mm in diameter and light brown. *S. stellata* strain Z/A grows in a chemically defined medium containing an appropriate carbon source (Table 21.29), 0.05% NH_4Cl, 1.0% Hutner's vitamin-free mineral base (Cohen-Bazire et al., 1957), and 0.001% phosphate. It grows over a wide pH range, from 4.5 through at least 9.0. No added vitamins are required.

S. stellata is positive for urease production and starch hydrolysis; it can produce H_2S from cystine; it can reduce nitrate to nitrite under either aerobic or anaerobic conditions; it is unable to liquefy gelatin, utilize citrate, hydrolyze casein, or produce indole, and it gives negative methyl red and Voges-Proskauer reactions.

S. stellata strain Z/A can produce both a subpolar, ensheathed, typically single flagellum and several lateral, ordinary (i.e. not ensheathed) flagella (Fig. 21.77). This flagellar development is characteristic of its swarmer cells grown on agar-solidified PYE medium at 25°C.

The mol% G + C of the DNA is 66 (Bd).

Type strain: ICPB 4130.

Table 21.29.

Carbon source utilization by **Seliberia stellata** *and* **Pseudomonas carboxydohydrogena**

Utilized as sole carbon source by *Seliberia stallata*[a]		
Arabinose	Glucose	Fumaric acid
Ribose	Maltose	Alanine
Xylose	Lactose	Arginine
Rhamnose	Mannose	Leucine
Trehalose	Cellibiose	Threonine
Fucose	Dextrin	Valine

Utilized as sole carbon source by *Pseudomonas carboxydohydrogena*[b]		
Acetate	Fumarate	Malate
Aspartate	Lactate	Succinate
Citrate	Pyruvate	

[a]Data are from S. V. Kelly, J. M. Schmidt and M. P. Starr, manuscript in preparation.

[b]Data are from Meyer et al., 1980; and from S. V. Kelly, J. M. Schmidt and M. P. Starr, manuscript in preparation.

Other organisms possibly related to Seliberia

A carbon monoxide-utilizing bacterium, originally named *Seliberia carboxydohydrogena* (Sanzhieva and Zavarzin, 1971) was reexamined by Meyer et al. (1980), who observed that <3.5% of the cells in autotrophically grown populations had a furrowed or helically sculptured surface. On the basis of its physiological traits, as well as the relatively weak support for close morphological similarity to the genus *Seliberia*, it was proposed that this bacterium be named *Pseudomonas carboxydohydrogena* Meyer, Lalucat and Schlegel 1980, 194 (also Palleroni 1984, 191).

Several *Seliberia*-like strains from aquatic (freshwater) sources and a few from soil have been enriched and isolated in pure culture, but these are not yet named. Ten strains have been characterized in some detail. A typical aquatic *Seliberia*-like strain (ICPB 4133) is shown in Figure 21.78. Their description is as for the genus, with the following additional characteristics: The aquatic *Seliberia*-like strains are unable to use any of 60 tested compounds as their sole carbon source; they appear to have complex growth factor requirements. They can be grown on the minimal medium described for *S. stellata* supplemented with 0.001% vitamin assay casamino acids (Difco) and 0.1% (v/v) Staley's vitamin solution (Staley, 1968). They grow dependably but sparsely on PYE medium (see "Enrichment and Isolation Procedures") (Schmidt and Swafford, 1981).

Growth of aquatic *Seliberia*-like strains is very sparse on all complex media so far tested. Grown on PYE agar, colonies are white, minute (0.5–1.0 mm in diameter) and very adherent to the agar medium surface. Growth in liquid PYE medium is granular and definitely not well dispersed, with a strong tendency for attachment to the submerged surfaces of glass culture vessels, so long as a shallow (about 1 cm deep) rather than deeper level of liquid medium is maintained. (The growth of *S. stellata* strain Z/A under similar conditions is well dispersed, with some rosettes visible microscopically but with no macroscopic granules present.) The aquatic *Seliberia*-like strains demonstrate an obligate requirement for oxygen, and they reduce nitrate under aerobic conditions but not anaerobically. They do not produce H_2S from cystine. Most of the aquatic *Seliberia*-like strains can hydrolyze urea, and all can hydrolyze starch.

All of the aquatic strains produce swarmers with a subpolar ensheathed flagellum, but only a few strains have been found to produce the lateral, ordinary (i.e. not ensheathed) flagella. Two of the aquatic strains, which have been examined with indirect immunoferritin surface labeling during growth, were found to exhibit unidirectional polar cell surface growth, with production of swarmers having de novo synthesized surface antigens. *S. stellata* exhibited the same kind of unusual growth and division pattern in such experiments (Schmidt and Starr, 1984). Nine of 10 aquatic *Seliberia*-like strains cross-react moderately to strongly with *S. stellata* strain Z/A in serological tests (tube agglutination and indirect immunofluorescence tests).

The mol% G + C of the DNA of the aquatic *Seliberia*-like strains is 63–65 (Bd).

Another bacterium with remarkable surface sculpturing is an unnamed bacterium with "screwlike" or "coiled rod" morphology, which is an epiphyte of the cyanophyte *Nodularia spumigenia* (Šmarda, 1985). Evidence suggesting a taxonomic relationship between *Seliberia* and this bacterium at present is either lacking or to the contrary.

Genus "**Metallogenium**" *Perfil'ev and Gabe 1961, 50*

G. A. Zavarzin

Me.tal.lo.ge′ni.um. Gr. n. *metallos* metal; Gr. v. suff. *genium* producing; M.L. neut. n. *Metallogenium* metal-producing.

Cells coccoid, 0.2–1.5 µm in diameter, usually in clusters, **sprouting with tapering filaments 0.2–0.02 µm in diameter** and 1–10 µm in length, **heavily encrusted by manganese dioxide.** A complicated life cycle includes cocci and cocci with tapering filaments radiating from the center and encrustated by oxides. The stage with radiating filaments is referred to as a trichosphere, microcolony, or coenobium. In this stage, *"Metallogenium"* is easily recognizable and identified by its peculiar morphology. **Oxidizes manganous compounds.** Multiplication is by a budding process. Cocci may also be found at the ends of the filaments, giving rise to daughter microcolonies around the periphery of the mother coenobium, much like the growth that occurs with strawberry plants. New coenobia are usually formed from one or several cocci sprouting by a straight filaments in liquid and irregularly bent ones in viscous media. Spherical buds are supposed to be motile, but the type of locomotion remains unknown. Aerobic. **Chemoorganotrophic or parasitic on mycelial fungi.** Optimum temperature: 28°C. Optimum pH: 6.8–7.2.

Widely distributed in plankton of freshwater lakes and in the bottom deposits where it is recognized as a causative agent of ore formation, in swamps, in soils, on decaying leaves and in desert varnish. It has not yet been reported in the marine environment. Structures indistinguishable from *"Metallogenium"* are recorded as microfossils from rocks more than 2 giga years old under the name of *Eoastrion* Barghoorn and Tyler 1967.

Type species: *"Metallogenium personatum"* Perfil'ev and Gabe 1961, 50.

Further Descriptive Information

The nature of *"Metallogenium"* remains a subject of much controversy. *"Metallogenium"* is the only representative of the group of metal oxide-accumulating microorganisms which has been cultivated in the laboratory. To this group belong *"Caulococcus"* and *"Kusnezovia."* These two genera have never been reported since their description (Perfil'ev and Gabe, 1961). *"Siderococcus"* resembles the coccoid stage of *"Metallogenium"* and was reported from the same environment. The name *"Metallogenium"* had been proposed by Perfil'ev at the Seventh International Geological Congress in 1937, but its description was published only in 1961 (Perfil'ev and Gabe, 1961) and was based on the observations of microcultures in rectangular capillary tubes. Its complicated life cycle begins with unicellular motile flagellated cocci 0.7–1.5 µm wide. The cell attaches to a solid surface and sprouts by a single or a few filaments which come to be encrusted by manganic oxides, forming a tapering sheath, which resembles *"Leptothrix echinata."* This stage, named by Perfil'ev "trichospheric," is usually referred to as a *"Metallogenium"* microcolony and is the only form by which *"Metallogenium"* can be easily identified. Perfil'ev observed budding on filaments and supposed it to be the mode of multiplication of *"Metallogenium"* similar to that of hyphomicrobia. In the next stage, microcolonies of *"Metallogenium"* become lobate and then indistinguishable. This cycle is illustrated in Figure 21.79. Zavarzin (1961, 1964a) isolated *"Metallogenium"* in a binary culture with a fungus (*Mycelium sterilium*) and observed its development in cultures and in slide microcultures. Under such conditions it was easy to observe the unicellular stage, which appears in the liquid medium as glistening cocci of various dimensions all over the column of broth, while the mycelium remains on the bottom. Flagella were never observed. The cocci sprout by thin filaments, which come to be covered with manganese dioxide, then make clusters and settle down as trichospheres. No cellular structures except for a very thin thread (not prostheca!) in the core of the manganese sheath were observed (Zavarzin, 1964a). The fungus could be cultivated in organic media with no indication of *"Metallogenium,"* but *"Metallogenium"* developed immediately when the same medium was supplemented with manganese (Epikhina and Zavarzin, 1963).

Dubinina (1969, 1984) and Balashova (1974) regarded *"Metallo-*

genium" as a free-living mycoplasma. Mycoplasma was isolated from a binary culture of *"Metallogenium"* and fungus. Typical "fried-egg" microcolonies developed in diluted mycoplasma medium. When supplied with manganous salts, mycoplasma formed a sheath of manganic oxides (Fig. 21.80). The same is true for *Acholeplasma laidlawii* in the presence of ferrous iron (Balashova and Zavarzin, 1972).

"Metallogenium" is reported to be capable of infecting and parasitizing various eucaryotic and procaryotic microorganisms (Dubinina, 1984). The fungi *Phoma alternaroides, Penicillium chrysogenum* and *Alternaria cuscutaci,* the yeast *Rhodotorula peneaus,* and bacteria *Bacillus megaterium* and *B. circulans* were infected by the coccoid stage of *"Metallogenium."* The infection is accompanied by (a) acquisition by the binary culture of a persistent capacity to oxidize manganese, (b) evolution of the characteristic filiform structures of *"Metallogenium"* and (c) inhibition of the growth of the inoculated cultures (inhibition manifests itself by fungi losing their capacity for spore formation, the upsetting of cell division processes, and lysis of the cells in the infected cultures). If the culture remained viable, the ability of binary cultures to oxidize manganese persisted over a period of several years.

This interpretation is challenged by investigators of *"Metallogenium"* who regard it as a nonliving structure either without further specification of its origin or as a phenomenon caused by the activity of microorganisms in manganese-containing media (Nealson, 1983). This interpretation is based on: (a) the inability to demonstrate cellular structures in thin sections of microcolonies of *"Metallogenium"* collected in natural habitats (Klaveness, 1977; Gregory et al., 1980; Czekalla et al., 1985), (b) a failure to cultivate *"Metallogenium"* (Gregory et al., 1980; Margulis et al., 1983), (c) the absence of any evidence of the chemical composition of biopolymers of *"Metallogenium,"* and (d) the formation of manganic oxides by autocatalytic processes. The *"Metallogenium"* phenomenon is explained as follows: The formation of a trichosphere might be initiated by the deposition of manganese oxides on the radiating fimbriae of an unknown bacterium (Gregory et al., 1980). The cell leaves through a hole shortly before it is completely closed. The cell divides outside the capsule, and the daughter cells again attach themselves (Czekalla et al., 1985). Such empty spaces or holes are well known in the iron and manganese oxidizers from the *Siderocapsaceae* group. Evidently, further work is needed for a better understanding of the *"Metallogenium"* phenomenon.

The ecology of *"Metallogenium"* has been extensively studied. Direct microscopic observations were used for counting in freshwater bodies where this organism causes blooms (for review, see Gorlenko et al., 1983) and develops in the bottom deposits (Perfil'ev and Gabe, 1961, 1964). In soils, it was observed by Aristovskaya (1965). A review of *"Metallogenium"* in the ancient environment is given by Awramik and Barghoorn (1977) and by Crerar et al. (1980).

"Metallogenium" was isolated from podzolic soils, chernozem, crust-chestnut solonetz on loams and chocolate clays, krasnozem on banded clays, and mountain-forest brown soils on granite (Aristovskaya and Zavarzin, 1971; Bolotina and Mirchink, 1975). *"Metallogenium"* is abundant in actively decomposing layers of leaf litter where it oxidizes the manganese washed out through the exodermis of plants (Bolotina and Mirchink, 1975). Leaching of manganese in binary cultures of *"Metallogenium"* and fungus was observed with rhodonite, olivine, hornblende, biotite, magnetite and pyrolusite.

Enrichment and Isolation Procedures

Due to the color of manganic oxides, the structures of *"Metallogenium"* are readily visible with brightfield light microscopy.

The following media are used for enrichment and maintenance of the binary culture of *"Metallogenium"* and fungi (Zavarzin, 1961): solid medium I (tap water, 1000 ml; agar, 15 g; and manganese acetate, 100 mg;

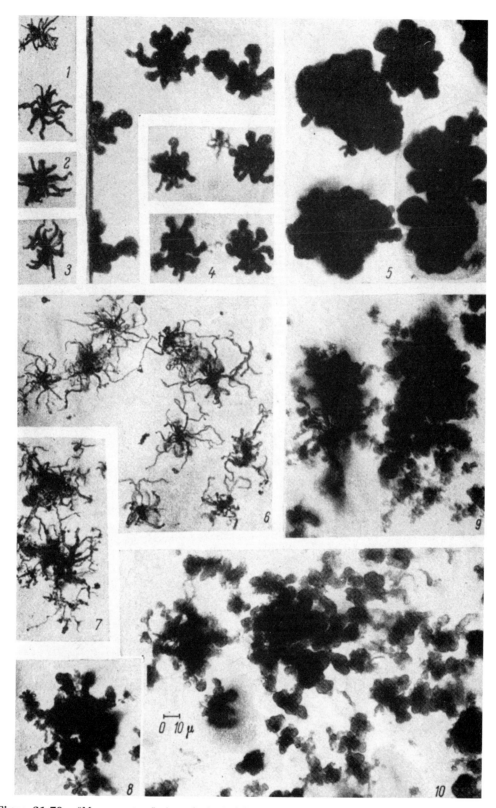

Figure 21.79. *"M. personatum"* microcolonies in different stages of manganese encrustation. Brightfield light microscopy. *1–3,* beginning of encrustation of trichosphaeric microcolonies; *4,* lobate microcolony; *5,* tuberculate microcolony; and *6–10,* stages of encrustation. *Bar,* 10 μm. (After Perfil'ev and Gabe, 1964.)

with autoclaving at 120°C for 20 min); and liquid medium II (starch, hydrolyzed by HCl from 20 to 1 g; manganese carbonate or powdered rhodochrosite, 0.5 g; and distilled water, 1000 ml). Incubation for 3–10 days at room temperatures is employed. The fungal growth should be maintained in subculturing. The binary culture has been stable for 26 years now.

For pure culture isolation (Dubinina, 1984) a medium for mycoplasma is used (hydrolyzed starch, 1 g; fresh acid yeast extract, 1 vol%; Difco PPLO broth, 10 vol%; catalase, 5 mg; horse serum, 1 ml; palmitic acid, 5 mg; and distilled water to 1000 ml (pH 7.2)). The use of freshly prepared medium is a prerequisite for *"Metallogenium"* growth. Even then, growth is not stable, and pure cultures usually die after 3–5 passages. Cocci are isolated by filtration through a 0.2-µm filter, centrifuged at $12,000 \times g$ for 15 min, and resuspended in 1 ml of freshly prepared medium. This suspension is inoculated with a minimal amount of a microorganism to be infected by *"Metallogenium."* An easier procedure is recommended by Balashova: The binary culture of *"Metallogenium"* and fungus is inoculated into 1.5% agar with 0.01% manganese acetate at 40°C, then overlayered by 0.5% starch. After incubation for 2 days, the coccoid stage from the liquid is inoculated into the medium (0.5% starch; 0.1% Difco horse serum; 0.1% yeast extract; and 0.5% $MnCO_3$). Subcultures are maintained in the same medium supplemented with penicillin and thallium acetate.

Differentiation of the genus "Metallogenium" from other genera

The genus *"Metallogenium"* is differentiated from other genera of manganese oxidizers on the basis of its morphology. From *"Leptothrix echinata"* and other organisms forming stellar microcolonies encrusted by oxides, it is differentiated by the cellular dimensions and the absence of chains of bacterial cells inside the filaments. It is differentiated from the genus *"Caulococcus"* by the shape of its microcolonies; however, this differentiation is arbitrary, and *"Caulococcus"* might also be a form of *"Metallogenium."* *"Kusnezovia"* is easily differentiated because of the peculiar structure of its coenobia. Cocci of *"Siderococcus"* with short "tails" closely resemble cocci of *"Metallogenium"* but are completely covered with ferric oxides.

Taxonomic Comments

"Metallogenium" represents a phenomenon with wide distribution in aquatic environments in both recent and ancient habitats. Its nature is, however, a subject of controversy. According to one group, it is a nonliving structure, possibly produced by microorganisms. Another group supposes it to be a free-living mycoplasma able to parasitize a variety of microorganisms.

Differentiation of the species of the genus "Metallogenium"

Differentiation of the species in the genus *"Metallogenium"* is arbitrary and might be caused by different methods of observation in the absence of the type culture of *"Metallogenium personatum."*

List of species of the genus "Metallogenium"

1. **"Metallogenium personatum"** Perfil'ev and Gabe 1961, 50.

per.so.na′tum. M.L. neut. adj. *personatum* masked, referring to coating by manganese oxides.

Polymorphic microorganism accumulating manganese and, to some extent, iron, minute coccoid microbe (about 0.5 µm) with a complicated life cycle which includes a unicellular stage of a motile flagellated microgonidium (about 0.8 µm) and various nonmotile microcolonies, usually sessile but sometimes planktonic. A single cell settles, multiplies and sprouts into a trichospheric microcolony formed by radial tapering filaments which are dark brown due to manganic oxides. Radial filaments after dissolution of oxides contain chains of cocci connected by thin filaments or thin filaments only with the reproductive cells on the ends. In the next stage, depending on the environment, microcolonies are zoogloeal, either lobate, amorphous, or reticulate (Fig. 21.79).

Motile coccoid cells are formed at all stages of development. Habitat: in the upper layer of bottom deposits, always close to the reductive horizon in freshwater lakes containing manganese. No culture available.

Type strain: represented by herbarium specimen All-Union Collection of Microorganisms VKM 1341.

2. **"Metallogenium symbioticum"** Zavarzin, 1961, 395.

sym.bi.ot′i.cum. M.L. neut. adj. *symbioticum* living together.
Description is the same as that of the genus. In contradistinction to *M. personatum*, cells within filaments were never observed. The core of the filament is represented by a very thin thread ("araia") 0.02 µm in diameter. The tapering envelope of this thread is formed by manganese dioxide identified as the mineral vernadite. Buds on the tips of filaments and flagellated cocci are never observed.

Multiplication is by coccoid cells (Fig. 21.81) which sprout into tapering filaments. The formation of filaments correlates with the beginning of manganese oxidation. Coccoid cells lack the cell wall and are surrounded by the cytoplasmic membrane (Fig. 21.71). They can be maintained in mycoplasma media forming typical "fried-egg" microcolonies. Parasitic for various eucaryotic and procaryotic microorganisms. Infected cultures acquire the ability to oxidize manganous compounds. Sporulation in infected fungi is suppressed, and partial lysis occurs. Pure cultures of *"M. symbioticum"* in the mycoplasma medium supplemented with $MnCO_3$ produce the typical cocci encrusted with manganese dioxide. In binary cultures, trichospheric microcolonies with irregularly bent, tapering filaments are formed.

Mesophilic, aerobic, chemoorganotrophic or parasitic. Optimal pH: 6.8–7.2. Rapidly oxidizes manganous compounds to manganic oxides. The oxidation has been ascribed to the destruction of peroxides formed during the respiratory process (Zavarzin, 1972).

Type culture: maintained by serial transfer in binary culture with a fungus in All-Union Collection of Microorganisms VKM 457.

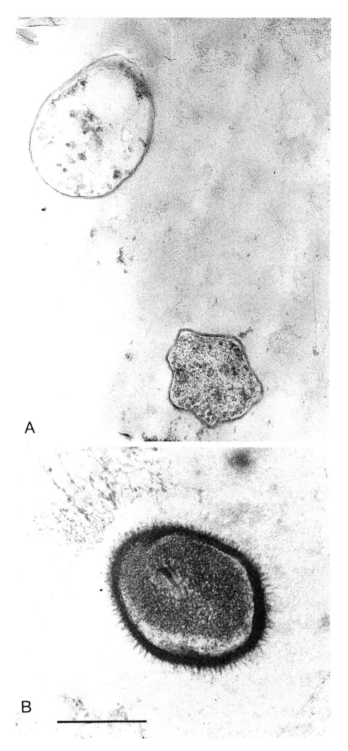

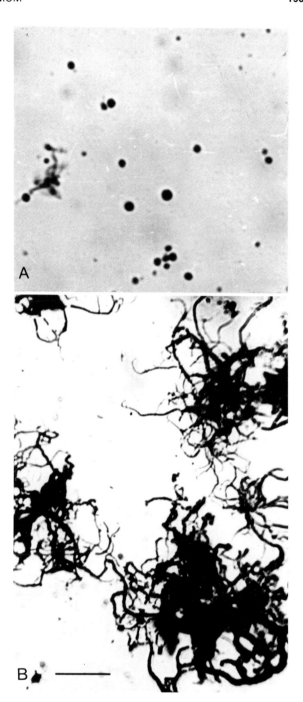

Figure 21.80. Pure culture of *"M. symbioticum"* in the medium for mycoplasma. Electron microscopy. *Bar,* 0.5 μm. *A,* thin section of *"M. symbioticum"* without manganese. Note the absence of the cell wall. *B,* *"M. symbioticum"* from the medium with manganese. Note thick layer of manganese dioxide in place of cell wall. (Courtesy of V. V. Balashova.)

Figure 21.81. *"M. symbioticum"* in the binary culture with the fungus. Brightfield light microscopy. *A,* coccoid cells in the very beginning of encrustation. *B,* filamentous stage of growth. *Bar,* 2 μm.

Genus **"Thiodendron"** *Perfil'ev and Gabe 1961, 162*

P. HIRSCH

(Not *Thiodendron* Lackey and Lackey 1961, 39)

Thi.o.den′dron. Gr. n. *thium* sulfur; Gr. n. *dendron* a tree; M.L. n. *Thiodendron* sulfur tree.

Vibrio-shaped cells spirally twisted and with both ends somewhat tapered, $0.4-1.0 \times 3-11$ μm; **bear thin threads ("stalks"** with a diameter of $0.15-0.25$ μm) on either one or both cell poles. The **stalks may be prosthecae;** they are straight or more or less flexuous, often are of considerable length, and occasionally appear to be branched dichotomously; they are arranged radially from a common center. The vibrio-shaped cells **may be motile** with flagella. Budding of the thin threads has been mentioned (Schmidt, 1981b); coccoid buds appear to grow out into Vibrio-shaped cells which then develop stalks.

Colonies concentrically layered, sometimes globular and grayish to bluish white with alternating lighter and darker zonation. The appearance is similar to that of thalli of the alga *Padina pavonia.* The layering is assumed to reflect rhythmical external **deposition of granular or colloidal sulfur** as a result of H_2S oxidation, but S^0 deposition is not always observed. In the water of natural sulfur springs, colonies may grow to a size of 4 cm in 3–4 days.

Gram reaction not recorded. This organism is presumably aerobic to microaerophilic. H_2S is required for growth. This organism was originally isolated in pure culture from a sulfur spring near Chokrakskoye in Russia. Also observed in peat mud, sand, or various freshwater samples.

Type species: *"Thiodendron latens"* Perfil'ev and Gabe 1961, 162.

Further Descriptive Information

The original description does not contain information on the mode of multiplication. Presumably the cells divided by binary fission, and a new "stalk" was grown between the daughter cells, thereby separating these. In this way, short chains of alternating cells and "stalks" arose. Budding as a mode of new cell formation has been mentioned by Schmidt (1981b).

Colonies of bacteria resembling the type species *"T. latens"* have been observed by Dr. P. Hippe, Göttingen (personal communication) on the walls of a vessel containing a mud and water sample from a pond, after storage in the laboratory for several months (Figs. 21.82 and 21.83). Growth on solid media was not possible, however. *"Thiodendron"* has also been observed in enrichments of groundwater bacteria (P. Hirsch, unpublished observations) and in samples and enrichments from the Solar Lake near Elat (Sinai; Hirsch, 1980). In the latter case, the *"Thiodendron"* cells came from depths of 0.1–1.0 m and were grown aerobically at 17–24°C.

Enrichment Procedures

Originally, *"Thiodendron"* was cultivated in continuously flowing, ultrafiltered sulfur spring water in an O_2/H_2S gradient (Perfil'ev and Gabe, 1961). Later, Perfil'ev (1969) cultivated *"Thiodendron"* from mud by adding 60% (v/v) potato extract. In the continuous flow chamber, the colonies reached a size of 4 cm within 3–4 days.

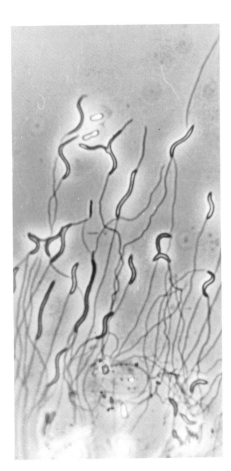

Figure 21.82 *"Thiodendron"* species observed in mud and water sample from a pond. Stalks are ~0.2 μm in diameter. (Courtesy of Dr. Hans Hippe.)

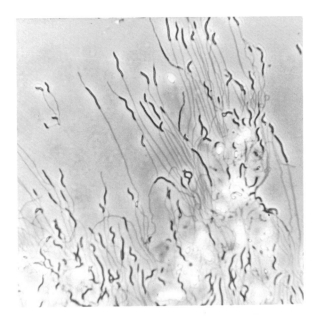

Figure 21.83. *"Thiodendron"* species observed in mud and water sample from a pond. Stalks are ~0.2 μm in diameter. (Courtesy of Dr. Hans Hippe.)

Differentiation of the genus "**Thiodendron**" from other closely related genera

A certain morphological similarity exists to other stalked bacteria. Unfortunately, it cannot as yet be clarified whether the observed appendages are secreted stalks or prosthecae. Since external sulfur deposits have not always been observed, "*T. latens*" could be related to *Prosthecobacter* species which usually have rather short prosthecae. Bipolar outgrowth of the appendages separates "*Thiodendron*" from *Asticcacaulis* species or *Planctomyces* species. The mode of attachment clearly differentiates "*Thiodendron*" from *Hyphomicrobium* and *Asticcacaulis* species. This genus is not clearly differentiated from *Caulobacter* species by the bipolar outgrowth of stalks, since aging *Caulobacter* cultures may show this property also (de Bont et al., 1970).

Taxonomic Comments

The organism described by Lackey and Lackey (1961) is clearly different from "*T. latens*," inasmuch as it lacks the stalks and, instead, grows embedded in a branching mucus tube.

Acknowledgments

Studies of Solar Lake and groundwater microorganisms were supported by grants from the Deutsche Forschungsgemeinschaft. Prof. M. Shilo, Jerusalem, provided laboratory space and many helpful discussions during the Solar Lake work.

List of species of the genus "**Thiodendron**"

1. "**Thiodendron latens**" Perfil'ev and Gabe 1961, 162.
la'tens. L. part. adj. *latens* concealed, hidden.

Description is the same as that of the genus. A pure culture does not exist.

2. SPINATE BACTERIA

K. B. Easterbrook

Spinate bacteria are so named because they characteristically produce pericellular nonprosthecate appendages termed spinae (Easterbrook and Coombs, 1976). These hollow structures are constructed of a helically wound (beta sheet) protein fibril cross-linked between successive turns (Coombs et al., 1976, 1978). Although this term was introduced to describe the appendage of a particular bacterium, "marine pseudomonad D71" (McGregor-Shaw et al., 1973; Easterbrook et al., 1973), a number of tubular appendages have been described on different bacteria. Such appendages may vary in length and, to a lesser extent, in diameter and may have dissimilar forms, but all appear similar in design and may accordingly be considered variants of a general class of nonprosthecate appendage distinct from flagella and pili. Spinae, as a class, might then include cylindric, cylindric with coniform base, and conic noncellular appendages (Easterbrook and Subba Rao, 1984).

At least in the two cases analyzed ("marine pseudomonad D71" and "*Agrobacterium* variant E59"), spina genes are concluded to be chromosomally borne, and the characteristics of spination and spina morphology are considered to be stable and taxonomically significant. Spinate bacteria are uniformly Gram-negative aerobes but are diverse in their metabolic activities. Current groupings of bacteria exhibiting comparable activities have a wide range of values for the mol% G + C of the DNA and are inadequately classified. Inside such groups, spinate bacteria in the future may well be found to constitute unique genera with more than (merely) spination in common. Certainly not all "*Methylocystis*" or "*Synechococcus*" species are spinate, and the characteristics of neither "marine pseudomonad D71" nor "*Agrobacterium* variant E59" conform precisely to those defining established genera.

Spinae are not then an indicator of a particular group but rather are, as the other nonprosthecate appendages, a reflection of adaptation to an ecological niche. This niche is presumably widely distributed, since spinate bacteria have been found from the arctic to the tropics (Easterbrook and Subba Rao, unpublished observations). Although a unique role has not been defined, a number of perhaps fortuitous functions—protective, inertial and interactive—have been suggested for spinae (Easterbrook and Sperker, 1983).

Spinae may be rendered visible in the light microscope by flagella staining techniques (Leifson, 1960), but visualization of their design and nonprosthecate nature requires electron microscopic techniques—negative staining and ultramicrotomy. The spinate phenotype is presumably expressed under growth conditions reflecting the ecological niche, and while "*Methylocystis*" strains are spinate in both liquid culture and on solid surfaces, other spinate bacteria may only be apparent as such when grown in liquid culture. The expression of spinae also appears controlled, to varying extents in different bacteria, by nutrient conditions and, in the case of "marine pseudomonad D71," by the environmental factors of pH, osmolarity and temperature (Easterbrook and Sperker, 1983).

The general properties of the different groups of spinate bacteria are those of the genera to which they have been provisionally allocated and appear elsewhere in this series. They are provided here in varying detail as available.

Heterotrophs

"*Marine Pseudomonad D71*" (McGregor-Shaw et al., 1973; NCMB 2018) is a Gram-negative aerobic coccobacillus or bacillus (0.7×1.5 μm) forming convex, round, unpigmented colonies with entire edges on agar. Catalase- and oxidase-positive. Chemoheterotroph utilizing a wide range of carbon compounds oxidatively (carbohydrates, organic acids and amino acids) but does not grow on C_1 compounds or produce acetic acid from alcohol. Utilizes NH_4^+, NO_3^- and amino acids but needs growth factors (niacinamide, biotin, thiamine) in defined media (Coughlin, 1980, Easterbrook and Alexander, 1983). May produce polyhydroxybutyrate. Growth requires Na^+ and occurs over a wide range of pH, temperature and salinity values but is optimal at pH 7, at 34°C and in 0.2 M NaCl. The organism produces alkali in unbuffered media with peptone as carbon and nitrogen sources. No extracellular enzymes or pigments are produced. No plasmids. The mol% G + C of the DNA is 57.7. In liquid culture, this organism may produce, depending on environmental parameters, either no appendages, a single polar flagellum (with 1.8-μm

wavelength) or an average of 12 pericellular spinae. Spination is maximal at pH > 7.5 and at 34°C but is depressed at > 0.4 Osm. The organism was isolated from rotting chondrus from Nova Scotia, Canada.

The relation between "marine pseudomonad D71" and listed *Pseudomonas* species is obscure. The structures described and illustrated by Leifson (1960) bear a striking resemblance to spinae and may well represent their first demonstration. However, spines were only observed in one enriched sample, and the bacterium actually isolated never produced spines, regardless of the medium used for growth. The relation then between the bacterium described under the name *P. spinosa* (see Vol. 1, "Family I. *Pseudomonadaceae*," p. 195) and deposited in the ATCC and the spinate organism initially observed in situ is uncertain. At any rate, the cultural characteristics described differ significantly from those of "marine pseudomonad D71"—particularly with respect to its inability to grow in 1% NaCl. Attempts in my laboratory to induce spination in the ATCC culture (14606) of *P. spinosa* by modification of the cultural conditions have failed. *P. echinoides,* despite its suggestive name, similarly does not produce spinae.

Spinate Bacteria Possibly Related to Agrobacteria

During a survey of the waters of the Baltic Sea and the Elbe River estuary, a number of bacteria with generally similar properties were isolated by Ahrens (Ahrens and Rheinheimer, 1967; Ahrens, 1968) and were originally described as new or marine strains of *Agrobacterium.* Spinate strains were described as being similar to "*Agrobacterium ferrugineum* or *stellulatum*" (Ahrens and Moll, 1971) but were subsequently considered misclassified and, in consequence, deleted from the genus in the eighth edition of the *Manual.* Maximal spination in these organisms occurred at 1% NaCl, and the degree of spination—percentage of spinate cells and spinae per cell—was greater at 20°C than at 30°C. The strain described here, provided by Dr. Rheinheimer, has a lower growth optimum than the original strain C8, and its spination appears to be less affected by growth temperature.

"*Agrobacterium variant E59*" (Moll and Ahrens, 1970) is a Gram-negative aerobic coccobacillus or bacillus (0.8×1.5 µm) forming round convex colonies with entire edges on agar, cream-colored becoming dark in the center. Catalase- and oxidase-positive. Chemoheterotroph utilizing a range of carbohydrates, organic acids and amino acids by respiratory metabolism. This organism utilizes NH_4^+ ions and amino acids but does not reduce nitrate. No H_2S production. Produces polymeric glucan (cellulose) but no slime. Growth is maximal at 20–25°C and pH 7 and does not require Na^+. No plasmids. The mol% G + C of the DNA is 53.5. Nonmotile. Produces in liquid culture an average of 12 spinae (cylindric with coniform base) which cross-react immunologically with spinae of "marine pseudomonad D71." Spination appears unaffected by environmental parameters but is better in defined medium than complex medium. This organism was isolated from the mouth of the Elbe River, Germany.

Spinate Methanotrophs

"*Methylocystis echinoides.*" (Gal'chenko et al., 1977) and "*Methylocystis*" strain IMET 10491 (Haubold, 1978) probably represent independent but identical isolates from lake mud (U.S.S.R.) and sewage (G.D.R), respectively, since electropherograms of strains were found by Gal'chenko and Nesterov (1981) to be identical.

Gram-negative aerobic mesophile. Type II internal membranes. Obligately dependent on C_1 compounds which are assimilated by the serine pathway. Utilizes NH_4^+, NO_3^- or molecular nitrogen. Convex smooth colonies are white to cream-colored, becoming pink. The mol% G + C of the DNA is 62.3 (61.1 for IMET 10491). Nonmotile. Produces numerous short cylindric spinae.

Azospirillum lipoferum (Nurmiaho-Lassila et al., 1981). A spiral structure with the design and dimensions of spinae has been observed in association with the single polar flagellum.

Miscellaneous unidentified bacteria with spinae have, in the past, been described in situ (Stefanov and Nikitin, 1965, Staley, 1968), and it is now apparent that they are a frequent occurrence in marine environments such as the coastal waters of the U.S. (Johnson and Sieburth, personal communication).

Phototrophs

"*Synechococcus*" strains (Perkins et al., 1981; Sarokin and Carpenter, 1981; Easterbrook and Subba Rao, 1984). A number of procaryotes with internal membranes have been observed in situ in coastal waters and have been isolated on phototrophic media. These have been assigned to "*Synechococcus*" group on the basis of morphological characteristics and have numerous short spinae (cylindric) which may be lost on solid surface culture. A procaryote that is possibly also a "*Synechococcus* sp." has been isolated from the Costa Rica Dome region; this carries conical appendages (spinae).

The morphology of spinate bacteria and spinae are illustrated in Figure 21.84. Spina dimensions are given in Table 21.30.

Table 21.30.
Structural characteristics of bacterial spinae

Organism	Spina type	Average no./ cell	Diameter (nm)	Length (µm)	Rib spacing (nm)
1. Heterotrophs					
A. "Marine pseudomonad D71"[a]	Cylindric (conic base)	12	42	0.5–3	11.5
"*Agrobacterium* variant E59"[b]	Cylindric (conic base)		42	0.5–4	11.9
Unidentified[c]	Cylindric (conic base)		60	0.7–1.9	8.5–9.5
Unidentified[d]	Cylindric (conic base)		65	2.7	12
B. "*Methylocystis echinoides*"[e]	Cylindric	300	40	0.3	6
"*Methylocystis*" strain IMET 10491[f]	Cylindric		70 (40)[g]		12 (8.6)[g]
2. Phototrophs					
A. "*Synechococcus*" sp.					
(a)[c]	Cylindric	30	44–65	2.7	6–9.2
(b)[h]	Cylindric		85	0.1–1	12–13
(c)[c]	Cylindric		180–230	0.15–0.35	11–13.8
(d)[i]	Cylindric		68		20
B. Unidentified[i]	Conic	30	70–75		8.5

[a] Data are from McGregor-Shaw et al. (1973).

[b] Data are from Moll and Ahrens (1970).

[c] Data are from Perkins et al. (1981).

[d] Data are from Johnson and Sieburth (personal communication, 1980).

[e] Data are from Suzina and Fikhte (1977).

[f] Data are from Haubold (1978).

[g] Measurements by Easterbrook on donated strain.

[h] Data are from Sarokin and Carpenter (1981).

[i] Data are from Easterbrook and Subba Rao (1984).

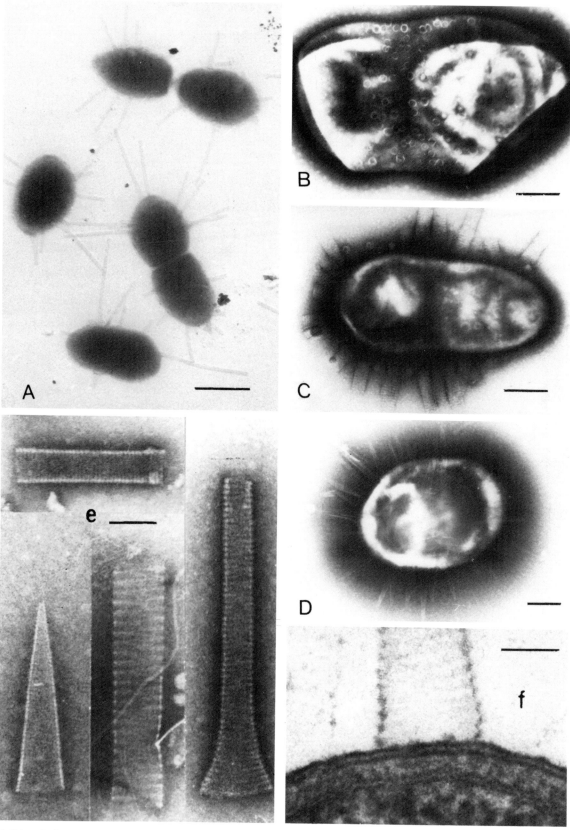

Figure 21.84. *A,* "marine pseudomonad D71." Metal (Pt/Pd)-shadowed. *Bar,* 1 μm. *B–D,* negatively stained spinate procaryotes "*Methylocystis*" IMET 10491 (*B*) and phototrophs with cylindric (*C*) and conic (*D*) spinae. *Bars,* 300 nm. *E,* isolated negatively stained spinae. *Clockwise from top:* "*methylocystis,*" "marine pseudomonad D71" and phototrophs. *Bar,* 100 nm. *F,* thin section of spina-outer membrane association. *Bar,* 50 nm. (Reproduced with permission from J. H. M. Willison, K. B. Easterbrook and R. W. Coombs, Canadian Journal of Microbiology *23:* 258–266, 1977, ©Research Council of Canada.)

Sheathed Bacteria

The sheathed bacteria grow as filaments. The cells comprising the filaments are enclosed within a tube of extracellular material referred to as a sheath. Typically, the sheath is transparent when viewed in wet mounts under the phase microscope. It appears much like a microscopic plastic tubule or pipe, usually but not always containing cells. Occasionally, the sheath is so thin and closely associated with the cells that it cannot be readily discerned by phase microscopy. The addition of 95% ethanol to the wet mount may help enable its visualization. Alternatively, it may be detected within the filament if there are gaps between cells (though lysed cells within a filament of ordinary chain-forming bacteria may give the false impression that a sheath is present).

Sheaths may appear yellow to dark brown, owing to the deposition of iron and manganese oxides.

Sheathed bacteria are found in aquatic habitats. They are a diverse group of organisms whose phylogeny is not yet understood. It is important to recognize that this grouping of sheathed bacteria is for deterministic purposes and does not reflect any evolutionary pattern.

Other sheathed procaryotic organisms are treated elsewhere in Volume III. For example, the genera *Herpetosiphon, Thioploca* and *Thiothrix* are included in Section 23, the "Nonfruiting Gliding Bacteria," and certain of the cyanobacteria (e.g. the genus *Lyngbya*) have sheaths.

Key to the genera of the Sheathed Bacteria

1. Single cells may be motile by means of a single polar flagellum or a tuft of subpolar flagella
    A. Sheaths rarely encrusted with iron and never encrusted with manganese oxides
        Genus *Sphaerotilus*, p. 1994
    B. Sheaths encrusted with iron or manganese oxides
        Genus *Leptothrix*, p. 1998
2. Single cells not motile by flagella
    A. Sheathed filaments attach to substrate
        1. Rod-shaped or cuboidal cells
            a. Longitudinal and transverse septation of cells
                Genus *Crenothrix*, p. 2006
            b. Transverse septation of cells only
                Genus "*Clonothrix*," p. 2008
        2. Disk-shaped cells
            Genus "*Phragmidiothrix*," p. 2005
    B. Sheathed filaments do not attach to substrate
        1. True branching of filaments
            Genus *Haliscomenobacter*, p. 2003
        2. Neither true nor false branching* of filaments
            Genus "*Lieskeella*," p. 2005

Genus Sphaerotilus Kützing 1833, 386 AL[†]

E. G. MULDER

Sphae.ro'ti.lus. Gr. n. *sphaera* a sphere; Gr. n. *tilus* anything shredded, floc, down; M.L. masc. n. *Sphaerotilus* spherical flock.

Straight rods, 1.2–2.5 × 2–10 μm, usually arranged **in single chains within sheaths** of uniform width, **which may be attached by** means of **holdfasts** to walls of containers, submerged plants, stones and other surfaces.[‡] Single or paired cells released from the sheaths are **motile by** means of **a bundle of subpolar flagella**, sometimes so intertwined as to give the appearance of a single large "unit flagellum." **Sheaths usually thin without encrustation by ferric and manganic oxides.** They cannot always be easily recognized when completely filled with cells. If parts of the sheaths are vacated by the cells, recognition of the organism cannot be misinterpreted (Fig. 22.1). Resting stages are not known. Gram-negative.[§]

Chemoorganotrophs; **metabolism respiratory**; never fermentative.

---

* False branching occurs when cells attach to an existing sheathed filament and develop into a new filament which appears as a branch. True branches are formed by an outgrowth of a filament.
† *AL* denotes inclusion of this name on the Approved Lists of Bacterial Names (1980).
‡ True, rather than false, branching of the filaments does not occur.
§ Has a propensity for storing poly-β-hydroxybutyrate in granules.

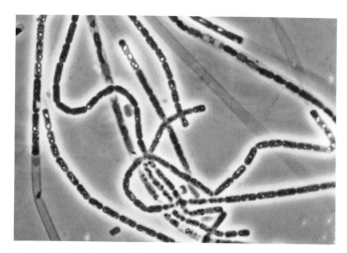

Figure 22.1. *S. natans* filaments from a rough colony grown on agar medium containing glucose and peptone at 1 g/l each. Partly filled and empty sheaths can be seen. Many cells contain globules of poly-β-hydroxybutyrate. × 1118. (Reproduced with permission from E. G. Mulder and W. L. van Veen, Antonie van Leeuwenhoek Journal of Microbiology and Serology *29:* 121–153, 1963.)

Can grow at very low concentrations of dissolved oxygen (below 0.1 mg/l). Temperature range: 10–37°C; optimum: between 20 and 30°C. Optimum pH: between 6.5 and 7.5. **Alcohols, several organic acids and sugars are used as sources of carbon and energy.** Ammonium salts and nitrates may serve as nitrogen source in the presence of vitamin B_{12} or methionine. Peptone, casamino acids and mixtures of aspartic and glutamic acids, and vitamin B_{12} or methionine give better results.

The mol% G + C of the DNA is 70 (Bd).

Type species: *Sphaerotilus natans* Kützing 1833, 386.

Further Descriptive Information

The only known species of the genus is *S. natans*.

Pure cultures, upon prolonged incubation, may sometimes show large, circular bodies resembling protoplasts. Their formation is probably due to the production of enzymes involved in the decomposition of the cell walls during the death phase. Incorporation of 0.4 g glycine per l nutrient medium favors this phenomenon (Phaup, 1968).

The surface of the sheaths has a smooth structure, contrasted with the rough structure of the sheath surface of *Leptothrix* species (Fig. 22.2). The sheaths of *S. natans* are covered with a cohering slime layer of variable thickness. For the composition of the slime, see Gaudy and Wolfe (1962), and for the composition of the sheath, see Romano and Peloquin (1963). More details on the structure of the sheath are given by Petitprez et al. (1969) and Hoeniger et al. (1973).

The normal habitat of *S. natans* is slowly running freshwater heavily contaminated with sewage or wastewater from paper, potato, dairy or other agricultural industries. The organism also occurs regularly in activated sludge, particularly when this material is settling poorly, so-called bulking.

S. natans is one of several types of filamentous bacteria that may cause bulking (Eikelboom, 1975). A ready settling of sludge flocs is one of the requisites for the successful operation of the activated-sludge process which includes the aerobic biological purification of sewage and industrial wastewater. After absorption of the soluble wastes by the sludge organisms, the sludge flocs should readily settle, so that flocs and purified water can be separated. When the sludge flocs are densely populated by *S. natans* or some other filamentous organism, they are voluminous with many trichomes protruding into the surrounding water, preventing a ready settling. This phenomenon is the cause of bulking sludge. The dominant growth of filamentous bacteria in activated sludge depends on two factors: (a) the low concentration of

available nutrients found in systems continuously fed with wastewater and (b) the low oxygen tensions which occur in such systems. Owing to the relatively high proportion of cell surface to cell contents of protruding filamentous bacteria compared with clumps of floc-forming bacteria, the former organisms occur in a more favorable position as to nutrient uptake and growth. The ability of *S. natans* to thrive at very low pO_2 values is an additional factor favoring the competition with floc-forming bacteria.

Although *S. natans* prefers a growth medium containing adequate amounts of easily assimilable organic nutrients, the organism is sporadically found in unpolluted water of brooklets, ditches and ponds where unknown compounds are the substrate. In the former habitat, the sheaths are thin and colorless; in the latter, particularly in the presence of soluble iron compounds, they may turn yellow-brown and sometimes become encrusted with ferric oxide. This characteristic can be clearly observed in a laboratory apparatus in which *S. natans* is grown in slowly running soil extract enriched with Fe (II). Under these conditions, the sheaths of *S. natans* resemble those of *Leptothrix ochracea*, and a number of authors (Pringsheim, 1949a, b; Stokes, 1954; and others) assume that both organisms are identical. More details concerning this hypothesis are included under "Differentiation of the Genera *Sphaerotilus* and *Leptothrix*."

Enrichment and Isolation Procedures

When slimy masses of the organism, attached to submerged surfaces in polluted, slowly running water, are available, direct isolation of *S. natans* may be tried. The same is true of activated sludge containing many filaments of the organism (bulking sludge). When the sheathed bacteria occur in low numbers in activated sludge or in nonpolluted water samples, the use of enrichment cultures is desirable (Mulder and Deinema, 1981). To that purpose, modifications of Winogradsky's hay infusion technique (1888) have been used. Extracted alfalfa straw (Stokes, 1954) or extracted pea straw (Mulder and van Veen, 1963, 1965) serve as the nutrient material. Most of the soluble organic matter should be removed to prevent the accumulation of undesirable organisms. This can be achieved by boiling and extracting the straw after it

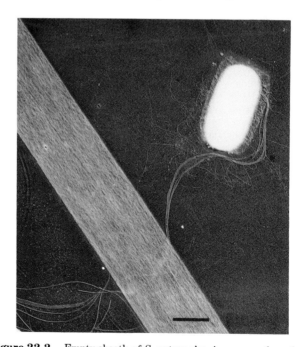

Figure 22.2. Empty sheath of *S. natans* showing a smooth surface, and a single cell with a tuft of subpolar flagella. Electron micrograph. *Bar,* 1 μm. (Reproduced with permission from E. G. Mulder and M. H. Deinema. 1981. *In* Starr, Stolp, Trüper, Balows and Schlegel (Editors), The Prokaryotes. A Handbook on Habitats, Isolation, and Identification of Bacteria. Springer-Verlag, Berlin, pp. 425–440).

has been cut into pieces of about 2 cm. In the case of alfalfa straw, a 1% suspension is extracted 3 or 4 times by boiling with large amounts of tap water. The extracted straw medium is distributed in 50-ml quantities in 125-ml Erlenmeyer flasks which are inoculated with about 10 ml of water from various sources. The preparation of the pea straw medium differs slightly from the preceding technique. The straw is extracted for 10 h at 100°C with tap water that is renewed every hour. One or 2 g of extracted pea straw (dry weight) in 25 ml of tap water is autoclaved twice (15 min at 110°C) and used as enrichment medium. After inoculation with small amounts of river or ditch water or activated sludge and incubation for about 1 week at 22–25°C, tufts of filaments of *S. natans* may be seen after microscopic observation.

Isolation may be achieved by streaking the enrichment cultures on previously dried agar plates containing low levels of nitrogen and carbon sources. Activated sludge containing many filaments of *S. natans* is streaked directly on such plates. Slimy masses of sheathed bacteria grown in slowly running, polluted water are washed several times with sterile water. Homogenization of the washed flocs by blending for a very short time may be advisable.

The use of a nutritionally poor agar medium limits the size of undesirable bacterial colonies, leaving large areas for the filamentous organisms. This medium has the following basal composition: KH_2PO_4, 27 mg/l; K_2HPO_4, 40 mg/l; $Na_2HPO_4 \cdot 2H_2O$, 40 mg/l; $CaCl_2$, 50 mg/l; $MgSO_4 \cdot 7H_2O$, 75 mg/l; $FeCl_3 \cdot 6H_2O$, 10 mg/l; $MnSO_4 \cdot H_2O$, 5 mg/l; $ZnSO_4 \cdot 7H_2O$, 0.1 mg/l; $CuSO_4 \cdot 5H_2O$, 0.1 mg/l; $Na_2MoO_4 \cdot 2H_2O$, 0.05 mg/l; cyanocobalamin, 0.005 mg/l; enriched with peptone (Brocapharm), 1 g/l; glucose, 1 g/l; and agar (Davis), 7.5 g/l of glass-distilled water. To inhibit the rapid spreading of contaminating bacteria, the excess surface moisture of the sterile agar plates should be evaporated by overnight storage of these plates at a temperature of 37–45°C.

Upon inoculation and incubation of these plates at 20–25°C, colonies of *S. natans* may be seen and tentatively identified within a few days by their characteristically flat, dull, cottonlike appearance. The edges of the colonies are irregular, owing to curly filamentous growth extend-

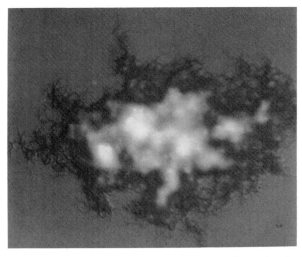

Figure 22.3. Rough colony of *S. natans*. × 22. (Reproduced with permission from E. G. Mulder and W. L. van Veen, Antonie van Leeuwenhoek Journal of Microbiology and Serology *29:* 121–153, 1963.)

ing in all directions (Fig. 22.3). Confirmation of the identification may be achieved by microscopic observation (Fig. 22.1).

Maintenance Procedures

Stock cultures of *S. natans* on agar slants of the previously described medium can be stored for about 3 months at 4°C. Addition of 2–3 ml of sterile tap water to the agar slants may prolong the viability for another 3 months. Preservation for longer periods is accomplished by common lyophilization techniques.

Differentiation of the genus **Sphaerotilus** from other genera

A survey of the main characteristics of the genera *Sphaerotilus*, *Leptothrix* and *Haliscomenobacter*, the three Gram-negative, sheath-forming bacteria known so far, is given in Table 22.1. *Sphaerotilus* is more closely related to *Leptothrix* than to *Haliscomenobacter*. This applies to the motility of separate cells when released from the sheaths, to the formation of poly-β-hydroxybutyrate as reserve material, to the accumulation of ferric oxide on the sheaths, and to the mol % G + C of the DNA. However, several other properties are clearly different. They include morphological as well as physiological characteristics, such as size of cells, flagellation, structure of sheath surface (see Figs. 22.2 and 22.4), ability of the *Leptothrix* species to oxidize Mn^{2+} to Mn^{4+} (MnO_2, see Fig. 22.5) which is absent in *Sphaerotilus,* and the pronounced response of *S. natans* to organic nutrients as contrasted with no or poor response of most *Leptothrix* species to added nutrients. The latter factor has important ecological consequences. *S. natans* thrives in water heavily contaminated with organic nutrients (wastewater); *Leptothrix* species are never found in such environments, except *L. cholodnii* which responds more clearly to added nutrients than the other *Leptothrix* species.

Taxonomic Comments

Despite the arguments in support of the classification of the Gram-

negative sheath-forming bacteria as reported in the eighth edition of the *Manual*, a number of authors are still following Pringsheim's proposal that the genus *Leptothrix* should be abolished (Pringsheim 1949a, b) and all the organisms isolated and described so far as *Leptothrix* species should be placed in *Sphaerotilus* under one common name, *Sphaerotilus discophorus*. In view of the pronounced differences between these *Leptothrix* species, this situation is regrettable and is leading to unnecessary confusion (see "Taxonomic Comments" under the genus *Leptothrix* on p. 2000).

Further Reading

Dondero, N.C. 1975. The *Sphaerotilus-Leptothrix* group. Annu. Rev. Microbiol. *29:* 407–428.
Mulder, E.G. and M.H. Deinema. 1981. The sheathed bacteria. *In* Starr, Stolp, Trüper, Balows, and Schlegel (Editors), The Prokaryotes. A Handbook on Habitats, Isolation, and Identification of Bacteria. Springer-Verlag, Berlin, pp. 425–440.
Pringsheim, E.G. 1949b. The filamentous bacteria *Sphaerotilus, Leptothrix, Cladothrix,* and their relation to iron and manganese. Philos. Trans. R. Soc. (London) Ser. B *233:* 453–482.
van Veen, W.L., E.G. Mulder and M.H. Deinema. 1978. The *Sphaerotilus-Leptothrix* group of bacteria. Microbiol. Rev. *42:* 329–356.

List of species of the genus **Sphaerotilus**

1. Sphaerotilus natans Kützing 1833, 386.[AL]

na′tans. L. part. adj. *natans* swimming.

Cell morphology is the same as that given for the genus. The organism may sometimes lose its sheath-forming capacity by mutation (Stokes, 1954). Colonies of sheathless cells are smooth (they have lost their filamentous edges). Discontinuation of sheath formation may also be

due to nongenetic factors, particularly nutritional conditions (Gaudy and Wolfe, 1961; Mulder and van Veen, 1963). When this organism is grown on a basal medium with glucose and peptone at 1 g/l each, normal hairy colonies are formed (Fig. 22.3), as contrasted with the smooth, almost circular colonies formed when 5 g of these nutrients are supplied. High concentrations of peptone are more effective in producing this

Table 22.1.

Main characteristics of the Gram-negative **Sheathed Bacteria**[a]

Characteristic	Sphaerotilus	Lepto-thrix	Haliscomeno-bacter
Cell dimensions			
Width (μm)	1.2–2.5	0.6–1.4	0.4–0.5
Length (μm)	2–10	1–12	3–5
Flagella			
Monotrichous polar	−	+[a]	−
Polytrichous subpolar	+	+[b]	−
Holdfasts	+	±[b]	−
Branchings	False	False[b]	Real
Structure of sheath surface[c]	Smooth	Rough	Smooth
Carbon source			
Glucose	+	+	+
Sucrose	+	+	+
Glycerol	+	+	−
Lactate	+	+	−
Nitrogen source			
NH_4^+	+	+	+
NO_3^-	+	+	+
Aspartic and glutamic acids	+	+	+
Casamino acids	+	+	+
Vitamin B_{12} requirement	+	+	+
Thiamine requirement	−	±	+
Optimum pH	6.5–7.5	6.5–7.5	7.0–8.0
Fe_2O_3 accumulation	+	+	−
Mn^{2+} oxidation	−	+	−
Carotenoid pigments	−	−	+
Reserve material			
Poly-β-hydroxybutyrate	+	+	−
Polysaccharide	+	−	+
Mol% G + C of DNA	70	69.5–71	49

[a]Symbols: −, 90% or more of strains are negative; +, 90% or more of strains are positive; ±, rarely observed.

[b]See also Table 22.2.

[c]Electron microscopic observations.

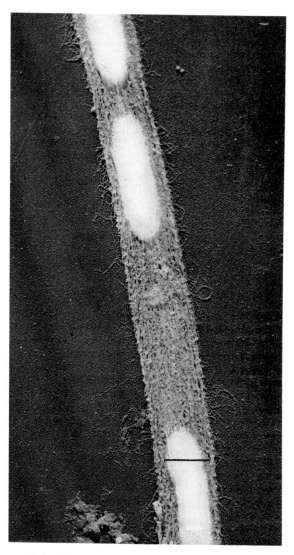

Figure 22.4. *L. cholodnii* showing rough surface (no manganese supplied). Electron micrograph. *Bar,* 1 μm. (Reproduced with permission from E. G. Mulder and M. H. Deinema. 1981. *In* Starr, Stolp, Trüper, Balows and Schlegel (Editors), The Prokaryotes. A Handbook on Habitats, Isolation, and Identification of Bacteria. Springer-Verlag, Berlin, pp. 425–440.)

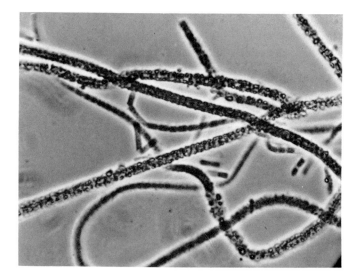

Figure 22.5. *L. cholodnii* sheaths encrusted with granulated MnO_2. × 1280. (Reproduced with permission from E. G. Mulder and W. L. van Veen, Antonie van Leeuwenhoek Journal of Microbiology and Serology *29:* 121–153, 1963.)

effect than are sugars. Smooth colonies consist of sheathless cells which have larger dimensions than cells in sheaths. Transfer of the former cells to a poor medium restores sheath formation.

False branching of the filaments occurs in every strain of *S. natans*, but it occurs in some strains more than others. Its occurrence depends on cultural conditions (relatively poor media) rather than on strain specificity (Pringsheim, 1949b).

Fructose, glucose, maltose, sucrose, galactose, ethanol, butanol, glycerol, mannitol, sorbitol, acetate, butyrate, β-hydroxybutyrate, pyruvate, lactate, malate, fumarate, succinate, citrate, alanine, aspartic acid, asparagine, glutamic acid and glutamine are utilized as carbon and energy sources for growth (Stokes 1954; Höhnl, 1955; Mulder and van Veen, 1963). Strains of *S. natans* differ widely in their capacity to dissimilate the above-mentioned carbon compounds. In contrast with most *Leptothrix* strains, *S. natans* utilizes relatively high concentrations of assimilable substrates from which it synthesizes considerable amounts of cellular material.

Cells may contain large amounts of poly-β-hydroxybutyrate either as numerous small globules or as a few large globules. Polysaccharides may also accumulate. The synthesis of both reserve compounds is stimulated by a high carbon/nitrogen ratio in the medium (Mulder and van Veen, 1963).

Genus *Leptothrix* Kützing 1843, 198[AL]

E. G. MULDER

Lep′to.thrix. Gr. adj. *leptus* fine, small; Gr. n. *thrix* hair; M.L. fem. n. *Leptothrix* fine hair.

Straight rods, 0.6–1.4 × 1–12 μm, **occurring in chains within a sheath** or free-swimming as single cells, in pairs or, in some species, as motile short chains containing up to 8 cells. One species has well-developed holdfasts (Table 22.2). Free cells are **motile** by means of **one polar flagellum;** one species has a subpolar tuft of several flagella. Most species may contain globules of poly-β-hydroxybutyrate as reserve material. **Sheaths** have a pronounced tendency to become **impregnated or covered with ferric and manganic** oxides. Resting stages are not known. Gram-negative.

Chemoorganotrophs; **metabolism respiratory;** never fermentative. Growth and manganese oxidation may proceed at low oxygen tensions. The temperature range extends from 10 to 35°C, with an optimum temperature for most strains around 25°C. Optimum pH: between 6.5 and 7.5 **A number of sugars,** including glucose, fructose and sucrose, **organic acids,** including lactic, malic and β-hydroxybutyric acids, **and glycerol are utilized** by most *Leptothrix* species **as carbon and energy sources.** Acetic and citric acids are not or are poorly utilized. Yield responses of *Leptothrix* species to consumed organic nutrients are generally considerably lower than those of *Sphaerotilus natans*. Although some species are able to utilize NH_4^+ and NO_3^-, most poorly growing strains do not assimilate inorganic nitrogen compounds. A mixture of aspartic and glutamic acids, casamino acids, peptone or other complex nitrogen compounds give better results. Excessive amounts of certain amino acids are inhibitory (Johnson and Stokes, 1965). Unless methionine is supplied, vitamin B_{12} should be added to the nutrient medium. For some strains, a requirement for biotin and thiamine has been reported (Rouf and Stokes, 1964). Adenine and guanine are also recorded in the literature as essential growth factors for some strains (Stokes and Johnson, 1965).

The mol% G + C of the DNA is 69.5–71 (Crombach et al., 1974).

Type species: *Leptothrix ochracea* (Roth 1797) Kützing 1843, 198.

Further Descriptive Information

Species respond in different ways to organic nutrients. "L. discophora" and L. lopholea, for instance, are hardly affected by any of the organic nutrients tested, whereas L. cholodnii behaves more or less similarly to S. natans in this respect. This behavior is in agreement with the occurrence of "L. discophora" in slowly running, unpolluted, iron- and manganese-containing ditch and well water, in contrast with S. natans, which thrives in polluted waters, and L. cholodnii, which is found in both unpolluted natural waters and in activated sludge.

Leptothrix species usually deposit large amounts of ferric and manganic oxides on and in their sheaths. This phenomenon can be easily seen in slowly running water rich in iron and manganese. The occurrence of flocculent masses of ferric and manganic oxides is often accompanied by masses of filamentous bacteria of various *Leptothrix* species (Figs. 22.6 and 22.7). The specific ability of these organisms to accumulate ferric iron was demonstrated by Rogers and Anderson (1976a, b) by growing *Sphaerotilus discophorus* (a *Leptothrix* species, presumably *L. cholodnii*) at different concentrations of $^{59}FeCl_3$. The amount of iron deposited on or in the sheaths increased with raised iron concentration of the medium. At the highest concentration used (4 mM), this amount was 10–100 times higher than the amount precipitated on the cells of a non-sheath-forming mutant and on a number of other nonsheathed bacteria, including "*Aerobacter aerogenes,*" *Escherichia coli* and *Pseudomonas denitrificans* The capacity of sheath-forming *Leptothrix* species to deposit large amounts of iron on their sheaths apparently enables these bacteria to grow at high concentrations of soluble iron compounds in the medium. The cells within the sheaths are protected against the soluble iron of the medium. This applies presumably also to *Sphaerotilus natans*, as was shown by Chang et al. (1979, 1980) who cultivated this organism in media with increasing amounts of different iron compounds and determined the iron deposited on and in sheaths and in cells, respectively, in connection with the growth inhibition of the organism. Although large amounts of iron were found on the sheaths which sharply increased with rising iron concentration of the medium, the iron content of the cells increased only slightly, so that relatively large iron concentrations were required to reach the critical concentrations at which the growth of the organism was inhibited by 90%.

The pronounced tendency of the sheath-forming bacteria to accumulate iron oxide on or in their sheaths is no proof that these organisms oxidize Fe^{2+} to Fe^{3+}. These bacteria grow in aerobic media at pH 6–7.5 where iron is readily oxidized nonbiologically. In manganese oxidation, these difficulties do not occur. Nonbiological oxidation occurs at pH

Table 22.2.
Differential characteristics of **Leptothrix** *species[a]*

Characteristic	L. ochracea	"L. pseudo-ochracea"	"L. discophora"	L. cholodnii	L. lopholea
Cell dimensions					
Width (μm)	1.0	0.8–1.3	0.6–0.8	0.7–1.3	1.0–1.4
Length (μm)	2–4	5–12	1–4	2–7	3–7
Flagella					
Monotrichous polar	+	+	+	+	−
Polytrichous subpolar	−	−	−	−	+
Holdfasts	−	−	−	−	+
False branchings	−	−	±		+
Loss of sheath formation by mutation	Unknown	Regular	Regular	Regular	Sporadic
Loss of Mn^{2+}-oxidizing capacity by mutation	Unknown	+	−	Regular	±
Response to increased concentration of organic nutrients	Unknown	±	−	+	−

[a]Symbols: +, 90% or more of strains are positive; −, 90% or more of strains are negative; and ±, rarely observed.

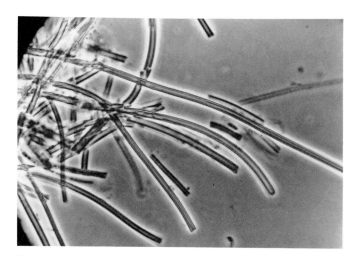

Figure 22.6. Broken empty sheaths of *L. ochracea* in crude culture in slowly flowing iron- and manganese-containing soil extract. Light micrograph, × 1186. (Reproduced with permission from E. G. Mulder and W. L. van Veen, Antonie van Leeuwenhoek Journal of Microbiology and Serology *29:* 121–153, 1963.)

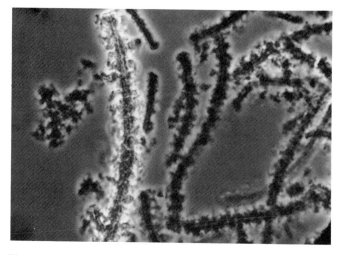

Figure 22.7. *"L. discophora"* grown under laboratory conditions in slowly running iron- and manganese-containing soil extract. Sheaths are covered with Fe (III) and Mn (IV) oxides. Light micrograph, × 1268. (Reproduced with permission from E. G. Mulder and W. L. van Veen, Antonie van Leeuwenhoek Journal of Microbiology and Serology *29:* 121–153, 1963.)

values above 9, conditions which are never found in environments where *Leptothrix* species are growing. In the presence of hydroxycarboxylic acids, nonbiological oxidation proceeds at pH values above 7.5 (Söhngen, 1914; Bromfield and Skerman, 1950; Mulder and van Veen, 1968). This type of reaction occurs in nutrient media containing relatively large amounts of Mn^{2+} and of neutralized hydroxycarboxylic acids such as citric and malic acids (0.5–10 g/l each). Microorganisms consuming these compounds raise the pH of the medium to about 8, whereupon the remaining acids exert a catalytic effect on Mn^{2+} oxidation. This reaction probably does not occur in the environments where the sheath-forming *Leptothrix* species are found, in that the levels of both Mn^{2+} and hydroxycarboxylic acids are too low. Biological oxidation of Mn^{2+} proceeds optimally between pH 6.5 and 7.5, values at which the bacteria of the *Sphaerotilus-Leptothrix* group grow optimally.

As to the possibly beneficial effect of biological manganese oxidation on the growth and functioning of *Leptothrix* species and other types of manganese-oxidizing microorganisms, various explanations have been offered.

Chemolithotrophy in Leptothrix *Species*

The concept of lithotrophy (autotrophy) in sheath-forming bacteria of the *Leptothrix* type has been the subject of controversy ever since it was put forward by Winogradsky in 1888. Cholodny (1926), Lieske (1919), Präve (1957), Habib Ali and Stokes (1971), and others agreed with this assumption but, as with Winogradsky, were unable to present convincing evidence to confirm that these bacteria can utilize the energy derived from the oxidation of Fe^{2+} or Mn^{2+}. Other workers, including Molisch (1910), Pringsheim (1949a, b), Mulder (1964), Dubinina (1978a, b), and van Veen et al. (1978), denied the lithotrophic character of these organisms. For studying lithotrophy in bacteria of the *Sphaerotilus-Leptothrix* type, biological oxidation of Mn (II) rather than of Fe (II) may be a better choice, in that it does not interfere with nonbiological oxidation. The beneficial effect of Mn (II) on the yield of cell nitrogen of *Leptothrix* species grown in media with organ nutrients has been ascribed by some authors to the utilization of the energy of oxidation for cell growth upon transfer of Mn^{2+} to Mn^{4+} (MnO_2) (Habib Ali and Stokes, 1971).

My colleagues and I have shown that the lower yield of cell nitrogen

of the cultures without Mn (II) is due to the loss of the proteinaceous catalyst which is excreted by the *Leptothrix* cells and is responsible for manganese oxidation. In the cultures with manganese, this protein forms an insoluble complex with MnO_2 on the sheaths which is not lost upon washing (van Veen et al., 1978). Data are recorded in Table 22.3.

Further evidence against the possible utilization of the energy of oxidation of Mn^{2+}* can be derived from Dubinina's experiments with *"L. pseudo-ochracea."* No additional assimilation of $^{14}CO_2$ was observed in media with added Mn^{2+}. This should have been the case if the manganese oxidation were an autotrophic process. The beneficial effect of Mn^{2+} which that author observed in cultures would be the removal by MnO_2 of H_2O_2 which is excreted in toxic amounts by *Leptothrix* species (Dubinina, 1978a, b).

Enrichment and Isolation Procedures

Enrichment of *Leptothrix* species can be achieved by imitating the conditions under which these organisms are found in massive amounts

Table 22.3.

Nitrogen content of cells and of manganic oxide-protein compounds produced in spent culture solutions of **L. cholodnii**

		Nitrogen (µg/25 ml of culture) in			
			Manganic oxide produced in		
Growth conditions	Time of harvest (days)	Washed cells	Spent culture solution[a]	Washing solution[a]	Total
Without MnCO₃	5	419	50	8	477
	8	349	70	12	431
With 0.3 g MnCO₃/l	5	467	18	5	490
	8	395	3	6	404

[a] Soluble protein precipitated upon treatment with Mn^{2+} and sodium malonate during 2 h at 40°C.

---

* With simultaneous assimilation of CO^{2+} as the main carbon source (autotrophy).

in nature, viz. slowly running water rich in soluble iron and manganese compounds but not contaminated with sewage. To that purpose, continuous-flow devices can be used successfully. They allow sheathed bacteria to attach to solid surfaces, whereas most of the unattached bacteria are washed out. My colleagues and I developed a special continuous-flow apparatus for growing *Leptothrix* species in artificial ditch water (see the drawing in Mulder and van Veen, 1963; Mulder and Deinema, 1981). This apparatus was used not only for enrichment and isolation purposes but also for growing pure cultures under more or less natural conditions.

One of the important principles of this technique is the preparation of iron- and manganese-containing soil extract. This is achieved by filling an iron cylinder with soil collected along a ditch or booklet in which *Leptothrix* species occur in large amounts. Such soils usually contain 10–20% of organic matter and are rich in ironstones and manganese. After adding 1–2 g ferric carbonate per kg soil, the cylinder is filled and the soil is saturated with tap water and kept for 3 weeks at room temperature. During this period, ferric compounds and MnO_2 are reduced. Tap water is then slowly let in at the bottom of the cylinder, and the iron- and mangagese-containing soil extract flows from the top of the cylinder.

This extract is sterilized by filtering through a Seitz filter and, subsequently, is continuously distributed into a series of Erlenmeyer flasks, fitted with outlets, which are inoculated with water containing many sheath-forming bacteria. To prevent a ready nonbiological oxidation of Fe^{2+}, the vessels are supplied with a sterile gas mixture consisting of 1% O_2, 5% CO_2 and 94% N_2. Within 2 weeks at room temperature, the slowly running culture media usually contain many brown flocs consisting of filaments of *Leptothrix* species covered with iron and manganese oxides.

Rouf and Stokes (1964) used a different enrichment method. With their method, a mixture of thoroughly extracted alfalfa hay, freshly precipitated $Fe(OH)_3$ and solid $MnCO_2$ is placed in glass cylinders which are almost entirely filled with water from rivers, ditches, etc. After incubation for about a week, reddish brown flakes may be seen on the sides of the cylinders near the surface of the water which probably will consist of sheaths of a *Leptothrix* species covered with iron and manganese oxides.

Isolation of various *Leptothrix* strains may be achieved by plating flocculent cell material directly from various natural environments. This method is preferable to the isolation via enrichment cultures, which often leads to the selection of only one strain.

The flocculent cell material is washed several times in sterile tap water and streaked on a solid medium of the following composition (in grams per liter of tap water): beef extract (Difco), 1.0; yeast extract (Difco), 0.075; sodium citrate, 0.15; vitamin B_{12}, 5×10^{-6}; $Fe(NH_4)_2(SO_4)_2$, 0.15; $MnCO_3$, 2.0; and agar (Davis), 7.5 (Mulder and van Veen, 1963; Mulder and Deinema, 1981). The medium of Rouf and Stokes (1964) has the following composition (in grams per liter of tap water): peptone, 5; ferric ammonium citrate, 0.15; $MgSO_4 \cdot 7H_2O$, 0.2; $CaCl_2$, 0.05; $MnSO_4 \cdot H_2O$, 0.05; $FeCl_3 \cdot 6H_2O$, 0.01; and agar, 12. The brown-black hairy colonies of *Leptothrix* species can be easily detected and are restreaked on fresh plates (Fig. 22.8).

Maintenance Procedures

Rubber-stoppered cultures on agar slants of the same composition as the isolation medium can be stored at room temperature or in the refrigerator at 4°C. They are subcultured every 3 months. Preservation for prolonged periods is accomplished by lyophilization.

Differentiation of the genera **Leptothrix** and **Sphaerotilus**

The main characteristics of both genera are summarized in Table 22.1. A discussion of these characteristics is reported in the corresponding section of the genus *Sphaerotilus*.

Taxonomic Comments

Pringsheim (1949a, b) has proposed abolishing the genus *Leptothrix* and transferring most of its species to the genus *Sphaerotilus* under one common species name, *S. discophorus*. One species, *L. ochracea*, would lose its name, since it would be a variation of the sewage organism *S. natans*. However, the evidence presented by Pringsheim in support of this nomenclature is inadequate, and this situation has led to confusion and error. The number of *S. discophorus* (*Leptothrix*) strains isolated and studied under laboratory and natural conditions was not mentioned but was apparently low. Although various "modifications" of *S. discophorus* are named, their description is poor, so that differentiation is not possible. As a result, the name *S. discophorus* is used in the literature for a variety of manganese-oxidizing and iron oxide-accumulating sheath-forming bacteria varying from such types as *L. cholodnii* to "*L. discophora*" (Stokes, 1954; Höhnl, 1955; Rogers and Anderson, 1976a, b). Some authors even use the name *S. discophorus* along with the names of various *Leptothrix* species without realizing that according to Pringsheim's nomenclature such organisms belong to *S. discophorus* (Caldwell and Caldwell, 1980).

The assumption that *L. ochracea* is a variation of the sewage organism *S. natans* is a further error in Pringsheim's scheme. It depends on the observation that pure cultures of *S. natans*, when cultivated in ferrous-ammonium-citrate-containing soil extract poor in organic nutrients, accumulate iron oxide in and on their sheaths and resemble *L. ochracea*. Pringsheim was unable to confirm his hypothesis that *L. ochracea* is a variation of *S. natans*. All of the efforts made to isolate *S. natans* from the iron oxide depositions in natural waters in which *L. ochracea* was seen microscopically have failed.

My colleagues and I have grown several strains of *Leptothrix* species and *S. natans* in slowly running iron (II)- and manganese (II)-containing soil extract under laboratory conditions and compared these organisms with crude cultures of *L. ochracea* growing under similar conditions

(Mulder and van Veen, 1963; Mulder and Deinema, 1981). Although in this medium *S. natans* in some respects resembled *L. ochracea*, both organisms were shown to be dissimilar for the following reasons: (a) the sheaths of *S. natans* were much longer, i.e. apparently less brittle, than those of *L. ochracea*; (b) the tendency of the cells to leave their sheath was much more pronounced in *L. ochracea* than in *S. natans*; and (c) *S. natans* was easily reisolated from its poorly growing iron-bacterium stage but not from the bulky enrichment culture of *L. ochracea*. All the efforts made so far by my colleagues and myself to isolate the latter organism either from natural or from laboratory enrichments have failed.

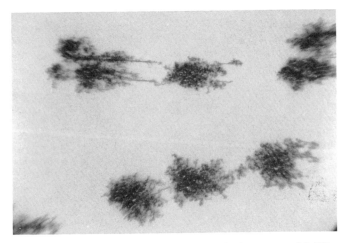

Figure 22.8. "*L. discophora*" filamentous colonies grown on $MnCO_3$-containing agar. Light micrograph, × 26. (Reproduced with permission from W. L. van Veen, E. G. Mulder and M. H. Deinema, Microbiological Reviews *42*: 329–356, 1978, ©American Society for Microbiology, Washington, D.C.)

Further Reading

(See also the list of papers and books on sheathed bacteria under "Further Reading" in the section on the genus *Sphaerotilus* on p. 1996.)

Ghiorse, W.C. 1984. Biology of iron- and manganese-depositing bacteria. Annu.

Rev. Microbiol. *38:* 515–550.

Mulder, E.G. and W.L. van Veen. 1968. Effect of microorganisms on the transformation of mineral fractions in soil. *In* Transactions of the Ninth International Congress on Soil Science, Adelaide, Australia, vol. 4, pp. 651–661.

Differentiation of the species of the genus **Leptothrix**

The most important differential characteristics of the species belonging to the genus *Leptothrix* are indicated in Table 22.2.

List of species of the genus **Leptothrix**

1. **Leptothrix ochracea** (Roth 1797) Kützing 1843, 198.[AL] (*Conferva ochracea* Roth 1797, Table V, Fig. 2.)

o.chra′ce.a. Gr. n. *ochra* yellow-ochre; M.L. adj. *ochracea* like ochre.

L. ochracea is the most common iron-storing ensheathed bacterium that probably occurs all over the world in slowly running ferrous iron-containing waters poor in readily decomposable organic matter. Its contribution to the oxidation of Fe^{2+} is uncertain, since (a) the organism normally grows at a pH value of 6–7, at which Fe (II) is readily oxidized nonbiologically, and (b) pure cultures of this bacterium have never been obtained. For the latter reason, its Mn (II)-oxidizing capacity, which probably occurs under natural conditions, has never been confirmed. The pronounced development and activity of *L. ochracea* in iron- and manganese-containing waters give rise to the accumulation and deposition of large masses of ferric oxide and, probably, MnO_2 which are thought to be responsible for the formation of bog ore (see, for instance, Ghiorse and Chapnick, 1983).

Authors who have studied and described *L. ochracea* under natural conditions were unable to obtain pure cultures (Cholodny, 1926; Charlet and Schwartz, 1954). Others who thought they had isolated *L. ochracea* had, in fact, described one of the other species of this genus (Winogradsky, 1888, 1922; Molisch, 1910; Lieske, 1919; Cataldi, 1939; Präve, 1957).

My colleagues and I observed the organism in natural environments and in the laboratory in crude culture of slowly running iron- and manganese-containing soil extract. The most typical characteristic of *L. ochracea* is the formation of large numbers of almost empty sheaths within a relatively short time. The mechanism of this procedure can be followed in a slide culture of the organism in an iron-containing soil extract medium under a phase-contrast microscope. In this way, the behavior of *L. ochracea* in crude culture can be observed continuously. It will be seen that chains of cells leave their sheath at the rate of 1–2 μm/min, continuously producing a new hyaline sheath connected with the old envelope (Fig. 22.9). Impregnation and covering of the sheaths with iron probably take place after the cells have left the envelopes. Aged golden-brown sheaths are brittle, so that they are easily broken into relatively short fragments (Fig. 22.6).

Isolation of *L. ochracea* has not been achieved, either from natural enrichments or, in the laboratory, from enrichment cultures of slowly running soil extract. In some instances, an organism resembling *L. ochracea* has been isolated, viz. "*L. pseudo-ochracea.*" *L. ochracea*, the type species of the genus, has never been isolated, so few details of the organism are available. "*L. pseudo-ochracea*" would be a better choice as a name for the type species.

2. **"Leptothrix pseudo-ochracea"** Mulder and van Veen 1963, 135.

pseu.do.o.chra′ce.a. Gr. adj. *pseudes* false; M.L. adj. *ochracea* specific epithet; M.L. adj. *pseudo-ochracea* not the true *L. ochracea.*

Cells are more slender than those of the other *Leptothrix* species (Table 22.2), and are very motile by one thin polar flagellum. Even chains of 6–10 cells after having left their sheath may show an undulatory locomotion. This characteristic may be responsible for the relatively large number of empty sheaths in culture, compared with the number found in other *Leptothrix* species, with the exception of *L. ochracea* which possesses even considerably more empty sheaths. In slowly flowing ferrous iron-containing soil extract, the sheaths become impregnated and slightly covered with ferric oxide and turn yellow-brown. In this respect,

the organism resembles *L. ochracea*. In media with added manganous compounds, the sheaths are covered with small granules of MnO_2. On manganese (II)-containing agar, the black-brown colonies are very filamentous and may exceed a width of 10 mm. On basal agar media containing 0.1% peptone and 0.1% glucose, the organism may grow in concentric rings.

The normal habitat of "*L. pseudo-ochracea*" is the slowly running, unpolluted, iron- and manganese-containing freshwater of ditches and brooklets. This species may also be found in slightly polluted water.

Type strain: none designated.

3. **"Leptothrix discophora"** (Schwers 1912) Dorff 1934, 31. (*Megalothrix discophora* Schwers 1912, 273.)

dis.coph′or.a. Gr. n. *discos* a disk; Gr. adj. *phoros* bearing; M.L. adj. *discophora* disk-bearing.

Cells are smaller than those of the other species described (Table 22.2). They may occur in narrow sheaths or be free-swimming; free cells are motile by a thin polar flagellum.

On glucose-peptone agar, the trichomes are thin and the colonies are small, often no more than 0.1–0.3 mm in diameter, with smooth edges. Increased supply of nutrients such as glucose, peptone, methionine, purine bases, vitamin B_{12}, biotin and thiamine hardly improve growth. When Mn (II) is supplied to this agar medium, the black-brown colonies will be somewhat larger (0.5–2 mm) and, sometimes, filamentous (Fig. 22.8). If widely spaced, they often are surrounded by a dark brown halo of pinpoint granules or by a diffuse light brown halo of oxidized manganese. The manganese-oxidizing and ferric oxide-storing capacities of this organism are very pronounced. In nutrient media containing Mn (II) salts, the sheaths are heavily but irregularly encrusted with MnO_2, giving rise to sheaths of sometimes 10 μm thickness (Fig. 22.10). In media with both manganese (II) and iron (II), as in slowly flowing soil

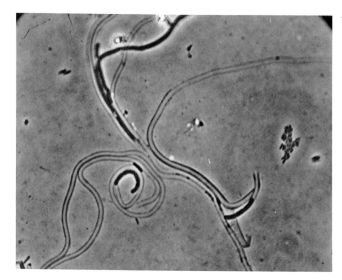

Figure 22.9. *L. ochracea* in iron- and manganese-containing soil extract. Cells are continuously leaving sheaths and forming new sheaths. Light micrograph, × 1268.

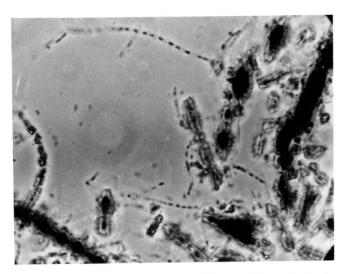

Figure 22.10. *"L. discophora"* in MnSO₄-containing nutrient solution. Young sheathed bacteria without encrustation and old sheaths, presumably empty, encrusted with thick layers of MnO₂ can be seen. Light micrograph, × 1203.

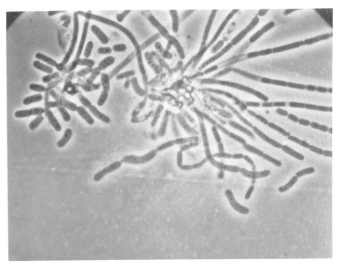

Figure 22.11. *L. lopholea* in culture solution. Many trichomes can be seen radiating from common holdfasts. Light micrograph, × 1316. (Reproduced with permission from E. G. Mulder and W. L. van Veen, Antonie van Leeuwenhoek Journal of Microbiology and Serology *29:* 121–153, 1963.)

extract, the sheaths become covered with a thick, dark brown, fluffy layer of ferric oxide and MnO₂ which may increase the diameter of the trichomes up to about 20–25 μm (Fig. 22.7). Under these conditions, the sheaths may taper toward the growing tips.

The normal habitat is slowly running, unpolluted, iron- and manganese-containing water of ditches, rivers or ponds.

Type strain: none designated.

4. **Leptothrix cholodnii** Mulder and van Veen 1963, 137.[AL]

cho.lod′ni.i. M.L. gen. n. *cholodnii* of Cholodny; named for N. Cholodny, a Russian bacteriologist.

For size of cells and flagellation, see Table 22.2. Cells are usually found in long chains inside the sheaths. Single motile cells may be seen outside the sheaths. In the presence of Mn²⁺, the cells become covered with granular MnO₂. At some sheath locations, the MnO₂ deposits may even exceed 10 μm.

L. cholodnii, in contrast with other *Leptothrix* species, responds to an increased supply of organic nutrients (Table 22.2). This results in relatively large colonies (up to 5 mm in diameter) on peptone-glucose agar. On manganese (II)-containing agar, black-brown hairy colonies, particularly when the organism is seeded densely, are formed.

Most strains display a strong tendency to dissociate spontaneously and to produce smooth rather than the usually rough colonies. Such mutant strains are largely sheathless and oxidize manganese slightly or not at all (Mulder and van Veen, 1963; Rouf and Stokes, 1964; Stokes and Powers, 1965).

In agreement with its nutritional requirements, *L. cholodnii* is found in slowly running iron- and manganese-containing unpolluted waters or in polluted waters, particularly in activated sludge.

Type strain: LVMW 99.

5. **Leptothrix lopholea** Dorff 1934, 33.[AL]

loph.o.le′a. Gr. n. *lophos* a crest; M.L. dim. fem. adj. *lopholea* somewhat crested or tufted.

L. lopholea resembles *S. natans* to a larger extent than do the other *Leptothrix* species. It is associated with polytrichous subpolar flagellation, formation of holdfasts, and false branching which may be found also in rich media. Cells usually develop short sheathed filaments radiat-

ing from a cluster of holdfasts, giving rise to many tiny flocs when the cells are grown in liquid media (Fig. 22.11).

Deposition of iron and manganese oxides is more pronounced on holdfasts than on filaments. On Mn (II)-containing agar media, encrustation of sheaths with MnO₂ is retarded, so that colonies at first are white and later become black-brown. The response in growth to an increased supply of organic nutrients is poor. Some strains show a good response, but they oxidize manganese more slowly.

This species may be isolated from slowly flowing, unpolluted or polluted freshwater and from activated sludge.

Type strain: LVMW 124.

Species Incertae Sedis

A. Organisms Probably Synonymous with the Species Described in This Edition

a. **"Leptothrix skujae"** Beger, in Beger and Bringmann 1953, 331.
Is presumably identical with *"L. discophora."*

b. **"Leptothrix thermalis"** (Molisch) Dorff 1934, 38.
Might be a thermophilic variety of *"L. discophora."*

c. **"Leptothrix sideropous"** (Molisch) Cholodny 1926, 25.
May be identical with or closely related to *L. lopholea.*

d. **"Leptothrix echinata"** Beger 1935, 401.
May be identical with or closely related to *L. lopholea.*

B. Insufficiently Described Organisms

e. **"Leptothrix major"** Dorff 1934, 35.
Sheathed bacterium with large cells, 1.4 × 5–10 μm, showing false branching. Sheaths, partly irregularly encrusted with ferric oxide, may be attached to submerged surfaces.

f. **"Leptothrix winogradskii"** Cataldi 1939, 64.
Cells 0.9 μm in diameter. Motile, presumably polarly flagellated; never attached. Colonies on iron-ammonium-citrate agar very filamentous.

g. **"Leptothrix pseudovacuolata"** (Perfil'ev) Dorff 1934, 36.

Is apparently not identical with "*L. discophora*," as was supposed in the eighth edition of the *Manual.* The so-called false vacuoles are not globules of poly-β-hydroxybutyrate, as was supposed in that edition, but indeed consist of gas vesicles that can be observed on the electron micrographs by Caldwell and Caldwell (1980, 41) of microbial iron deposits.

C. Probably Cyanobacteria

h. **"Leptothrix volubilis"** Cholodny 1924, 297.

i. **"Leptothrix epiphytica"** (Migula) Schönichen and Kalberlah 1900, 46.

May be cyanobacterium belonging to the genus *Lyngbya.*

Genus **Haliscomenobacter** *van Veen, van der Kooy, Geuze and van der Vlies 1973, 213*[AL]
(Streptothrix Cohn 1875, 186, sensu Mulder and van Veen 1974, 133)

E. G. MULDER

Ha.lis.co.me.no.bac′ter. Gr. v. *haliskesthai* to be imprisoned; Gr. n. *bacter* a rod or staff; M.L. masc. n. *Haliscomenobacter* imprisoned rod.

Thin rods, 0.4–0.5 × 3–5 μm, usually **in chains, enclosed by a** narrow, hardly visible **hyaline sheath. No ferric or manganic oxides are deposited** in or on the sheaths. **Branching of the filaments may** incidentally **occur** in stationary cultures. The branching cells disrupt the sheath and form a new sheath outside the envelop. Compared with the main filaments, the lateral branches are usually short. Cells outside the sheaths are seldom seen; **flagellation** and the motility of these cells have **not been observed.** Gram-negative.

Colonies on poor agar media are hardly visible macroscopically; they **are filamentous** and <0.5 mm in diameter. On a sucrose-peptone-yeast extract medium enriched with vitamin B₁₂ and thiamine, **pinkish,** smooth, slightly filamentous colonies of 1–3 mm in diameter develop. Liquid cultures turn pink, owing to the formation of carotenoid pigments.

Chemoorganotrophic, **aerobic.** Glucose, glucosamine, lactose, sucrose, starch and, to a lesser extent, mannitol are used as sources of carbon and energy; acetate, lactate, succinate, β-hydroxybutyrate, glycerol and sorbitol are not utilized. Inorganic nitrogen compounds (nitrate, ammonium salts) are moderately good nitrogen sources; amino acids and peptone give better results. Thiamine and vitamin B₁₂ are required for growth. Temperature range for growth: 8–30°C; optimum: approximately 26°C. The optimum pH is well above that of *Sphaerotilus* and *Leptothrix* species. Growth at pH 7.5 is much faster than that at pH 6.4.

The mol% G + C of the DNA is 49.

Type species: *Haliscomenobacter hydrossis* van Veen, van der Kooy, Geuze and van der Vlies 1973, 213.

Further Descriptive Information

H. hydrossis is widely distributed in activated sludge. It is one of those filamentous bacteria which sometimes occurs in large numbers in the sludge (Eikelboom, 1975; Wagner, 1982). They make the sludge flocs voluminous, while many trichomes, like tiny straight needles, protrude into the surrounding water. Both phenomena are responsible for the slow settling of the flocs (bulking). So far, no clear indications are available concerning the occurrence of the organism in large masses in certain sludges. It probably has to do with the substrate (type of wastewater) supplied. There are some indications that wastewater from meat industries and pig farms favors the dominating development of the organism in activated sludge.

H. hydrossis grows slowly. Maximum specific growth rates in continuous culture were approximately 0.05 h⁻¹ and 0.09 h⁻¹ for two different strains, corresponding to minimum doubling times of 14 and 9 h, respectively. These values are below those of most known bacteria occurring in wastewater and activated sludge (van Veen et al., 1982). The maintenance coefficients of these strains were low, 20 and 21 mg glucose (g biomass)⁻¹ h⁻¹, respectively. These values are far below those of most known bacteria and may contribute to the competitive ability of the organisms. The maximum yield coefficients (Y_G) found are 0.59 and 0.42 g biomass (g glucose)⁻¹, respectively.

Enrichment and Isolation Procedures

Bulking activated sludge which upon microscopic control is found to contain large masses of typical *Haliscomenobacter* filaments (Fig. 22.12)

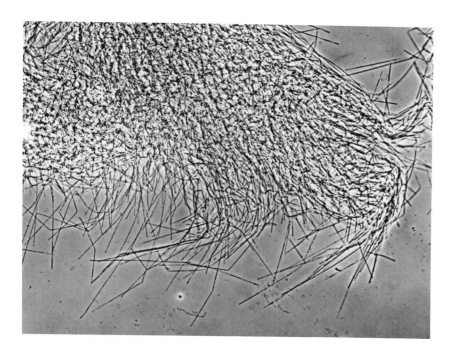

Figure 22.12. *H. hydrossis* flocculent growth of pure culture showing many needle-like filaments. Phase-contrast micrograph, × 1528. (Reproduced with permission from E. G. Mulder and M. H. Deinema. 1981. *In* Starr, Stolp, Trüper, Balows and Schlegel (Editors), The Prokaryotes. A Handbook on Habitats, Isolation, and Identification of Bacteria. Springer-Verlag, Berlin, pp. 425–440.)

is used as enrichment material. A sample of 0.1–0.5 ml of sludge is pipetted into tubes containing 10 ml of sterile tap water. The tubes are stirred for several minutes with a tube mixer, whereupon the flocs are allowed to settle. During moderate agitation of the floc suspensions, fragments of the threads are severed from the protruding filaments and will be seen in the supernatant. If upon microscopic observation insufficient amounts of separate filaments and free cells are present, the whole procedure is repeated. After settling of the flocs, a small amount of the supernatant is directly streaked on previously dried agar plates of the following composition (per liter of distilled water): glucose, 150 mg; $(NH_4)_2SO_4$, 50 mg; $Ca(NO_3)_2$, 10 mg; K_2HPO_4, 50 mg; $MgSO_4 \cdot 7H_2O$, 50 mg; KCl, 50 mg; $CaCO_3$, 100 mg; $FeCl_3 \cdot 6H_2O$, 5 mg; $MnSO_4 \cdot H_2O$, 2.5 mg; $CuSO_4 \cdot 5H_2O$, 0.1 mg; $ZnSO_4 \cdot 7H_2O$, 0.1 mg; $Na_2MoO_4 \cdot 2H_2O$, 0.05 mg; $CoCl_2 \cdot 6H_2O$, 0.05 mg; thiamine, 0.4 mg; vitamin B_{12}, 0.01 mg; and agar (Oxoid), 10 g. After incubation for some weeks at 17–20°C, small filamentous colonies may have developed which can hardly be recognized, even when viewed under the stereomicroscope. Low magnification ($\times$ 150) phase-contrast microscopy facilitates detection. Sterile capillary tubes are used to transfer cells to agar plates of the following composition (in grams per liter of distilled water) (S.C.Y. agar): sucrose, 1.0; casitone (Difco), 0.75; yeast extract (Difco), 0.25; Trypticase soy broth without dextrose (BBL), 0.25; thiamine, 4×10^{-4}; vitamin B_{12}, 10^{-5}, and agar (Oxoid), 10.

Maintenance Procedure

Stock cultures on the previously described S.C.Y. agar slopes, with 3 ml of sterile tap water added on the surface of the agar, are inoculated and kept at 20–25°C until turbid growth in the liquid layer. The organism remains viable during 3 months storage at 4°C and may be preserved for longer periods by common lyophilization techniques.

Differentiation of the genus **Haliscomenobacter** *from other genera*

A number of characteristics, summarized in Table 22.1, differentiate the genus *Haliscomenobacter* from the other two genera of Gram-negative, sheath-forming bacteria that have been grown in pure culture. It has been concluded that except for the presence of a sheath, *Haliscomenobacter* strains are entirely different from the bacteria of both of these other genera.

Taxonomic Comments

The reason for transferring this organism to a new genus is that the name *Streptothrix* (see the eighth edition of the *Manual*) is illegitimate. It was given earlier by Corda (1839) to a fungus and by Cohn (1875) to an actinomycete.

Further Reading

van Veen, W.L., D. van der Kooy, E.C.W.A. Geuze and A.W. van der Vlies. Investigations on the sheathed bacterium *Haliscomenobacter hydrossis* gen. n., sp. n., isolated from activated sludge. Antonie van Leeuwenhoek J. Microbiol. Serol. *39:* 207–216, 1973.

van Veen, W.L., J.M. Krul and C.J.E.A. Bulder. Some growth parameters of *Haliscomenobacter hydrossis* (syn. *Streptothrix hyalina*), a bacterium occurring in bulking activated sludge. Water Res. *16:* 531–534, 1982.

List of species of the genus **Haliscomenobacter**

1. **Haliscomenobacter hydrossis** van Veen, van der Kooy, Geuze and van der Vlies 1973, 213.[AL] (*Streptothrix hyalina* Migula 1895, 38, sensu Mulder and van Veen 1974, 133.)

hy.dross'is. Gr. n. *hydro* water; *Oss* town in the Netherlands; M.L. masc. adj. *hydrossis* from water of Oss.

Most of the characteristics are the same as those given for the genus (Fig. 22.13). Electron micrographs revealing details of cell structure have been presented by Deinema et al. (1977). They show that polysaccharides, not poly-β-hydroxybutyrate, are the reserve material of this organism. Extensive continuous-culture experiments have been carried out with *H. hydrossis* growing in a complex medium (trypticase soy, yeast extract, glucose) at different dilution rates (Krul, 1977, 1978). Owing to the pronounced proteolytic activity of the organism, a ready degradation of the complex nitrogen compounds took place. Amino acids from these compounds were used as both nitrogen and energy sources in the presence of glucose. Of these amino acids, glutamic acid, glycine, methionine, tryptophan, lysine and arginine were relatively easily taken up. The remaining amino acids accumulated in the free state at relatively high dilution rate, apparently owing to suppression of this uptake by glucose. At dilution rates below 0.015 h^{-1}, all the amino acids were taken up more or less completely.

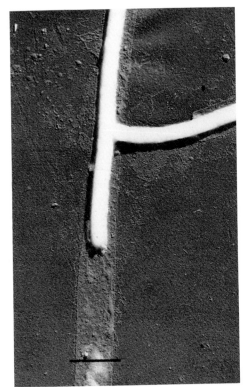

Figure 22.13. *H. hydrossis* branched filament with thin hyaline sheath. Electron micrograph. *Bar,* 1 μm. (Reproduced with permission from E. G. Mulder and M. H. Deinema. 1981. *In* Starr, Stolp, Trüper, Balows and Schlegel (Editors), The Prokaryotes. A Handbook on Habitats, Isolation, and Identification of Bacteria. Springer-Verlag, Berlin, pp. 425–440.)

Genus "**Lieskeella**" *Perfil'ev 1927, 335*

PETER HIRSCH

Lies.ke.el′la. M.L. dim. ending -*ella;* M.L. fem. n. *Lieskeella* named for H. Lieske, a German microbiologist.

Cells rod-shaped with rounded ends, 0.6 × 2–3 μm, **in chains.** Usually *two chains* (filaments) **are wound around one another to give a double spiral which is surrounded by a yellowish, slimy capsule,** often with heavy deposits of small ferric hydroxide granules. When the deposits are dissolved with dilute HCl, the cell chains fragment and the individual rods appear as a double zigzag band. **Cells show bipolar staining when treated with methylene blue.** Cells chains may aggregate in distinct layers or even in more or less solid skeins. The **filaments separate rapidly upon removal from the normal environment.**

There is **a slow but incessant motion** similar to that of the cyanophytes. Gram reaction has not been recorded. Presumably, these organisms are aerobic and chemoorganotrophic. Have not been obtained in pure culture.

Type species: *"Lieskeella bifida"* Perfil'ev 1927, 335.

Further Descriptive Information

Perfil'ev and Gabe (1961) point to an "extraordinary instability of the cells of this organism." The use of any of the usual fixatives, even greatly diluted, causes the threads to separate explosively into cells which instantaneously shorten, swell and burst into granular remains. A similar instability has been reported for *Toxothrix trichogenes,* which also glides slowly (Krul et al., 1970).

Originally found in the upper layers of mud in water bodies around Alt-Peterhof, Russia, it has also been observed (by Perfil'ev and Gabe, 1961) in several other locations in western Russia throughout the year, usually as thin layers of up to 15 chains. It has been found in the littoral zone of Kirstatellevyi Pond, Russia, at depths of 0.5–1.2 m and in the mud-water interface of Lake Windermere, England (V.B.D. Skerman, personal communication).

Differentiation of the genus "**Lieskeella**" *from other closely related taxa*

There are some morphological similarities to *Toxothrix trichogenes,* but this latter bacterium usually glides as a single filament of U shape, with the round middle section in front. The *Toxothrix* polymer is left behind the gliding filament rather than surrounding it, as in *"Lies-* *kella."* Morphologically similar *Leptothrix* species do not glide, and the filaments are usually straight; some species of *Leptothrix* live attached to surfaces.

List of species of the genus **Lieskeella**

1. "**Lieskeella bifida**" Perfil'ev 1927, 335.
bi′fi.da. L. adj. *bifida* cleft, divided.
Description of the species is the same as that for the genus.

Genus "**Phragmidiothrix**" *Engler 1883, 192*

PETER HIRSCH

Phrag.mi.di′o.thrix. Gr. n. *phragma* fence; Gr. n. *eidus* form, shape; Gr. n. *thrix* hair; M.L. fem. n. *Phragmidiothrix* fencelike hair.

Cells of variable size, usually small and **disk-shaped,** with a diameter 4–6 times the thickness of the cell. Cells are arranged as colorless, articulate and **unbranched filaments of over 100 μm in length. Filaments attached, forming** grayish-white **tufts.** The free end may be of larger diameter than the base, but there is no tapering in either direction; the diameter varies between 3 and 6 μm. Surrounded by a very **thin, delicate, gelatinous, colorless sheath** which is **not encrusted** with iron or manganese compounds. Cell walls are distinctive and of even thickness throughout the filament.

Multiplication is by cross-septation and, in certain regions of the filament, by both cross-septation and longitudinal septation, forming *Sarcina*-like aggregates of small, nearly cubical propagation cells. Septating cells may be of greater diameter, causing localized swelling of the filament; in areas septating in both planes, the filaments may be up to 6 μm in diameter (Fig. 22.14).

Type species: *"Phragmidiothrix multiseptata"* (Engler) Engler 1883, 192.

Further Descriptive Information

Engler (1883) reported outgrowths of slightly curved filaments of 4–10 cells, perpendicular to the main filament and seemingly a continuation of the adjacent cell. He suggested propagation cells in a particular row had grown out to form these thin, slightly curved, twiglike outgrowths.

Information on the physiology is lacking, but the organism is possibly anaerobic and tolerates H_2S. Has not been obtained in pure culture. Originally found attached to the surface of living *Gammarus locusta* collected from the anaerobic, H_2S-containing polluted area called "Weisser Grund" or "Todten Grund" in the Kiel Fjord, Germany. Apparently not rare; has been reported on seaweed from polluted water of the Northern Adriatic Sea (Beger, 1957).

Hirsch (unpublished observations) observed bacterial filaments resembling *"Phragmidiothrix"* in an anaerobic enrichment of polluted Long Island Sound water supplemented with seaweeds.

Differentiation of the genus **"Phragmidiothrix"** *from other closely related genera*

Multiplication by cross-septation and longitudinal septation is also found in *Crenothrix polyspora*, but in this species the filament clearly widens at the tip where multiple septation occurs (Völker et al., 1977). *C. polyspora* produces spherical "macrogonidia" and "microgonidia," while such forms have not been reported for *"Phragmidiothrix."*

A distinct morphological similarity can be seen with bacteria of the genera *Geodermatophilus* (Luedemann, 1968; Ishiguro and Wolfe, 1970) and *Blastococcus* (Ahrens and Moll, 1970). All of these show multiple septation, and *Blastococcus aggregatus* has been isolated from the Bay of Kiel, Germany. However, aggregates of the latter organism are usually short and contain only a few cells; motile swarmers are formed.

Acknowledgments

I am indebted to Dr. R. Schweisfurth (Homburg) for cell material of *Crenothrix* and to Dr. G. Rheinheimer (Kiel) for a culture of *Blastococcus aggregatus.*

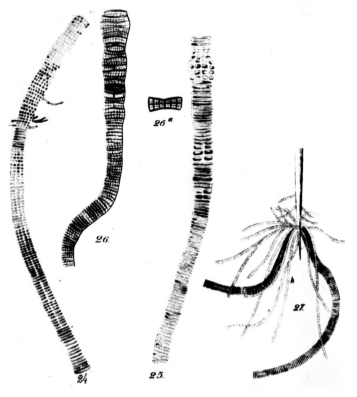

Figure 22.14. *"P. multiseptata." 24,* filament showing arrangement and septation of disk-shaped cells; *25,* part of filament showing enlarged end and individual disk-shaped cells of uneven diameter; *26,* part of filament with much cross-septation and longitudinal septation; *26ᵃ,* part of filament at higher magnification; *27,* a bristle of *Gammarus locusta* with two attached filaments of *"Phragmidiothrix"* (wide filaments) and several narrow filaments of young *"Beggiatoa alba."* Approximately × 330. (Reproduced from Engler, 1883.)

List of species of the genus **"Phragmidiothrix"**

1. **"Phragidiothrix multiseptata"** (Engler 1882) Engler 1883, 192. (*Beggiatoa multiseptata* Engler 1882, 19.)

mul.ti.sep.ta′ta. L. masc. n. *multus* much; L. adj. *septatus* fenced; M.L. fem. adj. *multiseptata* much fenced, with many septa.

Description of the species is the same as that for the genus.

Genus **Crenothrix** *Cohn 1870, 108*[AL]

Peter Hirsch

Cre′no.thrix. Gr. n. *crenus* a fountain, spring; Gr. n. *thrix* hair; M.L. fem. n. *Crenothrix* fountain hair.

Cells cylindrical to disk-shaped, 0.6–5.0 μm in diameter, dividing by cross-septation to **form sheathed filaments** up to 1 cm long and **often attached to a firm substrate. Filaments are unbranched** but may occasionally show what appears to be false branching. The **very thin sheaths** surrounding the filaments **may be colorless at the tip or encrusted with iron** (or manganese) **oxides at the base.**

Filaments may show increased cross-septation on one or both free ends to **form spherical propagation cells ("macrogonidia")** with the same diameter as the rod-shaped cells. Presumably, these macrogonidia are liberated from the sheath ends, and they may elongate and cross-septate to form new sheathed filaments. Some of the *Crenothrix*

filaments widen at the end(s), and here the **cells undergo cross-septation and longitudinal septation.** Numerous, small, **cubical cells arising in this fashion ("microgonidia") are rounded up and are also released from the filament tip.**

Gram-negative (Völker et al., 1977). Some cell chains show a gliding motility (Bump and Schweisfurth, 1981). This organism has not been grown on artificial media in pure culture. Found in stagnant and running waters containing low concentrations of organic matter, Fe^{2+} and traces of methane.

Type species: *Crenothrix polyspora* Cohn 1870, 108.

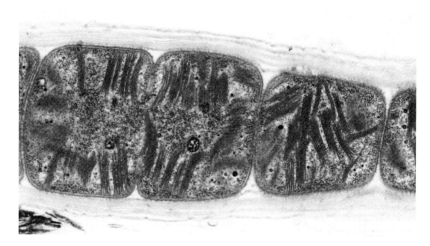

Figure 22.15. *C. polyspora* from natural materials. Electron micrograph of a thin longitudinal section through an ensheathed filament with perpendicular membrane stacks and the multilayered sheath shown (× 22,400).

Further Descriptive Information

The fine structure of *C. polyspora* was investigated by Völker et al. (1977). These authors observed, in all cells, lamellar membrane stacks arranged perpendicular to the cytoplasmic membrane and similar to those of methanotrophic bacteria (Fig. 22.15). There were no photosynthetic pigments. Some cells contained hexagonal bodies of unknown function, others (especially when older) had diagonally arranged fibrillar bundles within the cytoplasm. A sheath of sometimes considerable thickness was multilayered.

The diameter of the individual filaments when swollen may vary from 1–6 µm at the base to 6–9 µm at the tip. The reproductive cells ("gonidia") may be held together by a slimy substance to form a zoogloeal mass.

According to Cohn (1870), reproduction may also occur by outgrowth of swollen, terminal cells of ellipsoidal shape that are as much as 7 times long as wide; the short, colorless *Oscillatoria*-like filaments growing out of such swollen cells had a characteristic slow gliding motion and lacked a clearly defined sheath. Except for Bump and Schweisfurth (1981), most subsequent authors failed to mention this type of reproduction.

Cohn also indicated that the tip of the sheath was closed and retained the reproductive cells until rupture (see Figs. 9 and 10 in Cohn's original description). This author has found no evidence for closed sheaths.

Presumably, *C. polyspora* is aerobic (or microaerophilic), chemoorganotrophic, and probably oligotrophic, judging from its occurrence in certain springs, wells, ponds, etc. Despite using a large variety of organic compounds, Bump and Schweisfurth (1981) were unable to grow *C. polyspora*. The presence of an internal membrane system in *C. polyspora* indicates possible chemoautotrophy or methanotrophy.

Differentiation of the genus **Crenothrix** from other genera

The peculiar mechanism of gonidia formation and their nearly spherical shape (Fig. 22.16) differentiate this genus from other genera, as is shown in Table 22.4. In multiple and longitudinal septation, *Crenothrix* shows a certain resemblance to *Phragmidiothrix, Geodermatophilus, Dermatophilus* and *Blastococcus*. The latter three genera are Gram-positive actinomycetes and show motile swarmer cell formation.

Taxonomic Comments

Wolfe (1960) pointed out certain similarities between *C. polyspora* and the *Sphaerotilus* species, especially with respect to iron oxide deposition on the filament base. Cholodny (1926) believed *C. polyspora* to be identical with *Clonothrix fusca* Roze 1896, 325. However, the latter organism is characterized by tapering filaments.

Acknowledgments

Crenothrix cell material and some information on these organisms were kindly provided by Dr. R. Schweisfurth (Bad Homburg).

Table 22.4.

Differential characteristics of the genus **Crenothrix** *and other morphologically similar taxa[a]*

Characteristics	Crenothrix	Sphaerotilus	"Clonothrix"	"Phragmidiotrix"	Geodermatophilus
Filaments tapering	−	−	+	−	−
Filaments with false branches occasionally	+	+	+	−	−
Longitudinal septation may occur	+	−	−	+	+
Multiplication by formation of macrogonidia and microgonidia	+	−	−	−	−
Swarmer cells motile with flagella	−	+	−	−	+
Fe- and/or Mn-oxides deposited on filament sheath	∓	∓	∓	−	−
Gram reaction	−	−	ND	ND	+

[a]Symbols: −, 90% or more of strains are negative; +, 90% or more of strains are positive; ∓, rarely observed and then only as thin coatings; ND, not determined.

List of species of the genus **Crenothrix**

1. Crenothrix polyspora Cohn 1870, 108.[AL]

po.ly.spo′ra. Gr. adj. *poly* many; Gr. n. *sporus* a seed; M.L. n. *spora* a spore; M.L. fem. adj. *polyspora* many-spored.

Description of the species is the same as that for the genus.

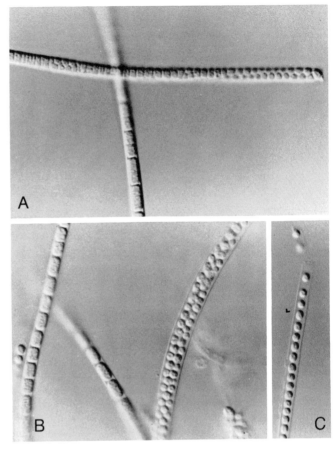

Figure 22.16. *C. polyspora* from a freshwater source. *A,* filaments with normal cross-septation and the beginning of longitudinal septation shown. *B,* normal filaments and the ensheathed and inflated part of a *Crenothrix* filament with microgonidia shown. *C,* macrogonidia released from the tip of an open filament. Nomarski interference contrast light micrographs (× 620).

Genus **"Clonothrix"** *Roze 1896, 329*

Peter Hirsch

Clo′no. thrix. Gr. n. *clon* twig; Gr. n. *thrix* hair; M.L. fem. n. *Clonothrix* twig hair.

Filaments 3–7 μm wide and up to 1.5 cm long, **attached or free,** surrounded by a more or less distinct sheath which **may be encrusted with iron or manganese oxides** giving a yellowish-brown color. **Filaments tapering;** they may be single or with false branches. Cells cylindrical, colorless or bluish, 2–2.5 × 12–18 μm, being larger at the base and smaller at the tip of the filament.

Reproduction is by separation of individual cells, followed by breakage of the sheath and release to the outside; such cells frequently attach themselves parallel to older cells and produce new filaments, giving rise to "pseudobranching." Most of these morphological features were noted in Roze's original drawings (Fig. 22.17).

These organisms have not been grown in pure culture on artifical media.

Type species: *"Clonothrix fusca"* Roze 1896, 330.

Further Descriptive Information

Rarely, apparently unicellular ampullike bodies are produced, subterminally, by a budding process from cells of certain filaments. These may serve as a means of propagation, but the mechanism is unknown.

Chemoorganotrophic and aerobic, with the ability to deposit Fe oxides on older parts of the filament. Originally, this organism was found attached to iron fittings in well water (at 14°C) containing *Aplococcus natans.* Hirsch (unpublished observations) found *"C. fusca"* in self-pumped cow troughs and in oligotrophic pond water rich in suspended clay particles. The filaments did not glide.

Differentiation of the genus **"Clonothrix"** from other morphologically similar taxa

The tapering filament tips, false branches and the brownish color of the filaments clearly differentiate *Clonothrix* from other filamentous bacteria, such as *Crenothrix*, *Sphaerotilus* and *Leptothrix*.

Taxonomic Comments

Schorler (1904) described an organism very similar to "*C. fusca*" Roze 1896 and independently gave it the same name. Beger and Bringmann (1953) compared "*C. fusca*" with *Glaucothrix putealis* and, on the basis of size and the occurrence of false branching in both, concluded that "*C. fusca*" Roze 1896 was a later synonym of "*G. putealis*" Kirchner 1876. However, a decision on this matter must be postponed until at least one organism has been cultivated and studied in greater detail. "*Clonothrix gracillima*" West and West 1898, 337, has filaments which never taper; it was isolated from a horse trough. Beger and Bringmann (1953) considered this organism to be a species of *Leptothrix*. "*C. tenuis*" Kolkwitz 1909, 144, was observed in sewage but never cultured.

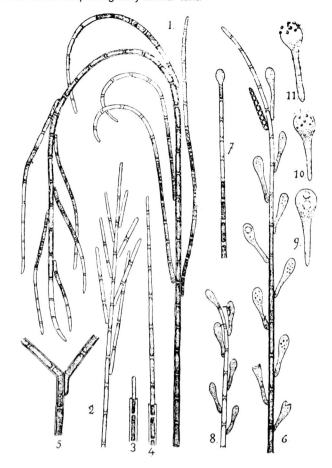

Figure 22.17. *C. fusca*, *1*, end of adult filament with false lateral branches; *2*, end of young filament with false branches; *3*, cell emerging from a broken filament; *4*, young filament growing from an adult filament; *5*, mode of insertion of two adult filaments, with the one on the right forming a false lateral branch; *6*, a filament carrying an ascending series of ampullike swellings; *7*, end of a filament terminating in an ampullike swelling; *8*, a filament terminating in swelling but also carrying a series of lateral swellings; *9–11*, buds with vacuoles and granules shown. Magnification: for *1–4* and *6–8*, approximately × 365; for *5* and *9–11*, approximately × 650. (Reproduced from Roze, 1896.)

List of species of the genus **"Clonothrix"**

1. **"Clonothrix fusca"** Roze 1896, 330.
fus'ca. L. fem. adj. *fusca* dark, tawny.
Description of the species is the same as that for the genus.

SECTION 23

Nonphotosynthetic, Nonfruiting Gliding Bacteria

John M. Larkin

The organisms in this section are morphologically and physiologically diverse and are not necessarily closely related. They are grouped on the basis of their ability to move upon a solid surface without any visible means of locomotion. In most instances the means of locomotion has been designated as "gliding," but in a few instances this may be questionable. *Agitococcus* has been described as moving by a twitching sort of gliding, *Achromatium* may have flagella, and *"Peloploca"* and *"Desmanthos"* are not motile. (The latter organisms are placed within this group because of obvious similarities with other organisms placed here which do move by gliding.)

None of the organisms within this section make fruiting bodies, but two genera, *Sporocytophaga* and *Chitinophaga*, produce microcysts that are similar to those made by the myxobacter *Myxococcus*. No organism in this group is capable of carrying out photosynthesis.

With the exception of some strains of *Beggiatoa*, which have been grown as chemoautotrophs, all the organisms in this section that have been obtained in pure culture are capable of chemoheterotrophic growth; however, some may be capable of mixotrophic growth, and perhaps even others, of chemoautotrophic growth. Some oxidize sulfide and presumably obtain energy from it, while another uses sulfate as an electron acceptor and produces sulfide. Pure cultures of some of the organisms described in this section have not been obtained.

This grouping of Gram-negative organisms is morphologically diverse and includes cocci, spirals, long flexible rods, filaments which may or may not be bound by a sheath, flexible gliding trichomes, and rosette formers. Some contain gas vesicles, and others contain sulfur inclusions. Many of the organisms are sufficiently distinctive morphologically to be easily recognizable to the generic level by light microscopy.

Key to the groups of Nonphotosynthetic, Nonfruiting Gliding Bacteria

I. Rod-shaped cells which grow singly and may range from short (i.e. <10 µm) to long (i.e. 10 to >100 µm) and filamentous. Filaments are rarely multicellular. Motility is by gliding, or the organisms are nonmotile. Colonies are usually yellow, orange or red due to the production of nondiffusible pigments. In the presence of sulfide, these organisms do not deposit sulfur. The mol% G + C of the DNA ranges from about 30 to 50.
Order I. *Cytophagales*, p. 2011

II. Rod-shaped cells which grow singly and may become very long (up to 70 µm). Motile by gliding. Colonies are cream, pink, or yellow-brown. May produce a brown, water-soluble pigment. Lyse a wide variety of microorganisms. The mol% G + C of the DNA ranges from 65 to 71.
Order II. *Lysobacterales*, p. 2082

III. Organisms typically grow as multicellular filaments. Motile by gliding. Colonies are white. In the presence of hydrogen sulfide, sulfur granules are deposited internally.
Order III. *Beggiatoales*, p. 2089

IV. Other families and genera
A. Rod-shaped cells which grow as flattened, multicellular filaments, with the long axis of the individual cells perpendicular to the long axis of the filament. From the oral cavity of warm-blooded vertebrates.
Family *Simonsiellaceae*, p. 2107

B. Rod-shaped cells which grow as multicellular filaments which may be single or aggregated into bands or bundles. Motile by gliding or nonmotile. May contain gas vesicles but do not contain sulfur inclusions. Probably anaerobic.
Family *"Pelonemataceae,"* p. 2112

C. Rod-shaped cells which grow as long (up to 500 µm), flexible, multicellular sheathed filaments. Unsheathed segments are motile by gliding.
Genus *Herpetosiphon*, p. 2136

D. Rod-shaped cells which form a long, U-shaped multicellular trichome. Movement is by gliding, with the rounded, central portion of the trichome forward. The ends of the trichome rotate, causing parallel tracks to be made on the substrate. The central portion of the trichome is occasionally raised off of the

surface temporarily and redeposited at another site. The polymer remaining in the tracks left by ends and the central portion may eventually become encrusted with iron oxide.

Genus *Toxothrix*, p. 2120

E. Rod-shaped cells which form long, unbranched, nonmotile multicellular filaments which may attach to a solid surface via a holdfast. Rosettes are produced. Gonidia are produced and are motile by gliding. Organism is usually of marine origin.

Genus *Leucothrix*, p. 2121

F. Rod-shaped cells which grow in motile multicellular filaments. No pigments are produced. In the presence of hydrogen sulfide, these organisms do not deposit sulfur inclusions.

Genus *Vitreoscilla*, p. 2124

G. Large rod-shaped cells which form long, flexible, gliding filaments. Strictly anaerobic, using sulfate and other oxidized sulfur compounds as electron acceptors and producing hydrogen sulfide.

Genus *Desulfonema*, p. 2128

H. Cells are single, large (>5 μm in diameter), coccoid or elongated. Normally contain sulfur globules and may contain calcium carbonate inclusions.

Genus *Achromatium*, p. 2131

I. Gram-negative coccus about 1–2 μm in diameter. Twitching, gliding motility. Aerobic.

Genus *Agitococcus*, p. 2133

Further Reading

Christensen, P.J. 1977. The history, biology, and taxonomy of the *Cytophaga* group. Can. J. Microbiol. *23:* 1599–1653.

Christensen, P. and F.D. Cook. 1978. *Lysobacter*, a new genus of nonfruiting, gliding bacteria with a high base ratio. Int. J. Syst. Bacteriol. *28:* 367–393.

Kuhn, D.A., D.A. Gregory, G.E. Buchanan, M.D. Nyby and K.E. Daly. 1978. Isolation, characterization, and numerical taxonomy of *Simonsiella* strains from the oral cavities of cats, dogs, sheep, and humans. Arch. Microbiol. *118:* 235–241.

Larkin, J.M. and W.R. Strohl. 1983. *Beggiatoa, Thiothrix,* and *Thioploca.* Annu. Rev. Microbiol. *37:* 341–367.

Reichenbach, H. 1981. Taxonomy of the gliding bacteria. Annu. Rev. Microbiol. *35:* 339–364.

Strohl, W.R., T.M. Schmidt, N.E. Lawry, M.J. Mezzino and J.M. Larkin. 1986. Characterization of *Vitreoscilla beggiatoides* and *Vitreoscilla filiformis* sp. nov., nom. rev., and comparison with *Vitreoscilla stercoraria* and *Beggiatoa alba.* Int. J. Syst. Bacteriol. *36:* 302–313.

ORDER I. **CYTOPHAGALES** LEADBETTER 1974, 99[AL]*

H. REICHENBACH

Cy.to.pha.ga′les. M.L. fem. n. *Cytophaga* type genus of the order; *-ales* ending to denote an order; M.L. fem. pl. n. *Cytophagales* the *Cytophaga* order.

Gram-negative rods, often pleomorphic, **motile by gliding or nonmotile.** usually yellow, orange or red due to cell-bound pigments. Morphologically differentiated resting cells in one genus only.

Chemoorganotrophs, aerobic, facultatively or obligately anaerobic. The **respiratory quinones are exclusively menaquinones. The fatty acid pattern is dominated by branched-chain and 2- and 3-hydroxy acids.**

The mol% G + C of the DNA is 30–66 (Bd, T_m).

Free-living bacteria in terrestrial and marine environments where they are very common and often occur in large numbers. Some may colonize or invade animals or the human body and may become pathogenic under certain circumstances; a few seem restricted to such habitats.

The most conspicuous, quasi-typical representatives of the order are the strictly aerobic, nonfermentative, yellow Gram-negative rods.

Further Comments

Much new data about organisms in the order *Cytophagales* described below and in the 8th edition of the *Manual* have accumulated since 1974. This information allows, for the first time, the presentation of a relatively clear, phylogenetic concept of the group.

The most interesting and momentous achievement has been the establishment, in the past few years, of 16S rRNA catalogs for many of the relevant organisms in this group. Although there are still inconvenient gaps, the published (Ludwig et al., 1983; Woese et al., 1984 a, b; Paster et al., 1985) and unpublished results (E. Stackebrandt and his colleagues, personal communications) allow important conclusions to be drawn, some of which were anticipated on the basis of other more conservative data, whereas others were quite unexpected. A substantial contribution to a better understanding of the taxonomy of the *Flavobacterium-*

Cytophaga complex had been made previously by the technique of DNA/rRNA hybridization (Bauwens and De Ley, 1981).

In several voluminous studies, large collections of organisms belonging to or thought to belong to this group of bacteria have been compared by DNA/DNA hybridization and by phenotypic analysis; these have included the terrestrial and marine *Cytophaga*-like bacteria (CLB) and *Flexibacter* (Christensen, 1973, 1977a; Behrens, 1978; Hirsch, 1980), *Lysobacter* (Christensen and Cook, 1978) and the *Flavobacterium-Cytophaga* complex (Owen and Snell, 1976; Bensoussan, 1977; Hayes, 1977; Price, 1977; Callies, 1979; Callies and Mannheim, 1980; Oyaizu and Komagata, 1981; Jooste, 1985). Although many questions remain, these studies are an essential first step in the direction of a sound taxonomy at the genus and species level. Several new genera that definitely or most likely belong to the *Cytophagales* have been proposed. These include *Capnocytophaga* (Leadbetter et al., 1979), *Chitinophaga* (Sangkhobol and Skerman, 1981), *Sphingobacterium* (Yabuuchi et al., 1981, 1983) and "*Taxeobacter*" (H. Reichenbach, unpublished data) (this is synonymous with the organism Myx 2105 in Paster et al., 1985). Important contributions on the chemical composition of many organisms of the *Cytophagales* have been published, providing essential data for the phenotypic characterization of the group as a whole and of subgroups within it. The new data include the respiratory quinones (Callies and Mannheim, 1978; Mannheim, 1981a; Oyaizu and Komagata, 1981; Collins et al., 1982), the fatty acid spectra (Rosenfelder et al., 1974; Moss and Dees, 1978; Dees et al., 1979, 1982; Holt et al., 1979b; Fautz et al., 1979, 1981; Oyaizu and Komagata, 1981; Collins et al., 1982), sphingolipids (Fritsche, 1975; Asselineau and Pichinoty, 1983; Yano et al., 1983), sulfonolipids (Leadbetter and Godchaux, 1981), pigments (Achenbach et al., 1978, 1981; Reichenbach et al., 1981; Weeks, 1981), and

*AL denotes the inclusion of this name on the Approved Lists of Bacterial Names (1980).

lipopolysaccharides (Sutherland and Smith, 1973; Rosenfelder et al., 1974). In a number of ecological studies, the wide distribution and often great abundance of organisms of the *Flavobacterium-Cytophaga* group in the natural environment and in sewage plants, where they obviously play an important role in the degradation and turnover of organic material, have been demonstrated (Güde, 1978a, b, 1980; Herman, 1978; Mullings and Parish, 1981; Reichardt, 1981; Reichardt et al., 1983; Yoshimizu and Kimura, 1983). These studies are necessarily impeded by the virtually complete absence of a reliable taxonomy and the unavailability of diagnostic keys, in particular of the *Cytophaga-Flexibacter* complex.

From the research cited above, the following taxonomic conclusions can be drawn. All former taxonomic schemes and phylogenetic speculations, including those in the 8th edition of the *Manual* (1974), in *The Prokaryotes* (Starr et al., 1981) and in several reviews (e.g. Soriano, 1973; Reichenbach, 1981) are incorrect: gliding motility has only limited significance as a taxonomically useful characteristic. There is no class *Flexibacteriae* which would collect all gliding bacteria. There is no relationship of any chemotrophic gliding bacterium with the cyanobacteria. Not even the unicellular gliding bacteria belong together, in spite of seemingly convincing chemosystematic conformity: the CLB and *Flexibacter* are not related at all to the myxobacters or to *Lysobacter*. Gliding bacteria appear in at least 7 of the 10 presently recognizable 16S rRNA main groups of the eubacterial genealogical tree. All families united in the order *Cytophagales* in the 8th edition of the *Manual* (1974), with the exception of the *Cytophagaceae*, belong elsewhere in different major groups, so that the order has to be redefined. Also, the genera of the former family *Cytophagaceae* are phylogenetically heterogeneous: *Herpetosiphon* belongs to the *Chloroflexus* group, and *Saprospira* does not appear to be a member of the *Cytophaga* cluster and may be better classified in a separate family and perhaps order.

The CLB together with several other organisms, some of them formerly classified with other groups, form 1 of the 10 main branches of the eubacterial phylogenetic tree. According to our present, still rather sketchy knowledge, the following organisms belong in this main group: the terrestrial and marine CLB, i.e. *Cytophaga*-like gliding bacteria with a mol% G + C of the DNA between 30 and 40; *Sporocytophaga myxococcoides*; *Flexibacter filiformis*; not unexpectedly, most of the species of *Flavobacterium* with a low mol% G + C ; most species of *Bacteroides* and some species of *Fusobacterium*; *Haliscomenobacter hydrossis*; *Saprospira grandis*; new, gliding *"Taxeobacter ocellatus"* (organism Myx 2105: Paster et al., 1985; H. Reichenbach, unpublished data); and a new anaerobic, flexible gliding rod, organism Pl-12fs (Paster et al., 1985; K. O. Stetter, unpublished data). *Capnocytophaga*, *Chitinophaga*, *Flexithrix* and *Sphingobacterium* are almost certainly additional members of the group.

The main groups in the genealogical tree of the eubacteria must be regarded to be equivalent to at least a whole phylum (Woese et al., 1984a, b), so that it is to be anticipated that not all organisms mentioned above can be united within a single order. This is also suggested by the rather low S_{AB} values found between several members of the group and by the distribution of signature sequences in the 16S rRNA catalogs, in addition to the phenetic differences. However, at the moment we do not yet know enough to clearly recognize the boundaries of the order *Cytophagales* or to define other orders. Also, it must be assumed that several more organisms will join the group in the near future, further differentiating the picture. Thus, to avoid later confusion, I shall try to define families where reasonably well-characterized subgroups become discernible, restrict the order *Cytophagales* essentially to two families which appear fairly closely related, and leave the remaining families and genera unconnected until more information is available.

Although this new taxonomy is now on a phylogenetically sound basis, we are left with the formidable, as yet largely unsolved task of finding new distinguishing phenotypic characteristics. In Table 23.1, characteristics are listed which may be useful in recognizing an organism as a member of the main group and of the order *Cytophagales*.

Table 23.1.

*Characteristics shared by organisms of the **Cytophaga-Flavobacterium-Bacteroides** 16S rRNA main group[a,b]*

Characteristic	Cytophagales[c]
Gram-negative	+
Unicellular rods	+[d]
Pleomorphic	d[e]
Gliding or nonmotile[f]	+
Fatty acid pattern dominated by	
Branched-chain acids[g]	+
2- and 3-Hydroxy acids[g]	+
Sphingolipids[h]	D
Sulfonolipids[i]	D
Menaquinones only[g]	+
Cell-bound pigments[j]	+
Strictly aerobic	+[k]
Strictly anaerobic	−

[a]In addition to S_{AB} values, the group members are recognized by characteristic oligonucleotide signatures in their 16S rRNA; e.g. the 3′-end terminates with CCAYAA; in all other organisms, however, it terminates with CCAYUA.

[b]Symbols: +, 90% or more of strains are positive; d, 11–89% of strains are positive; −, 90% or more of strains are negative; and D, different reactions in different taxa.

[c]The order as defined here comprises the families *Cytophagaceae* and *Flavobacteriaceae* including *Capnocytophaga*, *Flexithrix* and *Sphingobacterium* and the presently still isolated genera *Flexibacter* and *Microscilla*.

[d]The exceptions are: gliding *Saprospira* with screw-shaped multicellular filaments and nonmotile *Haliscomenobacter* with sheathed multicellular filaments. *Flexithrix* may, under certain conditions, form sheathed multicellular filaments.

[e]In addition, at least three organisms show a life cycle connected with a cellular shape change: *Sporocytophaga* forms spherical resting cells; *Flexibacter* may produce long agile thread cells in young cultures and short nonmotile rods in old ones; and *Flexithrix* grows as very long, sometimes sheathed filaments which shed gliding rods.

[f]Several gliding organisms have nonmotile stages (see Footnote e), and all glide only under certain environmental conditions. It thus seems conceivable that gliding will be demonstrated for several more of the nonmotile members. More important, however, are that no flagellated bacteria have been found so far to belong to this group and that no bacterium is known to glide at one time and to be flagellated at another.

[g]The fatty acid and quinone patterns have not yet been determined for all organisms of the group, but a sufficiently large number have been investigated so that the generalizations seem justified.

[h]Sphingolipids are known from certain flavobacteria *(Sphingobacterium)* and from *Bacteroides*.

[i]A special type of sulfonolipid, the capnoid, a kind of sphingolipid, seems to be common in *Cytophaga*, *Sporocytophaga* and *Flexibacter*. Capnoids are not found in gliding bacteria, but are found in unrelated *Beggiatoa*, *Vitreoscilla*, *Herpetosiphon* and *Lysobacter*.

[j]Virtually all members of the *Cytophagales* are, more or less, yellow to red. The pigments seem always to be carotenoids (mainly zeaxanthin, saproxanthin and flexixanthin) and/or flexirubin type pigments, but it must be emphasized that only a relatively few organisms have been thoroughly investigated. Organisms from outside the two families often are pink to brick red; in *Saprospira*, this color is due to the carotenoid saproxanthin.

[k]The few anaerobically growing species are facultative anaerobes or at least not particularly sensitive to oxygen, such as *Capnocytophaga*.

Key to the families and genera of the **Cytophagales**

1. Short to moderately long, more or less delicate rods, with the longer ones flexible; gliding; usually bright to golden yellow, rarely pink to red; strictly aerobic or facultatively anaerobic; probably all degrade some kinds of biomacromolecules like gelatin, starch, cellulose, pectin, agar and chitin; free-living in terrestrial and marine habitats, some may colonize fish; the mol% G + C of the DNA is 30–40.
   A. Family I. *Cytophagaceae*, p. 2013
   B. Other genera: *Flexibacter*, p. 2061
   Microscilla, p. 2071
   Chitinophaga, p. 2074
2. Short to moderately long rods; nonmotile, not gliding; yellow to orange; sometimes, however, rather pale; strictly aerobic, nonfermentative; many cannot degrade starch; free-living in terrestrial and marine environments, several live in humans and animals, are often found in clinical specimens, and may (rarely) become pathogenic; the mol% G + C of the DNA is 32–42.
   Family *"Flavobacteriaceae"*
   (*Flavobacterium* and its relationship to *Cytophaga* is discussed in Volume 1 of the *Manual*)
3. Strictly anaerobic, nonmotile, pleomorphic rods; these organisms live in the intestinal tract of humans.
   Family *Bacteroidaceae*
   (16S rRNA oligonucleotide cataloging indicates a relationship between *Bacteroides* and the *Flavobacterium-Cytophaga* group (Paster et al., 1985). The *Bacteroidaceae* appear in Volume 1 of the *Manual*.)
4. Genera of uncertain affiliation
   a. Screw-shaped multicellular filaments; gliding; unpigmented or pink to red; strictly aerobic; free-living in marine and freshwater habitats; the mol% G + C of the DNA is 35–48.
      Genus *Saprospira*, p. 2077
   b. Short to moderately long cylindrical rods with rounded ends, delicate in young cultures, but often expanding considerably later on, so that the population become pleomorphic; gliding; brick red; strictly aerobic; degrade biomacromolecules like gelatin, starch and chitin; free-living in soil; the mol% G + C of the DNA is 57–66.
      Genus *"Taxeobacter"*
      (This genus has not yet been formally proposed and is not treated in this edition of the *Manual*.)
   c. Straight thin rods, usually in chains, surrounded by a hyaline sheath; pink; nonmotile, not gliding; strictly aerobic; very common in activated sludge; the mol% G + C of the DNA is 49.
      Genus *Haliscomenobacter*
      (*Haliscomenobacter* is described in "Section 22, Sheathed Bacteria.")
   d. Strictly anaerobic; this organism is a gliding flexible rod.
      Organism Pl-12fs
(This organism has not been formally named and is not treated in this edition of the *Manual;* for further information consult Paster et al. (1985).)

Further Reading

Holdeman, L.V., R.W. Kelley and W.E.C. Moore. 1984. Genus I. *Bacteroides* Castellani and Chalmers 1919, 959. *In* Krieg and Holt (Editors), Bergey's Manual of Systematic Bacteriology, vol. 1. The Williams and Wilkins Co., Baltimore, pp. 604–631.
Holmes, B., R.J. Owen and T.A. McMeekin. 1984. Genus *Flavobacterium* Bergey, Harrison, Breed, Hammer and Huntoon 1923, 97. *In* Krieg and Holt (Editors), Bergey's Manual of Systematic Bacteriology, vol. 1. The Williams and Wilkins Co., Baltimore, pp. 353–361.
McMeekin, T.A. and J.M. Shewan. 1978. Taxonomic strategies for *Flavobacterium* and related genera. J. Appl. Bacteriol. *45:* 321–332.
Reichenbach, H. 1981. Taxonomy of the gliding bacteria. Annu. Rev. Microbiol. *35:* 339–364.
Reichenbach, H. and M. Dworkin. 1981. Introduction to the gliding bacteria. *In*

Starr, Stolp, Trüper, Balows and Schlegel (Editors), The Prokaryotes. A Handbook on Habitats, Isolation, and Identification of Bacteria. Springer-Verlag, Berlin, pp. 315–327.
Reichenbach, H. and M. Dworkin. 1981. The order *Cytophagales* (with addenda on the genera *Herpetosiphon, Saprospira,* and *Flexithrix*). *In* Starr, Stolp, Trüper, Balows and Schlegel (Editors), The Prokaryotes. A Handbook on Habitats, Isolation, and Identification of Bacteria. Springer-Verlag, Berlin, pp. 356–379.
Reichenbach, H. and O.B. Weeks (Editors). 1981. The *Flavobacterium-Cytophaga* Group. Verlag Chemie, Weinheim, F.R.G.
Shewan, J.M. and T.A. McMeekin 1983. Taxonomy (and ecology) of *Flavobacterium* and related genera. Annu. Rev. Microbiol. *37:* 233–252.
Weeks, O.B. 1981. The genus *Flavobacterium*. *In* Starr, Stolp, Trüper, Balows and Schlegel (Editors), The Prokaryotes. A Handbook on Habitats, Isolation, and Identification of Bacteria. Springer-Verlag, Berlin, pp. 1365–1370.

FAMILY I. **CYTOPHAGACEAE** STANIER 1940, 630,[AL] EMEND.

H. Reichenbach

Cy.to.pha.ga'ce.ae. M.L. fem. n. *Cytophaga* type genus of the family; *-aceae* ending to denote a family; M.L. fem. pl. n. *Cytophagaceae* the *Cytophaga* family.

Very **short to elongated rod-shaped cells,** the longer ones flexible, with rounded or tapered ends. Usually cells of different length are found in a single culture which thus often appears more or less pleomorphic. In one genus, very long filaments are also formed. **Gliding,** but nonmotile stages may occur. Spherical resting cells (microcysts) in one genus. Almost always pigmented, often very brightly so, usually **yellow,** rarely pink or red, always due to cell-bound pigments, which **often show a color shift** from yellow to shades of red, brown or purple

when the colonies are flooded **with alkali** (flexirubin type pigments).

Chemoorganotrophs, usually strictly aerobic, several species facultatively anaerobic or capnophilic. Virtually all are able to **degrade** one or several kinds of **biomacromolecules** such as proteins (e.g. milk casein, gelatin and keratin), starch, dextran, yeast cell-wall glucans, cellulose, pectin, agar or chitin. Many of them may also grow on simple defined media, e.g. with glucose and NH_4^+.

Very common in soil, freshwater, sewage plants, and seacoast habitats. Some may colonize fish and be pathogenic; one has been found to be allergenic for humans; several live in the mouth cavity of humans, may invade the body, and become pathogenic.

The mol% G + C of the DNA is 30-40.

Type genus: *Cytophaga* Winogradsky 1929, 577.

Further Comments

The family, as it is defined above, is once again very close to its original definition by Stanier (1940). The difference is the inclusion of the genera *Sporocytophaga, Capnocytophaga* and *Flexithrix,* with the latter two not known in 1940. As mentioned in the discussion of the order *Cytopagales,* there is now clear proof from RNA data that the other organisms classified with the family *Cytophagaceae* in the 8th edition of the *Manual* (1974) do not belong there.

Because of a shape change during microcyst formation which is very similar to that observed in *Myxococcus,* combined with gliding motility, *Sporocytophaga* was thought for some time to be a myxobacter. Its totally different G + C content, the presence of flexirubin type pigments (Reichenbach et al., 1981) and of capnoids (Godchaux and Leadbetter, 1983), and the recently demonstrated close correspondence between its 16S rRNA catalog and that of *Cytophaga johnsonae* (Paster et al., 1985) show unequivocally that its place is with the *Cytophaga*-like bacteria (CLB).

Although one would like to see DNA/rRNA hybridization data and an analysis of 16S rRNA catalogs, there seems to be little risk to include the genus *Capnocytophaga* in the family: gliding motility, cell morphology and composition, physiology, and G + C range would be well in agreement (e.g. Collins et al., 1982).

The case is less clear with *Flexithrix,* however, since less is known about this organism. Gliding motility, presence of zeaxanthin, and a G + C in the proper range may justify a tentative inclusion of the genus in the *Cytophagaceae.*

Gliding has been retained as a distinguishing characteristic of the family, separating it from the nonmotile, nongliding "*Flavobacteriaceae*" which otherwise resemble the *Cytophagaceae* in many respects, e.g. in their possession of capnoid lipids (Godchaux and Leadbetter, 1983) and flexirubin type pigments (Achenbach et al., 1981; Reichenbach et al., 1981; Weeks, 1981) as well as in their G + C range. The DNA/rRNA hybridization data (Bauwens and De Ley, 1981) and the 16S rRNA catalogs (Paster et al., 1985) show that the CLB form a cluster of relatively closely related organisms, clearly separated from the more heterogeneous flavobacteria. It is true that the CLB cluster also comprises four species of *Flavobacterium,* or perhaps "strains" would be the better term. This is not really a contradiction, however, since *F. pectinovorum* (Christensen, 1977b) and *F. uliginosum* (type strain ATCC 14397, personal observations) are unquestionably gliding bacteria and should probably be classified as *Cytophaga* species.

The case of *F. aquatile* is somewhat complicated (Holmes and Owen, 1979). It appears that the original strain as well as the lectotype and the quasi-neotype strain Taylor F36 (ATCC 11947) are gliding bacteria (Mitchell et al., 1967; Perry, 1973). On the other hand, it has been stated that at least some cells of strain F36 bear a flagellum (Webster and Hugh, 1979), although it seems that active swimming motions have not been observed. Could these flagella have been slime trails, as are sometimes observed on cells of gliding bacteria? Contrary to earlier reports, strain F36 contains menaquinones (Mannheim, 1981b), so that it could indeed be a *Cytophaga.*

The fourth case is also controversial at the moment. The type strain ATCC 15997 of *F. tirrenicum* is flagellated and motile beyond doubt (personal observation), as it should be according to the species description. It thus does not fit at all into the picture, and it would be very important to make sure that the DNA/rRNA hybridization data which suggest its relationship with the *Cytophaga-Flavobacterium* complex have been obtained with this strain.

As in the 8th edition of the *Manual,* several old genera of organisms belonging more or less clearly into the CLB are not found here among the *Cytophagaceae* because these genera must be regarded as invalid for various reasons. Authors studying an apparently new organism should, however, be aware of this literature to be in a position to do justice to the often careful work of earlier scientists. "*Promyxobacterium*" Imshenetski and Solntseva 1945 was created for nonfruiting gliding bacteria having cylindrical cells with rounded ends, in contrast with *Cytophaga* which was supposed to possess cells with tapered ends. The colonies of different strains were colorless, yellow, orange, pink, red, green or violet. It appears that quite different organisms were lumped together, including species of *Cytophaga, Lysobacter* and "*Taxeobacter.*" The descriptions are not precise enough to recognize the two described species again with certainty. A neotype is available for *P. flavum* and is discussed in connection with the genus *Cytophaga.* "*Flexiscilla*" Pringsheim 1951, found in decaying freshwater algae, seems to have been a facultatively anaerobic CLB. The only species had cells with tapered ends, 12-14 μm, and was never obtained in pure culture. Genus and species were regarded as provisional by Pringsheim himself. "*Bactoscilla*" Pringsheim 1951, with one species, formed gliding articulated chains of long slender rods, 0.4 μm wide. Isolated from freshwater, it was never kept in pure culture but seems to be different from any other described species. Its taxonomic position is obscure. This genus, too, was regarded by Pringsheim as provisional. "*Sphaerocytophaga*" Gräf 1961, with slender gliding rods, formed yellow colonies. It was isolated from the oral cavity of a human and grew only under anaerobic conditions, although it was not particularly sensitive to oxygen. The organism was assumed to be connected with occasional pathological conditions in the mouth and perhaps is identical with organisms later described as *Capnocytophaga.* "*Sphaeromyxa*" Bauer 1962, with slender gliding rods, was strictly aerobic, formed greenish-yellow colonies, and was found to be very common in sewage plants. The characteristic that distinguished it from other CLB was "spheroids" into which the rod cells transformed themselves in older cultures. These spheroids were evidently spheroplasts and thus of no taxonomic consequence. The organism was probably a *Cytophaga* species.

The genus *Flexibacter* Soriano 1945 (see also Soriano, 1947) was heterogeneous but comprises several organisms that are still more or less clearly recognizable (for details, see "Other Genera" for the genus *Flexibacter*). "*F. giganteus*" is almost certainly identical with *Herpetosiphon,* perhaps even the species *aurantiacus.* "*F. albuminosus*" was perhaps a *Lysobacter,* and "*F. aureus*" was probably a *Cytophaga.* The proposed type species, *F. flexilis,* seems not to be typical enough in its cell and colony morphology to be reliably identified, but "*F. elegans*" can be recognized rather clearly by its highly unusual cell form and extreme agility described quite appropriately by Soriano. "*F. elegans*" would therefore have been a better choice as the neotype species of the genus. Soriano's (but not Lewin's) "*F. elegans*" is very probably identical with organisms that have been studied during the past decade in several laboratories under the designation *Flexibacter* species and "*F. elegans.*" These organisms, however, show a cyclic change in cell morphology *not* described by Soriano. If all these bacteria are really identical, "*F. elegans*" Soriano would thus correspond to or be closely related to "*Myxococcus filiformis*" Solntseva 1940 and the recently described *Chitinophaga pinensis* Sankhobol and Skerman 1981. As already discussed in connection with the order *Cytophagales, Flexibacter* is removed from the family *Cytophagaceae* and provisionally classified as an isolated genus. It probably belongs in a family of its own. Marine *Microscilla* Pringsheim 1951 resembles *Flexibacter* in its cell morphology; some strains studied by Lewin (1969) also come close to "*F. elegans*" in their G + C values. *Microscilla* is therefore tentatively regarded as a genus related to *Flexibacter.*

The central problem of the family remains the subdivision of the genus *Cytophaga.* This problem still is essentially unresolved, in spite of considerable efforts in recent years (Christensen, 1973, 1977b; Behrens, 1978; Hirsch, 1980; Oyaizu and Komagata, 1981; Reichardt et al., 1983). The rather wide mol% G + C of the DNA of 30-45 already suggests that the genus is heterogeneous. This notion is further substantiated by DNA/DNA hybridizations which in many combinations are very weak or near 0 (Behrens, 1978; Pyle and Shotts, 1981). For example, NCIB strains 9059 and 10150 of *C. johnsonae* hybridize at 28% (with the same

method, intraspecies hybridization would be 75-100%) and thus can hardly belong in the same genus (H. Behrens, unpublished observations). The different collection strains designated as *C. johnsonae* do not even cluster particularly close together in the numerical analysis of phenotype data (Oyaizu and Komagata, 1981).

Although there is no doubt that the genus has to be broken up, difficulties arise because a clear delimitation of the individual species and their reliable phenotypic characterization is, with a few exceptions, presently out of reach. Before a revision of the genus can be made, a much larger number of strains has to be compared under inclusion of the powerful methods of molecular taxonomy. For the moment we can only fix the recognized species by naming generally available type strains. They are the only reliable references for further studies because the published phenotypic characterization of these "species" is hardly ever corroborated by a thorough comparative study, so that the reliability of the proposed distinguishing characteristics is usually doubtful. Although it is thus not justifiable to subdivide the genus now, I propose tentative subgenera to introduce some kind of structure into the genus, which can then be refined later. For this provisional subdivision of the genus, the following strategy has been adopted. The type species of the genus *Cytophaga* is the cellulose degrader, *C. hutchinsonii*, for which the genus had originally been created by Winogradsky (1929). The genus *Cytophaga* will be reserved for cellulose decomposers related to *C. hutchinsonii*. The species

has an unusually high mol% G + C of the DNA of 39, which sets it well apart from the remaining CLB, for those mostly show mol% G + C values around 34. This, as well as the case of *C. johnsonae* mentioned above, seems to indicate that a simple division of the genus on the basis of whether an organism is able or not to degrade polysaccharides, as proposed in the 8th edition of the *Manual*, may not be sufficient. As the degradative capabilities of CLB seem nevertheless to be characteristic for certain groups, they, together with the G + C values, are used as a first approach to the definition of subgenera. Further, ecological facts are considered in the subdivision of the genus, for it appears that at least the boundary between terrestrial and marine habitats is not easily crossed: DNA/rRNA hybridization (Bauwens and De Ley, 1981) and 16S rRNA data (Paster et al., 1985) show a clear separation of terrestrial and marine CLB, and the same is suggested by the distribution of flexirubin type pigments, which are very common in terrestrial CLB but which are only exceptionally found in strains isolated from marine environments (Reichenbach et al., 1981). Finally, chemosystematic data are exploited. The pattern of respiratory quinones particularly appears useful for the purpose of subdividing CLB (Callies and Mannheim, 1978; Oyaizu and Komagata, 1981).

Further Reading

See under "Order *Cytophagales.*"

Key to the genera of the family **Cytophagaceae** *and other genera*

I. Morphologically differentiated resting cells are not produced.
- A. Short to elongated (i.e. typically <15 μm in length) gliding rods
  - 1. Strictly aerobic, rarely facultatively anaerobic free-living species of terrestrial and marine habitats, with some colonizing fish
    - Genus I. *Cytophaga*, p. 2015
  - 2. Capnophilic, do not grow under a normal atmosphere; only known from the oral cavity of humans
    - Genus II. *Capnocytophaga*, p. 2050
- B. Very long (i.e. up to 50–100 μm or longer) gliding or nonmotile filaments
  - 1. Freshwater or soil organisms
    - Other genus *Flexibacter*, p. 2061
  - 2. Marine organisms
    - a. Sheaths not produced
      - Other genus *Microscilla*, p. 2071
    - b. Sheaths may be produced
      - Genus III. *Flexithrix*, p. 2058
II. Resting cells (microcysts) being produced
- A. Cellulose degrader
  - Genus IV. *Sporocytophaga*, p. 2061
- B. Chitin degrader
  - Other genus *Chitinophaga*, p. 2074

Genus I. **Cytophaga** *Winogradsky 1929, 577,*[AL] *emend.*

H. REICHENBACH

Cy. to′pha.ga. Gr. n. *cytos* vessel, container, cell, cell wall; Gr. n. *phagos* eater, devourer; M.L. fem. n. *Cytophaga* devourer of cell walls, i.e. cellulose digester.

Very short to moderately long rods, 0.3-0.8 × 1.5-15 μm, only rarely longer, with rounded or slightly tapered ends. The longer rods are **flexible.** Resting stages not known. **Motile by gliding. Gramnegative.**

On solid media with a low nutrient content (e.g. below 0.1% peptone), the **colonies are spreading swarms,** sometimes penetrating the agar, often very delicate and occasionally with a reddish or greenish iridescence. On substrates with a higher nutrient content (e.g. above 0.3% peptone), the colonies usually become compact, often convex, with a smooth or wavy edge, sometimes sunken into the agar.

Cell mass usually more or less intensely pigmented, **yellow, orange or red,** due to cell-bound carotenoids, flexirubin type pigments, or both. When covered with alakali (e.g. 20% KOH solution: flexirubin reaction), colonies may reversibly change their color from yellow to purple- or redbrown. Unpigmented species or strains also occur.

Strict aerobes or facultative anaerobes. Some may use NO_3^- as terminal electron acceptor.

Chemoorganotrophs. Metabolism respiratory or fermentative. In the latter case, acetate, propionate and succinate may be produced. Organic acids may, however, also arise during growth of strictly aerobic strains, particularly on sugar-containing media. All **decompose** one or several kinds of **organic macromolecules,** mainly various proteins and polysaccharides, including cellulose, agar, chitin, pectin and starch.

Optimum temperature: 20–35°C. Optimum pH: around 7.

Organisms common in soil, decomposing organic matter, freshwater and marine habitats.

The mol% G + C of the DNA is 30–45, with the mol% G + C of many strains occurring around 35.

Type species: *Cytophaga hutchinsonii* Winogradsky 1929, 578.

Further Descriptive Information

This is a rather heterogeneous assembly of organisms which certainly do not belong in one single genus (see "Taxonomic Comments"). In addition, as a consequence of a repeatedly modified taxonomic concept, the term *Cytophaga* has been used in the past with variable meanings and not always very critically, so that reports in the literature sometimes refer to organisms which may have been only remotely related with the old core of the genus, the aerobic cellulose degraders. It may thus be better to speak of *Cytophaga*-like bacteria (CLB) rather than of *Cytophaga* in the sense of a well-established genus. This group is very important ecologically because of their wide distribution, their large populations in nature, and their diversified and often unusual degradative capabilities. These organisms call for more thorough investigation!

Cell morphology. The cells of the CLB are rod-shaped, sometimes very short (≤1 µm), and usually moderately long (5–10 µm), although occasionally they are somewhat longer (15–20 µm). They may be stout but are more often slender, rather delicate, and almost rigid (Humphrey et al., 1979) to extremely flexible (e.g. *C. hutchinsonii*). Under phase-contrast microscopy they appear dark to light gray. The poles may be rounded or more or less tapering. The cell populations tend to be relatively uniform, at least much less pleomorphic than cultures of *Flexibacter*, and then mainly in later culture stages. Shape and particularly size may vary with the growth phase and the composition of the medium (see, for example, Stanier, 1947; Follett and Webley, 1965; Pacha and Porter, 1968; van der Meulen et al., 1974; Humphrey and Marshall, 1980; and Liebert et al., 1984). Thus cells from vigorously growing cultures tend to be longer than those from slowly growing or resting cultures. For example, *C. johnsonae* may become almost coccoid in stationary phase. Another, unclassified CLB averaged 6 µm during log phase and 2.2 µm during stationary phase. Still another measured 3.5 µm on nutrient agar, 4.4 µm in nutrient broth, and 8.9 µm in 1% peptone water (after 24 h at 23°C). It should be emphasized that this variability is minor in comparison with that observed with many *Flexibacter* strains. Only in late log or stationary phase cultures of CLB are very long threads often observed (see Fig. 23.6). These threads are, however, incompletely divided cells or cryptic cell chains with an irregular and somewhat broken contour. They are typically nonmotile and obviously result from a disturbance of cell growth and division, a phenomenon known from many bacteria and totally different from the thread cells in young *Flexibacter* cultures (Fig. 23.1). Also, certain types of nonmotile mutants of *C. johnsonae* have been found to grow in long filaments (Chang et al., 1984).

Many CLB are rather fragile and readily form spheroplasts. Although the phenomenon had already been observed and correctly interpreted by Winogradsky (1929), it created considerable confusion in the past because these spheroplasts were sometimes mistaken for microcysts. Several species and genera have been founded on this assumption: "*Sphaerocytophaga filiformis*" and "*S. fusiformis*" (Gräf, 1962), "*Sphaeromyxa xanthochlora*" (Bauer, 1962), and "*Sporocytophaga cauliformis*" (Gräf, 1962; Gräf and Stürzenhofecker, 1964). With *C. hutchinsonii* (and *Sporocytophaga myxococcoides*), the formation of spheroplasts could also be induced by incubation with penicillin, but efforts to stabilize them with 10% saccharose were not successful (Verma and Martin, 1967a). Spheroplasts and microcysts can usually be distinguished easily because the former lyse upon exposure to 0.04% sodium dodecyl sulfate and are often dark—or, at least, not bright—under phase contrast. The latter are resistant to elevated temperatures (up to about 60°C) and short bursts of ultrasound and can germinate. Recently, the formation of very peculiar coccoid cells of 0.8–1.2 µm in diameter in cultures of *C. johnsonae* which were starving at suboptimal temperatures has been described (Reichardt and Morita, 1982b). Although showing morphological and fine structural properties of spheroplasts, these cells were viable; had a slightly increased heat resistance compared with that of ordinary cells (thermal death point: 40 vs. 38°C); and when supplied with nutrients, grew out again into rods. Branched cells also have occasionally been observed with CLB (Garnjobst, 1945; Stanier, 1947). Their origin is obviously accidental, but they may still be motile.

The *fine structure of CLB* has been studied on only relatively few ex-

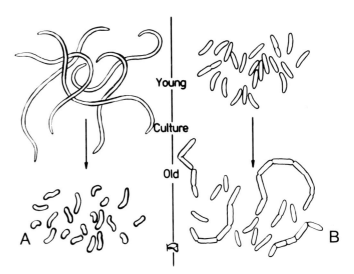

Figure 23.1. Morphological changes typical for many *Flexibacter (A)* and *Cytophaga (B)* species in aging cultures.

amples, mainly *C. johnsonae* and *C. columnaris (Flexibacter columnaris* or *Chondrococcus columnaris)*. The outer surface of CLB as shown by shadowing or negative contrast is unusual in that it appears granular, crenated or undulated, i.e. covered by a system of small cushionlike knobs or folds (Follett and Webley, 1965; van der Meulen at el., 1974; Bovallius, 1979; Humphrey et al., 1979; Strohl, 1979; Oyaizu et al., 1982; Reichardt and Morita, 1982b). This pattern seems to be typical for CLB, and interestingly it has also been observed on *Flavobacterium aquatile* (Follett and Webley, 1965) and *F. heparinum*, but it has not been observed on "flavobacteria" with a high mol% G + C (Oyaizu et al., 1982).

The cells may be surrounded by a thin, unstructured, more or less compact *slime layer*, or fine strands or fibrils may be seen radiating from the cell surface and connecting neighboring rods (Follett and Webley, 1965; Pate and Ordal, 1967b; Strohl and Tait, 1978; Bovallius, 1979; Humphrey et al., 1979; Strohl, 1979). Usually little or no slime is produced in liquid cultures, but when *C. hutchinsonii* (and *Sporocytophaga myxococcoides*) is grown in mineral salts medium containing 0.5% glucose, the cells are embedded in a dense network of slime fibrils. Also, *C. fermentans* may produce large quantities of slime (Collins, 1964). The unit fibril is about 3 nm wide. In some cases, the cells cannot be harvested by centrifugation unless the slime is precipitated with 10% $(NH_4)_2SO_4$ or is removed with diethylene glycol/water (1:1) or by repeated washing with 3% NaCl solution (Collins, 1964; Follett and Webley, 1965; Verma and Martin, 1967a, b). Sometimes, but not always (Humphrey et al., 1979), the slime is stainable by ruthenium red and thus can be assumed to be an acidic polysaccharide. For example, this is true of *C. columnaris* (Pate and Ordal, 1967b), but this organism also appears to produce, perhaps only under certain conditions, a second type of slime, a linear α-(1→4)-poly-D-galactosamine with half of the units *N*-acetylated (Johnson and Chilton, 1966). The slime of *C. hutchinsonii* seems to be an acidic heteropolysaccharide consisting of xylose, arabinose, mannose, glucose and glucuronic acid (Verma and Martin, 1967b). Efforts to digest this slime by using a variety of glycan hydrolases were without success (Martin et al., 1968). Slime of *C. fermentans* was found to contain glucose, glucosamine, mannose and rhamnose (Collins, 1964). In another, unclassified CLB, the slime appears to be a glycoprotein with 30% protein and with glucose, galactose and fucose as the sugar components (Humphrey et al., 1979). The slime probably plays a role during gliding as a temporary Stefan adhesive which allows easy translational motions but still keeps the cell attached to the surface. Calculations based on the rheological properties of isolated slime with a Newtonian viscosity of $\eta = 0.03$ Nsm^{-2} showed that horizontal drag would, indeed, remain 5 orders of magnitude below the force required to detach the cell (Humphrey et al., 1979).

Particularly when viewed in negative contrast, the cells of CLB are usually surrounded by substantial quantities of still another, quite differently appearing material: vesicles, coarse strands and uneven tubules which seem to be extruded from the cell and may become 0.5 µm long. These structures are contained by a unit membrane, which obviously derives from the outer membrane of the cell wall, and may be regarded as excessive extensions of the cushionlike surface structures mentioned above (Follett and Webley, 1965; Pate et al., 1967; Pate and Ordal, 1967a; Martin et al., 1968; Oyaizu et al., 1982). Indeed, *lipopolysaccharide* (LPS) components can be demonstrated within them, e.g. 2-keto-3-deoxyoctonate (Humphrey et al., 1979). Isolated and purified LPS from several CLB resembled essentially that of other Gram-negative bacteria (Sutherland and Smith, 1973). LPS yields are 0.4–3.4% of the dry weight. The predominant sugars are mannose, galactose, glucose, ribose, glucosamine and galactosamine; some cells also contain rhamnose. Although 2-keto-3-deoxyoctonate always seemed to be present, heptose was probably completely lacking in these cases, although in another CLB analyzed recently, heptose constituted fully one third of the carbohydrate of isolated endotoxin (Flaherty et al., 1984b). As the amino sugars remain after removal of the lipid A component, they seem also to be an integral part of the polysaccharide itself. Appendages resembling the stranded material discussed above have also been found on cells of *Flavobacterium aquatile* ATCC 11947 (but not on *F. meningosepticum*) and may have been mistaken earlier for flagella (Webster and Hugh, 1979; Thomson et al., 1981).

The cell wall of CLB is, in principle, typically Gram-negative but shows two peculiarities. One is that the outer membrane appears to be more flexible than usual. This may be of importance for gliding motility, allowing a close contact between cell surface and substrate (Humphrey et al., 1979), and perhaps the transmission of deformations of the cell body by the still-unknown machinery for locomotion. In cross-sections the outer membrane is usually somewhat wavy (Follett and Webley, 1965; Pate and Ordal, 1967a) which would be in accordance with the surface structures discussed above. Artifacts are possible, however, and a complete detachment of the outer membrane and opening of a very wide periplasmic gap would hardly reflect the natural state. In fact, it seems that the classical Ryter-Kellenberger fixation is not well-tolerated by CLB, resulting in a destabilization of membranes and ribosomes. Prefixation with glutaraldehyde gives apparently more reliable results and pictures similar to those of other Gram-negative bacteria (Pate and Ordal, 1967a). The second peculiarity are structures that may be connected with gliding motility. In *C. columnaris*, bundles of parallel fibrils with a triangular cross-section have been demonstrated. The fibrils are 10 nm wide and 16 nm apart, run directly under the outer membrane to which they are obviously attached, and form a steep helix around the rod cell, passing over the poles (Pate and Ordal, 1967b). The fibrils are lacking in nonmotile mutants (Glaser and Pate, 1973). In freeze-etch pictures of the same organism, small spherical particles 10–11 nm in diameter are seen on the inner surface of the outer membrane. When the cells are first fixed with glutaraldehyde, these particles appear arranged in lines, so that the fibrillar aspect could be a fixation artifact (Burchard and Brown, 1973). Further, small ring-shaped structures have been isolated from *C. columnaris* and *C. johnsonae* during an (unsuccessful) effort to extract actin-like proteins from these gliders (Pate and Chang, 1979). These rings are 20 nm across and 10 or, as double rings, 20 nm thick. They show a strong tendency to aggregate in the form of sheets or stacks and appear to be located in the cell surface, although their exact position remains to be determined. It has been proposed that these rings might be related to the ring structures at the base of flagella and would rotate, thereby propelling the cell.

The *peptidoglycan layer* is well distinguishable and 3–5 nm thick (Pate and Ordal, 1967a). The sacculus of *C. hutchinsonii* (and *Sporocytophaga myxococcoides*) could be isolated and appears to have a structure very similar to that of the enterobacteria, with 2,6-diaminopimelic acid as the diamino acid and a cross-linkage of about 70% (Verma and Martin, 1967a, b; Verma, 1970).

In *C. columnaris* the *cytoplasmic membrane* is 6.5 nm thick and asymmetric, with the outer leaflet staining more intensely (Pate and Ordal, 1967a). The membrane may fold in and form extended *intracytoplasmic membrane systems*—large membrane bodies bounded by a unit membrane and containing a sequence of concentric double membranes, with each consisting of two unit membranes attached to one another by their inner leaflet. The whole system may be connected to the cytoplasmic membrane via a stalklike membrane cylinder but apparently only rarely near a transverse septum. Intracytoplasmic membrane systems have also been found in other CLB (van der Meulen et al., 1974; Humphrey et al., 1979; Strohl, 1979). The "mesosomes" of *C. columnaris* are very labile structures. After Ryter-Kellenberger fixation, they appear as a system of convoluted tubes, and when the cells lyse or are broken, they are transformed into rod-shaped particles 30 nm wide and 50–1500 nm long and show an internal channel with periodic constrictions at a distance of 40 nm. In cross-section the particles show 12 globular subunits sitting on a central ring (Pate et al., 1967). These membrane particles have been named "rhapidosomes," but true rhapidosomes as defined for *Saprospira grandis* (Lewin, 1963) have a different structure and are, in fact, tails of defective phages (Reichenbach, 1967). The membrane particles of *C. columnaris* consist of lipid and protein in a similar pattern as found in the cytoplasmic membrane, only with fewer types of proteins (Kuhrt and Pate, 1973).

During cell division, well-developed *transverse septa* may be seen (Pate and Ordal, 1967a; Strohl and Tait, 1978; Liebert et al., 1984). In *C. columnaris*, small dense lamellar bodies of unknown composition have been very rarely found within cells (Pate and Ordal, 1967b). *Reserve material* or other kinds of inclusion bodies seem not to occur in CLB. CLB do not appear to produce fimbriae.

There are several studies on the *fatty acid composition* of CLB, often on a comparative basis with a taxonomic purpose (Walker, 1969; Fautz et al., 1979, 1981; Oyaizu and Komagata, 1981; Oyaizu et al., 1982; Yabuuchi and Moss, 1982; Godchaux and Leadbetter, 1984; Liebert et al., 1984). Although in detail the data are often somewhat at variance due to differences in the applied analytical techniques and the use of different strains of a specific taxon, still several generalizations can safely be made. The fatty acid pattern is always dominated by branched fatty acids, as was noted in the first study on fatty acids of a *Cytophaga* species, viz. *C. hutchinsonii* (Walker, 1969). The branch is usually at the penultimate carbon atom (*iso*-branched chain type), but smaller quantities of *anteiso*-branched chain fatty acids have also been reported (Oyaizu and Komagata, 1981; Yabuuchi and Moss, 1982; Liebert et al., 1984). Only in *C. hutchinsonii* have *anteiso*-branched chain fatty acids (mainly *anteiso*-17:0) been found as major constituents (Walker, 1969). It is, however, not always easy to distinguish between the two types of branching (Collins et al., 1982), so that it might be advisable to reinvestigate the latter case with modern instrumentation. The dominating fatty acid is usually *iso*-15:0 (15–43% of total fatty acids). Other branched acids are present in much smaller proportions, but straight-chain fatty acids may contribute substantially, mainly 15:0 (3–15%), 16:0 (1–23%) and particularly 16:1 (up to 35%). The position of the double bond in this acid has been determined in two cases and found to be between C_{11} and C_{12} (Walker, 1969; Oyaizu et al., 1982). Sometimes also, substantial amounts of monounsaturated branched fatty acids occur, mainly *iso*-17:1 (2–11%) and, more rarely, *iso*-15:1 (in unclassified marine CLB, Sy 126, about 20%; Fautz et al., 1981). More interesting is, however, the appearance of hydroxy fatty acids in unexpectedly high proportions (15–55% of total fatty acids; Fautz et al., 1979, 1981; Oyaizu and Komagata, 1981; Oyaizu et al., 1982; Yabuuchi and Moss, 1982). The hydroxyl usually stands in position 3, with 3-OH *iso*-17:0 (up to 29%), 3-OH *iso*-15:0 (up to 19%) and 3-OH *iso*-16:0 (up to 11%) as the main representatives. But substantial quantities of 2-hydroxy fatty acids have also been reported, mainly 2-OH *iso*-15:0 (up to 9%, in *C. arvensicola* up to 20%). Only a minor part of the hydroxy fatty acids of CLB are derived from the LPS, in which exclusively 3-hydroxy fatty acids—mainly 3-OH *iso*-15:0 (21–23%), 3-OH *iso*-17:0 (15–24%) and 3-OH *iso*-16:0 (12–19%)—have been found (Rosenfelder et al., 1974). The major part appears to come from the *capnoids*, a novel type of sulfonolipid discovered in *Capnocytophaga* but since found to be

widely distributed among CLB and other bacteria of the *Cytophaga* supergroup (Godchaux and Leadbetter, 1980, 1983, 1984). The core of these lipids is capnine, 2-amino-3-hydroxy-15-methylhexadecane-1-sulfonic acid, which is found in its free form only in *Capnocytophaga*, while in all other organisms investigated so far the amino group is connected to a variety of fatty acids via an amide linkage. Among the latter, hydroxy fatty acids dominate by far (70–90%), with the main species being the same as in whole cell hydrolysates. The capnoids (2–10 μmol produced per g wet cell mass) constitute up to 20% of the cellular lipids and are located in the cell envelope. Their biosynthesis has been studied in *C. johnsonae* and appears to proceed via a condensation of 13-methylmyristoyl-CoA with cysteic acid (White, 1984). Cyclopropane fatty acids (1–3%) are mentioned for CLB in only one report (Oyaizu and Komagata, 1981).

The fatty acid patterns of CLB closely resemble those of other bacteria of the emerging *Cytophaga-Bacteroides* supergroup: *Flexibacter* (Fautz et al., 1979; Godchaux and Leadbetter, 1984), *Capnocytophaga* (Holt et al., 1979; Collins et al., 1982; Dees et al., 1982; Godchaux and Leadbetter, 1984), *Sporocytophaga* (Holt et al., 1979) and the genera with low mol% G + C, *Flavobacterium* and *Sphingobacterium* (Moss and Dees, 1978; Fautz et al., 1981; Oyaizu and Komagata, 1981; Yabuuchi et al., 1983; Liebert et al., 1984). In some instances, there may be characteristic differences which would help to distinguish certain taxa. Thus, 2-hydroxy fatty acids are major components (10–35%) in the patterns of *Flexibacter*, *Sphingobacterium* and some flavobacteria, while they remain below 5% in *Cytophaga* (and certain *Flavobacterium*) species. As *C. arvensicola* shows an unusually high level of these compounds (up to 20%), this species might belong elsewhere.

Very little is known about *complex lipids* of CLB. *C. hutchinsonii* contains about 23% crude lipid (by dry weight), 50% of which is phosphatidylethanolamine; in addition, there are two glycolipids (Walker et al., 1968; Walker, 1969).

Another peculiarity of CLB is the exclusive presence of menaquinones as *respiratory quinones* (Callies and Mannheim, 1978; Oyaizu and Komagata, 1981; Oyaizu et al., 1982). The menaquinone content is 0.5–5 μmol/g cell protein; the menaquinone type is termed MK-6 in *C. arvensicola* and MK-7 in *C. heparina*. Again, this characteristic is shared by other bacteria of the supergroup: *Flexibacter* (MK-7: Kleinig et al., 1974), *Capnocytophaga* (MK-6: Collins et al., 1982) and the flavobacteria with low mol% G + C (Callies and Mannheim, 1978; most MK-6, some MK-7: Oyaizu and Komagata, 1981). Very likely all CLB with MK-7 can safely be excluded from the genus *Cytophaga*.

The *pigments* of CLB are cell-bound. Results of early reports suggest that in *C. succinicans* (Anderson and Ordal, 1961a) and *C. hutchinsonii* (Verma and Martin, 1967a) the pigments could be carotenoids. *C. lytica* is reported to contain the carotenoid, zeaxanthin (Lewin and Lounsbery, 1969). In *C. johnsonae*, *trans-* and *cis*-zeaxanthin constitute 15% of the total pigment, viz. 20 μg/g wet cell mass (Achenbach et al., 1978b). The rest of the pigment is a series of 18 flexirubin type pigments (Achenbach et al., 1978b, 1979b), a novel pigment type discovered in "*Flexibacter filiformis*" (Reichenbach et al., 1974; Achenbach et al., 1976, 1977). These pigments consist of an ω-phenyloctaenic acid chromophore connected

via an ester bond with a resorcinol which, in turn, is substituted with two hydrocarbon chains (Fig. 23.2). The hydrocarbons are highly variable, particularly in CLB, and this and the presence or absence of one or two chlorine atoms in the *meta* position on the phenyl ring is the basis for the appearance of a large variety of pigments even in one strain (Achenbach et al., 1978b, 1979a). Due to a phenolate reaction with alkali, colonies or bacterial cell mass containing flexirubin type pigments reversibly change color from yellow or orange to violet-red or purple-brown when exposed to KOH solution, and this test has been found positive with many CLB and other bacteria of the supergroup, viz. *Flexibacter, Sporocytophaga* and many flavobacteria (Hirsch, 1980; Humphrey et al., 1980; Reichenbach et al., 1981; Oyaizu et al., 1982; Jooste, 1985). The color reaction obtained with alkali had been observed long ago in cellulose-degrading CLB of somewhat uncertain affiliation, which could even have been *Sporocytophaga* strains (Walker and Warren, 1938; Fåhraeus, 1947). The former authors came to the conclusion that the pigment was not a carotenoid but an unsaturated aliphatic acid. It must be emphasized, however, that similar color reactions may also be given by other phenolate-forming chromophores, such as phenolic carotenoids (Kohl et al., 1983) which are the cause of a taxonomically useful color shift in *Brevibacterium linens* (Grecz and Dack, 1961; Jones et al., 1973). Apart from the cases cited above, the presence of flexirubin type pigments has been proven so far only for *Flavobacterium* species strain C 1/2 (Achenbach et al., 1981); moreover, it is strongly suggested in *Flavobacterium breve* and *F. odoratum* (Weeks, 1981). There is no question that *not* all CLB contain flexirubin type pigments. They are usually lacking in, for example, marine CLB (Reichenbach et al., 1981) but appear to be characteristic for certain species and perhaps groups of related species. The biosynthesis of flexirubin type pigments has been studied mainly in *Flexibacter*, with contributions from the study of *Flavobacterium* (Achenbach et al., 1979c, 1982, 1983). The pigments are assembled from tyrosine, acetate and, if branched side chains are present, leucine as major building blocks via two separately synthesized half-molecules. These, viz. ω-phenyloctaenic acid and a substituted orsellinic acid, are then joined in a late step.

Other types of pigments have also been reported for CLB. *C. diffluens* contains the carotenoid, saproxanthin, and *C. latercula*, an unknown red compound (Lewin and Lounsbery, 1969). In addition to cell-bound pigmentation, a greenish-reddish iridescence which is probably an interference phenomenon is sometimes observed on the swarm colonies of CLB (Reichenbach and Dworkin, 1981c). Diffusible brown to black pigments may also be produced, e.g. by the marine agar digesters "*C. krzemieniewskae*" (Stanier, 1941) and *C. uliginosa* (ZoBell and Upham, 1944).

Pigment production by CLB may be dependent on the growth conditions; e.g. *C. succinicans* cultivated anaerobically is colorless, whereas when it is grown aerobically, it is yellow-orange (Anderson and Ordal, 1961a). As a rule, on peptone-containing agar plates, CLB show their characteristic color.

Gliding motility is still regarded as an essential characteristic of CLB. It is part of the taxonomic definition and serves to distinguish these organisms from the flavobacteria. But unequivocal recognition of gliding in an organism is not always easy, and errors in this respect in the past have

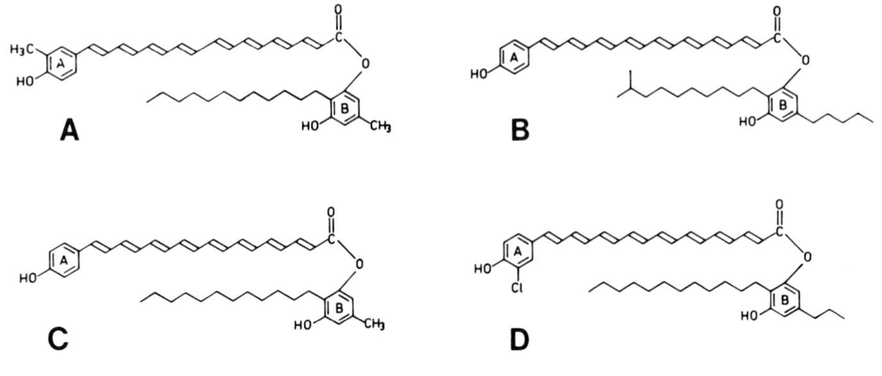

Figure 23.2. Examples for flexirubin type pigments from bacteria of the *Cytophaga* branch. *A*, parent compound, flexirubin, from *Flexibacter filiformis* Fx e1. *B*, variant typical for CLB, from strain Cy j1 *(C. johnsonae complex)*. *C* and *D*, variants from *Flavobacterium* species, strain C 1/2. Chlorinated compounds occur in all species.

resulted in several misnomers. Criteria for recognizing gliding motility—spreading of swarm colonies, the arrangement of the cells within the colony and at the colony edge, and microscopic observation of the movements of individual cells—have been established long ago, and methods have been described that allow an observer with some experience to demonstrate gliding relatively reliably (Lautrop, 1965; Perry, 1973; Reichenbach and Dworkin, 1981a). Problems may arise because gliding in CLB is strongly influenced by environmental conditions, e.g. nutrients, and because twitching motility (Lautrop, 1965) can be mistaken for gliding. Twitching may also result in a certain spreading of colonies, but the movements of individual cells are more erratic and jerky, with jumps of merely 0.5-1 μm at a time, not always in the direction of the long axis of the rod, and with a translocation speed of only 1-2 μm/min. Twitching is obviously connected with the possession of polar fimbriae (Henrichsen, 1975) which apparently have never been found on CLB.

Gliding of CLB may be rather swift, with speeds of 100-150 μm/min (Stanier, 1942; Garnjobst, 1945; Duxbury et al., 1980; Lapidus and Berg, 1982). Often, gliding movements are discontinuous. Thus *C. hutchinsonii* may move very fast for several cell lengths, stop for a while, and then continue in the same or the opposite direction. However, particularly when groups of cells are involved, gliding may also proceed smoothly for a longer time. During movement the rods may remain relatively stiff, whereas in other cases they vividly flex. They appear not to roll around their long axis or do so only occasionally, which can clearly be seen when branched cells or cells bent into a hook at one end are gliding (Garnjobst, 1945; Lapidus and Berg, 1982). The direction of movement can be reversed in several ways: (a) the cell bends until the anterior pole points into the opposite direction, (b) the cell swings around one of its poles and thus brings the leading end into a new direction, or (c) the trailing end becomes the leading one (Garnjobst, 1945; Lapidus and Berg, 1982).

In addition to gliding, CLB show several other kinds of highly characteristic movements, particularly when covered by a layer of liquid. As with gliding movements, contact with a surface is a prerequisite, and freely suspended cells are motionless. A gliding cell may detach itself except at one pole and swing around this pole into another direction or even for 360°. Or it may flip over or somersault. Often a cell oscillates or rotates in a conical orbit with one pole attached and the rest of the cell pointing away from the surface, perhaps 100-200 times successively, with 1-2 rotations/s (Garnjobst, 1945; Perry, 1973; Lapidus and Berg, 1982).

Gliding and spreading growth of CLB is usually inhibited by higher nutrient concentrations. Specifically, peptones and amino acids may completely block motility at "normal" concentrations of 1-2% (Garnjobst, 1945; Stanier, 1947; Christensen, 1977a; Duxbury et al., 1980). Sugars also may sometimes interfere with motility but do not always do so (Duxbury et al., 1980; Burchard, 1984). In *C. johnsonae* a wide variety of sugars blocks gliding regardless of whether the sugar can be taken up or metabolized (Wolkin and Pate, 1984). In this case, the sugars apparently cross-react with some surface component, perhaps slime, essential for contact with the substrate. Inhibition of gliding by certain ions, e.g. Na^+, may be explained in a similar way, while other ions, such as Ca^{2+}, Mg^{2+}, Zn^{2+} or K^+, seem to act on the machinery of gliding itself (Duxbury et al., 1980). Another critical factor seems to be humidity and the kind and concentration of gelling agent used, with high moisture and moderate agar concentrations usually favoring spreading of colonies (Glaser and Pate, 1973; Wolkin and Pate, 1984). For practical purposes, to elicit gliding motility in CLB, several substrates can be recommended: e.g. CA agar (*Cytophaga* agar) (Anacker and Ordal, 1959a) (tryptone (Difco), 0.05%; yeast extract, 0.05%; beef extract, 0.02%; sodium acetate, 0.02%; and agar, 0.9%; at pH 7.2); LY agar (yeast extract, 0.01%; phosphate buffer, 1 mM, pH 7.0; $(NH_4)_2SO_4$, 0.1%; $MgSO_4 \cdot 7H_2O$, 0.05%; $CaCl_2 \cdot 2H_2O$, 0.005%; standard trace elements; and agar, 1.5%); or yeast agar VY/2 (Reichenbach and Dworkin, 1981c) (baker's yeast, 0.5% by fresh weight of yeast cake; $CaCl_2$, 0.1%; cyanocobalamine, 0.5 μm/ml, which may be omitted for most organisms; and agar, 1.5%; at pH 7.2). (VY/2 agar al-

most always produces growth and spreading.) For marine organisms, of course, natural or artificial seawater has to be included. Also, many other formulations of similar composition have been used successfully.

In recent years, several CLB have been used to analyze gliding motility in considerable detail with the aim of elucidating its mechanism. Although this has not yet been accomplished, much has been learned (Glaser and Pate, 1973; Pate and Chang, 1979; Duxbury et al., 1980; Humphrey, et al., 1980; Lapidus and Berg, 1982; Burchard, 1984; Chang et al., 1984; Wolkin and Pate, 1984). The investigations into the fine structure of CLB mentioned above, studies using different kinds of motility mutants as well as metabolic inhibitors, and careful observations of moving cells and the movements of tiny latex beads on the surface of gliding and stationary rods allow the following conclusions to be made. Apparently, gliding is a complex phenomenon requiring an orderly interplay of several independent components. There is probably a machinery of gliding which consists of (a) a biochemical system providing the mechanical energy and (b) a mechanical apparatus translating this energy into a propulsive force. Further, there is some agent which mediates the contact of the cell with its substrate and is a prerequisite for the machinery of gliding to become effective. Experiments with metabolic inhibitors suggest that the required energy is not derived from ATP but directly from the membrane potential and proton motive force. The mechanical apparatus is still largely obscure. Electron microscopy so far has not provided a clear picture. Observations of the movements of latex beads suggest that there are moving tracks at the cell surface, but it has not yet been possible to elucidate the exact topology of these tracks, and in fact there may not even be a stable, well-defined system of such tracks. The slime at the cell surface plays an essential role as a mediator. As already mentioned, its properties may be influenced by environmental factors, particularly ions and chemical compounds, and its structure may be modified by mutation, both with serious consequences for gliding motility.

There are also effects on motility which are less easily explained. For example, in unclassified CLB, motility is inhibited by several antibiotics known to interfere with polypeptide synthesis, viz. chloramphenicol, tetracycline, amicetin, fusidic acid and others, and this occurs at concentrations which, although high, are not yet growth-inhibitory (Burchard, 1984). It must be emphasized, however, that chloramphenicol, for example, does not always have this effect in CLB (Duxbury et al., 1980).

The important role played by the cell surface is clearly shown by the peculiar fact that in *C. johnsonae* nonmotile cells are completely resistant to all known phages, regardless of whether motility is blocked by mutation, environmental conditions or metabolic inhibitors (Pate et al., 1979; Chang et al., 1984). Nonmotile mutants are also unable to digest chitin, although they still degrade starch, pectin, casein and gelatin; temperature-sensitive nonmotile mutants digest chitin only at the permissive temperature (Chang et al., 1984).

Serological studies have been performed on three CLB. The antigen pattern of fish-pathogenic CLB has been used to attack epidemiological and diagnostic questions (Anacker and Ordal, 1959a; Pacha and Porter, 1968; Shotts and Bullock, 1975; Becker and Fujihara, 1978). It appears that in *C. columnaris* there is a common species-specific antigen. In addition, there are several other major and minor antigens which occur in various combinations and have allowed subdivision of a collection of strains into four serotypes. All isolates from western Washington State belonged in one serogroup (I), which, however, also appeared in other regions. Otherwise, no correlation between serotype and geographical origin, species of host fish, or virulence was seen. Precipitating antisera against *C. columnaris* seem not to react with other CLB including nonpathogenic inhabitants of fish, so that such sera can be a valuable diagnostic tool. When heat-inactivated *C. columnaris* is inoculated into fish, high antibody titers (up to 1:5000) may be obtained, and occasional exposure to the bacterium in nature is apparently responsible for the development of immunity against infection (Fujihara and Nakatani, 1971; Schachte and Mora, 1973). In fact, it may be more convenient to produce diagnostic antisera in fish rather than in rabbits.

A LPS and weak endotoxin of an unclassified CLB ("*C. allerginae*") which lives on demister vanes in air humidification systems has been found to be very probably responsible for an occupational disease, hypersensitivity pneumonitis, and perhaps humidifier fever, in workers at textile plants (Flaherty et al., 1984a, b). Although the etiology has still to be unequivocally proven, all patients had antibodies against the antigen, as did 78% of healthy workers in the plant. Only 2% of control persons from outside had antibodies.

In an effort to serotype a collection of "*Sporocytophaga cauliformis*" strains from Lake Constance in Germany, antisera were produced in rabbits by subcutaneous and intravenous application (Gräf and Pfeiffer, 1967). In contrast to the former, the latter proved highly specific and were used to subdivide 389 isolates into 28 serotypes. When this system was applied to another 710 new isolates, 83% of the strains could be classified, while the remainder represented several additional serotypes. One serotype, IIa, was restricted to strains which were clearly distinguishable also by other characteristics (antibiotic-producing type II strains). These results may be added to those observations that indicate considerable heterogeneity of the species (see "Taxonomic Comments"). It was found that addition of homologous antiserum to gliding cells quickly stopped all motility and spreading growth on agar plates. The assumption that this was due to a specific interaction of the antiserum with the machinery of gliding motility is, however, disputable.

Phages have been reported for only a few CLB, but they appear to be rather common in nature and not particularly difficult to obtain (Anacker and Ordal, 1955; Kingsbury and Ordal, 1966; Stürzenhofecker, 1966; Pate et al., 1979). The seven phages studied by Kingsbury and Ordal (1966) were obviously all derived from lysogenic strains of *C. columnaris*. All known phages of CLB are of the head-and-tail type, with tails which are contractile, at least in the case of the *C. johnsonae* phages. All known phages form plaques. The polyhedral heads are between 60 and 145 nm wide; the tails are 100–165 nm long and 20–30 nm in diameter. Sometimes a neck and a base plate can be distinguished. Two groups of *C. johnsonae* phages bear a peculiar cylindrical knob on the distal end of their core. With one single strain of *C. johnsonae*, 28 phages were isolated which could be classified into 16 morphological groups. For one phage of *C. columnaris*, double-stranded DNA with a mol% G + C of the DNA similar to that of the host (41 vs. 43) has been demonstrated. In several cases, considerably higher phage yields are observed when infection is performed in the presence of $CaCl_2$ (1–4 mM). Burst sizes between 20 and 100 have been found. Multiplication of one phage of *C. columnaris* is blocked by streptomycin (70 μg/ml), although the host is completely resistant to the antibiotic. Apparently, the compound prevents the injection of the phage DNA (Kingsbury and Pate, 1966). The host ranges are always relatively narrow. Phages of *C. columnaris* attack only *C. columnaris* strains and, among these, only certain serotypes with a high probability (75% of strains). The various phages of *C. johnsonae* may infect different strains of *C. johnsonae* but not *Flexibacter*, *Vitreoscilla* or myxobacters and, as already mentioned, attack only motile cells (Pate et al., 1979). In spreading colonies of CLB taken from freshwater, pseudoplaques have been observed. They arise at sites where drops of condensation water have dried up on the agar surface (Stürzenhofecker, 1966).

In *C. columnaris*, bacteriocinlike lytic agents have been found and used for a bacteriocin typing (Anacker and Ordal, 1959b). As with the serotypes, no correlation was seen with geographical, ecological or epidemiological data.

On solid substrates, CLB typically form *spreading colonies or swarms*, an essential characteristic distinguishing them from flavobacteria with low mol% G + C. Unfortunately, however, the ability to glide is not always found in conjunction with swarming. Rather, basic motility (e.g. bending or transport of particles along the cell surface), cell translocation, and spreading of colonies have to be regarded as separate phenomena that are not linked under all conditions (Perry, 1973; Chang et al., 1984; Wolkin and Pate, 1984). Among 78 yellow isolates from sewage plants, only 25% formed swarms, although 70% clearly showed gliding motility (Güde, 1980). The prerequisites for spreading are not fully understood. They may have to do with the complexity of gliding motility as discussed above, particularly with the physicochemical properties of the matrix (slime) mediating the interaction of the gliding machinery with the substrate surface. Although different CLB may differ substantially in their specific requirements, spreading is usually controlled by three environmental factors: nutrients, humidity and temperature, which probably act chiefly on gliding itself. In general, low nutrient concentrations (particularly peptone) favor spreading (see, for example, Garnjobst, 1945; Bauer, 1962; and Agbo and Moss, 1979). With *C. johnsonae*, spreading is considerably reduced when the tryptone content of the medium is raised from 0.2 to 0.6% (Wolkin and Pate, 1984). For "spreading media" it is usually advisable to maintain the peptone concentration at 0.1% or less. Several examples for such media have already been given. The kind of nutrients added may also have a strong influence on spreading. *C. heparina* formed swarms on media containing yeast RNA but formed compact colonies on all other media tested (Mitchell et al., 1967). Moisture may influence spreading via the humidity of the atmosphere and the concentration and kind of gelling agent used. In general, humid conditions favor spreading (see, for example, Garnjobst, 1945; and Agbo and Moss, 1979). However, a decrease in agar concentration sometimes also reduces spreading, as occurs, for example, with *C. johnsonae* (Chang et al., 1984). Spreading of conditionally nonmotile mutants of *C. columnaris* (Glaser and Pate, 1973) and *C. johnsonae* (Chang et al., 1984) was particularly sensitive to the moisture conditions, perhaps because the mutations somehow affected the amount and structure of the slime. A temperature effect may be expected particularly in aquatic CLB, which often have a lower temperature optimum. *Flavobacterium aquatile* began to swarm after prolonged incubation at 15°C (Mitchell et al., 1967). Unclassified CLB U67 grows at 30°C but for spreading requires a reduced temperature, e.g. 25°C (Burchard, 1984). Also, temperature-sensitive nonmotile mutants are known (Chang et al., 1984). In contrast to the examples given above, peptone concentrations between 0.1 and 2.5% and agar concentrations between 0.75 and 2% do not greatly affect spreading of *C. aquatilis* (Strohl and Tait, 1978).

Colonies of CLB may spread with considerable speed and, under optimal conditions, may completely cover an agar plate within 1 week. For *C. johnsonae* a linear increase of the swarm diameter over 90 h with a rate of 0.5 mm/h at 25°C has been reported (Wolkin and Pate, 1984). This is, however, considerably less than the maximal speed of individual cells, with the reason for the discrepancy being that the movements of cells are neither continuous nor strictly outwardly oriented.

The *appearance of the colonies* of CLB varies considerably. They are almost always more or less intensely yellow to red. The spreading colonies are often relatively delicate and form a continuous sheet which ends at the edge in a corona of flamelike or tonguelike protrusions, sometimes with a network in between. The swarm sheet may be smooth or show some structure, such as flat mounds or blobs, warts, or a fibrous or fine feltlike surface. These structures arise through a discontinuous distribution of the cells within the swarm and local accumulation of slime. A parallel arrangement of the rod cells locally in thin swarm sheets may also be responsible for the kaleidoscopic iridescense occasionally observed (Anderson and Ordal, 1961a; Bauer, 1962; Reichenbach and Dworkin, 1981c). The swarm mat is always somewhat slimy, although copious amounts of slime are really the exception (Strohl and Tait, 1978). The slime is usually soft but may also become very tough, so that the swarm can be peeled off the agar as a pellicle or sticks tenaciously to the agar surface, as occurs, for example, in *C. columnaris* (Garnjobst, 1945) or in *C. uliginosa*. Sometimes, migrating microcolonies can be observed (Strohl and Tait, 1978). Colonies also may spread subsurface within the agar, which is usually the case with microaerophilic strains (Veldkamp, 1961). Particularly in soft agar, normal aerobic CLB, too, may form such colonies. Subsurface colonies are more or less dense clouds which usually are completely uniform but also may show some radial rhizoidal structure, as occurs, for example, with *C. columnaris*. Sometimes they are paler than surface colonies. For several CLB, colony variation has been reported (Stanier, 1942, 1947; Bachmann, 1955; Anderson and Ordal, 1961a; Veldkamp, 1961; Pacha, 1968; Oyaizu et al., 1982). No explanation can be offered for this phenomenon. Colonies of agar decomposers reside in craters sunk in the agar. The colonies of cellulose degraders on filter paper may also spread, producing essentially homogeneous, glassy, yellow or orange slimy areas within the paper. In the fine fabric of regenerated cellulose filters, such colonies appear as if punched into the white sheet. Nonspreading colonies remain small and are usually slightly elevated, with an entire edge and a smooth surface. Apart from their pigmentation they show nothing special which would allow them to be distinguished from the colonies of other bacteria. Colonies of certain nonmotile mutants of *C. columnaris* develop wrinkles in the form of seven radial spokes (Glaser and Pate, 1973).

In agitated *liquid cultures*, CLB usually grow as homogeneous, often intensely pigmented suspensions. When gently rotated, such suspensions appear silky. The medium does not become particularly viscous, but enough slime may be produced to make harvesting difficult (Verma and Martin, 1967a). When growing on fish tissue in liquid, *C. columnaris* forms short, sometimes branched, haystacklike columns projecting from the surface of the tissue and consisting of cells and slime (Ordal and Rucker, 1944; Becker and Fujihara, 1978). These columns were initially mistaken for fruiting bodies, resulting in a classification of the organism in the old myxobacterial genus "*Chondrococcus*." In static cultures also, CLB may spread along the surface of the liquid and along the glass walls and form star-shaped cell clusters (Garnjobst, 1945).

Cultures of CLB sometimes have a more or less characteristic *odor*. A sickening odor is described for *C. columnaris* on nutrient agar (Garnjobst, 1945). Many CLB produce a strong cheesy odor in peptone-containing liquid media. Plates with agar digesters may give off an agreeable fruity odor.

The basic *physiology* in many CLB is not particularly well studied, and virtually no exact data are available on most of the essential biochemical pathways, e.g. on electron transport systems or amino acid metabolism. In general, there appear to be no dramatic deviations from what is known for other comparable bacteria. Most CLB are strict aerobes. For some of these organisms, weak anaerobic growth has occasionally been stated. But this is certainly exceptional, and in the absence of rigorous proof it may be assumed that residual growth under semianaerobic conditions and acid production from carbohydrates in aerobic cultures have been misinterpreted. Several facultatively anaerobic CLB have been described (Stanier, 1947; Bachmann, 1955; Anderson and Ordal, 1961a; Veldkamp, 1961), and there may be more of these (Hirsch, 1980). The facultative anaerobes may ferment various sugars, mannitol, and polysaccharides such as starch or agar but usually do not ferment organic acids including amino acids (pyruvate in *C. succinicans* is an exception). The main fermentation products are always succinate and acetate, and usually propionate and formate arise. Small quantities of lactate and ethanol may also be found. *C. salmonicolor* including var. *agarovorans* produces gas, consisting of CO_2 and H_2, when fermenting glucose, but not all species do so (Veldkamp, 1961). Between 15 and 25% of glucose carbon is recovered as cell mass and slime. All facultatively anaerobic CLB require CO_2 for anaerobic growth and, at least in some cases (*C. salmonicolor*) also, for aerobic growth. When supplied as $NaHCO_3$, the optimum is between 0.3 and 1%. For *C. succinicans* it has been suggested that succinate arises via guanosine diphosphate-stimulated condensation of CO_2 with phosphoenolpyruvate, followed by a reduction which serves as an electron sink (Anderson and Ordal, 1961b). In fact, when lactate dehydrogenase is added to cell extracts, sugar phosphates can be converted to lactate in the absence of CO_2. The origin of the propionate produced by all other facultatively anaerobic CLB in substantial quantities has not been elucidated. Luxuriant anaerobic growth under nitrate respiration and gas production is reported for *C. johnsonae* var. *denitrificans* (Stanier, 1947). Some CLB may use fumarate as an electron acceptor for NADH oxidation under anaerobic conditions but are unable to grow in this way (e.g. *C. hutchinsonii, C. johnsonae* (Callies and Mannheim, 1978)). Strictly anaerobic CLB have not been found so far.

Comparative data on the metabolism of CLB are very incomplete and often difficult to evaluate because of differences in the methods applied and scanty descriptions of experimental details. It appears that all CLB grow on organic *N compounds* as the sole source of nitrogen and often also of carbon and energy. Even the cellulose decomposers grow more vigorously when the filter paper is placed on low-peptone (0.3%) agar rather

than on mineral salts agar, although in this case there is no growth without the addition of a suitable carbohydrate, preferentially cellulose. Peptones, yeast extract or casamino acids appear to be universally accepted, but glutamine, asparagine, glutamic acid or other single amino acids will often do. Almost all CLB grow on inorganic nitrogen. *C. psychrophila* seems to be an exception (Pacha, 1968). It appears that NH_4^+ is usually preferred to NO_3^-. Some CLB, e.g. *C. fermentans*, will not even accept NO_3^- (Bachmann, 1955). Urea is relatively rarely a suitable N source. Carbohydrates, particularly sugars, are the preferred *carbon and energy sources*. Various hexoses, pentoses, disaccharides and trisaccharides have been found suitable for many different strains of CLB. Almost all utilize glucose very well. However, the *C. diffluens* group does not grow on glucose but relies on other sugars, such as galactose or sucrose (Lewin and Lounsbery, 1969), and *C. psychrophila* seems not to utilize carbohydrates at all but to grow exclusively on organic N compounds (Pacha, 1968). Sugar alcohols, alcohols and organic acids are much inferior carbon sources. Malonate seems to be relatively often utilized (Hirsch, 1980), and sometimes mannitol, acetate or lactate are used as substrates (see, for example, Lewin and Lounsbery, 1969; and Christensen, 1977a). That single amino acids often serve as sole organic nutrient has already been mentioned. Particularly glutamic acid, glutamine and asparagine are widely accepted. Even under aerobic conditions, sugar metabolism usually results in acid production (see, for example, van der Meulen et al., 1974; and Oyaizu and Komagata, 1981). *C. johnsonae* has been shown to metabolize glucose via the Embden-Meyerhof-Parnas pathway (Reichardt and Morita, 1982a).

The most spectacular biochemical property of the CLB is their ability to *degrade* many different and sometimes rather recalcitrant *biomacromolecules*. In nature they probably always live on such compounds, and the CLB may well be one of the most important bacterial groups in the turnover of organic matter under aerobic conditions. There is a vast literature on such specialists, of which only a selection of introductory articles can be cited here. The organisms involved are often taxonomically ill-defined. Quite a few of them are also of biotechnological interest, and there may be even more of those, as several of the flavobacteria producing technically relevant enzymes may actually be CLB.

The genus *Cytophaga* was originally defined by Winogradsky (1929) to contain aerobic *cellulose-degrading* soil bacteria with long flexible cells probably motile by gliding. The first organism of this general type had already been characterized by Hutchinson and Clayton (1919) under the name *Spirochaeta cytophaga*. This bacterium produced, however, spherical resting cells and microcysts and was later renamed *Sporocytophaga myxococcoides*. For a long time there was a controversy about the nature of these coccoid cells, kindled by the fact that none of Winogradsky's organisms formed such microcysts but formed large numbers of spheroplasts which were correctly recognized by Winogradsky as a degeneration phenomenon. Indeed, *Cytophaga* cultures on cellulose tend to be very pleomorphic, and spheroplasts have been mistaken for microcysts again and again, making it difficult to know what kind of organism was really used in a particular study on cellulose decomposition. Fortunately, the specialized cellulose-degrading *Cytophaga* species, e.g. *C. hutchinsonii* and *Sporocytophaga* appear to behave very similarly physiologically, although taxonomically they are clearly distinguished as suggested by a gap in the mol% G + C of the DNA of 3–6. For some time, the cellulose-degrading CLB raised considerable interest, and a large number of publications on this topic appeared between 1930 and 1960 (see, for example, Winogradsky, 1929; Krzemieniewska, 1933; Stapp and Bortels, 1934; Imshenetski and Solntseva, 1936; Walker and Warren, 1938; Stanier, 1941, 1942; Fuller and Norman, 1943; Fåhraeus, 1947; Kadota, 1956; Imshenetski, 1959; and Meyer, 1961). These studies not only added new species but also extended their ecological range to marine habitats and resulted in a better understanding of the biochemistry of cellulose decomposition.

Much of the earlier work has been done with mixed cultures. Winogradsky himself never had pure strains. Indeed, the isolation of pure cultures of cellulolytic CLB is no easy task, and it was even thought that some of these organisms could not be purified because they depended on symbiotic companions (Stapp and Bortels, 1934; Politi, 1941). It seems, however, that with some patience it is possible to purify all of these organisms. Apparently cellulose can be degraded by CLB only in direct cell contact. With the new isolate, "*C. ureae*," and with carboxymethyl cellulose (CMC) as the substrate, it was shown that no cellulases are excreted and that there are two soluble exo-β-glucanases in the periplasm and in the cytoplasm, in addition to a membrane-bound endoglucanase which reduces the viscosity of CMC solutions. The periplasmic enzyme also attacks crystalline cellulose, releasing glucose as the only product (Chang and Thayer, 1977). Initially it was thought that CLB attack cellulose by oxidizing it to an acidic "oxycellulose" (Winogradsky, 1929). However, this oxycellulose is obviously only the slime produced in copious amounts from degradation products of cellulose. About 30% of the cellulose carbon may appear in this uronic acid-containing mucilage (Walker and Warren, 1938). It was also found that cellulose decomposition by CLB is stimulated considerably by certain ions, notably Ca^{2+}, Mn^{2+}, Fe^{2+} and Cu^{2+}, which together may increase the amount of decomposed cellulose from 20% to 50–70% (Bortels, 1956). Originally it was believed that cellulolytic CLB would obligatorily depend on cellulose. Later it was found that if sugars are autoclaved in mineral salts medium, products arise which are very toxic for CLB (Stanier, 1942). If the sugar is filter-sterilized, it may support luxuriant growth. Thus glucose and cellobiose are used by all tested strains; xylose, mannose and trehalose may also be used by some. Although the spectrum of utilizable sugars is always narrow for the specialized cellulolytic CLB, e.g. *C. hutchinsonii*, "*C. rubra*," "*C. rosea*," *C. marinoflava*, *Sporocytophaga myxococcoides*, there are others with a much wider substrate spectrum, e.g. "*C. krzemieniewskae*" and *C. diffluens*, marine organisms isolated as agar degraders but also attacking cellulose (Stanier, 1941). In addition to crystalline or precipitated cellulose, modified celluloses such as CMC or cellophane may also be used. However, activity on CMC not always reflects the presence of cellulases capable of degrading native cellulose (see, for example, Christensen, 1977b), and only strains able to decompose filter paper should be regarded as cellulose degraders. It appears that contrary to occasional reports the ability to degrade cellulose is not easily lost during cultivation on cellulose-free media (Fåhraeus, 1947; Chang and Thayer, 1977).

Another well-studied group of CLB are the *agar digesters*. They are common in marine environments from which they were first isolated and described by Stanier (1941), but several more have since been discovered. Some of these are facultative anaerobes (Humm, 1946; Veldkamp, 1961; Lewin and Lounsbery, 1969). Agarolytic CLB have also been isolated from freshwater (van der Meulen et al., 1974; Agbo and Moss, 1979). At least one of those, *C. flevensis*, could be a marine organism which has adapted to freshwater conditions during the gradual replacement of saltwater in its habitat on the Dutch coast after separation from the open sea. This would explain why it does not contain flexirubin type pigments otherwise quite common among freshwater CLB. Also, it has been isolated only from polders reclaimed from the sea in recent time. Finally, it still grows very well on full-strength seawater media. But freshwater agarolytic CLB need not necessarily be of marine origin. Agarolytic bacteria may either soften or totally liquefy agar gels. The respective CLB are of either type, with the marine species being the more active ones. One species, *C. fermentans*, produces gelase fields and craters on agar plates, but it seems at most to destroy the double-helical structure of the gel and to utilize only impurities in commercial agar (Bachmann, 1955). Like cellulose decomposition, agar degradation seems to be a stable characteristic. In all cases that have been investigated in more detail, agarase was an exoenzyme, although it could be relatively firmly attached to polysaccharide slime (Duckworth and Turkey, 1969). The enzyme was found to be inducible with agar, its degradation products, and melibiose. Sometimes also, other polysaccharides, such as starch and pectin, act as inducers (van der Meulen and Harder, 1976; Agbo and Moss, 1979). On rich media, and particularly in the presence of glucose or galactose, agarolysis is usually strongly repressed. The extracellular agarase was always found to be an endolytic enzyme producing oligosaccharides. With *C. flevensis* the smallest product was neoagarotetraose. There were two intracellular enzymes further degrading this sugar to the disaccharide and the two monosaccharides (van der Meulen and Harder, 1976). Agarase may attack other chemically related algal polysaccharides such as porphyran although with somewhat different hydrolysis products (Duckworth and Turvey, 1969). In general, however, agarase specificity appears rather narrow (van der Meulen et al., 1974). All agarolytic CLB may utilize a wide variety of sugars and attack, in addition to agar, one or several other polysaccharides, such as starch, alginate, pectin, inulin and cellulose. Some CLB, such as *C. diffluens* and "*C. krzemieniewskae*," depend on complex organic N compounds which they can also use as sources of carbon and energy (Stanier, 1941; Lewin and Lounsbery, 1969). As with the cellulose degraders, older cultures of agarolytic CLB often contain involution forms in large numbers, e.g. long filaments (Stanier, 1941).

Still another group of polysaccharide degraders of a more general interest are the *chitinovorous CLB*. The first strains of this kind were probably isolated by Johnson (1932), but the first study in depth is that of Stanier (1947), who also described the new species, *C. johnsonae*. Many more chitinoclastic strains have been found (Strohl and Tait, 1978; Reichardt et al., 1983), and their abundance and wide distribution in soil, freshwater and marine environments is now well-established. For some time, chitin degradation seemed so unusual that soil CLB with this property were automatically classified as *C. johnsonae*. This only resulted in taxonomic confusion, however, for many of the strains thus classified are not closely related and possession of a chitinase obviously has only limited taxonomic weight. The chitinases of CLB are always excreted and produce clear lysis zones around colonies on chitin agar. Chitin degradation is not particularly sensitive to the presence of other nutrients, e.g. 0.3% peptone, but higher nutrient levels, as in nutrient broth, or the presence of sugars such as glucose may totally repress the enzyme (Reichardt, 1975).

The chitinovorous CLB do not depend on chitin or on carbohydrates. All grow very well on complex organic N sources such as peptone or yeast extract, and these can also supply the required carbon and energy. Many may also subsist on NH_4^+ or NO_3^- as sole N compound, but marine strains appear to use only organic nitrogen (Reichardt et al., 1983). A variety of sugars is utilized, but some strains grow much better on disaccharides than on the corresponding monosaccharides (Stanier, 1947). Other polysaccharides, e.g. starch, are often degraded. Many strains have been found to be able to grow anaerobically (Reichardt et al., 1983), and nitrate respiration has been demonstrated for two (Stanier, 1947). At least some chitin-degrading CLB show a pronounced morphological cycle, becoming much shorter in old cultures, e.g. from 10–15 µm to 2 µm (Stanier, 1947).

Most CLB degrade starch (see, for example, Lewin and Lounsbery, 1969; Christensen, 1977a, b; and Reichardt et al., 1983). CLB have been found that also decompose glycogen (Ruschke, 1968; Gunja-Smith et al., 1970), pectin (Ruschke and Rath, 1966; Kamat and Bhat, 1967; Güde, 1973; van der Meulen et al., 1974; Agbo and Moss, 1979; Oyaizu et al., 1982), alginate (Stanier, 1941; Lewin and Lounsbery, 1969; Christensen, 1977b), carrageenan, arabinogalactan, galactomannan, xanthan, gum arabic (all in Agbo and Moss, 1979), dextran (Güde, 1980), laminarin (Bacon et al., 1970; Marshall, 1973), lutean (Bacon et al., 1970), xylan (Güde, 1973; Reichardt, 1974), inulin (Stanier, 1947; Veldkamp, 1961; van der Meulen et al., 1974; Oyaizu et al., 1982), bacterial succinoglycan (Oyaizu et al., 1982; Mendoza and Amemura, 1983), yeast cell wall β-glucan (Bacon et al., 1970), and heparin (Payza and Korn, 1956). In most cases, the participating enzymes are not known; in others, however, they are well-characterized and have, in fact, been used to elucidate the structure of macromolecules (e.g. heparin, succinglycan) or yeast cell walls. CLB break down *pectin* not by simple hydrolysis but by a trans-elimination reaction using a Ca^{2+}-dependent polygalacturonic acid lyase. The enzyme is inducible (e.g. by galacturonic acid), its synthesis is repressed by glucose, and it is free or cell-bound in varying proportions, depending on the physiological state of the organisms. It produces unsaturated oligouronides (Sundarray and Bhat, 1971; Kurowski and Dunleavy, 1976; Güde, 1978b). An *isoamylase* obtained from a CLB exhaustively hydrolyses all α-1,6 branch points on glycogen or amylopectin

(Gunja-Smith et al., 1970). A supposedly pure *laminarase* activity from the patent strain *Cytophaga* species NCIB 9497 turned out to consist of three enzymes of different specificity: an endo-β-1,3-D-glucanhydrolase degrading laminarin into oligosaccharides, an endo-β-1,4-D-glucanase producing oligosaccharides from CMC or lichenin, and a nonspecific β-1,3-D-glucanase releasing glucose, disaccharides and trisaccharides from laminarin and lichenin (Marshall, 1973). The same strain was later developed for producing, on a technical scale, enzymes for disruption of yeast cells (Asenjo and Dunnill, 1981). *Heparin* is broken down by *C. heparina* with the aid of a heparinase that produces free glucosamine-2,6-disulfate, a sulfamidase and a sulfoesterase which remove the sulfates from glucosamine (Dietrich, 1969). The *walls of baker's yeast* are attacked by a strain of *C. johnsonae* only after the yeast is autoclaved or treated with a thiol reagent. The involved enzymes are inducible (those of the strain mentioned above are constitutive and act on untreated yeast) and consist of two types of endo-β-1,3-(laminarases) and several β-1,6-glucanases (luteanases). Only one enzyme (one of the 1,3-glucanases) is able to disintegrate the yeast wall completely, and it produces oligosaccharides with 5 or more residues. The 1,6-glucanases solubilize mannan peptide (Bacon et al., 1970).

Polysaccharides are not the only biopolymers degradable by CLB. *Proteolytic activity* on gelatin, casein and other types of proteins is very common. More specialized enzymes that have been reported are, for example, keratinases with activity on autoclaved feathers and hair (Napier, 1966; Martin and So, 1969), (probably) enzymatic S-factor-releasing cholinesterase from plaice muscle (Bovallius, 1979), and an endopeptidase attacking *Staphylococcus epidermidis* peptidoglycan (Kawata et al., 1984). As mentioned above for certain polysaccharide-degrading enzymes, proteases may be associated with slime polysaccharides which could be a mechanism to stabilize enzymes and to prevent their free diffusion (Christison and Martin, 1971).

Very active extracellular *RNases* and *DNases* are also known from CLB and seem to be rather common (Mitchell et al., 1967; Greaves et al., 1970). A DNase of *C. johnsonae* was found to be an endoenzyme of type I, attacking only macromolecular DNA. Nucleotides, purine and pyrimidine bases, and orthophosphate are gradually released, and adenine may become deaminated to hypoxanthine (Graeves et al., 1970). Still *C. johnsonae* is not able to grow on nucleic acids as the sole source for C or P, and even the weak growth observed with DNA or RNA as the sole N source may have been due to impurities. The behavior with respect to P and N is not quite understandable, as the organism is able to grow on NH_4^+ and orthophosphate. Perhaps the release of the ions is too low, or a direct growth inhibition by nucleic acids, as has been observed on certain media, could be responsible. An interesting effect is that DNA or RNA in nutrient-rich media delay the autolysis which usually takes place soon after *C. johnsonae* has reached the stationary phase. In this case, the cells also retain their long and thin rod shape.

Phosphatases are almost always present (see, for example, Christensen, 1977b; Hirsch, 1980; and Reichardt et al., 1983). Hydrolysis of washing-powder polyphosphate to orthophosphate by CLB has been demonstrated (Ruschke and Köhn, 1970). Activity on tributyrin is often reported, sometimes also on Tweens (see, for example, Oyaizu et al., 1982; and Reichardt et al., 1983), but *lipases* of CLB have not yet been studied in detail.

Lytic activity on cellular systems appears less common among CLB (see, for example, Christensen, 1977a, b). Sometimes, hemolysis is observed (see, for example, Ruschke and Rath 1966; and Christensen, 1977a, b). Reports on lysis of cyanobacteria and algae by unclassified *Cytophaga* and "myxobacter" strains usually dealt in fact with *Lysobacter* (for a review, see Stewart and Daft, 1977), but at least in one case a CLB appears to have been responsible (Gromov et al., 1972). One strain of *C. johnsonae*, which could not attack living *Aerobacter aerogenes* and *Saccharomyces cerevisiae*, readily lysed and grew on the autoclaved microorganisms (Webley et al., 1967). Indeed, many CLB decompose autoclaved baker's yeast more or less completely, as can be seen from the clearing zones on VY/2 agar. Autoclaved cells of *Escherichia coli* are also often degraded (see, for example, Pacha, 1968; and Hirsch, 1980). Lysis

of filamentous fungi by CLB seems to be less common but has occasionally been reported (see, for example, Imshenetski and Solntseva, 1945; and Napier, 1966).

Vitamin requirements are rare for CLB and are known only for a few marine organisms. Thus *C. fermentans* depends on thiamine (Bachmann, 1955). Other strains do not need vitamins under anaerobic conditions but, when grown aerobically, are at least much stimulated by added vitamins (Veldkamp, 1961).

Marine CLB almost always require elevated salt concentrations, but the known species appear to be not particularly fastidious with respect to concentration and ionic composition. Usually, NaCl alone can satisfy the salt demand, and in the case of *C. fermentans*, NaCl can even be replaced by KCl (Stanier, 1941; Bachmann, 1955; Veldkamp, 1961). In any case, artificial instead of natural seawater would be satisfactory. The range of salt tolerance is usually between 1 and 5% NaCl, or one-half-strength to double-strength seawater, but a few marine strains would even grown at freshwater salt levels (Lewin and Lounsbery, 1969). Terrestrial species generally appear relatively sensitive to higher salt concentrations and rarely grow in the presence of >1% NaCl and often not even at that level. In special environments, such as estuaries, they may, however, be able to adapt to higher salt concentrations (Reichardt et al., 1983). On the other hand, marine species may gradually adapt to freshwater conditions (van der Meulen et al., 1974).

With respect to their *temperature range*, the CLB typically are mesophiles, often with a strong psychrotrophic tendency, but obligate psychrophiles have been described from antarctic environments (Inoue and Komagata, 1976). Many soil and marine species have temperature optima between 30 and 35°C, but the maximum is obviously never beyond 40°C (see, for example, Stanier, 1941; Veldkamp, 1961; Lewin and Lounsbery, 1969; and Oyaizu et al., 1982). The thermal death point was found to be 10 min at 48°C and 4 min at 50°C for a collection of species (Warke and Dhala, 1966). *C. flevensis* survives 10 min at 40° but does not survive at 45°C (van der Meulen et al., 1974). Freshwater species usually show a considerably lower temperature optimum, between 20 and 25°C. They are often psychrotrophs which become predominant in the bacterial flora of lakes and sewage plants during the cold season and can selectively be enriched in mixed cultures at low temperatures, e.g. 5°C (Ruschke and Rath, 1966; Pacha, 1968; Güde, 1973; 1978a, b; 1980; Reichardt and Morita, 1982a; Reichardt et al., 1983). Results of studies on the kinetics of glucose uptake, respiration and incorporation into macromolecules suggest a higher metabolic versatility of such CLB at lower temperatures (Reichardt and Morita, 1982a).

Many strains of this type grow rather well at 30°C when kept on plates but when grown in liquid media, require lower temperatures. There may be a very broad temperature range for near-optimal growth, e.g. 22–30°C in a strain of *C. johnsonae* (Reichardt and Morita, 1982b).

The optimal pH for CLB is always around 7. There is generally no growth below pH 5.5 and above pH 8–9.

The *sensitivity for various antibiotics* has been determined for many CLB. Because of differences in the applied methods, the results are not strictly comparable, and of course there also are differences between organisms. In general, it seems that CLB are relatively resistant to polymyxin B, the penicillins, sometimes also to the aminoglycosides and chloramphenicol; they are relatively sensitive to tetracyclines, actinomycin D and sulfafurazole (Warke and Dhala, 1966, 1968; van der Meulen et al., 1974; Christensen 1977b; Agbo and Moss, 1979; Reichardt et al., 1983). It was also reported that CLB are rather resistant to bile salts with, for example, a MIC of 6–20 mg/ml for sodium taurocholate (Warke and Dhala, 1968), to phenol and lysol (Warke and Dhala, 1966), and to Zn^{2+} salts (Mehra et al., 1967). In concentrations of 0.1–0.2%, the latter suppressed slime production and swarming. CLB were very sensitive to formalin and mercuric chloride (Warke and Dhala, 1966).

The *practical importance of CLB* is certainly still incompletely appreciated. In nature they obviously take an essential part in the degradation of biopolymers, and they appear to play the same role in the aerobic part of sewage plants, in particular on trickling filters during the cold season (Bauer, 1962; Güde, 1980). With these capabilities and their wide distribution they are probably also involved in the spoilage of food and goods. For example, before the age of plastics they were found to contribute substantially to the rotting of fishing nets on the seashore (Kadota, 1956). As already pointed out, CLB may be useful for the production of enzymes for industrial applications. Or the organisms could help to improve or to speed up certain complex processes such as the penetration of preservatives into wood (Kurowski and Dunleavy, 1976). Recently, new monobactam antibiotics have been obtained from a CLB (Cooper et al., 1983).

For a long time CLB have been considered to be responsible for a variety of freshwater fish diseases, often resulting in serious economic losses, e.g. columnaris disease, cotton wool disease, cold water disease, peduncle disease (perhaps identical with the former), (hemorrhagic) bacterial gill disease, saddleback disease of salmon, branchionephritis in eels, ulcer disease in cyprinids, and probably also fin and tail rot. Originally discovered and studied in the U.S., disorders of this type are known now from many countries and occur mainly in cultured fish or at least become particularly obvious there. Chief victims are salmonids, perhaps because they are especially sensitive to unfavorable changes in their habitat, but many other kinds of fishes are also attacked. Pathogenic CLB have been described for saltwater fishes or freshwater fishes in marine environments, e.g. (a) eroded mouth disease in rainbow trout (Anderson and Conroy, 1969) and in black and red sea breams (Hikida et al., 1979) and (b) black patch necrosis in sole (Campbell and Buswell, 1982). There is a vast and expanding literature on this topic, which cannot be discussed here in detail (for reviews, see Rucker et al., 1953; Colgrove and Wood, 1966; Anderson and Conroy, 1969; Bullock and McLaughlin, 1970; Collins, 1970; Pacha and Ordal, 1970; Bullock, 1972; Bohl, 1973; Wakabayashi and Egusa, 1974; and Becker and Fujihara, 1978). The relationship between these diverse diseases is still far from being clear, and the connections between the pathogenic organisms involved and saprophytic free-living strains are not known (see, for example, Pacha, 1968). Not even the exact etiology and pathology of the diseases are understood. There is, however, little doubt that there are several fish-pathogenic species of CLB with strains of graded infectivity. Sometimes, disease seems to depend on mixed infections, as occurs, for example, with a *Corynebacterium* (Marks et al., 1980). Not unexpectedly, environmental factors play an essential role in the development of disease. For example, unfavorably high or low temperatures and oxygen levels or the availability of Fe^{3+} may substantially aggravate symptoms (see, for example, Collins, 1970; Sniesko, 1974; Kuo et al., 1981; Morrison et al., 1981; and Chen et al., 1982). In fact, columnaris disease became a problem for salmonids only after the Columbia River had been warmed up by industrial activities; this disease is typically observed mainly in overstocked hatcheries or fish ponds.

Finally, as already mentioned, a CLB has recently been found to be the culprit in an allergenic lung disease of humans which is connected with humidifiers (Flaherty et al., 1984a, b; Liebert et al., 1984).

Certain facultatively anaerobic CLB that have regularly been isolated from human dental plaque have not been connected with pathogenic events so far (London et al., 1982). These organisms, which are not to be mistaken for *Capnocytophaga*, may ferment sugars with the formation of acidic end products. They bind very efficiently to the surface of the intact tooth root, apparently via the LPS vesicles protruding from the cell surface. In fact, they bind to hydroxyapatite beads 50- to 100-fold better than do *Capnocytophaga* and *Bacteroides*, so that they could pioneer the colonization of the tooth surface, mediating the attachment of other, more dangerous organisms.

Enrichment and Isolation Procedures

CLB are found in all climate zones worldwide. They regularly occur in places where biomacromolecules accumulate and are degraded: in soil, on rotting wood and other decaying plant material, in animal dung, on the carapaces of dead insects and crustaceans, etc. Cellulose-degrading CLB have even been isolated from the intestines of termites (Verona and Baldacci, 1939). CLB are very common in both freshwater and marine aquatic habitats, where they live on and in the sediment, on the surface of dead and living seaweeds and water plants, attached to plankton organisms, fish or other animals, or on suspended debris, which explains why they are often isolated in high numbers after the water has been agitated, for example, by a storm. But they may also occur free-living in great numbers in clean bodies of water. They have not yet been obtained from the open ocean, perhaps only for technical reasons. As is to be expected, CLB readily invade human-built habitats of a comparable setting, such as aquariums, sewage plants (Bauer, 1962; Güde, 1980), fish hatcheries, drinking water lines (Herman, 1978, 1981), and humidifiers (Herman, 1981; Flaherty et al., 1984a, b). No strains have been obtained so far from environments with extreme pH, salinity or high temperatures. As would be expected, metabolic specialists may show a more restricted distribution. Thus agar decomposers are very abundant along the seacoast but are found only rarely in freshwater environments (van der Meulen et al., 1974; Agbo and Moss, 1979). Cellulose-degrading CLB seem to prefer soils with a neutral to slightly acid pH, which has been explained by their stimulation or even dependence on Ca^{2+}, Fe^{2+}, Cu^{2+} and Mn^{2+}, ions which are more readily available in the lower pH range (Fåhraeus, 1947; Bortels, 1956). Often, CLB are present in their habitats in large populations, sometimes clearly dominating the total heterotrophic bacterial flora. *C. hutchinsonii* is reported to participate in the composting of cattle manure, with from 3×10^6 to 6×10^8 cells/g dry weight being dominant among the cellulose decomposers at the beginning of the process, together with *Sporocytophaga*. Their numbers decline during the thermophilic phase (42–53°C), but they survive and become dominant again during the maturation stage (Godden and Penninckx, 1984). Between 4 and 11% of all bacterial colonies obtained from Indian soils by plating on lean media were CLB (Warke and Dhala, 1968). In activated sludge, CLB may be present with from 10^6 to 3×10^7 cells/ml, constituting 7–10% of the total heterotrophic count. The comparable data for trickling filters are from 10^5 to 10^7 cells/ml or 12–15%. The share of CLB in the aerobic part of sewage plants becomes even higher when specialized bacterial groups are compared. Thus CLB constitute 40% of all cellulose-degrading bacteria and 20% of all chitin, pectin, dextran or xylan decomposers (Güde, 1980). From the water of a Canadian creek, from 2×10^4 to 3×10^5 CLB/ml were obtained by plating on media favorable for cytophagas, which was 10–25% of the total bacterial population growing on those media (Christensen and Cook, 1972). In lakes, CLB are found in the order of 10^3–10^5 cells/ml, with complex distribution patterns depending on temperature, depth, stratification, blooms of other organisms, and availability of certain nutrients (see, for example, Reichardt, 1974, 1981; and Lighthart, 1975). In eutrophic lakes in the southwest of Germany, CLB may constitute up to 97% of the total pectolytic bacterial flora. The highest numbers were observed in summer at the end of August with about 300 cells/ml (Güde, 1973; 1978b). Because CLB are so common in freshwater, their titers have been used as an indicator for the degree of eutrophication of water bodies (Gräf and Stürzenhofecker, 1965) or, as CLB seem to pass less easily through layers of sand and soil than do ordinary bacteria, for the pollution of aquifers by surface water (Gräf and Pelka, 1979). Between 10 and 30% of all bacteria isolated from fresh North Sea fish belong in the *Cytophaga-Flavobacterium* group (Shewan, 1971). On the Japanese coast, CLB and flavobacteria constitute 20–70% of the total bacterial flora isolated from the surface of red and green algae, with from 10^3 to 10^6 cells/cm². They are much less numerous on brown algae or directly in the seawater, where only 0–400 cells/ml, constituting 0–10% of the total count, have been found (Shiba and Taga, 1980). Specifically, freshwater strains often appear to be favored by low temperatures. Thus, in sewage plants, the share of CLB in the total heterotrophic bacterial count rises regularly by 30–200% during winter (Güde, 1980). Almost 50% of all bacteria isolated from the water of an oligotrophic lake in the southwest of Germany under 60 cm of ice and grown on peptone agar were CLB, i.e. about 60 cells/ml (Ruschke and Rath, 1966). In a eutrophic lake of the same region, an organism resembling *F. aquatile* was present all year round in the sediment but rose into the epilimnion during winter, with 10^5 cells/ml or 90% of the total heterotrophic count (Reichardt, 1974). In Maizuru Bay in Japan, CLB constituted up to 30% of the population of aerobic cellulose-decomposing bacteria during autumn, winter and spring, but they completely disappeared in summer. This was attributed, however, not to temperature but to the abundance of plankton organisms to which the CLB apparently attach. In fact, the count of cellulolytic CLB remained high all year round on immersed cotton fishing nets, on which they formed between 20 and 40% of the cellulolytic bacterial population, although the higher numbers occurred at the lower temperatures (Kadota, 1956).

The isolation and cultivation of CLB, in general, has been summarized repeatedly (Stanier, 1942; Veldkamp, 1965; Reichenbach and Dworkin, 1981c). In addition, there exist several systematic studies and numerous reports on the enrichment, isolation and enumeration of specialized groups (see, for example, Winogradsky, 1929; Stapp and Bortels, 1934; Jensen, 1940; Stanier, 1941, 1947; Anacker and Ordal, 1955; Bachmann, 1955; Veldkamp, 1955, 1961; Kadota, 1956; Imshenetski, 1959; Meyer, 1961; Bauer, 1962; Gräf and Stürzenhofecker, 1964; Wang et al., 1964; Anderson and Heffernan, 1965; Carlson and Pacha, 1968; Warke and Dhala, 1968; Fijan, 1969; Lewin and Lounsbery, 1969; Christensen and Cook, 1972; Güde, 1973; van der Meulen et al., 1974; Agbo and Moss, 1979; London et al., 1982; Reichardt et al., 1983; Godden and Penninckx, 1984; and Mullings and Parish, 1984).

The CLB are physiologically too heterogeneous to be isolated by one single method. Further, although several of the more specialized forms can be enriched to a certain degree, no conditions are known that would yield CLB exclusively or predominantly. Basically, there are three types of organisms. First, there are CLB that grow on peptone alone, often also on inorganic nitrogen compounds and a suitable carbon source, usually glucose. They are probably all proteolytic, as can be seen on skim milk agar (Christensen and Cook, 1972). As their metabolism resembles too closely that of many other heterotrophic bacteria, selectivity for them is not readily possible. Still, they may easily be isolated, since they are so common in nature, grow without problems on most bacteriological media, and may be readily recognized. Second, most cellulose degraders are specialists with relatively narrow growth requirements. Cellulose is their preferred carbon source. They may utilize inorganic or organic nitrogen, grow only poorly on mineral agar with glucose, and do not grow at all on peptone alone. They can be isolated only on native or modified cellulose. Third, between these extremes there is a large group of CLB that readily grow and can be isolated on general bacteriological media but that have special metabolic capabilities that allow for selective enrichment. Such is the case with the agar, chitin and pectin degraders, facultative anaerobes and others. Of course, there also may be more fastidious organisms occupying very special niches and requiring certain additives to their isolation media, such as the CLB from dental plaque or from sewage plants. High losses among primary isolates, e.g. 40% of the chitinoclastic bacteria obtained from estuarine environments (Reichardt et al., 1983), could reflect such special needs.

Efforts have been made to create selective conditions for CLB by adding compounds toxic for other organisms. Thus it is possible to eliminate molds effectively by adding 10–25 µg cycloheximide (or Acti-Dione) per ml (Carlson and Pacha, 1968), which was also used to control protozoa and algae and is tolerated by CLB even at 100 µg/ml (Lewin and Lounsbery, 1969). The antibiotic is especially valuable when cellulose degraders are being isolated, since the enrichment cultures are otherwise very often overgrown by fungi. Initially, it was attempted to curb molds in such cultures by keeping the filter paper saturated with water (Stanier, 1942) or by adding 0.01% potassium sorbate (Meyer, 1961). A high water content also suppresses growth of actinomycetes in enrichment cultures for cellulose (Stanier, 1942) or chitin decomposers (Veldkamp, 1965). C. columnaris was found to be relatively resistant to certain antibiotics (Fijan and Voorhees, 1969), and clearly better results were obtained when 5 µg of neomycin and 5–10 units of polymyxin B were added per ml of isolation medium (Fijan, 1969). The antibiotics may be valuable in this

case, in that fish, particularly when already dead, are colonized by many other bacteria, and the pathogen may be present in large numbers only at a few restricted sites. However, the method does not guarantee that the isolated CLB are really C. columnaris, for neomycin also allows the isolation of ordinary freshwater CLB (Carlson and Pacha, 1968), many of which are resistant to polymyxin B as well (Hirsch, 1980). For selective enrichment of CLB from soil, the addition of chloramphenicol (5 µg/ml) and penicillin G (sodium salt, 15 units/ml) to an alkaline (pH 9) plating medium has been recommended (Warke and Dhala, 1968). The same authors have also reported substantially better yields in CLB when the bile salts, sodium cholate and sodium taurocholate (5 mg/ml each), are added. Further, it was reported that Zn salts (e.g. 0.1% $ZnSO_4$) would reduce swarming and slime production and thus facilitate isolation of CLB (Mehra et al., 1967). It must be emphasized, however, that with the exceptions mentioned above, good results are generally obtained without such additives and it might actually be wise to avoid them, since nothing is known about the sensitivities of new organisms.

On plates used for isolation, CLB may be recognized by three properties: (a) spreading colonies, (b) yellow to red pigmentation and (c) cell shape and motility. It may be recalled that no one of these characteristics is fully reliable: spreading critically depends on the environmental conditions; there are weakly and unpigmented CLB and yellow to red bacteria in other groups; the cell shape is not characteristic enough to distinguish CLB from many other bacteria; and motility may temporarily be absent or too slow to be recognized. Thus it is essential to choose media for isolation which elicit these distinctive features with high probability.

The nonspecialized CLB can be obtained from soil and water by ordinary dilution plating. Addition of Tween 80 at 1–10 mg/l (Güde,1973; Shiba and Taga, 1980; Reichardt et al., 1983) or of Tween 20 at 1 µg/l (Christensen and Cook, 1972) to the dilution medium (e.g. distilled water, 0.9% NaCl, buffer solutions, diluted culture medium, seawater) improves the separation of the cells and their suspension and may result in a 2–4-fold increase in plate count. Primary isolation is almost always done on agar media with a low nutrient content to encourage spreading of CLB and to check growth of other, more fastidious heterotrophs. Numerous different formulations, usually on a peptone basis, have been used with good success, and it appears that the exact composition of the medium is not of particular importance. A few examples may suffice:

Mouton agar: meat broth diluted 1:10; and agar, 1.5% (Gräf and Stürzenhofecker, 1964; used for freshwater CLB)

PM (peptonized milk) agar: tryptone (Difco), 0.005%; yeast extract, 0.005%; beef extract, 0.002%; peptonized milk, 0.005%; Na-acetate, 0.002%; and agar, 1.5% (Carlson and Pacha, 1968; used for freshwater CLB)

T (tryptone) agar: tryptone, 0.02%; and agar, 1% (Lewin and Lounsbery, 1969; used for various CLB)

*PMYA II agar**: peptonized milk, 0.1%; yeast extract, 0.02%; Na-acetate, 0.002%; and agar, 1.5%

*TYA-agar**: tryptone, 0.1%; yeast extract, 0.02%; Na-acetate, 0.02%; and agar, 1.5%

*SM (skim milk) agar**: skim milk, 0.5%; yeast extract, 0.05%; and agar, 1.5% (Christensen and Cook, 1972)

CA (Cytophaga) agar[†]: tryptone, 0.05%; yeast extract, 0.05%; beef extract, 0.02%; Na-acetate, 0.02%; and agar 0.9% (Anacker and Ordal, 1955).

Much richer media have occasionally also been used:

PPES-II agar: polypeptone, 0.2%; soytone (Difco), 0.1%; yeast extract, 0.1%, proteose peptone (Difco), 0.1%; ferric citrate, 0.01%;

---

[*]High yields in counting freshwater CLB have been reported with use of this medium.

[†]Fish pathogens are isolated on this medium. At least for these organisms a slight reduction in the agar concentration seems to be favorable. Beef extract and Na-acetate, however, appear dispensable (Bootsma and Clerx, 1976), which may also be the case with the acetate in PM agar, PMYA agar and TYA agar.

and agar, 1.5% (Shiba and Taga, 1980; for bacteria on the surface of seaweeds; see also Oyaizu and Komagata, 1981)

On such media, spreading will usually be completely suppressed, although this can happen even on relatively lean media, e.g. Mouton agar (Pfeiffer, 1967). Sewage CLB have been obtained on the following medium:

NG (nitrate glucose) *agar*: KNO_3, 0.1%; KH_2PO_4, 0.1%; $CaCl_2$, 0.01%; $MgSO_4\cdot7H_2O$, 0.03%; NaCl, 0.01%; $FeCl_3$, 0.001%; glucose, 0.5%; and agar, 2% (Bauer, 1962)

When marine CLB are isolated, the media are prepared with fresh or aged (stored for at least 1 month in the dark) seawater, but artificial seawater also appears fully satisfactory, either commercial marine salts mixes or simplified formulations, e.g. NaCl, 2.5%; $MgSO_4\cdot7H_2O$, 0.5%; $CaCl_2\cdot2H_2O$, 0.1%; and KCl, 0.1% (Lewin and Lounsbery, 1969). My colleagues and I have always had excellent results with the following recipe: NaCl, 2.47%; $MgSO_4\cdot7H_2O$, 0.63%; $MgCl_2\cdot6H_2O$, 0.46%; $CaCl_2$, 0.1%; KCl, 0.07%; and $NaHCO_3$, 0.02% (Dawson et al., 1972). Even 3% NaCl will often do (Stanier, 1941; Bachmann, 1955; Veldkamp, 1961). For organisms from estuaries, bays and similar transitional environments, the salt concentrations have to be chosen according to the situation (0.75–2.5%; for example, in Anderson and Heffernan, 1965; Bullock, 1972; and Reichardt et al., 1983). The pH of the isolation media should be adjusted between 6.8 and 7.4 for soil and freshwater CLB and should be adjusted somewhat higher, around 7.6, for marine bacteria. An exceptionally high pH, around 9, has been recommended for the isolation of CLB from neutral to slightly acid soils (pH 4.2–7.2) from India (Warke and Dhala, 1968). Regarding the pH optima and maxima of most CLB, the general usefulness of this measure must be doubted. A remarkable tolerance to alkaline pH values has, however, been observed with cellulose-degrading CLB; at pH 8.5, for example, there was excellent growth with all tested strains (Stanier, 1942). The plates are incubated at 18–30°C, with lower temperatures (20–24°C) being an absolute requirement for many freshwater CLB and particularly for certain specialists such as *C. psychrophila* (18°C).

The colonies of CLB can be recognized after 2–10 days. Their appearance depends, of course, on the kind of organism and on the type of medium. They range from thin spreading swarms, visible only on the tilted plate or under the dissecting microscope, when oblique translucent illumination is applied, to small, smooth, more or less slimy, compact colonies, sometimes with a narrow swarming zone with flamelike extensions around them. *C. columnaris* typically forms rhizoid colonies with a tendency to penetrate into the agar. Pigmentation is more conspicuous the more compact the colonies are. In swarms, pigmentation often becomes apparent only after the cells have been scraped together. "Typical" colonies are bright yellow to orange, sometimes with a greenish hue, slightly iridescent or opalescent. The cell mass of many species turns deep red or brown when it is covered with a drop of 20% KOH solution, and it turns bright yellow again when the latter is replaced by 10% HC. For a first differentiation of CLB from other yellow bacteria, particularly flavobacteria, it may be of help to know that 91% of all CLB are sensitive to 0.1% sodium lauryl sulfate *and* show proteolytic activity on SM agar, while this combination of characteristics is shown by only 50% of flavobacteria and other bacteria (Christensen and Cook, 1972).

Finally, two unconventional methods for isolation of CLB may be mentioned. From marine environments, CLB can be obtained, among others, when the water sample (up to 40 ml) is passed first through a membrane filter of 0.45 μm and then through one with 0.22-μm pore size. The latter filter is incubated upside up on a suitable agar medium until colonies arise. From the 10^3 to 10^4 bacteria/ml of the original sample, 30 to <1 pass through the first filter, but not one passes through the second filter. Efforts to apply the method also for the isolation of bacteria from soil samples were unsuccessful (Anderson and Heffernan, 1965).

When patches or cross-streaks of living *Escherichia coli* on *WCX* (water-cycloheximide) *agar* ($CaCl_2$, 0.1%; agar, 1.5%; and cycloheximide, 25 μg/ml; at pH 7.2) are inoculated with small amounts of soil, as is done for the isolation of myxobacteria (Reichenbach and Dworkin, 1981b),

delicate swarms of other gliding bacteria, among them CLB, are often observed on the agar beyond the bacterial lawn. The organisms can be further enriched on the same substrate until sufficiently pure, so that transfers can be made from the swarm edge to a suitable growth medium.

Purification is easily achieved by making transfers from swarm edges and by dilution plating. This is done preferentially on somewhat richer media to speed up growth and make contaminants more conspicuous. Many standard bacteriological media with a peptone-glucose basis are suitable, but it is usually preferable to keep the overall concentration of the N compounds at or below 1%. My colleagues and I have always had good results, for example, with *CY agar* (casitone (Difco), 0.3%; yeast extract, 0.1%; $CaCl_2\cdot2H_2O$, 0.1%; and agar, 1.5%; at pH 7.2) or with *MYX agar* (Na-glutamate, 0.5%; yeast extract, 0.1%; $MgSO_4\cdot7H_2O$; glucose, 0.2% (autoclaved separately); and agar, 1.5%; at pH 7.2). Cultivation of these organisms is not a problem. The same media as above may be used, as solid or liquid media. An example of a simple liquid medium which we have found useful for many CLB is *FX A l.m.* (peptone from casein, tryptically digested, 1%; yeast extract, 0.2%; and $MgSO_4\cdot7H_2O$, 0.1%; at pH 7.2). Generation times may be as short as 1–2 h. Most CLB also grow well in completely defined media with casamino acids, glutamate, NH_4^+ or NO_3^- as the N source, and, if required, glucose or some other sugar as the carbon and energy source. An example of a simple medium which has successfully been used by us with many CLB is *MG* (mineral salts-glucose) *l.m.*: $(NH_4)SO_4$, 0.2%; $KHPO_4$, 0.07%; Na_2HPO_4, 0.14%; $MgSO_4\cdot7H_2O$, 0.02%; $FeSO_4$, 5 mg/l; $MnSO_4$, 5 mg/l; and glucose, 1% (autoclaved separately). We have found *VY/2 agar* (baker's yeast, 0.5% by fresh weight of yeast cake; $CaCl_2$, 0.1%; cyanocobalamine, 0.5 mg/l; and agar, 1.5%; at pH 7.2, autoclaved) a particularly useful medium because it elicits spreading growth with many CLB and the cultures usually remain viable for relatively long times.

Usually, the first step in the isolation of cellulose degrading CLB is an enrichment culture. Although some cellulose decomposers also attack agar (Stanier, 1940; Mullings and Parish, 1981), most appear to depend on cellulose (and a few sugars) for carbon and energy. In addition, the use of cellulose and a mineral salts solution introduces a substantial degree of selectivity into isolation and, in fact, is the only feasible way to obtain these organisms. Basically, three approaches have been tried over the years. With the first approach, filter paper (Stapp and Bortels, 1934; Meyer, 1961) or cellophane (Went and De Jong, 1966) is buried in soil, either in the laboratory or in the natural environment, and is re-collected after 1–2 weeks, and the responsible organisms are then isolated from areas of disintegration. A piece of filter paper may also be placed on a layer of moistened soil in a Petri dish and incubated until spots of decomposing cellulose appear. The latter method often yields fungi and actinomycetes (Stapp and Bortels, 1934; Jensen, 1940). Cotton fishing nets were suspended in seawater for 10 days, and rotting material was then placed onto cellulose agar for further enrichment (Kadota, 1956). Without such a seminatural enrichment, marine cellulolytic bacteria could not be isolated. With the second approach, pieces of filter paper are immersed in a mineral salts medium and inoculated with a small amount of soil or a water sample. Such a system is particularly clean and thus relatively selective. The disadvantages are: the aerobic CLB can develop only in a narrow zone near the air-liquid interface; contaminants tend to spread evenly through the culture; it is difficult to pick up material for transfers selectively from decomposing areas; and due to the uniformity of the system, only one kind of organism usually develops in each culture (Stanier, 1942). On the other hand, during an isolation of cellulose-degrading bacteria including CLB, from freshwater and soil, the yield of positive samples could be increased by an intermediary enrichment on wood pulp in a mineral medium (Mullings and Parish, 1984). With the third approach, the method of choice for enrichment and isolation of cellulolytic CLB is the use of plate cultures. For enrichment a thin and compact filter paper of high purity should be used as carbon and energy source. It has been stated that filter papers contain substances toxic for cellulolytic CLB (Fåhraeus, 1947; Imshenetski, 1959). But this seems no longer, or not in every case, to be true. At least my colleagues and I have never had problems using several types of ordinary round filters sterilized by autoclaving. The filters are placed on mineral salts agar and inoculated with soil, rotting plant material, or drops taken from water samples. If soil is used, a small quantity, about the size of a lentil or a pea seed, is placed in the center of a filter of 6-cm diameter, or the soil is sprinkled loosely over the whole filter area, or, better, the filter is inoculated in a regular pattern at different places with a few grains of soil, e.g. by stamping the soil on the filter with the flat end of a glass rod or by distributing the soil with a swab. To discourage the spreading of contaminants, several smaller pieces of filter paper may be distributed over the plate and inoculated separately. The plates are then incubated at a suitable temperature. For soil samples, 25-30°C is favorable, but some cellulolytic soil cytophagas seem to prefer lower temperatures (20-25°C). After 4-5 days the first glassy, translucent, yellow-to-orange spots may appear, indicating development of cellulolytic CLB. But often clear results are seen only after 1-2 weeks. Transfers are made as early as possible from the margins of the areas of cellulose decomposition to fresh plates with several small pieces of filter paper. The exact composition of the mineral agar has been regarded as not very critical (Stanier, 1942). In general, however, it appears that development of cellulolytic CLB is specifically stimulated if NH_4^+ instead of NO_3^- is used as the N source. Also, the addition of Mn^{2+} and Fe^{3+} in relatively high concentrations considerably speeds up development of CLB. Further, incorporation of cycloheximide substantially facilitates their isolation. My colleagues and I have found the following medium (ST6CX agar) very useful: $(NH_4)_2SO_4$, 0.1%; K_2HPO_4, 0.1%; $CaCl_2\cdot2H_2O$, 0.1%; $MnSO_4\cdot H_2O$, 0.01%; $FeCl_3\cdot6H_2O$, 0.02%; trace elements; cycloheximide, 25 mg/l; and agar, 1%; at pH 7.2. To prevent precipitation, the components are autoclaved separately in suitable combinations, and cycloheximide and trace elements are filter sterilized. Mn^{2+} and Fe^{2+} were in Winogradsky's medium (1929), although their importance for cellulose decomposition by CLB was demonstrated only much later (Fåhraeus, 1947; Bortels, 1956). A few examples of mineral media recommended for the isolation and cultivation of cellulolytic CLB follow:

Jensen (1940) *medium*: $(NH_4)_2SO_4$, 0.1%; K_2HPO_4, 0.1%; $MgSO_4$, 0.05%; NaCl, 0.02%; and $CaCO_3$, 0.2%.

Stanier (1942) *medium*: $(NH_4)_2SO_4$ or KNO_3, 0.1%; K_2HPO_4, 0.1%; $MgSO_4$, 0.02%; $CaCl_2$, 0.01%; and $FeCl_3$, 0.002%; at pH 7.0-7.5

Kadota (1956) *medium* number 7: $NaNO_3$, 0.05%; K_2HPO_4, 0.1%; $MgSO_4\cdot7H_2O$, 0.05%; and $FeSO_4\cdot7H_2O$, 0.001% in seawater, for isolation of marine cellulose degraders.

Many variations of the isolation procedure for cellulolytic CLB have been tried. Their merits often are difficult to judge in the absence of rigorous comparative studies. Therefore several alternatives shall be mentioned. Occasionally, filter paper was replaced with cellulose mats produced by *Acetobacter xylinum* (Mullings and Parish, 1981, 1984). The advantage seems to be that decomposition of this cellulose is faster, so that lysis zones appear earlier and the cellulose degraders can be transferred before everything is overgrown by contaminants. However, no other organisms were obtained than those on filter paper, and sometimes a general liquefaction of the mats made isolation from individual colonies impossible. Also, the preparation of the mats requires additional time and material. Cellophane has been used instead of filter paper and, in fact, is regarded as an excellent substrate by some (Stapp and Bortels, 1934; Imshenetski, 1959; Went and De Jong, 1966). But whether all cellulose degraders can really attack cellulose acetate is not certain. Results may depend on the kind of cellophane used. Apparently it is essential to boil the cellophane in water before use in order to remove inhibiting substances. Cellophane may be of advantage, however, if material exposed in natural habitats is to be examined directly under the microscope afterwards. Use of CMC obviously allows growth of many organisms which are unable to degrade native cellulose, so that the selectivity of the enrichment step is reduced. Other forms of cellulose which have been found useful, although more for physiological than other studies, are cotton cloth (Winogradsky, 1929), cotton wool and cellulose wadding (Fåhraeus, 1947). Cellulose agar has been recommended for plating diluted suspensions of decomposing natural material. Either finely powdered crystalline cellulose, cellulose precipitated after treatment with copper-ammonia or mineral acids (see, for example, Stanier, 1942; Kadota, 1956), cellulose dextrins (Fuller and Norman, 1942), or sulfite wood pulp is suspended in mineral agar and poured as a thin top layer onto a mineral agar base. The latter strategy prevents the cellulose from sedimenting to the bottom of the plate and thus out of reach of the bacteria and guarantees an early development of clearly recognizable lysis zones in the thin cellulose layer. Two other points are essential: (a) the cellulose must be finely divided and uniformly distributed and (b) the agar concentration has to be lowered to 0.8-1.0%, since CLB attack cellulose only when in direct contact (Stapp and Bortels, 1935; Jensen, 1940; Stanier, 1942). It is reported that by this method, cellulose degraders can be obtained which otherwise would not be seen (in this case, the organisms were not CLB, however); also, however, excessive growth of contaminants is favored (Imshenetski, 1959). Plating on cellulose agar has repeatedly been used to determine the numbers of cellulolytic bacteria in natural habitats (Kadota, 1956; Wang et al., 1964; Godden and Penninckx, 1984). To achieve high yields it is recommended to use high concentrations (7.5%) of (precipitated) cellulose in very thin layers (0.8 mm) of soft agar (0.4-0.5%; Wang et al., 1964). To improve selectivity, silica gel plates or beds of sand, both soaked with a mineral solution, were originally used as supports for the filter paper (Winogradsky, 1929; Krzemieniewska, 1933; Imshenetski and Solntseva, 1936). But the former are tedious to prepare, and the latter resemble liquid cultures with the drawbacks mentioned above. And in general, the advantages of these inorganic supports in comparison with agar are negligible, although some report that agar contains compounds inhibitory to cellulolytic CLB (Fåhraeus, 1947; Imshenetski, 1959). Indeed, *Sporocytophaga* grew only when agar was replaced by agarose (von Hofsten et al., 1971). But as in the case of filter paper, the observation cannot be generalized, for many investigators including my colleagues and I have obtained excellent growth on agar.

The purification of cellulolytic CLB may become a major problem. In fact, most of the early investigators never had pure strains, so that it was surmised that the organisms would grow only symbiotically (Stapp and Bortels, 1935). Of course, plating on cellulose agar would be the natural choice, but although this method has been used repeatedly for counting, it has not readily resulted in pure cultures. The reasons for this are not completely clear, and the statements in the literature are contradictory. It appears that individual cells do not easily grow out to form colonies, which would be understandable in that they first have to break down the substrate enzymatically and thus may starve before sufficient product has been set free. In any case, development is slow, plating efficiency is low with higher dilutions, and with low dilution, contaminants often find sufficient time to spread through the soft agar into developing colonies of cellulolytic CLB. Also, when a more intimate contact between cell and cellulose was created by applying the pour plate technique, results still varied from excellent (Stanier, 1942; Kadota, 1956) to poor (Stapp and Bortels, 1935). With either method, the CLB, if they develop, do not produce normal colonies but rather form transparent, often yellowish plaques, i.e. lysis zones, without any macroscopically recognizable structure. At later stages they may be covered with a yellow-to-pink slime (Jensen, 1940; Stanier, 1942; von Hofsten et al., 1971). Cellulolytic CLB also grow on mineral agar with glucose, provided the glucose is autoclaved separately or filter-sterilized, because otherwise toxic products specifically prevent any growth of these organisms (Stanier, 1942). However, from my and my colleagues experience the organisms grow on such media only if the plates are heavily inoculated. From higher dilutions as required during purification steps, no colonies develop from single cells (Meyer, 1961). Good results have recently been reported with mineral agar containing 1% glucose instead of the 0.1-0.5% usually applied (Mullings and Parish, 1984). My colleagues and I have sometimes had success with plating on CMC agar, *ST10 agar* ($(NH_4)_2SO_4$, 0.1%; K_2HPO_4, 0.1%; $MgSO_4\cdot7H_2O$, 0.1%; $CaCl_2\cdot2H_2O$, 0.1%; trace elements; casitone (Difco), 0.2%; agar, 0.6%; and CMC-Na salt of high viscosity (Sigma), 1.5%). After incubation for 4-8 days at 30°C, cellulolytic CLB form cloudy, greenish-yellowish, gradually spreading and finally relatively large (4–8-mm) spherical colonies within the substrate. Although such colonies are somewhat difficult to recognize, they often allow one to make transfers of pure material. Another strategy found very useful by my colleagues and myself is the following. First, fast-moving animals that are often present within the decaying cellulose of filter paper cultures are removed (Reichenbach, 1983): amoebae are killed by exposing the opened Petri dish upside down for 2–3 min to the vapors of a 5% NH₃ solution in a second dish. After another 3–5 min, material from colonies is transferred to a fresh filter paper plate. If nematodes are present, the plate is stored for 2–3 days at −80°C and transfers are made immediately after thawing. The real purification step is to allow the CLB to squeeze through a membrane filter of low pore size. First, a commercial filter pad consisting of regenerated cellulose is placed on mineral agar. This substrate is readily attacked by CLB, quickly yielding neat decomposition zones. On top of this is placed a second membrane filter of smaller diameter and with a pore size of 0.2–0.3 μm. This filter paper consists of cellulose nitrate (not degradable by CLB) and is inoculated with material from a filter paper culture. During this inoculation the margins of the pad should never be approached, in order to avoid spreading of contaminated liquid within the capillary space between the membranes. After 1–2 days incubation the top filter with the inoculum is removed. If the CLB are able to migrate through the membrane, then small yellow spots are seen on the regenerated cellulose pad or will develop in the following days. As different organisms penetrate the filter with different speeds, several pads should be inoculated and removed after different times to hit the shortest possible incubation time. There is no use to wait longer than 3 days, because by then many other bacteria start to grow through the filter. But also, short incubation times do not guarantee success: sometimes very small contaminants, often flagellated, are still present within the colonies of the cellulolytic CLB. Also, the extremely thin (0.1-μm) rods that have been found in *Sporocytophaga* cultures started from sewage (von Hofsten et al., 1971) could not be removed in this way. In most cases, however, at least the large number of different contaminants initially present can be reduced to one or two.

Pure cultures of cellulolytic CLB are easy to grow on the media described above. Vigorous growth is always obtained on filter paper placed on a peptone agar, e.g. C4 agar. As liquid media, a mineral base with cellulose powder or glucose will serve. The optimal glucose concentration appears to be around 0.5–0.75% (Stanier, 1942; Verma and Martin, 1967a). Other sugars can also be used, but the spectrum is rather restricted and varies with the organism. Besides glucose, cellobiose, mannose and xylose have been found to allow growth (Stanier, 1942). On some media, the organisms may fail to grow if the inoculum is low. At least some cellulolytic CLB seem to grow at relatively high temperatures (37°C, for example, in Meyer, 1961) and at an alkaline pH (Stanier (1942) obtained excellent growth at pH 8.5).

Many kinds of CLB with special degradative capabilities have been enriched more or less selectively by adding the special substrates to a suitable basal medium (see, for example, Payza and Korn, 1956; Martin and Soo, 1969; and Oyaizu et al., 1982). A few cases of more general interest are briefly discussed. Aerobic agar decomposers are easily obtained from marine environments such as fresh or decaying algae, mud or water samples (Stanier, 1941; Humm, 1946). The diluted or undiluted material is streaked onto mineral agar or, better, as some agar decomposers require a complex N source, onto agar with a small amount of peptone, e.g. yeast extract, 0.1%, and agar, 1.5%, in seawater. Most organisms would also grow at much higher peptone concentrations and could be isolated on nutrient agar, but this would stimulate excessive growth of contaminants. After 2–5 days at 20–25°C, thin yellow or pink, sometimes rapidly spreading colonies may be found sitting in shallow craters or surrounded by liquefied agar. If agar decomposition is weak, the colony can be visualized by flooding the plate with an I-KI solution. Colonies of agar degraders are then surrounded by a pale yellowish zone (Gran's gelase fields) in a violet-brown background. Purification can be achieved by dilution plating, preferentially on an agar medium with slightly elevated (0.3–0.5%) peptone concentrations. Some CLB liquefy agar vigorously, so that plating becomes problematical. In this case, the organism may be in-

oculated onto a membrane filter of 0.2–0.3 μm pore size placed on an agar plate. The filter is removed after 1–2 days as soon as or even before the first small colonies appear on the agar below. If agar degraders are rare in a habitat, as, for example, in freshwater, an introductory enrichment step may be necessary, as, for example, by incubating the sample for several days in a 0.1% agar solution with or without a N source (KNO₃ or (NH₄)₂SO₄, 0.1%; Stanier, 1941; van der Meulen et al., 1974; Agbo and Moss, 1979). Agarolytic CLB do not depend on agar. All appear to utilize a wide variety of sugars including glucose and galactose. Some can be cultivated on mineral media with agar or a sugar. For freshwater organisms, the following medium has been used: NH₄Cl, 0.05%; KH₂PO₄, 0.1%; MgSO₄·7H₂O, 0.05%; CaCl₂·2H₂O, 0.002%; trace elements; and agar, 0.1–0.5% for liquid cultures and 1.5% for solid plates (van der Meulen et al., 1974). It seems that all grow better if a complex organic N source is added, e.g. peptone; some even require it, and at least some grow with peptone alone without any carbohydrate (Stanier, 1941). On agar media, much acid is often produced, some of it perhaps sulfuric acid from the agar heteropolysaccharide, so that the addition of 2% CaCO₃ is advisable (Stanier, 1941, 1942).

From marine samples, facultatively anaerobic agarolytic (and nonagarolytic) CLB have also been obtained but appear to be relatively rare (Bachmann, 1955; Veldkamp, 1961). The organisms can be enriched in the following medium: NaCl, 3%; KH₂PO₄, 0.1%; NH₄Cl, 0.1%; MgCl₂·6H₂O, 0.05%; CaCl₂, 0.004%; NaHCO₃, 0.5%; Na₂S·9H₂O, 0.01%; M/250 Fe-citrate, 0.5 ml/100 ml; trace elements; yeast extract, 0.03%; and agar, 0.5%; at pH 7.0. Stoppered bottles completely filled with this medium are incubated for 3–5 days in the dark. Purification is achieved by plating and by incubating under anaerobic conditions or by agar shake culture. For nonagarolytic species, glucose (0.1%) is added. The organisms require CO₂. For cultivation under aerobic conditions the medium is enriched with yeast extract, corn steep and powdered nutrient broth (0.1% of each).

Pectolytic CLB are common in soil and freshwater and can specifically be enriched on pectate gel (Dorey, 1959; Güde, 1973). Pectin of a low degree of esterification, 2%, dissolved in water at 70°C and autoclaved for 10 min at 110°C, is poured as a thin layer on plates of *calcium agar* (K₂HPO₄, 0.05%; MgSO₄·7H₂O, 0.02%; NH₄Cl, 0.1%; CaCl₂·2H₂O, 0.2%; trace elements; and agar, 1.5%, in 0.1 M Tris buffer, pH 8.0). A pectate gel develops within 30 min and can be inoculated the next day by scattering soil crumbs on it or by plating diluted water samples. The cultures are incubated at 25°C. Those started from water samples may be kept at lower temperatures down to 5°C. Within 3–7 days (2–3 weeks at 5°C), pectolytic CLB may appear as yellow colonies sitting in depressions or in a pool of liquefied gel. Strains are purified by dilution plating on pectate gel or on a peptone-containing agar. It seems that no pectolytic CLB depends on pectin or even on carbohydrate and that all can grow exclusively on peptone. In fact, diauxic growth has been observed in a liquid medium containing pectin and yeast extract, with the latter being the preferred substrate (Güde, 1973). The pectolytic CLB are not yet particularly well characterized.

Chitinoclastic CLB are abundant in soil and aquatic habitats (Stanier, 1947; Güde, 1980; Reichardt et al., 1983). The organisms may be enriched on strips of chitin immersed in a mineral solution or by adding powdered chitin to a soil sample which then should be kept saturated with water to prevent actinomycetes from dominating. In general, however, it is sufficient to plate the sample after appropriate dilution on *chitin agar* (finely divided chitin, 1%; K₂HPO₄, 0.1%; MgSO₄·7H₂O, 0.1%; and agar, 1.5%). This agar is poured as a thin layer on top of water agar plates or on some agar with a low (0.1–0.3%) peptone content. The chitin should be reprecipitated from mineral acid suspensions before use in order to obtain a good dispersion and to achieve further purification, as described repeatedly (see, for example, Stanier, 1947; Veldkamp, 1955; and Hsu and Lockwood, 1975; the latter method gives especially good results). The plates are incubated at 25–30°C unless they are started from water samples (15–20°C). CLB may develop within 3–6 (−21) days as thin, translucent, orange, yellow or almost colorless, more or less rapidly spreading swarm colonies. Chitin decomposers are recognized by clear lysis zones which may, however, be restricted to the inner swarm area and may become conspicuous only in older cultures. Purification is achieved by dilution plating on chitin agar or on a peptone-containing agar. Growth is faster if the chitin agar is poured on a peptone-containing substrate, but at higher peptone concentrations, chitin degradation is sometimes suppressed. On the other hand, some chitinoclastic CLB develop only if a complex organic N source is available to them (Reichardt et al., 1983). It seems that no chitinoclastic CLB requires chitin or another carbohydrate for growth and that all grow well on peptone alone. Again, however, the full range of these organisms is not really known. Efforts to isolate chitinolytic CLB under anaerobic conditions failed (Stanier, 1947), but in suitable media many chitinoclastic CLB are able to grow anaerobically (Reichardt et al., 1983).

Maintenance Procedures

Depending on the organism and the culture medium, cultures of CLB have to be transferred at intervals of a few days to up to 1–3 weeks, if kept at 20–30°C, and of several months, if stored at 2–5°C. Most or all CLB seem to tolerate low temperatures fairly well (see, for example, Veldkamp, 1961; and Pacha, 1968). With some but not all tested strains, my colleagues and I have obtained growth after 15 months at 4°C. In general, media with a high peptone content are not suitable for maintenance, probably because of NH$_3$ production. Equally, media resulting in acid production should at least be buffered with CaCO$_3$, for example, if agar digesters are kept on agar media. For maintenance of aquatic CLB, in particular C. columnaris, CA agar with a reduced (0.4%) agar concentration is recommended (Anacker and Ordal, 1955; Anacker and Ordal, 1959a). Usually, CLB survive best on agar media which result in thin spreading growth, e.g. media with a low (0.1%) peptone concentration, or or yeast (VY/2) agar. Although cellulose degraders survive for at least 3 months on strips of filter paper immersed in a mineral salts solution, they die after 2–3 weeks on filter paper placed on an agar plate (Stanier, 1942; Mitchell et al., 1967). Although lyophilization has been regarded as a preservation method less suitable for CLB (Mitchell, et al., 1967), this can obviously not be generalized. C. columnaris can be lyophilized without problems (Anacker and Ordal, 1959a), and also the freeze-dried preserves of various culture collections (ATCC, NCIB, NCMB) apparently survive very well. I could readily start cultures from such preserves that had been prepared 4–10 years earlier, including strains of cellulolytic and marine CLB, and with very few failures. The only systematic study published on cryopreservation of CLB (Sanfilippo and Lewin, 1970) demonstrated that all five strains of CLB tested survived freezing in liquid nitrogen when suspended in growth medium supplemented or not with 10% glycerol. All five also survived storage at −196°C for at least 1 year in the glycerol medium. Addition of 10% dimethyl sulfoxide (DMSO) instead of glycerol was not tolerated by all. However, the cells were left in the DMSO medium for 24 h before freezing, and this storage was already

lethal for at least one strain. Some strains also survived freezing at −22°C in growth medium without additives for at least 21 weeks; others, however, died soon under such conditions. Freezing in liquid nitrogen has successfully been applied to fish pathogens (Hikida et al., 1979). My own experience with the maintenance of several hundred strains over more than a decade can be summarized as follows (for further details, see also Reichenbach and Dworkin, 1981c). The most reliable and easiest storage method is freezing in peptone-containing growth medium at −80°C or in liquid nitrogen. For terrestrial strains, my colleagues and I use CAS l.m. (casitone (Difco), 1%; and MgSO$_4$·7H$_2$O, 0.1%; at pH 6.8 unadjusted); for marine strains, SP5 l.m. (casitone, 0.9%; and yeast extract, 0.1%, in artificial seawater according to Dawson et al. (1972) as described above). For storage in liquid nitrogen, the media are supplemented with 5% DMSO. The cells are transferred from young plate cultures (1–3 days old) into the respective medium to give a dense suspension, which is then frozen either in small plastic screw-capped tubes filled with 1 ml (−80°C) or in sealed glass ampuls containing 0.5 ml (−196°C). The −80°C tubes are put directly into the deep freeze; the −196°C ampuls are precooled at 6°C for 15 min and then submerged into liquid nitrogen. So far there were no failures with either method, with the longest storage periods being up to 10 years in both cases. In most cases, drying in skim milk and storage at room temperature or at 2°C also gave satisfactory results. My colleagues and I first prepare plugs of freeze-dried skim milk in 5-ml glass ampuls. On these, 2–3 drops of a dense cell suspension in skim milk are placed, and the whole is dried at room temperature in a desiccator under vacuum. The dry ampuls are filled with nitrogen gas and sealed. Strains have been reactivated after more than 10 years. There were occasional failures, which may be related to poor standardization of the procedure, especially with respect to the age of the cultures used for drying, their growth medium and the density of the applied cell suspension. Storage for shorter periods, several months to a few years, is often possible at −25°C. Cells are suspended in 50 mM phosphate buffer (pH 7.2) and then mixed 1:2 (v/v) with precooled 87% glycerol to give a final glycerol concentration of 50%. Marine strains may be suspended in precooled (−25°C) SP5 l.m./87% glycerol (1:2, v/v). The suspensions are placed immediately into the deep freeze. As they do not become solid at the storage temperature, transfers to a suitable growth medium can be made repeatedly simply by taking out a few loopfuls of material without warming up the preserve. Another simple preservation method is to prepare light cell suspensions of barely visible turbidity in distilled water, in 0.9% or 0.5% NaCl solution, or in (artificial) seawater, seal them in ampuls, and store them at room temperature. My colleagues and I have found CLB still alive in such preserves after 7 years. However, although failures appear to be relatively rare, the method may result in a gradual shift in the genetic constitution of the strain, because the bacteria probably continue to grow very slowly under these conditions.

Differentiation of the genus **Cytophaga** from other genera

The species of the genus Cytophaga are distinguished from Flavobacterium by their gliding motility, from Flexibacter (and Microscilla) by their (much) shorter cells and, in general, by a lower G + C content. Several Flexibacter species show, in addition, a pronounced cyclic shape change. Lysobacter differs in its cell shape (stouter and more cylindrical, with rounded ends); in its pigmentation (in general, only light, white, yellowish, reddish or brownish, often also with brown or red, water-soluble, diffusing pigments); and in its much higher mol% G + C (62–70).

Taxonomic Comments

The genus Cytophaga was described in 1929 by Winogradsky for aerobic cellulolytic soil bacteria "probably motile" (by gliding). Later the genus was expanded to comprise gliding marine cellulose degraders as well as gliding agar and chitin decomposers with a similar cell morphology (Stanier 1940, 1941, 1942, 1947). At the same time the organisms were attached in the system of bacteria to the equally unicellular and gliding myxobacteria (Imshenetski and Solntseva, 1936; Stanier, 1940).

The genus Cytophaga continued to grow in the following years, absorbing all kinds of unicellular gliding bacteria with short to moderately long cells forming neither microcysts nor fruiting bodies. The result is the very heterogeneous assembly of species we are confronted with today. At the moment the taxonomy of the genus Cytophaga is completely unsatisfactory. There is a considerable overlap of characters with the genera Flavobacterium, Flexibacter and Microscilla. This has occasionally resulted in the wrong conclusion that everything should be lumped together or that the genus is a taxonomic dump and might be used in the same way as the genus Flavobacterium was used earlier. There are three sources for the present confusion: (a) almost all studies in the past were performed on only a few strains each; (b) these strains were usually isolated as specialists for the degradation of certain compounds or for some other conspicuous property; and (c) they were consequently easy to distinguish from other such specialists, so that barely one species has been described in sufficient detail to define it unequivocally. But anybody who isolates a larger number of strains from nature will discover quickly that there are many more organisms of this kind, many of them in between presently defined species. Many of these organisms are, in fact, not closely related. This can be deduced from the wide mol% G + C (30–45) and is clearly proven by low values in DNA/DNA hybridization (Behrens, 1978). Thus the correct conclusion is to invest more research into this group. The strategy, already adopted in a few cases, must be to compare larger collections of strains, beginning preferentially with the methods of molecular taxonomy to define groups of organisms which are reliably related, and then to look for distinguishing phenotypic characteristics, which may not necessarily be the same as found useful with the enterobacteria. For the time being, *all* species rest exclusively on the available type strains, and microbiologists should identify new isolates by direct comparison of the organisms they are studying with the type strains. The consequences of disobeying this rule are clearly shown by the example of *C. johnsonae* (for which only relatively recently a type strain was named). Many isolates have been identified with this species in different laboratories over the years. A careful phenotype analysis (Oyaizu and Komagata, 1981) and DNA/DNA hybridizations (Callies and Mannheim, 1980; H. Behrens, unpublished results) demonstrate, however, that several of these strains cannot belong in the same species and that some do not even belong in the same genus. From this must also be concluded that all data published about independent isolates of a species, particularly when the studies were performed in different laboratories, must be interpreted with extreme care: they might refer to totally different organisms. Of course, the *Cytophaga* problem has been realized for some time (e.g. Stanier, 1947; Mitchell et al., 1967; Lewin, 1969; Christensen, 1977b; Oyaizu and Komagata, 1981; Reichenbach and Dworkin, 1981c; Shewan and McMeekin, 1983), and efforts have been made to improve the situation by dividing the genus (Leadbetter, 1974). This had to be done on the basis of available data which were, and still are, not sufficient for this purpose. It was proposed to retain within the genus *Cytophaga* only those species that are able to degrade certain polysaccharides, mainly cellulose, agar and chitin, and to transfer those that cannot to the genus *Flexibacter*. But it must be doubted that this division line really separates the organisms according to their natural relationships. With regard to *C. salmonicolor*, for example, in the same environment an agar decomposer was found, a facultative anaerobe, which appeared to be very similar to the former, was also found. This strain has been classified as a variant, *agarovorans*, of the nonagarolytic species *salmonicolor* (Veldkamp, 1961). Perhaps the original systematic study came to an erroneous conclusion, but is there really a compelling reason that the two strains should be placed in different genera? Also, strains were discovered and described as new species, since they could degrade certain unusual polysaccharides, e.g. heparin (Payza and Korn, 1956) or succinoglycan (Oyaizu et al., 1982). Does this mean that the organisms belong in the genus *Cytophaga*, and if so, how can we be sure that the remaining *Flexibacter* species do not also attack some exotic polysaccharide? Still more arguments may be found in the comments on the genus *Flexibacter*.

An earlier effort to subdivide the "imperfect forms of myxobacteria" was founded on differences in cell shape: *Cytophaga* cells should have pointed ends, while the ends of the cells of the new (noncellulolytic) genus "*Promyxobacterium*" would be rounded (Imshenetski and Solnt-

seva, 1945). But this morphological difference is not clear enough to be really useful: The "*Promyxobacterium*" species themselves may have somewhat tapering ends (see Fig. 23.7), and even with the cellulolytic CLB, tapering is not always conspicuous. Finally, this characteristic may vary with culture medium and culture age.

In the absence of better data, there is no other choice except to return to the traditionally vague concept of the genus. This at least allows recognition of the organisms which *may* belong together. In this article, I try to define groups within the genus which are sufficiently distinct to give them, with some probability, the status of a subgenus. They may represent the nuclei of later genera. With a few exceptions, where the situation appears clear, I do not give names to these subgroups, in order to avoid later confusion. In structuring the genus, G + C data serve as a first lead, followed by physiological and ecological considerations. In several cases, hybridization data are also available.

Of course, the cellulose degraders around the type species *C. hutchinsonii* have to remain the core of the genus *Cytophaga*. The cellulolytic CLB seem to have several characteristics in common: they can utilize filter paper, i.e. "native" crystalline cellulose; they seem unable to grow in the complete absence of carbohydrate; and they have a relatively high mol% G + C of the DNA of around 40. However, far too little is known about them to be sure the group is uniform enough to be united in one genus. Actually there are some doubts, for besides the classical soil organisms there are marine cellulose degraders, strains that degrade agar in addition to cellulose, flexirubin-positive and flexirubin-negative strains, and differences in cell morphology and deviations in the mol% G + C of the DNA down to at least 35. The latter could, however, also be *Sporocytophaga* strains that do not produce microcysts under the conditions chosen and thus cannot readily be distinguished phenotypically from *Cytophaga* on the basis of current knowledge. Organisms that attack only CMC are not regarded here as truly cellulolytic.

With the agar degraders, the situation is even more complex. The *C. lytica* group, common organisms in marine environments, is distinct, but its relation to the other agarolytic CLB is uncertain and appears rather remote. The chitin and pectin degraders are most probably both heterogeneous groups. The same may be the case with the fish pathogens, which also seem not to be closely related to common saprophytic CLB in the same environment. Further, there are several "*Flavobacterium*" species for which gliding motility was established later and which have been transferred to the CLB, although their exact taxonomic position remains to be determined. There are many *Cytophaga* species for which strains seem to be no longer available and which therefore have no taxonomic status. Although in many cases the descriptions are so vague that the species could hardly be recognized, the species is listed below to give an idea of the range of organisms to be expected.

As mentioned above, the CLB were formerly classified with the myxobacters and consequently were often labeled as "myxobacters" or "myxobacteria." As we know today, the myxobacters are not related phylogenetically to the CLB (Ludwig et al., 1983; Paster et al., 1985), so indiscriminate application of these terms to CLB should be discontinued.

Further Reading

See under "Order *Cytophagales*."

Differentiation of the species of the genus **Cytophaga**

The distinguishing characteristics of the recognized species of the genus *Cytophaga* are compiled in Table 23.2.

List of species of the genus **Cytophaga**

1. **Cytophaga hutchinsonii** Winogradsky 1929, 578.[AL]

hut.chin.so′ni.i. M.L. gen. n. hutchinsonii of Hutchinson; named in honor of the English microbiologist H. B. Hutchinson, who, together with J. Clayton in 1919, gave the first unequivocal description of an aerobic cellulose-degrading gliding bacterium, *Sporocytophaga myxococcoides*.

Provisionally classified in subgenus *Cytophaga*.

Delicate flexible rods with slightly tapering ends, 0.3–0.5 × 2–10 μm, usually 0.4 × 2–5 μm (Fig. 23.3). On agar surfaces, the cells sometimes show very fast gliding, suddenly jumping forward with intense wriggling, although only for a few cell lengths at a time. Cell mass is bright yellow, turning a deep brown-red when covered with a 20% KOH solution. Colo-

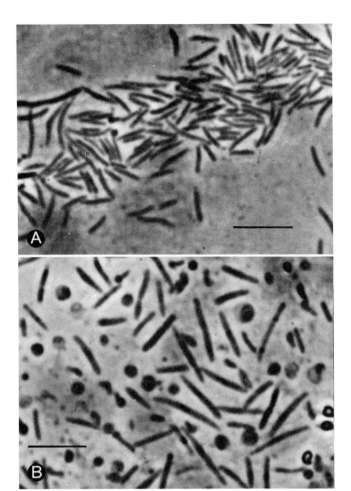

Figure 23.3. *A, C. hutchinsonii,* type strain. Cells from filter paper on peptone (CY) agar at 30°C. *B, Cytophaga* species, strain Cy ce14, from filter paper on CY agar at 30°C. The large and seemingly degenerated spindle-shaped cells are living and still very actively gliding. Phase contrast. *Bars,* 5 μm.

nies on filter paper are large, spreading, bright yellow, with the center soon becoming translucent, and somewhat slimy; colonies on glucose mineral agar are bright yellow, more or less compact to slightly spreading, with an entire or a wavy edge, and moderately raised to flat. In liquid media with cellulose or glucose, considerable amounts of slime may be produced, making the culture viscous and the harvesting of cells difficult.

Peptones, yeast extract, several amino acids including aspartic and glutamic acids, NO_3^- and NH_4^+ may serve as sole N source, but even with organic N compounds the addition of a carbohydrate is absolutely required. Cellulose, cellobiose and glucose are used; xylose, arabinose, galactose, fructose, mannose, mannitol and Na-pyruvate are not. Starch is not hydrolyzed (Mitchell et al., 1967).

Strictly aerobic. Catalase is reported as positive (Stanier, 1942) but is, at best, very weakly so. For further information, see Table 23.2.

C. hutchinsonii readily degrades crystalline cellulose (filter paper) on mineral media, preferentially with NH_4^+ and elevated concentrations of Mn^{2+} and Fe^{3+} (e.g. ST6 agar), but even more vigorously on peptone media (e.g. CY agar). In the latter case, the paper may be completely broken down within 6–10 days at 30°C. This species also grows on CMC (e.g. on CY agar with 1% CMC and the agar reduced to 0.6%). The organism is reported to be relatively insensitive to alkaline conditions up to at least pH 8.5 (Stanier, 1942).

Isolated from soils in various countries, reported as extremely common in California soils (Stanier, 1942).

The mol% G + C of the DNA of the neotype strain is 39 (Bd) (Mandel and Leadbetter, 1965) and 40 (T_m) (Callies and Mannheim, 1980).

Neotype strain: NCIB 9469 (ATCC 33406).

The origin of the neotype strain is not completely clear. Obviously it was supplied by R. Y. Stanier and was probably isolated from soil by himself rather than having been obtained from S. Winogradsky, who never had pure strains and apparently also never sent his strains to another laboratory. In the older literature, up to 1940, strains of *Sporocytophaga myxococcoides* are often labeled *C. "hutchinsonii"* (see, for example, Imshenetski and Solntseva, 1936; and Jensen, 1940), because at that time the status of coccoid cells in cultures of cellulolytic CLB was not clearly understood. Winogradsky (1929) incorrectly assumed that the spheroplasts common in older cultures of his *Cytophaga* strains were identical with the spherical cells observed by Hutchinson and Clayton (1919) in their cultures, while in reality the latter authors had a *Sporocytophaga* strain with spherical resting cells or microcysts under study. The question was settled definitely by H. Krzemieniewska (1933) who isolated both types of organisms and studied them side by side. Winogradsky's *C. hutchinsonii* was actually a misnomer. Another dispute was whether *Sporocytophaga* during cultivation would easily lose its ability to form microcysts (Imshenetski and Solntseva, 1936) and could thus be confused with *C. hutchinsonii*. Stanier (1942) is of the opinion that microcyst formation might become considerably reduced but as a rule is never completely abandoned, particularly if the cultures are well-aerated and incubated at elevated temperatures, i.e. 30–35° C. Krzemieniewska (1933) also emphasizes certain differences in the appearance of the two organisms, which otherwise resemble one another to a high degree: the cells of *C. hutchinsonii* are slightly shorter, and colonies on filter paper are bright yellow and remain so for a long time, while those of *Sporocytophaga* tend soon to become dirty yellow or brownish. The difference in pigmentation seems to be real, at least with many *Sporocytophaga* strains. Further, there seems to be a clear difference in the mol% G + C of the DNA, with 36 for *S. myxococcoides* (Mandel and Leadbetter, 1965). But it remains to be seen whether there is no overlap in the mol% G + C ranges.

But even when the name *C. hutchinsonii* was applied to true *Cytophaga* stains, this does not necessarily mean that the same species was studied. In fact, it may be questioned whether Stanier's *C. hutchinsonii* is really identical with Winogradsky's organism, for Stanier (1942) sharply disagrees that living *Cytophaga* cells have tapering ends, which he rather regards as a fixation artifact. And, in fact, his neotype strain does not show this property particularly well (Fig. 23.3). Yet there are cellulolytic CLB which, in the living state, have decidedly fusiform cells (Fig. 23.3), exactly as is shown on the figures in the articles of Winogradsky (1929) and other authors. In any case, there are certainly several more species of cellulolytic CLB, differing in cell shape and dimensions, color of colonies, flexirubin reaction, physiological characteristics, and ecology. In fact, many species have been described in the past. Unfortunately, in no case are the original strains still available, and although some of those species may be synonymous with *C. hutchinsonii*, others are certainly not. In most cases, the descriptions are not exact enough to recognize the organisms again, and comparative data, particularly that gathered with modern analytical methods, are essentially lacking, so that the organisms have first to be reisolated and studied again more carefully before taxonomic decisions can be made. At least one cellulolytic *Cytophaga* strain which is clearly different from *C. hutchinsonii* was found by my colleagues and myself to have a similarly high mol% G + C, viz. 40 (Bd), strain Cy ce14 (unpublished observations), so that it is conceivable that a new genus *Cytophaga* comprising only cellulolytic species with a mol% G + C of the DNA of around 40 will emerge. Also, for *C. aurantiaca* ATCC 12208, a mol% G + C of the DNA of 42 (Bd) has been established (Mandel and Leadbetter, 1965). It has been stated that DNA/DNA hybridization would indicate a relatively close relationship between *C. hutchinsonii* and *C. marinoflava* (mol% G + C of the DNA of 39) despite a considerable difference in genome size of 2.74×10^9 vs. 2.23×10^9 daltons (Callies and Mannheim, 1980). The same investigators also found appreciable hybridization with *Flavobacterium hepa-*

Table 23.2.
Differential characteristics of the species of the genus **Cytophaga**[a]

Characteristic	1. C. hutchinsonii	2. C. aurantiaca	3. C. lytica	4. C. marinoflava	5. C. uliginosa
Length of cells (μm)	2–5	3–5	1.5–3.5	1–3	1.2–4
Width of cells (μm)	0.4	0.3	0.4	0.5–0.6	0.4
Cell ends tapering	±	±	−	±	±
Color of cell mass	Bright yellow	Bright orange	Bright yellow	Yellow	Golden yellow
Flexirubin reaction[b]	+	−	−	−	+
Carotenoids present	•	•	Zeaxanthin	•	•
Suitable as nitrogen source					
Peptones	+	+	+	+	+
Casamino acids	+	•	+	•	•
Single amino acids	Glu, Asp	•	Glu	•	•
Urea	•	•	•	•	•
NH_4^+	+	+	•	•	•
NO_3^-	+	+	−[c]	•	•
Grows on peptone alone	−	−	+	+	+
NH_3 released from peptones	+	•	+	+	•
Glucose sole carbon and energy source	+	+	•	•	•
Acid from carbohydrates (aerobically)	+	•	•	+	+
Degradation of					
Gelatin	•	•	+	•	+
Casein	•	−	−	•	+
Starch	−	−	+	+	+
Cellulose (filter paper)	+	+	−	−	−
CMC	+	+	+	•	•
Agar	−	−	+	−	+
Carrageenan	•	•	•	•	•
Alginate	•	•	+	•	•
Pectin	−	•	•	•	•
Chitin	−	•	−	•	+
Inulin	•	•	•	•	•
Autoclaved yeast cells[e]	•	•	−	−	−
Hemolysis (kind of erythrocytes)	•	•	•	•	•
Lipases	•	•	•	T	−
DNase	•	•	•	•	•
Phosphatase	•	•	•	•	•
Urease	•	•	•	•	−
Indole produced	•	•	•	−	−
H_2S produced	•	•	+[d]	−	−
NO_3^- reduced [f]	•	•	−	+	+
Strict aerobe (a)/facultative anaerobe (f)	a	a	a	a	a
Catalase	−	−	+	+	+
Oxidase	+	+	+	+	+
Optimum temperature (°C)	30	20–25	22–30	20–30	20–30
Maximum temperature (°C)	•	•	35–40	<37	•
Highest NaCl concentration tolerated (%)	•	•	6	•	•
Growth on seawater media	−	−	+	+	+
Habitat	Soil	Soil	Marine	Marine	Marine
Mol% G + C of DNA of type strain (range of species)	39	42	33 (32–34)	37	42

[a]Symbols: ±, characteristic is not clearly positive or negative or varies with the culture condition; −, negative; +, positive; •, no information available; T, active against Tweens; and B, active against tributyrin.

[b]Color change from yellow to red, purple or red-brown when 20% KOH is added, and back to yellow again when the latter is replaced with 10% HCl.

[c]Characteristic variable: the type strain is negative, whereas other strains may be positive.

Table 23.2.—*continued*

Characteristic	6. *C. fermentans*	7. *C. salmonicolor*	8. *C. agarovorans*	9. *C. flevensis*	10. *C. saccharophila*	11. *C. diffluens*
Length of cells (µm)	2–10 (–30)	4–6 (2–30)	12–30 (8–50)	2–5	2.5–6	4–10 (–30)
Width of cells (µm)	0.5–0.7	0.3–0.5	0.3–0.4	0.5–0.7	0.5–0.6	0.5
Cell ends tapering	−	−	−	−	±	+
Color of cell mass	Bright yellow	Yellow to salmon	Pink to salmon	Yellow	Yellow	Orange
Flexirubin reaction[b]	•	•	•	−	+	
Carotenoids present	•	•	•	•	•	Saproxanthin
Suitable as nitrogen source						
Peptones	+	+	+	+	+	+
Casamino acids	•	+	+	+	•	+
Single amino acids	Glu, Asn	•	•	Glu, Asn	•	Glu
Urea	−	•	•	±	•	•
NH_4^+	+	+	+	+	+	•
NO_3^-	−	+	+	+	•	−[c]
Grows on peptone alone	•	+	+	+	+	+
NH_3 released from peptones	•	+	•	+	+	+
Glucose sole carbon and energy source	+	+	+	+	+	−[c]
Acid from carbohydrates (aerobically)	+	•	•	+	•	−[c]
Degradation of						
Gelatin	•	+	+	−	+	+
Casein	•	•	•	−	•	+
Starch	+	+	+	−	•	−[c]
Cellulose (filter paper)	−	•	•	−	+	+
CMC	•	•	•	•	−	−[c]
Agar	+	−	+	+	+	+
Carrageenan	•	•	•	−	+	•
Alginate	−	•	•	−	•	+
Pectin	•	•	•	+	+	•
Chitin	−	−	−	−	−	−
Inulin	•	•	•	+	•	•
Autoclaved yeast cells[e]	•	−	−	−	+	−
Hemolysis (kind of erythrocytes)	•	•	•	− (sheep)	•	•
Lipases	•	•	•	B	•	•
DNase	•	•	•	•	•	•
Phosphatase	•	•	•	+	+	•
Urease	•	•	•	−	•	•
Indole produced	•	•	•	−	−	•
H_2S produced	•	•	•	−	+	+[a]
NO_3^- reduced [f]	−	•	•	+	+	−[c]
Strict aerobe (a)/facultative anaerobe (f)	f	f	f	a	a	a
Catalase	+	+	+	−	−	−
Oxidase	•	•	•	+	−	+
Optimum temperature (°C)	30	28–37	28–37	25	25–30	25–30
Maximum temperature (°C)	•	•	•	<35	<37	<45[c]
Highest NaCl concentration tolerated (%)	•	3	3	•	2	6
Growth on seawater media	+	+	+	+	−	+
Habitat	Marine	Marine	Marine	Freshwater	Freshwater	Marine
Mol% G + C of DNA of type strain (range of species)	39	37	41	33/35	32 (32–36)	42 (40–42)

[d]Characteristic variable with different strains: the type strain is positive, whereas other strains may be negative.

[e]On yeast agar, e.g. VY/2 agar, if required with seawater.

[f]+: NO_3^-, reduced to NO_2^-; NH_3, reduced to NH_3.

Table 23.2.—*continued*

Characteristic	12. C. aprica	13. C. johnsonae	14. C. pectinovora	15. C. aquatilis	16. C. psychrophila	17. C. marina
Length of cells (μm)	6–30 (–50)	2–5 (–15)	1–5	2–6 (–15)	1.5–3.5 (–7.5)	2–5
Width of cells (μm)	0.5–0.7	0.3–0.4	0.4–0.5	0.4–0.6	0.4–0.5	0.4
Cell ends tapering	+	±	±	±	−	•
Color of cell mass	Orange	Yellow	Yellow	Yellow	Yellow	Yellow orange
Flexirubin reaction[b]	−	+	+	+	+	•
Carotenoids present	Saproxanthin	Zeaxanthin	•	•	•	•
Suitable as nitrogen source						
Peptones	+	+	+	+	+.	+
Casamino acids	+	+	+	+	+	+
Single amino acids	Glu	Glu, Asn	Glu, Asn	Glu	•	−
Urea	•	+	+	•	•	−
NH$_4^+$	•	+	+	+	•	−
NO$_3^-$	−	±	+	+	•	−
Grows on peptone alone	+	+	+	+	+	+
NH$_3$ released from peptones	+	+	+	+	+	+
Glucose sole carbon and energy source	−	+	+	+	−	−
Acid from carbohydrates (aerobically)	+	+	+	+	−	−
Degradation of	+	•+	+	+	+	+
Gelatin	−	+	+	+	+	+
Casein	+	+	+	+	−	−
Starch	−	−	−	−	−	−
Cellulose (filter paper)	+	+	+	+	•	−
CMC	+	−	−	−	•	•
Agar	•	•	•	•	•	•
Carrageenan	+	+	+	−	•	•
Alginate	•	+	+	+	−	•
Pectin	−	+	+	+	−	−
Chitin						
Inulin	•	+	+	•	•	•
Autoclaved yeast cells[e]	•	+	+	+	−	•
Hemolysis (kind of erythrocytes)	•	•	−(horse)/+(sheep)	−	•	•
Lipases	•	•	B	B/T	B	T
DNase	•	+	+	+	•	•
Phosphatase	•	+	+	•	•	•
Urease	•	+	−	−	•	+
Indole produced	•	−	−	−	−	−
H$_2$S produced	+	−	−	−	−	−
NO$_3^-$ reduced[f]	−[c]	−	+	NH$_3$	−	+
Strict aerobe (a)/facultative anaerobe (f)	a	a	a	f	a	a
Catalase	−	+	+	+	−	+
Oxidase	+	+	+	−	+	+
Optimum temperature (°C)	25–30	25–30	20–25	20–25	20	30
Maximum temperature (°C)	<40	<37	<37	30	<25	<37
Highest NaCl concentration tolerated (%)	6	1	1	2	0.8	•
Growth on seawater media	+	−	−	−	−	+
Habitat	Marine	Soil, freshwater	Soil	Freshwater	Freshwater	Marine
Mol% G + C of DNA of type strain (range of species)	35 (35–37)	33	34	32/34	32 (32)	31 (31–32)

[a]Symbols: ±, characteristic is not clearly positive or negative or varies with the culture condition; −, negative; +, positive; •, no information available; T, active against Tweens; and B, active against tributyrin.

[b]Color change from yellow to red, purple or red-brown when 20% KOH is added, and back to yellow again when the latter is replaced with 10% HCl.

[c]Characteristic variable: the type strain is negative, whereas other strains may be positive.

Table 23.2.—*continued*

Characteristic	18. *C. latercula*	19. *C. succinicans*	20. *C. columnaris*
Length of cells (μm)	1–5 (10–40)	4–6	2–12
Width of cells (μm)	0.3–0.4	0.5	0.4
Cell ends tapering	±	−	−
Color of cell mass	Orange red	Bright yellow	Golden yellow
Flexirubin reaction[b]	−	−	+
Carotenoids present	•	•	•
Suitable as nitrogen source			
Peptones	+	+	+
Casamino acids	+	+	+
Single amino acids	Glu	Glu	•
Urea	•	•	•
NH_4^+	•	+	−
NO_3^-	+	+	−
Grows on peptone alone	+	+	+
NH_3 released from peptones	+	+	+
Glucose sole carbon and energy source	+	+	−
Acid from carbohydrates (aerobically)	+	+	−
Degradation of	+	+	+
Gelatin	−	+	+
Casein	−	+	−
Starch	−	−	−
Cellulose (filter paper)	+	•	•
CMC			
Agar	+	−	−
Carrageenan	•	•	•
Alginate	+	•	•
Pectin	−	•	•
Chitin	+	−	−
Inulin	•	•	•
Autoclaved yeast cells[e]	±	+	+
Hemolysis (kind of erythrocytes)	•	•	•
Lipases	•	•	•
DNase	•	•	•
Phosphatase	•	•	•
Urease	•	•	•
Indole produced	•	•	−
H_2S produced	+	•	+
NO_3^- reduced [f]	−	+[c,d]	−
Strict aerobe (a)/facultative anaerobe (f)	a	f	a
Catalase	−	±	+
Oxidase	+		+
Optimum temperature (°C)	20–25	25	25–30
Maximum temperature (°C)	<35	>37	≤37
Highest NaCl concentration tolerated (%)	3.5	•	0.5
Growth on seawater media	+	−	−
Habitat	Marine	Freshwater	Freshwater
Mol% G + C of DNA of type strain (range of species)	34	38 (38)	30

[d]Characteristic variable with different strains: the type strain is positive, whereas other strains may be negative.

[e]On yeast agar, e.g. VY/2 agar, if required with seawater.

[f]+: NO_3^-, reduced to NO_2^-; NH_3, reduced to NH_3.

rinum (mol% G + C of the DNA of 45) but no hybridization at all with *C. johnsonae* and *C. pectinovorum.*

2. **Cytophaga aurantiaca** (ex Winogradsky 1929) nom. rev.

au.ran.ti′a.ca. M.L. fem. adj. *aurantiaca* orange-colored.

Provisionally classified in subgenus *Cytophaga.*

Slender flexible delicate rods with slightly tapering ends, 0.3–0.4 × 2–8 µm; may become larger and coarser in old cultures. The cells are able to perform swift gliding motions in a manner similar to that described for *C. hutchinsonii.* Cell mass is a bright orange; no color change is seen with KOH or HCl. Some data on LPS composition are available (Sutherland and Smith, 1973).

Colonies on filter paper spread slowly, may become very large, and are bright orange to orange-red.

Nutritional requirements are only partly known. Peptones, yeast extract, NH_4^+ and NO_3^- may serve as sole N source, but the addition of carbohydrate is a prerequisite for growth even in the presence of organic N compounds. Cellulose, e.g. filter paper, or CMC are suitable carbon and energy sources. The cellulolytic capabilities of *C. aurantiaca* are like those of *C. hutchinsonii.* Growth on mineral media with cellulose is much stimulated by Ca^{2+}, Mn^{2+} and Fe^{2+} (Bortels, 1956).

C. aurantiaca is more sensitive to higher temperatures than is *C. hutchinsonii.* Although it still grows at 30°C on agar plates with an optimal medium composition, e.g. filter paper on CY agar, it may fail to do so on minimal media or when a reactivated culture preserve is used for inoculum. It grows well at 20–25°C.

Strictly aerobic. Catalase completely negative, strong oxidase reaction. For further information, see Table 23.2.

Isolated from soil.

The mol% G + C of the DNA is 37 (Bd) (unpublished observation) and 42 (Bd) (Mandel and Leadbetter, 1965).

Neotype strain: NCIB 8628 (ATCC 12208).

The neotype strain was supplied by H. Bortels and is probably identical with his strain *C. aurantiaca* 51 (Bortels, 1956). At least no other strain has ever been mentioned in his articles. This strain was isolated by him from soil taken from the swampy edge of a pond in Germany. Of course, to be sure that the neotype strain is really the same as Winogradsky's organism is not possible. The latter was described as a very efficient cellulose degrader with slender rods with tapering ends, coarser than those of *C. hutchinsonii,* and 1 × 6–8 µm; colonies were bright pinkish orange; and it was isolated from soil in France. There is one obvious discrepancy between Winogradsky's description and the Bortels strain, viz. the cell dimensions. The latter has very fine and only moderately long rod cells, not much different from those of the *C. hutchinsonii* neotype (!) strain. Although somewhat longer and coarser cells may appear in older cultures or under certain culture conditions, e.g. when the organism worms its way through CMC agar, some doubts remain because Winogradsky observed large cells in young cultures and emphasized that the distinguishing characteristics of his strain remained stable over many transfers. Nevertheless, as Winogradsky's strain does not exist any more and the Bortels strain corresponds closely enough to the species description, the old species name is reactivated here with the only available strain as the neotype. There may not be too many alternatives, for Winogradsky mentioned that *C. aurantiaca* was less common than *C. hutchinsonii,* and only rarely do we find orange cellulose-degrading CLB. The mol% G + C of the DNA of the type strain has recently been reinvestigated by us and was consistently found to be considerably lower, viz. 37 (Bd), than that published previously, viz. 42 (Bd).

3. **Cytophaga lytica** Lewin 1969, 199.[AL] (*Pseudomonas iridescens* Stanier 1941.)

ly′ti.ca. Gr. v. *lyein* to loosen, dissolve; M.L. fem. adj. *lytica* loosening, dissolving.

Provisionally classified in subgenus *Agarophaga.*

Slender flexible rods, cylindrical with blunt ends, 0.3–0.4 × 1.5–10, usually 0.4 × 2–4 µm (Fig. 23.4), actively gliding.

Colonies pale yellow to orange, depending on the substrate, and typically bright yellow with an almost greenish iridescence or opalescence (e.g. on agar media with tryptone and yeast extract, 0.1% each). Main pigment is zeaxanthin (Lewin and Lounsbery, 1969); flexirubin-type pigments are lacking. On media with higher peptone concentrations (e.g. tryptone and yeast extract, 0.5% each), growth may be compact and elevated, but spreading swarm colonies which are sunken more or less completely into the agar, with a fibrous periphery, are more typical. The agar is softened but not liquefied.

Peptones, casamino acids or certain individual amino acids, e.g. glutamic acid, may serve as sole N source. At least some strains also grow on inorganic N (NO_3^-). Various sugars (glucose, galactose, sucrose) and, by some strains, also, acetate, lactate or glycerol are utilized. This species grows on casitone (0.9%)-yeast extract (0.1%) liquid medium without added carbohydrate; does not depend on agar.

Strictly aerobic marine organisms requiring elevated salt concentrations for growth. Further biochemical and physiological data may be found in Table 23.2.

Extremely common in tide pools, on the surface of (red) algae and in other coastal habitats around the world. Type strain was isolated from marine mud collected at Limon, Costa Rica.

The mol% G + C of the DNA of the type strain is 33 (Bd); other strains deviate but little (Mandel and Lewin, 1969).

Type strain: ATCC 23178 (LIM-21 Lewin).

Regarding the abundance of this organism in its natural habitat and the ease with which it is obtained, it would be peculiar had it not been observed by earlier investigators. In fact, nonmotile *Pseudomonas iridescens* Stanier (1941) looks very similar to *C. lytica,* particularly the description given of strains from the American Atlantic coast, which fits perfectly (Humm, 1946). DNA/rRNA hybridizations show that *C. lytica* is relatively closely related with *C. salmonicolor, C. marinoflava, C. (Flavobacterium) uliginosum* and *Flexibacter aurantiacus* var. *excathedrus,* while the connections to *C. johnsonae, Flavobacterium pectinovorum* and *F. aquatile* are somewhat more remote (Bauwens and De Ley, 1981). A relationship with *C. johnsonae, Sporocytophaga myxococcoides* and *C. (F.) uliginosum* is also demonstrated by 16S RNA oligonucleotide sequences (Paster et al., 1985). There are substantial differences in the pattern of shared signature sequences between *C. lytica* and most other organisms mentioned above. *F. uliginosum* corresponds in this respect to *C. lytica,* but the relatively low S_{AB} value between the two (0.52) seems to rule out a close relationship on the genus level. This conclusion is also supported by a large difference in the mol% G + C of the DNA. DNA/DNA hybridizations prove that many strains from widely separated places belong to the species *C. lytica* and that there is at least one other closely related species (Habicht and H. Reichenbach, unpublished data). The mol% G + C of the DNA given for the type strain above may be slightly too high, for we constantly find it to be 32 (Bd).

4. **Cytophaga marinoflava** (ex Colwell, Citarella and Chen 1966) nom. rev.

ma.ri.no.fla′va. L. adj. *marinus* marine; L. adj. *flavus* golden yellow; M.L. fem. adj. *marinoflava* yellow one from the sea.

Provisionally classified in group C.

Short, almost stout and somewhat stiff rods with rounded or slightly tapering ends; may become almost coccoid, often in pairs, 0.5–0.6 × 1–3 µm (Fig. 23.5). The cells may show very lively gliding movements but in a peculiar fashion. They move only one or two cell lengths in one direction, then either return on the same track or pivot around their center and then continue forward or backward. The movement is quite steady, certainly not Brownian, and is performed with considerable vigor, with the cells forcing their way through groups of other cells or any other obstacle. However, the rods move only when covered by a layer of liquid, e.g. in tiny pockets in the agar or around some crumb of material between agar surface and coverslip. When fixed to an agar surface the cells become completely immobilized. This may be the reason why no spreading growth is observed on any medium. The cell mass is bright yellow and does not change color with 20% KOH. The colonies are always small, punctiform (<2 mm), compact, flat or slightly raised, pale yellow, soft and somewhat

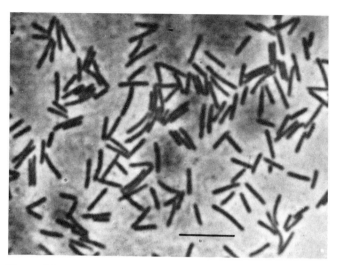

Figure 23.4. *C. lytica,* type strain. Cells from seawater-peptone (SP2) agar at 30°C. Phase contrast. *Bar, 5 μm.*

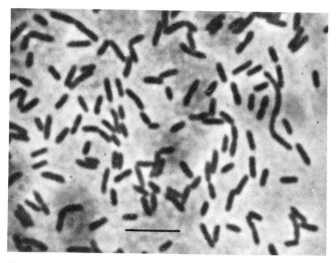

Figure 23.5. *C. marinoflava,* type strain. Cells from seawater-peptone liquid medium (SP5 l.m.) at 21°C. Phase contrast. *Bar, 5 μm.*

slimy. The heavy growth produced from streaks is pale to bright yellow and sometimes slightly greenish. No fluorescence is noted at 366 nm.

Peptones serve as sole N source and may also be used as sources of energy and C. Excellent growth is obtained on, for example, SP5 l.m. Under aerobic conditions, acid is produced from arabinose, xylose, glucose, galactose, fructose, sucrose, maltose, raffinose and trehalose, but it is not produced from rhamnose, sorbose, mannitol or salicin. Esculin and various Tweens are hydrolyzed. Arginine, lysine and ornithine decarboxylases are lacking. This species is resistant to polymyxin B, penicillin, aureomycin, kanamycin, dihydrostreptomycin and pteridin but is sensitive to tetracycline, terramycin, novobiocin, erythromycin, chloramphenicol and vibriostat 0/129. For further data, see Table 23.2.

Strict aerobe. Growth is not stimulated by fumarate under oxygen-limited conditions (Callies and Mannheim, 1980). The catalase and oxidase reactions are positive but may be weak. Marine organism growing at elevated (at least up to seawater level) salt concentrations, which need may be served simply by NaCl. The latter is not replaceable by KCl or 0.8 M sucrose. After a lag period of up to 1 week (25°C), excellent growth may take place on media without additional salt, e.g. on 1% peptone + 0.1% yeast extract or on MYX agar. Wide temperature range: 4–30°C; excellent growth is obtained at 30°C.

Only one strain is available, which was isolated from water collected on the open North Sea off Aberdeen, Scotland.

The mol% G + C of the DNA is 37 (Bd) and 39 (T_m); genome size is 2.26 × 10^9 daltons (Callies and Mannheim, 1980).

Type strain: NCMB 397 (ATCC 19326).

Isolated originally as an "unidentified flavobacterium" and a host for marine bacteriophages (Spencer, 1960), the organism was later classified as a new *Cytophaga* species, although gliding motility was not observed at that time. The way the organism moves is unusual, indeed, compared with other cytophagas. Later authors report that acid is produced from lactose (Callies and Mannheim, 1980). DNA/DNA hybridization shows considerable homology with *C. hutchinsonii* which seems peculiar (see there). DNA/rRNA hybridization indicates that the organism belongs into the *C. lytica* group (Bauwens and De Ley, 1981). Of course, *C. marinoflava* cannot be closely related with *C. lytica* because of the large mol% G + C difference between the two.

5. **Cytophaga uliginosa** (ZoBell and Upham 1944) comb. nov. (*Agarbacterium uliginosum* ZoBell and Upham 1944, 263; *Flavobacterium uliginosum* (ZoBell and Upham) Weeks 1974, 360[AL]).

u.li.gi.no'sa. L. fem. adj. *uliginosa* wet, swampy.

Provisionally classified in group D.

Rather short cylindrical rods with blunt ends, 0.4–0.5 × 1.2–4 μm (Fig.

23.6), may show fast gliding movements. Cell mass golden yellow, turns instantly rust brown with KOH and bright yellow again with HCl. Colonies golden yellow, with a very tenacious slime, either compact, raised and often sitting in shallow craters or, more rarely, spreading (e.g. on chitin agar with 0.1% casitone, 0.02% yeast extract and 0.5% reprecipitated chitin in seawater agar). One certain media, e.g. seawater agar with 0.1% tryptone, 0.1% yeast extract and 0.2% glucose (SAP5 agar), a brown water-soluble pigment is produced which may also tinge the bacteria cell mass. Agar is softened but not liquefied. Upon addition of I-KI solution, large gelase fields develop around the colonies.

Good growth on peptones without agar or any other carbohydrate. Glucose, maltose, lactose, sucrose, xylose and salicin are metabolized with acid production; glycerol and mannitol are not. Starch is not hydrolyzed. Chitin is slowly (8–10 days, 30°C) but completely degraded, however, only directly under the colony.

Strictly aerobic marine organism requiring elevated salt concentrations. Temperature optimum: 20–25°C; but good growth is obtained at 30°C. Further biochemical and physiological data are given in Table 23.2.

Isolated from marine bottom sediment; only one strain is known.

The mol% G + C of the DNA is 42 (Bd).

Type strain: ATCC 14397 (ZoBell 553).

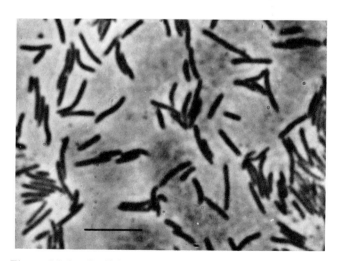

Figure 23.6. *C. uliginosa,* type strain. Cells from seawater-peptone liquid medium (SP5 l.m.) at 30°C. Phase contrast. *Bar, 5 μm.*

The mol% G + C of the DNA was formerly stated to be 32 (T_m) (Weeks, 1974); my colleagues and I have, however, found it to be 42 (Bd), with two cultures of the type strain obtained independently at different times from NCMB (1981) and ATCC (1985). Gliding of *C. uliginosa* can be easily observed microscopically and was apparently recognized first by M. Hendrie (personal communication, 1981). Also, spreading growth may be observed on certain media (see above). When originally isolated, the strain liquefied agar, but this property was gradually lost during cultivation. Softening of agar is, however, stable and still very striking with the presently available strain. About the phylogenetic relationship of *C. uliginosa*, see under *C. lytica*.

6. Cytophaga fermentans Bachmann 1955, 549.[AL]

fer.men'tans. L. part. adj. *fermentans* fermenting.

Provisionally classified in group E.

Slender flexible rods with rounded ends, 0.5–0.7 × 8–15 µm, up to 50 µm in old cultures, actively gliding. Cell mass from aerobic cultures on peptone media is bright yellow, but on minimal media or from anaerobic cultures, it is unpigmented. Colonies are spreading thin films with yellow blobs, in shallow craters. An unstable variant with small (1–2-mm) compact colonies may appear in the same culture.

Peptones, glutamine, asparagine and NH_4^+ serve as sole N source; NO_3^-, urea and various amino acids do not. Xylose, arabinose, glucose, fructose, mannose, sucrose, lactose, maltose, cellobiose, raffinose, mannitol and starch are suitable carbon and energy sources, but galactose, rhamnose, trehalose, sorbose, dulcitol, glycerol, agar, alginate, cellulose, chitin, ethanol, and any of the tested amino acids and other organic acids including acetate are not. In mineral salts-glucose media, permanent growth is possible only if thiamine, CO_2 and relatively high concentrations of Fe^{3+} (0.5 mg/l) are supplied. It is stated that the organism grows on mineral salts-yeast extract (1%) media only in presence of agar or of an agar extract. But although agar is softened and obviously attacked (large gelase fields), it is not used as a C source, nor is there really a dependence on it.

Facultative anaerobe. Ferments glucose with production of acetate, propionate and succinate. Large quantities of (nitrogen containing) slime also arise.

Marine organism required elevated (at least 1%) salt concentrations, which need may be served simply by 3% NaCl or KCl. Good growth between room temperature and 30°C. For further data, see Table 23.2

Isolated from marine mud; only one strain is available.

The mol% G + C of the DNA is 39 (Bd) and 41 (T_m) (Mandel and Leadbetter, 1965).

Type strain: ATCC 19072.

7. Cytophaga salmonicolor Veldkamp 1961, 339.[AL]

sal.mo.ni'co.lor. L. masc. n. *salmo*, gen. *salmonis* salmon; L. masc. n. *color* color; M.L. adj. *salmonicolor* salmon-colored.

Provisionally classified in group F.

Slender flexible cylindrical rods with rounded or slightly tapering ends, 0.3–0.5 × 2–30, usually around 6 µm (Fig. 23.7), gliding rather slowly. Color of cell mass originally described as pink to salmon but usually rather pale yellow. In aerobic cultures on media with a low nutrient content the colonies are yellowish to salmon-colored, either flat and spreading or convex with a smooth edge, somewhat slimy, and up to 1 cm in diameter. Agar around colonies never depressed or softened. In anaerobic agar shake cultures, the colonies are pinkish, small (1–2 mm), spherical or disk-shaped.

Peptones, casamino acids, NH_4^+ or NO_3^- are suitable N sources. This species may grow aerobically solely on the expense of complex N compounds, while for anaerobic growth a fermentable carbohydrate has to be added. The following compounds were found suitable: arabinose, xylose, glucose, galactose, mannose, fructose, sucrose, lactose, maltose, cellobiose, trehalose, raffinose, inulin and starch. Rhamnose, sorbose, sugar alcohols and agar are not utilized. Anaerobic growth is possible on mineral salts media with, for example, glucose or galactose but depends on a sufficient supply of CO_2 (0.3% $NaHCO_3$). Growth under such condi-

tions is much stimulated by the addition of vitamins. Aerobically, no growth occurs on simple defined media. Filter-sterilized galactose (0.1%) strongly inhibits growth on agar media under aerobic conditions, but glucose does not.

Facultative anaerobe. Fermentation products from glucose are formate, acetate, propionate, succinate, lactate, CO_2, H_2 and traces of ethanol.

Marine organism requiring elevated salt concentrations, but NaCl (1–3%) alone is sufficient for this purpose. Good growth between 28 and 37°C and at pH 7.0–7.5. Further data may be found in Table 23.2.

Only one strain is known, isolated from marine mud off the coast of California.

The mol% G + C of the DNA is 37 (Bd) (unpublished result).

Type strain: ATCC 19041.

DNA/rRNA hybridization shows that *C. salmonicolor* is related to *C. lytica* (for details, see Bauwens and De Ley, 1981). The cells of this organism are clearly coarser than those of most other bacteria described here, so that it is questionable whether there are really close phylogenetic connections.

8. Cytophaga agarovorans (Veldkamp 1961) comb. nov. (Cytophaga salmonicolor var. agarovorans Veldkamp 1961, 340).

a.gar.o.vo'rans. Malayan n. *agar* agar, gelling polysaccharides from seaweeds; L. v. *vorare* to devour; M.L. part. adj. *agarovorans* agar-consuming.

Provisionally classified in group G.

Moderately long to very long, thin, thread cells with slightly tapering or rounded ends, 0.3–0.4 × 8–50, usually 12–30 µm (Fig. 23.8), very flexible and rapidly gliding, particularly under oxygen limitation. Colonies in aerobic cultures pink to salmon-colored, spreading or compact, usually not exceeding 1 cm in diameter, with a tendency for the cells to penetrate into the plate. The agar around the colonies shows wide gelase fields, is softened, and may even become liquified when lower agar concentrations (0.6%) are used. In anaerobic agar shake cultures on mineral media with 1% agar and 0.1% yeast extract (or a vitamin mixture), large spherical pink colonies arise, surrounded by completely liquified agar. The same medium does not allow growth under aerobic conditions unless it is supplemented with corn steep liquor and nutrient broth (0.1% each). In contrast to the former organism, *C. agarovorans* is inhibited on agar media by glucose as well as by galactose under aerobic and semianerobic conditions. Agar is also suitable as a fermentation substrate. On media with reduced (1%) agar concentration, the catalase reaction may become negative.

Facultative anaerobe. Good growth is obtained in a normal aerobic atmosphere, but if the vitality of the inoculum is impaired (old cultures, culture preserves), anaerobic conditions should be applied.

Only one strain is known, isolated from the same environment as the former organism.

The mol% G + C of the DNA is 41 (Bd) (unpublished observation).

Type strain: ATCC 19043.

It was stated in the original description that this organism is identical with the former in most respects, with the exception that it is able to degrade and utilize agar. But there is a substantial difference in cell shape and mol% G + C, and it may be doubted that the two organisms are really so closely related as thought initially. In fact, *C. salmonicolor* var. *agarovorans* might be better classified as a *Microscilla*.

9. Cytophaga flevensis van der Meulen, Harder and Veldkamp 1974, 340.[AL]

fle.ven'sis. L. n. *Flevum* is a former inner sea in The Netherlands which is now the IJsselmeer, a freshwater lake; M.L. adj. *flevensis* from the IJsselmeer.

Provisionally classified in group H.

Relatively short stout rods with rounded ends, 0.5–0.7 × 2–5 µm (Fig. 23.9), may become almost coccoid in old cultures; in liquid cultures, it sometimes occurs in pairs and chains; slowly gliding. Cell mass bright yellow; pigment extracts show a β,β-carotene spectrum; no color change

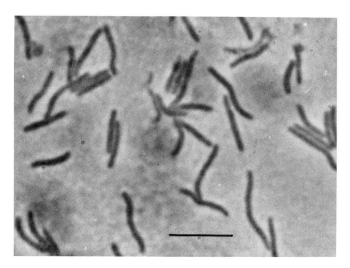

Figure 23.7. *C. salmonicolor,* type strain. Cells from seawater-peptone liquid medium (SP5 l.m.) at 30°C. Phase contrast. *Bar,* 5 μm.

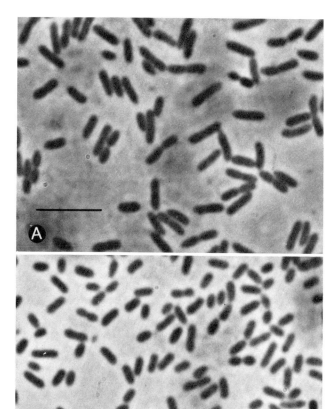

Figure 23.9. *C. flevensis,* type strain. Cells from starch-peptone liquid medium after 20 h at 21°C *(A)* and at 30°C *(B).* At the higher, suboptimal temperature the culture has a considerably lower density and more delicate cells. Phase contrast. *Bar,* 5 μm.

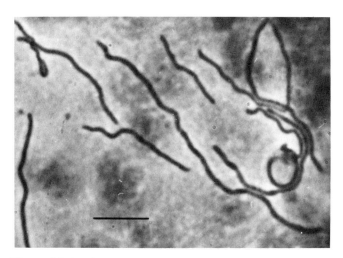

Figure 23.8. *C. agarovorans,* type strain. Cells from seawater-peptone (SAP5) agar at 30°C. Phase contrast. *Bar,* 5 μm.

is seen with alkali. Colonies usually compact, convex, with an entire edge, initially faintly yellow and iridescent and, later, bright yellow. Occasionally, spreading colonies appear on nutrient agar after 1–2 weeks of incubation, or spreading fans emerge locally from the otherwise compact colony (e.g. on CY agar). The colonies are sitting in shallow craters which arise through partial decomposition of the agar by an inducible extracellular agarase. Cultures may develop an agreeable fruity odor.

Peptones, casamino acids, NH_4^+ and NO_3^- are good N sources; less so are glutamate, arginine and urea. This species grows on peptone alone, although less vigorously than in the presence of carbohydrate, and over several transfers only if the peptone concentration is sufficiently high, e.g. 1% casein peptone. Excellent growth on nutrient agar. Grows also on mineral salts media supplemented with a suitable C compound, preferentially a sugar, such as xylose, arabinose, glucose, galactose, mannose, rhamnose, lactose, saccharose, maltose, isomaltose, melibiose, raffinose, but also on galacturonic acid, agar, agarose, agaropectin, inulin and pectin. Fucose, ribose, cellobiose, trehalose, amino sugars, alcohols, sugar alcohols, various amino acids and other organic acids do not support growth. Sugars are metabolized with acid production. Proteins such as casein, single-cell protein, and gelatin are not hydrolyzed. No lysis of bacteria and cyanobacteria. Resistant to novobiocin, penicillin G, poly-

myxin B and streptomycin; sensitive to chloramphenicol, tetracycline, erythromycin, nalidixic acid, nitrofurantoin and sulfafurazole. Catalase has been reported positive but is, in fact, negative (gas production with H_2O_2 delayed and moderate).

Strictly aerobic. Growth occurs between 0 and 30°C, with the optimum occurring around 25°C. Survives 10 min at 40°C but not at 45°C. Grows very well on media with full strength seawater, e.g., SP2 agar or VY/2 agar (Reichenbach and Dworkin, 1981c) with artificial seawater. For further information, see Table 23.2.

Isolated from freshwater and wet soil collected in the IJsselmeer area, The Netherlands.

The mol% G + C of the DNA is 35 (T_m) and 33 (Bd) (unpublished observations).

Type strain: ATCC 27944 (A-34 van der Meulen, Harder and Veldkamp).

The organism could be obtained so far only from the IJsselmeer area, an old bay of the North Sea. Its ability to grow on seawater media suggests that it was originally a marine bacterium. Perhaps there are connections to the *C. lytica* group.

10. **Cytophaga saccharophila** (ex Agbo and Moss 1979) nom. rev.
sac.cha.ro.phi′la. G. n. *sacchar,* gen. *saccharos* sugar; G. v. *philein* to love; M.L. fem. adj. *saccharophila* sugar-loving.

Provisionally classified in group I.

Short to moderately long rods with slightly tapering ends, usually somewhat curved, 0.5–0.7×2–$6\ \mu m$, may become almost coccoid in older cultures. The organism shows a strong tendency to pleomorphism, particularly in agar cultures, where cells of very different length, width and shape may be found. On carbohydrate-containing media, including all agar media, the rods tend to become fatter than on pure peptone media. On the latter (e.g. with 1% casein peptone), the rods are sometimes much more slender and delicate, only 0.3–$0.4\ \mu m$ wide, and extremely flexible (Fig. 23.10). Both types of cells may be seen to be slowly but actively gliding. Cell mass bright to golden yellow, turns into copper-red with 20% KOH, and again bright yellow with HCl. The reaction is, however, not easy to observe on all media; it is very obvious on, for example, MYX agar. Colonies on nutrient agar small (1–2 mm), compact, convex, glistening, slimy, sitting in shallow depressions, and surrounded by large gelase fields. The agar becomes softened but is never liquefied. On certain media, e.g. water agar, CY agar or chitin agar, spreading colonies develop.

Peptones and NH_4^+ serve as sole N source. Good growth on nutrient agar. This species grows on peptone alone but is much stimulated by the addition of a carbohydrate, e.g. glucose. The following C compounds are used as sole carbon and energy source: xylose, arabinose, glucose, galactose, mannose, fructose, rhamnose, lactose, sucrose, maltose, cellobiose, melibiose, trehalose, raffinose, stachyose, agar, agarose, starch, pectin, carrageenan, arabinogalactan, gum arabic, xanthan and galactomannan. The agarase is extracellular and inducible by agar and several other polysaccharides, e.g. starch, pectin and arabinogalactan. It is completely repressed in the presence of glucose or galactose. Two of the six original isolates lost the ability to attack agar during subcultivation. Strongly proteolytic (casein, single-cell protein). Resistant to polymyxin B, chloramphenicol, neomycin; sensitive to tetracycline, streptomycin, fucidin, novobiocin, vibriostat 0/129 and benzylpenicillin. Catalase and oxidase are reported to be positive but appear to be negative. For further data, see Table 23.2.

Strictly aerobic. Growth occurs between 4 and 30°C. Although there is still good growth at 30°C, lower temperatures (20–25°C) are clearly preferred, particularly in liquid cultures. This species tolerates NaCl up to 2%, but no growth occurs on seawater media.

Isolated from the River Wey, a lowland river in England, but was obtained relatively rarely.

The mol% G + C of the DNA is 32 (Bd) (unpublished observation) and 36 (T_m) (Agbo and Moss, 1979.) The mol% G + C of the DNA was recently determined by my colleagues and myself via density gradient centrifugation and was found to be substantially below the T_m value given in the species description.

Type strain: NCIB 2072 (024 Agbo and Moss).

11. **Cytophaga diffluens** (ex Stanier 1940, 623; emend. Lewin 1969, 197) nom. rev.

dif'flu.ens. L. part. adj. *diffluens* flowing away.

Provisionally classified in group K.

Slender flexible rods with tapering ends, 0.5×4– 30, usually below or around $6\ \mu m$ (Fig. 23.11), gliding. Cell mass orange due to the carotenoid saproxanthin (Lewin and Lounsbery, 1969). Colonies usually fast-spreading, filmlike, light pink to deep orange, and sunken into the agar, which later may become completely liquefied. Agar cultures often develop an agreeable fruity odor.

Peptones, casamino acids and glutamate may serve as N source. Some strains grow on NO_3^-; the type strain, however, does not. Peptones may be used also as the sources of carbon and energy. Galactose and acetate and, with some strains, also glucose and sucrose stimulate growth.

Strict aerobe. Marine organism requiring elevated salt concentrations, but NaCl (1.5–5%) may be substituted for seawater. The type strain shows a relatively high temperature tolerance (grows still at 40°C), while the other strains do not grow beyond 30 or 35°C. For further data, see Table 23.2.

All strains were isolated from sand and mud collected in the littoral at different places around the world. Type strain from Bombay, India.

The mol% G + C of the DNA is 42 (Bd) (Mandel and Lewin, 1969).

Neotype strain: NCMB 1402 (B-1 Lewin).

This organism was originally described by Stanier (1940, 1941), whose strain is, however, no longer available. The strains isolated by Lewin seem to conform to the earlier description to such a degree that revival of the species with a neotype strain, as suggested by Lewin, appears justified. Stanier's organism had the same color, was a strict aerobe, had the same temperature and salt range, grew only on organic N, was a vigorous agar decomposer, and attacked alginate but not chitin. It differed in that a wider variety of sugars stimulated growth, it reduced NO_3^-, it did not produce H_2S, and it did not attack starch, but it did degrade filter paper, while Lewin's strains attack only CMC. But Stanier's strain, too, was hardly a typical cellulose decomposer, growing on, for example, peptone alone. Lewin isolated seven strains which appear very similar by the admittedly restricted range of characteristics given in the description. They fall into a narrow mol% G + C range and may, indeed, belong in the same species. Two "variants" are clearly separated by their mol% G + C of the DNA and cannot belong into this species. Although var. *carnea* is lost, var. *aprica* is still available and is described below as a species of its own.

12. **Cytophaga aprica** (Lewin 1969) comb. nov. *(Cytophaga diffluens* var. *aprica* Lewin 1969, 197).

a'pri.ca. L. fem. adj. *aprica* sunlit, sun-loving.

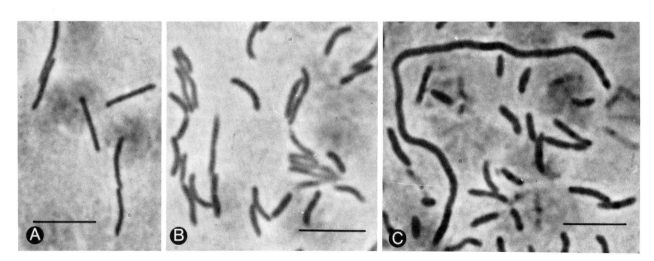

Figure 23.10. *C. saccharophila,* type strain. In pure peptone liquid medium, the cells are longer and more slender *(A)* than in starch-peptone liquid medium *(B),* both at 21°C. On peptone (CY) agar at 30°C, they become much fatter and more pleomorphic *(C).* Phase contrast. *Bars,* 5 μm.

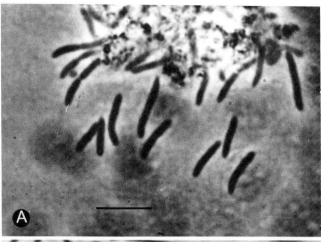

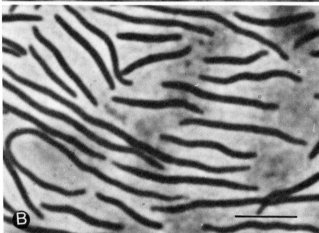

Figure 23.11. *C. diffluens*, type strain. Cells from seawater-peptone liquid medium (SP5 l.m.) grown at 30°C *(A)* or at 21°C *(B)*. Phase contrast. *Bars*, 5 μm.

Provisionally classified in group L.

Long rods to very long threads, slender, flexible, with pointed ends, 0.5–0.7 × 6–30 μm and longer (Fig. 23.12), slowly gliding and bending. The cell populations are always heterogeneous with respect to length, and this occurs also in liquid cultures at all stages. The long threads seem to be divided by cross-walls into long segments. The cells are rather sensitive to environmental changes, degenerating in slide mounts quickly into ghosts and spheroplasts. Cell mass orange. Colonies spreading, orange, producing large gelase fields and deep craters in the agar plate. The agar is softened but not liquefied. Excellent growth in pure peptone media, e.g. SP5 l.m. at 21°C as well as at 30°C, with a slight preference for lower temperatures.

In most of the characteristics given in the scant species description, the organism is identical with *C. diffluens*. In addition to its cell morphology, it differs, however, in two other important properties: it is resistant to 0.01% sodium lauryl sulfate and has a considerably lower mol% G + C of the DNA.

Three strains have been isolated from marine mud and sand collected at widely separated sites. The type strain comes from Kailua, Hawaii.

The mol% G + C of the DNA is 35 (Bd) (Mandel and Lewin, 1969).

Type strain: ATCC 23126 (JL-4 Lewin).

This organism is almost certainly not closely related with the CLB. It somewhat resembles *C. agarovorans* and, like that organism, might probably be better classified as a *Microscilla*.

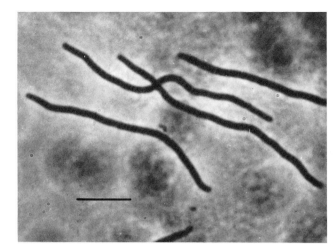

Figure 23.12. *C. aprica*, type strain. Cells from seawater-peptone liquid medium (SP5 l.m.) at 21°C. Phase contrast. *Bar*, 5 μm.

13. **Cytophaga johnsonae** Stanier 1947, 306.[AL] *(Cytophaga johnsonii* [sic] Stanier 1957, 860.)

john.so'nae. M.L. gen. fem. n. *johnsonae* of Johnson; named in honor of the American microbiologist D. E. Johnson, who made an earlier study on chitinoclastic gliding soil bacteria.

Provisionally classified in subgenus *Chthonophaga*.

Slender flexible rods, usually with tapering ends, of variable length, 0.3–0.4 × 1.5–15 μm (Fig. 23.13 and 23.14). Long rods (6–12 μm) predominate in young cultures; short ones (1–3 μm) and almost coccoid cells predominate at later stages. Cell mass bright yellow to orange, turning quickly purple-brown with KOH and bright yellow again with HCl. Colonies are either large spreading yellow swarms sometimes almost greenish iridescent (on many media, e.g. VY/2, starch, pectin agar) or, on rich media (e.g. with 1% peptone), compact, convex, glistening, usually bright to golden yellow, with their margin entire or somewhat spreading, flat, and with flamelike protrusions. Deep orange and pale yellow variants may arise with, for example the type strain.

Peptones, casamino acids, glumate, asparagine, urea or NH$_4$⁺ are good N sources, NO$_3$⁻ is less so (type strain: Christensen, 1977b; Oyaizu and Komagata, 1981), and NO$_2$⁻ and glycine are not used. This species may exclusively grow very well on organic N compounds, e.g. on pure peptone or yeast extract media. NH$_3$ is released from organic N compounds. This species grows on mineral salts media with NH$_4$⁺ and a suitable carbon and energy source, preferentially a carbohydrate: arabinose, xylose, glucose, galactose, mannose, lactose, maltose, sucrose, cellobiose, raffinose, starch, inulin or chitin. Sugar alcohols and organic acids including acetate are generally not utilized, but some strains (for an evaluation of such observations, see below) grow on succinate, fumarate or malate. Some strains grow much better on disaccharides than on the respective monosaccharides. Sugars are metabolized with acid production. Strong proteolytic activity. Degrades various polysaccharides. Chitin decomposition is fast and complete, e.g. on CHIT 3 agar (yeast extract, 0.05%; reprecipitated chitin, 0.5%; MgSO$_4$·7H$_2$O, 0.1%; and agar, 1.2%; as top layer on CY agar; 4 days at 30°C), but is restricted essentially to the colony area.

Strict aerobe. The report that the type strain metabolizes glucose fermentatively (Christensen, 1977b) seems erroneous (Callies and Mannheim, 1980; Oyaizu and Komagata, 1981). The type strain uses neither NO$_3$⁻ nor fumarate (Callies and Mannheim, 1978) as electron acceptor but was reported to produce gas from NO$_2$⁻ (Christensen, 1977b). Other strains, however, grow anaerobically, with NO$_3$⁻ reducing the latter to NO$_2$⁻ and even to N$_2$. Stanier (1947) distinguished a var. *denitrificans* which grew luxuriantly under such conditions, producing copious amounts of gas. The catalase reaction is slightly delayed and moderately

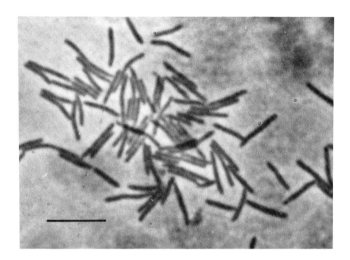

Figure 23.13. *C. johnsonae*, type strain. Cells from peptone liquid medium at 30°C. Phase contrast. *Bar*, 5 μm.

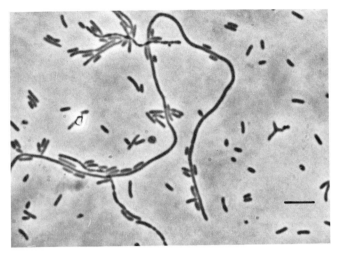

Figure 23.14. *Cytophaga* species, *johnsonae* complex, strain Cy j1. Cells from yeast (VY/2) agar after 4 weeks at 30°C. Typical aspect of an aged culture, with cell chains, threads and a branched cell. Many cells were, however, still actively gliding. Phase contrast. *Bar*, 5 μm.

strong. Tolerant to 1% but not to 3% NaCl. For further data, see Table 23.2.

Organisms of this general type are common in soil, compost, mud and freshwater.

The mol% G + C of the DNA is 33% (Bd) (Mandel and Leadbetter, 1965).

Cotype strain: ATCC 17061 (Hopkins Marine Station Culture Collection HMS MYX 1.1.1 van Niel).

The type strain is probably an authentic strain, although its origin is not completely clear. It seems to come from Stanier's original collection and would then have been isolated from a soil sample from Rothamsted Experimental Station in England. The strain was used in several studies by different laboratories. The mol% G + C of the DNA of 37 (T_m) is obviously incorrect (Callies and Mannheim, 1980); my colleague and I found a mol% G + C of the DNA of 34 by the same technique (H. Behrens and H. Reichenbach, unpublished observation). Callies and Mannheim (1980) give a genome size of 3.14 × 10⁹ daltons. DNA/rRNA hybridizations show a relatively close relationship between *C. johnsonae* (type), *Flavobacterium aquatile* ATCC 11947 and *C. pectinovorum* (type). This group is clearly distinguished from the *C. lytica* group (Bauwens and De Ley, 1981). There are some discrepancies in the pattern of utilizable sugars reported by different authors (Stanier, 1974; Christensen, 1977b; Callies and Mannheim, 1980). Many strains resembling Stanier's organism in their general appearance have, in the past, been labeled *C. johnsonae*, but that all these organisms were really the same must be doubted. The distinguishing characteristic of chitin degradation is not restricted to *C. johnsonae* among the CLB, and the remaining characteristics listed in the species description are not sufficient to characterize the organism reliably. Unfortunately, this cannot be corrected at the moment, and the warnings uttered above are particularly true for this species. A few examples illustrate this. A chitinoclastic bacterium regarded as very similar to *C. johnsonae* and assumed to "belong undoubtedly to this species group" (Veldkamp, 1955) was later found to have a mol% G + C of the DNA of 71 (NCIB 8501) (Mitchell et al., 1967). It has then provisionally been classified as a *Polyangium* species (NCIB Catalogue of Strains) but appears rather to be a *Lysobacter*. On the basis of a phenotype analysis, *C. pectinovorum* was assigned to *C. johnsonae* (Christensen, 1977b). However, by applying the same procedure but by using somewhat different characteristics, other authors find only a moderate relationship between the two type strains (Oyaizu and Komagata, 1981). The same authors demonstrate an even lower relationship between the type strain of *C. johnsonae* and other named strains of the "same" species. DNA studies show only very low hybridization (10%) between the two type strains of *C. johnsonae* and *C. pectinovorum* (Callies

and Mannheim, 1980). In the same study, DNA homology between *C. johnsonae* and *C. hutchinsonii* was 0%. The *C. johnsonae* strain which my colleague and I used for many of our studies, Cy j1, (NCIB 10150, DSM 425, and C4 Webley) shows only 22% DNA homology with the type strain and 28 with *C. pectinovorum* (H. Behrens and H. Reichenbach, unpublished observation). This is far below the species (75% and better) and even below the genus level (50% and better). The same study also demonstrated considerable heterogeneity between the other 50 environmental strains of CLB involved, all with a mol% G + C of the DNA of around 34. The 16S RNA oligonucleotide catalog identifies Cy j1 clearly as a member of the *Cytophaga* group, relatively close to *Sporocytophaga myxococcoides* and *F. aquatile*, more remote to *C. lytica* and *C. uliginosa* (Paster et al., 1985). Thus the data obtained with Cy j1 in for example, pigment studies can be regarded as representative for the group of soil and freshwater CLB but not specifically for *C. johnsonae*. It is also quite uncertain whether Stanier's strains, especially the denitrifying variant, really all belonged in one and the same species, so that the deviations of individual strains mentioned in the species description could well refer to different species.

14. **Cytophaga pectinovora** (Dorey 1959) comb. nov. (*Flavobacterium pectinovorum* Dorey, 1959, 94; *Cytophaga johnsonae* sensu Christensen 1977b).

pec.ti.no.vo′ra. M.L. n. *pectin* methylated polygalacturonic acids in plant cell walls, from Gr. adj. *pectos* tightly attached, firmly fixed, curdled; L. v. *vorare* to devour; M.L. fem. adj. *pectinorora* pectin-devouring.

Provisionally classified in group N.

Slender rods with slightly tapering or rounded ends, 0.4–0.5 × 1–5 μm (Fig. 23.15). On rich media, e.g. liquid media either with 1% peptone or with 0.25% peptone and 0.5% starch, the cell population becomes heterogeneous, and much longer forms (15–25 μm) may appear. Originally described as nonmotile, the cells of the type strain were later observed to move by gliding (Lund, 1969; Christensen, 1977b). Cell mass bright to golden yellow, turning copper-red with 20% KOH and golden yellow again with HCl. The shape of the colonies depends critically on the temperature. At 30°C, the colonies are compact on all media, flat to slightly raised, with an entire or lobed margin, bright to golden yellow, often with a dry, tenacious slime, making it difficult to remove the inoculum from the loop. At 22°C, large, spreading swarms develop on many media, e.g. on CY and on VY/2 (yeast) agar.

Peptones, casamino acids, glutamate, asparagine, urea, NH₄⁺ and

NO$_3^-$ serve as N sources. This species grows well on peptone alone and shows excellent growth on nutrient agar. NH$_3$ is released from casamino acids and peptones. This species also grows on mineral media with arabinose, xylose, glucose, maltose, sucrose, lactose, cellobiose, inulin or pectin as the sole carbon and energy source but does not grow on glycerol, mannitol or salicin. Carbohydrates are utilized under aerobic conditions with acid production. On pectate gels, the colonies produce depressions, and the gel may later become liquefied due to extracellular inducible pectinase. Polygalacturonase but not pectin methyl esterase could be demonstrated (Dorey, 1959). Various proteins (casein, gelatin, single-cell protein) are digested.

Strict aerobe. Catalase-positive, but reaction slightly delayed and of moderate intensity. Tolerates 1% NaCl but is completely inhibited by 3%. Good growth occurs at 30°C, but lower temperatures (20–25°C) are preferred. Survives 10 min at 40°C but not at 45°C. An unusually wide pH range (pH 5–10) is reported (Christensen, 1977b). For further data, see Table 23.2.

Isolated from soil in southern England.

The mol% G + C of the DNA is 34 (Bd) (unpublished observation) and 36 (T_m) (Callies and Mannheim, 1980).

Type strain: NCIB 9059 (ATCC 19366; number 81 Dorey).

The mol% G + C of the DNA as given initially (33) (Mitchell et al., 1967) appears slightly too low. My colleague and I have found a mol% G + C of the DNA of 34 (by both Bd and T_m) (H. Behrens and H. Reichenbach, unpublished observations). The eight isolates studied by Dorey were identical with the type strain in almost all characteristics. One strain differed in that it did not utilize pentoses, two strains produced H$_2$S, and several strains could not use urea as N source. But as the ability to degrade pectin is not uncommon among CLB, the strains could still have belonged to different species. More recently, *F. pectinovorum* was reclassified as *C. johnsonae* (Christensen, 1977b). As already mentioned in the comments on *C. johnsonae*, it must be doubted that this is justified. DNA/DNA hybridization between the type strains is very low: 10% (Callies and Mannheim, 1980). My colleague and I have found only 25% homology between strains that hybridize at species level, each (>80%) with the two type strains (H. Behrens and H. Reichenbach, unpublished observations). Both values suggest a relationship between *C. johnsonae* and *C. pectinovora* below genus level. In fact, there are also phenotypic differences between the two type strains, although the taxonomic relevance of those cannot be judged at the moment: *C. pectinovora* clearly differs in its cell shape from *C. johnsonae*, has a much lower temperature optimum, develops spreading swarms only around 20°C, produces a very sticky dry slime, grows only modestly on VY/2 (yeast) agar but grows vigorously, much better than *C. johnsonae*, on glucose-nitrate

agar. At 30°C, it attacks chitin rather sluggishly, particularly on peptone-containing media, e.g. on CHIT 3 agar (see *C. johnsonae*), in spite of good growth. Only when chitin agar is poured on top of plain water agar does a clear lysis zone gradually develop, but growth is very poor. Chitin decomposition is, however, quite efficient at 22°C on both media.

15. **Cytophaga aquatilis** Strohl and Tait 1978, 302.[AL]

a.qua′ti.lis. L. fem. adj. *aquatilis* living in water.

Provisionally classified in group O.

Slender flexible rods with slightly tapering or rounded ends, 0.4–0.6 × 1.5–15, usually 2–6 µm (Fig. 23.16). Almost coccoid forms and long irregular filaments may also occur, with the latter occurring as, for example degenerative forms in liquid cultures at 30°C. Slowly but actively gliding. Cell mass yellow to orange, turning copper-brown with 20% KOH and bright yellow again with HCl. Colonies either compact, soft and somewhat slimy or thin spreading swarms, e.g. on VY/2 (yeast) agar or on CY agar; yellow to orange under aerobic conditions and, when grown anaerobically, light cream-colored or unpigmented. Slime stains with ruthenium-red.

Peptones, casamino acids, NH$_4^+$ or NO$_3^-$ serve as N source. This species grows well on peptone alone. NH$_3$ is released from peptones. Arabinose, xylose, glucose, galactose, mannose, fructose, lactose, maltose, sucrose, cellobiose, raffinose, glycerol, dulcitol and mannitol are fermented with acid production; sorbose, sorbitol and inositol are not. The same compounds that are fermented are also metabolized aerobically with more or less acid production. Strong proteolytic activity. Ornithine and lysine decarboxylase and phenylalanine deaminase are absent. Esculin and glycogen are degraded. Chitin is efficiently decomposed. Several Gram-positive and Gram-negative bacteria are lysed, cyanobacteria are not. Resistant to ampicillin, methicillin, lincomycin, polymyxin B and vancomycin (the latter inhibits gliding, however); sensitive to bacitracin, erythromycin, the aminoglycosides, chloramphenicol, nalidixic acid, novobiocin, the tetracyclines, and sulfathiazole.

Facultative anaerobe requiring growth factors in peptone or yeast extract for anaerobic growth. Anaerobic growth either fermentative with one of the carbohydrates mentioned above and yeast extract or under NO$_3^-$ reduction. Aerobically grown cells show a strong catalase reaction. Temperature range: 5–30°C; but at 30°C the cultures degenerate quickly, and sustained growth is not possible. Tolerates NaCl up to 2%; no growth occurs on seawater media. For further data, see Table 23.2.

Isolated from the gills of salmon affected by bacterial gill disease in a fish hatchery in Michigan, U.S.A., but etiological connections are not certain.

The mol% G + C is of the DNA is 34 (Bd).

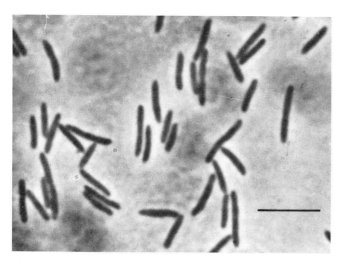

Figure 23.15. *C. pectinovora,* type strain. Cells from peptone liquid medium at 30°C. Phase contrast. *Bar,* 5 µm.

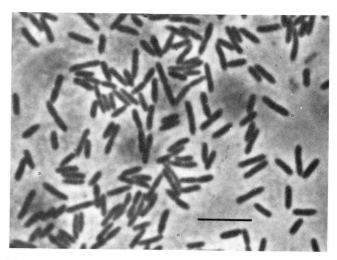

Figure 23.16. *C. aquatilis,* type strain. Cells from peptone liquid medium at 21°C. Phase contrast. *Bar,* 5 µm.

Type strain: ATCC 29551 (strain N; Strohl and Tait).

This is one of a still unknown number of ill-defined freshwater species of CLB. Strohl and Tait isolated four more strains from fish taken in the same area. These strains resembled the type strain almost exactly in all characteristics tested and were assumed to belong to the same species. The species is regarded as common, but apparently no efforts were made to isolate it directly from environmental samples. The type strain shows only low DNA homology, with seven strains of CLB isolated from aqueous habitats and having mol% G + C of the DNA of around 34 (H. Behrens and H. Reichenbach, unpublished observations). Some data reported by later authors (Oyaizu and Komagata, 1981) are not fully in accordance with the species description: oxidase was found positive but was really at best very weakly so; no fermentative activity was found with glucose in the OF test; and NO_3^- respiration was negative, which was, however, perhaps due to the dependence of the organism on yeast extract under anaerobic conditions. In the species description the occurrence of rotating and migrating microcolonies on media with a low nutrient content (no formulation given) is mentioned. This I could never observe, and it would indeed be very unusual for a *Cytophaga*. My colleague and I have recently determined for the type strain a mol% G +C of the DNA of 32 (Bd), so that the mol% G + C of the species may be slightly lower than that given above.

16. **Cytophaga psychrophila** (ex Borg 1960) nom. rev.

psy.chro′phi.la. Gr. adj. *psychros* cold; Gr. v. *philein* to love, to like; *psychrophila* liking it cold.

Provisionally classified in group P.

Slender flexible rods with rounded ends, in growing cultures 0.4–0.5 × 1.5–7.5, usually around 3.5 µm (Fig. 23.17); gliding. Cell mass golden yellow, turns orange-brown to dark red with 20% KOH. Colonies on CA agar bright yellow with a thin spreading margin. Deeply colored nonspreading variants with an entire edge also occur.

Grows on peptones or vitamin-free casein hydrolysate but is unable to utilize any carbohydrate. Actively proteolytic. Decomposes autoclaved cells of *Escherichia coli* and several other bacteria. Xanthine and esculin are not hydrolyzed. Sensitive to tetracyclines, bacitracin, chloramphenicol, dihydrostreptomycin, neomycin, erythromycin and penicillin; some isolates are also sensitive to polymyxin B.

Strict aerobe. Tolerates 0.8% but not 2% NaCl. Grows well between 4 and 23°C but not at 25°C. For further data, see Table 23.2.

Isolated from salmonid fishes affected by cold water disease, for which the organism may be responsible as the etiological agent.

The mol% G + C of the DNA is 33 for the type strain and strain NCMB 1947 (Bd) (unpublished observations) and 32 (Bd) for strain PSY (ATCC 23108) (Mandel and Lewin, 1969).

Cotype strain: DSM 3660 (NCMB 1947).

So far, no type strain has been named for this organism. Up to recently, only two strains supposed to represent *C. psychrophila* were available at public culture collections. Both were supplied by E. J. Ordal, in whose laboratory the pioneering studies on the organism were performed. Nothing at all is known about the origin of strain PSY (ATCC 23108; NCMB 1455). Presently, this strain is labeled *Flexibacter aurantiacus* (see below). The second strain, NCMB 1947, reportedly was isolated from Coho salmon *(Oncorhynchus kisutch).* However, in the literature on *C. psychrophila* I could not find any strain isolated from that source, so the identity of NCMB 1947 is equally obscure. Very recently, I obtained from the collection of Dr. R. F. Pacha a preserved culture of strain 143a which is one of the original isolates of Borg and can be regarded as typical for the species (Pacha, 1968; see below). This culture preserved from February 1967 was viable and has since been deposited at several culture collections. It was isolated from Minter Creek Hatchery in the State of Washington, U.S.A. The 10 isolates studied by Pacha (1968), all from outbreaks of cold water disease in the Western U.S. and including two of the original strains of Borg, appeared very similar phenotypically. The only variations observed were differences in salt tolerance (6 grew at 1% NaCl), in tyrosine degradation (2 were positive) and in sensitivity to polymyxin B (4 were positive) and sulfadiazine. Serologically all 10 iso-

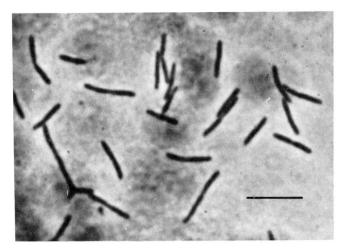

Figure 23.17. *C. psychrophila,* type strain. Cells from peptone liquid medium at 21°C. One cell is branched. Phase contrast. *Bar,* 5 µm.

lates cross-reacted to a high titer. There was no cross-reaction with *C. columnaris* and with saprophytic CLB isolated from the surface of various fishes (Pacha and Porter, 1968; Bullock, 1972). There is a high serological cross-reaction between isolates from Western cold water disease and from peduncle disease of brook trout in the Northeastern U.S. (Bullock, 1972). Fish pathologists believe that the two diseases are caused by the same etiological agent, viz. *C. psychrophila.* Although this may in fact be the case, DNA reassociation studies still show considerable heterogeneity among isolates from cold water fishes (Pyle and Shotts, 1980). Also, cold and warm water strains in general are clearly separated. Unfortunately, the simple phenotypic differentiation scheme proposed for CLB from fish (Pyle and Shotts, 1980) does not differentiate according to the DNA reassociation groups. *C. psychrophila* seems clearly to be distinguished from *C. columnaris,* which is regarded as the well-defined and monotypical etiological agent for columnaris disease (Bullock, 1972), by its much lower temperature range and by completely different surface antigens. The DNA reassociation studies support the taxonomic separation of the two. Saprophytic aquatic CLB differ from *C. psychrophila* (and *C. columnaris)* in that they usually metabolize carbohydrates (see, for example, Pacha and Porter, 1968). Cold water disease affects mainly young fish and particularly coho salmon, and losses during outbreaks may be >50% (Pacha and Ordal, 1970). The disease abates when the temperature rises to at least 13°C.

There is some confusion with *Flexibacter aurantiacus* (see also there), because one of the two available strains (PSY Lewin 1969) was originally supplied as *C. psychrophila* and, indeed, is likely to belong to this taxon. However, DNA/rRNA hybridization indicates that *F. aurantiacus* is not a member of the *Cytophaga* complex (Bauwens and De Ley, 1981), which would be difficult to reconcile with the present species concept. The strain used for the hybridization is not identified, but probably it was the type strain (DWO Lewin 1969; ATCC 23107), so that the explanation for the contradiction might be that the two *F. aurantiacus* strains are fundamentally different organisms.

17. **Cytophaga marina** (Hikida, Wakabayashi, Egusa and Masumura) comb. nov. (*Flexibacter marinus* Hikida, Wakabayashi, Egusa and Masumura 1979, 421).

ma.ri′na. L. fem. adj. *marina* belonging to, living in the sea.

Provisionally classified in group Q.

Slender flexible rods, 0.4 × 2–5 µm, occasionally longer (30 µm); tend to become shorter in older cultures; gliding.

Colonies spreading, with an irregular edge, yellow-orange. Pigment extracts show a β,β-carotene type spectrum.

Peptones and casamino acids serve as N source; glutamate, urea, NH_4^+

and NO_3^- do not. This species grows on peptone alone. NH_3 is released from peptone. None of the 24 carbohydrates tested was utilized. It also grows well on nutrient agar with seawater. Esculin is not hydrolyzed. Dead cells of several bacterial species are lysed.

Strict aerobe. Temperature range: 14–35°; optimum: 30°C. Marine organism depending on natural or synthetic seawater (at least one-third strength), no growth with NaCl alone. For further data, see Table 23.2.

Isolated from black and red sea bream *(Acanthopagrus schlegeli* and *Pagrus major)* in Japan.

The mol% G + C of the DNA is 31 (T_m); the mol% G + C range for eight isolates is 31–32.

Type strain: NCMB 2153 (B-2; Hikida et al., 1979).

The organism is found in mouth erosions and rotten tails of sea breams and seems to be the etiological agent responsible for these disorders. It attacks mainly juvenile fish and may cause serious losses (up to 30% of the population). A similar organism has been isolated from other sea fish in Japan (Kusuda and Kimura, 1982). It differs mainly in its ability to degrade starch and chitin, although it cannot utilize carbohydrates either. The eight isolates from sea breams studied by Hikida et al. (1979) appear as a homogeneous group and seem to belong in the same species. *C. marina* may be a marine counterpart to the freshwater fish pathogens, *C. psychrophila* and *C. columnaris,* which it also resembles in its failure to metabolize carbohydrates, its strong proteolytic activity, and its low mol% G + C.

18. **Cytophaga latercula** Lewin 1969, 200.[AL]

la.ter′cu.la. L. n. *laterculus* a small brick; M. L. fem. adj. *latercula* bricklike, brick-red.

Provisionally classified in group R.

Short to moderately long rods, in young growing cultures relatively delicate with slightly tapering or rounded ends 0.3–0.4 × 1–5 μm (Fig. 23.18); in older cultures, long fine threads may also appear. Liquid cultures growing close to the temperature maximum at 30°C show a completely different aspect: long and relatively course, irregularly bent threads or filaments, 0.5–0.6 × 10–40 μm (Fig. 23.18). Upon plating and incubation at 21°C, the short slender rods return. Cell mass brick-red. The pigment extract has a maximum at 465 nm (hexane) which seems to distinguish the organism from other orange or red species. Colonies small, compact, convex, with an entire edge, soft, slimy, intensely orangered, surrounded by large gelase fields and producing shallow depressions in the agar.

Peptones, casamino acids, glutamate and NO_3^- serve as N source. This species grows on peptone alone. Glucose, galactose and sucrose are suitable C sources; glycerol, acetate and lactate are not used. Agar is softened but not liquefied. Chitin is slowly degraded. Autoclaved yeast cells are attacked but not completely decomposed.

Strict aerobe. Marine organism, stenohaline. At 30°C, there is still excellent growth, but the cultures degenerate quickly. For further data, see Table 23.2.

Only one strain known, isolated from the outflow of a marine aquarium in La Jolla, California.

The mol% G + C of the DNA is 34 (Bd) (Mandel and Lewin, 1969).

Type strain: ATCC 23177 (SIO-1 Lewin).

Gliding is not unequivocally established for this organism. With the presently available strain, I could never observe gliding cells nor spreading colonies under any condition. The organism differs from all other cytophagas in its color and its compact colonies, although the peculiar change in cell morphology at elevated temperatures may be observed also in other species, e.g. *C. aquatilis.* It corresponds in its cell shape to the typical *Cytophaga* species rather than to the *C. diffluens* and *C. salmonicolor* group.

19. **Cytophaga succinicans** (ex Anderson and Ordal 1961) nom. rev. *(Flexibacter succinicans* (Anderson and Ordal) Leadbetter 1974, 106.)

suc.ci′ni.cans. L. n. *succinum* amber; M. L. n. *acidum succinicum* succinic acid (derived from amber); M. L. pres. part. *succinicans* forming succinic acid.

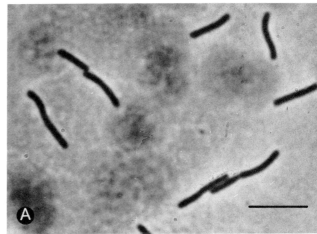

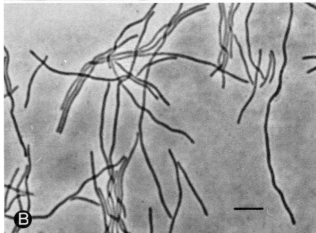

Figure 23.18. *C. latercula,* type strain. Cells from seawater-peptone liquid medium (SP5 l.m.), grown at 21°C *(A)* or at 30°C *(B).* Phase contrast. *Bar,* 5 μm.

Provisionally classified in group S.

Slender, relatively rigid rods with rounded ends, 0.5 × 4–6 μm, becoming shorter and slightly fatter (0.7 × 2 μm) in old cultures; gliding. Some strains were found to have considerably longer cells, up to 40 μm, although typically shorter. Cell mass white when grown anaerobically, yellow-orange under aerobic conditions, probably due to a β,β-carotenoid. No color change with 20% KOH.

Colonies on peptone agar, e.g. CA agar, are large (10–15 mm), thin, spreading swarms, often with a greenish iridescence. Nonspreading variants may occur. On yeast agar, e.g. VY/2 agar, colonies are thin, spreading swarms, yellow; yeast cells are decomposed; and a clear lysis zone appears. On certain media, e.g. with 1% glutamate + 0.5% glucose, the colonies remain small and compact and are unpigmented or very pale greenish yellow even under aerobic conditions.

Peptones serve as N source, one strain (of the three studied) used casein hydrolysate. Glutamate and KNO_3 may also serve as sole N source. This species grows aerobically on peptone alone but grows anaerobically only when a fermentable carbohydrate and CO_2 (15–25 mM $NaHCO_3$) are also present. All strains readily fermented glucose, galactose, maltose, mannose and starch but lactose only with a long lag period (6–38 days); individual strains also used arabinose, sucrose, cellobiose and trehalose; none used xylose, fructose, sorbose, raffinose, melezitose, cellulose, inulin, salicin, sugar alcohols, malate or lactate. Fermentation products are succinate, acetate and formate. Gelatin is slowly liquefied. Single cell protein and casein are hydrolyzed. One strain reduced NO_3^- to NO_2^-.

Facultatively anaerobic. Catalase-variable, often negative, sometimes moderately positive. Oxidase-positive but weakly so.

Temperature optimum: 25°C; grows at 2°C and, at least on plates, also at 30°C but not at 37°C. For further data, see Table 23.2.

Isolated from salmon and water from aquaria containing salmonid fish in the Western U.S., not pathogenic.

The mol% G + C of the DNA is 36 (Bd) (unpublished observation) and 38 (T_m) (Johnson and Ordal, 1968).

Cotype strain: DSM 4002 (strain 8; Anderson and Ordal, 1961a).

C. succinicans is clearly distinguished from other species of CLB: it is a facultative anaerobe with a requirement of CO_2 and has a terrestrial habitat and a negative flexirubin reaction.

No type strain was named in the species description, nor in recent years has a reference strain been available at a public culture collection. Through the courtesy of Dr. J. T. Staley, preserved cultures of the three strains on which the species description is based could be located at the former laboratory of E. J. Ordal. These cultures proved to be viable, and the strains have since been deposited at several culture collections. I propose to use strain 8 as the cotype, because most of the data on which the species description rests are specifically connected with this strain. The strain was isolated from the eroded caudal fin of a chinook salmon fingerling with furunculosis disease in December 1954 at the fish hatchery of the University of Washington. There are slight differences between the three strains, e.g. in their ability to grow on NO_3^- or glutamate as the sole N source, in their lytic activity and in their catalase reaction, and it has not been established whether they really belong to one species.

Although a mol% G + C of the DNA of 38 (T_m) is reported for all three strains (Johnson and Ordal, 1968), my colleagues and I have determined a mol% G + C of the DNA of 36 for strain 8, 35 for strain 14, and 34 for strain 16 (Bd) (unpublished observations).

20. Cytophaga columnaris (ex (Davis) Garnjobst 1945) nom. rev. (*Bacillus columnaris* Davis 1922, 263; *Chondrococcus columnaris* (Davis) Ordal and Rucker 1944, 18; *Flexibacter columnaris* (Davis) Leadbetter 1974, 107.)

co.lum.na′ris. L. n. *columna* column, pillar; M.L. fem. adj. *columnaris* rising like a column or pillar.

Provisionally classified in group T.

Slender flexible rods with rounded ends, 0.3–0.5 × 2–12 μm, may become longer (12–20 μm) in aging cultures; gliding. Cell mass yellow to orange, becoming deep red with KOH and bright yellow again with HCl.

Colonies growing on the surface of agar plates, e.g. CA agar, are thin spreading swarms with a warty center and conspicuous radial, branching veins up to 5 cm in diameter, sticking tenaciously to the agar surface, so that they can hardly be removed with the inoculation loop. Their color ranges from pale greenish yellow to orange. When growing subsurface, e.g. in CA soft agar, the colonies are globular with an irregular rhizoidal outer zone. This species prefers media with reduced (0.5–0.9%) agar content and sometimes refuses to grow on dry and firm agar surfaces. Cultures on nutrient agar produce a sickening odor. In liquid media the cells may form dense star-shaped clusters. When freshly isolated and suspended in water which contains tiny pieces of fish tissue, the bacteria collect into columnlike masses at the edge of the tissue. These columns were formerly mistaken for myxobacterial fruiting bodies, and the spheroplasts within them, for myxospores.

Peptones and casein hydrolysate serve as N source; NH_4^+ and NO_3^- do not. This species grows on peptone alone. Carbohydrates are not metabolized; agar, starch and cellulose are not attacked. Reasonable growth on nutrient agar, good growth on CA agar. Gelatin is liquefied. Single-cell protein and casein are vigorously hydrolyzed. Autoclaved bacterial and yeast cells are decomposed. NO_3^- is not reduced to NO_2^-. H_2S-positive, indole-negative. For further data, see Table 23.2.

Strict aerobe. Catalase-positive. Temperature range: 4–30°C and, for some isolates, up to 37°C; optimum: 25–30°C. Tolerates 0.5% but not 1% NaCl.

Isolated from lesions in skin and connective tissue of a wide variety of fishes.

The mol% G + C of the DNA is 30 (T_m) for strain NCMB 1038 (Mitchell et al., 1967).

Neotype strain: NCMB 2248 (1-S-2cl; Anacker, 1956).

Until recently, there was only one strain accessible in a public culture collection, viz. NCMB 1038. This strain was isolated from the kidney of a diseased chinook salmon *(Oncorhynchus tschawytscha)* from the Snake River in the State of Washington, U.S.A., in July 1955 (Anacker, 1956). The strain belongs to serological group I and bears the antigens 1, 2 and 8. It had only low virulence for chinook salmon after experimental infection. Strain NCMB 1038 subsequently lost rhizoid growth and firm adherence to agar, but a substrain retained these typical characteristics. This substrain was given a new number, NCMB 2248, and I propose to use this strain as a neotype because it comes from a laboratory which studied *C. columnaris* over many years and obviously regarded this strain as representative for the species. It is not known whether the strain is still pathogenic. However, the pathogenicity of *C. columnaris* appears to be a property only of certain strains, and a highly pathogenic type strain would not be desirable anyway because of epidemiological problems and safety regulations. Very recently, Dr. R. E. Pacha, Ellensburg, Washington, kindly sent me two preserved cultures from his collection. The cultures proved to be viable, and the strains have since been deposited at several culture collections and can be used as further representatives of the species for which they appear to be quite typical. Strain C-lla was isolated from a sockeye salmon from Chilko Lake, British Columbia, and was included in a comparative study on CLB from fish (Pacha and Porter, 1968). Strain 2-B58-5b (1) comes from Bonneville Dam, Washington, and is highly pathogenic or at least originally was so. Apparently nothing has been published about this strain. A mol% G + C of the DNA of 33 (Bd) was found for both strains (unpublished observations).

C. columnaris is clearly a distinct, separate species, although its relatedness to other aquatic CLB is still to be elucidated. The organism can easily be recognized by its peculiar swarm colonies not found in this form with any other *Cytophaga* species, as well as its extremely strong casein hydrolysis and very low mol% G + C.

C. columnaris is regarded as responsible for columnaris disease. High losses are reported particularly with salmonid fishes. Pathogenicity seems to increase dramatically with the water temperature, specifically above 18°C. *C. columnaris* appears serologically well separated from other aquatic CLB (see also *C. psychrophila),* although several serological groups can be distinguished within the species (Anacker and Ordal, 1959a). Also, DNA homology studies support an isolated position of *C. columnaris* (Pyle and Shotts, 1980).

Organisms regarded as *C. columnaris* have been studied in many laboratories over the years, but it must be assumed that very different species were involved. This is clearly shown by G + C differences of 6 mol% between three strains of different origin (Mitchell et al., 1967) and by very low DNA hybridization between a bona fide *C. columnaris* and various fish-pathogenic CLB (Pyle and Shotts, 1980). The description given here rests entirely on data about strains isolated from salmonid fishes in the U.S. (mainly from Ordal and Rucker, 1944; Garnjobst, 1945; and Becker and Fujihara, 1978).

Other Species

A considerable number of additional *Cytophaga* species have been described in the past. No strains seem to be available for the following species. Further, several of them were never isolated in pure culture; their descriptions are often too vague to permit recognition. Also, some may be identical with other, established species. At least for the moment these species should be abandoned.

i. *"Cytophaga rubra"* Winogradsky 1929, 598.

Cellulose degrader. Distinguished from *C. hutchinsonii* by its shorter (3 μm) and stouter cells, its brick-red colonies and its less vigorous attack on filter paper. Isolated from soil in France.

ii. *"Cytophaga lutea"* Winogradsky 1929, 599.

Cellulose degrader. Rods longer (6-8 μm) than those of *C. hutchinsonii,* sharply pointed. Colonies bright yellow. Isolated from soil in France, rare.

iii. *"Cytophaga tenuissima"* Winogradsky 1929, 599.

Cellulose degrader. Rods more delicate than those of the aforementioned species. Colonies with a greenish or olive tint. Isolated once from raw humus of a Swedish forest soil.

iv. *"Cytophaga silvestris"* Stapp and Bortels 1934, 55.

Cellulose degrader. Resembled *Sporocytophaga myxococcoides* in cell shape and size (0.2-0.3 × 3-7 μm) and in its pigmentation (grayish, dirty yellow) but did not form microcysts. Perhaps a *Sporocytophaga* strain that refused to produce microcysts under the conditions tested ("symbiotic" culture). Isolated from forest soil in Germany.

v. *"Cytophaga anularis"* Stapp and Bortels 1934, 56.

Cellulose degrader. Slender rods with tapering ends, 0.2-0.3 × 2.5-5 μm, tend to bend into rings of 1-1.2 μm in diameter. Bright yellow. Isolated from forest soil in Germany.

vi. *"Cytophaga crocea"* Stapp and Bortels 1934, 60.

Very efficient cellulose degrader (20-28°C). Slender rods with tapering ends. Golden yellow. Relatively high thermal death point: 49°C. Isolated from forest soil in Germany.

vii. *"Cytophaga flavicula"* Stapp and Bortels 1934, 62.

Cellulose degrader. Slender rods with tapering ends, pale yellow, with a relatively low optimum temperature of 20-24°C; and no cellulose decomposition occurs at 28°C. Isolated from forest soil in Germany.

viii. *"Cytophaga winogradskii"* Verona 1934, 732.

Vigorous cellulose degrader. Slender flexible rods with tapering ends, 0.3-0.5 × 6.5-8.5 μm, producing glassy spots in filter paper. As coccoid Gram-positive cells (0.8-1 μm in diameter) were observed to accumulate in aging cultures, the strain might have been a *Sporocytophaga*, although the nature of the cocci was not really elucidated.

ix. *"Cytophaga haloflava"* Kadota 1956, 51.

Marine cellulose degrader. Flexible rods with rounded ends and of very variable length, 0.3-0.5 × 2.5-10 μm, gliding. Growth on filter paper bright yellow. Cellulose, cellobiose, trehalose and glucose are used as C source; all other sugars tested, sugar alcohols, lactate, gluconate, agar, alginate, starch and inulin are not. Agar is not attacked. NO_3^-, NH_4^+, NO_2^-, urea, aspartate, histidine and peptones are suitable as N source. No growth on peptones alone, no NH_3 from peptones. NO_3^- is reduced to NO_2^-. Strict aerobe. Salinity range: 1-5%. Temperature range: 15-30°C; optimum: 20-25°C. Isolated from fishing nets in Japan (eight strains). This organism is most likely a species of its own.

x. *"Cytophaga haloflava* var. *nonreductans"* Kadota 1956, 52.

This organism is distinguished from the former by its inability to reduce NO_3^- to NO_2^- and to use the latter as N source. Isolated from seawater and fishing nets in Japan (22 strains).

xi. *"Cytophaga rosea"* Kadota 1956, 54.

Marine cellulose degrader. The organism resembles *C. marinoflava* in most characteristics mentioned above but differs in the following: growth on filter paper is pink; NO_2^- is produced from NO_3^- but is not used as the N source, nor is histidine; cellulose, cellobiose and glucose are the only suitable C sources; and the organism is stenohaline: no growth at 1 or 5% NaCl. Isolated from cotton cords immersed in seawater in Japan (10 strains). This organism is probably a species of its own.

xii. *"Cytophaga krzemieniewskae"* Stanier 1940, 623, emend. 1941, 547 (*"Cytophaga krzemienwskii"* Stanier 1940, 623).

Marine cellulose and agar digester. Long flexible rods with rounded or

slightly tapering ends, 0.5-1.5 × 5-20, usually around 12 μm, gliding. Colonies are thin, fast-spreading swarms, initially pale pink, later dark brown due to the production of a dark brown water-soluble pigment. Only peptones serve as N source. Xylose, glucose, galactose, lactose, maltose and cellobiose are metabolized with acid production; arabinose and sucrose are not. Cellulose, starch and alginate are decomposed; chitin is not. Agar and gelatin are liquefied. NO_3^- is reduced to NO_2^-. Strict aerobe. Catalase reaction is weak. Salinity range: 1.5-5% NaCl. Temperature range: 15-30°; optimum: 25°C. Isolated from the Pacific Ocean off California. This species resembles *C. diffluens* in many respects and is hardly closely related with the core of the genus *Cytophaga.*

xiii. *"Cytophaga sensitiva"* Humm 1946, 64.

Marine agar digester. Slender flexible rods with rounded or slightly tapering ends, 0.8-1.0 × 7-20 μm, gliding. The light orange colonies are thin fast-spreading swarms sunken into the agar, with large gelase fields. Agar is liquefied. Good growth on plain seawater agar. Appears to be sensitive to higher nutrient concentrations (e.g. 0.4% peptone is already inhibitory), but good growth is obtained on media with 0.1% peptone, 0.05% beef extract, 0.05% glucose, and traces of yeast extract and ferric phosphate, with or without agar. Peptones and NO_3^- serve as N source. Isolated from the brown alga, *Dictyota dichotoma*, and from seawater from the Atlantic coast off North Carolina.

xiv. *"Cytophaga albogilva"* Fuller and Norman 1943, 566.

Soil organism attacking chemically modified cellulose. Flexible rods with pointed ends, 0.3-0.5 × 4.5-7.5 μm, gliding. The colonies remain relatively small, 2-4 mm in diameter, and are flat, with an irregular edge, and cream to pale yellow (starch agar). Peptones, NH_4^+ and NO_3^- serve as N source. Glucose, galactose, lactose, maltose, sucrose, gum arabic, pectin, starch and hemicellulose are utilized, but acid is not produced. The organism grows on cellulose dextrins but not on filter paper. Gelatin is liquefied. NO_3^- is not reduced to NO_2^-. Strict aerobe. Optimum temperature: 22-30°C. No growth with 3% NaCl. Isolated from soil in the U.S.A.

xv. *"Cytophaga deprimata"* Fuller and Norman 1943, 566.

Soil organism attacking chemically modified cellulose. Flexible rods with pointed ends, 0.3-0.5 × 5.5-10 μm, gliding. Colonies 2-5 mm in diameter; flat, with an irregular edge and a thin, spreading margin; sunken into the agar surface in shallow pits; faint, later bright yellow to orange (starch agar). Peptones, NH_4^+ and NO_3^- serve as N source. Glucose, maltose, sucrose, lactose, pectin, starch and hemicellulose are utilized, but acid is not produced. Slow growth on cellulose dextrins, no growth on filter paper. Gelatin is liquefied. NO_3^- not reduced to NO_2^-. Strict aerobe. Temperature optimum: 25-30°C. No growth with 3% NaCl. Isolated from soil in the U.S.A.

xvi. *"Sphaeromyxa xanthochlora"* Bauer 1962, 392.

Strictly aerobic organism from sewage treatment plants. Slender flexible rods with rounded ends, in young cultures 0.3 × 7-10 μm, in older ones more variable in length, 3-40 μm; gliding. Colonies on low-nutrient agar are large, thin, spreading swarms with a rhizoid internal structure, greenish yellow, iridescent. On high-peptone agar, colonies are compact, convex and with a lobed edge. Peptones, NH_4^+ and NO_3^- serve as N source. This organism grows on peptone alone. It also grows in mineral media with one of the following sugars: xylose, arabinose, glucose, galactose, fructose, malatose, mannose, trehalose and starch. One of two studied strains did not utilize pentoses and fructose. Rhamnose, saccharose and sugar alcohols are not used. Acid is not produced. Filter paper is not attacked. Gelatin is liquefied. NO_3^- is reduced to NO_2^-. Optimum temperature: 25°C. Isolated from trickling filters in Germany. Spheroplasts were misinterpreted as a novel propagative stage ("spheroids"). The organism is a CLB and may belong into the large *C. johnsonae* complex.

xvii. *"Cytophaga antarctica"* Inoue and Komagata 1976, 168.

Nonmotile psychrophilic organism, classified as a *Cytophaga* because of its rugged cell surface on electron micrographs. Slender rods with rounded ends, 0.4–0.6 × 1.3–3.5 μm. Colonies circular, smooth, convex and orange. Peptone is used as N source. No acid produced from carbohydrates aerobically or anaerobically. Acetate but no other organic acid is utilized. NH₃ released from peptone. Gelatin, starch and cellulose are not attacked. Strict aerobe. Catalase-negative, oxidase-positive. Optimum temperature: 12°C; maximum: 20°C; minimum: below 0°C. No growth with 3% NaCl. The mol% G + C of the DNA is 37 *(Tₘ)* and, with two more strains, 36. Isolated from soil in Antarctica. A type strain was designated and deposited under IAM 12025 (13-0-d; Inoue and Komagata, 1976) but is not available at any public collection. If the organism had not been gliding, it would have to be classified as a *Flavobacterium*.

xviii. *"Sporocytophaga flava"* Pfeiffer 1967, 258.

Facultatively anaerobic freshwater saprophyte. The organism resembles *"Sporocytophaga cauliformis"* type 2 (see below) but differs in its tendency to form compact colonies, in the absorption spectrum of crude pigment extracts, and in its ability to grow anaerobically, although it does not metabolize sugars. Isolated from Lake Constance, Germany.

xix. *"Flexibacter aureus"* Soriano 1945, 93.
See under *"Flexibacter,"* *"Other Species."*

Species Incertae Sedis

For the following species, strains are available in publicly accessible culture collections.

a. **"Sporocytophaga cauliformis"** Gräf 1962, 144.

cau.li.for′mis. Gr. n. *caulos* stalks, tem; L. n. *forma* form, shape; M.L. adj. *cauliformis* stalk-shaped, stalked.

Slender flexible rods with slightly tapering ends, 0.4 × 2–5 μm, gliding. Colonies compact with a spreading margin or, on low nutrient agar, large, spreading swarms (e.g. on VY/2 agar), yellow to orange, sometimes almost greenish iridescent, turning purple-brown with 20% KOH and bright yellow again with HCl. Peptones may serve as N source. This organism grows on peptone alone. NH₃ is released from peptone. No acid from sugars. Starch is degraded, cellulose is not. Yeast cells are decomposed. Indole-, H₂S- and urease-negative; no NO₂⁻ from NO₃⁻.

Strict aerobe. Catalase-negative, oxidase-positive. Temperature range: 5–30°C; optimum: 22°C; no growth is obtained at 37°C.

Isolated from freshwater in Germany.

The mol% G + C of the DNA is 35 (Bd) (unpublished observation).

Type strain: NCIB 9488.

There are a number of problems with this species. First, a variety of degenerative phenomena were misinterpreted as special morphological forms (stalk-shaped appendices, spheroids), and the organism was consequently classified in the wrong genus. It is, however, unquestionably a member of the CLB. Second, later, a large number of freshwater isolates were studied (Gräf and Stürzenhofecker, 1964), and the data were confused with the previously described species, *"S. cauliformis."* Among these isolates two types could be distinguished. Type 2 is supposed to represent the new species, *"S. cauliformis."* It is catalase-negative and does not produce acid from sugars. Type 1 resembles the former in many respects but shows a strong catalase reaction and produces acid from sugars. Serologically there is no cross-reaction between the two types. They also differ substantially in their mol% G + C. Also, for type 1, a type strain is still available: NCIB 9484, with a mol% G + C of the DNA of 31 (Bd) (unpublished observation). Both organisms obviously belong to the large group of freshwater CLB, perhaps somewhere within the *C. johnsonae* complex, and probably represent species of their own. Before they can reliably be classified, however, a thorough comparative study is required.

b. **Flavobacterium heparinum** Payza and Korn 1956, 854.^{AL}
(Cytophaga heparina (Payza and Korn) Christensen 1980, 473.^{VP‡})

he.pa.ri′num. Gr. n. *hepar* liver; M.L. neut. adj. *heparinum* connected with degrading heparin, acidic mucoheteropolysaccharides with sulfate groups from various animal tissues.

Small short rods with rounded or slightly tapering ends, may become almost coccoid, 0.3–0.4 × 1–3 μm. Although originally described as motile, the organism is not flagellated. The cells may show gliding motility, however, when covered by a layer of liquid (Perry, 1973; compare with *C. marinoflava).* Colonies circular, soft, with a lobed margin. On certain media, spreading growth may develop, e.g. on agar containing yeast RNA (Mitchell et al., 1967). Sliding may be observed on low nutrient media (Oyaizu et al., 1982). The color of the colonies varies from gray and pale yellow to lemon-yellow and yellow-orange. The cells tend to be less pigmented at higher temperatures (30°C) than at lower temperatures (21°C). With the addition of KOH the color becomes slightly deeper, but with the addition of HCl the effect is reversed; which is not the typical flexirubin reaction.

Peptones, casamino acids, asparagine, urea and NH₄⁺ serve as N source; glutamate and NO₃⁻ do not. This organism grows on peptone alone. NH₃ is released from peptone. It also grows on mineral media (NH₄⁺) with arabinose, xylose, glucose, fructose, maltose, sucrose, cellobiose, raffinose or heparin, but it does not grow with ribose, inulin, pectin, cellulose, CMC, chitin, agar or alginate. Acid is produced from arabinose, glucose, galactose, fructose, maltose, cellobiose, trehalose, glycerol and mannitol but not from ribose, sorbose, rhamnose, raffinose, salicin and ethanol. Filter paper, CMC, pectin, chitin, agar, gelatin and autoclaved yeast cells are not attacked. This organism grows on heparin as the source of nitrogen, carbon, sulfur and energy. Heparin is degraded by inducible enzymes (Payza and Korn, 1956). Growth on heparin is inhibited by agar (Payza, 1956). Good growth occurs on nutrient agar. Sheep erythrocytes are hemolyzed; Tweens are degraded. No NO₂⁻ from NO₃⁻. Urease- and idole-negative, phosphatase-positive. Resistant to chloramphenicol, dihydrostreptomycin and penicillin; sensitive to polymyxin B and actinomycin D.

Strict aerobe. Nitrate respiration is negative; fumarate does not stimulate anaerobic growth. Catalase-positive; the oxidase reaction is weak. Temperature range: 5–30°C; optimum: 20–25°C; no growth is obtained at 0 and 37°C. Tolerates 3% but not 5% NaCl. Isolated from soil. Only one strain known.

The mol% G + C of the DNA is 42 (Bd) (unpublished observation) and 45 *(Tₘ)* (Perry, 1973; Callies and Mannheim, 1980); the genome size is 2.23 × 10⁹ daltons.

Type strain: ATCC 12125 (NCIB 9290).

The original description is so meager that it is almost nonexistent. Unfortunately the data supplied by later authors are not always in agreement (Mitchell et al., 1967; Callies and Mannheim, 1980; Christensen, 1980; Oyaizu and Komagata, 1981; Oyaizu et al., 1982). Thus the mol% G + C of the DNA for the type strain vary between 40 (Oyaizu and Komagata, 1981), 42 (Mitchell et al., 1967) and 45–46 (see above). My colleagues and I have recently determined a mol% G + C of the DNA of 42 (Bd). Controversial results are further given for: starch and esculin hydrolysis; H₂S production; DNase reaction; fermentative attack on glucose; acid production from xylose, lactose and sucrose; and growth at 37°C.

It was proposed to transfer this species to the genus *Cytophaga* (Christensen, 1980). For the following reasons this appears, however, not to be justified. The organism contains MK-7 as respiratory quinone, while the cytophagas seem always to contain MK-6 (Oyaizu and Komagata, 1981). DNA/rRNA hybridization demonstrates that *F. heparinum* is, at best, a border case of the *Cytophaga-Flavobacterium* complex (Bauwens and De Ley, 1981). The 16S rRNA catalog shows that the organism is not closely related to the cytophagas, although it clearly

---

‡*VP* denotes that this name, although not on the Approved Lists of Bacterial Names (1980), has been validly published in the official publication, *International Journal of Systematic Bacteriology.*

belongs into the large *Cytophaga* supergroup and is relatively close to the new genus, "*Taxeobacter*," strain Myx 2105 (Paster et al., 1985). Also, a phenotype analysis seems to indicate that there is no direct connection to *Cytophaga* (Oyaizu and Komagata, 1981). Why there should be a high DNA homology (24%) with *C. hutchinsonii* remains to be explained (Callies and Mannheim, 1980). Another open consideration is whether it is justified to lump *F. ferrugineum* and *F. sewanense* with the species *F. heparinum* (Oyaizu et al., 1982). In any case, the molecular data cited above clearly suggest that *F. heparinum* represents a species of its own, belonging to a genus other than *Cytophaga*.

c. **Cytophaga arvensicola** Oyaizu, Komagata, Amemura and Harada 1983, 438.[VP] (Effective publication: Oyaizu et al. 1982, 385.)

ar.ven.si′co.la. L. adj. *arvensis* belonging to, living in the fields; L. n. *incola* inhabitant; M.L. fem. adj. *arvensicola* dwelling in the fields.

Relatively stout to slender rods, 0.4 × 0.6-2.0 (−4.0) μm. The type strain did not show motility under any condition, but with five of nine isolates, sliding or gliding was observed, preferentially on rich media at 30°C. Also, segregants exhibiting spreading growth appeared in two isolates. Cell mass is yellow-orange; flexirubin reaction is positive.

Peptones and NH_4^+ serve as N source. This organism grows on peptone alone. All strains grew in mineral media (NH_4^+) with xylose, arabinose, glucose, fructose, cellobiose, maltose, sucrose, raffinose or succinoglycan. Starch, cellulose, heparin, chitin, agar and alginate were not suitable; with ribose, pectin, CMC and inulin, results were variable with different strains. Acid is produced from various sugars under aerobic but not anaerobic conditions. H_2S, indole, urease and nitrate respiration-negative. Tweens are not hydrolyzed. DNase and esculin hydrolysis-positive. The type strain reduces NO_3^- to NO_2^- and does not attack gelatin and starch, but these characteristics vary with different strains. All strains degrade succinoglycan, a polysaccharide produced by *Rhizobium* and *Agrobacterium* species.

Strict aerobe. Catalase- and oxidase-positive. All strains grow at 37°C; many also grow at 5°C; none grow at 42°C. Tolerates 1% but not 5% NaCl.

Isolated from soil and the rhizosphere of cucumber roots in Japan. Appears to be a major member of the rhizosphere.

The mol% G + C of the DNA is 47 (Bd) (unpublished observation) and 46 (T_m) with a range of 43-46 for nine isolates.

Type strain: IAM 12650 (DSM 3695, M64; Oyaizu et al, 1982). This species contains MK-7 as respiratory quinone, as does *C. heparina*, which it also resembles in other respects (Oyaizu et al., 1982). *C. arvensicola* differs from *C. heparina* in its positive flexirubin reaction, in the exceptionally high share (20-34%) of the $\triangle^{11}C_{16:1}$ species in its fatty acid spectrum, in its failure to hydrolyze Tweens and in its ability to decompose succinoglycan. There also is a difference in the mol% G + C of 5, although the absolute figures appear to be slightly higher than those stated originally (viz. 45 vs. 40). What has been said about the phylogenetic relationship of *C. heparina* may apply also to this species.

d. **"Promyxobacterium flavum"** Imshenetski and Solntseva 1945, 224.

fla′vum. L. neut. adj. *flavum* golden yellow.

Cell populations tend to be pleomorphic, from short stout, often almost coccoid rods, 0.6-0.7 × 1.0-2.5 μm, to slender flexible rods, 0.4-0.5 × 2.5-6.0 μm, with rounded or slightly tapering ends (Fig. 23.19). In older cultures the stout form may prevail. All cell types are growing and dividing. Gliding.

Colonies either compact, somewhat slimy, soft, with a lobed edge and a more or less spreading margin, bright to golden yellow; or, on lean media such as VY/2 agar, large, filmlike, spreading swarms, yellow, often with a greenish iridescence. Variants with a dry, folded surface may occur. The cell mass turns purple or pinkish brown with the addition of 20% KOH and turns bright yellow again with the addition of HCl.

According to the original species description, proteins, peptones, alanine, asparagine, tyrosine, urea, NH_4^+ and NO_3^- are good N sources; much less so are lysine and NO_2^-; glycine and cysteine do not serve as N

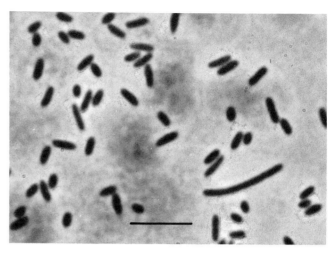

Figure 23.19. "*Promyxobacterium flavum*," type strain. Cells from yeast (VY/2) agar, grown for 4 days at 30°C. Phase contrast. *Bar*, 5 μm.

source. Xylose, glucose, galactose, fructose, maltose, starch, dextrin, glycogen and acetate are utilized as C source; very weakly so are arabinose, lactose and inulin; sucrose, raffinose, cellulose, glycerol, mannitol and dulcitol do not serve as C source at all. Gelatin is liquefied, NH_3 is produced, and H_2S is weakly positive. This organism is indole-negative.

Although most of these characteristics have not yet been verified for the neotype strain, observations of Vozniakovskaya and Rybakova (1969) and of my own indicate that proteins, peptones and NO_3^- may serve as sole N source, and glucose may serve as the carbon and energy source. Acid may be produced from glucose. Gelatin, proteins (e.g. single-cell protein), starch, hemicellulose and pectin are degraded, chitin and cellulose are not. Autoclaved yeast cells are slowly decomposed. No growth is obtained on media with full-strength seawater.

Strict aerobe. The neotype strain is catalase-negative but shows a weakly positive oxidase reaction. Good growth at 30°C.

Isolated from soil in Russia.

The mol% G + C of the DNA is 33 (Bd) (unpublished observation).

Neotype strain: YKM B-1553 (All-Union Collection of Microorganisms, Moscow (DSM 3577)).

The original strains of Imshenetski and Solntseva are lost. A strain labeled "*Promyxobacterium flavum*," available at the All-Union Collection of Microorganisms of the U.S.S.R., has been isolated by Vozniakovskaya and Rybakova (1969; strain no. 19) from the rhizosphere of a tomato plant in Russia. The strain was identified by the authors on the basis of published data after a rather scant biochemical study. To decide whether the strain really represents the original species, however, is not possible. Although Imshenetski and Solntseva mention that the new species uses NO_3^- and NH_4^+ as a N source, Vozniakovskaya and Rybakova state that strain no. 19 does not grow on a mineral medium with NH_4NO_3 and glucose. However, I observed reasonable growth over several transfers on a mineral agar with KNO_3 and glucose. As there is no obvious contradiction to the original species description, the strain may be accepted as a neotype. The morphological description given above rests on the neotype strain. There is, however, full agreement with the original species description, except that the cells were stated to be slightly fatter.

The organism is probably a member of the *Cytophaga* group, but its exact taxonomic position remains to be determined. Its most remarkable feature is its pleomorphism.

e. **"Cytophaga xantha"** Inoue and Komagata 1976, 169.

xan′tha. Gr. adj. *xanthos* yellow; M.L. fem. adj. *xantha* yellow.

Short rods with rounded ends, 0.4-0.5 × 1-2 μm; in older cultures, elongated and threadlike forms often occur. Neither flagellated nor gliding.

Colonies on peptone agar are compact, circular, convex, with an entire edge, and bright yellow to orange-yellow; no color change is exhibited with the addition of KOH.

Peptones and NO_3^- serve as N source. This organism grows on peptone alone. NH_3 is released from peptone. Acid is produced aerobically from xylose, glucose, sucrose and maltose but not from arabinose, galactose, lactose and glycerol. Formate, acetate, lactate and hippurate are assimilated; succinate, fumarate, citrate, propionate, protocatechuate and p-hydroxybenzoate are not. Starch is degraded; cellulose and hemicellulose are not. Gelatin is liquefied. Autoclaved yeast cells are attacked but not completely decomposed. NO_3^- is not reduced to NO_2^-. Indole-negative, H_2S-positive.

Strict aerobe. Catalase- and oxidase-positive. Optimum temperature: 15–20°C; maximum: 25°C; minimum: below 0°C. The organism grows well on full-strength seawater media, but no growth is obtained in peptone-glucose broth with 3% NaCl.

Isolated from soil in Antarctica.

The mol% G + C of the DNA is 39 (T_m).

Type strain: NCMB 2069 (IAM 12026; 5-0-c; Inoue and Komagata).

The organism was classified as a *Cytophaga* because of the peculiar surface structure of its cells and its yellow pigmentation, in spite of the absence of gliding motility. Under the present concept it would better be classified as a *Flavobacterium*. But even this rests on a weak basis before more is known about the organism, e.g. its quinone and fatty acid pattern.

f. **"Cytophaga allerginae"** Liebert, Hood, Deck, Bishop and Flaherty 1984, 936.

al.ler.gi'nae. Gr. n. *allos* stranger, someone else; Gr. n. *ergon* work, act, deed; M.L. gen. fem. n. *allerginae* connected with, causing an allergy.

Slender flexible rods with rounded ends, 0.3 × 3–5 μm in young cultures, up to 9 μm in older ones, gliding.

Colonies spreading, edge with fingerlike projections; bright yellow; flexirubin test is positive.

Good growth is obtained on peptone-containing media. Acid is produced aerobically from arabinose, glucose, maltose and cellobiose but not from sucrose and lactose, although β-galactosidase was positive. Glucose is not fermented. Gelatin, casein, starch, CMC and chitin are degraded; cellulose alginate and agar are not. Phenylalanine, deaminase, arginine dihydrolase, lysine and ornithine decarboxylase, DNase, urease and lecithinase are lacking. Indole, H_2S and NO_3^- reduction-negative. Resistant to ampicillin, penicillin, cephalotin, polymyxin B, bacitracin and the aminoglycosides; sensitive to carbenicillin, chloramphenicol and tetracycline.

Appears to be essentially an aerobe, although it is stated that some growth takes place anaerobically on peptone-glucose-NO_3^- media, which is somewhat astonishing as neither glucose is fermented nor nitrate is reduced. Catalase- and oxidase-positive. Temperature range: 10–30°C; no growth occurs at 4 and 37°C. pH range: 5.5–9.5. Tolerates 1.5% but not 3% NaCl.

Isolated from the water of an air-cooling system in the U.S.

The mol% G + C of the DNA is 35 (T_m).

Type strain: ATCC 35408 (WF-164; Liebert et al., 1984).

The organism was isolated as the causative agent for an allergenic

pneumonitis in a textile plant (Flaherty et al., 1984a, b). Its DNA shows high homology (78%) to that of *C. aquatilis*. Although this value cannot be fully appreciated because comparative hybridizations with representatives of other species are not supplied, it still could indicate a close, perhaps intraspecific relationship. For this reason the species is listed for the time being as of uncertain position. In the composition of its LPS the organism is more or less identical with other CLB but is clearly distinguished from *Flavobacterium breve* and *F. meningosepticum:* the latter contrast in having a much higher share of the ribose and no heptose.

Addendum

A few names brought into connection with the genus *Cytophaga* need a brief comment.

a. *"Cytophaga succinogenes":* obviously erroneously for *C. succinicans* (Ko et al., 1977).

b. *"Cytophaga ureae"* Thayer, strain ATCC 29474 (WTHC 2421; Chang and Thayer, 1975, 1977), a cellulose-degrading soil organism "resembling *C. johnsonae.*" A formal description is not available.

c. *"Flexibacter sancti"* Lewin 1969, 199. See under *"Flexibacter,"* "Species Incertae Sedis."

d. *Flavobacterium aquatile* Bergey et al. 1923, 100.[AL] The neotype strain of the genus *Flavobacterium* (strain Taylor F36; ATCC 11947) has been shown to swarm at 15°C and to glide (Mitchell et al., 1967; Perry, 1973) and would thus have to be regarded as a *Cytophaga* species. Indeed, DNA/rRNA hybridization indicates that it is relatively close to *C. johnsonae* (Bauwens and De Ley, 1981), and a comparison of 16S RNA catalogs shows that it belongs in the core of the *Cytophaga* complex. Both techniques also show that *F. aquatile* is quite distant from other bona fide *Flavobacterium* species, e.g. *F. breve.* The taxonomic implications of this situation are to be resolved in connection with the revision of the *Cytophaga* complex.

e. *"Flavobacterium keratolyticum"* Kitamikado and Ito. Reclassified as *"Cytophaga keratolytica"* (Imai, K. 1985. IFO Res. Commun. *12:* 120–121). The organism does not glide and has MK-7 as respiratory quinone and a mol% G + C of the DNA of 40.

f. *"Cytophaga caryophila"* Preer, Preer and Jurand 1974, 156 (Bacteriol. Rev. *38:* 113–163). The alpha symbiont of *Paramecium aurelia*, was transferred to the genus *Holospora* (Preer, J.R. and L.B. Preer. 1982. Int. J. Syst. Bacteriol. *32:* 140–141).

g. *"Cytophaga anitrata,"* proposed for *Bacterium anitratum* Schaub and Hauber 1948 (Lautrop, H. 1961. Int. Bull. Bacteriol. Nomencl. Taxon. *11:* 107–108), now *Acinetobacter calcoaceticus.*

h. *"Cytophaga lwoffi,"* proposed for *"Moraxella lwoffi"* Audureau 1940 (Lautrop, H., 1961. Int. Bull. Bacteriol. Nomencl. Taxon. *11:* 107–108), now *Acinetobacter lwoffii.*

Genus II. **Capnocytophaga** *Leadbetter, Holt and Socransky 1982, 266*[VP] *(Effective publication: Leadbetter, Holt and Socransky 1979, 13)*

S. C. HOLT AND S. A. KINDER

Cap' no. cy. to' pha. ga. Gr. n. *capnos* smoke; Gr. n. *cytos* hollow vessel or cell; Gr. v. *phagein* to eat; M.L. n. *Cytophaga* eater, digester; M.L. n. *Capnocytophaga* eater in carbon dioxide.

Short to elongate flexible rods or filaments, 0.42–0.6 μm in diameter and 2.5–5.7 μm in length. Ends of **cells usually round to tapered.** Cells can be pleomorphic. Capsules and sheaths not formed. Resting stages not known. No flagella; **motile by gliding.** Gram-negative.

Facultative anaerobic. Growth occurs in air **with 5% CO_2.** Optimum temperature: 35–37°C. Some strains are reported to grow aero-

bically without CO_2. **Primary isolation** and initial in-vitro growth **require CO_2.**

Chemoorganotrophic, with **fermentative** type **metabolism.** This organism utilizes variable carbohydrates as fermentable substrates and energy source. Fermentation of glucose yields chiefly **acetate and succinate** as **major acidic end products**; trace amounts of isovalerate.

Polysaccharides such as dextran, glycogen, inulin, or starch **may be fermented**. Catalase- and oxidase-negative, *o*-nitrophenyl-β-D-galactoside (ONPG), and benzidine-positive.

Found in association with animal and human hosts. Although the pathogenicity of these organisms is unknown, they are **frequent isolates from oral sites** and are also recovered from pulmonary lesions and abscesses, as well as from healthy oral and nonoral sites in their hosts.

The mol% G + C of the DNA of the strains is 33–41 (T_m).

Type species: *Capnocytophaga ochracea* Leadbetter, Holt and Socransky 1982, 266.

Further Descriptive Information

Capnocytophaga ochracea, C. gingivalis and *C. sputigena* are members of the class *Flexibacteriae*, characterized by gliding motility on solid surfaces (Fig. 23.20). They are members of the family *Cytophagaceae*.

Cells can be single, short or elongate flexible rods (Fig. 23.21); long filaments and pleomorphic cells have also been observed when these organisms have been grown in liquid. In liquid culture, cells also grow in characteristic tight masses (Fig. 23.21*E*). When grown on Trypticase soy agar containing 5% (v/v) sheep's blood (TS-blood agar), prepared by Baltimore Biological Laboratories (BBL), cells formed flat, thin colonies (Figs. 23.20 and 23.22) which, when viewed by oblique illumination, had uneven edges which could form fingerlike projections, characteristic of gliding motility (Fig. 23.22). Gliding motility is consistent with the strains of the genus being actinomycin D-sensitive (Dworkin, 1969). Laboratory-prepared TS-blood agar did not reproducibly support this typical spreading or gliding motility; hence, spreading is medium-dependent. Macroscopically, colonies (after incubation for 24 h at 35–37°C) were very small to pinpoint; between 48 and 96 h the colonies were convex and 2–4 mm in diameter. Some colonies appear to pit the agar, and they are all nonhemolytic (Fig. 23.23). Blood was not required for cell growth or gliding motility; the harder the agar surface, the more characteristic the cell spreading or gliding motility. (See Leadbetter et al. (1979) for a discussion of the effects of medium and agar concentration on gliding motility.) Cultures have a characteristic sour, bitter almond odor.

The salient staining, growth and genetic characteristics and the salient physiological characteristics of the genus *Capnocytophaga* are listed in Tables 23.3 and 23.4, respectively. Pigmentation of colonies on an agar surface varied from white-gray to pink and orange-yellow. However, when these were centrifuged into pellets, all strains were yellow to orange. Benzidine-positive pigmentation was not inhibited by the carotenoid inhibitor diphenylamine. The three type species contained menaquinones (vitamin K_2) as their sole respiratory quinones.

A detailed study of the fine structure of the genus *Capnocytophaga* was carried out by Holt et al. (1979C) and Poirier et al. (1979). The typical fine structural appearance of *Capnocytophaga* species is shown in Fig. 23.24. The cell envelope is typical of Gram-negative bacteria. The outer membrane has a tendency to slough material from its surface (Fig. 23.25), also typical of Gram-negative microorganisms. When cells are removed from agar surfaces and prepared for electron microscopy, they are held together by an extracellular material (Fig. 23.26), with the external most layer of *Capnocytophaga* species staining positively with ruthenium red (Fig. 23.27). Cell division resembles that seen in other Gram-negative bacteria, characterized by a constriction of the central region of the cell.

There have been several studies reported on several enzymes of *Capnocytophaga* (see Table 23.5; and Laughon et al., 1982; Nakamura and Slots, 1981; Poirier and Holt, 1983a–c; Lillich and Calmes, 1979; and Takeshita et al., 1983). *Capnocytophaga* species displayed significant aminopeptidase activity, exhibiting leucine, valine and cystine aminopeptidases by the API ZYM system (Analytab Products, Plainview, N.Y.) (Laughon et al., 1982; Slots, 1981), as well as being positive for α-glucosidase. Although the API ZYM pattern was distinct for the aminopeptidases, the *Capnocytophaga* species varied enough in the other enzymatic reactions tested to make these chromogenic assays of only limited value for correlating API ZYM reactions with key phenoty-

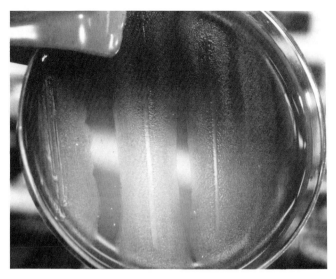

Figure 23.20. *Capnocytophaga* strain grown on blood agar plate and photographed by oblique illumination. Cells spread from a central streak line in opposite directions. (Courtesy of M. Newman, University of California School of Dentistry, Los Angeles.)

pic characteristics. *Capnocytophaga ochracea* possessed high levels of phosphoenolpyruvate carboxykinase, which is the only CO_2 (HCO_3)⁻-fixing enzyme in the genus (Kapke et al., 1980). Cell-free extracts of *C. ochracea* also contained a NAD-specific glutamate dehydrogenase, as well as high levels of acid and alkaline phosphatase. Detectable levels of the malic enzyme, pyruvic acid carboxylase, phosphoenolpyruvate (PEP) carboxylase, or PEP carboxytransphosphorylase were not observed. Glucose is transported into *C. ochracea* by a PEP/phosphotransferase system, and the glucose was catabolized to PVA by the Embden-Meyerhof-Parnas Pathway (Lillich and Calmes, 1979). Although key enzymes of the Entner-Doudoroff, hexose phosphoketolase or Warburg-Dickens pathways have not been found, definitive proof of their absence from *Capnocytophaga* will require the tracing of the distribution of specifically labeled glucose carbons to their specific end products.

Information has been published on the chemical composition of the lipopolysaccharide of *Capnocytophaga* after phenol/water and butanol/water preparative procedures, as well as the biological activity of these molecules (Poirier et al., 1983c). The lipid chemistry of the genus has also been reported (Holt et al., 1979a, b; Dees et al., 1982). Cellular fatty acid analysis of the strains of *Capnocytophaga* revealed the predominant fatty acids to be saturated, *iso*-branched chain, 15-carbon, 13-methyltetradecanoate, and a saturated, *iso*-branched chain, 3-hydroxy-13-methyl-3-hydroxytetradecanoate. Small amounts of a 15-methyl-3-hydroxyhexadecanoate were also found. The major phospholipid was phosphatidylethanolamine and an ornithine-amino lipid, as well as lesser amounts of lysophosphatidylethanolamine. *Capnocytophaga* species also contained the unique sulfonolipid, 1-deoxy-15-methylhexadecasphingamine-1-sulfonic acid or *capnine* (Godchaux and Leadbetter, 1980).

In-vitro agar dilution testing of *Capnocytophaga* species to a variety of antimicrobial agents (Sutter et al., 1981; Forlenza et al., 1981) has been reported (Tables 23.6 and 23.7). Essentially all isolates were sensitive at a minimum inhibitory concentration (MIC_{90}) of at least 1 μg/ml for penicillin, ampicillin, carbenicillin, erythromycin, clindamycin and tetracycline. Doses of tetracycline, metronidazole, cefoxitin and chloramphenicol of between 1 and 3.12 μg/ml were effective bacteriocidal agents, killing 90% of the examined strains. For *Capnocytophaga* strains, the MIC_{90} was only 25 and 50 μg/ml, respectively, for cephalothin and cefazolin, while the MIC_{90} was 3.12 μg/ml for cefamandole. The aminoglycoside antibiotics (i.e. streptomycin, kanamycin, gentamicin,

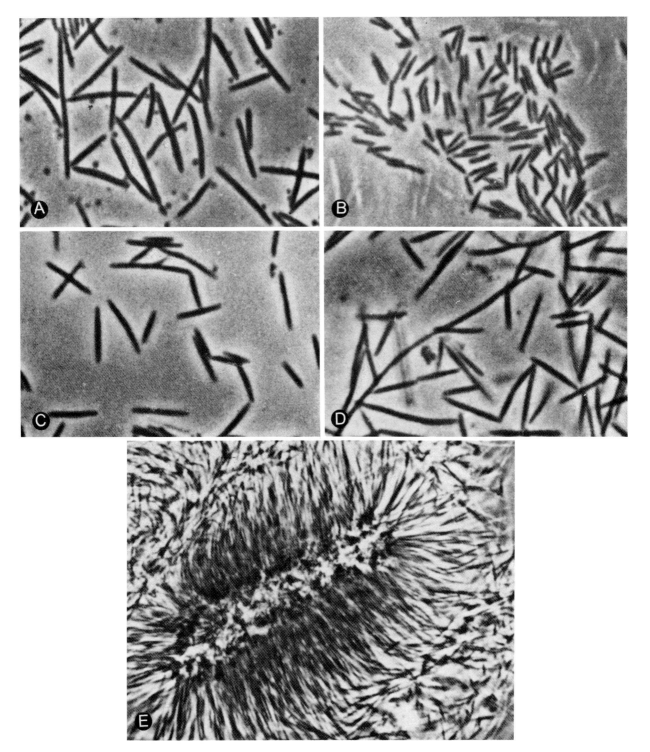

Figure 23.21. Phase-contrast photomicrographs of representative strains of *Capnocytophaga* species. Strains *A–D* were grown on Trypticase soy agar + 5% sheep's blood; *E* was grown in Trypticase soy broth. *A, C. sputigena* strain 4 (ATCC 33612). *B, C. ochracea* strain 25 (ATCC 33596). *C, C. gingivalis* strain 27 (ATCC 33624). *D* and *E*, *Capnocytophaga* strain 60-38.1 grown on liquid and on plate, respectively. (Reproduced with permission from S. C. Holt, E. R. Leadbetter and S. S. Socransky, Archives of Microbiology. *122:* 17–27, 1979, ©Springer-Verlag, Berlin.)

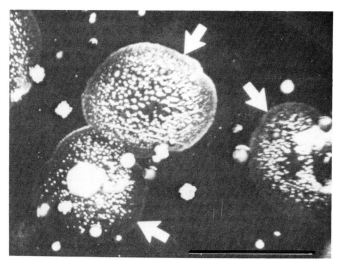

Figure 23.22. Diluted sample of subgingival plaque after 48 h of growth on TS-blood agar prepared by BBL. *Arrows, Capnocytophaga* species displaying characteristic gliding morphology. *Bar*, 1 cm. (Reproduced with permission from M. G. Newman, V. L. Sutter, M. J. Pickett, U. Blachman, J. R. Greenwood, V. Grinenko and D. Citron, Journal of Clinical Microbiology. *10:* 557–562, 1979, ©American Society for Microbiology, Washington, D.C.)

Table 23.3.
Salient characteristics of **Capnocytophaga** *spp.*

Characteristic	Reaction
Gram reaction	−
Benzidine reaction	+
Colony pigmentation (yellow-orange)	+
Bitter almond odor	+
Surface translocation; gliding motility	+
Fusiform to rod-shaped cells	+
CO_2 required for initial growth	+
Growth at 35–37°C on	
Blood agar	+
In air	−[a]
Air + 5% CO_2	+
7.5% H_2 + 80% N_2	+
80% N_2 + 10% H_2 + 10 CO_2	+
Thayer-Martin agar	+
Chocolate agar	+
Blood agar + 50 µg/ml	
Bacitracin + 100 µg/ml	+
Polymyxin B	
MacConkey agar	−
Actinomycin D inhibition	+[b]
Mol% G + C of DNA (T_m)	34–40

[a] Some strains are positive after initial cultivation.

[b] Some strains are resistant.

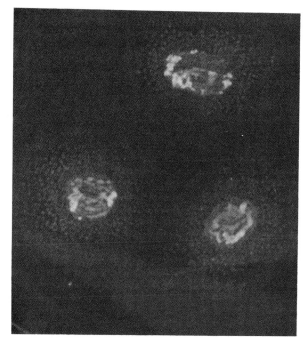

Figure 23.23. *Capnocytophaga* strain grown on blood agar plate. Colonies are flat, with concentrically spreading growth from a central point of inoculation. × 3.5. (Reproduced with permission from R. E. Weaver, D. G. Hollis and E. J. Bottone. 1985. Gram-negative fermentative bacteria and *Francisella tularensis*. *In* Lennette, Balows, Hausler and Shadomy (Editors), Manual of Clinical Microbiology, 4th Ed. American Society for Microbiology, Washington, D.C.)

Table 23.4.
Salient physiological characteristics of **Capnocytophaga** *spp.[a, b]*

Characteristic	Reaction
Oxidase	−
Catalase	−
Indole	−
Nitrate reduction (NO_3 to NO_2)	D
Acid from	
Glucose	+
Lactose	+
Maltose	+
Mannitol	−
Mannose	+
Sucrose	+
Xylose	−
Acid end products	
Acetic	Trace
Succinic	Major
Propionic	Trace
Hydrolysis of	
Esculin	+
Starch	D[c]
Dextran	D[c]
Gelatin	D[d]

[a] Data are from Socransky et al. (1979); see this reference for additional characteristics.

[b] Symbols: −, 90% or more of strains are negative; D, different reactions in different taxa; +, 90% or more of strains are positive.

[c] Only hydrolyzed by *C. ochracea*

[d] Only hydrolyzed by *C. sputigena*

Figure 23.24. Thin section of *C. ochracea* strain 25 (ATCC 33596). The outer membrane encloses a periplasmic space, with the cytoplasmic membrane limiting the electron-opaque ribosomes in the cytoplasmic region. The peptidoglycan is closely adherent to the outer aspect of the cytoplasmic membrane. An electron-opaque "fuzz" covers the surface of the outer membrane. Stained with uranyl acetate-lead citrate. *Bar*, 0.25 µm.

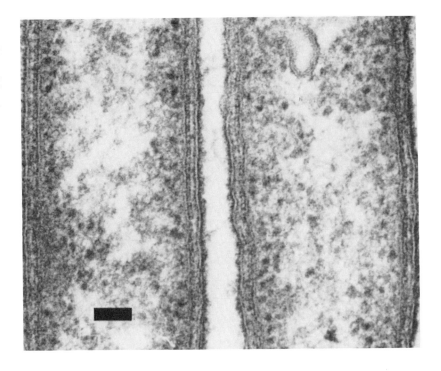

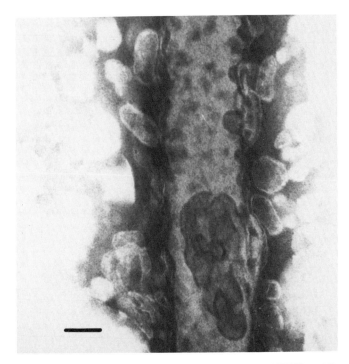

Figure 23.25. Negative-stained *C. ochracea* strain 25 (ATCC 33596). Numerous outer membrane fragments were in the process of being removed from the cell surface. A large mesosome is apparent. Negative stain, (NH₄)MoO₄, at pH 7.2. *Bar*, 0.5 µm.

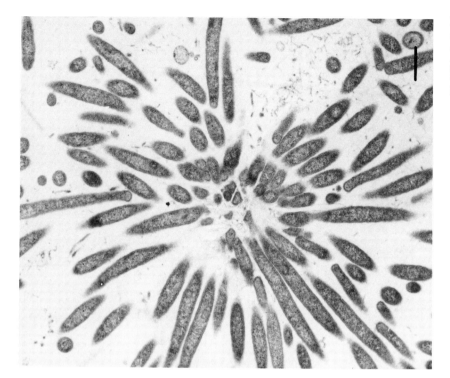

Figure 23.26. Thin section of *C. sputigena* strain 4 (ATCC 33612). Cells were grown on BBL TS-blood agar, at 37°C for 48 h. Agar square was cut from the plate and fixed in glutaraldehyde-osmium tetroxide by standard techniques. The cells were thin-sectioned parallel to the cell-covered agar surface. *Bar*, 2.5 μm.

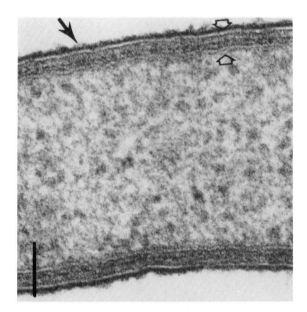

Figure 23.27. Thin section of ruthenium red-fixed *C. ochracea* strain 25 (ATCC 33596). The ruthenium red has stained the extracellular polysaccharide (*arrow*). The large periplasmic space (*open arrows*) encloses the outer membrane, the electron-opaque periplasm and the inner cytoplasmic membrane. *Bar*, 0.25 μm.

Table 23.5.
Enzymatic activities of human oral **Capnocytophaga** *strains[a, b]*

Enzyme	C. gingivalis	C. ochracea	C. sputigena
C_4 esterase	1	1	1
C_8 esterase lipase	1	2	2
C_{14} lipase	0,1	1	0,1
Leucine aminopeptidase	2	2	2
Valine aminopeptidase	2	2	2
Cystine aminopeptidase	2	2	2
Trypsin	0	0,1	0,1
Chymotrypsin	0,1	1	1
Acid phosphatase	2	2	2
Alkaline phosphatase	2	2	2
Phosphoamidase	1	1	1
α-Galactosidase	0	0	0
β-Galactosidase	1	1	1
β-Glucuronidase	0	0	0
α-Glucosidase	2	2	2
β-Glucosidase	1	1	1
N-Acetyl-β-glucosaminidase	0	1	1
α-Mannosidase	0	0	0
α-Fucosidase	0	0	0
ONPG	0	2	2

[a] Data have been modified from Kristiansen et al. (1984) and Laughon et al. (1982).

[b] Numbers indicate color intensities of chromogenic reactions: 1, weak activity; 2, strong activity; 0,1, no activity to weak activity; and 0, no activity.

Table 23.6.

Antimicrobial susceptibility of **Capnocytophaga** *strains[a]*

Antimicrobial agent	MIC[b] (µg/ml)			MBC[c] (µg/ml)		
	Range	For % of strains		Range	For % of strains	
		50	90		50	90
Penicillin	< 0.20– 0.39	< 0.20	< 0.20	< 0.20– 0.78	< 0.20	0.20
Ampicillin	< 0.20– 0.39	< 0.20	< 0.20	< 0.20– 0.78	< 0.20	0.39
Oxacillin	0.78– 25.00	6.25	25.00	6.25– 25.00	25.00	25.00
Carbenicillin	< 0.50– 2.00	0.50	< 0.50	< 0.50– 2.00	< 0.50	1.00
Cephalothin	1.56–>50.00	12.50	25.00	3.12–>50.00	12.50	50.00
Cefazolin	0.78–>50.00	6.25	50.00	3.12–>50.00	12.50	>50.00
Cefamandole	< 0.20– 25.00	0.78	3.12	0.78–>50.00	3.12	50.00
Cefoxitin	< 0.20– 6.25	0.39	1.56	< 0.20– 6.25	0.78	3.12
Erythromycin	< 0.20– 50.00	< 0.20	0.78	< 0.20– 50.00	< 0.20	0.78
Tetracycline	< 0.20– 1.56	< 0.20	0.78	< 0.20– 1.56	0.20	1.56
Chloramphenicol	< 0.20– 6.25	0.39	6.25	0.78– 12.50	6.25	6.25
Clindamycin	< 0.20– 0.39	< 0.20	< 0.20	< 0.20– 0.39	0.20	< 0.20
Metronidazole	< 0.25– 8.00	< 0.25	2.00	< 0.25–> 8.00	0.50	2.00
Vancomycin	< 0.20– 50.00	< 3.12	25.00	12.50–>50.00	50.00	50.00
Amikacin	12.50–>50.00	<50.00	>50.00	All–>50.00	>50.00	>50.00
Gentamicin	25.00–>50.00	<50.00	>50.00	All–>50.00	>50.00	>50.00
Tobramycin	All–>50.00	<50.00	>50.00	All–>50.00	>50.00	>50.00

[a] Data are from Forlenza et al. (1981). Thirteen isolates were tested.

[b] MIC, lowest antibiotic concentration at which turbidity was visible after 48 h (anaerobic incubation).

[c] MBC, value calculated from plates inoculated with 0.01 ml of broth from each clear MIC tube onto BBL TS-blood agar plates. Designated as lowest antibiotic concentration at which these plates were devoid of bacterial growth after 48 h (anaerobic incubation).

Table 23.7.

Antimicrobial susceptibility of **Capnocytophaga** *strains[a]*

Antimicrobial agent	Range[b]	MIC$_{50}$[c]	MIC$_{90}$[c]
Penicillin G	0.5–2	1	2
Cephalexin	1–128	4	64
Cefaclor	0.5–8	2	8
Cephradine	2–128	4	128
Cefamandole	0.5–64	16	32
Cefoxitin	1–8	2	8
Cefoperazone	0.5–32	8	32
Moxalactam	0.125–8	1	8
Erythromycin	0.125–4	0.5	1
Clindamycin	≤0.062–4	0.062	0.125
Chloramphenicol	2–8	4	8
Metronidazole	2–128	4	16
Tetracycline	0.25–2	0.5	1
Bacitracin	2–16	8	16
Colistin	64–>128	>128	>128
Kanamycin	128–>128	>128	>128
Nalidixic acid	32–>128	>128	>128
Vancomycin	4–128	32	64

[a] Data are from Sutter et al. (1981). Twenty-seven isolates were tested.

[b] Concentrations are in µg/ml, except for penicillin G and bacitracin, which are in units/ml.

[c] MIC$_{50}$ and MIC$_{90}$, minimal concentrations required to inhibit 50 and 90%, respectively, of the tested strains. Units are as described in Footnote b.

neomycin) did not inhibit the growth of the *Capnocytophaga* species tested, even at concentrations of 50 µg/ml.

Immunological analysis of the antigenic components of the *Capnocytophaga* species has revealed the presence of two cell envelope-associated antigens: a *group-specific antigen*, which has been found in all species so far examined, and a *type-specific antigen*, which has been found only in clinical isolates (Murayama et al., 1982; Stevens et al., 1979). An exopolysaccharide has been recovered from the surface of *C. ochracea* strain 25, which upon DEAE-Sepharose CL-SB column purification exhibited immunoregulatory properties (Bolton and Dyer, 1983; Dyer and Bolton, 1985).

The mol% G + C of the DNA for the members of the genus was 34–40 (T_m) (Tables 23.3 and 23.8).

Capnocytophaga species may be found as part of the normal microbiota of humans and primates. They are routinely recovered from periodontal lesions as well as from soft-tissue infections and bacteremias. They are frequently recovered from individuals diagnosed with juvenile periodontitis. The members of the genus are also recovered from a variety of lesions and/or abscesses from compromised hosts. The genus has been isolated from patients with hematological malignancy and profound neutropenia. These patients routinely have oral mucosal ulcerations, which may be the portal of entry of *Capnocytophaga* into the bloodstream. *Capnocytophaga* species have also been recovered from sputum and throat samples, spinal fluid, vagina, cervix, amniotic fluid, trachea and eyes.

Enrichment and Isolation Procedures

The genus can be isolated selectively, by streaking onto Thayer-Martin selective medium or on TS-blood agar containing bacitracin (50 µg/ml) and polymyxin B (100 µg/ml) (see Table 23.3; and Mashimo et al., 1983). *Capnocytophaga* species have also been isolated by standard laboratory procedures employing TS-blood agar-based media (Leadbetter et al., 1979; Forlenza et al., 1980; Gilligan et al., 1981), blood agar or chocolate agar. *Capnocytophaga* species do not grow on MacConkey agar. The plates are incubated 3–5 days at 35–37°C in an anaerobic chamber (5% CO_2 + 10% H_2 + 85% N_2) or in Brewer jars (under 5% CO_2 + 95% air atmosphere). *Capnocytophaga* species grow as a flat, concentrically spreading film from a central colony or point of inoculation (Figs. 23.20, 23.22 and 23.23). Colonies have also been observed to sometimes pit the agar.

The colonies are easily removed from the agar surface, diluted in sterile phosphate-buffered saline or in a reduced transport fluid (Syed and

Table 23.8.

Mol% G + C of the DNA from **Capnocytophaga** *spp.,* **Bacteroides ochraceus,** *and* **CDC group DF-1**[a]

Group	Mol% G + C of DNA (T_m)
Capnocytophaga ochracea	39
C. gingivalis	40
C. sputigena	34
Bacteroides ochraceus	39.6
CDC DF-1	41.4

[a]Data are from Newman et al. (1979) and Williams et al. (1979).

Loesche, 1972), and restreaked to Thayer-Martin or TS-blood agar. Pure isolates can be obtained by employing this procedure.

Maintenance Procedures

Capnocytophaga species can be maintained on TS-blood agar or TS agar. The characteristic spreading morphology is best observed and maintained on BBL TS-blood agar plates or on TS agar (3% w/v agar concentration). After suitable incubation in an anaerobic environment with at least 5% CO_2 or in Brewer jars (5% CO_2 + 95% air), stock cultures can be maintained on agar slants or Petri dish agar surfaces in Brewer jars at room temperature or in the refrigerator. Cultures can also be frozen in liquid nitrogen or freeze-dried by standard bacteriological procedures.

Taxonomic Comments

A comparison of *Capnocytophaga ochracea* ATCC 33596 (strain 25 of Leadbetter et al., 1979) with *Bacteroides ochraceus* (VPI 5567, VPI 5568, VPI 5569), and the Centers for Disease Control (CDC) biogroup DF-1 by DNA homology and phenotypic characteristics (see Tables 23.8 and 23.9; and Williams et al., 1979; and Newman et al., 1979) designates these latter two bacteria as *C. ochracea* (Leadbetter et al., 1979). One DF-1 strain was designated *C. gingivalis* (Williams et al., 1979). The original isolate of Loesche, *Bacteroides oralis* var. *elongatus* (strain SS31), is extant as *B. ochraceus* (originally ATCC 27872). DNA homology (Williams and Hammond, 1979), serological cross-reactivity (Stevens et al., 1979; and B. F. Hammond, personal communication) and phenotypic characteristics (Socransky et al., 1979) have designated *B. oralis* var. *elongatus* as *C. ochracea*.

Further Reading

Calmes, R., G.W. Rambicure, W. Gorman and T.T. Lillich. 1980. Energy metabolism in *Capnocytophaga ochracea*. Infect. Immun. *29*: 551–560.

Table 23.9.

DNA homology in **Capnocytophaga** *spp.,* **Bacteroides ochraceus,** *and* **CDC group DF-1**[a]

	Capnocytophaga			Bacteroides ochraceus (VPI 5567)	CDC DF-1
Characteristic	ochracea	gingivalis	sputigena		
Percent hybridization with DNA from:					
C. ochracea	100	4	22	76–86	14–87
C. gingivalis	14	100	11	6–12	7–12
C. sputigena	23	9	100	15–22	9–23

[a]Data are from Williams et al. (1979).

Collins, M.D., H.N. Shah, A.S. McKee and R.M. Kroppenstedt. 1982. Chemotaxonomy of the genus *Capnocytophaga* (Leadbetter, Holt and Socransky). J. Appl. Bacteriol. *52*: 409–415.

Fung, J.C., M. Berman and T. Fiorentino. 1983. *Capnocytophaga*: a review of the literature. Am. J. Med. Technol. *49*: 589–591.

Hawkey, P.M., H. Malnick, S.A. Glover, N. Cook and J.A. Watts. 1984. *Capnocytophaga ochracea* infection: two cases and a review of the published work. J. Clin. Pathol. *37*: 1066–1070.

Holdeman, L.V., E.P. Cato and W.E. Moore. 1984. Taxonomy of anaerobes: present state of the art. Rev. Infect. Dis. *6*: S3–S10.

Newman, M.G. and T.N. Sims. 1979. The predominant cultivable microbiota of the periodontal abscess. J. Periodontol. *50*: 350–354.

Newman, M.G. and S.S. Socransky. 1977. Predominant cultivable microbiota in periodontosis. J. Period. Res. *12*: 120–128.

Parenti, D.M. and D.R. Snydman. 1985. *Capnocytophaga* species: infections in nonimmunocompromised and immunocompromised hosts. J. Infect. Dis. *151*: 140–147.

Shurin, S.B., S.S. Socransky, E. Sweeney and T.P. Stossel. 1979. A neutrophil disorder induced by *Capnocytophaga*, a dental microorganism. N. Engl. J. Med. *301*: 849–850.

Slots, J. and R.J. Genco. 1984. Black-pigmented *Bacteroides* species, *Capnocytophaga* species, and *Actinobacillus actinomycetemcomitans* in human periodontal disease: virulence factors in colonization, survival, and tissue destruction. J. Dent. Res. *63*: 412–421.

Stevens, R.H., M.N. Sela, J. Shapiro and B.F. Hammond. 1980. Detection of fibroblast proliferation inhibitory factor from *Capnocytophaga sputigena*. Infect. Immun. *27*: 271–275.

Van Palenstein Helderman, W.H. 1981. Microbial etiology of periodontal disease. J. Clin. Periodontol. *8*: 261–280.

Winn, R.E., W.F. Chase, P.W. Lauderdale and F.K. McCleskey. 1984. Septic arthritis involving *Capnocytophaga ochracea*. J. Clin. Microbiol. *19*: 538–540.

List of species of the genus **Capnocytophaga**

The common characteristics of the three species of *Capnocytophaga* are indicated in Tables 23.3 and 23.4. Characteristics which are useful for distinguishing the three species are listed in Tables 23.4 and 23.5.

1. **Capnocytophaga ochracea** Leadbetter, Holt and Socransky 1982, 266.[VP] (Effective publication: Leadbetter, Holt and Socransky 1979, 14.)

o. chra.′ ce. a. Gr. n. *ochra* yellow; M.L. adj. *ochracea* of color of ocher, yellow.

The characteristics are the same as those described for the genus. Macroscopic morphological features are depicted in Figures 23.20, 23.22 and 23.23; phase-contrast microscopic characteristics are seen in Figure 23.21, while electron microscopic characteristics are seen in Figures 23.24–23.27. The majority (92%) of strains of *C. ochracea* produce acid from lactose; a variable number (11–89%) are capable of fermenting galactose with acid production. Only 8% of the strains were capable of reducing nitrate. A majority of strains so far analyzed produce acid from amygdalin, esculin and glycogen, as well as hydrolyze starch and dextran.

The mol% G + C of the DNA of the type strain is 39 (T_m).

Type strain: ATCC 33596 (strain 25 of Leadbetter et al., 1979).

2. **Capnocytophaga gingivalis** Leadbetter, Holt and Socransky 1982, 266.[VP] (Effective publication: Leadbetter, Holt and Socransky 979, 14.)

gin.gi.va′lis. M.L. adj. *gingivalis* of the gum.

The physiological and morphological characteristics are the same as those described for the genus (Tables 23.3 and 23.4). It does not produce acid end products from lactose or galactose; only 8% of the strains of *C. gingivalis* examined reduced nitrate. *C. gingivalis* is physiologically inactive, compared with *C. ochracea*; does not ferment amygdalin, salicin, cellobiose, esculin or glycogen; and did not hydrolyze starch.

The mol% G + C of the DNA of the type strain is 40 (T_m).

Type strain: ATCC 33624 (strain 27 of Leadbetter et al., 1979).

3. **Capnocytophaga sputigena** Leadbetter, Holt and Socransky 1982, 266.[VP] (Effective publication: Leadbetter, Holt and Socransky 1979, 14.)

spu. ti. ge′ na. M.L. fem. adj. *sputigena* sputum-produced.

The physiological and morphological characteristics are the same as those described for the genus (Tables 23.3 and 23.4).

C. sputigena possessed a variable ability to ferment lactose, fructose and dextran. The strains examined were unable to ferment galactose.

Eighty percent of the *C. sputigena* strains examined hydrolyzed esculin; none of the examined strains were capable of utilizing cellobiose, glycogen or starch.

The mol% G + C of the DNA of *C. sputigena* type strain is 34 (T_m).

Type strain: ATCC 33612 (strain 4 of Leadbetter et al., 1979).

Genus III. **Flexithrix** Lewin 1970, 513[AL]

H. REICHENBACH

Flex′i.thrix. L. adj. *flexilis* flexible; Gr. n. *thrix* hair; M.L. fem. n. *Flexithrix*, flexible hair.

Very long nonmotile filaments, multicellular, uniseriate and sheathed; may release, as a second form, flexible gliding cells. Gram-negative. Depending on the culture conditions, the organism may grow alternatively in the one or the other form. For example, liquid cultures in relatively rich media contain exclusively flexible rods which give the suspension a silky appearance when shaken. In such cultures,

the organism may be mistaken for a *Microscilla* or a *Flexibacter*.

Chemoorganotroph with respiratory metabolism. There is only one species with one single strain known, and this is a marine organism with a mol% G + C of the DNA of 37.

Type species: *Flexithrix dorotheae* Lewin 1970, 511.

List of species of the genus **Flexithrix**

1. **Flexithrix dorotheae** Lewin 1970, 511.[AL]

do.ro.the′ae. M.L. gen. fem. n. *dorotheae* of Dorothy; named to commemorate a deceased technical assistant, Dorothy White.

Morphology as described above. The filaments may become more than 500 µ*m* long and are about 1 µm wide. A hyaline sheath may be recognized, either as an empty cuff at the filaments' ends or if the cells have locally separated, in the middle of the filaments. Occasionally, false branching occurs. The sheath appears to consist of a mixture of acid heteropolysaccharide (arabinose, xylose, galactose, mannose, uronic acids) and an unusual poly α-L-glutamine (Kandler et al., 1983). The peptidoglycan is of the mDpm-direct type (A1γ; Kandler et al., 1983).

Gliding cells 5–15 µm long and 0.4–0.6 µm wide, with rounded or slightly tapering ends (Fig. 23.28), may move with considerable speed (1–2 µm/s), usually bending and looping vividly at the same time. Often, thread cells are observed (Fig. 23.29) which are much longer (30–60 µm), lack recognizable cross-walls and a sheath, and may still be very agile. Thread cells may fragment into a series of shorter cells. All free cells are

extremely flexible, and the longer ones are usually bent several times and even tightly coiled, particularly when growing within the agar (Fig. 23.30). Whether or not sheathed filaments appear depends on the medium. In liquid media with a high glucose content and NH_4^+ as the nitrogen source, only free cells are found, while in media with a low glucose content, tangled filaments develop. The ability to form sheaths may be lost completely during prolonged cultivation, for I have not observed sheathed filaments in cultures of type strain ATCC 23163, although very long thread cells were often present in large number.

The shape of the colonies varies with the medium composition and, in particular, with its gel strength. On media of moderate gel strength (1% agar and less), the colonies tend to sink into the substrate, and only shallow pits may remain at the surface. Satellite colonies may arise in the vicinity of large colonies, obviously started by gliding cells released from the filamentous mass. Spreading of the colony is only moderate, however, and typical swarm colonies as with *Cytophaga* do not arise. On media of higher gel strength (1.5–2% agar), the colonies are convex and smooth

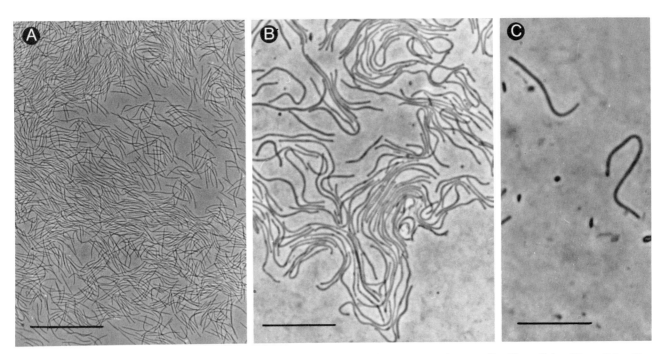

Figure 23.28. *Flexithrix dorotheae* gliding cells from agar cultures. Slide mounts, phase contrast. *A*, survey. *Bar*, 50 µm. *B*, *bar*, 12 µm. *C*, *bar*, 10 µm.

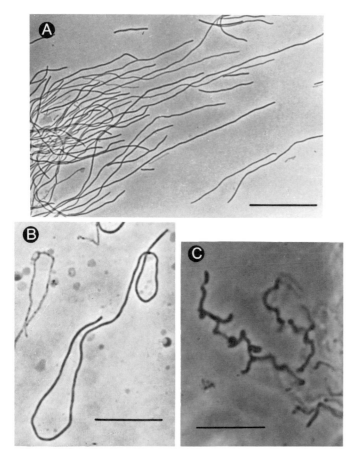

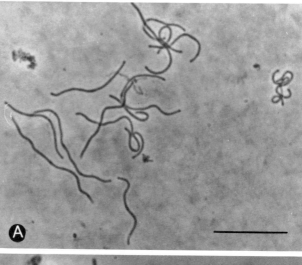

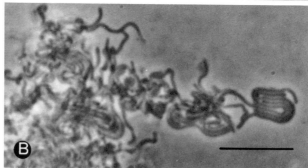

Figure 23.29. *F. dorotheae* thread cells. Phase contrast. *A*, cells from seawater agar with 0.1% sodium glutamate and 0.1% glucose, slide mount. *Bar*, 24 μm. *B*, thread cell at higher magnification. *Bar*, 12 μm. *C*, twisted thread cells within the agar. The "branches" are either narrow lateral loops or different superimposed cells. Organism growing on a thin agar layer in a chamber culture, in situ. *Bar*, 10 μm.

Figure 23.30. *F. dorotheae* coiled cells. Phase contrast. *A*, cells from an agar plate, slide mount. As soon as the cells become released from the agar during the mounting procedure, they tend to stretch themselves out. *Bar*, 12 μm. *B*, organism growing on a thin agar layer in a chamber culture, in situ. *Bar*, 10 μm.

(Fig. 23.31). The edge is usually entire, but flamelike protrusions occasionally do appear. There is little gliding and spreading; the colonies increase only slowly in size and usually remain relatively small. From the base of such surface colonies, some cells always penetrate into the upper layers of the substrate (Fig. 23.32). If there is filamentous growth, the colonies may appear fibrous. When there are long flexible cells, often a fountainlike pattern is observed in the marginal region of the colony, which is caused by a parallel arrangement of wavy thread cells (Fig. 23.33). Local cell patterns are also responsible for a peculiar mottled appearance of the colonies in dark field (Fig. 23.34).

Colonies and cell mass from liquid cultures are intensely golden yellow due to (3R,3'R) zeaxanthin, which may constitute up to 0.08% of the dry mass (Aasen and Liaaen-Jensen, 1966; Aasen et al., 1972). Pigment synthesis is stimulated by light.

Strictly aerobic, apparently using only O_2 as the terminal electron acceptor. Catalase- and oxidase-negative. Glutamate, peptones, ammonium (optimum: 0.02% NH$_4$Cl) and nitrate (optimum: 0.02% NaNO$_3$) are useful nitrogen sources (in that order). Various sugars (e.g., glucose, galactose, sucrose) and glutamate may serve as carbon and energy sources (glutamate at the same time as a nitrogen source). Glycerol and acetate are not utilized. No requirement for organic growth factors. Production of indole, H_2S and NH_3 is negative. No nitrite from nitrate. In litmus milk, no acid production, no coagulation, no reduction of litmus. Gelatin, starch, alginate and cellulose not degraded, but carboxymethyl

cellulose is depolymerized, and agar is attacked (becomes soft around the colony). Obligately marine, tolerating variation of salt concentration between one-half- and double-strength seawater. Simple artificial seawater allows good growth. Grows at temperatures up to at least 35°C, but not at 40°C, and at pH 7-9.

Isolated from marine silt from the coast of Kerala, India, by streaking samples on seawater agar with 0.01% tryptone (Difco), 0.01% yeast extract and 1% agar. Colonies with irregular edges and a rough fibrous appearance were restreaked on seawater agar with successively increasing concentrations of tryptone and yeast extract (first 0.03%, then 0.1% each). Excellent growth was obtained on seawater-peptone media (e.g. 0.5% tryptone, 0.5% yeast extract) or on the following defined medium (FT1 medium): Na-glutamate, 1%; Na-glycerophosphate, 0.01%; Tris(hydroxymethyl)aminomethane, 0.2%; glucose, 0.2% (autoclaved separately); NaCl, 2.4%; MgSO$_4$·7H$_2$O, 0.8%; KCl, 0.07%; CaCl$_2$·2H$_2$O, 0.05%; and trace elements (any standard solution); at pH 8.0, with or without agar (1–1.5%).

Cultures at room temperature die within a few weeks. Frozen in growth medium without additives at −22°C, the organism survives only for 4–5 weeks, but with 10% glycerol added and frozen at -196°C, the organism was still alive after 1 year (Sanfilippo and Lewin, 1970). Cells that were frozen in liquid nitrogen in medium SP5 (casitone (Difco), 0.9%; yeast extract (Difco), 0.1%; NaCl, 2.47%; KCl, 0.07%; MgSO$_4$·7H$_2$O, 0.63%; MgCl$_2$·6H$_2$O, 0.46%; CaCl$_2$·2H$_2$O, 0.12%; and NaHCO$_3$, 0.02%; at pH 7.2,

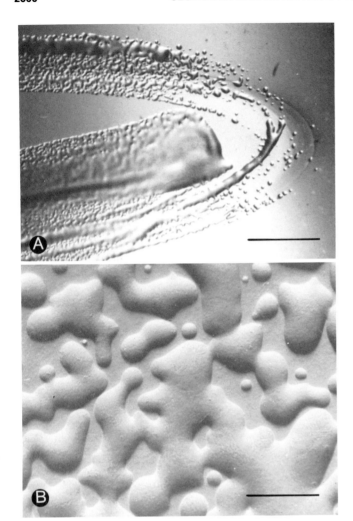

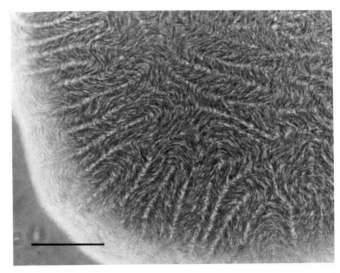

Figure 23.33. *F. dorotheae* surface colony with curly arrangement of the highly flexible cells. After 6 days at room temperature, the organism grows on a thin agar layer in a chamber culture. Phase contrast. *Bar*, 50 μm.

Figure 23.31. *F. dorotheae* surface colonies on medium of high gel strength (1.5% agar). *A*, growth along a streak of the inoculation loop, after 8 days at 30°C. *Bar*, 4 mm. *B*, colonies under oblique illumination, 8 days old. *Bar*, 230 μm.

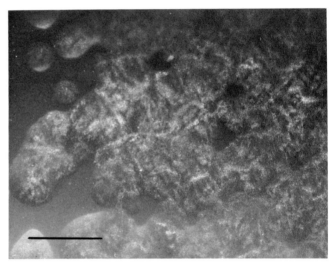

Figure 23.34. *F. dorotheae* surface colonies in dark field, appearing mottled because the cells are locally arranged in an ordered pattern. *Bar*, 230 μm.

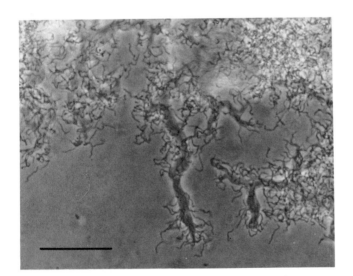

Figure 23.32. *F. dorotheae* cells penetrating into the substrate. The organism grows on a thin film of agar in a chamber culture (2 days old). Starting from flamelike sheets of densely packed bacteria on the surface, many cells invade the agar like rootlets. Phase contrast. *Bar*, 40 μm.

autoclaved), without additives or a special freezing program, my colleagues and I found to be still alive after 6 years. If cells were dried without freezing on lyophilized skim milk and stored at 2°C under an atmosphere of N₂, my colleagues and I could reactivate the organism after 6 years with a moderate survival rate. It also survived long storage periods at −80°C (suspended in medium SP5).

The mol% G + C of the DNA is 37 (Bd) (Mandel and Lewin, 1969).

Type strain: ATCC 23163 (QQ-3 Lewin).

Taxonomic Comments

F. dorotheae has been isolated only once. However, when sheathed filaments are lacking, the organism is said to closely resemble so-called *Microscilla aggregans* which appears to be relatively common in seashore habitats. Also, it seems that organisms with a morphology similar to *F. dorotheae* are not uncommon in soil, but whether they are taxonomically related cannot be decided at the moment.

Genus IV. **Sporocytophaga** Stanier 1940, 629[AL]

E. R. LEADBETTER

Spo.ro.cy.toph'aga. M.L. n. *spora* a spore; M.L. fem. n. *Cytophaga* generic name; M.L. fem. n. *Sporocytophaga* sporing *Cytophaga*.

Flexible rods with rounded ends 0.3–0.5 × 5–8 μm, occurring singly. Spheroplasts and distorted cells occur in older cultures. A resting stage, the microcyst, is formed. Motile by gliding. Gram-negative.

Chemoorganotrophs. Metabolism is respiratory, with molecular oxygen used as terminal electron acceptor. **Cellobiose, cellulose, glucose and, for some strains, mannose are the only known sources of carbon and energy.** Agar and chitin are not known to be attacked. Either ammonium or nitrate ions, or peptone, urea or yeast extract, can serve as sole nitrogen source. Amino acids, peptones, yeast extract or nutrient agar (Difco) cannot serve as sole carbon and energy sources. No organic growth factor requirements are known.

Catalase-positive.

Strict aerobe. Temperature optimum: ~30°C.

The mol% G + C of the DNA of the two strains examined was 36. (B).

Type species: *Sporocytophaga myxococcoides* (Krzemieniewska) Stanier 1940, 629.

Further Comments

Only one species of the genus has been extensively examined. *S. myxococcoides* was shown by Stanier (1942) to grow on glucose sterilized by filtration and by Kaars Sijpesteijn and Fahraeus (1949) to grow on glucose autoclaved separately from other components of the medium, thus, apparently, refuting the assertion that growth of the organism is obligately linked to cellulose utilization. Recent studies (Leadbetter, unpublished observations) indicate that the organism, when isolated from nature, is unable either to oxidize or to utilize glucose but that putative mutants able to do so arise in the population. These "mutants" are able to attack immediately either cellulose or glucose, irrespective of the substrate in which they are grown. These observations thus confirm and extend those of Kaars Sijpesteijn and Fahraeus (1949).

Recent studies of S. *myxococcoides* have demonstrated that the organism is able to form microcysts when either glucose or cellulose is the carbon and energy source (Leadbetter, 1963; Gallin and Leadbetter, 1966).

List of species of the genus **Sporocytophaga**

1. **Sporocytophaga myxococcoides** (Krzemieniewska) Stanier 1940, 630.[AL] (*Cytophaga myxococcoides* Krzemieniewska 1933, 400.)

myx.o.coc.coi'des. M.L. masc. n. *Myxococcus* a generic name; Gr. n. *eidus* shape; M.L. adj. *myxococcoides* resembling *Myxococcus*.

Single, often flexible rods with rounded ends 0.3–0.5 × 5–8 μm. Spheroplasts and abnormally long forms may occur in old cultures. The resting stage, the microcyst, is spherical and about 1.5 μm in diameter. Both the growing (vegetative) rod and the microcyst have noticeably smaller dimensions when cultures are grown on cellulose rather than on glucose.

Electron microscopic studies indicate that the vegetative cell has a fine structure typical of Gram-negative bacteria, while the microcyst has a thick, fibrillar capsule exterior to a highly convoluted cell wall.

Growth on cellulose (filter paper)-salts agar (or silica gel) or glucose-salts agar is gummy, and liquid cultures become viscous as a result of extracellular slime production. Filter paper on the agar or silica gel surface is eventually dissolved around colonies so that translucent areas result. Colonies on glucose-salts agar medium are raised.

Other characteristics are the same as those of the genus.

Other Species

The following may be species of *Sporocytophaga*. They are incompletely characterized.

a. "*S. cauliformis*" Knorr and Gräf in Gräf 1962, 124.

b. "*S. congregata*" subsp. *maroonicum* Akashi 1960, 899.

c. "*S. ellipsospora*" (Imshenetski and Solntseva) Stanier 1942, 190.

d. "*S. ochracea*" Ueda, Ishikawa, Itami and Asai 1952, 545.

OTHER GENERA

Genus **Flexibacter** Soriano 1945, 92,[AL] emend.

H. REICHENBACH

Flex.i.bac'ter. L. adj. *flexilis* flexible; M.L. masc. n. *bacter* from Gr. neut. n. *bacterion* little stick or rod; M.L. masc. n. *Flexibacter* flexible rod.

Rod-shaped cells of variable length, typically 10–50 μm long, slender, 0.2–0.6 μm wide, flexible, and with tapering or rounded ends. **Gliding, but nonmotile stages may occur. In some species,** there is a **(cyclic) change in cell morphology.** In young liquid cultures or on plates at the edge of spreading colonies or swarms, the cells are thread-like, 20–50 μm and more in length, and very agile, actively twisting and bending. As these cells have no cross-walls or, at best, very few cross-walls, they will be called thread cells to distinguish them from multicellular filaments. In aging cultures or behind the swarm edge, the cells become shorter and shorter until only short, stout, nonmotile and phase-dark rods are left, clearly fatter than the thread cells, sometimes almost coccoid. **Cell mass** usually **yellow to orange,** sometimes very pale or even colorless. The pigments are cell-bound and often **carotenoids and/or of the flexirubin type.** In the latter case, the colonies show an immediate and **reversible color change to red-brown or purple when covered with alkali solution** (e.g. 20% KOH; reversed by 10% HCl). **Gram-negative.**

Chemoorganotrophs. Strictly aerobic or facultatively anaerobic. Peptones and amino acid mixtures serve as nitrogen sources. Various sugars are utilized. Some grow on simple defined media, e.g. with glucose and NH_4^+. Cellulose and agar are not attacked, but chitin and starch are often degraded.

Organisms widely distributed and common in soil and freshwater. The recognized species are listed in Table 23.10.

The mol% G + C of the DNA is 37–47. Strains very probably belonging to the genus *Flexibacter* but not yet attributed to defined species extend the mol% G + C of the DNA to 50.

Type species: *Flexibacter flexilis* Soriano 1945, 92.

Further Descriptive Information

The most distinguishing characteristic of *Flexibacter* is the occurrence *in young cultures* of long slender thread cells, which are often 40–60 µm long and very flexible. In some species, they are extremely delicate, only 0.2–0.3 µm wide, but in other species their width never exceeds 0.5–0.6 µm. These thread cells usually have tapering ends and either no cross-walls at all or only very few ones separating long segments, with each containing several nucleoids. They may show an impressive agility, vividly gliding and bending. They also may penetrate into the agar and sometimes tightly coil up there. In older cultures, the thread cells tend to break up into shorter units which may, however, still be rather long (10–15 µm). In some species, a pronounced and cyclic shape change takes place during which the cells become very short, sometimes almost coccoid. At the same time they become clearly stouter and darker in phase contrast, and below a certain length they become nonmotile. The short cells grow out into thread cells again when transferred into fresh medium. Conditions may be found under which the organisms grow mainly as long or short cells. On plates, the different stages of the morphological cycle may be observed simultaneously within one single colony as one proceeds from the swarm edge (thread cells) toward the center. Depending on the substrate, the colonies of *Flexibacter* may be large, more or less delicate, fast-spreading swarms as are often seen on yeast agar (e.g. VY/2 agar; Reichenbach and Dworkin, 1981c) or on media with low concentrations (0.01%) of peptone or yeast extract. Usually the swarm forms a coherent sheet, often with a pattern of flat slimy mounds on its surface and a network or flamelike protrusions at its edge. On rich substrates, growth may become solid, slimy and convex, with little or no indication of gliding.

Most *Flexibacter* strains are colored, either yellow or orange. Pigmentation often depends on the medium and may be bright and intense on one substrate and pale or even lacking on another. In general, rich substrates also stimulate pigment formation. There also are unpigmented strains; some of these, however, show a blue-green iridescence on certain substrates. The pigments are cell-bound and are either carotenoids (mainly saproxanthin or zeaxanthin) or flexirubins, a novel pigment type known so far only from *Flexibacter, Cytophaga, Sporocytophaga* and *Flavobacterium* species. Some strains contain both pigment types. In those strains, the flexirubins are located in the outer membrane, while the carotenoids are found in the cytoplasmic membrane (Fig. 23.35). Due to a phenolate reaction, the color of the flexirubin type pigments is much deeper at alkaline than at acid pH, which can be used for the color test mentioned above. The test is, however, not entirely specific for flexirubin type pigments, in that other pigments with a phenolic chromophore, e.g. the phenolic carotenoids of *Brevibacterium linens*, may react in the same way (Kohl et al., 1983). The occurrence of these different kinds of pigments with different *Flexibacter* species could be taken to indicate a heterogeneity of the genus. It seems, however, that in this case pigments are not a reliable guide to taxonomy. For example, the unusual carotenoid saproxanthin is the main pigment of *Saprospira grandis* (Aasen and

Liaaen-Jensen, 1966a, b), but while the 16S rRNA catalog of *F. filiformis* strain Fx e1 shows a clear, albeit remote, relationship to *S. grandis*, strain Fx e1 contains flexirubins and no carotenoids at all. On the other hand, the neotype strains of *F. flexilis* and of *F. elegans* appear to contain saproxanthin (Fager, 1969). As already mentioned, Fx e1 produces exclusively flexirubins, but its 16S rRNA catalog does not indicate a direct relationship to *Cytophaga*-like bacteria (CLB) and flavobacteria with flexirubin type pigments.

The fatty acid and quinone patterns have been determined for a few *F. filiformis* strains only. In all cases, these were predominantly acids with branched chains (mainly *iso*-C_{15}), often hydroxylated in the 2- or 3-position (mainly 2-OH nC_{16}, 2-OH *iso*-C_{15}, 3-OH *iso*-C_{15}, and 3-OH *iso*-C_{17}). A substantial quantity of monounsaturated $nC_{16:1}$ was also present. The respiratory quinones are always menaquinones, almost exclusively MK-7 (for references, see "Taxonomic Comments"). The lipopolysaccharide of strain Fx e1 (formerly Fx 1/2) resembles that of many other Gram-negative bacteria. It contains the usual 3-hydroxy fatty acids and, as sugars, mainly mannose, rhamnose, galactose, xylose, glucose, heptose, glucosamine and 2-keto-3-de-oxyoctonate (Rosenfelder et al., 1974).

The mol% G + C of the DNA of *Flexibacter* is somewhat above that of the CLB: roughly between 40 and 50.

All *Flexibacter* utilize complex organic nitrogen sources such as peptones, yeast extract and casamino acids, but the addition of a sugar, e.g. glucose, may stimulate growth in such media substantially or even be a prerequisite for growth. Apparently, the organic nitrogen compounds cannot always be utilized as carbon and energy sources, as, for example, is the case with *F. elegans* NZ-1 or with *F. filiformis*-like strain FS-1 (Simon and White, 1971). Nitrogen can often also be supplied in form of simpler organic compounds such as glutamate or other single amino acids, sometimes even as NH_4^+. Several sugars have been found to be metabolized, e.g. glucose, galactose, cellobiose, mannose, saccharose, lactose, maltose and arabinose; sugars such as ribose, rhamnose and sorbose seem not to be used. As a rule, organic acids are not accepted as the carbon source. Typically, sugar metabolism results in acid production, even with strictly aerobic strains. In a synthetic medium with NH_4^+ and glucose, *F. filiformis* strain Fx e1 produced acetate (0.042 mmol), lactate (0.023 mmol) and succinate (0.014 mmol), each per millimole of glucose utilized, in shake cultures without pH control. In casitone medium with glucose, no lactate was produced, but acetate (0.17 mmol), succinate (0.061 mmol/mmol glucose), isobutyrate and isovalerate were formed. The latter two acids were also produced in casitone medium without sugar and obviously arise from the amino acid metabolism (H. Fink and H. Reichenbach, unpublished results). Generation times are typically between 1.6 (in complex medium at 35°C) and 6.3 h (in NH_4^+-glucose medium at 30°C). Starch and chitin may or may not be degraded; no strain is known to decompose cellulose; all seem to hydrolyze gelatin. Most *Flexibacter* are strict aerobes, but there also appear to exist facultative anaer-

Figure 23.35. Localization of flexirubin pigments and carotenoids in the cell envelope of *Flexibacter filiformis*.

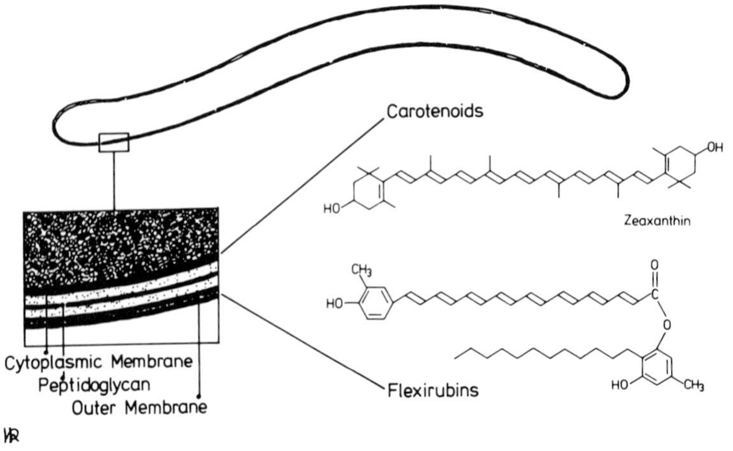

obes using either organic compounds, e.g. from glucose metabolism, or NO_3^- as terminal electron acceptors. Catalase is usually negative, oxidase is positive. All *Flexibacter* species are mesophiles with the optimum temperature between 24 and 35°C. They seem to be typical soil organisms but may also be isolated from freshwater. In general, they are sensitive to elevated salt concentrations, but *F. elegans* strain NZ-1 tolerates full-strength seawater.

Enrichment and Isolation Procedures

Specific enrichment conditions for *Flexibacter,* in general, are not known. The organisms have been obtained from soil, dung of herbivorous animals, rotting plant material, ditch water and other freshwater environments. Samples are transferred to (a) agar media with a low nutrient content, such as plain water agar prepared either with distilled water + 0.1% $CaCl_2$ or with filtered pond water, or (b) agar containing 0.02% of a peptone, e.g. tryptone (Difco). To suppress growth of molds, cycloheximide at 25–100 mg/l may be added to these media (Lewin and Lounsbery, 1969). Soil suspensions in water or water samples from nature may be plated in the usual way, but often it is better to apply them undiluted as solid soil crumbs or drops of water, for the frequency of the flexibacteria may be too low to allow dilution. *Flexibacter* is often obtained when soil is inoculated onto streaks of living *Escherichia coli* on water agar, as is done for the isolation of myxobacteria. In all these cases, *Flexibacter* forms thin, spreading colonies within one to several days which can be discovered under a dissecting microscope, especially when oblique translucent light is applied. Under ordinary illumination the very delicate swarms may be virtually invisible. A microscope with a low power objective and phase contrast would also do. With some experience, spreading colonies can even be seen with the naked eye as dull dots on the glistening surface of the tilted plate. *Flexibacter* strains may finally be distinguished from other gliding bacteria by their characteristic cell morphology and motility. Material from the swarm edge is then transferred to a suitable growth medium by cutting out tiny pieces with the tip of a fine injection needle or a drawn-out glass rod. Final purification is easily achieved by dilution and plating on a pure peptone or a peptone-glucose agar. *Flexibacter* can also be obtained by plating samples on richer peptone media, e.g. CY agar (Reichenbach and Dworkin, 1981c). Although growth is then faster, recognition becomes more difficult, because the colonies do not spread but are convex and compact. Under such circumstances, *Flexibacter* may be distinguished by the color of the colonies, which may be pink, orange or golden yellow (in the latter case, flexirubin-positive (KOH)), and by the cell morphology, which often, however, becomes characteristic only after a transfer is made to a medium which allows spreading growth. Certain N_2O-reducing specialists (Adkins and Knowles, 1984) can be enriched in soil by incubating the sample, after depletion of NO_3^- with N_2O and acetylene. The organisms are obtained later by plating on nutrient or plate count agar.

All *Flexibacter* grow well on a variety of peptone-glucose, peptone or amino acid media at neutral pH and at optimal temperatures between 24 and 35°C (strains from freshwater may prefer or even require temperatures at the lower end of the scale). Examples for suitable media are CY, FX A, HP6 (Reichenbach and Dworkin, 1981c) and MYX agars. The recipe for the latter is: Na-glutamate, 0.5%; yeast extract (Difco), 0.1%; $MgSO_4 \cdot 7H_2O$, 0.1%; glucose (autoclaved separately), 0.2%; and agar, 1.5%; at pH 7.2. The same media may also be used without agar for liquid cultures. In liquid media, the organisms grow dispersed. As already mentioned, some strains cannot grow on peptone media unless a sugar is added. Sometimes, slightly reduced nutrient concentrations are preferred to those used in standard bacteriological media such as nutrient agar. Many strains also grow on simple defined media, e.g. (in g/l): KH_2PO_4, 0.7; $Na_2HPO_4 \cdot 2H_2O$, 1.4; $(NH_4)_2SO_4$, 2.0; $MgSO_4 \cdot 7H_2O$, 0.2; $FeSO_4$, 0.005; $MnSO_4$, 0.005; and glucose, 10; at pH 7.0. A very good substrate to elicit spreading growth is yeast agar containing autoclaved cells of baker's yeast (VY/2 agar; Reichenbach and Dworkin, 1981c). Often, large swarms also develop on media with very low nutrient content (e.g. 0.01% yeast extract).

Maintenance Procedures

Agar cultures on rich peptone media usually die within 1 or 2 weeks (30°C), but on media with a low nutrient content (e.g. VY/2 agar or agar with 0.05 and 0.3% casitone (Difco)), cultures have been found viable in several instances after 4 months (30°C) and 13 months (4°C), respectively. In dry soil samples, *F. filiformis* survives for up to 2 years; however, my colleagues and I could never isolate the organism from older samples. All *Flexibacter* can reliably be preserved by storage at −80°C or in liquid nitrogen. Cells from young plate cultures are suspended in a peptone-containing liquid medium (e.g. CAS l.m.: casitone (Difco), 1%; and $MgSO_4 \cdot 7H_2O$, 0.1%), and 0.5–1-ml amounts are either put directly into the deep freeze or precooled at 6°C for 15 min and then put into the liquid nitrogen tank. Alternatively, vigorously growing liquid cultures can be used. Addition of a cryoprotective (10% DMSO or glycerol) appears to be required in some cases for storage at −196°C (Sanfilippo and Lewin, 1970). My colleagues and I routinely add 5% DMSO to liquid nitrogen cultures and nothing to −80°C cultures. The longest period we could test so far at −80°C was 9 years, and we have never had any failures with this method. For storage in liquid nitrogen, survival for 1 year was reported for all *Flexibacter* strains tested (Sanfilippo and Lewin, 1970), but the organisms would probably survive a much longer time. Drying in skim milk is usually well-tolerated. The cells are suspended in skim milk, then two or three drops are placed on a plug of freeze-dried skim milk in an ampul and dried in vacuo at room temperature. The ampuls are finally flooded with nitrogen gas, sealed, and stored at room temperature. Such preserves we could reactivate after 8 years, the longest period tested. The results are, however, somewhat variable with different strains and different preserves of the same strain. Probably the growth stage of the culture used for drying is critical. The lyophilized cultures of the ATCC obviously also survive quite well. Cell suspensions of *F. filiformis* in 1% NaCl solution or in distilled water and stored in sealed ampuls at room temperature we have found living after 7 years. The cell density of the initial suspension should not be too high (turbidity just well-visible).

Differentiation of the genus **Flexibacter** from other genera

Terrestrial *Flexibacter* is distinguished from marine *Microscilla,* its closest ally, by its habitats. From *Cytophaga* it can be differentiated by its characteristic cell morphology and motility. The cytophagas usually have very short to moderately long rod-shaped cells. The occasional appearance of somewhat longer threads is restricted to old cultures, and these threads also do not show any motility. The filamentous gliding soil and freshwater bacteria such as *Herpetosiphon* and *Vitreoscilla* differ from *Flexibacter* in their multicellular structure which becomes clearly recognizable upon drying or staining. Further, their filaments are usually much longer than the *Flexibacter* thread cells, and their movements are much slower.

Taxonomic Comments

The genus *Flexibacter* was created by Soriano (1945; see also 1947) to accommodate five species of gliding bacteria he discovered. The definition of the genus was mainly a morphological one and not very restrictive: "Bacteria with a flexible body that move by gliding are not screw-shaped [like spirochetes], do not form fruiting bodies [like myxobacteria], do not contain sulfur granules [like *Beggiatoa*], and cannot degrade cellulose [like *Cytophaga*]." Not surprisingly, the genus was heterogeneous from the very beginning as far as can be said today without any of the original strains available (see comments to the family *Cytophagaceae*).

Two of Soriano's species may, however, have been related: the type species, *F. flexilis,* and *F. elegans. F. flexilis* is perhaps not recognizable with certainty from its description by Soriano, but organisms resembling it morphologically have been reisolated (Lewin and Lounsbery, 1969). On the basis of these strains and of others seemingly related to them, an emended definition of *Flexibacter* has been proposed (Lewin, 1969):

"Gliding flexible rods or filaments, 5–50 µm long and 1 µm or less wide; no cross walls recognizable in the light microscope; neither branched, nor sheathed [n]or helical; fruiting bodies, spores or microcysts not formed; pink, red, orange or yellow due to cell-bound pigments; do not attack cellulose, agar or alginate, but hydrolyze gelatin; living mostly along fresh water banks and in hot springs, two species, however, marine."

Microscilla could be more or less distinguished from this type of *Flexibacter* only by its, in average, longer filaments (20–100 µm), alginate degradation in some species, and its marine habitats.

This new definition of *Flexibacter* was again not completely satisfactory. Although it allowed one to name a series of new isolates, it was still based to a large part on negative characteristics. Indeed, the genus was still heterogeneous. This could be surmised from the wide mol% G + C of the DNA of its species, 30–47, and has since also been directly shown by DNA/RNA hybridization (Bauwens and De Ley, 1981). By this technique it was shown that *F. roseolus*, *F. ruber* and *F. aurantiacus* (mol% G + C of the DNA of 35–38, 36 and 31, respectively) clearly belong together, but that they have no relationships with the rest of the *Flavobacterium-Cytophaga* group. *Flexibacter aurantiacus* var. *excathedrus*, on the other hand, was closely related to *Cytophaga lytica*.

The situation was further complicated in the eighth edition of the *Manual* (1974). Under the need to subdivide the genus *Cytophaga*, the definition of *Flexibacter* was again emended, by adding physiological characteristics which became the governing characteristics ultimately distinguishing *Flexibacter* from *Cytophaga*, while cell morphology and flexibility were reduced to minor qualities shared more or less by both: "Chemoorganotrophs, usually strictly aerobic, but one species facultatively anaerobic with fermentative metabolism; polymers such as agar, alginate, cellulose and chitin not attacked." Two or three one-time *Cytophaga* species were now included in the genus *Flexibacter*, while most of the former *Flexibacter* species were given the status *species incertae sedis*. *F. elegans* fell into oblivion. Two marine species were retained in the revised genus. The mol% G + C of the DNA was still wide, viz. 31–43.

For several reasons, this definition, too, does not appear sound. The organisms collected in this revised genus *Flexibacter* are almost certainly not all closely related to one another. For one thing, the type species, *F. flexilis* differs quite considerably in its cell morphology from that of the *Cytophaga*-like bacteria (CLB) including the two former *Cytophaga* species transferred to the redefined genus. Particularly in young cultures, there are long (at least 10–20 µm), slender and very flexible cells. Long cells also may occasionally be observed in CLB (but then in old cultures) or for some time after a transfer has been made from an old culture, obviously due to a disregulation in cell division, as is known from many bacteria. Long thread cells also are typical for the second of Soriano's *Flexibacter* species, *F. elegans*.

Then there are problems with the distinguishing physiological characteristic, viz. the inability to degrade polysaccharides. Apart from the fact that the definition remains somewhat vague in this point ("polysaccharides such as . . ."), the selection also seems arbitrary (β-glycosides only?), and the mentioned polysaccharides are so heterogeneous that it is difficult to see why organisms able to attack them should be phylogenetically related. In addition, two of the substances would probably make ecological sense to marine organisms only. In other words, this characteristic was useful as long as the genus definition had to remain merely operational, but it should be replaced by more reliable characteristics. In fact, among the CLB with a mol% G + C of the DNA of around 34 many strains have been found that cannot degrade any of the polysaccharides mentioned above but quite efficiently break down starch or pectin. On the other hand, *F. flexilis* degrades starch, and *F. filiformis* is a potent chitin decomposer. Yet the latter is definitely not closely related to, for example, *Cytophaga johnsonae* but belongs in another subgroup within the *Cytophaga-Flavobacterium* complex. It is therefore proposed to eliminate the lack of polysaccharide degradation from the genus definition of *Flexibacter* and to establish the genus entirely on cell morphology, G + C range, and habitat, as has been done above. The marine

organisms of this general type would then all be gathered within the genus *Microscilla*. Future research will show whether these genera are really uniform and reflect the natural relationships of the organisms in question. As is already suggested by the wide G + C range, they are very probably still heterogeneous and will have to be subdivided. Before this can be done, however, more data on the molecular taxonomy of these bacteria are desperately needed.

Although the type species, *F. flexilis*, seems not to have been studied any more in recent years, many new data have become available about organisms apparently identical with or closely related to Soriano's *F. elegans*, which is now, however, renamed *F. filiformis* for reasons discussed below. The outstanding feature of these bacteria is a cyclic shape change. In young liquid cultures about 6–10 h after inoculation or on plates at the edge of the swarm colony, there are thread cells, 20–50 µm long, with, at best, very few cross-walls, and extremely agile, gliding, bending and twisting like little worms. When the culture ages, in liquid cultures after a few hours, on plates in the direction to the center of the swarm, these thread cells fragment until finally only very short, sometimes nearly coccoid rods are left. These short rods are somewhat fatter, darker, more rigid, and become nonmotile as soon as they come below a certain length. When transferred to fresh medium, they soon grow out to form thread cells again, and a new cycle begins. Conditions may be found under which the organism grows continuously in the one or other morphological state (Simon and White, 1971; Poos et al., 1972; Reichenbach et al., 1974; Costenbader and Burchard, 1978; Hirsch and Reichenbach, 1981). These *Flexibacter* strains thus resemble the *Arthrobacter* group in many aspects.

The organisms just described fit perfectly into the *Cytophaga-Flavobacterium* complex with respect to their fatty acid pattern (Fautz et al., 1979, 1981) and respiratory quinones (Kleinig et al., 1974). Their main pigment is flexirubin, a new pigment type originally discovered in *Flexibacter filiformis* (formerly *F. elegans*) Fx e1 but since found in several slightly modified chemical structures with many other members of the *Cytophaga-Flavobacterium* complex (Reichenbach et al., 1974, 1981; Achenbach et al., 1976–1978). The flexirubin type pigments thus seem to be useful chemosystematic markers. They are located in the outer membrane of the cell wall (Irschik and Reichenbach, 1978). The mol% G + C of 10 strains of the *F. filiformis* complex was 45–47 (T_m, Bd) (Behrens, 1978). The 16S rRNA catalog of strain Fx e1 showed that this bacterium is not directly related with typical cytophagas. Although it clearly belongs in the *Cytophaga-Flavobacterium* complex, it is in a separate branch with connections to *Flavobacterium ferrugineum* (Paster et al., 1985; see comments to the order *Cytophagales*). These bacteria are probably identical with, or at least closely related to, Soriano's *Flexibacter elegans*, although Soriano did not mention the cyclic shape change, perhaps because he did not observe it or because he mistook the short cells as contaminants. The organisms are so common in nature, however, that with the isolation techniques he applied and the habitats he studied, Soriano must have obtained them. Furthermore, he described the typical and apparently unique thread cells very appropriately: "filamentous thin rods, 0.4–0.5 × 20–50 µm . . ., very active flexibility and motility of the cells which often move with the twisted central part of the body going ahead, forming elegant capricious figures. . . ." The cultures also looked identical: "good yellowish growth on 1% peptone agar." No other of Soriano's *Flexibacter* species fits the *F. filiformis* strains so precisely.

I discovered, unfortunately somewhat belatedly, that an organism corresponding to the above-mentioned bacteria in almost every respect had already been described in 1940 by Solntseva under the name of "*Myxococcus filiformis*." As the final stage of cell shortening was mistaken for myxospores, the bacterium was classified as a myxobacter in spite of the absence of fruiting bodies and the presence of considerable physiological differences. As a most peculiar and distinguishing characteristic of the new species, long threadlike cells are mentioned, often 45 µm long, occurring only in young cultures. This was specifically emphasized and regarded as quite different from the behavior of ordinary bacteria. Such thread cells later gradually shorten and finally end up as very short rods or cocci, 1.4 × 1.4 µm. Although the thread cells are gliding and bending, the shorter cells are nonmotile. The slimy colonies, golden yellow on several media, show a pattern of flat slimy mounds, which also is very typical for the *Flexibacter* strains mentioned above. "*M. filiformis*" grows well with organic nitrogen sources, including complex ones, but also with NH_4^+ or NO_3^- in combination with various sugars, often with acid production, all of which again are typical for the flexibacters. "*M. filiformis*" appears to be a strict aerobe. When it is compared with the *Flexibacter* strains mentioned above, two differences are noticed which may, however, be of minor importance. Young cells of "*M. filiformis*" from potato agar showed a slime capsule (overall diameter of 1.5 μm) when they were contrasted via India ink; and starch was readily hydrolyzed, which is not the case with all of the above-mentioned flexibacters.

To confuse things further, a strain isolated in the 1960s from a hot spring in New Zealand was identified as *F. elegans* Soriano and proposed as a neotype (strain NZ-1, ATCC 23112; Lewin, 1969; Lewin and Lounsbery, 1969; Fager, 1969). Although again no mention is made of a cyclic shape change, nor of the peculiar motility, the strain shares several characteristics with the organisms discussed above. Its cells may be > 50 μm long; it is catalase-negative and decomposes gelatin, but it does not degrade starch; and it has mol% G + C of the DNA of 47. In spite of the habitat from which it was obtained, the organism is not a thermophile. There are, however, also differences. The organism does not degrade chitin, which most of the *F. filiformis* strains do (Hirsch, 1980). It can grow on full-strength seawater media, which is not the case with any of the other strains. Its pigments are different, the cell mass is bright orange, like that of *F. flexilis*, due to a carotenoid with an absorption maximum at 478 nm (Lewin's pigment type III), reportedly saproxanthin (group 17 of Fager (1969)). In contrast, the other strains are golden yellow and contain flexirubin and, if carotenoids are also present, then mainly zeaxanthin and never saproxanthin.

Examination of the ATCC 23112 strain corroborates the existence of thin *Flexibacter* thread cells which are very flexible and agile, moving as described above. The strain does not show a cyclic shape change, is certainly not identical with the above-mentioned organisms, and is probably not identical with *F. elegans* Soriano. It appears to be a rather rare bacterium, at least it has been found only once and then in a special habitat, whereas Soriano's organism was common soil inhabitant. As a type strain is available, however, it is proposed to regard this as *F. elegans* Lewin, non Soriano. No strains are available for "*M. filiformis*" Solntseva and "*F. elegans*" Soriano. These two are regarded as the same organism

and identical with the bacteria discussed above. As the former name antedates the latter, it is suggested to reclassify the bacteria which so far have often been labeled *F. elegans* Soriano as *F. filiformis*, with strain Fx e1 (DSM 527) as a neotype.

The recently described *F. canadensis* was isolated from soil (Christensen, 1980). It forms long and very thin and flexible thread cells measuring 0.3 × up to 60 μm. Usually the population consists of rods of only moderate length, and there is no cyclic shape change. In particular, the edge of swarming colonies contains exclusively rather short, actively gliding cells. The colonies are essentially unpigmented and white, but they may show a blue-green iridescence. This organism differs from all other bacteria discussed so far in that it is a facultative anaerobe and seems to prefer a reduced oxygen tension, although it grows very well in a normal atmosphere too. It has a comparatively low mol% G + C of the DNA of 37 and may, indeed, not be a *Flexibacter* species; rather, it may belong to the CLB. It is treated here as a *species incertae sedis*.

Not long ago, an organism resembling *F. canadensis* in some respects had been isolated because of its peculiar physiological capability to reduce N_2O in the presence of sulfide and of otherwise inhibitory concentrations of acetylene (Adkins and Knowles, 1984). It was provisionally classified as a *Cytophaga*, but it shows a cyclic shape change as described for "*F. filiformis*". In contrast to *F. canadensis*, its extremely delicate thread cells are typically found in young cultures and are very agile. It also is essentially unpigmented, may show a blue-green iridescense on certain media, is a facultative anaerobe, prefers a reduced oxygen tension, and reduces NO_3^-. This organism has been obtained from soil and may turn out to be a new *Flexibacter* species.

Another recently described species, "*F. chinensis*" (Qinsheng et al., 1984) has been isolated from freshwater. It has thin, moderately long (4–16 μm) rods, which, however, in liquid media may reach >60 μm; moves by gliding; forms pink and, later, orange colonies with a pale iridescense; is a faculative anaerobe; and has a mol% G + C of the DNA of 34. A cyclic shape change is not mentioned. It is probably not closely related to the flexibacters mentioned above, for it has a very low G + C content. A decision about its taxonomic position is not possible on the basis of available data. It is included below as a species of uncertain affiliation.

Further Reading

See under "Order *Cytophagales*."

Differentiation of the species of the genus **Flexibacter**

The distinguishing characteristics of the species of the genus *Flexibacter* are compiled in Table 23.10. Several more species of uncertain affiliation are listed at the end of the species descriptions.

List of species of the genus **Flexibacter**

1. **Flexibacter flexilis** Soriano 1945, 92,[AL] emend. Lewin 1969, 199.
flex'i.lis. L. adj. *flexilis* pliable, flexible.

Long flexible thread cells with tapering, occasionally crooked ends, 0.5 × 10–60, usually 10–20 μm (Fig. 23.36). Motile by gliding but not particularly active. On some media the colonies become spreading swarms, typically with long branched extensions at the edge (Fig. 23.37). On many substrates a tough slime develops which may effectively prevent the formation of a pellet upon centrifugation. Cell mass orange, reportedly due to the carotenoid saproxanthin (Fager, 1969), but pigmentation on many media is very pale.

Peptones or casamino acids may serve as sole nitrogen source, but not glutamate or NO_3^-, since several amino acids are essential (arginine, isoleucine, leucine, methionine, valine and threonine). Grows well on peptone alone. Sugars such as glucose or sucrose may stimulate growth. Thiamine is required. In litmus milk there is no acid production or coagulation, and litmus is reduced. For further biochemical characteristics, see Table 23.10.

Strictly aerobic. Optimum temperature: around 25°C; but at 30°C growth is still good. Optimal pH: around 7.

Isolated from various freshwater environments in the Americas.

Several strains have been shown by numerical phenotype analysis to group together (Fager, 1969; Lewin, 1969; Lewin and Lounsbery, 1969), but confirmation by DNA hybridization would be desirable. The mol% G + C of the DNA is 40–43 (Bd) (Mandel and Lewin, 1969). All strains are available at the ATCC. Also one of the two described variants, var. *pelliculosus* (Lewin and Lounsbery, 1969) is still there (ATCC 23098). Its mol% G + C is 39 (Bd). It differs from the main group in that it degrades carboxymethyl cellulose (CMC) and grows on glutamate or NO_3^- as sole nitrogen source. Its relation to the other strains should be reinvestigated. A strain described as var. *algavorum* (Gromov et al., 1972) is hardly a variant of *F. flexilis*, since it has a mol% G + C of the DNA of only 36 (T_m) and is catalase-positive. The organism has long, nonseptated, slender, flexible cells, 7–10 up to 200 μm long, and is gliding. The cell mass is orange, due to a carotenoid, perhaps saproxanthin. The organism grows on media containing low concentrations of a peptone (0.1%) and yeast extract (0.1%) and apparently requires growth factors, probably polypeptides and vitamins. Addition of glucose or acetate does not stimulate growth. Agar, starch and cellulose are not degraded, but gelatin is

Table 23.10.

Differential characteristics of the species of the genus **Flexibacter**[a]

Characteristic	1. *F. flexilis*	2. *F. elegans*	3. *F. filiformis*
Length of threads (μm)	10->50	1.0->80	
Width of threads (μm)	0.5	0.4	0.6-0.4
Cyclic shape change	−	−	+
Color of cell mass	Orange[b]	Bright orange	Golden yellow
Flexirubin reaction[c]	+	−	+
Carotenoids present	Saproxanthin	Saproxanthin	Zeaxanthin
Relation to oxygen	Aerobe	Aerobe	Aerobe
Growth on peptones alone	+	−	+
Suitable as sole nitrogen source			
Peptones	+	+	+
Casamino acids	+	+	+
Glutamic acid	−	−	+
NH_4^+	−	−	+
NO_3^-	−	−	+
Sugars metabolized	+	+	+
Acid from glucose	+	+	+
Degradation of			
Gelatin	+	+	+
Casein	•	•	+
Starch	+	−	−
Chitin	−	−	+
Yeast cells[d]	−	−	+
Indole produced	−	−	−
H_2S produced	+	−	−
NO_3^- reduced	−	−	−
Catalase	−		−
Oxidase	+	+	+
DNase	•	•	−
Growth on seawater media	−	+	−
Highest NaCl concentration tolerated (%)	•	2.4	0.3
Optimum temperature (°C)	40–45	40–45	40–45
Highest temperature permitting growth (°0)	40–45	40–45	40–45
Optimum pH	7	7	7
Habitat	Freshwater	Freshwater	Soil/freshwater
Mol% G + C of DNA	40–43	•	46–47
Mol% G +C of DNA of type strain	41	48	47

[a]Symbols: −, 90% or more of strains are negative; +, 90% or more of strains are positive; •, no information available.

[b]On many media very pale.

[c]Color change from yellow to red, purple to red-brown when alkali is added.

[d]In yeast agar, e.g. VY/2 agar.

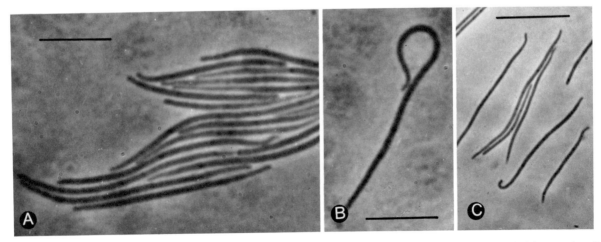

Figure 23.36. *F. flexilis* type strain cells on starch-casitone agar. Culture 2 days old. Phase contrast. *A*, characteristic arrangement on agar surfaces. *Bar*, 6 μm. *B*, high flexibility typical of the organism. *Bar*, 6 μm. *C*, hooked ends may often be observed. *Bar*, 12 μm.

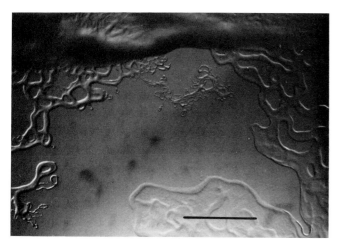

Figure 23.37. *F. flexilis* swarm edge on agar with 0.01% yeast extract. *Bar*, 1.6 mm.

liquefied. The bacterium is strictly aerobic and grows at 25°C. The most conspicuous property of the organism is its capability for slow lysis of cyanobacteria, e.g. lawns of *Anabaena, Phormidium* and *Nostoc* species. Ordinary bacteria are not attacked. The strain was isolated from a pond in Leningrad, U.S.S.R. It is available at the All-Union Collection of Microorganisms in Moscow (BKM 1001).

The mol% G + C of the DNA of the neotype strain is 41 (Bd).

Neotype strain: ATCC 23079 (CR-63 Lewin 1969).

2. **Flexibacter elegans** (ex Lewin 1969, non Soriano 1945, 92) nom. rev.

e'le.gans. L. adj. *elegans* refined, fashionable, elegant.

Very long, fine filaments with rounded ends, 0.4–0.5 × 50 μm, often much longer, rarely shorter down to 10–20 μm (Fig. 23.38). In old cultures, filaments are sometimes found which fragment at regular intervals (7–12 μm) (Fig. 23.39). This suggests a subdivision by crosswalls, and cross-walls can, in fact, be seen with the electron microscope. On solid substrates the filaments tend to form loops and coils (Fig. 23.38), but suspended in liquid medium they appear relatively straight and somewhat stiff. Motile by gliding, with threads from young cultures actively bending and twisting. On some solid media the colonies are spreading. A very tenacious slime may develop on agar media. The cell mass is bright orange, reportedly due to the carotenoid saproxanthin (Fager, 1969).

Grows with peptones or casamino acids but not with glutamate or NO₃⁻ as sole nitrogen source. Requires threonine. On media containing only a peptone, growth is often poor or absent but may be much stimulated by the addition of a sugar such as glucose. In litmus milk, there is no acid production, coagulation, or reduction of litmus. Further biochemical characteristics are listed in Table 23.10.

Grows on media containing full-strength seawater and at least equally as well without any sea salt added; it is not regarded as a marine organism. Strictly aerobic. Good growth occurs around pH 7 and at 30°C; maximum temperature: 40–45°C.

Only one strain is known. It was isolated from a hot spring in New Zealand. The organism is almost certainly not identical with *F. elegans* Soriano. It has different pigmentation and habitats (see "Taxonomic Comments").

The mol% G + C of the DNA is 48 (Bd).

Neotype strain: ATCC 22112 (NZ-1 Lewin).

3. **Flexibacter filiformis** (Solntseva 1940) comb. nov., emend. (*Myxococcus filiformis* Solntseva 1940, 221; *Flexibacter elegans* Soriano 1945, 92, non Lewin 1969, 200).

fi.li.for'mis. L. n. *filum* thread; L. n. *forma* shape; M.L. adj. *filiformis* threadlike.

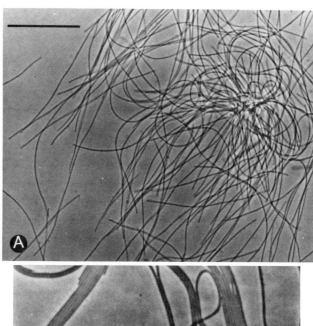

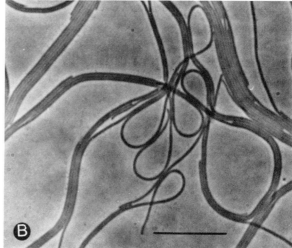

Figure 23.38. *F. elegans* type strain threads from glutamate-yeast extract-glucose medium. Phase contrast. *A*, in liquid. *Bar*, 24 μm. *B*, on an agar surface. The threads tend to align parallel to one another and to stick together. *Bar*, 12 μm.

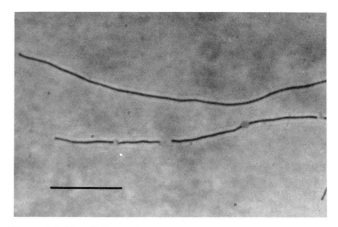

Figure 23.39. *F. elegans* fragmenting thread, which suggests segmentation. Phase contrast. *Bar*, 12 μm.

Organism with a cyclic shape change. Cell populations usually highly pleomorphic. In young cultures, long and very flexible thread cells with tapering ends, 0.4–0.5 × 30–80 μm, sometimes even longer (Fig. 23.40). Later the thread cells fragment so that even shorter cells appear when the culture ages. Finally, only short, often curved, sometimes almost coccoid rods are present which are clearly fatter and, under phase contrast, darker than the thread cells, measuring 0.5–0.6 × 7–1.0 μm or less (Fig. 23.41). The short cells may still continue to grow and divide as such. Usually they grow out into thread cells again when brought into fresh medium. The morphological cycle is controlled by environmental factors, particularly nutrients and temperature, and may be manipulated experimentally. On agar plates, particularly on media that allow swarming, the different morphological forms are, as a rule, found within one (usually the same) colony, with the longer cells near the edge of the swarm. The thread cells have no cross-walls, or very few ones, 10–30 μm apart, recognizable with the electron microscope (Poos et al., 1972). Each compartment appears to contain several nucleoids. The thread cells are extremely agile, gliding, bending and twisting; but below a certain length (about 6 μm) the cells become completely nonmotile. On solid media with a low nutrient content (e.g. 0.01% yeast extract) or on yeast agar (e.g. VY/2 agar) the colonies are fast-spreading delicate swarms (Fig. 23.42). On VY/2 agar the colonies have a characteristic surface pattern of circular or elongated flat mounds. On agar media with peptone concentrations above 0.3% the colonies become more and more compact, with a convex surface and a smooth edge. Such colonies often contain only short rods. On yeast agar the cell mass is usually pale yellow, whereas on peptone media it is intensely golden yellow. This color changes quickly into purple or red-brown when alkali (e.g. 20% KOH solution) is added, and it returns to bright yellow when acid (e.g. 10% HCl) is added. The color reaction is due to the presence of flexirubin pigments (Fig. 23.35), which are the main pigments of the organism. Many strains also contain substantial quantities of the bright yellow carotenoid, zeaxanthin. Rarely, strains are also found which are very pale or totally unpigmented.

Peptones or a simpler organic nitrogen compound, NH_4^+ or NO_3^-, may serve as sole source of nitrogen. Various sugars are used as carbon and energy sources and are usually metabolized with the production of acids. Acetate produced in this way is reused later; other organic acids, however, are not utilized. In litmus milk, there is no acid production or coagulation; litmus is reduced and casein is hydrolyzed. There is no growth on seawater media. This organism is resistant to polymyxin B and penicillin G. Further biochemical data are listed in Table 23.10.

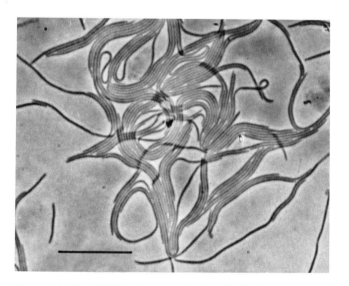

Figure 23.40. *F. filiformis* type strain thread cells from a swarm colony on yeast agar near the swarm edge. Phase contrast. *Bar*, 12 μm.

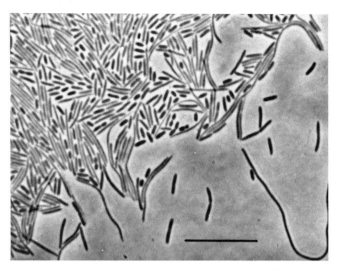

Figure 23.41. *F. filiformis* heterogeneous cell population from an area behind the swarm edge. Phase contrast. *Bar*, 12 μm.

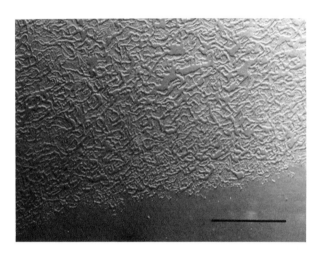

Figure 23.42. *F. filiformis* swarm edge on agar with 0.01% yeast extract. *Bar*, 1.4 mm.

Strictly aerobic. Optimum temperature: around 35°C; this organism still grows well at 38°C. Optimum pH: around 7.

Isolated from soil, decaying plant material, dung of herbivorous animals, and freshwater habitats in many different places. Rather common. The neotype strain was isolated in 1966 from soil collected on the island of Upolu, Samoa.

Several strains belonging or closely related to this species have been studied in recent years in various laboratories (Simon and White, 1971; Poos et al., 1972; Kleinig et al., 1974; Reichenbach et al., 1974; Rosenfelder et al., 1974; Achenbach et al., 1976, 1977; Behrens, 1978; Costenbader and Burchard, 1978; Irschik and Reichenbach, 1978; Fautz et al., 1979, 1981; Hirsch, 1980; Hirsch and Reichenbach, 1981; Paster et al., 1985). One of these strains, Fx e1, proposed as the neotype strain of the species, has formerly been classified as *F. elegans*. As pointed out in the "Taxonomic Comments," this organism is probably identical with Soriano's *F. elegans*, but it appears preferable to change its name to *F. filiformis*. The description given here rests exclusively on this neotype strain. Other strains that have been studied may deviate in certain characteristics. It has yet to be shown by a thorough comparative study, including DNA/DNA hybridizations, whether these differences are of taxonomic relevance. The mol% G + C of the DNA for 13 strains is 46–47

(Bd, T_m) (Behrens, 1978). One strain, however, which otherwise closely resembles the former strains, has a mol% G + C of the DNA of 50. This suggests that there are still more species of the general type of *F. filiformis*, a conclusion also supported by the facultative anaerobe mentioned in the general description of the genus.

The mol% G + C of the DNA of the neotype strain is 47 (Bd, T_m).

Neotype strain: DSM 527 (ATCC 29495; Fx e1 Reichenbach).

Other Species

No strains are available for the following species; at least two of them have never been grown in pure culture, and all descriptions are very scant. The species are probably not recognizable with reasonable certainty and have to be abolished, at least for the moment.

i. "*Flexibacter albuminosus*" Soriano 1945, 93.

Fine rods of moderate length, 0.3–0.4 × 4–10 μm, gliding. Growth on 1% peptone agar is dirty white; a dark diffusible pigment is produced. Isolated from mud and ditch water in Argentina. This organism was perhaps a *Lysobacter*.

ii. "*Flexibacter aureus*" Soriano 1945, 93.

Rather short rods, 0.3–0.4 × 3–5 μm, gliding. Growth on 1% peptone agar is golden yellow. Isolated from mud and ditch water in Argentina. This organism was probably a CLB.

iii. "*Microscilla agilis*" Pringsheim 1951, 142.

Thread-shaped cells without recognizable cross-walls, 0.6–0.8 × 12–70 μm, very agile, gliding and twisting. Isolated from decaying plant material in a ditch in England. This may have been a *Flexibacter* of the *filiformis* type.

iv. "*Microscilla flagellum*" Pringsheim 1951, 143.

Long thread cells, barely 0.4 μm wide, extremely agile, gliding and lashing. Common in floating masses of cyanobacteria and plant debris in freshwater in England. This organism may have been a *Flexibacter*.

v. "*Flexibacter giganteus*" Lewin 1969, 199.

Apparently, no strains are available. Long flexible threads, 0.5 × up to 50 μm, gliding. Cell mass is pink, due to carotenoids. Grows on peptones and casamino acids but not on glutamate or NO_3^- as sole nitrogen source. Degrades starch and gelatin. Catalase-negative. Does not reduce NO_3^-. No halotolerance. Strict aerobe with an optimum temperature of 20–25°C and an optimum pH of 7. Isolated from freshwater in Costa Rica. The mol% G + C of the DNA (32) seems to rule out a relationship with the *Flexibacter* species.

vi. "*Flexibacter giganteus*" Soriano 1945, 93.

Rather thick and very long filaments, 0.75–0.9 × 100 μm and longer, slowly gliding. Swarm colonies orange-red, with small elevations. Isolated from mud and ditch water in Argentina. This organism is probably not identical with the former species (dimensions, color) but very likely was a *Herpetosiphon aurantiacus*. It has therefore been suggested to rename the latter organism "*H. giganteus*" (Reichenbach and Golecki, 1975), but as more than one species may be hidden in the *H. aurantiacus* complex, it is not possible to be sure about the identity of the two species, and the idea should be abandoned.

vii. "*Promyxobacterium lanceolatum*" Imshenetski and Solntseva 1945, 225.

Relatively fat rods with slightly tapering ends. In young cultures the cells measure 0.8–1.8 × 2.6–5.5 and up to 26 μm, gliding. When the culture ages the cells shorten down to 1.4–1.8 μm and become nonmotile. Colonies on agar media are slimy, shiny, with a folded surface, grayish white, and difficult to remove from the agar. Peptones, several amino acids, urea, NO_3^- or NH_4^+ may serve as sole nitrogen source. Dextrin and gelatin are degraded. Aerobic. Optimum temperature: 25–30°C. Isolated

from soil in Russia. In some of its characteristics the organism distantly resembles the flexibacters, but the description is too vague to allow any reliable identification.

Species Incertae Sedis

For all species listed below, strains are available. The published information does not allow a reliable classification or an identification of newly isolated strains with them, before a careful comparison with the type strains is made. The taxonomy of these interesting organisms deserves and urgently needs to be reinvestigated.

a. **Flexibacter aurantiacus** Lewin 1969, 200.[AL]

au.ran.ti′a.cus. M.L. adj. *aurantiacus* orange-colored.

Rods of moderate length, 5–20 μm, gliding. Cell mass yellow. Peptones, casamino acids, glutamate or NO_3^- may serve as sole nitrogen source. Various sugars are metabolized. Degrades CMC, starch and gelatin but not cellulose. Catalase-positive, no reduction of NO_3^-. Tolerates seawater. Maximum temperature: 30°C. One strain was isolated from garden soil in Minneapolis.

The mol% G + C of the DNA is 32.

Type strain: ATCC 23107 (DWO Lewin/Dworkin).

It was inferred that this strain is identical with *Cytophaga aurantiaca* Winogradsky 1929, 597 (ATCC Catalogue 1976), but there is no basis for such an assumption, particularly as Winogradsky's organism is an efficient cellulose decomposer. Also, the suggestion that the organism might be related to or identical with "*Sphaeromyxa xanthochlora*" Bauer 1962, 392, must be regarded as casual and is of no consequence, as that organism is no longer available. A second strain, ATCC 23108 (PSY Lewin) was formerly classified as *Cytophaga psychrophila* and very probably is a representative of that species (see comments on *C. psychrophila*). More recently, it has been shown by rRNA/DNA hybridization that *F. aurantiacus* is relatively closely related to *F. roseolus* and *F. ruber*, but that all three do not belong in the *Cytophaga-Flavobacterium* complex (Bauwens and De Ley, 1981). Unfortunately, the strain on which this study has been performed is not identified. Probably it was the type strain, ATCC 23107 (DWO). In any case, the low G + C content of both *Flexibacter aurantiacus* strains would not fit *Flexibacter*. A variant, *F. aurantiacus ex-cathedrus* Lewin 1969, 200 (ATCC 23086), isolated from a pool in Costa Rica, was demonstrated by the same hybridization technique to be a member of the *Cytophaga* group and is thus not related at all to the type. This variant also differs from the type in its pigments. It does not use NO_3^- as sole nitrogen source, does not degrade CMC, is catalase-negative, has no salt tolerance, has a maximum temperature of 40–45°C, and has a mol% G + C of the DNA of 35. A second supposed variant, *co-pepodarum* Lewin 1969, 200, is also still available (NCMB 1394). It is a marine organism isolated from an offshore crustacean. Its pigments are different from those of the type, it does not grow with NO_3^- as sole nitrogen source, does not degrade CMC and starch, is catalase-negative, and has a mol% G + C of the DNA of 33.

b. **Flexibacter roseolus** Lewin 1969, 199.[AL]

ro.se′o.lus. L. adj. *roseus* rose-colored; L. dim. adj. *roseolus* with a rosy tinge.

Very long threads, >50 μm. Cell mass is red, due to the carotenoid, flexixanthin, demonstrated in strain CR-141 (Aasen and Liaaen-Jensen, 1966b). Peptones or casamino acids may serve as sole nitrogen source, but glutamate or NO_3^- may not. Gelatin is degraded, starch is not. Catalase-negative. This organism does not reduce NO_3^-. Tolerates seawater. Maximum temperature: 40°C. Isolated from a hot spring in Costa Rica.

The mol% G + C of the DNA of the type strain is 38. A second strain from the same source, ATCC 23087 (CR-141 Lewin), has a mol% G + C of the DNA of 35 and hardly belongs to the same species.

Type strain: ATCC 23088 (CR-155 Lewin).

This organism appears not to belong to the *Cytophaga-Flavobacterium* complex (see *Flexibacter aurantiacus*).

c. **Flexibacter ruber** Lewin 1969, 199.[AL]

ru'ber. L. adj. *ruber* red.

Very long threads, >50 μm, gliding. Cell mass is red, reportedly due to the carotenoid, flexixanthin. Peptones, casamino acids, glutamate or NO_3^- serve as sole nitrogen source. Various sugars are metabolized with acid production. Degrades starch and gelatin. Catalase-negative. Reduces NO_3^-. No halotolerance. Maximum temperature: 40–45°C. One strain was isolated from a hot spring in Iceland.

The mol% G + C of the DNA is 37.

Type strain: ATCC 23103 (GEY Lewin).

This organism does not appear to belong to the *Cytophaga-Flavobacterium* complex (see *Flexibacter aurantiacus*).

d. **Flexibacter sancti** Lewin 1969, 199.[AL]

sanc'ti. L. n. *sanctus* saint; L. gen. n. *sancti* of Saint; named perhaps in honor of Dr. *Santos* Soriano, from whose laboratory the type strain was supplied (etymology is not clear).

Rather short cylindrical rods with slightly tapering ends, 0.5 × 2–5 μm and up to 15 μm (strain MIC: 10–50 μm). Cell mass on peptone agar is golden yellow, reportedly due to the carotenoid, zeaxanthin (Lewin & Lounsbery, 1969), but it turns instantly purple-red when alkali is added, so that, supposedly, flexirubin type pigments are present. On yeast agar (e.g. VY/2 agar), delicate swarms develop, and yeast cells are attacked. On solid media, a tough sticky slime is produced. Grows with peptones, casamino acids or NO_3^- but not with glutamate as sole nitrogen source. Various sugars are metabolized, with the production of acid. Degrades CMC, starch and gelatin. Catalase-negative. Reduces NO_3^-. No halotolerance. Maximum temperature: 35°C. Stated to resemble *Cytophaga johnsonae* in most respects, except that it does not degrade chitin (Lewin, 1969). But a mol% G + C difference of >10 makes a classification with the CLB impossible. The three strains attached to this species (type strain; ATCC 23090 (BA-23 Lewin/Cataldi); and ATCC 23097 (MIC Lewin/Holt)) differ substantially in several respects and may not really belong together. Isolated from soil (or similar material) in Argentina and the U.S.A.

The mol% G + C of the DNA is 46–47.

Type strain: ATCC 23092 (BA-3 Lewin/Cataldi).

e. **Flexibacter canadensis** Christensen 1980, 431.[VP]

ca.na.den'sis. M.L. adj. *canadensis* Canadian.

Elongated rods, thin and flexible, with slightly tapering ends, 0.4–0.5 × 2–12 μm; tend to become longer, up to 60 μm, in older cultures or on less suitable substrates (Figs. 23.43 and 23.44). In ordinary cultures the cell population is, therefore, considerably heterogeneous. In addition to the typical fine rods, somewhat coarser and darker cells are often observed. The latter are about 0.6 μm wide and of different lengths. Vigorously growing young cultures and the advancing edge of fast-spreading swarm colonies, e.g. on yeast agar, typically consist of short to moderately long fine rods. This organism thus does not show the typical *Flexibacter* morphology. Motile by gliding, with the short rods being the more agile.

On solid substrates with a low nutrient content, e.g. skim milk or yeast agar, large whitish swarms develop. On media with a higher concentration of organic compounds, growth becomes compact, pale pink or dirty white. Colonies often show a yellow-green-blue iridescense. In the dissecting microscope, tiny shining flakes with an intense red iridescence are sometimes seen.

Facultative anaerobe, microaerophilic with an optimum around 10% O_2 but still grows very well in shake cultures under a normal atmosphere. Gelatin, casein, peptones, casamino acids, glutamate, aspartate or NH_4^+ may serve as sole nitrogen source, but NO_3^- or urea may not. Grows on peptone alone. Various sugars and glycerol are metabolized aerobically with acid production. Glucose may be utilized oxidatively or fermentatively. Catalase- and oxidase-positive. DNase, indole and H_2S production; NO_3^- reduction-positive. Tweens and tributyrin not attacked. Pectin slowly degraded. Casein, gelatin and starch are hydrolyzed but not chitin and CMC. Bacterial cells, fungal hyphae and yeast cells in yeast

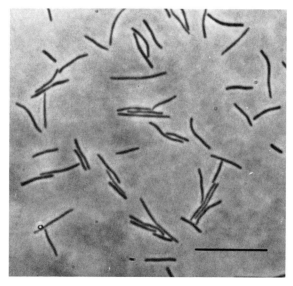

Figure 23.43. *F. canadensis* actively gliding cells from the edge of a 3-day-old swarm on yeast agar. Note the difference in typical *Flexibacter* morphology between the *F. canadensis* of this micrograph and that of Figure 23.44. Phase contrast. *Bar*, 11 μm.

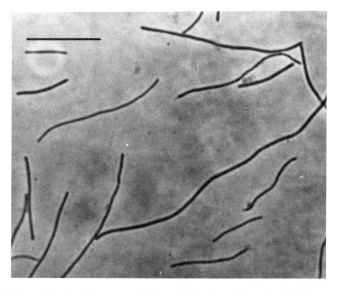

Figure 23.44. *F. canadensis* elongated cells and threads on 0.3% peptone agar. The variability in cell width is well-recognizable. Phase contrast. *Bar*, 11 μm.

agar are not decomposed. Resistant to penicillin. No growth on seawater media.

Grows between 10 and 40°C; optimum temperature: around 30°C. A pH range of 5–10 is reported, with the optimum between 6 and 8.

Isolated from soil in Canada.

The mol% G + C of the DNA is 37 (T_m) (corroborated by my colleagues and myself by Bd (unpublished observation)).

Type strain: ATCC 29591 (UASM 9D Christensen).

Morphology and G + C seem to exclude this organism from the genus *Flexibacter*. It may be related to certain organisms that are, at the moment, probably incorrectly, classified in the genus *Cytophaga*, but in absence of supporting data there is no point in transferring it. There also is some similarity to the following species.

f. "**Flexibacter chinensis**" Qinsheng, Shanghao and Dasi 1984, 7.
chi.nen′sis. M.L. adj. *chinensis* Chinese (erroneously spelled chinenses in the original description).

Slender flexible rods, 0.4-0.5 × 4-16 μm; in liquid media they are usually >60 μm long; gliding. Cell mass on agar media pink, later becoming orange and, on the third day, colorless. Colonies with a pale iridescence. Facultative anaerobe. Peptones, casamino acids, NH_4^+, or NO_3^- may serve as sole nitrogen source. Various sugars are metabolized with acid production. Starch is degraded but not cellulose, CMC, chitin, agar or gelatin. NO_3^- is reduced. No halotolerance. Optimum temperature: around 30°C. Resistant to actinomycin D, polymyxin B and E, mito-mycin C, erythromycin, neomycin and chloramphenicol. One strain, isolated from a mat of freshwater cyanobacteria in China.

The mol% G + C of the DNA is 34 (T_m).

Type strain: FCA, deposited at the Institute of Hydrobiology of the Academia Sinica at Wuhan but not available outside of China.

Its morphology and its low G + C content seem to exclude this organism from *Flexibacter*. It may be related to *F. canadensis*.

A thorough comparative study with other relevant species would be essential before its exact taxonomic position can be assessed. Also, the taxon cannot be accepted before the type strain is generally accessible.

Genus **Microscilla** Pringsheim 1951, 140, emend. Lewin 1969, 194[AL]

H. REICHENBACH

Mic.ro.scil′la. Gr. adj. *micros* small; L. n. *oscillum* swing; M.L. fem. n. *Microscilla* small swinging organism.

Long thin flexible threadlike rods usually measuring from 10 to >100 μm. **Motile by gliding. Cell mass** more or less intensely **orange or yellow.**

Strictly aerobic chemoorganotrophs. All grow on peptones as sole source of nitrogen. Chitin and cellulose are not attacked, but other polysaccharides including carboxymethyl cellulose (CMC) may be decomposed.

Marine, from coastal habitats. Do not grow below half-strength seawater (only some strains of *M. tractuosa* tolerate lower salt concentrations).

The **mol% G + C of the DNA is 37–44** (Bd).

Type species: *Microscilla marina* Pringsheim 1951, 140.

Further Descriptive Information

Virtually nothing has been added to our knowledge of these organisms since their original description (Pringsheim, 1951; Fager, 1969; Lewin, 1969; Lewin and Lounsbery, 1969). Their characterization is fragmentary, and in attempting to name a new isolate it is therefore indispensable to compare the latter carefully with the type strains of the *Microscilla* spp., which fortunately are all still available. In particular, next to nothing is published about the morphological details of the organisms. Only Pringsheim, in his description of *M. marina*, mentions that the thread cells were only 0.5-0.6 μm wide and, although they became >100 μm long, showed no segmentation. These thread cells were extremely agile, swiftly gliding, bending and twisting, exactly as described for *Flexibacter*. On agar media with low nutrient content, large delicate swarm colonies developed, with tongues at the edge, consisting of a fine network of widely separated thread cells with denser local aggregates in between. All strains are pigmented; the pigments are cell-bound and appear to be carotenoids. Their identification with saproxanthin and zeaxanthin seems to rest entirely on a comparison of electron spectra and chromatographic data (Lewin and Lounsbery, 1969). A chemical char-acterization was not published for any of the organisms treated below.

All *Microscilla* strains grow on full-strength seawater, and only a few tolerate salt concentrations below half-strength seawater. Usually, inorganic nitrogen seems insufficient as sole nitrogen source, but all strains grow on peptones, and many also grow on simpler organic nitrogen compounds such as glutamate. Most utilize glucose, apparently with the exception of *M. marina;* some also are stimulated by acetate. Polysaccharides may or may not be degraded; those which are, are typically found in marine environments. All species appear to be strict aerobes. The optimum temperature seems to be 25-30°C in all cases.

Enrichment and Isolation Procedures

The microscillas live in coastal sediments and on and in between marine plant material. From these sources they can be obtained as described for *Flexibacter*, except that seawater media have to be used. Artificial seawater is sufficient for their cultivation. All described species have been grown in pure culture on media containing 0.1-0.5% of a peptone, e.g. tryptone (Difco), and 0.1-0.5% yeast extract (Difco). The higher concentrations may not be suitable for all strains, e.g. Pringsheim's *M. marina* was inhibited at concentrations of >0.2%. Glucose (0.5%) or acetate (0.1%) may have an enhancing effect.

Maintenance Procedures

The microscillas appear not to be particularly delicate. On lean media, cultures may stay alive for several weeks; on rich media, they may die within 1 week. Suspended in 0.5% tryptone-0.5% yeast extract-seawater medium, all tested strains survived freezing in liquid nitrogen for at least 1 year (Sanfilippo and Lewin, 1970). In this case, 10% glycerol was added as cryoprotective, but DMSO (10%) was tolerated equally well, and the additives may not even be required. Most strains also survived storage at −22°C for at least 5 months.

Differentiation of the genus **Microscilla** from other genera

Microscilla is the marine counterpart to *Flexibacter*, from which it is distinguished by its generally absolute dependence on seawater. It differs from the marine *Cytophaga*-like bacteria (CLB) in its much longer (from 10 to >100 μm) fine, flexible and, at least in some species, very agile threads. The color of the cell mass for flexibacters is usually more orange than that for the CLB, and flexibacters have a somewhat higher mol% G + C of the DNA (37-44) than do the CLB.

Taxonomic Comments

The genus *Microscilla* was created by Pringsheim (1951) for actively gliding organisms which produce narrow trichomes without perceptible septation. Besides the marine type species, *M. marina*, two freshwater species were also included. They would be regarded as *Flexibacter* species under the present concept but must, in fact, be given up as invalid (see *Flexibacter*). Pringsheim himself realized the close relationship between Soriano's *Flexibacter* and the *Microscilla* but made no effort to distinguish between the two in his genus definition. Pringsheim's strains are no longer available.

The genus was later revived by Lewin (1969) during his effort to bring order into a vast assembly of strange, mainly marine bacteria. The definition was emended, and the following characteristics were considered to be in common with *Flexibacter:* "Flexible but not helical rods or filaments . . . 1 μm or less in width; crosswalls not apparent . . .; not branched or sheathed; without flagella; . . . gliding . . .; Gram negative; without photosynthetic pigments or intracellular sulfur granules; unable to attack cellulose. . . ." The following characteristics were considered to be specific for *Microscilla:* "Filaments usually 20–100 μm or longer; color . . . yellow or orange; do not digest cellulose or agar, although some liquefy alginate and gelatin. Habitat: marine shores." Five new species and a variant were added to *M. marina*. Lewin's *M. marina* may not be identical with Pringsheim's species of this name. As Pringsheim's strain is no longer available, the neotype strain of *M. marina* may serve as the type strain of the genus.

The essential point in Lewin's definition is the restriction of the genus to marine organisms, because otherwise there is hardly a difference from *Flexibacter*. This concept is followed in the genus definition presented here, as it appears reasonable to assume that, in general, marine and terrestrial organisms are well-separated. However, both definitions very probably do not delimit a genus of phylogenetically related organisms. Thus, the occurrence of strains with a very low mol% G + C of the DNA of around 30 is suspicious. The present concept therefore restricts the genus to organisms with a mol% G + C of the DNA of above 37, again approaching *Flexibacter*. As with *Flexibacter* and *Cytophaga*, degradation of certain polysaccharides is not regarded as an essential characteristic of the genus *Microscilla*. In this respect, the former definition was not strictly followed as, for example, "*M. furvescens*" is reported to attack agar. In summary, it is obvious that too little is known about the bacteria classified as *Microscilla* (and *Flexibacter*). Probably, the phenetic analysis on which the species are based, did not define reliable taxa. A thorough comparative study on the available strains, preferentially under addition of newly isolated organisms and including modern molecular taxonomy, is the prerequisite for progress in this field.

Differentiation of the species of the genus **Microscilla**

The distinguishing characteristics of the species of the genus *Microscilla* are compiled in Table 23.11. Several more species are of uncertain affiliation. As type strains are available for all of them, they are described as *species incertae sedis*.

List of species of the genus **Microscilla**

1. **Microscilla marina** Pringsheim 1951, 140, emend. Lewin 1969, 201.[AL]

ma.ri′na. L. adj. *marinus* of the sea, marine.

Threads may become very long, >150 μm, but exact morphological description of the neotype strain is lacking. For morphological details of the original Pringsheim strain, see above. This species appears to utilize lactose, but not glucose or galactose. Other distinguishing characteristics are listed in Table 23.11.

Only one strain, isolated from the outflow of the marine aquarium in La Jolla, California.

The mol% G + C of the DNA is 42 (Bd).

Type strain: ATCC 23134 (S10-8 Lewin).

2. "**Microscilla aggregans**" Lewin 1969, 197. (Flexibacter aggregans (Lewin 1969) Leadbetter 1974, 106.[AL])

ag′gre.gans. L. v. *aggregare* to flock or band together; L. pres. part. *aggregans* assembling, aggregating.

Long flexible threads, 0.5 × 20 to >100 μm; further morphological details are not reported. Various sugars are metabolized; some strains also utilize acetate and glycerol. Further distinguishing characteristics are listed in Table 23.11.

It must be doubted that the five strains assigned to this species by phenotype analysis (Fager, 1969; Lewin, 1969; Lewin and Lounsbery, 1969) really belong together, for they cover a mol% G + C range of 37–42 and also vary in several characteristics. In addition, a variant is described, var. *catalatica* Lewin 1969, 197 (type strain ATCC 23190 (HI-3 Lewin)) which is the only *Microscilla* strain with a positive catalase reaction. It further differs from the other *M. aggregans* strains in its particularly low mol% G + C (35), in a relatively low maximum temperature (30°C), in H_2S production and in its inability to metabolize any of the tested sugars and to grow on a nitrogen source other than peptone. It is doubtful that this organism belongs in this species.

All strains come from marine sand samples collected at widely separated places; the type strain is from a beach in Ghana.

Table 23.11.
Differential characteristics of the species of the genus **Microscilla**[a]

Characteristic	1. *M. marina*	2. "*M. aggregans*"	3. "*M. furvescens*"	4. "*M. sericea*"	5. "*M. tractuosa*"
Length of threads (μm)	>150	20->100	10–50	30->100	5->50
Color of cells mass	Orange	Yellow	Orange	Orange	Orange
Main carotenoid[b]	Saproxanthin	Zeaxanthin	Saproxanthin	Saproxanthin	Saproxanthin
Salinity range (S[c])	1–2	½–2	•	½–2	0–2[d]
Maximum temperature (°C)	30–35	35–45	•	30–35	30–45
Suitable as sole nitrogen source					
Peptones	+	+	+	+	+
Casamino acids	±	+	+	−	+
Glutamate	−	+	+	−	+
NO_3^-	−	±	+	−	−
Utilization of glucose	−	+	+	+	+
Degradation of					
Gelatin	+	−	+	+	±
Starch	−	−	+	+	±
Alginate	−	−	+	+	−
CMC	−	±	+	−	−
Agar	−	−	+	−	∓
NO_3^- reduced	−	−	−	−	∓
Mol% G + C of DNA	•	37–42	•	38–39	35–40
Mol% G + C of DNA of type strain	42	37	44	39	37

[a]Symbols: •, no information available; +, 90% or more of strains are positive; ±, most strains are positive; −, 90% or more of strains are negative; and ∓, most strains are negative.

[b]Type of carotenoids inferred from electron spectra of crude extracts and chromatographic data (Lewin and Lounsbery, 1969).

[c]Expressed as manifolds of seawater (S); 0 = freshwater.

[d]Some strains do not grow below ½ S.

The mol% G + C of the DNA of the type strain is 37 (Bd).
Type strain: ATCC 23165 (NN-13 Lewin).

3. **"Microscilla furvescens"** Lewin 1969, 201.

fur.ves′cens. L. adj. *furvus* pitch black, dark; M.L. pres. part. *furvescens* becoming black.

Long threads, 10–50 μm, morphology not described in detail. Various sugars are utilized; acetate is not. This species excels in degrading organic polymers. Further distinguishing characteristics are listed in Table 23.11.

One strain, isolated from marine sand from Samoa.

The mol% G + C of the DNA is 44 (Bd).

Type strain: ATCC 23129 (TV-2 Lewin).

4. **"Microscilla sericea"** Lewin 1969, 201.

se.ri′cea. L. adj. *sericus* made of silk, silken; M.L. adj. *sericeus* silklike, silky.

Long threads, 30 to >100 μm, morphology not described in detail. Various sugars and glycerol are utilized. For further distinguishing characteristics, see Table 23.11.

Two strains, isolated from the outflow of the marine aquarium in La Jolla, California.

The mol% G + C of the DNA is 38 and, for the type strain, 39 (Bd).

Type strain: ATCC 23182 (SIO-7 Lewin).

5. **"Microscilla tractuosa"** Lewin 1969, 199. (*Flexibacter tractuosus* (Lewin) Leadbetter 1974, 106.[AL])

trac.tu.o′sa. L. v. *trahere* to draw, drag; perf. part. *tractus* drawing, dragging; M.L. adj. *tractuosus* drawn or clumped together.

Threads 0.5 × 10 to >50 μm, morphological details not reported. Most strains, including the type strain, tolerate freshwater. Usually sugars and glycerol are utilized; a few strains reduce NO_3^-. Further distinguishing characteristics are compiled in Table 23.22.

The mol% G + C of the DNA of the eight strains attributed to the species varies between 35 and 40; these strains also differ in several other characteristics, and may not all belong together.

All strains have been isolated from coastal sediments all around the world, the type strain comes from Vietnam.

The mol% G + C of the DNA of the type strain is 37 (Bd).

Type strain: ATCC 23168 (H-43 Lewin).

Species Incertae Sedis

a. **"Microscilla arenaria"** Lewin 1969, 197.

a.re.na′ria. L. adj. *arenarius* coming from or living on sand.

Threads becoming >20 μm long, further morphological details not reported. Cell mass orange, supposedly due to saproxanthin.

Does not grow at salt concentrations below half-strength seawater. Peptones or casamino acids serve as sole nitrogen source, various sugars, acetate and lactate are utilized. Degrades CMC, starch and alginate but does not attack agar and gelatin. Catalase-negative. Produces H_2S. Does not reduce NO_3^-. Maximum temperature: 30–35°C.

Only one strain, isolated from marine sand in Mexico.

The mol% G + C of the DNA is 32.5 (Bd).

Type strain: ATCC 23161 (HJ-1 Lewin).

In the relatively unspecific characteristics used for classifying *Microscilla,* this organism resembles the genus, but its low G + C content makes it unlikely it belongs to the genus.

b. **Flexibacter litoralis** Lewin 1969, 199.[AL]

li.to.ra′lis. L. adj. *litoralis* from the shore.

Threads 0.5–0.7 × >180 μm, agile, gliding and bending, apparently without cross-walls. Cells mass is brick-red, supposedly due to flexixanthin.

Does not grow at salt concentrations below half-strength seawater. Only peptones serve as sole nitrogen source; this organism requires many amino acids and thiamine. Sugars and organic acids are not utilized. Starch and gelatin are degraded; agar, alginate and CMC are not. Catalase-negative. No H_2S production or NO_3^- reduction. Maximum temperature: 30–35°C.

Only one strain, isolated from the outflow of the marine aquarium in La Jolla, California.

The mol% G + C of the DNA is 31 (Bd).

Type strain: ATCC 23117 (SIO-4 Lewin).

Because of its dependence on seawater and its low G + C content, the organism does not fit *Flexibacter;* the latter characteristic also excludes it from *Microscilla.*

c. **Flexibacter polymorphus** Lewin 1974, 393.[AL]

po.ly.mor′phus. Gr. adj. *polys* many; Gr. n. *morphe* form, shape; M.L. adj. *polymorphus* of many shapes, variable in form.

Long flexible filaments, 1.1 μm wide and up to several hundred μm long, with cross-walls 3.5–7 μm apart. The cross-walls are recognizable under the phase-contrast microscope, the cells may be separated by mild lysozyme digestion. In media containing 0.1% $NaHCO_3$, much finer and shorter filaments, 0.6 × 10–40 μm, in addition to the long ones, appear. The long filaments tend to form loose but regular left-handed helices. At a pH above 8, the cells contain optically refractile granules, presumably some lipid material. Sometimes, inflated and branched filaments also do occur. The fine structure of the cell envelope has been studied in considerable detail (Ridgway and Lewin, 1973, 1983; Ridgway et al., 1975; Ridgway, 1977a). The outer membrane of the otherwise conventional Gram-negative cell wall is covered by a dense layer of goblet-shaped structures, each apparently consisting of five morphological subunits and four different proteins. The proteins seem not to contain polysaccharide. The goblets may be a pore apparatus for the extrusion of a fibrillar polymer, presumably polysaccharide, which seems to be required for the attachment of the organism to the substrate surface. The filaments are very actively gliding with speeds up to 12 μm/s (23°C). Experiments with inhibitors of energy metabolism suggest that ATP is not involved in generating the mechanical energy (Ridgway, 1977b). The cell mass is orange, due to a light-induced carotenoid.

The salinity range is 20–75°/$_{oo}$. Tryptone, casamino acids or glutamic acid may serve as sole nitrogen source, but NH_4^+ or NO_3^- does not. An additional C source such as glucose is not required, but cobalamine is needed. The organism grows without problems on fully defined media on the basis of glucose with artificial seawater. *F. polymorphus* is relatively delicate. Cultures autolyze within a few days at 25°C and have to be transferred in short intervals (e.g. 3 days at 23°C). Cellulose, starch, agar, alginate and gelatin are not digested. Catalase and H_2S production are negative. Maximum temperature: above 32°C; faster growth occurs at 32°C (generation time: 2 h) than at 22°C (generation time: 6 h), but cultures are more stable at lower temperatures. The pH range for growth is 7–8.5.

One strain, isolated from a *Beggiatoa* mat on a decaying ascidian, off Baja California.

The mol% G + C of the DNA is 29 (Bd).

Type strain: ATCC 27820.

Its dependence on seawater media, the width of the filaments, their multicellular nature, and the very low G + C content exclude this organism from the genus *Flexibacter,* with the latter three characteristics from *Microscilla.*

Genus **Chitinophaga** *Sangkhobol and Skerman 1981, 285ᵛᵖ*

V. B. D. SKERMAN

Chi.ti.no′pha.ga. M.L. n. *chitinum* chitin; Gr. v. *phagein* to devour; M.L. fem. n. *Chitinophaga* chitin destroying.

Flexible rods with rounded ends, 0.5–0.8 μm × ~40 μm when fully developed (Fig. 23.45*A, left side*). Occur singly. **A resting stage (microcyst), 0.8–0.9 μm in diameter, is formed** but is not highly refractile (Figs. 23.45*C* and 23.46). **Macroscopic fruiting bodies are not formed. Motile by gliding and flexing. Gram-negative, aerobic.** Optimum temperatures: 23–24°C; maximum: 37–40°C; minimum: 10–12°C. Optimum pH of growth: 7; maximum: 8–10; minimum: 4.

Chemoorganotrophic, oxidative or fermentative. Acid but no gas produced from some carbohydrates. **Chitin is hydrolyzed, but cellulose and agar are not.** Congo red is not absorbed. Cell masses are yellow.

The mol% G + C of the DNA is 43–46 (T_m).

Type species: *Chitinophaga pinensis* Sangkhobol and Skerman 1981, 285.

Further Descriptive Information

Growth of the organisms on an unsupplemented lake water medium of low nutritional status is thin spreading and apparently colorless. Pigment is visible in masses of cells scraped from the medium. In the central area of the colony the cells transform to a mass of poorly refractile spherical microcysts. Growth on chitin agar is more copious, and colonies do not spread to the same extent as on the lake water medium.

Enrichment and Isolation Procedures

Although it is a popular practice to attempt to enrich populations by growth on specific substrates, the strains of *Chitinophaga* were all isolated by inoculation of water samples from the littoral zones of freshwater lakes and creeks onto a medium prepared by the addition of 1.5% of an optically clear agar to lake water which had been freed of optically visible particles by filtration through an 0.45-μm membrane filter. The pH was not adjusted. The medium was sterilized at 121°C for 15 min.

This medium contains adequate nutrients for the development of mi-

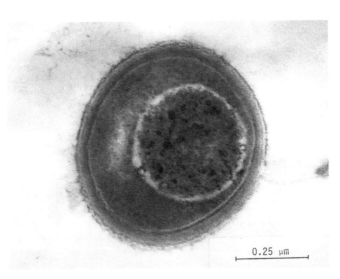

Figure 23.46. Thin section of the microcyst of *C. pinensis* UQM 2036. (Reproduced with permission from V. Sangkhobol and V. B. D. Skerman, International Journal of Systemic Bacteriology *31:* 285–293, 1981, ©International Union of Microbiological Societies.)

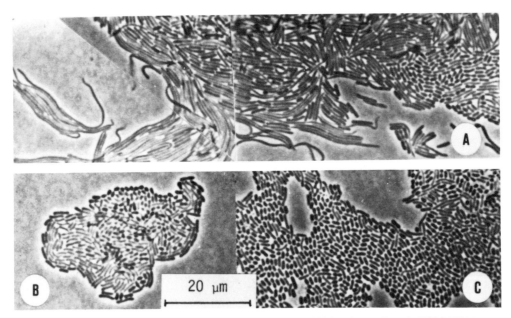

Figure 23.45. Transition from the filamentous gliding cells of *Chitinophaga pinensis* UQM 2034 to myxospores on lake water peptone-yeast extract agar. *A,* various stages, from the long filamentous cells found at the margin of a band of growth to stages immediately preceding the formation of spherical myxospores. *B* and *C,* advanced stages in which some spherical myxospores and some short rods in the final stage of division are visible. In *B* is shown also an isolated microcolony near the center of a band of growth where competition between numerous small colonies forced an early transition to myxospores. Long filaments are no longer visible. (Reproduced with permission from V. Sangkhobol and V. B. D. Skerman, International Journal of Systematic Bacteriology *31:* 285–293, 1981, ©International Union of Microbiological Societies.)

crocolonies of most organisms which constitute the resident populations of freshwaters. Supplementation tends to produce overgrowth that makes isolation more difficult.

The medium is inoculated by allowing ~0.05 ml to flow across the surface of the medium which is then exposed at 22°C for 10 min in a sterile chamber to remove surface moisture and thereby limit the spread of motile cells.

Petri dish cultures are examined periodically from ~8 to 24 h by using a × 10 phase objective, and typical gliding filaments are isolated with a microloop (Skerman, 1968) before overgrowth of colonies of other microorganisms occurs. Without a doubt, initial enrichment in a chitin-supplemented medium would enhance the development of the cells, but it could conceivably enhance other chitin-hydrolyzing bacteria at the expense of the slower growing *Chitinophaga* cells.

Selected cells are transferred to a lake water agar supplemented with

0.01% peptone (Difco) and 0.01% yeast extract (Difco) which supports more luxuriant growth. Cultures are stored on casitone-yeast extract agar (CYEA) containing 0.5% casitone (Difco), 0.3% yeast extract (Difco), 0.1% magnesium sulfate and 1.5% agar (Difco).

Maintenance Procedures

Cultures may be preserved by lyophilization or by liquid nitrogen storage. For lyophilization, cultures grown on CYEA for 48 h at 22°C are suspended in *Mist Desiccans* containing (per liter distilled water): Bacto peptone (Difco), 12 g; and glucose, 30 g (Greaves, 1956), freeze-dried, and stored in ampuls under oxygen-free nitrogen at 4°C. For liquid nitrogen storage, cells from CYEA are suspended to a density of 10^9 cells/ml in filtered lake water containing 10% glycerol. This suspension, distributed and sealed in 0.5-ml amounts in 0.7-ml ampuls is precooled to −20°C for 2 h before storage in liquid nitrogen.

Differentiation of the genus **Chitinophaga** from other genera of unicellular gliding organisms

Some characteristics by which the genus *Chitinophaga* may be differentiated from other genera of unicellular gliding organisms are given in Table 23.12 It seems clear from the data on the mol% G + C of the DNA that the genus *Lysobacter* bears little relationship to the other genera. Within the latter the roughly similar ranges of the mol% G + C of the DNA give no clue of the distribution of G + C in the DNA molecules. Any attempt at further definition of the relationships between these genera must await more critical evidence, particularly the composition of the 16S rRNA. For the moment it appears that the genus *Chitinophaga* may find a place in the family *Cytophagaceae*, but there seems little merit in

the inclusion in the same family of the genera *Saprospira* and *Herpetosiphon* or in the inclusion in the family *Cytophagaceae* of multicellular gliding organisms of the order *Cytophagales*, as was done in the eighth edition of the *Manual*.

Further Comments

Five strains of the single species have been isolated from widely separated localities in Australia. They differed only in some minor properties and are combined into one species *Chitinophaga pinensis*

List of species of the genus **Chitinophaga**

1. **Chitinophaga pinensis** Sangkhobol and Skerman 1981, 285.[VP] pi′nen.sis. M.L. n. *pinus* genus of pine trees; M.L. adj. *pinensis* pertaining to pines.

Cell morphology and properties as for the genus. The combined characteristics for the five strains are given in Table 23.13.
Type strain: UQM 2034 (DSM 2588; NCTC 11800).

Table 23.12.
Some characteristics differentiating the genus **Chitinophaga** *from other genera of unicellular gliding organisms*[a]

Characteristic	Lysobacter	Cytophaga	Flexibacter	Capnocytophaga	Sporocytophaga	Chitinophaga
Production of fruiting bodies	−	−	−	−	−	−
Production of myxospores (microcysts)	−	−	−	−	+	+
Hydrolysis of						
Agar	−	+	−	−	Etching	−
Chitin	+	−	−	?	−	+
Cellulose	−	±	−	?	+	−
Catalase	+	±	−	−	+	+
Length (~μm)	Varied	10	5–100	2.5–4.2	5–8	≤40
Mol% G + C of DNA	65–70	33–42	31–43	33–41	36	43–45
Require 10% CO_2 for growth	−	−	−	+	−	−

[a]Symbols: −, negative; +, positive; ?, characteristic unknown; and ±, different species give different reactions.

Table 23.13.
Morphological and physiological characteristics of strains of **Chitinophaga pinensis**[a]

Characteristic	UQM 2034	UQM 2035	UQM 2036	UQM 2037	UQM 2096	Sporocytophaga myxococcoides UQM 1962
Dimensions in µm of vegetative cells						
Length	40	40	40	40	40	5–8
Diameter	0.5–0.8	0.5–0.8	0.5–0.8	0.5–0.8	0.5–0.8	0.3–0.6
Microcyst diameter (µm)	0.8–0.9	0.8–0.9	0.8–0.9	0.8–0.9	0.8–0.9	1.0–1.5
Rounded cell ends	+	+	+	+	+	+
Yellow pigment[b]	+	+	+	+	+	
Gram stain	−	−	−	−	−	−
Gliding	+	+	+	+	+	+
EDS[c] growth in broth	+	+	+	+	+	No growth
Generation time (h)[d]	16		15.75			
Physiological characteristics						
Grows aerobically	+	+	+	+	+	+
Temperature range for growth (°C)	12–40	10–37	10–39	10–37	10–39	
Optimum temperature (°C)	24	23	24	23	24	30
pH range	4–10	4–10	4–8	4–10	4–8	
Salt tolerance (%)	0.0–1.5	0.0–2.0	0.0–2.0	0.0–2.0	0.0–1.0	
Biochemical characteristics						
Hydrolysis of						
Chitin	+	+	+	+	+	−
Cellulose	−	−	−	−	−	+
Starch	−	−	−	−	−	
Alginate	−	−	−	−	−	
Agar	−	−	−	−	−	Agar etching
Casein	+	+	+	+	+	−
Gelatin liquefaction	+	+	+	+	+	
Phenylalanine deaminase	−	−	−	−	−	−
Tryptophan deaminase	−	−	−	−	−	
Nitrate reduction	−	−	−	−	−	
Urease test	+	+	+	+	+	
Oxidative and fermentative production of acid from carbohydrates[e]						
Glucose	Slow, oxidative	Slow, oxidative	Fermentative	Fermentative	Slow, oxidative	
Lactose	Slow, oxidative	Slow, oxidative	Fermentative	Fermentative	Slow, oxidative	
Sucrose	Slow, oxidative	Slow, oxidative	Fermentative	Fermentative	Slow, oxidative	
Miscellaneous biochemistry						
Catalase	+	+	+	+	+	+
Oxidase	−	−	−	−	−	−
H$_2$S production	−	−	−	−	−	
Indole production	−	−	−	−	−	
Congo red adsorption	−	−	−	−	−	
DNA hydrolysis	−	−	−	−	−	
Hemolysis of horse red blood cells	+	+	+	+	+	
Benzidine test for iron porphyrins	+	+	+	+	+	
Lipase–Tween 80	+	+	+	+	+	
Lipase–Tween 40	+	+	+	+	+	
Lipase–Tween 20	+	+	+	+	+	
Antibiotic resistance						
Tetracycline (10 µg)	S	S	S	S	S	
Streptomycin (10 µg)	S	S	S	S	S	
Neomycin (10 µg)	R	R	R	R	R	
Kanamycin (30 µg)	R	R	R	R	R	

Table 23.13.—*continued*

Characteristic	UQM 2034	UQM 2035	UQM 2036	UQM 2037	UQM 2096	*Sporocytophaga myxococcoides* UQM 1962
Penicillin G (4 units)	R	R	R	R	R	
Erythromycin (5 µg)	R	R	R	R	R	
Chloramphenicol (25 µg)	S	S	S	S	S	
Sodium lauryl sulfate tolerance						
0.01%	R	R	R	R	R	
0.1%	S	S	S	S	S	
Ability to lyse cells of						
Escherichia coli	–	–	–	–	–	
Pseudomonas aeruginosa	–	–	–	–	–	
Bacillus subtilis	–	–	–	–	–	
Staphylococcus aureus	+	+	+	+	+	
Micrococcus lysodeikticus (INV)[f]	–	–	–	–	–	
Mol% G + C of DNA (T_m)	44.58 ± 0.94	45.47 ± 0.37	43.82 ± 0.70	42.92 ± 0.20	43.80 ± 0.28	

[a]Data are taken from Tables 2 and 3 of the article by Sangkhobol and Skerman in the *International Journal of Systematic Bacteriology* (*31:* 285–243, 1981, ©International Union of Microbiological Societies). Symbols: +, positive; –, negative; S, susceptible; and R, resistant.
[b]Yellow color matches color harmony chip 3ga.
[c]EDS, easily dispersible sediment.
[d]On lake water-peptone-yeast extract agar at 22°C.
[e]Observation period of 3 weeks.
[f]INV, invalid name.

Genus *Saprospira* Gross 1911, 202[AL]

H. REICHENBACH

Sap.ro.spi′ra. Gr. adj. *sapros* rotten, putrid; Gr. n. *spira* a spiral; M.L. fem. n. *Saprospira* spiral associated with decaying matter.

Helical filaments, multicellular, unbranched and without sheaths, 10–500 µm long, filaments 0.5–3 µm wide. Length of cells 1.5–5.5 µm. Gram-negative. **Move by gliding** in longitudinal direction; simultaneously the screws rotate around their long axes. Resting stages not known. Colonies often have a regular pattern of stripes. **Strictly aerobic organotrophs** requiring amino acid mixtures, peptones or proteins as nitrogen source and often, perhaps always, as carbon and energy sources. Most strains are pigmented: pink, yellow, orange or brick-red. Aquatic organisms living in bottom sediments in marine and freshwater environments.

The mol% G + C of the DNA is 33–48 (Bd, T_m).

Type species: *Saprospira grandis* Gross 1911, 202.

Further Descriptive Information

The saprospiras have rarely been studied, and relatively few strains have been grown in pure culture. Consequently, little information is available. The helices of *Saprospira* are rather lax and are usually coiled dextrally; their width is 1.5–2.5 (to 9) µm, and their pitch, 2–10 (to 40) µm. Both characteristics are somewhat variable within one (the same) culture, but particularly under different culture conditions. The filaments may even completely uncoil and then become nonmotile. Uncoiling is common in liquid cultures and in chamber cultures under space limitation and may be irreversible. The length of the screws depends to a considerable extent on the culture conditions; the screws are usually much (3 times and more) longer in liquid culture than on agar plates. In contrast to the dimensions of the helices, the diameter of the filaments seems to be a rather constant feature for each strain. The helices move by gliding, with speeds of up to 180 µm/min. The end cells of the filaments are rounded. There seems to be no polarity within the filament. The cells divide along the entire length of the filament, independently from one another and without apparent pattern. The filaments multiply by breaking somewhere, probably at sites where by chance an individual cell has died, forming a necridium. In slide mounts the helices become rather fragile, particularly when taken from a shake culture, often disintegrating after a short time through spheroplast formation of the cells. Gross (1911) mentioned the appearance in aging cultures of "spores": The cells round up, concomitantly decreasing in diameter, and develop thick walls, and the filament disintegrates into short cylindrical units. Gross did not observe germination of these "spores," nor have other investigators corroborated thus far the phenomenon. In old chamber cultures of *S. grandis* the ends of the filaments often develop into large optically refractile bulbs 1.4–3 µm in diameter (Reichenbach, 1980; Reichenbach and Dworkin, 1981c). The meaning of these structures is not clear. Possibly they result merely from a degeneration of the end cells. Terminal but dark inflations of up to 5 µm in diameter have also been described for "*S. flammula*" (Lewin, 1965b).

The nutritional requirements of all *Saprospira* species are complex. All strains studied in pure culture depend on organic nitrogen in the form of amino acid mixtures, e.g. casamino acids, peptones or proteins. Vitamins and, sometimes, unknown growth factors present in yeast extract, yeast nucleic acid hydrolysate or tryptone (Difco), a tryptic digest of casein, may be required. Only "*S. thermalis*" and "*S. toviformis*" grow on casamino acids and minerals without supplements. The addition of carbon and energy sources usually has no stimulatory effect. However, "*S. toviformis*" utilizes lactate, *S. thermalis* utilizes glucose and glycerol, and some strains of *S. grandis* respond favorably to acetate, glucose or galactose. Cellulose, alginate, agar and chitin are generally not degraded, but starch is hydrolyzed by "*S. thermalis*," and carboxymethyl cellulose, by

"*S. toviformis*" and some strains of *S. grandis*. All saprospiras liquefy gelatin.

Temperature range for growth: 6–37°C; optimum temperature usually 30–35°C; for "*S. toviformis*" it is 25°C. Optimum pH: around 7. Light has no growth-promoting effect.

Most saprospiras grow well on solid media and in liquid media; slow-growing "*S. albida*" prefers semisolid media (0.25% agar). On solid substrates with relatively high nutrient content the colonies remain rather small, round and convex; at low nutrient concentrations they become flat with flamelike or rhizoidal protrusions. But even the flat colonies tend to remain very moderate in size and do not develop into large thin swarms, as is typical for most gliding bacteria. The colonies, in particular the flat ones, often show a striking pattern of fine stripes, which is due to a strictly parallel arrangement of the filaments with the windings of the screws more or less exactly "in phase." The stripes are formed by the alternating ascending and descending parts of the windings and arise optically through differences in light reflection and scattering. The phenomenon is also observed with other helical organisms such as *Methanospirillum* (Ferry et al., 1974) or *Spirulina*. In liquid media the saprospiras usually grow as silky suspensions; only "*S. toviformis*" grows in clumps. Liquid cultures of "*S. thermalis*" in glucose-containing media become viscous due to slime production (Lewin, 1965a). The marine species grow perfectly well in simplified artificial seawater.

Most saprospiras are more or less brightly colored. The pigments are probably always carotenoids; in the case of *S. grandis* the main pigment (97% of the total) has been shown to be the monocyclic carotene-3,1'-diol, saproxanthin (Aasen and Liaaen-Jensen, 1966a). "*S. albida*" appears colorless, but the cell pellets obtained by centrifugation show a pale pinkish tinge (Lewin, 1965b). The supernatant of liquid cultures of "*S. toviformis*" turns yellow; the chemistry of this phenomenon is not understood (Lewin, 1970).

All *Saprospira* species have been found in aquatic environments; one strain of "*S. albida*" was isolated from soil (Lewin, 1965b), so that it seems that at least the freshwater species may occasionally invade terrestrial habitats. *S. grandis* has been isolated from coastal sediments worldwide and seems to be a very common organism. Saprospiras also inhabit the aerobic parts of sewage plants in fair numbers.

Enrichment and Isolation Procedures

Gross (1911) originally enriched *S. grandis* and "*S. nana*" by filling large dishes with bottom sand and seawater from the Mediterranean and floating cover glasses on the water surface. Overnight, the saprospiras attached themselves firmly to the glass surface. R. A. Lewin (personal communication) has collected them on glass slides immersed at a depth of 1000 m off the coast of California. Other specific enrichment techniques for *Saprospira* species are not known. To isolate these organisms, samples from bottom sediments from the seacoast, rivers or lakes are placed as streaks or spots on the surface of dry low-nutrient agar plates, e.g. seawater agar, perhaps with 0.1% NH_4Cl and 0.002% sodium acetate or with 0.03% casein peptone and 0.01% yeast extract. Corresponding media may be used for freshwater species. The crude cultures are incubated at room temperature or 30°C and checked under a dissecting microscope from time to time for spreading colonies. *Saprospira* colonies may easily be recognized by their stripes. *S. grandis* grows in a very wide temperature range, and it may be favorable to incubate the plates at 6°C. The desired organism grows still reasonably well at this temperature, while the development of contaminants is much restricted. Transfers are made from the crude cultures to increasingly rich media, and finally pure cultures may be obtained by plating of cell suspensions. By that time, other gliding bacteria and agar liquefiers (a serious problem with marine samples) should be eliminated, for otherwise well-separated colonies are not easily obtained. More details about isolation procedures and composition of suitable media may be found in Lewin (1962, 1965b) and in Reichenbach and Dworkin (1981c).

Maintenance Procedures

Cultures of *S. grandis* die within a few days (30°C) or weeks (at room temperature). *S. grandis*, "*S. toviformis*" and some strains of "*S. thermalis*" could be preserved in liquid nitrogen for 1 year; in most cases, addition of 10% glycerol has been essential; "*S. flammula*" and "*S. albida*" did not survive (Sanfilippo and Lewin, 1970). *S. grandis* strain Sa g1 survives for at least 2 years when stored at −80°C in peptone-yeast extract medium (e.g. SP5 liquid medium) (Reichenbach and Dworkin, 1981c). The same strain did not survive drying in skim milk.

Differentiation of the genus **Saprospira** from other genera

Helical multicellular filaments and gliding motility distinguish *Saprospira* from all other genera. Should uncoiled nonmotile strains, as observed in culture, also occur in nature, they would not be recognizable as saprospiras. Straight but gliding filaments from marine habitats, classified as *Microscilla marina*, are perhaps identical with *S. grandis* (Lewin, 1962). From pure cultures of *S. grandis*, stable variants have also been isolated that no longer form filaments but grow as 1–4-celled segments (Lewin, 1962).

Taxonomic Comments

On the basis of the 16S rRNA oligonucleotide pattern of *S. grandis* strain Sa g1, the genus is not closely related to any other bacterium including the cyanobacteria. There may be a very remote relationship with the *Cytophagales* (E. Stackebrandt, personal communication).

Following a proposition of Lewin (1962), nonphototrophic helical multicellular filamentous bacteria with gliding motility are classified in the genus *Saprospira*. The genus had been defined earlier by Gross (1911), and his *S. grandis* is very probably identical with Lewin's strains. Only the "spore" formation described by Gross and included in the species definition of *S. grandis* has not been observed again and had to be discarded from the description. The present taxa rest, of course, on Lewin's more recent and more detailed investigations and his neotype strain. Lewin later described several more species, viz. "*S. thermalis*" (1965a, freshwater), "*S. flammula*" (1965b, freshwater) and "*S. toviformis*" (1970, marine), and revived another old species, "*Spirulina albida*" Kolkwitz (1909), as "*Saprospira albida*" (1965b, freshwater). Although the assumption is supported by correspondences in several morphological and

physiological characteristics, it is not certain whether all these organisms are really related to one another, as no molecular taxonomic data are available. The mol% G + C range of 35–48 would at least not rule out a relatively close relationship. Unfortunately, except for *S. grandis*, the type strains of all species have been lost, so that these species were not included in the Approved Lists of Bacterial Names. However, the organisms have been fairly well characterized, and there is no doubt that they really exist. I list their distinguishing characteristics below to help with their identification if they are isolated again.

Saprospiras seem to have been observed already before Gross (1911) and Kolkwitz (1909). In 1875, van Tieghem collected from the water course of an old mill in Northern France a white scum which, under the microscope, turned out to consist of tightly coiled helical filaments bending and moving by rotating around their long axes. The organism may have been identical with "*S. albida*", and van Tieghem (1880) named it "*Spirulina alba*" because he thought that it was an apochlorotic blue-green alga, as Kolkwitz later assumed for his organism. The idea that there are apochlorotic cyanobacteria has been popular until recently (see, for example, Lewin, 1962; Pringsheim, 1963; Reichenbach, 1981; and Reichenbach and Dworkin, 1981a). In the light of the 16S rRNA data mentioned above and produced for other organisms of this kind, it seems that this concept has to be abandoned.

At about the same time, Warming (1875) observed a very large colorless helical filamentous organism slowly moving through algal mats which he had collected at the Danish coast. He named this organism "*Spirochaete gigantea*," but from his description, particularly of its movements, it seems quite likely that it was a *Saprospira*. This organism appears never to have been observed again. It may be mentioned that Gross, too, mistook his saprospiras for free-living saprophytic spirochetes.

Differentiation of the species of the genus **Saprospira**

In the genus *Saprospira* there is only one acknowledged species, *S. grandis,* but several more species have been described.

Further Information

A scientific film on *S. grandis* is available showing the movements, growth of uncoiled filaments and colony formation (Reichenbach et al., 1975/1976; Reichenbach, 1980).

Their distinguishing characteristics are compiled in Table 23.14.

List of species of the genus **Saprospira**

1. **Saprospira grandis** Gross 1911, 202, emend. Lewin 1962, 560.[AL]

gran′dis. L. adj. *grandis* large.

Helical flexible filaments of constant width, 0.8–0.9 (to 1.2) µm depending on the strain, but variable in length; usually shorter in plate cultures (15–130 µm) than in liquid media (20–500 µm) (Fig. 23.47). The pitch and width of the screws may vary considerably even in one (the same) culture. The filaments may even uncoil entirely during culture (Fig. 23.48). Stable variants have also been reported that grow as single cells or 2–4-celled segments (Lewin, 1962). The filaments are composed of cylindrical cells, 1–5.5 µm long depending on the strain and the culture; within one filament the longest cells are twice as long as the shortest ones. The cross-walls may be difficult to distinguish in young cultures but become well-recognizable in old and drying filaments (Fig. 23.49). End cells of the filaments are rounded.

Colonies on poor media are thin and spreading and remain relatively small, often with a pattern of parallel fine stripes (Figure 23.50). Colonies on rich media are round convex, thick and slimy, relatively small, deep orange to red (Figs. 23.51 and 23.52). In liquid media, *S. grandis* grows in homogeneous suspension; upon shaking, the cultures show a silky appearance. In peptone-yeast extract medium the generation time is 2–2.8 h (at 30°C) (Lewin, 1962, 1972).

The cell mass is orange to red, due to carotenoids, mainly saproxanthin (Aasen and Liaaen-Jensen, 1966a).

Grows on peptones, casamino acids and defined amino acid mixtures; in addition, unknown growth factors, e.g. with yeast extract, have to be supplied. Glucose, galactose, sucrose and acetate are growth stimulatory for some strains. Gelatin is liquefied. Starch, agar, alginate and carboxymethyl cellulose are not decomposed. In litmus milk, coagulation occurs, but acid is not produced, the curd is usually not digested, and litmus is not reduced. Tyrosine is degraded to colored products. H_2S is not produced from cysteine-containing media. Nitrate is not reduced to nitrite. Catalase-negative. Strictly aerobic.

Optimum temperature: 30–37°C; still some strains grow fairly well at 3–6°C. Optimum pH: around 7.

Most strains depend on seawater for growth and tolerate between one-half-strength and double-strength seawater. Some strains are reported to grow on freshwater media also (Lewin and Lounsbery, 1969).

Isolated from sand, mud and decaying organic material collected at seacoasts in temperate and warm climate zones all around the world.

The mol% G + C of the DNA is 46–48 (Bd, T_m).

Neotype strain: ATCC 23119 (WH Lewin).

Species Incertae Sedis

No strains are available for the following organisms. Several of them also have never been studied in pure culture. The descriptions suggest more or less strongly that the organisms exist in nature and belong to the genus *Saprospira* or a similar genus. In most cases, however, their exact specific status has to be established.

a. **"Saprospira nana"** Gross 1911, 202.

A marine organism. Filaments shorter and more delicate than with *S. grandis.* Cells relatively long, often occupying one whole winding of the screw. Therefore the remains of the necridia may form long "beaks" at the ends of the filaments. May fragment to single cells. In liquid cultures, filaments often in thick tufts. Isolated from bottom sand collected in the Mediterranean near Sorrento, Italy.

b. **"Saprospira toviformis"** Lewin and Mandel 1970, 510.

A marine organism, closely resembling *S. grandis* but clearly different from it by the lower mol% G + C, viz. 37 (T_m) to 38 (Bd). It has other distinguishing characteristics. It moves only very slowly. The cell mass is rather yellow-orange. It grows on casamino acids alone and does not require growth factors. Growth is stimulated by lactate but is inhibited by higher concentrations of peptone (1% and more). It grows in clumps in liquid media, and the culture supernatant turns yellow (tryptone-yeast

Table 23.14.

Differential characteristics of the species of the genus **Saprospira**[a]

Characteristic	1. *S. grandis*	a. "*S. nana*"	b. "*S. toviformis*"	c. "*S. gigantea*"	d. "*S. albida*"	e. "*S. thermalis*"	f. "*S. flammula*"
Length of cells (µm)	1–5.5	1.5–3	1–2.5		2–3	2–5	2–3
Diameter of filaments (µm)	0.8–1.2	0.5	0.8	1.5–3	0.8–1.2	1	1
Width of helix (µm)	1.4–2		1.5	5–9	1.5–2	1.5–2.5	1.5
Pitch of helix (µm)	4–10	2.3–3	4–9	25–40	3–7	7–17	3–4
Length of filaments (µm)	6–500	36	10–500	400	10–500	10–500	10–500
Growth factors required	+		−		+	−	+
Starch degraded	−		−		?	+	?
Optimal temperature (°C)	30–37		25		30	35	30 (?)
Color of cell mass	Orange-red		Orange-yellow		Pinkish tinge	Pink	Bright orange
Mol% G + C of DNA	46–48		38		42–47	35–37	48
Habitat	Marine	Marine	Marine	Marine	Freshwater	Freshwater	Freshwater

[a]Symbols: +, 90% or more of strains are positive; −, 90% or more of strains are negative; and ?, no information available.

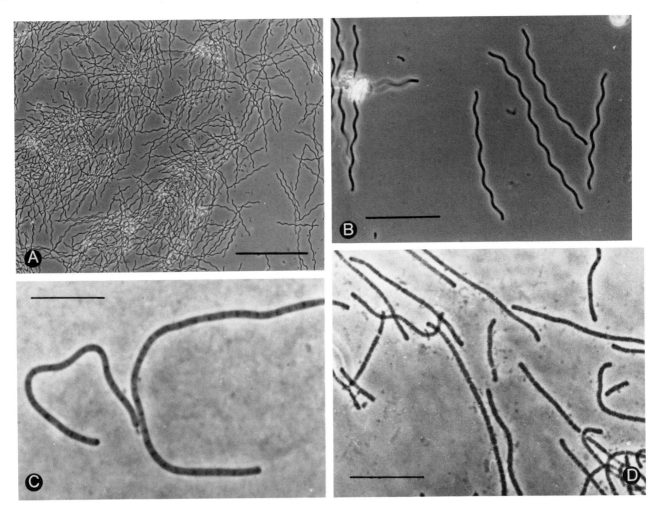

Figure 23.47. *S. grandis* filaments. *A*, filaments from a liquid culture, survey at low magnification. Although the pitch and, particularly, the length of the screws are variable, the width and the diameter of the filaments are essentially constant. Phase contrast. *Bar,* 80 μm. *B*, filaments at higher magnification. Phase contrast. *Bar,* 25 μm. *C*, living fila-ments from an agar culture. At high magnification with an objective of high resolution, the cross-walls become clearly recognizable. Zeiss Axio-mat, phase contrast. *Bar,* 10 μm. *D*, when the slide mount is briefly heated on a flame, the filaments decay into their individual cells. Phase contrast. *Bar,* 15 μm.

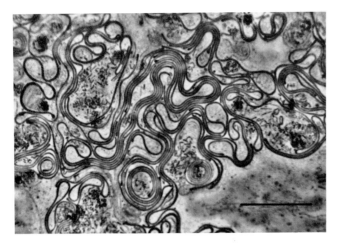

Figure 23.48. *S. grandis* uncoiled filaments on a thin agar layer in a chamber culture. Phase contrast. *Bar,* 50 μm.

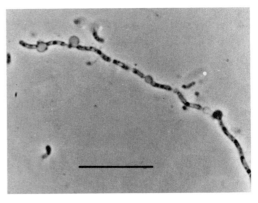

Figure 23.49. *S. grandis* decaying filament with spheroplastlike in-flations and cell-like compartments. Phase contrast. *Bar,* 16 μm.

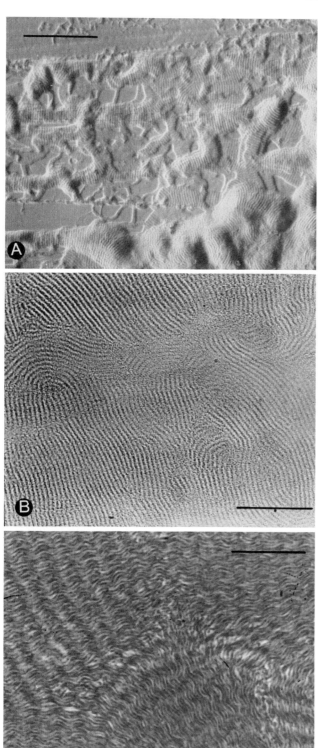

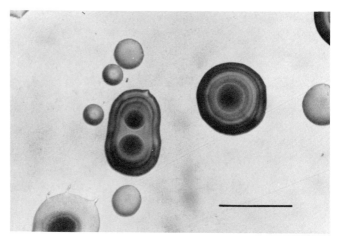

Figure 23.51. *S. grandis* compact colonies on agar medium with "high" peptone content (0.1% peptone from casein + 0.02% yeast extract). Plating of an enrichment culture with *S. grandis* (small smooth colonies) and a spirillum (large colonies with concentric rings). *Bar,* 1200 μm.

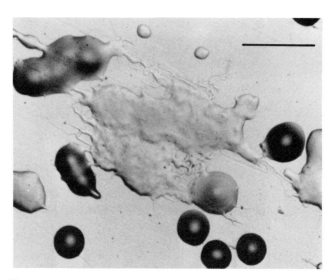

Figure 23.52. *S. grandis* spreading colony on agar medium with "low" peptone content (0.03% peptone from casein + 0.01% yeast extract). Enrichment culture; the round dark colonies are contaminants. *Bar,* 1200 μm.

Figure 23.50. *S. grandis* striped colonies. *A,* spreading colony, survey picture. The gliding filaments preferentially follow scratches in the agar surface produced by the inoculation loop. Oblique illumination. *Bar,* 250 μm. *B,* central part of a large colony. Brightfield. *Bar,* 125 μm. *C,* at high magnification the strict alignment of the filaments becomes recognizable. Phase contrast. *Bar,* 25 μm.

extract medium). It does not tolerate one-half-strength seawater. Optimum temperature: 25°C; the organism fails to grow at 35°C. Obtained from sand collected at a tide pool in Campbell's Bay, New Zealand; one strain only.

c. **"Saprospira gigantea"** (Warming) Reichenbach 1980, 11. (*Spirochaete* [sic] *gigantea* Warming 1875, 374.)

A marine organism which is distinguished by its large dimensions. Long flexible sinistrorotatory helical filaments with truncated ends, moving sluggishly under rotation around its long axis. Without flagella, sulfur granules and pigments. Probably composed of cells, for dead filaments decay into cell-like fragments. Although described as a spirochete, the mentioned characteristics indicate another kind of organism. As it is unpigmented, it seems not to be a *Spirulina*, with which Warming was, of course, well-acquainted. Thus it would be a likely candidate for the genus *Saprospira*. Found repeatedly among oscillatorias and algae at the Danish coast near Copenhagen and at other places.

d. **"Saprospira albida"** (Kolkwitz) Lewin 1962, 561. (*Spirulina alba* van Tieghem 1880, 177. *Spirulina albida* Kolkwitz 1909, 137. *Saprospira flexuosa* Dobell 1912, 137. *Achroonema spiroideum* Skuja 1948, 31.)

A freshwater organism distinguished from all other species by being almost unpigmented. Lewin (1965b) mentions a pale pinkish tinge of the centrifuged cell mass, attributable to small amounts of a nonpolar pigment, presumably carotenoid (R. A. Lewin, personal communication). Organisms of this kind have been described repeatedly, although it is, of course, impossible to decide whether all authors were dealing with the same species. The most detailed description is given by Dobell (1912). Lewin (1965b) is the only author who studied pure cultures and reports biochemical data. His strains depended on complex growth media with growth factors and grew best in semisolid media. The organisms described by Kolkwitz (1909), Dobell (1912) and Lewin (1965b) are quite similar with respect to dimensions and motility. Dobell is in doubt about subdivision of the filaments into cells (as is Kolkwitz) but mentions propagation by simultaneous division into multiple fragments, which obviously suggests a cellular organization. The same kind of multiplication is also described by Gross (1911); still, this seems to be at least not the ordinary way of propagation. Dobell and several other authors report the presence of tiny granules in the cytoplasm which are metachromatic but are not sulfur. The bacterium of van Tieghem (1880) differs in that it is very densely coiled. "*Achroonema spiroideum*" has a lax helix, which is, however, not uncommon for *Saprospira* in liquid media, and moves remarkably fast (600 μm/min) "in the way of *Oscillatoria* and *Spirulina*." Further, the filaments are very delicate (0.3–0.5 μm wide) and consist of rather long (3–15 μm) cells. An organism described by Lauterborn (1916, 408) as "*Pelonema spirale*" from mud collected in *Chara* ponds in the Rhine valley is distinguished by tiny gas vacuoles (?granules) and, according to the genus definition, should be nonmotile. Otherwise it resembles a *Saprospira*. Lewin's strains were obtained from a hot spring (no thermophile!), a fish pond, a small river, and (one strain) soil. The other organisms were found on mud from the bottom of various freshwater bodies, in mats of blue-green bacteria, and in plankton, in Europe and North America. The organism is also quite common in activated sludge.

e. **"Saprospira thermalis"** Lewin 1965a, 139.

A freshwater organism. Differs from *S. albida* by its intense pink color, its growth on casamino acids without additional growth factors, and its much lower mol% G + C. Isolated from a hot spring in Iceland (no thermophile!) and from the banks of a streamlet in Costa Rica.

f. **"Saprospira flammula"** Lewin 1965a, 138.

A freshwater organism. Differs from "*S. albida*" mainly by its bright orange color. Grows better when 0.3% NaCl is added to the medium. Obtained from mud collected in a hot spring in New Zealand (no thermophile!). One strain only. The organism has been surmised to be a freshwater strain of *S. grandis* (Lewin, 1974), but truly marine, i.e. not simply halotolerant, bacteria seem not so easily to adapt to freshwater conditions.

This section may be closed appropriately with the concluding remarks of Dobell from the description of "*S. flexuosa*": "It is to be hoped that now [that] attention has been called to these interesting organisms, other investigators will study them. It is possible that there are many undescribed species inhabiting both fresh and salt water." Hopefully, these investigations will be carried out with more effect.

ORDER II. **LYSOBACTERALES** CHRISTENSEN AND COOK 1978, 372[AL]

PENELOPE CHRISTENSEN

Lys.o.bac.te.ra′les. M.L. masc. n. *Lysobacter* type genus of the order; -*ales* ending to denote an order; M.L. fem. pl. n. *Lysobacterales* the *Lysobacter* order.

Rod-shaped, Gram-negative cells, some of which may be up to 70 μm long, and which are **motile by means of gliding. Fruiting bodies and microcysts are not produced.**

The mol% G + C of the DNA is 65–70 (T_m).

Type genus: *Lysobacter* Christensen and Cook 1978, 372. There is only one family and one genus.

Taxonomic Comments

Early in the history of these investigations, the possibility was raised that these organisms were actually members of the *Myxobacterales* that had lost their ability to fruit. This position has been rejected now that close to 100 freshly isolated strains have been observed and none has ever been seen to produce fruiting bodies when appropriate techniques are used. Other workers believe that the genus *Lysobacter* should be placed as a suborder within the *Cytophagales* (Reichenbach, 1981), a position which would indicate a closer relationship to cytophagas than to the fruiting *Myxobacterales* and which would stress the relative importance of the ability to fruit over the mol% G + C of the DNA. As further gliding bacteria are discovered, so our concept of the whole group broadens. The recently described *Chitinophaga* has a midrange mol% G + C of the

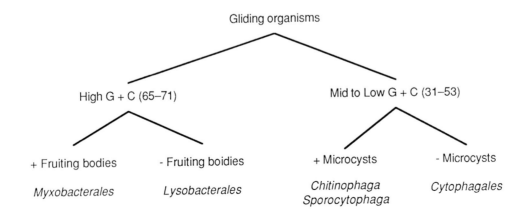

DNA, yet it produces abundant microcysts but no fruiting bodies, and the authors refer to it as a "myxobacter," using this term to cover all slime-forming, gliding bacteria (Sangkhobol and Skerman, 1981.) The mol% G + C of the DNA and the microcysts of *Chitinophaga* are features which resemble those of *Sporocytophaga* (of the *Cytophagales*), although its cell morphology and polysaccharase potential differ from the latter genus. I prefer to use the mol% G + C of the DNA as the primary differentiator, followed by production of fruits or microcysts, providing a classification which produces less confusion, especially for the novice, as indicated in the accompanying figure on page 2082.

All workers in the field agree that much taxonomic work remains to be done, starting with the urgently needed descriptions of the numerous unnamed gliding organisms, many of which probably have ecological significance. Until more of the dramatis personae are known, inevitably the taxonomic boundaries will be poorly constructed, and the *Cytophagales*, in particular, will remain a heterogeneous collection of creatures.

FAMILY I. **LYSOBACTERACEAE** CHRISTENSEN AND COOK 1978, 372[AL]

PENELOPE CHRISTENSEN

Lys.o.bac.te.ra′ce.ae. M.L. masc. n. *Lysobacter* type genus of the family; -*aceae* ending to denote a family; M.L. fem. pl. n. *Lysobacteraceae* the *Lysobacter* family.

Description is the same as for the order.

Type genus: *Lysobacter* Christensen and Cook 1978, 372. There is only one genus.

Genus I. **Lysobacter** *Christensen and Cook 1978, 372*[AL]

PENELOPE CHRISTENSEN

Lys.o.bac′ter. Gr. adj. *lysis* loosing; M.L. n. *bacter* masc. equivalent of Gr. neut. n. *bactrum* a rod; M.L. masc. n. *Lysobacter* the loosing rod; intended to mean the lysing rod.

Thin rods, 0.2–0.5 × 1.0–15 (sometimes up to 70) μm, which are Gram-negative, nonflagellated, **gliding, flexing,** and aerobic. **Colonies are highly mucoid, cream-colored, pink or yellow-brown;** many strains also produce a brown, water-soluble **pigment. Nonfruiting, no microcysts** produced. Growth in broth culture is silky. Most strains are resistant to actinomycin D. This organism **degrades chitin** and often other polysaccharides, but it does not degrade filter-paper cellulose, and it infrequently degrades agar. Strongly proteolytic and characteristically **lyses a variety of microorganisms** (Gram-negative and Gram-positive bacteria including actinomycetes, blue-green and green algae, yeasts and filamentous fungi) and also nematodes.

Habitat: soil and freshwater.

The mol% G + C of the DNA is 65.4–70.1 (T_m).

Type species: *Lysobacter enzymogenes* Christensen and Cook 1978, 374.

Further Descriptive Information

Thin, flexible, gliding, Gram-negative rods, 0.2–0.5 × 1.0–15 (sometimes up to 70) μm (Figs. 23.53–23.55). Colonies are slimy or mucoid, with the rubbery ones of *L. gummosus* being particularly difficult to handle, and are white, cream-colored, yellow, pink or brown; many strains also produce a brown, water-soluble pigment, especially in older cultures. The nature of *Lysobacter* pigments is not known, but they are not carotenoids or flexirubins (Reichenbach et al., 1981.) Colonies of *L. brunescens* spread in the typical *"Cytophaga"* fashion, but those of *L. antibioticus* and *L. enzymogenes* are more mucoid, and it is believed that this conceals the typical spreading. All strains of the latter two species have been observed to produce a thin, advancing fringe of cells at the edge of the colony on one or more media, however. *L. gummosus* has never been observed to spread, and this seems to be associated with both the shorter cells and the large amount of gum produced on every medium on which it has been grown.

Liquid cultures show a characteristic silkiness when gently tapped, and this is correlated with the presence of longer cells. Silkiness is not often seen with *L. gummosus* where the heavy gum seems to preclude lengthy cells. Liquid cultures of all four species are somewhat viscous, and *L. gummosus* is so much so that a 2-day-old tube culture may be inverted without spillage.

Aerobic. Mesophilic. The optimum temperature for growth of these organisms is relatively high (20–40°C) for soil and water organisms; pH range for growth: 5–10; growth of most strains is reduced by 1% NaCl.

Chemoorganotrophic. Metabolism is usually respiratory; molecular oxygen is used as the terminal electron acceptor. NO_3^-, NH_4^+, glutamate and asparaginate are used as sole nitrogen sources, but urea is used by only a few strains. In general, the addition of yeast extract to a salts-glucose-nitrate agar or to a chitin-only medium stimulates growth. Chitin, but not filter-paper cellulose or agar, is hydrolyzed; some species degrade alginate, pectate, starch and/or carboxymethyl cellulose (CMC). One of the extracellular enzymes of *L. enzymogenes* strain ATCC 27796, previously known as "myxobacter AL-1," was the first enzyme with both β-1,4-gluconase and chitosanase activities to be described (Hedges and Wolfe, 1974). This enzyme attacks amorphous forms of cellulose such as CMC but does not attack crystalline cellulose. This was the first enzyme with chitosanase activity to be purified to homogeneity, and it could be useful for the characterization of fungal cell walls and as a tool for the classification of fungi. It has been shown to be capable of attacking some fungal cell walls to release glucosamine. The enzyme has a mol. wt. of 28,900–31,000 and contains large amounts of the basic amino acids, lysine and arginine, in its 230 residues.

Strongly proteolytic. The enzymes of two strains of *L. enzymogenes* have been the subjects of intensive study. One strain, ATCC 27796, known formerly as "myxobacter AL-1," excretes firstly a bacteriolytic enzyme designated "AL-1 protease I", with a mol. wt. of 14,300 and containing 136 amino acids. In contrast to many exocellular enzymes, this protein contains a disulfide bond, 1 mol of hexose, a relatively high content of aromatic amino acids, and an $E_{1cm}^{1\%}$ of 15.8 at 280 μ (Jackson and Wolfe, 1968). This enzyme was found to cleave the pentaglycine bridge in the cell wall of *Staphylococcus* and other bacteria and to remove peptide moieties from the peptidoglycan (Katz and Strominger, 1967; Tipper et al., 1967). Secondly, ATCC 27796 produces another extracellular protease ("AL-1 protease II"), which crystallizes as fine needles and has a mol. wt. of 17,000, with 157 amino acid residues (Wingard et al., 1972). This enzyme does not possess cell wall lytic activity and has a unique specificity for lysine residues, exhibiting peptide bond cleavage on the amino side of lysine.

It was not realized, at the time, that the AL-1 protease reported on by Jackson and Matsueda (1970) in *Methods in Enzymology* was from the same species of bacterium as the α-lytic protease described in the paper immediately following it in that publication (Whitaker, 1970). The "myxobacterium *Sorangium*"/"myxobacter 495" (now ATCC 29487) has since been classified as *L. enzymogenes,* and it was upon this strain that Whitaker's group did the initial enzymological characterization of α- and

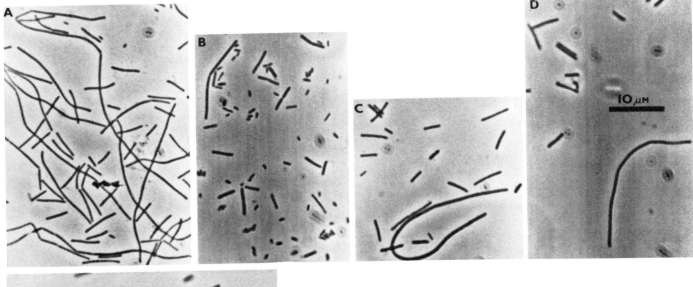

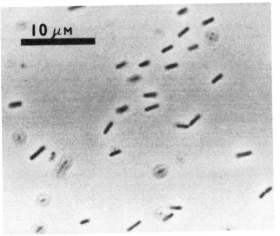

Figure 23.53. *Top (A–D): cells of L. enzymogenes* from skim-acetate broth cultures. *A,* ATCC 29487, 44 h. *B,* ATCC 21123, 44 h. *C,* ATCC 29485, 44 h. *D,* ATCC 29488, 60 h. All micrographs are at the same magnification. (Reproduced with permission from P. J. Christensen and F. D. Cook, International Journal of Systematic Bacteriology *28:* 383, 1978, ©International Union of Microbiological Societies.) *Left: cells of L. gummosus* from skim-acetate broth culture, ATCC 29489, 44 h. (Reproduced with permission from P. J. Christensen and F. D. Cook, International Journal of Systematic Bacteriology *28:* 390, 1978, ©International Union of Microbiological Societies.)

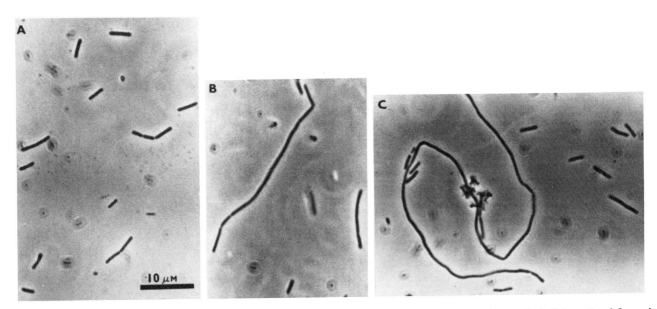

Figure 23.54.   Cells of *L. antibioticus* from skim-acetate broth cultures. *A,* ATCC 29479, 66 h. *B,* UASM 4593, 32 h. *C,* UASM 4578, 72 h. All micrographs are at the same magnification. (Reproduced with permission from P. J. Christensen and F. D. Cook, International Journal of Systematic Bacteriology *28:* 389, 1978, ©International Union of Microbiological Societies.)

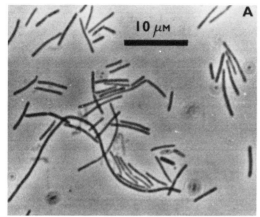
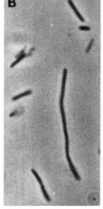
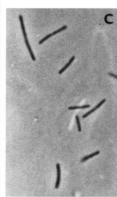
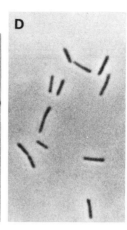

Figure 23.55. Cells of *L. brunescens* from skim-acetate broth cultures. *A,* ATCC 29483, 60 h. *B,* ATCC 29482, 60 h. *C,* UASM 4541, 44 h. *D,* UASM CB 5, 30 h. All micrographs are at the same magnification. (Reproduced with permission from P. J. Christensen and F. D. Cook, International Journal of Systematic Bacteriology *28:* 391, 1978, ©International Union of Microbiological Societies.)

β-lytic proteases (Whitaker, 1965, 1967; Whitaker et al., 1965a, b). The proteases of "495" (now ATCC 29487) have provided much fruitful work for biochemists interested in the three-dimensional structure of microbial proteases compared with mammalian examples. Although the classification of the zinc-containing α-lytic protease is uncertain, β-lytic protease was shown to be a serine protease with the active site amino acid sequence Asp-Ser-Gly (Whitaker et al., 1966; Whitaker and Roy, 1967). This is the same sequence as that of the mammalian pancreatic serine protease and was the first microbial serine protease isolated which was not a member of the Thr-Ser-Met family. The subsequent elucidation of the complete polypeptide sequence showed 198 amino acids in a single polypeptide chain which contains three intrachain disulfide bridges and has an overall mol. wt. of 19,869 (Olson et al., 1970). In a 2.8-Å resolution crystallographic study of α-lytic protease, the three-dimensional structure of the enzyme was determined, and a detailed description of the active site was facilitated. Comparisons with other microbial serine proteases (viz. *Streptomyces griseus* proteases A and B) support the possibility that they arose from a common ancestral gene (Brayer et al., 1979). Recent work includes further study of the active site and comparison with mammalian elastase (Bauer et al., 1981), investigation of the molecular structure at 1.8-Å resolution (M. N. G. James, personal communication), and D. Agard's isolation of the α-lytic protease gene, sequencing, and point-specific mutations (M. N. G. James, personal communication.)

The nucleases of *L. enzymogenes* strain ATCC 29487 (formerly "myxobacter 495") have been characterized by von Tigerstrom (1980, 1981, 1983), with the two major ones being extracellular RNAase and DNAase. The RNAase consists of one polypeptide chain with a mol. wt. of 46,000–47,000, most active at pH 8.0–8.5 and in the presence of Mg^{2+}. The nonspecific nuclease has a mol. wt. of 22,000–28,000, is most active at pH 8.0, and requires Mg^{2+} or Mn^{2+}.

Catalase, oxidase, and phosphatase are produced; work is in progress on the phosphatases of *L. enzymogenes* (R. G. von Tigerstrom, personal communication). The indole, methyl-red, and Voges-Proskauer tests are negative.

Lyses Gram-negative, Gram-positive bacteria including actinomycetes, yeasts and filamentous fungi, blue-green and green algae, and nematodes. Lysobacters do not attack Gram-negative bacteria as vigorously as they do Gram-positive bacteria. As lysobacters themselves are Gram-negative, this may be a self-protective feature.

All strains known at present have been isolated from soil or freshwater habitats; I know of no studies aimed at finding them elsewhere, but this would probably be a fruitful area for investigation. Their polysaccharolytic and proteolytic abilities suggest a role in the degradation of biological structural and storage materials. The significance of their lytic abilities toward other organisms has yet to be fully assessed. It is quite possible that marine members of the genus will be found or that these organisms may have medical significance. They were probably confused with "eubacteria," in the past, when encountered on regular plating media; nutritionally dilute media are needed in order for lysobacters and other gliding bacteria to be recognized, since they do not exhibit spreading on plate count agar (PCA)!

The mol% G + C of the DNA is 65.4–70.1 (T_m).

One species, *L. antibioticus,* elaborates a potent, wide-spectrum antibiotic named "myxin," a 1-hydroxy-6-methoxyphenazine (Cook et al., 1971; Behki and Lesley, 1972). It is manufactured by Hoffman and Roche, but there are two important drawbacks to its widespread medical usage: it has too wide a spectrum, especially for internal use, and it is explosive when dry. Its use is restricted to topical application for resistant fungal skin problems.

Enrichment and Isolation Procedures

Lysobacters have the unusual ability to hydrolyze chitin, and their isolation is facilitated by providing chitin as a suspension, in ground mushrooms, or in autoclaved yeast cells. The simplest method is to enrich soil samples with one of the above sources of chitin, incubate it for at least 1 month, then plate it out on yeast cell agar (Smit and Clark, 1971) which consists of 0.5% baker's yeast in a 1.5% agar medium. The number of colonies capable of lysing autoclaved yeast cells increases dramatically with such enrichment procedures (Christensen and Cook, 1978). Water samples can be plated directly onto yeast cell agar.

Maintenance Procedures

Lysobacters grow profusely on PCA (plate count agar from, for example, Difco), SAA (skim-acetate agar: 0.5% skim milk, 0.05% yeast extract, and 0.02% sodium acetate in 1.5% agar) or broth, or CCA (Cook's *Cytophaga* agar: 0.2% tryptone in 1.0% agar) (Christensen and Cook, 1972). The more dilute the medium, the greater the expression of the spreading morphology, thus CCA is recommended for this purpose and also because on this medium organisms do not appear to lose their polysaccharolytic and proteolytic potential. On PCA, colonies of lysobacters are often indistinguishable from nongliding bacteria. Ordinary plating techniques are sufficient with incubation at room temperature for the species so far known; however, difficulty can occur with *L. gummosus* because of its intensely rubbery colonies, and for this species it is recommended that young cultures (<24 h) be used when it is possible. Lyophilization is successful, and cultures are readily obtainable from these preparations, which are recommended for long term storage. Caution is advised on two aspects, however: (a) colony morphology may change slightly after freeze-drying, and (b) strains of *L. enzymogenes* do not exhibit as strong a microbial lytic action and do not maintain as high a level of certain proteolytic enzymes, after they have been maintained in the laboratory on skim milk media for some time, as do cells not freeze-dried, and this may also apply to lyophilized cultures.

Procedures for Testing for Special Characteristics

In order to differentiate lysobacters from the *Myxobacterales*, it is nec-

essary to demonstrate the absence of fruiting bodies. At least two methods should be attempted, as, for example, inoculation onto sterile *wild* herbivore pellets in water agar (Smit and Clark, 1971) and induction of myxospores following addition of 0.5M glycerol during exponential growth (Dworkin and Gibson, 1964.)

Suitable methods for demonstration of polysaccharide degradation, antimicrobial lytic action, and susceptibility to actinomycin D have been published by Christensen (1977b).

Differentiation of the genus **Lysobacter** from other genera

Table 23.15 contains properties that are useful for distinguishing the genus *Lysobacter*.

Differentiation of the species of the genus **Lysobacter**

Characteristics useful for distinguishing among the species of *Lysobacter* are given in Tables 23.16 and 23.17.

List of species of the genus **Lysobacter**

1. **Lysobacter enzymogenes** Christensen and Cook 1978, 378.[AL]
en.zy.mo′ge.nes. Gr. n. *zyme* leaven; M.L. *n.enzymum* enzyme; Gr. v. *gennaio* to produce; M.L. adj. *enzymogenes* enzyme-producing.

Two distinct colony forms are known: a dirty-white, mucoid colony and a yellowish, nonmucoid one. The mucoid colony produces nonmucoid mutants, but the yellowish, nonmucoid form does not produce revertants to the dirty-white, mucoid form. The colony descriptions given here and in Table 23.16 cover the whole range of colony forms observed. The forms are identical in other properties.

On CCA, 5-day-old colonies are dark cream-colored, with Munsell notation 2.5Y 6-8/4-8 and 5-10YR 6-8/4-8; circular to irregular; usually with a smooth surface but occasionally with a rough surface; edge may be entire, undulate, lobate or erose; elevation typically effuse with a raised or convex center, occasionally flat; transparent or translucent; no brown, water-soluble pigment is produced.

On SAA, 5-day-old colonies are dark cream-colored, with Munsell notation 2.5-7.5Y 6.5-8.5/4-6 and 7.5-10YR 5.5-7/5-7; circular to irregular; with a smooth or rough surface; edge may be entire, undulate or

erose; elevation typically effuse with a raised, convex or umbonate center, occasionally flat; transparent, translucent or opaque; no brown, water-soluble pigment is produced.

On PCA, 5-day-old colonies are deep yellow-cream-colored or creamy-brown, with Munsell notation 1.5-5Y 3-7/4-8; more or less circular; usually with a smooth surface; edge may be entire, undulate or erose; elevation usually convex but may be effuse with a convex or raised center or may be umbonate; translucent or opaque; some brown, water-soluble pigment may be produced.

Older cultures of the majority of strains produce copious, dark-brown, water-soluble pigment on most media.

The mol% G + C of the DNA is 65.4-70.1 (T_m).

Type strain: ATCC 29487 (UASM (University of Alberta Soil Microbiology Lab) 495). Other strains: ATCC 27796 (UASM AL-1), ATCC 29488 (UASM 13B) and ATCC 29485/6 (colony types of UASM 18L).

2. **Lysobacter gummosus** Christensen and Cook 1978, 388.[AL]
gum.mo′sus. L. adj. *gummosus* slime (gum)-producing.

Table 23.15.

Characteristics useful in differentiating the genus **Lysobacter** *from similar taxa[a,b]*

Characteristic	Cytophaga	Sporocytophaga	Lysobacter	Myxobacterales	Chitinophaga
Mol% G + C of DNA	29–42	36	65–70	67–71	43–46
Fruiting bodies	−	−	−	D	−
Microcysts (myxospores)	−	+	−	+	+
Colony color	Y, O or R	Y	W, C, Y, Br, Pi, R	G, Y, O, Br, Pi, R, Pu, nearly B1	Y
Brown, water-soluble pigment produced	In one Pi sp. only	−	In all except one sp. W-Y	D	−
Optical properties of colony	Mainly Tp	Not reported	Tl or Op except one Y-Br sp.	Tp, Tl, or Op	Tl
Degradation of					
Filter-paper cellulose	D	+	−	D	−
Agar	D	Etching	−	D	−
Chitin	One Y sp. only	−	+	D	+
Antimicrobial lytic action	A few strains	Not reported	+	D	+[c]
Susceptibility to actinomycin D	+	Not reported	3 of 4 spp.	+	Not reported

[a]Symbols: −, 90% or more of strains are negative; D, different reactions in different taxa; and +, 90% or more of strains are positive.

[b]Abbreviations: Bl, black; Br, brown; C, cream-colored; G, gray; O, orange; Op, opaque; Pi, pink; Pu, purple; R, red; Tl, translucent; Tp, transparent; W, white; and Y, yellow.

[c]Only reported against one organism (Sangkhobol and Skerman, 1981).

Table 23.16.
Differential characteristics of the species of the genus **Lysobacter**[a–c]

Characteristic	1. *L. enzymogenes*	2. *L. gummosus*[b]	3. *L. antibioticus*	4. *L. brunescens*
Broth culture viscous	+	+ heavy	+	−
Colonies				
Type of growth	Sloppy, mucoid	Pulvinate, gummy	Sloppy, mucoid	Spreading, thin
Surface smooth	+ or −	+	+	+ or −
Opacity	Tp, Tl or Op	Tl or Op	Tl or Op	Tp or Tl
Color	Dark C to deep Y-C	Pale Y-G to Y-G	Pi to Br-Pi or O-Br	Y to Ch
Brown, water-soluble pigment produced	None to moderate	−	Weak to heavy	Weak to heavy
Myxin crystals in old cultures	−	−	Usually +	−
Urea as nitrogen source	+ or −	+	−	−
Acid from				
Cellobiose	+	+	+	−
Sucrose	+	+	−	−
Lactose	+	+	d	−
Lipase-Tween 20	+	+	d	−
Hydrolysis of				
Alginate	+ or −	−	d	−
CMC	+	+	+	−
Pectate	+	+	−[d]	+
SYS or NBS starch	−	−	−[e]	+
Potato starch	+ or −	−	−[f]	+
Sheep erythrocytes	α, β or γ	α	β or α	γ or −
H_2S produced	d	−	−	+
Citrate as sole carbon source	+	+	+	−
Growth on				
MacConkey's	+, colorless or −	−	d, colorless	−
EMB	+, Pi	+, Pi	+, Pi	−
Completely inhibited by 0.1% SLS	+ or −	−	+	+
Susceptible to				
Chloramphenicol (30 μg)	d	−	−	+
Penicillin G (10 U)	−	−	−	d
Actinomycin D	d	d	−	+
Habitat	Soil	Soil	Soil	Freshwater

[a]Data are from Christensen and Cook (1978, 373–392), to which the reader is referred for details of tests.
[b]Symbols: +, 90% or more of strains are positive; −, 90% or more of strains are negative; and d, 11–89% of strains are positive.
[c]Abbreviations: Br, brown(ish); C, cream-colored; Ch, chocolate; EMB, eosin methylene blue; G, gray; NBS, nutrient broth-starch; O, orange; Op, opaque; Ri, Pink(ish); SLS, sodium lauryl sulfate; SYS, salts-yeast extract-starch; Tl, translucent; Tp, transparent; and Y, yellow(ish).
[d]Growth but no liquefaction.
[e]Only one strain recorded on SYS.
[f]Only one strain recorded.

On CCA, 5-day-old colonies are pale yellowish-gray, with Munsell notation 5Y 8/2; circular; with a smooth surface; entire edge; elevation pulvinate; translucent; no water-soluble pigment produced; gummy.

On SAA, 5-day-old colonies are pale yellowish-gray, with Munsell notation 5Y 8/2; circular; with a smooth surface; entire edge; elevation pulvinate; opaque; no water-soluble pigment produced; very gummy.

On PCA, 5-day-old colonies are yellow-gray, with Munsell notation 5Y 7/4; circular; with a smooth surface; entire edge; elevation pulvinate; opaque; no water-soluble pigment produced; very gummy.

Older cultures are intensely gummy and do not produce a water-soluble pigment. In very old cultures, the viscosity of the colony may decrease dramatically, although viable cells can still be recovered from this thin slime.

The mol% G + C of the DNA is 65.7 (T_m).

Type strain: ATCC 29489 (UASM 402).

3. **Lysobacter antibioticus** Christensen and Cook 1978, 387.[AL]

an.ti.bi.o′ti.cus. Gr. pref. *anti* against; Gr. n. *bios* life; M.L. adj. *antibioticus* against life, antibiotic.

On CCA, 5-day-old colonies are pinkish brown, with Munsell notation 1–10YR 2.5–7/4–8; circular to irregular; with a smooth surface; edge usu-

ally erose, may be entire, undulate or filamentous; elevation usually flat or raised, sometimes effuse with a convex center; translucent or opaque; some or much brown, water-soluble pigment is produced.

On SAA, 5-day-old colonies are pinkish brown, with Munsell notation 2.5Y 7/5 and 1.5–7.5YR 3-6/4–8; more or less circular; with a smooth surface; edge usually erose, may be entire or filamentous; elevation usually raised, may be effuse, flat or convex; translucent or opaque; some or much brown, water-soluble pigment is produced or may be absent.

On PCA, 5-day-old colonies are orange-brown, with Munsell notation 1–2.5Y 4-6/3-4 and 5–10YR 2-5/2–6; more or less circular; with a smooth surface; edge usually entire, may be erose or undulate; elevation convex or raised; usually opaque; weak to heavy, brown, water-soluble pigment is produced.

Older cultures on most media produce copious, brown, water-soluble pigment, and deep-red crystals of the antibiotic myxin may be observed within the highly mucoid colonies.

The mol% G + C of the DNA is 66.2–69.2 (T_m).

Type strain: ATCC 29479 (UASM 3C). Other strains: ATCC 29480 (UASM L17) and ATCC 29481 (UASM 4045).

4. **Lysobacter brunescens** Christensen and Cook 1978, 390.[AL]

Table 23.17.

Other characteristics of the species of the genus **Lysobacter**[a-c]

Characteristic	1. *L. enzymogenes*	2. *L. gummosus*	3. *L. antibioticus*	4. *L. brunescens*
Cell dimensions (μm)	$0.3-0.5 \times 4-50$	0.4×2	$0.4 \times 4-40$	$0.2-0.5 \times 7-70$
Flexing[d]	+	−	+	+
Gliding[d]	+	+ short jerks	+	+
Silkiness in broth culture[d]	+	+	+	+
Fruits induced by				
Glycerol	−	−	−	−
Pellets	−	−	−	−
Partial inhibition by 1% NaCl	d	−	+	+
% NaCl causing complete inhibition	3 or below	3	3	2 or below
Preferred atmosphere	Air or 10% O$_2$	Air	Air or 10 % O$_2$	Air or 10% O$_2$
Growth range temperature (0°C)	5–40	10–40	2–40	4–50
Growth optimum temperature (0°C)	25–35	20	25–33	30–40
Initial pH for growth	5->10	6->10	5->10	<5->10
Nitrogen sources				
Nitrate	+	+	+	+
Ammonia	+	+	+	+
Glutamate	+	+	+	+
Asparaginate	+	+	+	d
OF test (glucose)				
Oxidation	+	+	+	+
Fermentation	−	−	d	d
Acid from				
Glucose	+	+	+	+
Glycerol	d	−	−	−
Mannitol	d	−	−	−
Lipase-Tween 40	+	+	+	d
Lipase-Tween 60	+	+	+	+
Lipase-Tween 80	+	+	+	d
Hydrolysis of				
Agar (gelase)	+ or −	−	−[e]	+
Agar tubes	−	−	−	−
Cellulose (filter paper)	−	−	−	−
Chitin	+	+	+	+
Gelatin liquefaction	+	+	+	+
Complete peptonization of milk (days)	1–3	1	1	1
Casein—growth and NH$_3$ produced	+, +	+, +	+, +	+, +
Penassay—growth	+	+	+[e]	+
Casitone—growth and NH$_3$ produced	+, +	+, +	+, +	+, +
Casamino acids-salts—growth and NH$_3$ produced	+, +	+, −	+, −[e]	+, −
Grows well on 0.2% tryptone	+	+	+	+
Catalase	+	+	+	+
Oxidase	+	Unable to test	+	+
Phosphatase	+	+	+	+
Indole	−	−	−	−
Methyl red	−	−	−	−
Voges-Proskauer	−	−	−	−
Reduction of NO$_3^-$ to NO$_2^-$	−	−	d	−
Reduction of NO$_2^-$ to gas	−	−	−	−
Growth reduced by 0.01% SLS	+ or −	−	−	d
Susceptible to				
10 μg streptomycin	−	−	d	d
300 U polymyxin B (Kirby-Bauer)	d	d	−	d
300 U polymixin B (Christensen)	+	+	+	+
Antimicrobial lytic action				
Gram-negative bacteria				
Escherichia coli	d	−	d	d
Pseudomonas aeruginosa	d	−	−	d
Serratia marcescens	d	−	d	d
Gram-positive bacteria				
Arthrobacter sp.	+	+	d	d
Bacillus subtilis	+	+	d	d

Table 23.17.—*continued*

Characteristic	1. *L. enzymogenes*	2. *L. gummosus*	3. *L. antibioticus*	4. *L. brunescens*
Actinomycetes				
UASM 4432	+	+	−	−
UASM 4441	+	+	d	d
Fungi				
Rhizopus sp.	+	d	d	d
Penicillium notatum	+	+	d	d
Sclerotinia sclerotiorum	d	+	+	d
Baker's yeast	+	+	d	+
Alga				
Chlorella sp.	d	+	+	+

[a]Data are from Christensen and Cook (1978, 372–392), to which the reader is referred for details of tests.

[b]Symbols: +, 90% or more of strains are positive; −, 90% or more of strains are negative; and d, 11–89% of strains are positive.

[c]Abbreviations: OF, oxidation/fermentation; and SLS, sodium lauryl sulfate.

[d]Flexing, gliding and silkiness are more readily observed with longer cells.

[e]Only one strain recorded on nutrient broth.

bru.nes′cens. L. v. *brunesco* to become dark brown; L. part. adj. *brunescens* becoming dark brown.

On CCA, 5-day-old colonies are brownish yellow, with Munsell notation 2.5–5Y 3-4/4-8 and 10YR 4-5/6-8; irregular; with a rough surface; edge usually filamentous, may be lobate, undulate or erose; elevation effuse with umbonate or convex center; transparent; amounts of brown, water-soluble pigment vary from moderate to absent.

On SAA, 5-day-old colonies are yellow-brown, with Munsell notation 2.5Y 4.5/6 and 7.5–10YR 4-6/6-8; usually irregular, occasionally circular; usually with a rough surface; edge typically erose or filamentous, may be entire, undulate or lobate; elevation effuse or raised, with convex or umbonate centers; transparent or translucent; weak to moderate amounts of brown, water-soluble pigment are produced.

On PCA, 5-day-old colonies are deep yellow-brown, with Munsell notation 1-2.5Y 3-4/4-6 and 10YR 3-4/4-6; circular to irregular; smooth or rough surface; edge usually entire or undulate, sometimes erose or filamentous; elevation effuse with convex or umbonate center, or raised, or convex; translucent; production of brown, water-soluble pigment is moderate to heavy.

Older cultures on all media produce copious, dark-brown, water-soluble pigment.

The mol% G + C of the DNA is 67.6–67.8 (T_m).

Type strain: ATCC 29482 (UASM D). Other strains: ATCC 29483 (UASM 2) and ATCC 29484 (UASM 6).

ORDER III. **BEGGIATOALES** BUCHANAN 1957, 837[AL]

WILLIAM R. STROHL

Beg.gi.a.to.a′les. M.L. fem. n. *Beggiatoa* type genus of the order; *-ales* ending to denote an order; M.L. fem. pl. n. *Beggiatoales* the *Beggiatoa* order.

Cells of widely varying sizes **occur mostly in filaments.** Filaments usually demonstrate flexing or bending and usually can be considered as distinct multicellular units. Gram-negative. **Colorless;** chlorophyll, phycobiliproteins, and carotenoid pigments are not produced. When in contact with a substrate, the motile organisms **glide over the surface in a slow wavy type of motion. No flagella or other motility organelles are proven.** Gliding motility is usually in a direction parallel with the length of the filaments. Multiplication is by transverse binary fission of both singly occurring cells and cells throughout the length of filaments. Cells within filaments may be visible or not visible. Filament dispersion may be via disintegration or sacrificial cell death. Sheaths and holdfasts may be formed. Resting cell forms not known.

Sulfur is deposited in the presence of hydrogen sulfide. Poly-β-hydroxybutyric acid (PHB) and polyphosphate (volutin) often occur.

Aerobic or microaerophilic.

Chemoorganotrophic and chemolithotrophic nutrition known; **mixotrophic nutrition postulated** for several organisms. **Metabolism respiratory.** Normally found in freshwater and marine environments and in waterlogged soils.

FAMILY I. **BEGGIATOACEAE** MIGULA 1894, 238[AL]

WILLIAM R. STROHL

Beg.gi.a.to.a′ce.ae. M.L. fem. n. *Beggiatoa* type genus of the family; *-aceae* ending to denote a family; M.L. fem. pl. n. *Beggiatoaceae* the *Beggiatoa* family.

Colorless cells typically arranged in filaments. Cells in living filaments usually are not visible when viewed by phase microscopy. Cells and filaments are **motile by gliding** and usually are flexible. **Colorless;** carotenoid, phycobiliproteins, and chlorophyll pigments are not formed.

Resting stages are not known. Holdfasts and/or sheaths may be found. **Gram-negative.**

Autotrophic and chemoorganotrophic metabolism have been demonstrated. **Mixotrophic metabolism has been postulated** for several of these organisms. **Metabolism is respiratory**, with molecular oxygen used as the terminal electron acceptor. Nitrogen fixation has been demonstrated for several strains of *Beggiatoa*. **Sulfur globules (inclusions) are deposited when cells are grown in the presence of hydrogen sulfide**. PHB or polyphosphate bodies often occur intracellularly.

Aerobic or microaerophilic.

Found in **freshwater and marine sediments** and attached to submerged objects.

The mol% G + C of the DNA is 37–52 (T_m, Bd). Species that have been examined via 5S rRNA sequences are phylogenetically distant from the cyanobacteria.

Type genus: *Beggiatoa* Trevisan 1842, 56.

Taxonomic Comments

The genera of *Beggiatoaceae* are separated on the basis of major morphological differences such as the types of filaments formed, stable formation of spirals and coils in nature, deposition of sulfur, and formation of sheaths, holdfasts and/or rosettes. Members of this family are among the few bacteria to be recognized and differentiated mostly on the basis of their morphology (Table 23.18). Because many of these organisms can be recognized in situ and because many of them have also been difficult to purify, several population and ecological studies on these organisms (Uphof, 1927; Lackey et al., 1965; Jørgensen, 1982) have been carried out.

The family *Beggiatoaceae* was placed in "The Gliding Bacteria," Part 2 of the eighth edition of the *Manual* under the order *Cytophagales* (Leadbetter, 1974c), a heterogeneous group of nonfruiting gliding bacteria (Reichenbach, 1981; Reichenbach and Dworkin, 1981a). Suggestions since then have been made to alter the taxonomic status of the family within "The Gliding Bacteria" (Reichenbach, 1981; Reichenbach and Dworkin, 1981a). Because of the close morphological similarity to cyanobacteria of the genus *Oscillatoria*, the beggiatoas have often been considered as colorless cyanobacteria (Pringsheim, 1949b, 1963; Reichenbach, 1981). Similarities also exist in the gliding motility (Burchard, 1980), the life cycles (Strohl and Larkin, 1978a) and the ultrastructure (Drawert and Metzner-Küster, 1958; Maier and Murray, 1965; Strohl et al., 1982) of the beggiatoas and oscillatorians. These factors, coupled with the discovery that certain filamentous cyanobacteria can oxidize sulfide (Garlick et al., 1977), further supported the claims of taxonomic similarity. One suggestion has been to place the sulfide-oxidizing apochlorotic "cyanobacteria" (including *Beggiatoa, Thioploca, Thiothrix*, "*Thiospirillopsis*" and *Achromatium*) into the order *Beggiatoales* under the class "*Cyanomorphae*" (Reichenbach and Dworkin, 1981a). In that classification, the non-sulfide-oxidizing "organoheterotrophic apochlorotic cyanobacteria" (i.e. *Vitreoscilla, Leucothrix, Herpetosiphon, Simonsiella, Alysiella* and *Saprospira*) would be in the order "*Leucotrichales*" under the same class (Reichenbach and Dworkin, 1981a).

Recent evidence, however, suggests that the beggiatoas are not as physiologically or phylogenetically similar to the cyanobacteria as was formerly thought. Larkin and Strohl (1983) pointed out several physiologi-

Table 23.18.
*Morphological differentiation of genera in **Beggiatoaceae***[a]

Characteristic	*Beggiatoa*	*Thiothrix*	*Thioploca*	"*Thiospirillopsis*"
Gliding motility[b]	+	+	+	+
Filament formation	+	+	+	+
Sulfur deposition[c]	+	+	+	+
Sheath formation	−	+	+	−
Holdfast formation	−	+	−	−
Rosette formation	−	+	−	−
Permanently spiraled/coiled	−	−	−	+

[a]Symbols: +, 90% or more of strains are positive; and −, 90% or more of strains are negative.
[b]Only the gonidia of *Thiothrix* glide (Larkin and Shinabarger, 1983); individual filaments of *Thioploca* glide (the entire sheath does not glide (Maier, 1974)).
[c]When cells are grown in the presence of hydrogen sulfide.

cal differences between the beggiatoas and oscillatorians. Analysis of the 16S rRNA of a strain labeled *Beggiatoa leptomitiformis* indicated that it belonged to the gamma subgroup of the purple bacteria (Woese et al., 1985a). Similarly, analyses of 5S rRNA sequences showed that *Beggiatoa alba, Thiothrix nivea* and *Vitreoscilla beggiatoides* are phylogenetically related to the gamma subgroup of the purple bacteria (Stahl et al., 1987). The cyanobacteria tested form a cohesive natural assemblage which is distant phylogenetically from the purple bacteria, distinct enough so that Woese et al. (1985b) proposed that the cyanobacteria and purple bacteria belonged to separate phyla.

Acknowledgements

I wish to thank John M. Larkin, Thomas M. Schmidt and David A. Stahl for discussions concerning the taxonomy of these organisms.

Further Reading

Larkin, J.M. and W.R. Strohl. 1983. *Beggiatoa, Thiothrix*, and *Thioploca*. Annu. Rev. Microbiol. *37*: 341–367.
Nelson, D.C. 1989. Physiology and biochemstry of filamentous sulfur bacteria. *In* Schlegel and Bowien (Editors), Autotrophic Bacteria. Science Tech Publishers, Madison, Wisconsin, in press.
Wiessner, W. 1981. The family *Beggiatoaceae. In* Starr, Stolp, Trüper, Balows and Schlegel (Editors), The Prokaryotes. A Handbook on Habitats, Isolation, and Identification of Bacteria. Springer-Verlag, Berlin, pp. 380–389.

Key to the genera of family **Beggiatoaceae**

1. Cells arranged in single filaments that move by gliding motility. Gliding is usually rapid. Sulfur is deposited in periplasmically located envelopes when cells are exposed to hydrogen sulfide. Filaments may be bent or straight but are not permanently coiled or spiral. Sheaths, holdfasts and rosettes are not formed. PHB and polyphosphate may be deposited. Heterotrophic and autotrophic growth are proven, and mixotrophic growth is postulated for different strains. Both freshwater and marine forms are known to occur. The mol% G +C of the DNA is 37–51 (T_m, Bd).

Genus I. *Beggiatoa*, p. 2091

2. Cells arranged in filaments that are found singly within sheaths. Sheaths containing filaments do not glide, but hormogonia formed by division do glide. Holdfasts attach ensheathed filaments to objects in aquatic habitats. Rosettes are formed. Filaments are not permanently coiled. PHB and polyphosphate may be deposited. Several strains thus far studied require a reduced sulfur source for growth; thus mixotrophic metabolism for these organisms has been postulated. Some strains also grow heterotrophically. Both freshwater and marine forms are known to occur. The mol% G+C of the DNA, based on two strains isolated from the same location, is 52 (T_m).

Genus II. *Thiothrix*, p. 2098

3. Cells arranged in filaments that are found singly or multiply within sheaths. Individual filaments glide. Sulfur inclusions are formed. Large vacuoles may be formed, particularly in larger strains. No holdfasts or rosettes are formed. Filaments are not permanently coiled. Both freshwater and marine forms are known to occur. Not grown in pure culture.

Genus III. *Thioploca*, p. 2101

4. Cells are usually not visible in filaments; filaments are permanently coiled or spirally wound. Not grown in pure culture.

Genus IV. "*Thiospirillopsis*," p. 2106

Genus I. **Beggiatoa** *Trevisan 1842, 56*^{AL}

WILLIAM R. STROHL

Beg.gi.a.to'a. M.L. fem. n. *Beggiatoa* a genus of bacteria; named in remembrance of F. S. Beggiato, a physician of Vicenza who authored the *Delle Terme Euganea*.

Colorless cells, ~1-50 μm in diameter and ~2-10 μm in length, occur in filaments with diameters of from ~1 to > 50 μm. **Organisms may exist as single cells or in filaments** containing up to 50 or more cells. Cells in filaments are cylindrical and are longer than they are wide in the thinner strains (≤7 μm in diameter). In wider strains (≳7 μm in diameter), cells are usually disk-shaped and typically are wider than they are long. **Filaments occur singly or in cottony masses** in which each filament retains its individuality. Reproduction is by transverse binary fission of cells within filaments; divisions are made by septation, in which the peptidoglycan and cytoplasmic membranes close like the iris of a diaphragm. Filament dispersion is via sacrificial cell death (necridial cells) and filament breakage or via simple disintegratioh. With some strains, the disintegration of filaments occurs until mostly single or double cell units (hormogonia) exist; a hormogonium then may grow to become a filament. **Cells contain inclusions of sulfur when they are grown in the presence of hydrogen sulfide** and, with some strains, thiosulfate. Intracellular inclusions of poly-β-hydroxybutyric acid (PHB) or polyphosphate may be present. Resting stages are not known. **Attachment holdfasts or sheaths are not present.** Capsules are not formed, but filaments usually produce a slime matrix.

Gram-negative. Hormogonia and filaments are motile by gliding; no motility organelles are known. Gliding is relatively rapid (1-8 μm s^{-1}) and is often accompanied by flexing and bending of the filaments. Gliding motility determines the nature of growth and colony formation; on agar media containing relatively few nutrients, spiral colonies are usually produced.

Aerobic or microaerophilic. Anaerobic growth is not known.

Chemoorganotrophic and facultatively autotrophic. Some strains may also grow mixotrophically. Only a marine strain has thus far been proven to grow autotrophically. **Metabolism is respiratory**, with molecular oxygen used as the terminal electron acceptor. Internally stored sulfur may also serve as an electron acceptor for short term maintenance in the absence of oxygen. Nitrate, nitrite or sulfate does not substitute as the terminal electron acceptor for anaerobic growth in strains thus far studied. H$_2$S or thiosulfate may be used as the electron donor for chemolithotrophic metabolism. Acetate is oxidized to CO$_2$ by all freshwater strains tested. Several C$_2$, C$_3$, and C$_4$ organic acids and, sometimes, their amino acid equivalents are utilized as sole carbon and energy sources for heterotrophic growth. Growth factors are not required by most strains; some strains may require vitamin B$_{12}$. Gelatin and starch are not hydrolyzed. Dinitrogen is fixed by a variety of strains. Nitrate, nitrite, ammonium, dinitrogen or certain amino acids are used as sole nitrogen source. Oxidase-positive, **catalase-negative.**

Freshwater, estuarine and marine strains are known. **Beggiatoas are gradient organisms existing in horizontal layers in sediments at the interface between the underlying anoxic sulfide-liberating zone and the overlying oxic zone.** Growth may occur between 0 and 40°C. Thermophilic strains have not been characterized, although some beggiatoas have been observed in high temperature runoffs associated with thermal springs.

The mol% G + C of the DNA is 37-51 (T$_m$, Bd).

Type species: *Beggiatoa alba* Trevisan 1842, 56.

Further Comments

Use of Filament Diameter as a Differentiation Criterion

In the eighth edition of *Bergey's Manual*®, six species were recognized: *B. alba* (type species), "*B. arachnoidea*," "*B. gigantea*," "*B. leptomitiformis*," "*B. minima*" and "*B. mirabilis*"; all were differentiated on the basis of filament diameter alone (Leadbetter, 1974c). There also were 18 listed as *species incertae sedis*, differentiated on the basis of filament diameter, habitats and other general characteristics. Until the recent characterization of *B. alba* (Mezzino et al., 1984), species designation in *Beggiatoa* had been solely on the basis of filament diameter, general morphology, or habitat.

B. alba was originally described in 1803 as "*Oscillatoria alba*," an organism characterized by "white filaments, of diameter of 1/800th of the length, distance between septa equal to diameter, extremities rounded and not pointed" (Vaucher, 1803). The length of *Beggiatoa* filaments is variable (Strohl and Larkin, 1978a, b), however, so the diameter of the first observed "*O. alba*" cannot be calculated. Trevisan (1842) described the genus *Beggiatoa*, in which "*O. alba*" (Vaucher) was included as a species. The two original species of *Beggiatoa*, *B. alba* and "*B. leptomitiformis*," were differentiated by their filament tips being rounded and pointed, respectively (Trevisan, 1842, 1845), not by filament diameter as in more recent years.

The differentiation of *Beggiatoa* species by filament diameter has evolved during the past 50 years. The filament width of *B. alba*, the only species of *Beggiatoa* listed in the 1931 edition of Lehmann and Neumann's manual, was given as 1-3 μm (Lehmann and Neumann, 1931). Cataldi (1940) later claimed that her *Beggiatoa* strains, which measured 5.5-6.3 μm in width, fit the description for *B. alba* as given in the fifth edition of *Bergey's Manual*. *B. alba* was given a filament diameter of 2.5-5.0 μm in the seventh (Buchanan, 1957) and eighth (Leadbetter, 1974c) editions of the *Manual*. Thus the use of filament diameter to differentiate species of *Beggiatoa* has been both arbitrary and inconsistent.

The use of filament diameter is a problem primarily with the smaller strains, i.e. those having diameters ≤5 μm. Several "smaller" (~2.0-5.0 μm in diameter) beggiatoas having about the same filament diameters varied widely in their physiological characteristics (Pringsheim, 1964; Strohl and Larkin, 1978b). The filament diameter of strains maintained in axenic culture may change with time (Strohl et al., 1986a) and is also somewhat dependent on growth conditions. Moreover, the measurement of filament diameters may include inherent errors caused by optics, micrometer standardization techniques, and interpretation. The percentage of strains near the cutoff points between species as cited in the eighth edition of the *Manual* (Leadbetter, 1974) is much greater in strains with filament diameter ≤5 μm than for strains of much greater diameters. Finally, the restriction of sizes to various groupings (Buchanan, 1957; Leadbetter, 1974c) was due to lack of better information on pure cultures of *Beggiatoa*.

On the other hand, good historical logic and experimental evidence exist for using filament diameter as a differentiation tool for certain beggiatoas. In various field investigations, beggiatoas have been observed ranging from <1 to >50 μm in diameter. Klas (1936) found that two size ranges of marine beggiatoas, i.e. 14.8–21.4 μm (18.4-μm average) and 26.4–49.2 μm (34.4-μm average), existed among trichomes from environmental samples. Likewise, Jørgensen (1978) found clusters in the size classes of 3–5 μm, 8–17 μm, and >23 μm among marine beggiatoas he observed. In contrast to the difficulty of distinguishing several species among freshwater strains between ~1 and 5 μm in diameter, it would not be expected that two strains, one averaging 4.0 μm in diameter and the other averaging 34.0 μm in diameter, could be the same "species." Examples such as these demonstrate the interesting but confusing state of affairs with *Beggiatoa* taxonomy and have prompted the deletion of all but *B. alba*, the type species, from acceptance (Skerman et al., 1980). This should induce future descriptions of new *Beggiatoa* species to include physiological as well as morphological data. In subsequent descriptions, filament width should be considered as a single characteristic among several characteristics which differentiate the various species. Among the marine beggiatoas, however, size classes probably do exist which are descriptive for a given "species." This, it is hoped, will be confirmed with the purification and characterization of large marine beggiatoas.

Cell Structure and Cycle

Beggiatoa is a multicellular bacterium with filaments containing from a few cells to perhaps 50 or more cells. The filaments are capable of gliding on agar surfaces to form various patterns of waves and concentric rings (Fig. 23.56). The cells within the filaments are separated by the membranes and the first cell wall layer (Fig. 23.57; Strohl and Larkin, 1978a). Cell division occurs by septation of those two inside layers (Fig. 23.57). Nearly one fourth of the cells in a trichome may be dividing simultaneously (Hinze, 1901). The outer cell wall layers do not take part in septation (Strohl et al., 1982) and are longitudinally continuous with the length of the filament. Beggiatoas do not contain a classical sheath but do exude large quantities of extracellular neutral polysaccharide slime (Strohl and Larkin, 1978b; Larkin and Strohl, 1983).

Filament dispersion occurs via sacrificial cell death (necridia formation) and filament breakage (Strohl and Larkin, 1978a) in a manner similar to that observed in *Oscillatoria*. Filament dispersion may also occur via simple separation of an end cell to produce a hormogonium (Wiessner, 1981), or the filaments may divide by simple fragmentation (Pringsheim, 1949b). Fragmentation, however, is often associated with filament death.

Beggiatoas stain Gram-negatively (Strohl and Larkin, 1978b), but they contain a cell envelope which is much more complex than typical Gram-negative bacteria (Fig. 23.58; Maier and Murray, 1965; Strohl et al., 1982; Strohl et al., 1986a). *Cell wall layer A* is probably a peptidoglycan layer, and *layer B* is a unit membranelike layer positionally similar to the lipopolysaccharide layer of Gram-negative bacteria (Fig. 23.58; Strohl et al., 1982). Depending on the strain and the method of fixation, two or three further external layers may be observed (Drawert and Metzner-Küster, 1958; Maier and Murray, 1965; Strohl et al., 1981a, 1982), the most external of which usually has a fibrillar pattern (Drawert and Metzner-Küster, 1958; Strohl et al., 1982).

Beggiatoa cells are known to contain at least three types of inclusions: PHB (Pringsheim and Wiessner, 1963; Strohl and Larkin, 1978b; Strohl et al., 1982), polyphosphate (Maier and Murray, 1965; Strohl and Larkin, 1978b) and sulfur (Lawry et al., 1981; Strohl et al., 1981a). It is this final inclusion which separates organisms of the genus *Beggiatoa* from those in *Vitreoscilla* (Leadbetter, 1974c; Strohl el al., 1986a).

Several investigators have observed sulfur inclusions in thin sections of fixed and dehydrated *Beggiatoa* trichomes (Morita and Stave, 1963; Maier and Murray, 1965; Lawry et al., 1981; Strohl et al., 1981a). The sulfur is dissolved away during dehydration with ethanol or acetone, leaving empty, electron-translucent spaces (Strohl et al., 1981a). Sulfur inclusions are located in pockets formed by invaginations of the cytoplasmic membrane; thus they are external to the cytoplasm but internal to the cell wall (Maier and Murray, 1965; Strohl et al., 1981a). Sulfur inclusions within these cytoplasmic membrane invaginations may be bounded by envelopes typically composed of a single dense layer (Fig. 23.59; Strohl et

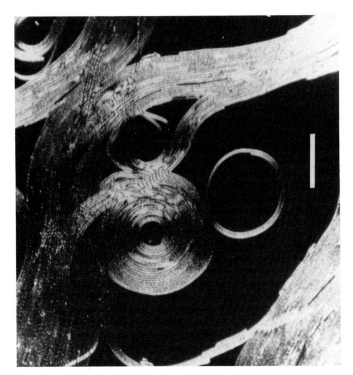

Figure 23.56. Light micrograph of a *Beggiatoa* colony on a 1.4% agar surface, taken through a dissecting microscope. *Bar*, 50 μm.

al., 1981a). Unusual pentalaminar sulfur inclusion envelopes were observed in cells of *B. alba* strain B15LD (Strohl et al., 1981a; Strohl et al., 1982). Rudimentary pentalaminar envelopes were observed in cells of B15LD grown in the total absence of reduced sulfur, indicating that a "primer" envelope was always present (Strohl et al., 1982). This may partially explain the rapidity with which sulfur inclusions appear after exposure of *Beggiatoa* cells to sulfide (Winogradsky, 1887; Burton and Morita, 1964; Schmidt et al. 1986).

Under certain growth conditions, PHB comprised over 50% of the cell dry weight of *B. alba* (Güde et al., 1981). Furthermore, ~50% of the [^{14}C]acetate assimilated by heterotrophically grown cells was incorporated into PHB (Strohl et al., 1981b). The amount of PHB in the cells is usually proportional to the amount of acetate in the growth medium (Kowallik and Pringsheim, 1966). Cultures containing PHB were shown to survive in media containing sulfide but lacking organic nutrients (Kowallik and Pringsheim, 1966), suggesting a survival role for the endogenous metabolism of PHB during carbon starvation. Furthermore, a *B. alba* strain that contained massive PHB inclusions was able to survive up to 7 days of starvation in a mineral salts medium lacking a carbon and an energy source (W. R. Strohl, unpublished observation).

Genetics

Little has been done to characterize the beggiatoas genetically. The molecular mass of the *B. alba* genome, as characterized by C_0t analysis, is 2.02×10^9 (3.03×10^3 kilobase pairs; Genthner et al., 1985). Thus the *B. alba* genome is approximately the same size as the genome of *Escherichia coli* (Genthner et al., 1985). Three *Beggiatoa* strains contained plasmids with molecular masses of ~12–13 × 10^6 (Minges et al., 1983); however, no function was ascribed to these plasmids. No phages specific for infection of *Beggiatoa* species have been found, either in sediment samples or endogenously in the genome of four strains tested (W. R. Strohl, unpublished data). No mutants or strains containing auxotrophic markers have yet been described for any *Beggiatoa* species.

Physiology

Winogradsky (1887) developed his theory of chemoautotrophy based

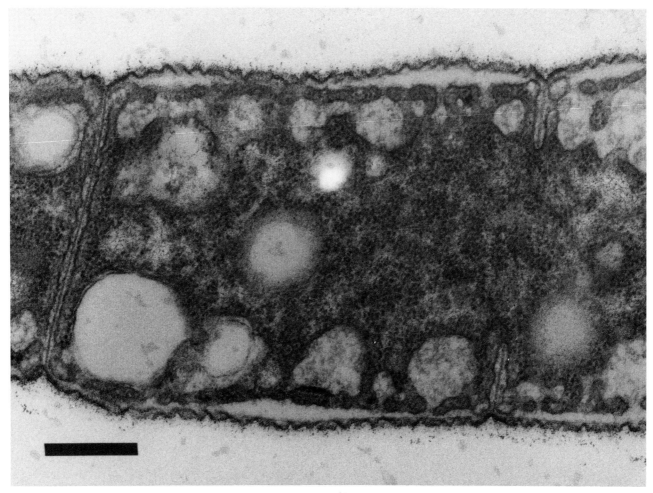

Figure 23.57. Thin-section micrograph of *B. alba* strain B18LD, showing the separation of cells in the filament by the cytoplasmic membranes and the peptidoglycan layer. A newly forming septation is also visible. The outer cell walls, not well preserved via a modified Ryteron Kellenberger fixation technique (Strohl and Larkin, 1978b), are continuous with the length of the filament. *Bar*, 0.5 μm. (Reproduced with permission from W. R. Strohl and J. M. Larkin, Current Microbiology *1:* 151–155, 1978, ©Springer-Verlag, New York.)

on his observations of sulfide oxidation by beggiatoas in slide cultures. The beggiatoas were considered as autotrophs until the mid-1900s when Cataldi (1940), Faust and Wolfe (1961), Scotten and Stokes (1962), Burton and Morita (1964) and Pringsheim (1964) described heterotrophic growth for various strains of *Beggiatoa*. At that point, controversy began between various investigators concerning the role of sulfide oxidation in *Beggiatoa* metabolism. Pringsheim and his colleagues claimed that *Beggiatoa* was a facultative autotroph with the ability to grow autotrophically, with sulfide used as the sole energy source, or heterotrophically, with acetate used as sole carbon and energy sources (Kowallik and Pringsheim, 1966). Burton and Morita (1964) claimed that sulfide oxidation was responsible for the detoxification of peroxides produced during *Beggiatoa* growth. Because sulfide was oxidized in the presence of organic carbon, Pringsheim (1967, 1970) later rescinded his claim of autotrophy and suggested that the beggiatoas were capable of "mixotrophic" growth, obtaining their carbon from acetate and CO_2 and their energy from sulfide oxidation (and perhaps from acetate oxidation). *B. alba* B18LD has been postulated to grow mixotrophically, with sulfide or thiosulfate serving as a supplemental energy source (Güde et al., 1981; Strohl and Schmidt, 1984). *B. alba* can grow heterotrophically, albeit with much less apparent efficiency (Güde et al., 1981). It has been suggested, however, that *B. alba* B18LD, as well as other freshwater strains of *Beggiatoa*, may not couple sulfide oxidation with energy conservation (Nelson and Castenholz, 1981a; Kuenen and Beudeker, 1982).

Thus controversy still exists concerning the role of sulfide oxidation in the metabolism of freshwater *Beggiatoa* strains (Kuenen and Beudeker, 1982; Nelson and Jannasch, 1983; Strohl and Schmidt, 1984). Nelson and his colleagues have recently proven facultatively autotrophic growth for a marine strain of *Beggiatoa* (Nelson and Jannasch, 1983; Nelson et al., 1986b).

Some aspects of the *Beggiatoa* sulfur metabolism have recently been clarified. Sulfide oxidation to sulfur by *B. alba* is constitutive (Schmidt et al., 1986) and does not promote an increase in growth rate (Güde et al., 1981) or in the rate of protein synthesis (Schmidt et al., 1986). Sulfide oxidation by *B. alba* is oxygen-dependent (Vargas and Strohl, 1985b; Schmidt et al., 1987) and is inhibited by several electron transport inhibitors (Strohl and Schmidt, 1984), suggesting that sulfide oxidation is coupled with oxygen via the electron transport system. Once sulfur is formed by *B. alba*, it is apparently not further oxidized to sulfate, as evidenced by isotopic and chemical studies (Strohl and Larkin, 1980; Schmidt et al., 1987) and by a lack of (sulfuric) acid production (Williams and Unz, 1985). The inability of freshwater strains to oxidize sulfur to sulfate may be more widespread than was originally thought. Freshwater strains, however, can reduce stored sulfur back to sulfide under anaerobic conditions (Nelson and Castenholz, 1981a; Schmidt et al., 1987). A marine strain of *Beggiatoa*, on the other hand, produced acid from sulfur, indicating that it was capable of sulfate production (Nelson and Jannasch, 1983).

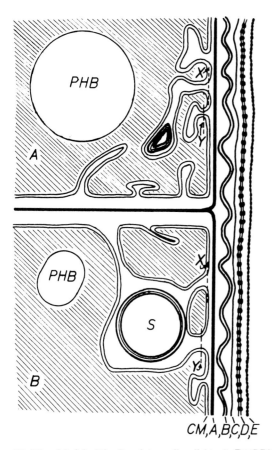

Figure 23.58. Model of the *Beggiatoa* cell wall (strain B15LD). (Reproduced with permission from W. R. Strohl, K. S. Howard and J. M. Larkin, Journal of General Microbiology *128*: 73–84, 1982, ©Society for General Microbiology, London.)

Freshwater strains of *Beggiatoa* grow heterotrophically (Pringsheim, 1964; Strohl and Larkin, 1978b; Nelson and Castenholz, 1981b; Strohl et al., 1981b; Larkin and Strohl, 1983), and they typically utilize acetate as sole carbon and energy sources (Larkin and Strohl, 1983; Strohl et al., 1986b). Several *Beggiatoa* strains have been shown to grow on C_2, C_3, and C_4 organic acids, although none of the beggiatoas described thus far grows on C_5 or C_6 organic acids or on hexose sugars (Burton and Morita, 1964; Nelson and Castenholz, 1981b; Mezzino et al., 1984; Williams and Unz, 1985). A small amount of CO_2 is fixed by freshwater strains of *Beggiatoa*, but it is assimilated by heterotrophic metabolism mechanisms, not by the Calvin-Benson cycle (Nelson and Castenholz, 1981b; Strohl et al., 1981b). Recently, low levels of ribulose-1,5-biphosphate carboxylase/oxygenase (RuBisCO) activity have been observed in extracts of the freshwater strains OH-75-2a and *B. alba* B18LD (Nelson et al., 1989). Moreover, a gene probe derived from the gene encoding the large subunit of *Anacystis nidulans* RuBisCO hybridized strongly to DNA isolated from strain OH-75-2a (Nelson et al. (1989). During autotrophic growth by the marine strain, CO_2 is fixed by ribulose-1,5-bisphosphate carboxylase (Nelson and Jannasch, 1983). It is probable that *Beggiatoa* strains utilize the glyoxylate and tricarboxylic acid cycles during growth on acetate (Nelson and Castenholz, 1981b; Larkin and Strohl, 1983), although definitive proof for these is still lacking. *B. alba* appeared to contain *c* type, *a* type, and CO-binding cytochromes, as well as ubiquinone 8 and NAD(P)H dehydrogenases, indicating that it possesses a respiratory electron transport chain to which acetate and sulfide oxidation can be coupled (Strohl and Schmidt, 1984; Strohl et al., 1986b). More recently, Schmidt and his colleagues have reinvestigated the cytochromes of *B. alba* B18LD and have found only a CO-binding

flavocytochrome *c* (T. M. Schmidt, manuscript in preparation). Similarly, Prince et al. (1988) have determined that a sample of marine *Beggiatoa* filaments contained only *c* type cytochromes. These *c* type cytochromes from marine *Beggiatoa* filaments did not appear to bind CO (Prince et al., 1988).

Ammonia is a nitrogen source used by every *Beggiatoa* tested thus far (Larkin and Strohl, 1983). Recent evidence has indicated that the glutamine synthetase (GS)-glutamate synthase (GOGAT) pathway is the primary route for ammonia assimilation by *B. alba* B18LD (Vargas and Strohl, 1985a). Glutamate dehydrogenase activity was not observed, and a low alanine dehydrogenase activity was not observed, and a low alanine dehydrogenase activity was observed under "high" ammonia conditions (Vargas and Strohl, 1985a). Other nitrogen sources that supported growth of *B. alba* B18LD were nitrate, nitrite, urea, aspartate and, to a lesser degree, asparagine, alanine and thiourea (Vargas and Strohl, 1985a). Glutamate, aspartate or asparagine supported the growth of certain other beggiatoas, indicating they could be used as sole nitrogen, carbon and energy sources (Pringsheim, 1964).

Beggiatoa can utilize nitrate (Nelson et al., 1982; Vargas and Strohl, 1985b; Williams and Unz, 1985) or nitrite (Vargas and Strohl, 1985b) as sole nitrogen source. The product of nitrate reduction by *B. alba* was not N_2 or N_2O but ammonia, indicating that it has an assimilatory type nitrate reduction mechanism (Vargas and Strohl, 1985b). *B. alba* B18LD is unable to grow anaerobically by using nitrate as an electron acceptor, and nitrate reduction is not coupled with sulfide oxidation (Vargas and Strohl, 1985b).

Nine strains of *Beggiatoa* were shown to fix dinitrogen at rates of 3–12 nmol/min/mg protein when grown in slush agar tubes in which the redox, sulfide and oxygen gradients had been established (Nelson et al., 1982). The gradient cultures were required to provide proper redox conditions for N_2 fixation (Nelson et al., 1982). Nitrate or ammonia inhibited the fixation of nitrogen, and sulfide was required by some of the beggiatoas to fix nitrogen (Nelson et al., 1982). Polman and Larkin (1988) recently found that ammonia and urea inhibited the activity of *B. alba* B18LD nitrogenase in vitro, whereas nitrate, nitrite, glutamine, and asparagine did not. Nitrite and nitrate, however, were found to inhibit in vivo nitrogenase induction. On the other hand, glutamine stimulated nitrogenase activity of *B. alba* B18LD (Polman and Larkin, 1988).

Ecological Niche—The Sulfide/Oxygen Interface

Beggiatoas exhibit four physiological characteristics which describe their ecological niche. First, they appear to be oligotrophic organisms which generally do not tolerate or utilize high concentrations of organic (W. R. Strohl, unpublished observations) or nitrogenous (Vargas and Strohl, 1985b) nutrients. Low concentrations (e.g. ≤ 20 mM) of organic acids and, in some cases, amino acids are apparently optimal for the growth and metabolism of beggiatoas.

Second, beggiatoas are respiratory organisms that couple the oxidation of organic acids (Scotten and Stokes, 1962; Strohl et al., 1986b) and/or sulfide (Jørgensen and Revsbech, 1983; Strohl and Schmidt, 1984; Vargas and Strohl, 1985b), with the reduction of oxygen as the terminal electron accepting step. Stored elemental sulfur can be utilized as an alternative electron acceptor under strictly anaerobic conditions (Nelson and Castenholz, 1981a; Schmidt et al., 1987). Because the pool of sulfur would be limiting, however, the sulfur is probably used only as an electron acceptor in situ for maintenance purposes while the filaments glide to a new sulfide-oxygen interface.

Third, beggiatoas are microaerophilic bacteria (Larkin and Strohl, 1983) that exhibit a phobic response to oxygen (Møller et al., 1985). Microaerophilic bacteria have been described as "aerobic or facultative anaerobic bacteria, which under aerobic conditions use O_2 as hydrogen acceptor in a respiratory way of energy production and show optimal growth at low oxygen tensions" (Stouthamer et al., 1979). Beggiatoas apparently produce hydrogen peroxide in potentially autolytic quantities (Burton and Morita, 1964); however, peroxide accumulation has not been quantitated. High levels of nutrients usually induce fast autolysis of *Beggiatoa* (Faust and Wolfe, 1961; Scotten and Stokes, 1962; Strohl and

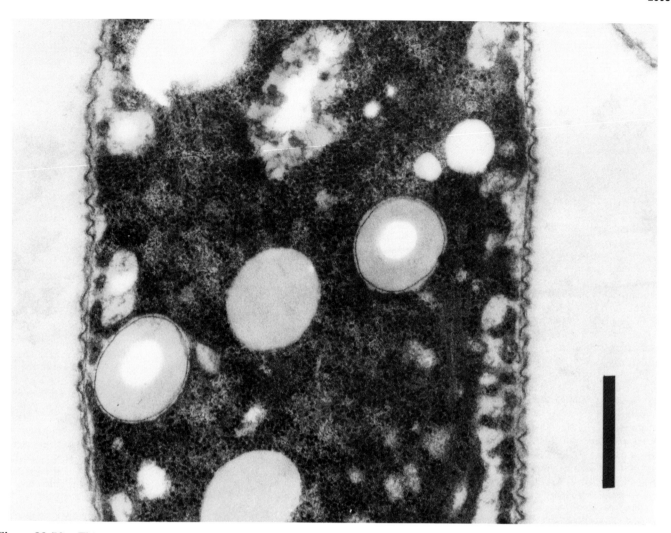

Figure 23.59. Thin-section micrograph of *B. alba* B18LD fixed via the modified Ryter-Kellenberger technique, showing sulfur inclusions and the 4-nm-thick sulfur inclusion envelopes. *Bar*, 0.5 μm.

Larkin, 1978b), which may be directly related to the amount of peroxide produced. Catalase is not produced to degrade the potentially toxic peroxides (Burton and Morita, 1964; Joshi and Hollis, 1976; Strohl and Larkin, 1978b; Nelson and Castenholz, 1981a). Addition of catalase to growth medium may enhance growth yields (Burton and Morita, 1964) or survival of certain *Beggiatoa* strains (Strohl and Larkin, 1978b).

Finally, beggiatoas are gradient organisms that live in sediments, in which they occupy the horizontal interface between sulfide emanating upward from below and oxygen diffusing downward from above (Jørgensen, 1982; Jørgensen and Revsbech, 1983; Nelson et al. 1986a). Jørgensen and his colleagues (Jørgensen, 1982; Jørgensen and Revsbech, 1983; Møller et al., 1985; Nelson et al., 1986a) have described the sulfide/oxygen interface location of *Beggiatoa* mats and plates, in situ and in vivo, respectively. In marine *Beggiatoa* mats, gradients of oxygen and sulfide were created by the beggiatoas above and below the horizontal mats, respectively (Jørgensen and Revsbech, 1983). In creating such concentration gradients, the beggiatoas apparently do not encounter high concentrations of most nutrients at their surface, a phenomenon probably preferential to their oligotrophic nature. Oxygen in high concentrations, especially if coinciding with concentrations of carbon nutrients, is apparently toxic to the beggiatoas, probably due to peroxide or other toxic product formation. Thus the vertical gradient effect which permits only minute amounts of oxygen to the organisms is seemingly ideal for them

(Nelson et al., 1986a). Stimulation of certain enzymes, such as nitrogenase (Nelson et al., 1982) and ribulose-1,5-bisphosphate carboxylase (Nelson and Jannasch, 1983), may depend on the attributes of the gradient effect (i.e. gradients of oxygen and sulfide in which the organism selects its best position). Beggiatoas also exhibit a photophobic response (Nelson and Castenholz, 1982), which, in conjunction with an aerophobic response (Møller et al., 1985), explains the diurnal vertical migration of *Beggiatoa* filaments in nature.

Enrichment and Isolation Procedures

Keil (1912) isolated *Beggiatoa* by washing the filaments repeatedly with sterile stream water. The washed filaments were placed in Petri dishes containing stream water and were incubated under a bell jar containing the gases H_2S (7.8 Pa), O_2 (147 Pa), CO_2 (245 Pa) and H_2. It has been suggested that Keil's methods have been only isolation procedures to be specifically designed to enrich for and isolate autotrophic strains.

Cataldi first observed *Beggiatoa* during her studies with iron bacteria (Cataldi, 1940) and for *Beggiatoa* enrichment, therefore, used the extracted hay technique that Winogradsky had developed for enrichment of iron bacteria. Recent investigators (Joshi and Hollis, 1976; Strohl and Larkin, 1978b) have successfully used various modifications of Cataldi's boiled hay procedure. Burton and Lee (1978) used an alternative procedure in which gallon jars were filled with raw sewage and aerated for 3 days, after which bundles of *Beggiatoa* filaments were observed on the surface.

For enrichment of salt marsh or estuarine beggiatoas, a marine salt mix can be added to a typical hay enrichment to approximate 50% seawater (Strohl and Larkin, 1978b). An excellent enrichment procedure for marine beggiatoas uses the sulfuretum concept of Baas-Becking (1925). A 1-2-inch layer of sea sand is covered by a 1-inch layer of sulfide-emanating mud and a few inches of 50–80% seawater. Then some decaying leaves (or boiled hay) and ~1 g l⁻¹ CaSO₄ are added. Two thirds of the tank is darkened by wrapping in aluminum foil, and a light is shined on the remaining third so that a natural sulfur cycling takes place between the photosynthetic and the dark zones as well as between the aerobic and reduced zones. Combined cyanobacterial, photosynthetic bacterial, and *Beggiatoa* mats develop in about 2 weeks and remain stable for months.

Depending on the nutritive conditions of the hay enrichments and the agar plates upon which the beggiatoas are isolated, it is likely that a wide variety of different nutritional types of beggiatoas may be obtained (Strohl and Larkin, 1978b). Cataldi (1940) used the gliding motility of *Beggiatoa* to isolate them. She placed washed filaments from enrichments into the center of a Petri dish containing 0.1% yeast extract, 0.6% ethanol and 1.2% agar. After 48 h, the contaminant-free trichomes at the edge of the plates were picked up by a Pasteur pipette and were placed into liquid medium (Cataldi, 1940). Most investigators have used various modifications of Cataldi's isolation procedures (Faust and Wolfe, 1961; Scotten and Stokes, 1962; Pringsheim, 1964; Burton and Lee, 1978; Strohl and Larkin, 1978b). The following is a general isolation procedure for *Beggiatoa* strains. Filaments from enrichments are washed 5 times with sterile basal salts containing 5 mM neutralized sodium sulfide. Tufts of filaments are transferred from one wash bath to the next via microforceps. The tufts of filaments are teased and prodded to remove as much macroscopic contaminating material as possible. The washed tufts are placed onto a dry 1.6% agar plate for about 1 min to adsorb away as much of the excess fluid away as possible. They can be touched with a corner of filter paper to further remove excess fluid (Burton and Lee, 1978). The tufts of filaments are then removed from the "drying plate" and placed onto prescored (Burton and Lee, 1978), freshly prepared 1.4% agar plates containing 2 mM sodium sulfide, 0.01% each of yeast extract and sodium acetate, and basal salts (Vargas and Strohl, 1985a). After 5–48 h, the plates can be observed by using a dissecting microscope for any contaminant-free filaments, which, along with a small amount of the agar beneath them, are removed by using flame-sterilized 23–26-gauge needles. It is usually best to wait for at least 24 h, so that the filaments which are contaminated are overgrown and those which are pure are far away from contaminants, making them easy to isolate.

For growth of most freshwater beggiatoas, a defined medium can be constructed that contains the following nutrients: 0.2–10.0 mM sodium acetate, succinate, or malate as carbon source, ~2.0 mM ammonium or nitrate as nitrogen source (Vargas and Strohl, 1985a), and standard basal salts (Vargas and Strohl, 1985a). An apparent requirement for high concentration of calcium and a low concentration of phosphate are notable. A reduced sulfur source such as sulfide or thiosulfate at concentrations of 1–2 mM can be added to the heterotrophic medium above. Increasing carbon nutrients shortens the survival time of the organism, which may be

due to higher levels of the peroxides produced. A good general purpose medium for growth, isolation and maintenance of most freshwater beggiatoas is one modified from the MY medium described by Larkin (1980). It contains 0.01% each of sodium acetate, yeast extract, and nutrient broth (Difco, Detroit, Michigan), 2 mM neutralized sodium sulfide nonahydrate, and basal salts (Vargas and Strohl, 1985a). For routine maintenance, sodium sulfide can be added prior to autoclaving, after which the medium should appear gray due to production of FeS. About 90% of the sulfide is lost upon autoclaving (Vargas and Strohl, 1985a). The medium should be inoculated immediately after cooling so that some of the sulfide can be used before it is chemically oxidized or volatilized. For critical experiments, the sulfide should be neutralized and then autoclaved separately under a nitrogen atmosphere in sealed Wheaton serum bottles. It then can be added to the medium just prior to inoculation.

Maintenance Procedures

The best media for general maintenance of freshwater beggiatoas are usually low nutrient media with adequate sulfide or thiosulfate concentrations and relatively low oxygen concentrations. The modified MY medium described above is a good general medium for maintenance of freshwater beggiatoas. Biphasic cultures can be constructed by overlaying a 1.6% agar plug of MY medium, modified by increasing the sulfide concentration to 4 mM, with MY liquid medium or with MY and 0.2% agar slush medium. Normally, cultures will survive about 1 month under any of these conditions. For growth and maintenance of marine cultures, refer to methods described by Nelson et al. (1982) and Nelson and Jannasch (1983).

Beggiatoa strains have been preserved for long term viability by freezing them in the presence of 20–30% glycerol at −70°C or −196°C. Survival at −196°C is at least several months for the strains tested.

Further Reading

Jørgensen, B.B. 1982. Ecology of the bacteria of the sulphur cycle with special reference to anoxic-oxic interface environments. Philos. Trans. R. Soc. Lond. [Biol.] 298: 473–497.

Larkin, J.M. and W.R. Strohl. 1983. *Beggiatoa, Thiothrix,* and *Thioploca.* Annu. Rev. Microbiol. 37: 341–367.

Nelson, D.C. and H.W. Jannasch. 1983. Chemoautotrophic growth of a marine *Beggiatoa* in sulfide-gradient cultures. Arch. Microbiol. 136:262–269.

Nelson, D.C. 1989. Physiology and biochemistry of filamentous sulfur bacteria. *In* Schlegel and Bowien (Editors), Autotrophic Bacteria. Science Tech Publishers, Madison, Wisconsin, in press.

Strohl, W.R. and J.M. Larkin. 1978. Enumeration, isolation, and characterization of *Beggiatoa* from freshwater sediments. Appl. Environ. Microbiol. 36: 755–770.

Strohl, W.R. and T. M. Schmidt. 1984. Mixotrophy of *Beggiatoa* and *Thiothrix. In* Strohl and Tuovinen (Editors), Microbial Chemoautotrophy. Ohio State University Press, Columbus, pp. 79–95.

Wiessner, W. 1981. The family *Beggiatoaceae. In* Starr, Stolp, Trüper, Balows and Schlegel (Editors), The Prokaryotes. A Handbook of Habitats, Isolation, and Identification of Bacteria. Springer-Verlag, Berlin, pp. 380–389.

Acknowledgments

I sincerely thank Thomas M. Schmidt for our many discussions on the taxonomy and characteristics of *Beggiatoa* during the preparation of this manuscript. Ingeborg Geffers assisted in the preparation of the electron micrographs.

List of species of the genus **Beggiatoa**

1. **Beggiatoa alba** (Vaucher, 1803) Trevisan, 1845.[AL]
al′ba. L. adj. *albus* white.

Filaments measure about 1.5–4.0 μm in diameter and are of uniform width. Filament diameter may vary with growth conditions. Cells are generally 3.0–9.0 μm long, with filament lengths averaging from 60 to 120 μm. Ends of the filaments are rounded. Necridia and hormogonia may be produced. Circuitans type colonies usually are formed. Sulfur is deposited in inclusions external to the cytoplasmic membrane but within the cell wall, when the organism is grown in the presence of sulfide or thiosulfate. PHB and polyphosphate deposits may be present.

Chemoorganotrophic growth is obtained by using acetate, fumarate, lactate, malate, pyruvate, succinate or ethanol as sole carbon and energy sources. The oxidation of sulfide, thiosulfate or hydrogen has been proposed to be coupled with energy conservation for chemolithotrophic metabolism, although this has yet to be proven. Ammonia, nitrate, nitrite or urea is used as sole source of nitrogen.

Organisms grow by respiratory metabolism, with molecular oxygen used as the terminal electron acceptor. Microaerophilic to aerobic. Maintenance under anaerobic conditions, with sulfur used as the terminal electron acceptor, may occur.

Gelatin, starch and casein are not hydrolyzed. Filaments are catalase-negative, and N,N,N',N'-tetramethyl-p-phenylenediamine (TMPD) cytochrome oxidase-positive. No growth is observed in the presence of 0.05% sodium dodecyl sulfate or 1.5% NaCl. Strains thus far have been isolated only from freshwater sediments.

The mol% G + C of the DNA is 40–43 (T_m).

Neotype strain: LSU strain B18LD (ATCC 33555). B18LD was isolated from an enrichment obtained from a rice paddy in Lacassine, Louisiana, U.S.A. This strain, along with other *B. alba* strains, was recently described in detail (Mezzino et al., 1984).

Other Beggiatoas

Several other strains of *Beggiatoa* have been isolated and partially characterized in recent years. In this section, the currently existing, partially characterized strains of *Beggiatoa* are presented with data from the literature or data which are as yet unpublished. All of these strains are colorless and filamentous, and they glide and deposit sulfur in the presence of sulfide. Several of these strains may eventually be characterized as new species of *Beggiatoa*, but only after more thorough classification efforts are made. In Table 23.19, the salient characteristics of these organisms are compared.

Table 23.19.

Comparison of the salient characteristics of several unspeciated **Beggiatoa** *strains*[a]

Characterisitic	Beggiatoa strains							
	L1401-4	L1401-13	L1401-15	PD-1	SM-1	75-2a	MS-81-6	U1
Investigator[b]	E.P.	E.P.	E.P.	K.M.	S.M.	D.N.	D.N.	T.W.
Source of isolate[c]	FW	FW	FW	FW	FW	FW	M	FW
Mol% G + C of DNA[d]	nd	nd	50 (T_m)	61 (T_m)	nd	nd	nd	nd
Colony type[e]	C	L	C	L	C	C	nd	nd
Optimal growth temperature (°C)[f]	20–25	20–25	20–25	25–30	20–25	35–38	nd	20–28
Deposition of								
Sulfur on								
Sulfide	+	+	+	+	+	+	+	+
Thiosulfate	nd	nd	nd	nd	+	+	nd	+
Cysteine	−	−	−	−	−	nd	nd	nd
Polyphosphate	+	+	+	nd	nd	nd	nd	+
PHB	+	+	+	+	+	+	nd	+
Filament diameter (μm)[g]	2.0	2.5	2.5	1.0	2.5	2.0	4.5	1.5
Heterotrophic growth	+	+	+	+	+	+	+	+
Autotrophic growth	−	−	−	−	−	−	+	nd
Utilization of								
Succinate	nd	nd	nd	+	nd	−[i]	nd	−[i]
Malate	nd	nd	nd	+	nd	−[i]	nd	−[i]
Fumarate	nd	nd	nd	+	nd	−[i]	nd	+[i]
Pyruvate	nd	nd	nd	+	nd	+	nd	+[i]
Ethanol	nd	nd	nd	+	nd	+	nd	+
Gelatin hydrolysis	−	−	nd	nd	−	nd	nd	−
Growth with sole N source								
NH₃	+	+	+	+	+	+	nd	nd
NO₃⁻	nd	nd	nd	+	nd	+	nd	+
N₂	nd	nd	nd	nd	nd	+	+	nd
Growth on aspartate or glutamate as sole C and N sources	+	+	nd	+	nd	nd	nd	nd
Growth on glucose as sole C and energy sources	−	−	−	+	−	−	nd	−
Oxidase	nd	nd	nd	+	+	nd	nd	−
Catalase	nd	nd	nd	−	−	−	nd	−
Reference or source[h]	*1*	*1, 2*	*1, 3*	*4*	*5*	*6*	*7*	*8*

[a]Symbols: nd, not determined; +, 90% or more of strains are positive; and −, 90% or more of strains are negative.

[b]Investigators (who isolated strains): E.P., Ernst Pringsheim; K.M., Kevin Marshall; S.M., Siegfried Maier; D.N., Douglas Nelson; and T.W., Terry Williams.

[c]Sources: FW, freshwater; and M, marine.

[d]Data are from M. J. Mezzino and J. M. Larkin.

[e]Colony types: C, circuitans; L, linguiformis. See Pringsheim (1964), Strohl and Larkin (1978b), and Mezzino et al. (1984) for further descriptions.

[f]Optimal temperatures are approximations.

[g]Filament diameters are given to the nearest 0.5 μm because of limited resolution and accuracy of phase microscopy.

[h]References and sources: *1*, Pringsheim, 1964; *2*, Strohl et al., 1981a; *3*, M. J. Mezzino, M.S. thesis, Louisiana State University, Baton Rouge, Louisiana; *4*, K. C. Marshall, gift and unpublished observations; *5*, S. Maier, gift, isolated from the Ohio Wesleyan University Campus, Delaware, Ohio, and unpublished observations; *6*, Nelson and Castenholz, 1981a, b, and Nelson et al., 1982; *7*, Nelson and Jannasch, 1983; and *8*, Williams and Unz, 1985.

[i]Data are taken from Nelson, 1989.

Genus II. **Thiothrix** *Winogradsky 1888, 39*[AL]

J. M. LARKIN

Thi'.o.thrix. Gr. n. *thium* sulfur; Gr. n. *thrix* hair; M.L. fem. n. *Thiothrix* sulfur hair.

Rods, about 1.0–1.5 μm in diameter, which exist in **multicellular** rigid **filaments** of uniform diameter **within a sheath** and which **produce gonidia from the open end of the sheath**. Rosettes may be produced. The closed end of the sheath may have a holdfast. Capsules are not produced. Resting stages are not known. Gram-negative. The **gonidia are motile by gliding**. No flagella are present, but a tuft of fimbria may be present on one end of the gonidium.

Aerobic or microaerophilic. Optimum temperature: 25–30°C; maximum: about 32–34°C; minimum: about 6–8°C. Isolates, to date, are mixotrophic, requiring any of several small organic compounds as well as a reduced inorganic sulfur source (see "Other Organisms"). **Sulfur globules are deposited** within invaginations of the cytoplasmic membrane when cells grow in the presence of a reduced inorganic sulfur compound. **By light microscopy the sulfur globules appear to be internal**. Cytochrome oxidase-positive. Catalase-negative.

Found in sulfide-containing flowing water and in activated-sludge sewage systems.

The mol% G + C of the DNA is 52 (T_m).

Type species: *Thiothrix nivea* Winogradsky 1888, 39.

Further Descriptive Information

Cells are rigid. The sheath appears to be made up of several layers which may pull apart in preparation (Fig. 23.60). The cell wall appears to be typically Gram-negative. Sulfur globules are deposited within invaginations of the cytoplasmic membrane and are therefore external to the cytoplasm, as in *Beggiatoa*. Poly-β-hydroxybutyrate (PHB) and polyphosphate may be produced. Several strains, including the type, fix nitrogen, as demonstrated by acetylene reduction (J. K. Polman and J. M. Larkin, unpublished observations). Minges et al. (1983) reported that *T. nivea* strain JP3 contained an 8.1 Md plasmid, and Polman and Larkin (unpublished observation) have detected a much larger plasmid in strains JP1 and JP2. Gonidia glide at a rate of about 1–2 μm/min and appear to twitch as they move. In freshly collected material there may be many rosettes (Fig. 23.61), but the ability to form rosettes may be lost in the laboratory, resulting in a culture composed of filaments of various lengths. The loss of rosette-forming ability is accompanied by the loss of the polar fimbriae (Larkin, unpublished observation). A life cycle (Fig. 23.62) has been proposed (Larkin and Shinabarger, 1983) in which gonidia released from the open end of the sheathed filament may remain and accumulate, at the site of their release, for the eventual formation of a rosette which is attached to the original filament. The filament may then continue to grow past the rosette. Alternatively, the gonidia may grow into filaments or, presumably, can aggregate to form rosettes by virtue of their motility. Initial attachment of the gonidia involves the fimbriae, with holdfast material being produced after attachment.

Thiothrix is found in flowing sulfide-containing waters with a pH of near neutrality (Bahr and Schwartz, 1956) and an oxygen concentration of about 10% of saturation (Keil, 1912; Bahr and Schwartz, 1956; Bland and Staley, 1978). It may be the dominant filamentous sulfide-oxidizing organism in suitable waters (Lackey et al., 1965). The ability of *Thiothrix* to attach to objects and to itself undoubtedly allows it to remain situated in a suitable location in flowing water. *Thiothrix* may also be found in activated-sludge–sewage systems where its presence is associated with bulking (Farquhar and Boyle, 1971, 1972).

Enrichment and Isolation Procedures

Thiothrix-containing material is placed in a Petri dish and observed with a dissecting microscope with transmitted light. Tufts of filaments are picked up with fine-tipped forceps and transferred to a Petri dish containing about 5–10 ml of a salt solution* (SS) (Strohl and Larkin, 1978a). The tufts are agitated with the forceps and then transferred to another Petri dish containing the same solution. This is repeated

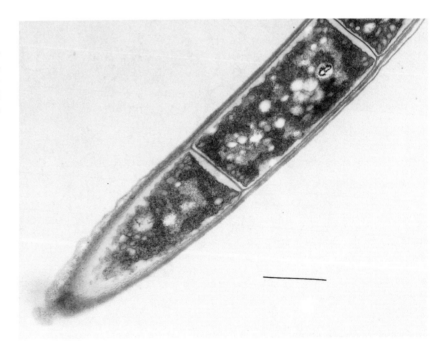

Figure 23.60. Thin section of *T. nivea* strain JP2 grown on MY agar. PHB granules are seen near the center of the cells, and smaller sulfur globules are near the periphery, especially adjacent to the septa. The cell wall, sheath and holdfast are also visible. Prepared according to Kellenberger et al. (1958) and poststained with lead acetate and uranyl acetate. *Bar*, 1 μm.

---

*Salt solution contains: NH$_4$Cl, 0.02%; K$_2$HPO$_4$, 0.001%; MgSO$_4$, 0.001%; CaSO$_4$, 20 ml/l of a saturated solution; and trace element solution, 5 ml/l. pH is about 7.5 (Trace element solution contains: ZnSO$_4$·7H$_2$O, 0.001%; MnSO$_4$·4H$_2$O, 0.002%; CuSO$_4$·5H$_2$O, 0.0000005%; H$_3$BO$_3$, 0.001%; Co(NO$_3$)$_2$, 0.0001%; Na-molybdate, 0.0001%; EDTA, 0.02%; and FeSO$_4$·7H$_2$O, 0.07%.)

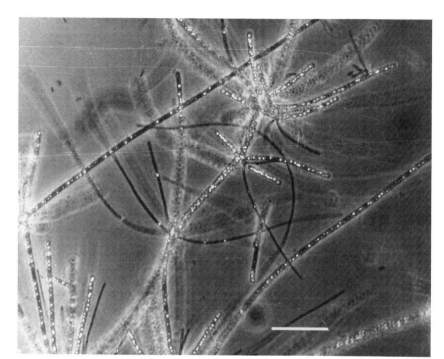

Figure 23.61. Phase micrograph of *T. nivea* from a freshwater sulfide-containing spring. *Bar*, 10 μm.

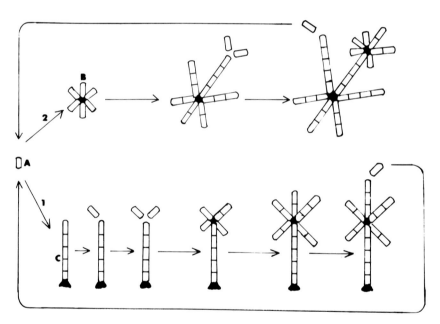

Figure 23.62. A proposed life cycle for *T nivea*. A gonidium (*A*) may aggregate with other gonidia to form a rosette (*B*), or it may grow into a filament (*C*). Additional rosettes may form on the initial rosettes and on the filaments, from gonidia which remain at the site of their release. (Modified from J. M. Larkin and D. L. Shinabarger, International Journal of Systematic Bacteriology *33*: 841–846, 1983.)

through four or five transfers. A few drops from each dilution is transferred with a Pasteur pipette to either MP agar (SS plus 0.0001% sodium acetate, 0.03% Na₂S and 1.5% agar; Strohl and Larkin, 1978a) or MY agar (SS plus 0.01% each of sodium acetate, nutrient broth powder, and yeast extract, plus 0.03% Na₂S, and 1.5% agar; Larkin, 1980) in separate Petri dishes. Each dish is held on an angle so that the drops will flow across the agar surface. The excess is then withdrawn from the other side

with the pipette. The dishes are incubated at about 25–30°C and are examined daily with a dissecting microscope in transmitted light. Colonies with a hairy or filamentous edge are transferred with sterile toothpicks to fresh media and are restreaked until pure.

Isolation of the strains listed under "Other Organisms" was accomplished by dilution and washing of the filaments in a mineral salts solution,[†] followed by streaking on glucose-sulfide[‡] or LT[§] medium. Before

---

[†]Mineral salts solution contains (per liter): (NH₄)₂SO₄, 0.5 g; MgSO₄·7H₂O, 0.1 g; CaCl₂·2H₂O, 0.05 g; K₂HPO₄, 0.11 g; KH₂PO₄, 0.085 g; FeCl₃·6H₂O, 0.002 g; EDTA, 0.003 g; and vitamin mix (Eikelboom, 1975), 1.0 ml. pH is about 7.5.
[‡]Glucose-sulfide medium contains (per liter): glucose, 0.15 g; (NH₄)₂SO₄, 0.5 g; Ca(NO₃)₂, 0.01 g; K₂HPO₄·7H₂O, 0.05 g; KCl, 0.05 g; CaCO₃, 0.1 g; Na₂S·9H₂O, 0.187 g; vitamin mix, 1.0 ml; and agar, 15.0 g, when needed. pH is about 7.5.
[§]LT medium contains: mineral salts with vitamins; sodium lactate, 0.75 g/l; Na₂S₂O₃·5H₂O, 0.25 g/l; HEPES buffer, 0.01 M; and agar, 15.0 g/l, when needed. pH is about 7.5.

the solid media are streaked for isolation, some samples were enriched by adding a small amount of sample to a tube containing a butt of glucose-sulfide agar overlaid with mineral salts.

Maintenance Procedures

Cultures can be maintained in semisolid (0.15% agar) deeps of either MP or MY medium, with transfers at intervals of about 3–4 weeks. Other methods of preservation have not been tested.

Procedures for Testing Special Characteristics

Utilization of Sole Carbon Sources

Carbon sources are added to MP broth without acetate to a final con-

centration of 0.05%. Growth must occur through three successive transfers to be considered positive.

Utilization of Sole Nitrogen Sources

MP broth without the ammonium salt and supplemented with the appropriate nitrogen source in concentrations of 0.02 or 0.05% is used.

Utilization of Sole Sulfur Sources

The sulfate salts in MP broth are replaced by the chloride salts. Sulfur sources to be tested are added at concentrations of 0.03%.

Differentiation of the genus Thiothrix from other genera

Thiothrix and *Beggiatoa* are separated from each other by the presence of a sheath, the production of rosettes, and the lack of gliding motility of the filaments of *Thiothrix*. *Thiothrix* and *Thioploca* are separated by the production of rosettes and the lack of gliding filaments of *Thiothrix* and by the presence of multiple filaments within a single sheath of *Thioploca*. *Thiothrix* may be differentiated from *Leucothrix*, which it resembles morphologically, by the presence of a sheath and the ability to deposit sulfur globules. *Thiothrix* is found in both freshwater and marine environments, whereas *Leucothrix* has been reported only from marine habitats. Moreover, *Thiothrix* produces gonidia from only the end of a filament, whereas the entire filament of *Leucothrix* may segment into gonidia.

Taxonomic Comments

It is not certain how closely *Thiothrix* may be related to the other gen-

era of filamentous sulfur-oxidizing bacteria. A significant number of cultures of *Beggiatoa* and *Thiothrix* have been available for only a few years, and comparative studies between the two genera have not been undertaken. The lack of pure cultures of *Thioploca* has prevented adequate comparison with that genus.

Winogradsky (1888) believed that *Thiothrix* might be autotrophic, but if autotrophic strains exist, they have not yet been isolated.

Acknowledgments

I thank Terry Williams for supplying all of the information used to compile the "Other Organisms" section. Rod Nelson prepared the electron micrograph.

Further Reading

Larkin, J.M. and W.R. Strohl. 1983. *Beggiatoa, Thiothrix,* and *Thioploca.* Annu. Rev. Microbiol. 37: 341–367.

List of species of the genus Thiothrix

1. **Thiothrix nivea** (Rabenhorst 1865) Winogradsky 1888, 39.[AL] (*Beggiatoa nivea* Rabenhorst 1865, 94.)

ni′ve.a. L. adj. *nivea* snow-white

The description of the genus and the data in Table 23.20 contain the features of this species.

Neotype strain: JP2 (ATCC 35100).

Other Organisms

R. Richard and the team of R. Unz and T. Williams have isolated six strains of *Thiothrix*-like organisms from bulking activated sludge-wastewater treatment plants. Unz and Williams (unpublished data) have carried out an extensive characterization of these strains. The isolates probably represent more than one species, and because their existence may cause a broadening of the definition of the genus in the future, their features are presented here.

All strains are multicellular filaments which may have a sheath. They produce gonidia from the open end of the sheath, deposit sulfur internally in the presence of reduced inorganic sulfur, produce PHB and polyphosphate, and form rosettes.

i. *Thiothrix* sp. strains A1 and A3.

These strains resemble *T. nivea* in requiring reduced inorganic sulfur for growth and are probably mixotrophic. Rods within the filaments are about 0.7–1.5 μm in diameter. Growth occurs at 4 and 33°C and over a pH range of 6.5–8.5. No growth occurs at 37°C. Oxidase-positive. Catalase-negative.

Gelatin and casein are hydrolyzed. Starch, Tween 80 and urea are not hydrolyzed.

Pyruvate, succinate, acetate, lactate or propionate is used as sole carbon source if $Na_2S_2O_3$ is present. Slight growth occurs with malate. No growth occurs with the following: mannoheptulose, glucose, galactose, mannose, sorbose, fructose, rhamnose, fucose, ribose, xylose, arabinose, glyceraldehyde phosphate, maltose, sucrose, lactose, trehalose, melibiose, gentiobiose, cellobiose, melizitose, raffinose, starch, inulin, sali-

cin, esculin, amygdalin, mannitol, inositol, glycerol, erythritol, sorbitol, gluconate, glucuronate, galacturonate, Tween 80, tributyrin, methanol, ethanol, *n*-propanol, *n*-butanol, isoamyl alcohol, *n*-amyl alcohol, phenol, citrate, α-ketoglutarate, formate, butyrate, hydroxybutyrate, valerate, caproate, oleate, benzoate, *m*-toluate or glycollate.

Table 23.20.
Characteristics of the species of the genus **Thiothrix**[a]

Characteristic	1. *T. nivea*
Utilization as sole carbon source[b]	
Acetate, malate, pyruvate, oxalacetate	+
Formate, citrate, *cis*-aconitate, succinate, fumarate, phosphoenolpyruvate, carbonate, glyoxalate, methylamine, propionate, lactate, glucose, lactose, fructose, sucrose, maltose, ribose, mannose, arabinose, cellobiose, rhamnose, raffinose, sorbose, melibiose, xylose, ethanol, methanol, propanol, glycerol, erythritol, asparagine, cysteine, methionine, serine, glutamate, aspartate	−
Use as sole nitrogen source[b]	
Ammonia, nitrate	+
Nitrite, N_2	−
$NO_3^- \rightarrow NO_2^-$	+
NO_2^- reduction	−
Use as sole sulfur source	
Sulfide, thiosulfate	+
Sulfite, sulfate, tetrathionate, 2-mercaptoethanol	−

[a]Symbols: +, 90% or more of strains are positive; and −, 90% or more of strains are negative.

[b]With sulfide or thiosulfate present.

Ammonia, nitrate, asparagine, glutamine, aspartate, glutamate or glucosamine is used as sole nitrogen source. Nitrite, alanine, glycine, phenylalanine, lysine, cystine, leucine, proline and cysteine cannot serve as sole nitrogen source. Utilization of methionine as sole nitrogen source varies between the strains. Nitrate is reduced to nitrite. Sulfide and thiosulfate serve as sole sulfur source.

ii. *Thiothrix* sp. strains I and Q.

Heterotrophic. Strains do not require a reduced inorganic sulfur compound. Rods within the filaments are about 1.2–2.5 μm in diameter. Growth occurs at 4 and 28°C and over a pH range of 6.5–8.5. No growth occurs at 33°C. Oxidase-positive. Weakly catalase-positive.

Gelatin is hydrolyzed. Starch, casein, Tween 80 and urea are not hydrolyzed.

Fructose, sucrose, melizitose, pyruvate, succinate, malate, acetate, lactate or propionate is used as sole carbon source. No growth occurs with the following: mannoheptulose, glucose, galactose, mannose, sorbose, rhamnose, fucose, ribose, xylose, arabinose, glyceraldehyde phosphate, maltose, lactose, trehalose, melibiose, gentiobiose, cellobiose, raffinose, starch, inulin, salicin, esculin, amygdalin, mannitol, inositol, glycerol, erythritol, sorbitol, gluconate, glucuronate, galacturonate, Tween 80, tributyrin, methanol, ethanol, *n*-propanol, *n*-butanol, isoamyl alcohol, *n*-amyl alcohol, phenol, citrate, α-ketoglutarate, formate, butyrate, hydroxybutyrate, valerate, caproate, oleate, benzoate, *m*-toluate or glycollate.

Ammonia, nitrate, proline, cysteine, asparagine, glutamine, aspartate, glutamate or glucosamine is used as sole nitrogen source. Nitrite, alanine, glycine, phenylalanine, lysine, cystine, leucine or methionine cannot serve as sole nitrogen source. Nitrate is reduced to nitrite.

iii. *Thiothrix* sp. strain TH3.

Heterotrophic. Does not require a reduced inorganic sulfur compound. Rods within the filaments are about 0.7–1.5 μm in diameter. Growth occurs at 10 and 37°C and over a pH range of 6.0–8.5. No growth occurs at 4 or 45°C. Oxidase-positive. Catalase-positive.

Urea is hydrolyzed. Gelatin, starch, casein and Tween 80 are not hydrolyzed.

Succinate, malate, acetate, lactate, propionate, ethanol or propanol is used as sole carbon source. Growth on α-ketoglutarate is poor. No growth occurs with the following: mannoheptulose, glucose, galactose, mannose, sorbose, fructose, rhamnose, fucose, ribose, xylose, arabinose, glyceraldehyde phosphate, maltose, sucrose, lactose, trehalose, melibiose, gentiobiose, cellobiose, melizitose, raffinose, starch, inulin, salicin, esculin, amygdalin, mannitol, inositol, glycerol, erythritol, sorbitol, gluconate, glucuronate, galacturonate, Tween 80, tributyrin, methanol, *n*-butanol, isoamyl alcohol, *n*-amyl alcohol, phenol, pyruvate, citrate, formate, butyrate, hydroxybutyrate, valerate, caproate, oleate, benzoate, *m*-toluate or glycollate.

Ammonia, nitrate, nitrite, lysine, cystine, leucine, methionine, proline, cysteine, asparagine, glutamine, aspartate, glutamate or glucosamine is used as sole source of nitrogen. Alanine, glycine or phenylalanine cannot serve as sole nitrogen source. Glutamate can serve as both a carbon and a nitrogen source. Nitrate is reduced to nitrite.

iv. *Thiothrix* sp. strain TH1.

Heterotrophic. Does not require a reduced inorganic sulfur compound. Rods within the filaments are about 1.2–2.5 μm in diameter. Growth occurs at 10 and 37°C and over a pH range of 6.5–8.5. No growth occurs at 4 or 45°C. Oxidase-positive. Catalase-positive.

Gelain is hydrolyzed. Casein, starch, Tween 80 and urea are not hydrolyzed.

Glucose, fructose, ribose, maltose, sucrose, trehalose, melizitose, amygdalin, mannitol, inositol, ethanol, *n*-propanol, *n*-butanol, pyruvate, α-ketoglutarate, succinate, malate, acetate, lactate, propionate, butyrate, hydroxybutyrate or valerate is used as sole carbon source. Growth is poor with galactose, glycerol, isoamyl alcohol or caproate. No growth occurs with the following: mannoheptulose, mannose, sorbose, rhamnose, fucose, xylose, arabinose, glyceraldehyde phosphate, lactose, melibiose, gentiobiose, cellobiose, raffinose, starch, inulin, salicin, esculin, erythritol, sorbitol, gluconate, glucuronate, galacturonate, Tween 80, tributryin, methanol, *n*-amyl alcohol, phenol, citrate, formate, oleate, benzoate, *m*-toluate or glycollate.

Ammonia, nitrate, cysteine, asparagine, glutamate, aspartate, glutamate or glucosamine is used as sole nitrogen source. Nitrite, alanine, glycine, phenylalanine, lysine, cystine, leucine, methionine or proline cannot serve as sole nitrogen source. Glutamate can serve as both a carbon and a nitrogen source. Nitrate is reduced to nitrite.

Genus III. **Thioploca** Lauterborn 1907, 242[AL]

SIEGFRIED MAIER

Thi.o.plo′ca. Gr. neut. n. *thion* sulfur; Gr. fem. n. *ploke* a braid, a twist; M.L. fem. n. *Thioploca* sulfur braid.

Flexible, uniseriate filaments made up **of numerous cells,** generally **with** numerous **sulfur inclusions, occur in** parallel or braided **fascicles, enclosed by a common sheath** of variable width. The **number of filaments within a sheath is variable.** Within one sheath, filaments may be of fairly uniform or of greatly differing diameters. The sheath is frequently encrusted with detritus. Individual **filaments show independent gliding** movement, and they may emerge from the end of or from breaks in the sheath. The long filaments are of **uniform diameter;** their **terminal segments** may be **tapered or rounded.** Not isolated in pure culture.

Type species: *Thioploca schmidlei* Lauterborn 1907, 242.[AL]

Further Descriptive Information

Thioploca can be described as a colonial, undifferentiated multicellular procaryote. An individual consists of a single row of cylindrical or slightly barrel shaped cells, a uniseriate filament. The individual cells of a filament are not always distinguishable in the microscope (Fig. 23.63). Several filaments inhabit a common sheath. Coupled with the gliding motility of the filaments, the gross morphology of *Thioploca* resembles that of the oscillatorian *Hydrocoleum* and *Microcoleus*. However, instead of the pigments of the oscillatorians, the cells of *Thioploca* contain numerous sulfur inclusions (Figs. 23.63 and 23.64). All these features are readily apparent in wet mounts of living samples observed with the microscope, making it possible to identify *Thioploca* on sight. The species have been differentiated solely on filament diameter (Maier, 1974).

Since none of the thioplocas have been isolated in pure culture, information about the species is rather scant. The appearance of the cell wall in the electron microscope is that of a Gram-negative structure (Maier and Murray, 1965; Maier and Gallardo, 1984b). Only the inner, single, electron-dense wall layer (peptidoglycan?), together with the cytoplasmic membrane, participates in cell division and eventually completely encloses each cell of the filament. Numerous membrane intrusions traverse the cytoplasm. Vacuoles in *T. ingrica* are more or less filled with electron-dense material (Maier and Murray, 1965), while in the large marine species, a large, "empty," membrane-bound vacuole (Maier and Gallardo, 1984b) results in a thin peripheral cytoplasm with sulfur inclusions (Figs. 23.65 and 23.66). This arrangement may be the solution to the transport problem for the large procaryotic cells. The "cytoplasmic" sulfur inclusions are deposited within the membrane intrusions and are thus, in strict terms, extracellular (Maier and Murray, 1965; S. Maier and H. Völker, unpublished observations).

When the sheathed fascicles are washed from the sediment, they may appear as tangled threads at low magnification (Fig. 23.67). Filaments and sheaths become apparent at higher magnification. The large marine

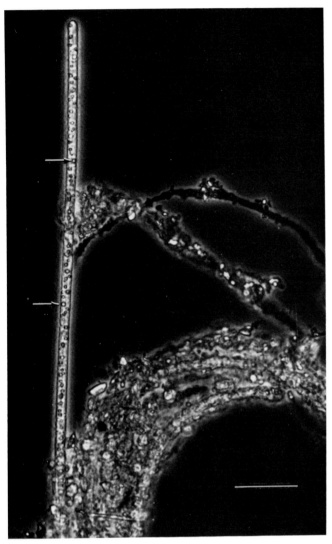

Figure 23.63. Filament of *Thioploca ingrica* gliding from a break in the mineral encrusted sheath. Phase contrast. Note rounded terminal segment and sulfur inclusions (*arrows*). *Bar*, 25 μm.

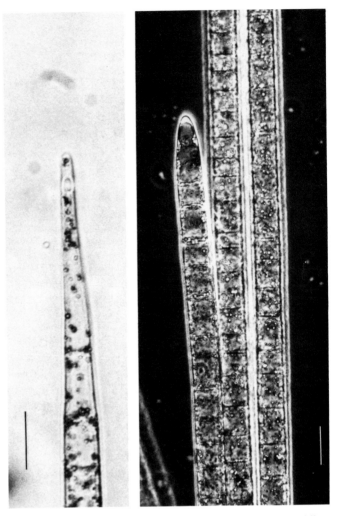

Figure 23.64. Terminal segments of filaments of *Thioploca chileae*. Vacuolation is most apparent in the tapered terminal cells. *Left*, brightfield; *right*, phase contrast. *Bar*, 20 μm.

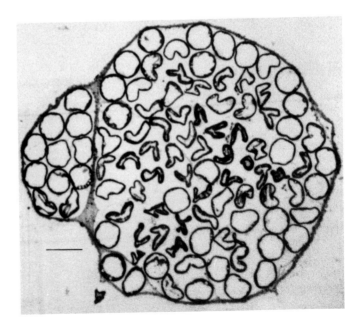

Figure 23.65. Transverse thick section of *T. chileae*. The collapsed filaments are senescent or poorly fixed. Osmium-DMSO prefix, Kellenberger, Epon, toluidine blue. *Bar*, 25 μm.

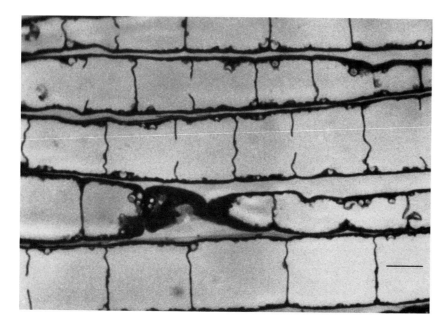

Figure 23.66. Longitudinal thick section of *T. chileae*. Kellenberger, Epon, toluidine blue. *Bar*, 10 μm.

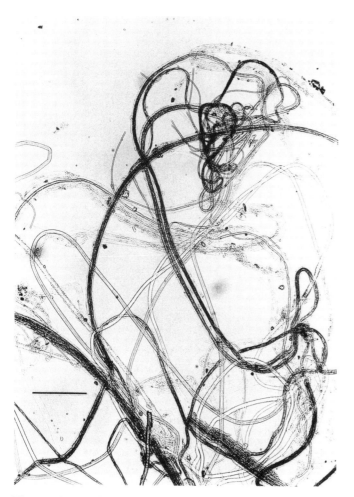

Figure 23.67. Tangled bundles of sheathed *T. ingrica* washed from the sediment. *Bar*, 200 μm.

species (Table 23.21) are easily visible with the unaided eye (Fig. 23.68); details are visible only by microscopic examination (Fig. 23.69). In these large forms, branching of the sheath (Fig. 23.68, left end of upper fascicle), sheathed bundles within a sheath (Fig. 23.69), or composite sheaths (Fig. 23.65) are also encountered.

The diameters of the filaments within the common sheath are generally rather uniform. However, Koppe (1924) described "*T. mixta*," because the common sheath contained filaments of mixed diameters (1.0 and 6–8 μm). Similar associations of filaments have been encountered in Lake Erie (C. I. Randles, personal communication) with diameters of 1.0 and 2.0–4.5 μm and on the Chilean continental shelf of any combination of filaments with diameters of 2.5–5.0, 12–20 and 30–43 μm. Whenever different species exist in sufficient density in the same sediment, such combinations are possible, since the filaments do emigrate from their sheath under environmental pressures, only to reestablish their colonial habit in a more favorable horizon, as already suggested by Kolkwitz (1955). Therefore, "*T. mixta*" must be considered a colonial association of two species.

Little is known about the growth and nutrition of the thioplocas. Historically, a chemolithotrophic nutrition had been assumed (Kolkwitz, 1955; Perfil'ev, 1964). Recently, Maier and Gallardo (1984a) investigated the nutrition of two marine thioplocas by autoradiography. In the presence of sulfide, both species incorporated acetate, mixed amino acids, glycine, glucose, thymidine and carbonate but did not incorporate glutamate, methane and methanol, with or without sulfide. Thus, methylotrophy (Morita et al., 1981) has been excluded, and a mixotrophic nutrition based on sulfide oxidation under reduced oxygen tension has been indicated (Maier and Gallardo, 1984a). These experiments were carried out at 8 and 18°C. *Thioploca* was recovered from sediments with temperatures ranging from 5 to 20°C (Kolkwitz, 1912; Maier and Preissner, 1979; Rosenberg et al., 1983) and from a thermal spring (Anagnostidis, 1968).

The importance of the relative concentrations of hydrogen sulfide and oxygen had been pointed out previously (Maier, 1963) and is corroborated by observations in the field (V. A. Gallardo, personal communication) and in the laboratory (Maier, 1980, and unpublished data). Indeed, the organism is microaerophilic and occurs in the upper layers of sediments in fresh, brackish and/or marine waters at the interphase between the oxidizing horizon and the reducing horizon with low concentrations

Table 23.21.
Differential characteristics of the species of the genus **Thioploca**[a]

Characteristic	1. *T. schmidlei*	2. *T. ingrica*	3. "*T. minima*"	4. *T. araucae*	5. *T. chileae*	6. "*T. marina*"
Habitat and sediments						
Freshwater	+	+	+	−	−	−
Brackish water	+	+	−	−	−	−
Marine water	−	−	−	+	+	+
Size (μm)						
Filament diameter	5.0–9.0	2.0–4.5	0.8–1.5	30–43	12–20	2.5–5.0

[a]Symbols: +, positive; and −, negative.

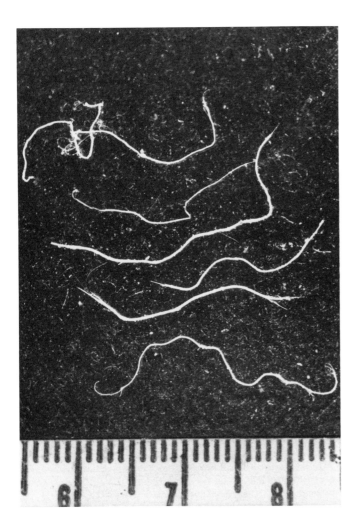

Figure 23.68. Sheathed fascicles of marine thioplocas (centimeter scale).

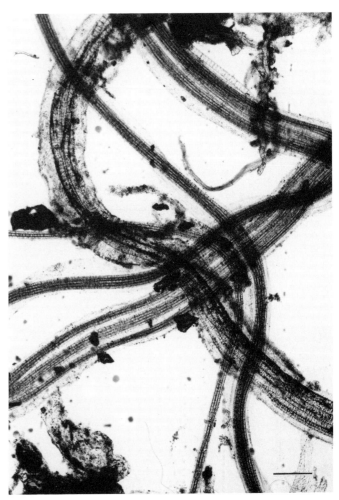

Figure 23.69. Microscopic (brightfield) appearance of washed sheathed bundles of marine thioplocas. *Bar*, 200 μm.

of hydrogen sulfide. Perfil'ev (1964) contends that the sheathed filaments show a horizontal orientation in the reducing horizon, changing to vertical in the oxidizing layer. The motility of the filaments would allow transport of sulfide from the lower to the higher horizon where oxygen is available for oxidation. Constant movement of individuals through the boundary of aerobic and anaerobic layers has also been observed in *Beggiatoa* and *Thiovulum* (Jørgensen and Revsbech, 1983). Perfil'ev (1964) suggested that the detritus adhering to the sheath in the oxidizing horizon contained iron and manganese oxides. The actual concentration of oxygen in the overlying water does not seem to be too important, since

values from near saturation (Kolkwitz, 1912) to very low levels (Gallardo, 1977) have been reported. The consequent oxygen gradient within the sediment becomes the important factor. Thus, the recent increase of oxygen concentration in the Peru-Chile subsurface countercurrent in the wake of "el niño" has resulted in a displacement of thioplocas to a lower horizon (V. A. Gallardo, personal communication). A sulfide gradient within the sediment has also been reported (Henrichs, 1980). Although oxygen and hydrogen sulfide react spontaneously, there is a narrow overlap between these zones (Jørgensen and Revsbech, 1983). In addition, low concentrations of dissolved carbohydrates and free amino acids are present in interstitial water from *Thioploca*-containing sediments (Henrichs, 1980), thus mixotrophy would be possible.

Thioploca has been found in Central Europe (Lauterborn, 1907; Visloukh, 1911; Kolkwitz, 1912, 1955; Bavendamm, 1924; Koppe, 1924; Perfil'ev, 1964; Maier and Preissner, 1979), Greece (Anagnostidis, 1968), Lake Erie (C. I. Randles, personal communication), the southern Pacific from central Chile (Gallardo, 1977) to latitude 6.5°S in northern Peru (Rosenberg et al., 1983) and the northern Pacific off the coast of California (R. Iturriaga, personal communication). In some of these locations, thioplocas have declined in numbers or have disappeared (Maier and Preissner, 1979).

Maintenance Procedures

Although thioplocas have not been isolated in pure culture, *T. ingrica*

has been maintained for years in the laboratory in undisturbed sediment samples (~½-gal) in 1-gal jars overlaid with tap water at 8–20°C in the dark. At approximately yearly intervals a few stems of extracted grass (Scotten and Stokes, 1962) may be stuck into the sediment. *Thioploca* often colonize these stems, which makes harvesting easier. However, too much grass or too frequent additions will destroy the culture. Sections of the colonized grass stem can be used to inoculate hay enrichments modified from the *Beggiatoa* enrichment (Maier, 1980). Briefly, 0.2 or 0.3 g of pulverized extracted hay is autoclaved in 60 ml of tap water in 125-ml Erlenmeyer flasks and inoculated with 4–10 ml of *Thioploca*-free sediment. After 4–5 weeks of undisturbed incubation at room temperature, *Thioploca* bundles are added and incubation is continued. Ramifying bundles of *Thioploca* can be seen through the bottom of the flask with an inverted microscope after 2–4 weeks.

Differentiation of the genus **Thioploca** from other taxa

Besides the colonial sheathed cyanobacteria, *Hydrocoleum* and *Microcoleus*, which can easily be distinguished by pigmentation and habitat, differentiation of *Thioploca* from *Beggiatoa* can present a problem, since *Thioploca* can and does leave its sheath under environmental stress. Free filaments of the two genera are then indistinguishable microscopically, except possibly for the frequently encountered attenuated terminal segments in *Thioploca*. However, blunt filament tips are also encountered in *Thioploca* (Fig. 23.63), and tapering terminal segments have been reported in *Beggiatoa* (Pringsheim, 1963). Enrichment, even enumeration, from small numbers is possible for *Beggiatoa* (Strohl and Larkin, 1978b) but not for *Thioploca* (Maier, 1980). Although there are ultrastructural differences between *B. alba* (Strohl et al., 1981a, 1982) and *T. ingrica* (Maier and Murray, 1965), the nature of the ultrastructural preparations precludes their use for the differentiation of a few questionable filaments. However, when *Thioploca* is recovered in its normal growth state from the surface layers of sediments, the filaments are surrounded by their common sheath, and simple microscopic observation of living ma-

terial (Figs. 23.63 and 23.64 and 23.67–23.69) allows definitive identification. The normal growth state of *Beggiatoa*, on the other hand, is represented by veils of free filaments on the surface of sediments which contain more hydrogen sulfide than do *Thioploca*-containing sediments (Kolkwitz, 1912; S. Maier, unpublished data).

Taxonomic Comments

The gliding "sulfur bacteria" have long been claimed to be apochlorotic *Cyanophyceae* (cyanobacteria) (Pringsheim, 1963). But in the eighth edition of the *Manual* (Buchanan and Gibbons, 1974), the *Beggiatoaceae* are included in "Division II, The Bacteria," rather than in "Division I, The Cyanobacteria." Yet, there are recent advocates for the cyanobacterial affinity of the *Beggiatoaceae* (Reichenbach and Dworkin, 1981a) as well as substantive counterarguments (Larkin and Strohl, 1983). Final judgment should be reserved until sufficient numbers of pure cultures from the *Beggiatoaceae* and the filamentous cyanobacteria can be compared in much more detail than is possible now.

Differentiation of the species of the genus **Thioploca**

In the eighth edition of the *Manual*, four species of *Thioploca* were recognized (Maier, 1974). Because of lack of detailed information and pure cultures, only *T. schmidlei* is retained in the Approved Lists of Bacterial Names (Skerman et al., 1980). My own observations suggest that none of the marine thioplocas survive in freshwater and that filament diameters

form well-defined and nonoverlapping clusters, allowing definitive separation of species, even though knowledge of other characteristics is as yet scarce. Consequently, three more species of *Thioploca* have been validly described (Maier, 1984; Maier and Gallardo, 1984b). This information is presented in Table 23.21, which includes valid as well as invalid species.

List of species of the genus **Thioploca**

1. **Thioploca schmidlei** Lauterborn 1907, 242.[AL]
schmid'le.i. M.L. gen. n. *schmidlei* of Schmidle.
Identified from fresh and brackish waters of various localities in Central Europe and Greece.

2. **Thioploca ingrica** Maier 1984, 344.[VP]
in'gri.ca. M.L. adj. *ingrica* pertaining to Ingria, ancient district of Leningrad, Russia.
Identified from fresh and brackish waters of various localities in Central Europe and Lake Erie.

3. **"Thioploca minima"** Koppe 1924, 630.
mi'ni.ma. L. sup. adj. *minima* least, smallest.
Identified from freshwaters of various localities in Central Europe and Lake Erie.

4. **Thioploca araucae** Maier and Gallardo 1984b, 417.[VP]
a.rau'cae. M.L. gen. n. *araucae* of Arauco.
Identified from the Pacific South American continental shelf.

5. **Thioploca chileae** Maier and Gallardo 1984b, 417.[VP]
chi'le.ae. M.L. gen. n. *chileae* of Chile.
Identified from the Pacific South American continental shelf.

6. **"Thioploca marina"** (Maier and Gallardo, unpublished data).
ma.ri'na. L. adj. *marina* marine.
Identified from the Pacific South American continental shelf.

Genus IV. "**Thiospirillopsis**" Uphof 1927, 81

WILLIAM R. STROHL

Thi.o.spi.ril.lop'sis. M.L. neut. n. *Thiospirillum* a genus of bacteria; Gr. n. *opsis* appearance; M.L. fem. n. *Thiospirillopsis* that which has the appearance of *Thiospirillum*.

Colorless sulfur bacteria occurring in spirally wound filaments. Continuous cell envelope; cells may or may not be visible in filaments. **Exhibit a creeping motility combined with rotation,** so that the trichomes move forward with a corkscrew motion. The tips may oscillate. This organism resembles *Spirulina* among the oscillatorian cyanobacteria. Not grown in pure culture.

Type species: "*Thiospirillopsis floridana*" Uphof 1927, 83.

Further Comments

Some strains of *Beggiatoa*, when grown under certain culture conditions, may take on the appearance of having spirally wound filaments (Fig. 23.70). Although the conditions are not entirely delineated, they include shaking at fast rotation rates (>250 rpm) and relatively high aeration. These beggiatoas return to normal "straight" filaments, however, if they are cultured further under different conditions. In nature, however, the spirals of "*Thiospirillopsis*" species appear to be inherent, not transient. Until strains of "*Thiospirillopsis*" are isolated and studied in pure culture, it is not possible to know how stable the spiral formation is.

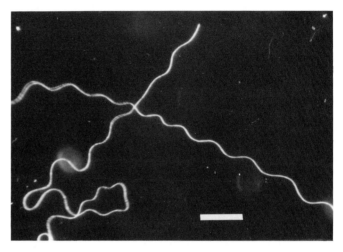

Figure 23.70.   Darkfield phase micrograph of *Beggiatoa alba* B18LD grown in liquid culture for 24 h at about 275 rpm, showing the phenotype sometimes observed when *Beggiatoa* species are grown under rapid rotary shaking conditions. *Bar,* 50 μm.

List of species of the genus "**Thiospirillopsis**"

1. "**Thiospirillopsis floridana**" Uphof 1927, 83.
flo.ri.da'na M.L. adj. *floridanus* pertaining to Florida.

Filaments 2–3 μm in diameter. Segments about 3–5 μm long; segmentation is difficult to observe without special precautions. The spiral windings are regular.

Source: Found in sulfur spring water at Wekiwa Springs, Palm Springs, and Warm Mineral Springs, Florida, and in freshwater sediment samples from Campus Lake, Baton Rouge, Louisiana.

Further comments. A very similar organism has been observed at Pacific Grove, California, in a marine aquarium where hydrogen sulfide had been generated by sulfate reduction. Lackey et al. (1965) also reported rare observation of "*Thiospirillopsis*" from Florida spring sources. Recently, a similar organism was observed in enrichments obtained from a small, shallow freshwater lake on the campus of Louisiana State University (Fig. 23.71, *A* and *B*). The genus "*Thiospirillopsis*" may, therefore, be more widespread than is generally believed.

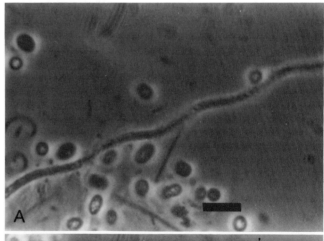

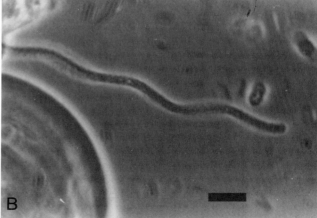

Figure 23.71.   *A* and *B* phase micrographs of "*Thiospirillopsis*" in an enrichment culture derived from samples from Campus Lake, Louisiana State University, Baton Rouge, Louisiana. *Bar,* 10 μm.

OTHER FAMILIES AND GENERA

FAMILY **SIMONSIELLACEAE** STEED 1962, 615[AL]

JOHN M. LARKIN

Si.mon.si.el.la′ce.ae. M.L. fem. n. *Simonsiella* type genus of the family; *-aceae* ending to denote a family; M.L. fem. pl. n. *Simonsiellaceae* the *Simonsiella* family.

Multicellular filaments that are **flat rather than cylindrical. The width of an individual cell is greater than its length. Gliding motility** when the flat side of the filament is in contact with a surface. Chemoorganotrophic. Aerobic. Some may produce acid aerobically from carbohydrates. Optimum temperature: 37°C. **Found in the oral cavity of warm-blooded vertebrates.**

The mol% G + C of the DNA ranges from 40 to 55 (Bd.).

Key to the genera of the family **Simonsiellaceae**

I. Filament has rounded ends and is often segmented into groups of eight cells.
Genus I. *Simonsiella*
II. Filament ends are square. Cells are paired within the filament.
Genus II. *Alysiella*

Genus I. **Simonsiella** *Schmid* in *Simons 1922, 504*[AL]

JOHN M. LARKIN

Si.mon.si.el′la. M.L. dim. ending *-ella*; M.L. fem. n. *Simonsiella* (organism of) Simons; named for H. Simons, who studied the species of this genus.

Organisms that exist in characteristic **muticellular filaments** which are often segmented into groups of eight cells. **The long axis of an individual cell is perpendicular to the long axis of the filament.** The diameter of the filaments (the width of the individual cells) may vary from about 2.0 to 8.0 μm, and the length of filaments may vary from about 10.0 to over 50.0 μm. Individual cells within the filaments may be from about 0.5 to 1.3 μm long. In thin sections cut perpendicular to the long axis of the filament, the **cells are flattened and curved to yield a crescent-shaped, convex-concave (dorsal-ventral) asymmetry. The ends of the individual filaments are rounded.** Gram-negative. **Motile by gliding** of the entire filament in the direction of the long axis. Aerobic. Chemoorganotrophs.

The mol% G + C of the DNA ranges from 41 to 55 (Bd.).

Type species: *Simonseilla muelleri* Schmid *in* Simons 1922, 504.

Further Descriptive Information

The filaments of *Simonsiella* are distinctive, and members of this genus can be recognized by their morphology alone (Figs. 23.72–23.74). The dorsal-ventral flattening of the filaments is quite striking, as is the fact that the individual cells of the filament are wider than they are long if the long axis of the filament is considered to represent the length of the cells. The cells toward either end of the filament decrease in width, and the terminal cells may be rounded, giving the filaments a tapered appearance with rounded ends. In isolated colonies, some of the filaments may be turned on their sides, which shows the flattening quite clearly. From the convex (bottom) side of the filaments there are numerous fine fibrils (Fig. 23.74) which appear to be involved in the adhesion of the filaments to a surface and perhaps in locomotion (Pangborn et al., 1977). In thin sections, the cells appear to have a typical Gram-negative cell wall structure.

Individual filaments glide over the agar surface only when the broad, ventral surface is in contact with the agar. Movement of the filaments over the agar leaves depressed tracks in the agar surface (Fig. 23.73), perhaps indicating a change in the structure of the agar (Pangborn et al., 1977). No flagella or other organs of locomotion have been demonstrated. The speed of gliding varies from about 5 to 24 μm/min (Buchanan and Kuhn, 1978). Colonies on BSTSY agar (see "Enrichment and Isolation Procedures") may have a pale yellow pigmentation. Most, but not all, strains produce a zone of hemolysis on agar containing horse, sheep or rabbit blood. No resting stage has been detected.

All isolates of *Simonsiella* are chemoorganotrophic, and the nutrition of the isolates (as well as their classification) parallels their source of ori-

gin. Those isolates from sheep (*S. crassa*) are generally the most physiologically active, being both proteolytic and saccharolytic. In contrast, the isolates from dogs (*S. steedae*) are neither proteolytic nor saccharolytic. Kuhn et al. (1978) have described 49 isolates of *Simonsiella*. All strains are aerobic, possess cytochrome oxidase, and produce catalase. Good growth occurs between 3 and 40°C, is optimal at 37°C, and does not occur at 45°C. Growth occurs in 1% NaCl but not in 2% NaCl. No strains hydrolize starch or agar or produce urease or indole. No strains produce acid from cellobiose, dulcitol, erythritol, galactose, glycerol, inositol, lactose, mannose, melibiose, melizitose, raffinose, rhamnose, salicin, sorbitol, sorbose or xylose. Some species may produce acid from other carbohydrates. A rich medium is best for growth, and the addition of serum to the medium has been found to be necessary for some strains and to be advantageous for all other strains (Kuhn et al., 1978).

All reports and isolations of *Simonsiella* indicate that they are strictly inhabitants of the oral cavity of warm-blooded vertebrates, where they are apparently not pathogenic.

Kuhn et al. (1977, 1978) have isolated nearly 50 strains of *Simonsiella* from dogs, cats, sheep and humans. On the basis of morphology, physiology and the mol% G + C of the DNA, the strains could be separated into distinct groups which correlated with their source of origin. Three of these groups (dogs, sheep and humans) have been designated as separate species, while the isolates from cats need additional characterization before any decisions about species designations can be made (Kuhn et al., 1978; Kuhn and Gregory, 1978).

The cell-bound fatty acid profiles of 48 strains of *Simonsiella* matched the general pattern of Gram-negative bacteria, in which high percentages of even-numbered saturated and monounsaturated fatty acids occur (Jenkins et al., 1977). Tetradecanoic acid was the predominant saturated fatty acid, followed by hexadecanoic acid. 9-Hexadecanoic and 9-octadecanoic acids were the predominant monounsaturated fatty acids. Results of stepwise discriminant analysis of the mean relative percentages of tetradecanoic, hexadecanoic and 9-octadecanoic acids demonstrated that 85% of the isolates (with two cat strains and one dog strain being the exceptions) were correctly identified in their source-of-origin groups.

Enrichment and Isolation Procedures

At the present time, there are no enrichment procedures for *Simonsiella*. Isolation directly from the oral cavity has been achieved by several people, however. The easiest method for isolation of *Simonsiella* was described by Kuhn et al. (1978). A sterile cotton swab is rubbed over the pal-

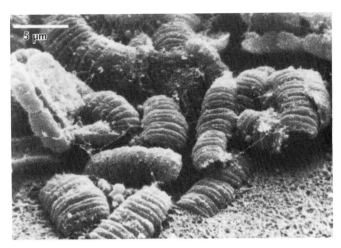

Figure 23.72.   Scanning electron micrograph of the edge of a colony of *Simonsiella* obtained from a cat. (Micrograph taken by J. Pangborn; reproduced with permission from J. Pangborn, D. A. Kuhn and J. R. Woods, *Archives of Microbiology 113:* 197–204, 1977, ©Springer-Verlag.)

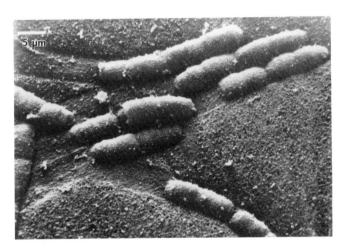

Figure 23.73.   Scanning electron micrograph of a culture of *S. steedae* ATCC 27411 growing on BSTSY agar (see "Enrichment and Isolation Procedures"). The depressed tracks where the organism has glided over the surface of the agar are clearly shown. The dorsal surface of the filaments are covered with a capsular material that obscures the individual cells. (Micrograph taken by J. Pangborn; reproduced with permission from J. Pangborn, D. A. Kuhn and J. R. Woods, *Archives of Microbiology 113:* 197–204, 1977, ©Springer-Verlag.)

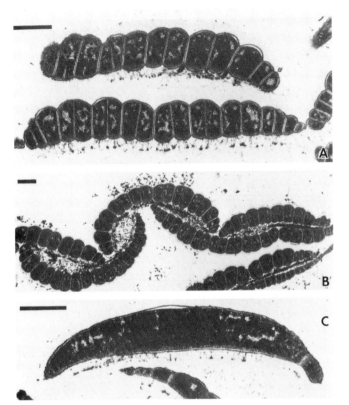

Figure 23.74.   Transmission electron micrograph of thin sections of *S. steedae.* The multicellular nature of the filaments and the dorsal-ventral differentiation are shown. *A,* strain ATCC 27411 from an agar surface. *B,* strain ATCC 27396 showing a curvature of the filaments which often causes them to stand on their edge in a colony. *C,* section of strain ATCC 27411 cut perpendicular to the long axis of the filament. The dorsal-ventral, convex-concave curvature which results in a crescent-shaped transverse section is shown. Notice the fine fibrillar structures on the ventral surface of all of the filaments. (Micrograph taken by J. Pangborn; reproduced with permission from J. Pangborn, D. A. Kuhn and J. R. Woods, *Archives of Microbiology 113:* 197–204, 1977, ©Springer-Verlag.)

ate, tongue or inner surface of the cheeks of the animal and immediately rolled over the surface of a thin layer of BSTSY agar (tryptic soy broth without dextrose (Difco), 27.5 g; yeast extract (Difco), 4 g; agar, 15.0 g; water, 900 ml; and sterile bovine serum, 100 ml, which is added after autoclaving and cooling the other ingredients to 45°C) in a plastic Petri dish. Without delay, the dish is then placed into a 37°C incubator for about 6–10 h. During this short incubation period the filaments glide away from the oral epithelial cells and multiply. The Petri dish is then scanned via a microscope with a magnification of up to × 125 or a dissecting microscope. Isolated filaments or microcolonies are fished from the agar surface and transferred to fresh plates of BSTSY agar. Suitable

instruments for transfer could include a dissecting needle, inoculating needle, toothpick, dental probe, light bulb filament or other fine-tipped instrument. Macroscopically visible colonies generally appear within 16–24 h after transfer. Although this method was used to isolate nearly 50 strains of *Simonsiella*, some strains did not grow on this medium and could not be isolated.

Steed (1962) isolated *Simonsiella* from sheep with a medium consisting of Oxoid nutrient agar plus 10% horse or ox serum. This medium was not suitable for the isolation of strains from humans (Kuhn et al., 1978). Berger (1963) used blood agar to detect and isolate *Simonsiella*, but this medium suffers from the opaqueness of the blood, which prevents easy observation of the colonies with a microscope.

Maintenance Procedures

Freshly isolated cultures should be grown at 37°C and transferred about every 2–3 days to the same medium on which they were isolated. Older cultures must be transferred at intervals of about 1 week.

Refrigeration of cultures is not recommended for preservation, but they can be preserved by freezing in liquid nitrogen or by lyophilization.

Procedures for Testing Special Characteristics

The procedures for characterizing *Simonsiella* were first described by Steed (1961) and later modified by Kuhn et al. (1978). The procedures generally parallel those that are commonly used for other taxa, except that for *Simonsiella* most media contain 10% serum. All incubations are carried out at 37°C. The procedures below are from Kuhn et al. (1978).

Casein Hydrolysis

BSTSY agar containing 2% skim milk is inoculated, incubated for 3 days, and examined for evidence of hydrolysis.

Starch Hydrolysis

TSY agar (BSTSY agar without serum) containing 5% soluble starch is inoculated, incubated for 4 days, and then flooded with Lugol's iodine.

Gelatin Hydrolysis

TSY broth containing 10% serum and 12% gelatin is inoculated and tested for liquefaction after 5 days of incubation by chilling the tube to 4°C.

Peptonization of Litmus Milk

Litmus milk (Difco) containing 10% serum is inoculated and examined for peptonization over a 14-day incubation period.

Action on Carbohydrates

A medium is poured into Petri dishes, inoculated, and examined after 48 h for the production of acid (yellow color). It consists of the following ingredients: phenol red broth (Difco), 1.6%; yeast extract (Difco), 0.2%; agar (Difco), 1.5%; phenol red (Hartman Leddon Co., Philadelphia, Pennsylvania), 0.007%; serum, 10%; and carbohydrate, 1%.

Indole Production

BSTSY broth containing 1% tryptone is inoculated, incubated for 3 days, and examined for evidence of indole production with Kovac's reagent.

Nitrate Reduction

TSY broth containing 0.2% KNO_3 in a Durham tube assembly is inoculated and examined for 5 days by the dimethyl-α-naphtholamine/sulfanilic acid method of Branson (1972).

Differentiation of the genus **Simonsiella** *from other closely related taxa*

The unusual morphology of the *Simonsiella* filament serves to differentiate the genus from all other procaryotic organisms. *Alysiella* resembles *Simonsiella*, but filaments of *Alysiella* do not show the unusual dorsal-ventral differentiation and do not have rounded ends, and the individual cells are paired within the filament.

Caryophanon filaments may be mistaken for *Simonsiella* in stained preparations. However, in live preparations the cylindrical form of *Caryophanon* and the flattened shape of *Simonsiella* are easily distinguished. Also, *Caryophanon* are motile by flagella; they do not glide.

Taxonomic Comments

The citation "Schmid *in* Simons" following the generic name in the title is the result of Simons (1922) crediting the name *Simonsiella* to G. Schmid. However, no record can be found that Schmid published the name *Simonsiella*.

When Simons (1922) first described the genus *Simonsiella* from the human oral cavity, he named two species, *S. muelleri* and *S. crassa,* which he differentiated on the basis of the width of the filaments. Later, Steed (1962), examining strains from sheep, and Berger (1963), examining strains from guinea pigs, named their isolates *S. crassa* and *S. muelleri,* respectively, because of the similarity in filament width to those known species. When Kuhn et al. (1978) carried out an extensive investigation of 49 isolates from humans, dogs, cats and sheep, they determined that

each animal had its own species and that filament width was not a suitable indicator for the differentiation of species.

Simonsiella has been reported from the oral cavity of many warm-blooded vertebrates including cats, chickens, cows, dogs, goats, guinea pigs, humans, horses, pigs, rabbits and sheep. Only those from cats, dogs, humans and sheep have been described in detail (Steed, 1962; Kuhn et al., 1978). When those from other animals are well-studied, it may be necessary to revise the number of species within this genus and the means of differentiation among the species. Moreover, some *Simonsiella* have been refractory to isolation, possibly indicating that they were a different strain or species (Kuhn et al., 1978) from those that grew and were isolated on BSTSY agar.

Kuhn et al. (1978) characterized several strains from cats but have not yet determined their place within this genus or provided a specific epithet.

Further Reading

Kuhn, D.A. 1981. The genera *Simonsiella* and *Alysiella. In* Starr, Stolp, Trüper, Balows and Schlegel (Editors), The Prokaryotes. A Handbook on Habitats, Isolation, and Identification of Bacteria. Springer-Verlag, Berlin, pp. 390–399.

McCowen, R.P., K.J. Cheng and J.W. Costerton. 1979. Colonization of a portion of the bovine tongue by unusual filamentous bacteria. Appl. Environ. Microbiol. *37:* 1224–1229.

Differentiation of the species of the genus **Simonsiella**

Some differential features of the three recognized species of *Simonsiella* are shown in Table 23.22.

List of species of the genus **Simonsiella**

1. **Simonsiella muelleri** Schmid *in* Simons 1922, 504.[AL]

muel′le.ri. M.L. gen. n. *muelleri* Müller; named for R. Müller, who first described these organisms.

See table 23.22 and the generic description for many features.

The long axis of the cells (width of filament) varies from 2.1 to 3.5 μm, with an average of about 2.5–3.2 μm; the short axis (length of individual cell) varies from about 0.5 to 0.9 μm, with an average of about 0.8 μm.

Casein, gelatin, esculin and hippurate are not hydrolyzed. No change occurs in litmus milk. The ability to reduce nitrates varies among strains, with about half of them being positive; when reduction occurs, nitrite is

produced, and a few strains produce N_2 gas. H_2S production is variable and inconsistent.

Found in the oral cavity of humans.

The mol% G + C of the DNA of 16 of 18 strains varies from 40 to 42 (Bd). Two other strains had a mol% G + C of 44 and 50 (Bd).

Neotype strain: ATCC 29453 (ICPB 3636).

2. **Simonsiella crassa** Schmid *in* Simons 1922, 509.[AL]

cras′sa. L. fem. adj. *crassa* thick.

See Table 23.22 and the generic description for many features.

Table 23.22.

Characteristics differentiating the species of the genus **Simonsiella**[a]

Characteristic	1. *S. muelleri*	2. *S. crassa*	3. *S. steedae*
Acid from			
Glucose	+	+	−
Maltose	+	+	−
Trehalose	−	+	−
Ribose	−	+	−
Fructose	−	+	−
Sucrose	−	+	−
Mannitol	−	+	−
Growth at			
27°C	+	+	−
43°C	−	+	−
pH 6.0	+	+	−
pH 8.0	−	+	−
Source	Humans	Sheep	Dogs

[a]Symbols: +, 90% or more of strains are positive; −, 90% or more of strains are negative.

The long axis of the cells (width of filament) varies from 1.9 to 3.6 μm, with an average of about 2.9–3.5 μm; the short axis (length of individual cell) varies from 0.7 to 0.9 μm, with an average of about 0.8 μm.

Steed (1962) reported that her isolates produced acid from inulin and that four of six isolates produced acid from arabinose. Kuhn et al. (1978) reported negative results with both carbohydrates for her isolates, as well as for one of Steed's strains. The discrepancy may be due to differences in the method of testing.

Gelatin and casein are hydrolyzed. Litmus milk is peptonized. Nitrate is reduced to nitrogen gas. MR-negative. VP-negative. Steed reported that all of her isolates produced H_2S, but Kuhn et al. (1978) stated that H_2S production is variable and inconsistent.

Found in the oral cavity of sheep.

The mol% G + C of the DNA ranges from 44 to 45 (Bd).

Neotype strain: NCTC 10283 (ATCC 27504, ICPB 3651).

3. **Simonsiella steedae** Kuhn and Gregory 1978, 13.[AL]

stee'dae. M.L. gen. n. *steedae* of Steed; named for P. Steed (Glaister) who first isolated axenic cultures of *Simonsiella* and erected the family *Simonsiellaceae*.

See Table 23.22 and the generic description for many features.

The long axis of the cells (width of filament) varies from 2.5 to 7.1 μm, with an average of about 3.1–3.8 μm; the short axis (length of individual cell) varies from 0.7 to 1.3 μm, with an average of about 1.1 μm.

Casein, gelatin, esculin and hippurate are not hydrolyzed. No change in litmus milk. Most strains reduce nitrate to nitrite without gas production. H_2S production is variable and inconsistent.

Found in the oral cavity of dogs.

The mol% G + C of the DNA ranges from 48 to 52 (Bd).

Holotype strain: ATCC 27409 (ICPB 3604).

Genus II. **Alysiella** *Langeron 1923, 116*[AL]

JOHN M. LARKIN

A.ly.si.el'la. Gr fem. n. *alysion* small chain; M.L. dim. ending -*ella*; M.L. fem. n. *Alysiella* small chain.

Organisms that exist in characteristic **flat, ribbonlike multicellular filaments. The long axis of the individual cells is perpendicular to the long axis of the filament. The cells within the filament are paired,** and in axenic culture the filament often breaks up into groups of two or four cells. The width of an individual cell (the width of a filament) is about 2.0–3.0 μm, and the length of a cell is about 0.6 μm. The length of the filament is quite variable. The filament does not show either a dorsal-ventral differentiation or a convex-concave curvature in transverse cross-section. The **ends of the individual filaments are square.** Gram-negative. **Motile by gliding** of the entire filament in the direction of the long axis. Aerobic. Chemoorganotrophic.

The mol% G + C of the DNA of the one strain examined is 44 (Bd).

Type species: *Alysiella filiformis* (Schmid *in* Simons) Langeron 1923, 118.

Further Descriptive Information

The filaments of *Alysiella* are distinctive, and members of this genus can be recognized by their morphology alone (Fig. 23.75). The filament is flat and ribbon-shaped rather than cylindrical and consists of continuous pairs of cells (Fig. 23.76 and 23.77). The individual cells are several times greater in width than in length. Fibrils are produced from only one side of the filament (Fig. 23.77), and the fibrils appear to be involved in anchoring the filament to epithelial cells of the oral cavity (Kaiser and Starzyk, 1973; McCowen et al., 1979). Cells anchored in this way give rise to a typical palisade arrangement (Fig. 23.75).

Gliding motility occurs when the flat surface of the filament is in contact with an agar surface. No organs of locomotion have been detected. Colonies on Oxoid nutrient agar containing 10% horse or ox serum are nonpigmented and about 1.0–1.5 mm in diameter (Steed, 1962). On BSTSY agar (see *Simonsiella* for ingredients), the colonies are about 1.0–2.0 mm in diameter and exhibit a pale yellow pigmentation (Kuhn, 1981). No resting stage has been detected.

All reports of *Alysiella* indicate that it is restricted to the oral cavity of warm-blooded vertebrates, where they are apparently not pathogenic.

Enrichment and Isolation Procedures

At the present time there is no enrichment procedure for *Alysiella*. Direct isolation from the oral cavity can be achieved, however, Steed (1962) isolated *Alysiella* from sheep and rabbits with oral swabs that were plated directly onto Oxoid nutrient agar containing 10% horse or ox serum. After 6 h the microcolonies were transferred to new media via a micromanipulater.

McCowan et al. (1979) isolated *Alysiella* from cows by impressing a portion of tongue on the agar surface and then spreading the organisms or by washing a portion of tongue in phosphate-buffered saline, homogenizing the tongue with a Waring blender, and plating the resulting suspension on agar. They used both Tryptose-blood agar (Difco Laboratories) with 10% sheep blood or an agar consisting of the following ingredients: nutrient agar (Difco), 2.5%; sodium acetate, 0.01%; and yeast extract (Difco), 0.5%.

Kuhn (1981) suggests that *Alysiella* can be isolated on BSTSY agar by using the procedures that she used for isolating *Simonsiella*. (See the description of the genus *Simonsiella*.)

Maintenance Procedures

Alysiella should be grown at 37°C, and freshly isolated cultures should be transferred at intervals of 2–3 days. Older cultures must be transferred at weekly intervals.

Refrigeration is not recommended for preservation of cultures, but they can be preserved by freezing in liquid nitrogen or by lyophilization.

Procedures for Testing Special Characteristics

The procedures that should be used for characterizing isolates of *Alysiella* are identical with those used for *Simonsiella*, and they are presented in the description of that genus.

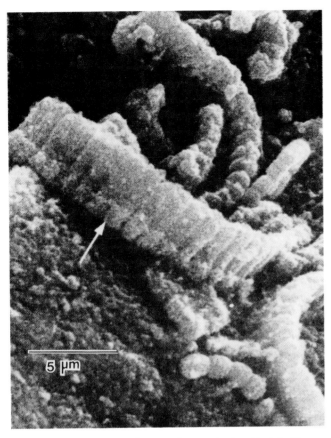

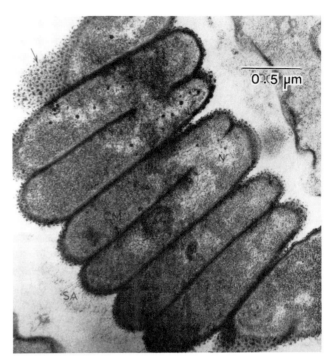

Figure 23.76. Longitudinal electon micrograph of *Alysiella* from the oral cavity of a rabbit. The paired nature of the cells within the filament is typical of the genus. (Reproduced with permission from G. E. Kaiser and M. J. Starzyk, Canadian Journal of Microbiology *19:* 325–327, 1973, © National Research Council of Canada.)

Figure 23.75. Scanning electron micrograph of an *Alysiella* filament attached to the epithelium of the bovine tongue. The *arrow* indicates the fringe of fibers that attach the bacterial filament by its side to the substrate. The palisade organization of the filament is characteristic of *Alysiella*. (Reproduced with permission from R. P. McCowen, K.-J. Cheng and J. W. Costerton, Applied and Environmental Microbiology *37:* 1224–1229, 1979, © American Society for Microbiology.)

Figure 23.77. Section of *Alysiella* from the bovine tongue, showing ruthenium red-stained fibrils emanating from one side of the filament only. (Reproduced courtesy of J. W. Costerton.)

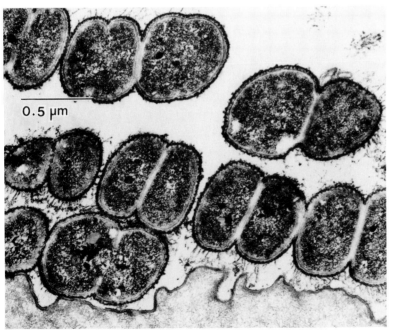

Differentiation of the genus **Alysiella** from other closely related taxa

The unusual morphology of the *Alysiella* filaments serves to differentiate the genus from all other procaryotic organisms. *Alysiella* filaments differ from *Simonsiella* in consisting of continuous pairs of cells instead of being segmented into units of eight cells, and the terminal cells are not rounded. In addition, *Alysiella* has a fringe of fibers on the side of the filament rather than on the bottom as in *Simonsiella*, and the former does not show the dorsal-ventral, convex-concave curvature of the latter.

Taxonomic Comments

Alysiella has been reported from the oral cavity of many animals including chickens, sheep, horses, cows, goats, pigs, rabbits and guinea pigs. Isolates have only been obtained from guinea pigs (Berger, 1963), sheep (Steed, 1962), and cows (McCowan et al., 1979), and only a few strains from sheep have been described in detail. Strains from other animals have resisted isolation. It is probable that as strains from other animals are isolated, there will prove to be additional species, just as with *Simonsiella*.

Differentiation of the species of the genus **Alysiella**

Only a single species of *Alysiella* is presently recognized.

List of species of the genus **Alysiella**

1. **Alysiella filiformis** (Schmid *in* Simons 1922) Langeron 1923, 118.[AL] (*Simonsiella filiformis* Schmid *in* Simons 1922, 509.)

fi.li.for'mis. L. n. *filum* thread; L. n. *forma* shape; M.L. adj. *filiformis* filiform.

See the generic description for additional features.

Alysiella is aerobic, possesses cytochrome oxidase, and produces catalase. Good growth occurs between 33 and 40°C, with an optimum temperature at 37°C. Growth also occurs at 43°C but not at 27°C. This organism grows in the presence of 1% but not 1.5% NaCl. Grows at pH 7.3 and 9.0 but not at 6.0.

Acid is produced from fructose, glucose, maltose, sucrose and trehalose. No acid is produced from the following: arabinose, cellobiose, dulcitol, erythritol, galactose, glycerol, inositol, lactose, mannose, melibiose, melizitose, raffinose, rhamnose, salicin, sorbitol, sorbose or xylose. Variable results occur on inulin and ribose. A rich medium containing 10% serum is best for growth.

A slight hydrolysis of gelatin may occur, but agar, casein, starch, esculin and hippurate are not hydrolyzed. No change occurs in litmus milk. Indole, MR, VP and reduction of nitrates are negative. Urease is not produced. H_2S production is variable and inconsistent. Hemolytic on rabbit or horse blood agar.

Neotype strain: NCTC 10282 (ATCC 29469; ICPB 3653).

FAMILY "**PELONEMATACEAE**" SKUJA 1956, 81

P. HIRSCH

Pel.o.ne.ma.ta'ce.ae. M.L. neut. n. *Pelonema* type genus of a family; *-aceae* ending to denote family; M.L. fem. pl. n. *Pelonemataceae* the *Pelonema* family.

Cells cylindrical or short rods, colorless, arranged in unbranched filaments, usually visible without staining. Filaments straight, flexuous, or spirally coiled, with or without a polymer sheath, occurring singly or aggregated in bands or bundles. Single filaments of two genera may show a gliding movement combined with rotation around the longitudinal axis. Cells may contain gas vesicles, but the cells are always unpigmented and lack sulfur globules.

Reproduction is by binary fission of the cells and by fragmentation of the filaments or even of the aggregates. Some species in one genus appear to form arthrosporelike resting cells.

Characteristics differentiating the genera of the "*Pelonemataceae*" from other morphologically similar genera are given in Table 23.23.

Aquatic, heterotrophic. Have not been cultivated.

Further Comments

Gliding occurs only in "*Achroonema*" species and (rarely) in "*Pelonema*" species. The position of these organisms in the present classification, based only on morphological grounds, is therefore in some doubt.

Genus I. "**Pelonema**" Lauterborn 1916, 408

P. HIRSCH

Pel.o.ne'ma. Gr. adj. *pelos* dark-colored, hence anaerobic mud; Gr. n. *nema* thread; M.L. neut. n. *Pelonema* mud filament.

Cells colorless, more or less cylindrical, **usually with gas vesicles** in the center. Cells arranged in **multicellular, unbranched straight** or loosely flexuose **filaments** of uniform thickness, which may or may not be constricted at the cross-walls (Figs. 23.78 and 23.79). Filaments of **some species** occasionally show a **slow gliding motility.** Propagation by fragmentation of filaments. Resting cells unknown.

Anaerobic and presumably heterotrophic. **Found in the hypolimnion and on the sediment surface of** deeper **lakes or** stratified **ponds.** Pure cultures are not available.

Type species: "*Pelonema tenue*" Lauterborn 1916, 408.

Further Descriptive Information

Skuja (1956) suggested that "*Pelonema*" cells be centrifuged, with their gas vesicles thereby removed, in order to recognize better the cross-walls and cell length. In most species, gas vesicles are initially unevenly distributed; Skuja (1956) describes this state of the gas "vacuole" (the area occupied by gas vesicles) as "fissured." Later, all gas vesicles are concentrated in the central, axial region of the cell. "*Pelonema*" filaments observed in the laboratory may show slightly inflated cells, possibly due to inflation of the gas vesicles. If viewed with a phase microscope, gas vacuoles may appear to be pinkish, depending on the microscope adjustments.

Table 23.23.

Characteristics differentiating the genera of the family **"Pelonemataceae"** *from other morphologically similar bacteria[a]*

Characteristic	Genus I. "Pelonema"	Genus II. "Achroonema"	Genus III. "Peloploca"	Genus IV. "Desmanthos"	Haliscomenobacter	Chloroflexus	Thioploca	Leptothrix	"Toxothrix"	Crenothrix	"Clonothrix"	Flexithrix
Filaments												
Single	+	+	−	−	+	+	−	+	+	+	+	+
In bands or bundles	−	−	+	+	+	−	+	−	−	−	−	−
Straight or wavy	+	D	+	+	+	+	+	+	+	+	+	+
Coiled (but not wavy)	−	D	D	−	−	−	−	−	−	−	−	−
Constricted at cross-walls	D	D	D	−	+	−	−	+	−	+	+	+
With arthrospores (resting cells)	−	D	−	−	−	−	−	−	−	−	−	−
With gas vesicles	+	D	D	−	−	−	−	−	−	−	−	−
Photosynthetic	−	−	−	−	−	+	−	−	−	−	−	−
Truly branching	−	−	−	−	+	−	−	−	−	−	−	−
Gliding	±[b]	+	−	−	−	+	−	−	+	±[c]	−	+
Holdfasts	−	−	−	+	−	−	−	D	−	±[d]	−	−
Sheaths	−	D	D	+	+	−	+	D	−	+	−	+

[a]+, positive; −, negative; and D, different reactions in different taxa.
[b]Three of six species are positive.
[c]Has been claimed for propagative stages.
[d]Rarely observed.

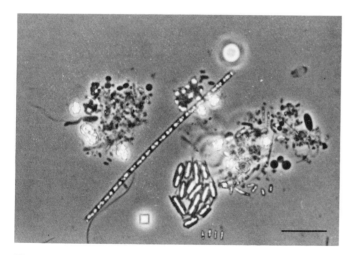

Figure 23.78. *"Pelonema pseudovacuolatum"* sensu Skuja 1956. The sample came from Wintergreen Lake (Michigan) on August 26 from a 5-m depth (anaerobic hypolimnion). *Bar,* 1 μm.

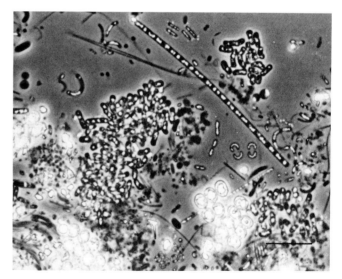

Figure 23.79. *"P. pseudovacuolatum"* sensu Skuja 1956. Sample was collected on August 5 from Wintergreen Lake (Michigan) from a 4.5-m depth (anaerobic hypolimnion). Other organisms shown are *Thiopedia rosea* and *Brachyarcus* species. *Bar,* 1 μm.

"Pelonema pseudovacuolatum" has successfully been enriched in test tubes containing 0.005% Na₂S and autoclaved lake or pond mud. This anaerobic culture was kept at 20–40 lx and 14–18°C (Hirsch, 1981c).

The habitat of *"Pelonema"* species appears to be the anaerobic hypolimnion of eutrophic lakes or ponds. Hirsch (1981b) listed a number of sightings in Lake Plußsee (Holstein; in 24–31-m depth), Wintergreen Lake (Michigan; in 4–4.5-m depth), and in a Michigan forest pond (Augusta; in a 0.5–0.6-m depth). *"Pelonema"* species occurred in these cases in April, July, August, or November at water temperatures ranging from 7 to 17°C and always in the presence of low concentrations of sulfide.

Taxonomic Comments

As morphological characteristics are the only ones to identify *"Pelonema"* species, proper differentiation of these from other, morphologically similar bacteria may not always be possible. *Chloronema* species, recently described by Dubinina and Gorlenko (1975) and belonging to the *Chloroflexaceae,* show close morphological similarity to *"Pelonema"* species. The often only faintly greenish pigmentation of these organisms could be easily overlooked.

Until *"Pelonema"* species are available in pure culture, the classification of Skuja (1974) should be maintained.

Differentiation of the species of the genus "Pelonema"

The differential characteristics of *"Pelonema"* species are indicated in Table 23.24.

List of species of the genus "Pelonema"

1. **"Pelonema tenue"** Lauterborn 1916, 408.
ten′u.e. L. neut. adj. *tenue* thin, slender.
Cells 1.8–2.2 × 3–19 μm, cylindrical, containing gas vesicles. Cells arranged in straight or slightly flexuous filaments up to 300 μm long and only slightly constricted at cross-walls. Filaments may occasionally glide at a rate up to 60 μm/min. Found in deeper fresh and brackish water, in the hypolimnion and on sediments of lakes.

2. **"Pelonema aphane"** Skuja 1956, 92.
aph′an.e. Gr. adj. *aphanes* invisible, transparent; M.L. adj. *aphane* invisible, transparent.
Cells 1–1.7 × 5–16 μm, cylindrical, with central gas vesicles which are initially irregularly dispersed and later arranged along the cell's axis. Cells in filaments up to 600 μm long and only slightly constricted at the cross-walls. Filaments may rarely show a very slow gliding motility. Found in deep hypolimnion and on sediment of freshwater lakes. During vernal circulation, *"P. aphane"* may be also found in upper water layers.

3. **"Pelonema pseudovacuolatum"** Lauterborn 1916, 408.
pseu.do.va.cu.o.la′tum. Gr. adj. *pseudes* false; M.L. dim. n. *vacuolum* a vacuole; M.L. adj. *pseudovacuolatum* false vacuolated.
Cells 1.5–2.0 × 1.5–4.0 μm, cylindrical or slightly barrel-shaped, colorless with central gas vesicles. Arranged in straight or slightly and irregularly coiled filaments with none or only minute constrictions at cross-walls (Figs. 23.78 and 23.79). Filaments do not glide. Found in deeper freshwater pools and on sediment of eutrophic lakes or ponds; occasionally present in plankton.

4. **"Pelonema subtilissimum"** Skuja 1956, 91.
sub.til.is′si.mum. L. sup. adj. *subtilissimum* finest, very slender.
Cells cylindrical, small (0.6–0.7 × 1.5–6.0 μm), with irregularly formed central gas vesicles. Cells arranged in straight filaments of uniform diameter and 15–120 μm long, with no constrictions at the cross-walls (Fig. 23.80). Filaments not motile. Found in deep hypolimnion of Blankvatn, a relic lake near Oslo, Norway.

5. **"Pelonema hyalinum"** Koppe 1924, 625.
hy.a.lin′um. Gr. adj. *hyalines* glassy; M.L. adj. *hyalinum* glassy.
Cells 2 × 4–6 μm, hyaline, with central gas vesicles. Cells arranged in filaments of >200 μm in length. Filaments not or only very slowly motile and not constricted at cross-walls. Found on or in sediment of deep freshwater lakes.

6. **"Pelonema spirale"** Lauterborn 1916, 408.
spi.ra′le. Gr. n. *spira* a spiral; M.L. adj. *spiralis* spiral.
Cells 1–1.5 μm wide, with irregularly distributed gas vesicles that give the appearance of several small, elongated gas "vacuoles." Cells arranged in spirally twisted filaments 40–160 μm long, with a wave length of 8–14 μm. Filaments weakly constricted at cross-walls (Fig. 23.81).
Found in the bottom mud of a German freshwater pool rich with *Chara* species.

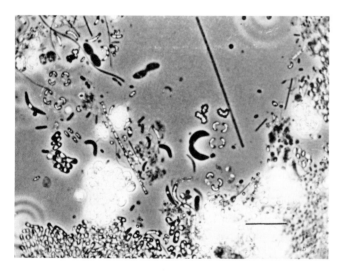

Figure 23.80. *"P. subtilissimum"* (gas-vacuolated filament *left of center*) and *"Achroonema angustum"* (dark, straight filament without gas vesicles on the *upper right side*). Sample of anaerobic hypolimnion of Wintergreen Lake (Michigan) on August 5, taken from a 4.5-m depth. *Bar,* 1 μm.

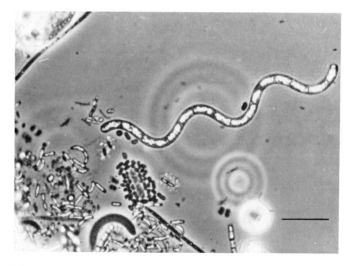

Figure 23.81. *"Pelonema"* species, probably *"P. spirale."* This organism may be identical with *Chloronema giganteum* Gorlenko, a green bacterium. Sample collected on August 11 from the anaerobic hypolimnion of Cassidy Lake (Michigan) from a 7-m depth. Also shown (on *lower left side*) is *Chlorochromatium aggregatum* consortium. *Bar,* 1 μm.

Table 23.24.
Differential characteristics of the species of the genus "Pelonema"[a]

Characteristic	1. "P. tenue"	2. "P. aphane"	3. "P. pseudovacuolatum"	4. "P. subtilissimum"	5. "P. hyalinum"	6. "P. spirale"
Cell width (μm)	2.0 (1.8–2.2)[b]	1.0–1.7	2.0 (1.5–2.0)[b]	0.6–0.7	2.0	1.0–1.5
Cell length (μm)	8–12	5–16	4.0	1.5–6.0	4–6	?
Constriction at cross-walls[c]	+	+	±	−	−	+
Length of filament (μm)	300	600	?	120	>200	40–60
Gliding of filament (μm/min)	Up to 60	Very slow; rarely	−	−	Weakly	?

[a]Symbols: ?, not known; +, positive; ±, occasionally present; and −, negative.
[b]Data are from Skuja (1956).
[c]If positive, constriction only weakly.

Genus II. "Achroonema" *Skuja 1948, 30*

P. HIRSCH

A.chro.o.ne′ma. Gr. adj. *achroos* colorless; Gr. n. *nema* filament; M.L. neut. n. *Achroonema* colorless filament.

Cells have a delicate, smooth, sometimes distinctly porous cell wall; protoplasm homogeneous, granular, or differentiated into lighter peripheral and darker central portions. **Cells range from 0.3–0.5 to 5–6.8 μm in width; they are arranged in multicellular, colorless, unbranched filaments** that are always **more or less motile** and may be up to 5 mm long. **Filaments straight** or nearly so **or in very loose spirals;** in some species, filaments are **constricted at cross-walls.** Three species appear to form **arthrosporelike resting cells; one species contains gas vesicles in older cells.** Multiply by fragmentation of filaments. Aquatic. Have not been cultivated.

Type species: *"Achroonema spiroideum"* Skuja 1948, 31.

Further Descriptive Information

The morphology of filaments varies with the species. Filaments may be more or less straight or coiled in loose spirals; and they may be shorter (up to 350 μm long) or longer (up to 5 mm long), narrower (0.3–0.5 μm wide) or wider (5–6.8 μm). Motility varies with the species, from very motile to not or only slightly motile by gliding.

"Achroonema" species are presumably chemoorganotrophic; their presence in hypolimnia of freshwater lakes indicates possibly anaerobic metabolism and possible psychrophily.

Most *"Achroonema"* species were found in lakes at 11–22-m depths; only some came from ponds or brooks (Skuja, 1948; Hirsch, 1981c).

Differentiation of the genus "Achroonema" from other morphologically similar taxa

As the lack of special properties may presently be the best characteristic of *"Achroonema"* species, this genus has to be compared with a large number of other filamentous bacteria (Table 23.25 of the *"Pelonemataceae"*).

grounds. It is quite possible, therefore, that some of the species may be identical with species of other genera, as, for example, *"A. lentum"* falls into the size range of *"Pelonema aphane"* or *"Pelonema pseudovacuolatum."*

Taxonomic Comments

The genus *"Achroonema"* has been described largely on morphological

Differentiation of the species of the genus "Achroonema"

Some differential features of the *"Achroonema"* species are listed in Table 23.25. For habitats, see Hirsch (1981c). Skuja (1948, 1956, 1974)

also considered the density and structures of the protoplasts important.

List of species of the genus "Achroonema"

1. **"Achroonema spiroideum"** Skuja 1948, 31.
spi.ro.i′de.um. L. n. *spira* spiral; L. adj. suff. *-oideus* form of; L. adj. *spiroideum* having a spiral form.

Cells 0.3–0.5 × 3–15 μm. Filaments up to 250 μm long, wound in loose spirals and not constricted at the indistinct cross-walls. Filaments very motile (~600 μm/min). From 11- to 14-m hypolimnion of lakes and in slime of planktonic organisms.

2. **"Achroonema angustum"** (Koppe) Skuja 1956, 84. (*Oscillatoria angusta* Koppe 1924, 641.)
an.gus′tum. L. adj. *angustum* slender.

Cells 0.7–1.2 × 2.5–8 μm, forming nearly straight filaments without marked constrictions at the cross-walls. Filaments motile. Found in hypolimnion of lakes or in lake bottom mud.

3. **"Achroonema proteiforme"** Skuja 1956, 84.
pro.te.i.for′me. Gr. comp. adj. *proteros* earlier, premature; L. n. *forma* shape, form; M.L. n. *proteiforme* earlier form.

Cells 1.3–1.6 × 3–13 μm, with some large granules partly in a single row. In filaments 200–600 μm long and without constrictions at cross-walls. Filaments may be lightly and irregularly coiled. Filaments are motile (50–60 μm/min). From bottom mud of lakes and ponds.

4. **"Achroonema profundum"** (Kirchner) Skuja 1956, 85. (*Oscillatoria profunda* Kirchner 1896, 101.)
pro.fun′dum. L. adj. *profundum* of the depths.

Cells 2 × 2–6 μm, in straight or slightly twisted filaments which are not constricted at the rather obscure cross-walls; filaments nearly straight or slightly twisted. Filaments motile. From lake hypolimnion.

5. **"Achroonema splendens"** Skuja 1956, 88.
splen′dens. L. part. adj. *splendens* brilliant.

Cells 3.4–4.2 × 4–10 μm, in straight filaments up to 1000 μm long and not constricted at the distinct cross-walls; filaments motile (200–500 μm/min). From sediments or H_2S-containing pond water; probably thiophilic.

Table 23.25.
*Characteristics differentiating "**Achroonema**" species[a]*

Characteristic	1. "A. spiroideum"	2. "A. angustum"	3. "A. proteiforme"	4. "A. profundum"	5. "A. splendens"	6. "A. sporogenum"	7. "A. inaequale"	8. "A. lentum"	9. "A. simplex"	10. "A. articulatum"	11. "A. macromeres"	12. "A. gotlandicum"
Cell width (µm)	0.3–0.5	0.7–1.2	1.3–1.6	2	3.4–4.2	2.5	2–2.7	1.4–2	1.8–2	2–3.5	5–6.8	2.5–3
Cell length (µm)	3–15	2.5–8	3–13	2–6	4–10	2.5–4	1.5–3	3–12	1.5–3	2.8–13	4–19	9–12
Filaments												
Coiled	+	–	–	–	–	–	–	–	–	–	–	–
Straight or slightly bent	–	+	+	+	+	+	+	+	+	+	+	+
Constricted at cross-walls	–	–	–	–	–	+	+	+	+	+	+	+
With gas vesicles	–	–	–	–	–	–	–	+	–	–	+	–
With resting cells ("spores")	–	–	–	–	–	+	+	+	–	–	–	–
Motility (µm/min)	600	+[b]	50–60	+	200–300	•	135	±	±	30–50	80–150	+
Filament length (maximal) (µm)	250	•	600	•	1000	•	•	•	•	100–350	5000	•

[a]Symbols: +, positive; –, negative; ±, motility is very slow or absent; and •, no data are available.
[b]Exact data are not available, but "fast" motility has been observed.

6. **"Achroonema sporogenum"** Skuja 1956, 87.

spor.o′ge.num. M.L. n. *spora* a spore; Gr. v. *gennano* produce; M.L. adj. *sporogenum* producing spores.

Cells 2.5 × 2.5–4 µm; in nearly straight filaments which show distinct constrictions at the cross-walls; the cells appear to be nearly separated. Filaments are motile. Resting cells ("spores") are formed; these are short, cylindrical or barrel-shaped with flattened or occasionally rounded ends, 2.5–2.8 × 2.7–5 µm, with a relatively thick, brown cell wall. There may be up to three resting cells in a row. Originally observed among decaying leaves of water plants in a rivulet near Riga, Latvia.

7. **"Achroonema inaequale"** Skuja 1956, 86.

in.ae.qua′le. L. adj. *inaequale* unequal, referring to unequal thickness of sporiferous filaments.

Cells 2–2.7 × 5–3 µm, in straight filaments which are more or less constricted at the distinct cross-walls. Filaments may be slightly and irregularly flexuous; they are motile (~135 µm/min).

Resting cells ("spores") are formed. These are short, barrel-shaped or discoid, up to 3.5–4 µm wide × 2.5–4.5 µm long, with relatively thin colorless and smooth walls. From hypolimnion of eutrophic lakes.

8. **"Achroonema lentum"** Skuja 1956, 85.

len′tum. L. adj. *lentum* slow.

Cells 1.4–2 × 3–12 µm, in filaments slightly constricted at the cross-walls, straight or slightly flexuous. Filaments show only very slow motion, if at all.

Resting cells ("spores") 2–2.5 × 5–10 µm, cylindrical with rounded ends and thin colorless walls, usually occur singly.

From the hypolimnion or sediment of lakes and deep ponds.

9. **"Achroonema simplex"** Skuja 1956, 85.

sim′plex. L. adj. *simplex* simple.

Cells short, barrel-shaped, 1.8–2 × 1.5–3 µm, in straight or slightly flexuous filaments with distinct constrictions at the cross-walls. Filament motility very slow. From hypolimnion of lakes, especially beneath the bottom mud.

10. **"Achroonema articulatum"** Skuja 1956, 89.

ar.ti.cu.la′tum. L. adj. *articulatum* divided into joints, articulate.

The cylindrical cells have slightly rounded ends; they are 2–3.5 × 2.8–13 µm, and the protoplasm is differentiated into the lighter periphery and the darker axial portion. In filaments that are straight and 100–350 µm long, with definite constrictions at the thick and hyaline cross-walls. Filaments show slow motility (30–50 µm/min). From deeper waters, generally from hypolimnion of lakes. May be found in the upper water layers during the period of vernal circulation.

11. **"Achroonema macromeres"** Skuja 1956, 90.

ma.cro.me′res. Gr. adj. *macros* large; Gr. n. *meros* part; M.L. n. *macromeres* large parts.

Cells cylindrical or slightly barrel-shaped, 5–6.8 × 4–19 µm, with a distinctly porous wall and lighter peripheral protoplasm differentiated from darker axial protoplasm. Filaments straight or slightly flexuous, fragile, of varying lengths from a few cells to 5 mm long. There are more or less constrictions at the cross-walls. Filaments are motile (80–150 µm/min). Older cells may contain gas vesicles. From the hypolimnion of lakes, pools and other stagnant waters. May be found in the epilimnion during periods of vernal circulation.

12. **"Achroonema gotlandicum"** Skuja 1956, 88.

got.lan′di.cum. Swed. n. *gotland* Gotland, a Swedish island; L. adj. suff. *-icum* belonging to; *gotlandicum* belonging to Gotland.

Cylindrical cells are 2.5–3 × 9–12 µm, in straight or slightly flexuous filaments which are not fragile and which are more or less constricted at the cross-walls. Motility is medium-fast. From hypolimnic water of Lake Sigwaldeträsk on Gotland.

Genus III. **"Peloploca"** Lauterborn 1913, 99

P. HIRSCH

Pel.o.plo'ca. Gr. adj. *pelos* dark-colored, hence anaerobic mud; Gr. n. *plokē* braid, wickerwork; M.L. fem. n. *Peloploca* mud braid.

Cells rod-shaped, 0.3–1.0 × 0.6–10 μm, arranged in filaments of variable length and **with or without common sheath.** Cells of **some species contain gas vesicles.** There may or may not be constrictions at cross-walls. **Filaments bound together laterally to form rigid bundles or flat ribbons** which may be straight, undulate in one plane, or spirally wound; the ends may appear more or less fibrous. Not motile. Gram reaction not recorded.

Propagation by fragmentation of bundles or ribbons.

Aquatic, nonmotile but free floating or in sediment surface layers. Have not been cultivated.

Type species: *"Peloploca undulata"* Lauterborn 1913, 90.

Further Descriptive Information

Cells are always rod-shaped, but the cell length (within a filament) may vary. Most *"Peloplaca"* species are found in the anaerobic hypolimnion of stratified lakes or ponds, hence an anaerobiotic life style of these bacteria can be assumed (Hirsch, 1981c).

Gas vesicles have been observed in *"P. taeniata," "P. undulata"* and *"P. pulchra."* In the latter case, Skuja (1956) assumed these to be located in the polymer layer covering the cell surface. This appears to be quite unlikely. Hirsch (1981c) observed *"P. pulchra"* in Lake Plußsee (Holstein, Germany) and found the gas vesicles to occur *within* cell filaments.

"P. undulata" has recently been found in hypolimnetic samples from Cassidy Lake and Wintergreen Lake (both in Michigan, U.S.A; Hirsch, 1981c). Additional sightings came from samples from a lake in Holstein. In all these cases, the ribbon consisted of two types of filaments: thinner, dark filaments without gas vesicles and thicker, bright ones filled completely with gas vesicles. The bright filaments alternated with one or two dark filaments on either side. It was assumed, therefore, that *"P. undulata"* represents a consortium of two different organisms (Hirsch, 1981c, 1984). Not one of the components has been found alone.

The normal habitat of *"Peloploca"* species is the anaerobic hypolimnion of ponds and lakes (Hirsch, 1981b). Usually, H₂S is found in *"Peloploca"*-containing water samples, and observed temperatures are in the range of 4–17°C (Hirsch, 1981c).

Differentiation of the genus **"Peloploca"** from other closely related taxa

The arrangement of *"Peloploca"* cells in filaments which aggregate to form flat bands or three-dimensional bundles differentiates the species of this genus from most other similar genera. *"Desmanthos"* filament bundles lack gas vesicles and live attached to surfaces. *Thioploca* species contain elemental sulfur storage granules. Other morphologically similar genera are compared with *"Peloploca"* in Table 23.26 (*"Pelonemataceae"*).

Taxonomic Comments

The presence, in the type species *"Peloploca undulata,"* of two morphologically different filaments raises a question: Which of the two should be the *Peloploca*? Consortia consisting of two or more species cannot carry normal, binary names. However, on the other hand, a decision cannot be made as yet, with our present lack of knowledge. It is suggested, therefore, that the name *"Peloploca undulata"* be retained but that it be used with the addition "consortium."

Table 23.26.
Characteristics differentiating the species of the genus **"Peloploca"**[a]

Characteristic	1. *"P. undulata"*	2. *"P. taeniata"*	3. *"P. fibrata"*	4. *"P. pulchra"*	5. *"P. ferruginea"*
Cell width					
0.3–0.6 μm	−	−	+	+	+
0.6–1.0 μm	+	+	−	−	−
Cell length (μm)	6–10	3–4	2–10	0.8–2.0	0.6–1.5
Gas vesicles	+	+	−	+[b]	−
Cell aggregates with visible common capsule	−	+	(+)	+	+
Cell aggregate a flat band, often wavy or loosely spiral	+	+	+	−	−
Cell aggregate a bundle	−	−	−	+	+
Constrictions at cross-walls	−	+	(+)	(+)	(+)

[a]Symbols: −, negative; +, positive; and (+), barely visible.

[b]According to Skuja (1956), the gas vesicles of *"P. pulchra"* occur outside of the cells within the polymer capsules.

List of species of the genus **"Peloploca"**

1. **"Peloploca undulata"** (consortium) Lauterborn 1913, 99.

un.du.la′ta. L. fem. adj. *undulata* wavy.

Cells 0.8–1.2 × 6–10 μm, colorless, in filaments not constricted at cross-walls. Joined in bands up to 10 μm wide and 150 μm long, usually as a single ribbon but occasionally as multiple bands. These bands consist of thinner, darker filaments without gas vesicles, which alternate with thicker filaments that are completely filled with gas vesicles. Often two dark filaments alternate with one bright (gas-vacuolated) filament (Fig. 23.82). Skuja (1956) described the aggregates as "parallel striped."

Probably heterotrophic and anaerobic. Found in deep freshwater pools and lakes in the hypolimnion close to the sediment surface.

2. **"Peloploca taeniata"** Lauterborn 1913, 99.

taen.i.a′ta. L. n. *taenia* a band; M.L. adj. *taeniata* stripped, banded.

Cells 0.6–1.0 × 3–10 μm, colorless with central gas vesicles, in uniform filaments, minutely but distinctly constricted at the thickened cross-walls and thin sheath. Filaments form bands 9–15 μm wide, 1–3 μm thick and up to 1 mm long, flat, straight or slightly twisted, flexible but not fragile, and often with pointed ends. The filaments have a common capsule up to 5 μm thick (Fig. 23.83).

Probably anaerobic and heterotrophic. Found in the hypolimnion of lakes and in deeper fresh and brackish waters, in quarries, near the sediment surface.

3. **"Peloploca fibrata"** Skuja 1956, 95.

fi.bra′ta. L. adj. *fibrata* fibrous.

Cells 0.4–0.6 × 2.0–10 μm, colorless without gas vesicles, in uniform, fragile filaments, not constricted or with only minute constrictions at the indistinct cross-walls. Filaments form rigid bands or bundles up to 17 μm wide, up to 3 μm thick and up to 600 μm (rarely 1 mm) long. There is a common capsule clearly visible (see Fig. 4 in Hirsch (1981c)). Multiplication is by fragmentation of the filament aggregate. Filaments of an aggregate do not all have the same length.

Anaerobic and presumably heterotrophic. Found in the hypolimnion of lakes, often at great depths, close to the sediment surface.

4. **"Peloploca pulchra"** Skuja 1956, 96.

pul′chra. L. adj. *pulcher, pulchra* beautiful.

Cells 0.4–0.6 × 1.6–2.4 μm, colorless, containing no gas vesicles. In uniform filaments, often slightly constricted at the sites of the indistinct cross-walls, and with a colorless or slightly brownish sheath, 0.5–0.6 μm thick; 4–15 filaments in rigid, regularly and slightly curved or spirally twisted bundles 3–20 μm wide, 3–15 μm thick and up to 400 μm in length; the curves are 30–57 μm in length with an amplitude of 3–20 μm. Propagation by fragmentation of individual bundles.

Anaerobic and presumably heterotrophic. Found in deeper freshwater pools and in the hypolimnion and sediment of eutrophic ponds and deeper lakes.

5. **"Peloploca ferruginea"** Skuja 1956, 94.

fer.ru.gin′e.a. L. adj. *ferruginea* dark red, rust-colored.

Cells 0.3–0.5 × 0.3–1.5 μm, colorless, without gas vesicles, in uniform filaments minutely constricted at the indistinct cross-walls. Filaments with an often brownish sheath containing iron oxide hydrate and which is 0.6 μm thick. They are aggregated in rigid, sigmoidally curved and loosely twisted bundles of two to seven filaments, 3–10 μm wide and up to 300 μm long. Propagation by fragmentation of the bundles.

Anaerobic and presumably heterotrophic. Found in hypolimnion of eutrophic deeper lakes in Sweden.

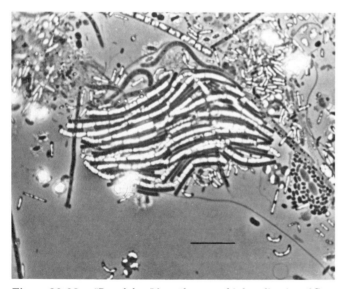

Figure 23.82.   *"P. undulata"* from the anaerobic hypolimnion of Cassidy Lake (Michigan) from a 7-m depth. The sample was collected in August. Gas-vacuolated cell filaments alternate with one to two filaments without gas vesicles. *"P. undulata"* is a consortium of two different organisms. *Bar,* 1 μm.

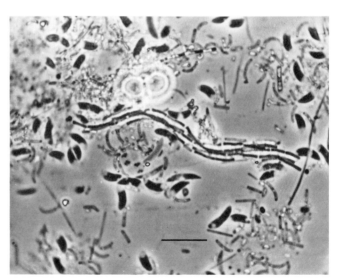

Figure 23.83.   *"Peloploca"* species, possibly *"P. taeniata,"* from the anaerobic hypolimnion of Lake Pluβsee (Holstein) from a 30-m depth. The sample was collected in July. The two cell types of this consortium are clearly visible; those with gas vesicles alternate with cells without gas vesicles. *Bar,* 1 μm.

Genus IV. **"Desmanthos"** *Skuja 1958, 442*

P. HIRSCH

Des.man′thos. Gr. n. *desmos* bundle; Gr. n. *anthos* flower; M.L. neut. n. *Desmanthos* flower(-like) bundle.

Colorless cells in unbranched, more or less straight **filaments** which are **thicker at the base than at the apex; filaments in bundles, the base of which is enclosed in a common hyaline, gelatinous sheath of variable thickness;** the filaments at the top are free and divergent (Fig. 23.84). Bundles are attached by a holdfast or are partially buried in bottom mud. **Propagation by fragmentation of filaments** and probably by longitudinal separation of the bundle-filaments. Motility not observed. Have not been cultivated.

Type species: *"Desmanthos thiokrenophilum"* Skuja 1958, 442.

Differentiation of the genus **"Desmanthos"** *from other morphologically similar taxa*

Certain morphological similarities exist with *"Clonothrix"* and *Thioploca* species. However, the former organisms do not live together as bundles, and *Thioploca* species store sulfur granules and show gliding motility.

List of species of the genus **"Desmanthos"**

1. **"Desmanthos thiokrenophilum"** Skuja 1958, 442.
thio.kre.no′phi.lum. Gr. n. *thium* sulfur; Gr. n. *krene* a spring; Gr. adj. *philus* loving, fond of; M.L. adj. *thiokrenophilum* fond of sulfur springs.

Bundles are composed of up to 10 filaments which are 50–160 µm long and measure about 0.5 µm in diameter at the top and up to 1.5 µm in diameter at the base, with a rounded conical basal cell. Cells in the middle of the filament are more or less isodiametrical but may be about 4 times longer than wide. Bundles are 6–8 µm thick at sheathed base; at tips, filaments are divergent. Cells have a colorless protoplast, occasionally differentiated into a light center and a somewhat darker periphery. Do not form gas vesicles. Have not been cultivated.

Habitat: Found in some sulfur springs at Kemeri, Latvia.

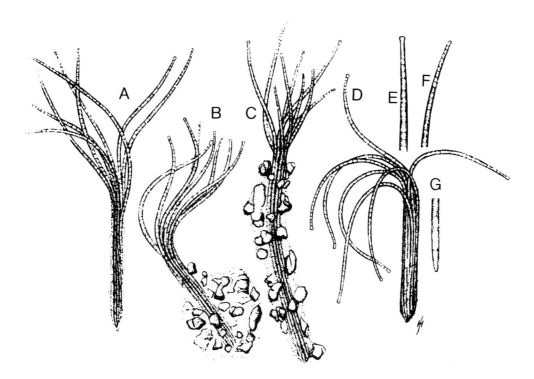

Figure 23.84. *"Desmanthos thiokrenophilum"* reproduced from Skuja (1958). *A–D* show filament bundles with varying amounts of terminal polymer which, in some cases, allowed the incorporation of small mineral particles. *E–G* show ends of filaments.

OTHER GENERA

Genus **Toxothrix** Molisch 1925, 144[AL]

P. Hirsch

Tox'o. thrix. Gr. n. *toxon* a bow; Gr. n. *thrix* a thread; M.L. fem. n. *Toxothrix* bent thread.

Cells cylindrical, colorless, 0.5–0.75 x 3–6 µm, **in filaments (trichomes) up to 400 µm long.** A dense body **(polyphosphate?)** is often located at either end of the cell (Fig. 23.85A). Gram reaction not recorded.

Filaments often U-shaped (Fig. 23.85A and B) and **rotating while slowly moving forward with the rounded part in the lead;** a **mucoid substance,** excreted from several sites on the trailing ends, **is deposited as a double track** ("railroad track") **of twisted strings** each 0.2 µm wide (Fig. 23.85D). **Fan-shaped structures may be deposited laterally** along the tracks, as the arms of the U move from side to side, and between the tracks, as a result of the middle section being lifted and then touched down again (Fig. 23.85C; Krul et al., 1970).

Oxidized iron may be deposited on the mucoid threads, rendering them yellowish brown and brittle and giving them a diameter of 2.5 µm.

Have not been obtained in pure culture, but chemoorganothrophic and psychrophilic cultures have been maintained for long periods at 5 and 10°C. **Filaments are extremely fragile during laboratory examination, and explosive disintegration of filaments has been observed after short periods under the microscope.**

Grow attached to surfaces and develop best at reduced oxygen tensions (Hässelbarth and Lüdemann, 1967) and slightly below neutrality (pH 5.1– 7.7). Originally found in water reservoir near the Biological Station at the Dnjepr River in the U.S.S.R. Widely distributed in cold iron springs, brooks, forest ponds and lakes containing ferrous iron and with reduced oxygen tension (Hirsch, 1981a).

Type species: *Toxothrix trichogenes* (Cholodny) Beger *in* Beger and Bringmann 1953, 332.

Further Descriptive Information

The normal trichome does not appear to have cross-walls when viewed with the phase microscope (Fig. 23.85A). Cholodny (1924) thought the organisms had a thin, tubular sheath which split repeatedly longitudinally, thus giving rise to the "twisted thread rope." However, Krul et al. (1970) followed the formation of the double tracks and fan-shaped structures on living, undisturbed and actually growing specimens.

Toxothrix trichogenes has been reported to have been cultivated by Teichmann (1935). Hirsch (1981a) kept natural samples containing *Toxothrix* in the laboratory for several months; *Toxothrix* cells survived if the samples contained sediment and organic detritus and were kept cold (5°C) and dark.

The appearance of *Toxothrix* throughout the year (except for May and

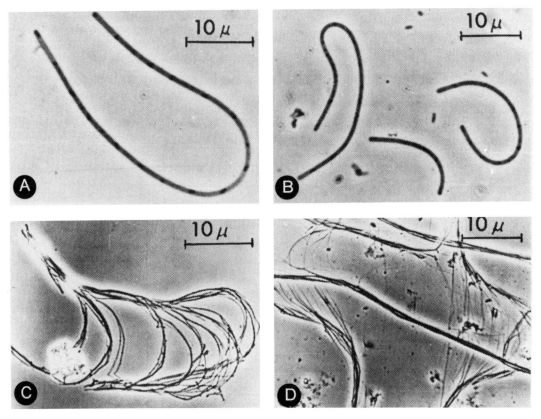

Figure 23.85.   *Toxothrix trichogenes* observed in a small iron spring catch basin. *A* and *B*, laboratory wet mounts of living trichomes during the first minute. Phase-contrast micrographs. *C* and *D*, excreted polymer coated with iron oxides, from which, through the peculiar type of motion, arose fan-shaped structures (*C*) or double tracks (*D*). (*A–D* are reproduced with permission from J. M. Krul, P. Hirsch and J. T. Staley, Antonie van Leeuwenhoek Journal of Microbiology *36:* 409–420, ©1970 by Martinus Nijhoff Publishers. Reprinted by permission of Kluwer Academic Publishers.)

June) has been reported (Hirsch, 1981a). Usually, it is found where *Gallionella ferruginea* grows and in waters with Fe^{2+} at 1–2.7 mg/l. But *Toxothrix* cells, contrary to *Gallionella* cells, prefer habitats with a slightly

higher concentration of organic compounds. An iron spring catch basin with cold, Fe-containing water and decaying leaves appears to be the optimal *Toxothrix* habitat.

Differentiation of the genus **Toxothrix** from other morphologically similar taxa

In the absence of Fe deposition, the *Toxothrix* filaments closely resemble *Herpetosiphon*, *Haliscomenobacter* or "*Achroonema*" filaments. But *Herpetosiphon* filaments are extremely long (300–1200 µm) and vary in their cell diameter. Also, there are transparent sections at the filament tips (called necridia) which are not present in *Toxothrix*. Strains of *Haliscomenobacter* are not known to glide or to show true branches, and their optimum pH is 7.0–8.0; also, they do not deposit iron oxides. "*Achroonema*" filaments do not glide in a U-shaped way but remain straight and fairly rigid.

Taxonomic Comments

Balashova (1968) has pointed out that in some respects *Toxothrix* resembles *Gallionella*. The great differences in cell shape do not seem to support this view. Beger and Bringmann (1953, p. 333) described "*Toxothrix gelatinosa*" on the basis of smaller filaments (diameter with slime threads: 1.5–1.7 µm) and the fan-shaped arrangements of individual filaments in a gelatinous matrix. However, the individual cell size (0.5 x 3 µm) falls within the range given for *T. trichogenes*.

List of species of the genus **Toxothrix**

1. **Toxothrix trichogenes** (Cholodny) Beger *in* Beger and Bringmann 1953, 332.[AL] (*Leptothrix trichogenes* Cholodny 1924, 296.)

tri.cho'ge. nes. Gr. n. *thrix* hair; Gr. v. suff. - *genes* producing; M.L. adj. *trichogenes* hair-producing.

Description is the same as for the genus.

Genus **Leucothrix** Oersted 1844, 44[AL]

T. D. BROCK

Leu′co.thrix. Gr. adj. *leucus* clear, light; Gr. n. *thrix, trichis* hair; M.L. fem. n. *Leucothrix* colorless hair.

Long filaments composed of short cylindrical or ovoid cells (gonidia), cross-walls clearly visible, **colorless, unbranched;** typically uniform filaments may taper from base to apex, under some conditions showing an apical beady chain of gonidia connected end to end. In nature, filaments **usually attached to solid substrates by means of inconspicuous holdfasts; stalks absent. Filaments do not glide** but may wave sporadically from side to side. **Dispersal by means of gonidia** (single cells arising from cells of the filaments by rounding up, often released primarily from apices, but they may also be formed in an intercalary fashion); **gonidia often** but not always **show jerky gliding motion** on solid substrates. **Rosette formation** is a key diagnostic characteristic of the genus but is found rarely in nature, although it is frequently seen in a laboratory culture. The rosettes may be formed of gonidia or, after gonidial growth, of several or more filaments attached at their bases. Filaments in a laboratory culture often form true knots; these structures also occur in nature, although rarely. The organism morphologically resembles some filamentous cyanobacteria but does not form photosynthetic pigments. **Strictly aerobic, heterotrophic. Aquatic; usually marine,** although one freshwater strain has been isolated. Most strains require NaCl for growth; optimum concentration: about 1.5% NaCl; grows at concentrations of 0.3–6.0% NaCl. Most strains do not require growth factors. Optimum temperature: 25°C; maximum: 30–35°C; minimum: 0°C, forming visible colonies within 1–2 weeks. Strains from tropical waters are more stenothermal, not growing below 15°C. Catalase-positive.

The mol% G + C of the DNA of the more than 46 strains examined is 46–51 (Brock and Mandel, 1966; Kelly and Brock, 1969a).

Type species: *Leucothrix mucor* Oersted 1844, 44.

Further Descriptive Information

Habitat. Leucothrix was first obtained in pure culture by Harold and Stanier(1955). It is found widely in the littoral zone in marine environments, growing primarily as an epiphyte of plants (Brock, 1966) or animals (Johnson et al., 1971). Bland and Brock (1973) carried out a quantitative survey of the distribution of *Leucothrix* in the Friday Harbor, Washington State area, and found it associated with many species of seaweeds, although the density varied widely. The red alga *Bangia fuscopurpurea*, a filamentous species living in the high intertidal region, was unusually heavily colonized, having *Leucothrix* populations 10–30 times

larger than those on other algal species. Brock (1966) showed that *Leucothrix* could grow on nutrients produced or liberated from algae. Although *Leucothrix* is also able to colonize artificial substrates (plastic strips) in the marine environment, Bland and Brock (1973) showed that growth was much poorer on these strips than on seaweeds.

Johnson et al. (1971) showed that *Leucothrix* was able to grow extensively on benthic crustacea and fish eggs. Since that report, *Leucothrix* has frequently been found to cause infestations of crustaceans that have been under cultivation in high-density aquaculture situations (Shelton et al., 1975; Couch, 1978; Fisher et al., 1978; Solangi et al., 1979). *Leucothrix* has generally been considered to be nonpathogenic, with its heavy colonization of benthic crustacea generally being seen as a result of high crowding in aquaculture situations. Couch (1978) reported that mortality of shrimp was proportionate to the extent of growth of *Leucothrix* on their gills. He suggested that the mortality may have been due to the massive growth of the bacterium over the gill cuticle, blocking the normal gas diffusion across the gill surfaces. *Leucothrix* infections of marine animals can be prevented by treatment with penicillin, streptomycin and neomycin (Fisher et al., 1978).

Leucothrix has frequently been associated with activated sludge systems, where it has been implicated in the phenomenon of bulking, as well as in self-purification and biological waste treatment processes (Cyrus and Sladka, 1970). In most such cases, brackish water was involved (Eikelboom and van Buijsen, 1981), although one strictly freshwater strain of *Leucothrix* has been isolated from petrochemical wastewater undergoing activated sludge treatment (Poffe et al., 1979). Even this strain grows well at seawater salinity and thus may be considered to be simply more euryhaline than are other isolates.

Life cycle. A simplified life cycle of *Leucothrix mucor* is shown in Figure 23.86. Rosette and gonidia formations are not obligatory, with the organism growing quite well indefinitely in the filamentous form. Gonidia formation may occur in nature, ensuring the dispersal of the organism. Photomicrographs of various stages of the life cycle have been published by Brock (1981).

Structure. Electron microscopic studies of *Leucothrix* have been presented by Brock and Conti (1969), Snellen and Raj (1970) and Raj (1977). The filaments of *Leucothrix* are multicellular, with the individual gonidia being separated by well-defined cross-walls (Fig. 23.87). Gonidia in a filament are capable of cell division without any basal-apical differ-

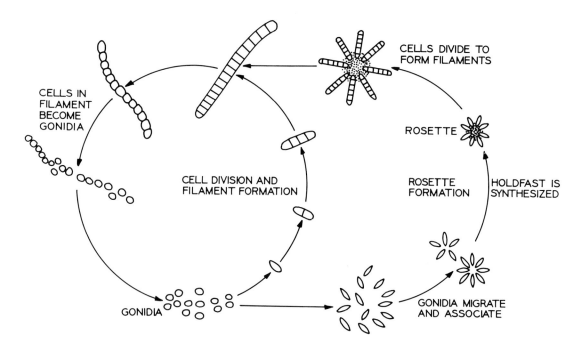

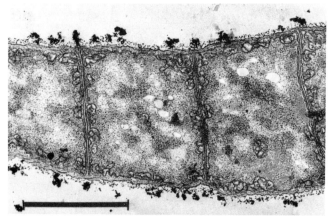

Figure 23.87. Electron micrograph of a thin section of a portion of a filament of *L. mucor. Bar*, 1 μm.

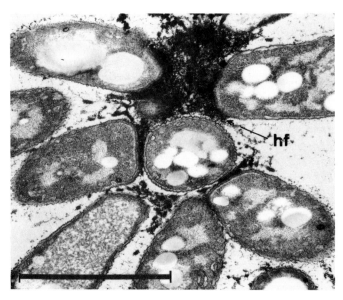

Figure 23.88. Electron micrograph of a *Leucothrix* rosette, with the electron-dense holdfast materials (*hf*) shown. *Bar*, 1 μm. (Reproduced with permission from T. D. Brock and S. F. Conti, Archiv für Mikrobiologie *66:* 79–90, 1969, ©Springer-Verlag.)

entiation (Brock, 1967). Filaments are of variable length, often much greater than 100 μm, with a diameter of 2–3 μm or more. The filaments are colorless, unbranched and nonmotile (although occasionally waving back and forth) and lack a sheath (Fig. 23.87). The cell envelope shows structural features characteristic of the Gram-negative bacterial envelope. Filaments often grow intertwined or in dense tangles. One of the intriguing characteristics of *Leucothrix* is the ability of most strains to form true knots (Brock, 1964). The function of knot formation is unknown, and it may actually be an accidental process, but it seems to be characteristic of most *Leucothrix* strains as part of the growth process. Swollen cells often form apparently at random along filaments. Larger structures (bulbs) usually form in knotty cultures, possibly as the result of fusion of cells in the region of knots. Filaments are found in nature attached to solid substrates by inconspicuous holdfasts. Such a holdfast can be easily seen in the electron microscope as an electron-dense material, possibly a polysaccharide, peripheral to the outer wall layer (Fig. 23.88); it can also be seen in the fluorescence microscope when the fluo-

rochrome dye primulin is used; when viewed in blue light, the holdfast fluoresces red, whereas the cell wall fluoresces yellow. Gonidia are formed by rounding up of cells of the filaments, and the gonidia retain all of the envelope structures observed in filaments. At a low concentration of an organic energy source, filaments do not grow very long and form gonidia more readily. Gonidial formation is also increased if growth rate is slowed by anaerobiosis, starvation, or reducing the temperature of incubation (Pringsheim, 1957; Bland and Brock, 1973). Gonidia move by a jerky sort of gliding motility, which can only be seen well when observations are made in slide cultures. Single gonidia may move for extended periods of time, but if the gonidial density is high enough, gonidia appear to be attracted to each other by homotaxis, and they form aggregates, which ultimately results in rosette formation. Free gonidia appear to lack holdfast material, but they form it after aggregation. Once a gonidium has attached to a surface by its holdfast, it remains attached indefinitely. Gonidia grow into filaments if conditions are favorable.

Nutrition. Leucothrix is a versatile heterotroph, being able to grow on a variety of organic energy sources including sugars, amino acids, sugar alcohols and organic acids. Walker et al. (1975) reported utilization of a mixed hydrocarbon substrate by the type strain, ATCC 25107. Both inorganic and organic nitrogen sources are utilized, but *Leucothrix* is unable to fix N_2 (Mague and Lewin, 1974). Most strains do not require growth factors, although a stenothermal strain required vitamin B_{12} for growth. Inorganic nutrition has been studied by Snellen and Raj (1970).

Physiology and metabolism. The physiology and the metabolism of *Leucothrix* have been extensively reviewed by Raj (1977). *Leucothrix* is a strict aerobe, with an optimum temperature for growth of 25–30°C, an optimum pH for growth of 7.6, and an optimum salinity of 1.5°/$_{oo}$. Bland and Brock (1973) showed that *Leucothrix* was able to withstand several hours of drying without an apparent reduction in viability, consistent with the fact that the organism extensively colonizes *Bangia fuscopurpurea*, an alga found high in the intertidal zone and frequently subject to drying during low tides. Radiorespirometric studies have shown that *Leucothrix* oxidizes carbohydrate substrates via the Entner-Doudoroff pathway, in conjunction with the tricarboxylic acid (TCA) cycle, and via the Embden-Meyerhof pathway, with some simultaneous operation of the pentose phospate pathway (Raj, 1977). The operation of the TCA cycle is consistent with the finding of isocitrate and malate dehydrogenases (Kelly and Brock, 1969a). The organism is catalase-positive (Poffe et al., 1979). The electron transport pathway has been studied by Biggins and Dietrich (1968) using spectrophotometric methods. The terminal electron transport system is a particulate cytochrome chain containing cytochrome b_{562}, cytochrome c_{552} and cytochrome b_{558}. The cytochrome b_{558} was proposed to be functionally equivalent to cytochrome o, and it operated as the terminal oxidase. Cytochrome b_{558} had high CO-binding properties. The activity of the oxidase system is markedly affected by the degree of aeration during growth. Although several strains of *Leucothrix* have been tested for ability to oxidize hydrogen sulfide, these tests have been negative (Harold and Stanier, 1955). However, K. Eimhjellen of the Technical University in Trondheim found sulfide-oxidizing ability and deposition of elemental sulfur in a pure culture of *Leucothrix* isolated at Pacific Grove, California (Brock, 1981). He was also able to demonstrate oxidation of thiosulfate to either tetrathionate or sulfate, and this latter oxidation was followed manometrically. Eimhjellen's strain was obviously different from those studied by Harold and Stanier (1955). In light of recent pure culture isolations of *Thiothrix*, more work on sulfide and thiosulfate oxidation by *Leucothrix* is in order.

Enrichment and Isolation Procedures

Although any marine type seawater salts base can be used in the formation of a culture medium, pH control and the avoidance of metal precipitation are easier in a Provasoli type culture medium (Provasoli, 1963). The salts formulation (Brock, 1966) given in Table 23.27 has proved quite effective. The low phosphate concentration in this salts base is critical, as media of more typical phospate concentrations are frequently inhibitory. Most strains have no vitamin requirements and are able to use glutamate as sole sources of carbon, nitrogen and energy. If a richer culture medium is desired, 0.1% tryptone plus 0.1% yeast extract can be used. In the initial isolation step, it is best to keep the concentration of organic materials low to avoid problems with overgrowth by unicellular bacteria. Although Harold and Stanier (1955) describe a procedure for enrichment of *Leucothrix* by using rotting seaweeds, direct isolation from fresh seaweeds is preferable. Rapidly growing, highly motile unicellular bacteria are frequently a problem when isolation of *Leucothrix* from rotted materials is attempted. An effective way of obtaining cultures of *Leucothrix* is to place relatively clean seaweeds taken directly from the sea onto on agar medium (Table 23.27) which will support the

Table 23.27.
Culture medium for **Leucothrix**

Ingredient	Amount
Basal salts	
NaCl	11.75 g
MgCl$_2$·6H$_2$O	5.35 g
Na$_2$SO$_4$	2.0 g
CaCl$_2$·2H$_2$O	0.75 g
KCl	0.35 g
Tris(hydroxymethyl)aminomethane	0.5 g
Na$_2$HPO$_4$	0.05 g
Deionized water (pH 7.6)	1000 ml
Organic ingredients	
Monosodium glutamate	1 g
or	
Tryptone	1 g
+	
Yeast extract	1 g

growth of *Leucothrix*. The plates are incubated overnight at 20–25°C and examined within 12–18 h for the presence of *Leucothrix* colonies. This examination is best done by using × 125 magnification (× 12.5 eyepiece and × 10 objective) with a long-working-distance condensor. It is important to use short incubation periods in order to find *Leucothrix* colonies before they have become overgrown by motile contaminants. A *Leucothrix* colony is recognized by its coiled rope or thumbprint morphology. Colonies are immediately picked by touching them with a sterile insect pin and transferring them in patches to fresh agar plates of the same composition. One advantage of isolating *Leucothrix* in this way is that the precise habitat of the organism can be recognized; such information is of considerable value in studies on the molecular evolution of the organism (Kelly and Brock, 1969a). Transfer of agar cultures to liquid medium frequently presents problems. It has been observed that if a small inoculum is used in a large volume of liquid medium, growth often does not occur, whereas if the inoculum is placed in a small volume of medium, such as 1–2 ml, heavy growth occurs overnight. Once satisfactory growth has been obtained in an initial small-volume liquid culture, it is possible to make transfers to large volumes of liquid medium. In liquid medium, growth is best when flasks are shaken gently, such as on a wrist-action shaker or slowly on a rotary shaker. When a rotary shaker is used, growth rate is increased if the flasks contain small internal baffles, made by pushing in the sides of the flasks during heating with an oxygen flame.

Maintenance Procedures

Once rapidly growing liquid cultures have been obtained (see above), there are no special maintenance problems. Cultures in the early stages of growth can be stored in the refrigerator for several months, after which they may consist mostly of gonidia. Cultures can also be lyophilized, with the best suspension medium being skim milk. When a lyophilized culture is rehydrated, it is preferable if the dry plug is placed in 1–2 ml of liquid medium and 0.1 ml of this suspension is placed in another tube of 1–2 ml of liquid medium. Both tubes are incubated for 1 or 2 days. If there is no visible growth in the dilution, 0.1–0.2 ml of the tube containing the original rehydrated culture should be transferred to another tube containing 1–2 ml of medium, followed by another incubation period. Only after good growth has been obtained in a small volume of medium should large-volume cultures be prepared. Contamination is easy to recognize, since *Leucothrix* cultures never show uniform turbidity. Microscopic examination of a culture should permit ready determination of the presence of contaminants. If contaminants do become established, they will generally grow better than the *Leucothrix* and will quickly take over the culture. Streaking onto a seawater agar medium containing tryptone and yeast extract is also a satisfactory way of recognizing many contaminants.

Identification

Leucothrix is identified simply on the basis of morphological examination with the light microscope. There is no need for conventional diagnostic tests. In the extensive isolations of Kelly and Brock (1969a), all of the isolates recognized morphologically had virtually the same physiological properties. The morphological properties described at the beginning of this article are generally found in any strain isolated.

Differentiation of the genus **Leucothrix** *from other genera*

The taxonomic relationship between *Leucothrix* and *Thiothrix* is being resolved, now that pure cultures are available (Larken and Strohl, 1983). A *Thiothrix* filament or rosette which has lost its sulfur granules cannot be distinguished superficially from a *Leucothrix* filament. There are, however, some significant differences. *Thiothrix* has a sheath; *Leucothrix* does not. *Leucothrix* uses a wide variety of organic compounds for growth; *Thiothrix* uses only a few. *Thiothrix* requires the presence of sulfide or thiosulfate to grow and is probably a mixotroph; *Leucothrix* needs neither and seems to be a rather versatile heterotroph. *Leucothrix* is largely restricted to marine habitats; *Thiothrix* is found in rapidly flowing sulfide-containing freshwater; and *Leucothrix* filaments may break up into many gonidia, while *Thiothrix* produces gonidia only from the open end of the sheath. If more strains of *Leucothrix* similar to Eimhjellen's strain, which oxidizes sulfide and deposits sulfur, are found, the taxonomic distinction between these two genera may not be tenable. At present, it is preferable to maintain the two genera until detailed studies (preferably at the molecular level) have been carried out.

Taxonomic Comments

It has been popular to consider *Leucothrix* to be a colorless cyanobacterium (Pringsheim, 1957; Raj, 1977). However, this is not really a useful designation, since the cyanobacteria as a group are extremely heterogeneous. Certainly, *Leucothrix* has morphological resemblances to some of the filamentous cyanobacteria, but it can hardly be considered related to the many unicellular cyanobacteria. There is no evidence that *Leucothrix* is a cyanobacterium which has lost its photosynthetic pigments. As far as chemoorganotrophic growth is concerned, *Leucothrix* is much more versatile nutritionally than any cyanobacterium that has been studied. However, the DNA base ratio of a number of *Leucothrix* strains (mol% G + C of 46–51) is in the range found by Edelman et al. (1967) for filamentous cyanbacteria (mol% G + C of 42–51).

List of species of the genus **Leucothrix**

1. **Leucothrix mucor** Oersted 1844,44.[AL]
mu. cor. L. n. *mucor* mold; M.L. n. *mucor* a genus of molds.
The characteristics are the same as those described for the genus.

Occur in marine habitats.
Neotype strain: number 1 (Brock, 1969) (ATCC 25107).

Genus **Vitreoscilla** *Pringsheim 1949, 70*[AL]

WILLIAM R. STROHL

Vit.re.os.cil'la. L. adj. *vitreus* glassy, clear; L. n. *oscillum* a swing; M.L. fem. n. *Vitreoscilla* transparent oscillator.

Organisms exist in **colorless filaments,** which contain cells with diameters of 1 to about 3 μm and lengths of 1–12 μm; **cells may be clearly delimited and barrel-shaped or may be undelimited and cylindrical (similar to *Beggiatoa*).** Filaments may contain from 1 to >40 cells. Cell walls of *V. stercoraria* are composed of the amino acids alanine, glutamate, and diaminopimelic acid with approximate molar ratios of 2:1:1. Cell division is by transverse binary fission; dispersion is by fragmentation of filaments or by sacrificial cell death and necridia formation in species similar to the beggiatoas. Resting stages are not known. **Sheaths or holdfasts are not produced. Gram-negative. Motile by gliding;** no locomotor organelles known. **Aerobic to microaerophilic. Chemoorganotrophs. Metabolism is respiratory** with molecular oxygen as sole known terminal electron acceptor. **Sulfur inclusions are not formed** from hydrogen sulfide or thiosulfate. Nutritional requirements vary among species, with the simplest organic requirement being acetate as sole carbon and energy sources and with the more complex requirements being for groups of amino acids. The larger *Vitreoscilla* species show similarities to certain *Beggiatoa* strains, with the exception to their inability to deposit sulfur when exposed to hydrogen sulfide.

The mol% G + C of the DNA ranges from 42 (T_m, Bd) to 63 (T_m).
Type species: *Vitreoscilla beggiatoides* Pringsheim 1949, 70.

Further Descriptive Information

The genus *Vitreoscilla* consists of two morphological types. One type is characterized by *V. beggiatoides*, the type species, and *V. filiformis*. They are ultrastructurally similar to *Beggiatoa* in having continuous outer layers of the filaments (Figs. 23.89 and 23.90), extra cell wall layers outside of the "lipopolysaccharide-like" layer (Strohl et al., 1986a), large accumulations of poly-β-hydroxybutyrate (PHB; sometimes >50% of dry cell mass), and membrane invaginations in the cytoplasm. If these filaments are mechanically broken up into individual cells, the cells die, an indication that these are truly multicellular bacteria like the beggiatoas. The cells within a filament of these species divide via septation, with only the cytoplasmic membrane and peptidoglycan layers invaginating like the closure of an iris diaphragm as in *Beggiatoa* (Strohl and Larkin, 1978a). In thin-section transmission electron micrographs, cells of *V. beggiatoides* and *V. filiformis* appear very similar to cells of *Beggiatoa* (Strohl et al., 1986a). Furthermore, the sacrificial cell death-life cycle described for beggiatoas (Strohl and Larkin, 1978a) appears to apply to *V. beggiatoides* and may occur with *V. filiformis* strains.

The other morphological type of *Vitreoscilla* is exemplified by *V. stercoraria*. This species has discontinuous outer layers (Figs. 23.91 and 23.92), and the filaments appear like chains of bacilli. The cells are held together by a ruthenium red-staining material, but they can be mechanically broken apart without accompanying massive cell death. Multicellular filaments seemingly are formed only because the cells do not completely detach after division. Reports have indicated that certain growth conditions promote growth of *V. stercoraria* as single cells (Brzin, 1966a, b). Ultrastructurally, *V. stercoraria* contains a typical Gram-negative cell envelope, with the addition of an external, ruthenium red-staining surface layer (Fig. 23.91; Strohl et al., 1986a).

For all vitreoscillas, the growth conditions determine the shape and characteristics of the colonies. On agar media containing low amounts of nutrients, wavy, curly or spiral colonies are produced from which trichomes glide radially outward from the central colony area. On solid media containing high nutrient concentrations, the trichomes spread very little and can form droplike colonies resembling those of most eubacteria.

The species of this genus formerly have been differentiated on the basis of trichome size alone, although certain nutritional differences among them are now known (Strohl et al., 1986a). Most strains grow best on media with very low nutrient concentrations (e.g. 0.05–0.1% peptone,

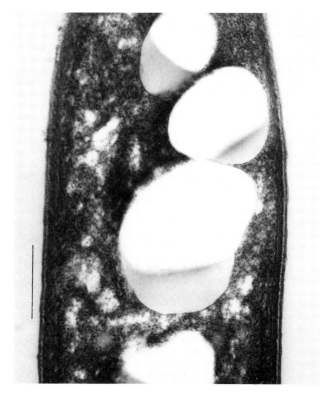

Figure 23.89. Thin-section electron micrograph of *V. beggiatoides* strain B23SS with continuous cell wall and extra cell wall layers. Also note the large depositions of PHB. *Bar*, 0.5 μm. (Reproduced with permission from W. R. Strohl, T. M. Schmidt, N. H. Lawry, M. J. Mezzino and J. M. Larkin, International Journal of Systematic Bacteriology *36*: 302–313, 1986a, ©International Union of Microbiological Societies.)

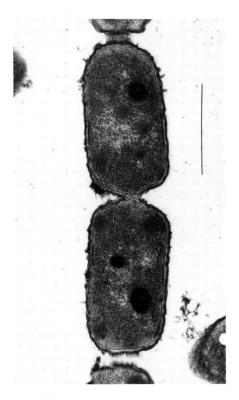

Figure 23.91. Thin-section electron micrograph of ruthenium red-stained *V. stercoraria* strain VT-1, with chains of cells, held together by connecting material, and the Gram-negative cell envelope shown. *Bar*, 1 μm.

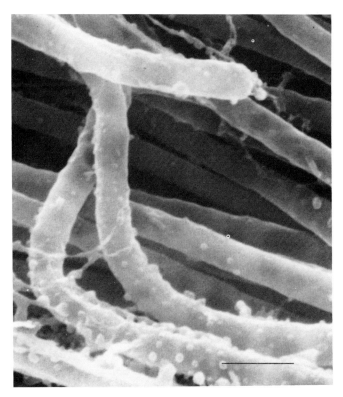

Figure 23.90. Scanning electron micrograph of *V. beggiatoides* strain B23SS, with continuous cell envelope and slimelike matrix shown. *Bar*, 5 μm.

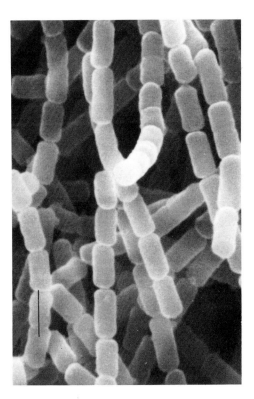

Figure 23.92. Scanning electron micrograph of *V. stercoraria* strain VT-1, with the discontinuous cell walls and the connecting material between the cells shown. *Bar*, 1 μm.

acetate, etc.), but strains similar to *V. stercoraria* grow luxuriantly on rich media (0.5% peptone (w/v)). *Vitreoscilla* filaments resemble those of certain cyanobacteria, but the vitreoscillas do not possess pigments and are phylogenetically distinct from cyanobacteria (Reichenbach et al., 1986).

The division of vitreoscillas on the basis of their nutrition parallels their structural differences. The *Beggiatoa*-like species can grow on a simple defined medium containing acetate, ammonium, and basal salts. *V. filiformis* is more nutritionally diverse than *V. beggiatoides*, but neither species tolerates high concentrations of nutrients or nutritionally rich media well. Neither species can grow to great cell masses, with 50–80 mg l⁻¹ dry cell mass about maximum. These organisms can withstand moderate concentrations of sulfide, even though they do not form sulfur depositions from it. On the other hand, *V. stercoraria* is an obligate amino acid utilizer with fairly complex nutritional requirements (Mayfield and Kester, 1972, 1975). *V. stercoraria* grows very well in nutritionally complex and rich media, and it achieves much higher cell masses during growth than do the *Beggiatoa*-like vitreoscillas.

Cultures of *V. beggiatoides* and *V. filiformis* are able to oxidize both the methyl and carboxyl carbons of acetate to CO_2 (Strohl et al., 1986b). The rate of acetate oxidation is very high, as it is with the beggiatoas. These organisms may use the glyoxylate bypass cycle when growing on acetate, but little of this has been investigated. *V. stercoraria* contains all of the enzymes of the tricarboxylic and glyoxylate bypass cycles (W. R. Strohl and G. W. Luli, unpublished data). The activities of the enzymes isocitrate lyase and malate synthase are stimulated significantly by the addition of 1% sodium acetate to the *V. stercoraria* growth medium (W. R. Strohl and G. W. Luli, unpublished data). This is in apparent contradiction to Pringsheim's original statement that acetate did not stimulate growth of *V. stercoraria* (Pringsheim, 1951).

According to recent results, certain unclassified *Vitreoscilla* strains, similar morphologically to *V. stercoraria* (Costerton et al., 1961; Nichols et al., 1986; Strohl et al., 1986a), may now be considered as strains of *V. stercoraria*. Strain VT-1 was physiologically identical with *V. stercoraria* ATCC 15218, the type strain of the species (Strohl et al., 1986a). *Vitreoscilla* strains 389 and 390 (Costerton et al., 1961) were recently found to be nearly 100% related by DNA homology to *Vitreoscilla stercoraria* strain ATCC 15218 (Nichols et al., 1986). On the other hand, "*Filibacter limicola*", an organism morphologically similar to *V. stercoraria*, has been shown to be completely unrelated to the vitreoscillas (Clausen et al., 1985; Nichols et al., 1986).

Phylogenetically, *V. stercoraria* belongs to the *Rhodocyclus tenuis* subgroup of the beta subdivision of the purple bacteria, as determined by the analysis of 16S rRNA (Woese et al., 1984b, 1985b). Recent analyses of 5S rRNA sequences have shown that *V. beggiatoides* belongs phylogenetically to the gamma subdivision of the purple bacteria, similar to *Beggiatoa alba* and *Thiothrix*, whereas *V. stercoraria* and *V. filiformis* strains belong to the beta subgroup of the purple bacteria (Stahl et al., 1987).

V. beggiatoides and *V. filiformis* strains are apparently devoid of small plasmids such as the 12.3 and 12.8 × 10⁶ M_r plasmids observed in *Beggiatoa alba* (Minges et al., 1983). Strains of *V. stercoraria* contained small plasmids with an apparent 1.4 × 10⁶ M_r (Minges et al., 1983). No functions has yet been ascribed to these plasmids.

Vitreoscillas generally are found in dung (*V. stercoraria* types), in soil, in water with decaying plant material, and in association with oscillatorian mats (Pringsheim 1949b, 1951). *V. beggiatoides* (group B strains; Strohl and Larkin, 1978b) was isolated from a sandy, lightly sulfide-emanating sediment which also included sulfur-containing beggiatoas.

Enrichment and Isolation Procedures

For *V. beggiatoides* and *V. filiformis* and similar vitreoscillas, enrichment and isolation procedures are basically the same as for *Beggiatoa* (Pringsheim, 1964; Strohl and Larkin, 1978b; W. R. Strohl in the article on *Beggiatoa* in this volume). The media used, however, should reflect the type of *Vitreoscilla* being sought (i.e. lack of sulfide in media; type and amount of organic supplements). A medium which is excellent for the isolation and maintenance of these types of vitreoscilla is "MY medium,"

but without the added reduced sulfur source, described in the article on *Beggiatoa* (this volume).

For isolation of *V. stercoraria*, small samples of dung may be placed directly onto plates containing a nutritionally rich medium. After several days, trichomes gliding away from the inoculum can be observed with a dissecting microscope. Those filaments can be retrieved with a flame-sterilized 26-gauge needle, as with *Beggiatoa*. A good medium for this purpose is 0.1-CAYTS medium, which contains 0.1% each of casitone, tryptone, sodium acetate and yeast extract.

Maintenance Procedures

These organisms can survive about 3 weeks on plates of standard media employed for their growth. Generally, the lower the amount of nutrients in the media, the longer the time of survival. Care should be taken to transfer from the edges of the spreading colonies, so as to transfer the youngest and most active filaments. *V. stercoraria* can be lyophilized. *V. beggiatoides* and *V. filiformis* cannot be lyophilized, but they can be stored at −70°C or −196°C in the presence of 20–30% glycerol.

Procedures for Testing Special Features

Because the larger species of *Vitreoscilla* are distinguished from beggiatoas on their inability to deposit sulfur, it is critical that the tests for sulfide oxidation and sulfur deposition be sensitive and reproducible. Investigators frequently have viewed the filaments with a phase microscope and assumed that refractile objects are sulfur. In fact, the strains now included in *V. filiformis* were once considered to be *Beggiatoa* strains (Pringsheim, 1964; Kowallik and Pringsheim, 1966) because the phase-bright bodies (presumably polyphosphate) in these organisms were interpreted as sulfur.

One method for determining if inclusions contain sulfur is a chemical analysis of ethanol-extracted (Jørgensen and Fenchel, 1974) or carbon disulfide-extracted (Nelson and Castenholz, 1981) filaments. These analyses should be compared with analyses of non-sulfur-depositing organisms (i.e. *Escherichia coli*) and sulfur-depositing organisms (*Beggiatoa* species) as controls. A more sensitive method for analyzing sulfur deposition is through the oxidation of ³⁵S-labeled Na_2S to internal ³⁵S⁰ (Strohl and Schmidt, 1984; Strohl et al., 1986a; Schmidt et al., 1986). Controls should be included for the adsorption of $Na_2^{35}S$ by autoclaved cells and $Na_2^{35}S$ assimilation by known sulfide-oxidizing organisms (i.e. *Beggiatoa* species) and non-sulfide-oxidizing organisms (i.e. *V. stercoraria*). Once it is demonstrated that labeled sulfide is assimilated, it should be at least 50–70% extractable by washing with warm ethanol and ~90% extractable by the ethanol treatment, followed by a wash with ethanol/diethyl ether (1:1) (W. R. Strohl, unpublished data).

Taxonomic Comments

A taxonomic problem exists with the genus *Vitreoscilla*. *V. beggiatoides* was designated as the type species of the genus with the intent that the vitreoscillas were *Beggiatoa*-like organisms that did not deposit sulfur from hydrogen sulfide (Pringsheim, 1949b, 1951). Until recently, however, the only well-characterized species of *Vitreoscilla* was *V. stercoraria*, since no other species from Pringsheim's collection survived (Koch, 1964). Thus strains did not exist for the type species of the genus until the recent description (Strohl et al., 1986a) of strains that fit the original description of *V. beggiatoides*. *V. stercoraria* does not seem to related closely to *V. beggiatoides* or *V. filiformis*. *V. stercoraria* is morphologically, ultrastructurally, nutritionally, physiologically, and ecologically very different from the other species (Strohl et al., 1986a) (Table 23.28; Figs. 23.89–23.92). Because *V. beggiatoides* is the type species and the intent of the genus was to contain non-sulfur-depositing beggiatoa-like organisms, it seems that *V. stercoraria* should be removed from the genus. This may be objectionable, however, because all of the literature on *Vitreoscilla* since Pringsheim's original descriptions are concerned with *V. stercoraria*-like cultures (cf. Strohl et al., 1986a, and references therein) because of the previous lack of well-characterized pure cultures of other species.

Ackowledgments

I thank Thomas M. Schmidt for his helpful discussion on the taxonomy of this genus and for his skillful assistance in preparation of much of the up-to-date data on these organisms. I also thank David Stahl for discussions concerning 5S rRNA analyses that he and his colleagues performed.

Further Reading

Strohl, W.R., T.M. Schmidt, N.H. Lawry, M.J. Mezzino, and J.M. Larkin. 1986a Characterization of *Vitreoscilla beggiatoides* and *V. filiformis* sp. nov., nom rev., and comparison to *V. stercoraria* and *Beggiatoa alba*. Int. J. Syst. Bacteriol. *36:* 302–313.

List of species of the genus **Vitreoscilla**

1. **Vitreoscilla beggiatoides** Pringsheim 1949, 70.[AL]

beg.gi.a.toi′des. M.L. fem. n. *Beggiatoa* a generic name; Gr. n. *idos* shape, form; M.L. adj. *beggiatoides* Beggiatoa-like.

Cells colorless and cylindrical, existing in filaments with a diameter of about 2.5–3.0 µm and a length of up to several hundred micrometers. Filaments continuous; ends of filaments rounded. Necridia and hormogonia produced. Motile by gliding; gliding relatively fast with speeds of ~3 µm s⁻¹. Produce either circuitans type (low nutrients in media) or linguiformis type (high nutrients in media) colonies. Trichomes often glide

singly, away from other trichomes. Resting stages not known. Sheaths and holdfasts not formed. Gram-negative.

Sulfur not deposited when grown on sulfide; sulfide at ~1 mM, however, is apparently not inhibitory. PHB is always present when cells are cultured on acetate-containing media; PHB often makes up >50% of the cell dry weight. Polyphosphate bodies are often present.

Chemoorganotrophic. Acetate, ethanol, and some C_4 organic acids are utilized as sole carbon and energy sources. Ammonium and nitrate are used as nitrogen source.

Metabolism is respiratory, with molecular oxygen used as the terminal electron acceptor. Microaerophilic to aerobic. No growth anaerobically.

Gelatin, starch and casein are not hydrolyzed. Catalase-negative. Cytochrome oxidase-positive. Growth in 0.5% but not 1.0% NaCl. Sensitive to the antibiotics polymyxin B, neomycin, and furadantin/macrodantin; resistant to the antibiotics bacitracin and streptomycin.

Found in sandy but lightly sulfide-emanating sediments of *freshwater* streams.

The mol% G + C of the DNA of strain B23SS is 42.

Neotype strain: ATCC 43189 (B23SS).

2. **Vitreoscilla filiformis** Strohl 1986, 310.[VP]

fi.li.for′mis. L. n. *filum* a thread; L. n. *forma* shape; M.L. adj. *filiformis* thread-shaped.

Cells colorless, existing in flexible filaments with a diameter of about 1.0–1.5 µm and, when cells are grown in liquid media, a length of up to several hundred micrometers. Filament width may vary slightly. Filament walls continuous; ends of filaments rounded. Slight indentations of the trichomes may sometimes be observed at septal regions between cells. Hormogonia are sometimes produced. Motile by gliding; gliding is relatively slow at ~0.1–0.5 µm s⁻¹. Produce linguiformis type colonies. Resting stages not known. Sheaths and holdfasts not formed. Gram-negative. Sulfur is not deposited when cells are grown in the presence of sulfide. PHB and condensed phosphate deposits may be present.

Chemoorganotroph. Can grow by using many 2-, 3-, 4-, and 6-carbon organic acids, several amino acids, ethanol, or glucose as sole carbon and energy sources. Organic and inorganic forms of nitrogen can be used as nitrogen source. Nitrate is reduced to nitrite.

Metabolism respiratory, with oxygen used as the terminal electron acceptor. Aerobic to microaerophilic. No growth anaerobically.

Gelatin and starch are weakly hydrolyzed. Casein is not hydrolyzed. Catalase-negative, cytochrome oxidase-positive. No growth occurs in the presence of 0.5% NaCl. Sensitive to the antibiotics bacitracin, streptomycin, furadantin/macrodantin and polymyxin B.

Found in freshwater sediments, usually in association with decaying matter.

The mol% G + C of the DNA ranges from 59 to 63 (T_m).

Type strain: ATCC 43190 (strain L1401-2).

3. **Vitreoscilla stercoraria** Pringsheim 1951, 136.[AL]

ster.co.ra′ri.a. L. fem. adj. *stercoraria* pertaining to dung.

Cells colorless, usually existing in flexible chains with a diameter of about 1.0 µm and, when grown in liquid media, a length of up to about 100 µm. Deep constrictions separate the individual cells, yielding discontinuous filaments. Cells can occur singly, especially if grown at temperatures of ~22°C. Sausage-shaped cells are 1.0 × 1.5–12 µm and are connected in filaments by extracellular material. Division is by binary fission. The cell wall peptidoglycan contains alanine, glutamate and diaminopimelic acid with a molar ratio of 2:1:1. Resting stages not known.

Table 23.28.
Differentiation of the species of the genus **Vitreoscilla**[a]

Characteristic	1. *V. beggiatoides*	2. *V. filiformis*	3. *V. stercoraria*
Type strain	B23SS	L1401-2	ATCC 15218
Colony type	L, C	L	L
Filament type[b]			
Continuous cell wall	+	+	−
Discontinuous cell wall	−	−	+
Filament diameter (µm)	2.5–3.0	1.0–1.5	1.0
Mol% G + C of DNA	42	59–63	50–51
Habitat			
Freshwater sediments	+	+	−
Cow dung	−	−	+
Obligately requires amino acid mixtures	−	−	+
Growth on			
Nutrient agar	−	−	+
Acetate plus salts	+	+	−
Use as sole carbon and energy sources			
Glucose	−	+	−
Citrate	−	+	−
Lactate	−	+	−
Glutamate	−	+	−
Succinate	+	+	−
Acetate	+	+	−
Utilization of nitrate as sole nitrogen source	+	+	−
Cytochromes			
CO-binding types	+	+	+
c type	+	+	−

[a]Symbols: L, linguiformis type colonies; C, circuitans type colonies (see Pringsheim (1964) and Strohl and Larkin (1978b) for a description of these colony types); +, 90% or more of strains are positive; and −, 90% or more of strains are negative.

[b]Cells within filaments having continuous cell walls share the outer cell wall layers, and only shallow constrictions are noticed between cells (cf. Figs. 23.89 and 23.90). Strains containing discontinuous filament cell walls consist of chains of individual cells held together by "connective material" (cf. Figs. 23.91 and 23.92).

Sheaths and holdfasts not formed. Gram-negative. Sulfur is not deposited when cells are grown in the presence of sulfide. PHB and condensed phosphate deposits may be present.

Chemoorganotroph. Growth on casamino acids plus acetate. Requires amino acids; arginine, tyrosine, tryptophan, and glutamine are required for good growth. Combinations of amino acids from the glutamate and aspartate families plus arginine are required minimally for growth.

Metabolism respiratory, with oxygen used as the terminal electron acceptor. Cytochrome o is present; cytochromes a and c and the non-CO-binding b are not present. Aerobic. No growth microaerophilically or anaerobically. Catalase-positive and N,N,N',N'-tetramethylphenylenediamine (TMPD) cytochrome oxidase-negative. Gelatin, casein, and starch not hydrolyzed.

Usually isolated form cow dung.

The mol% G + C of the DNA is 50–51 (Bd).

Type strain: ATCC 15218.

Genus **Desulfonema** *Widdel 1981, 382*[VP] *(Effective publication: Widdel 1980, 378)*

FRIEDRICH WIDDEL

De.sul.fo.ne′ma. L. pref. *de* from; L. n. *sulfur* sulfur; Gr. n. *nema* thread; M.L. neut. n. *Desulfonema* thread-forming sulfate reducer.

Cells arranged in **uniseriately multicellular, flexible filaments with gliding motility.** Filaments are **3–8 μm in diameter** and sometimes about 1 mm in length; the nearly cylindrical cells are 2.5–13 μm long. Cross-walls are visible (Figs. 23.93–23.95). Granules of poly-β-hydroxybutyric acid are commonly stored. Filaments are always **attached to surfaces that are necessary as substrata for gliding moving.** Gram stain may be positive (unequally stained), but electron microscopy of ultrathin sections exhibits **cell walls characteristic of Gram-negative bacteria**; the outer membrane has a wavy structure. **Cytochromes** are present.

Strictly anaerobic chemoorganotrophs or chemolithotrophs, metabolism respiratory, growth by fermentation not observed. **Sulfate and other oxidized sulfur compounds serve as electron acceptors and are reduced to hydrogen sulfide. Fatty acids and other organic acids are used as electron donors** and carbon sources; **oxidation of electron donors is complete** and results in carbon dioxide.

Temperature range: 10–36°C. **Anoxic media** containing a reductant and **vitamins are necessary** for growth. Marine forms usually require brackish water or seawater concentrations of NaCl, MgCl₂ and, in some cases, CaCl₂. Gliding movement and growth are promoted by addition of insoluble substrata such as agar or inorganic precipitates.

The mol% G + C of the DNA is 34–42 (T_m).

Type species: *Desulfonema limicola* Widdel 1981, 382.

Further Descriptive Information

The multicellular filaments of *Desulfonema* species are not sheathed; however, remaining cell walls of lysed cells within a filament can simulate a sheath. Filaments of *D. limicola* do not glide regularly; the most conspicuous motility characteristic of this species is a twitching or jerky swinging of the filaments when they creep out of sediment particles. The gliding movement of *D. magnum* is more regular, and a speed of about

4 μm s⁻¹ is reached. Gliding filaments reverse the direction of their movement if they meet obstacles; a reversion of the gliding direction may also occur without obvious reason. Gliding filaments often form trails from sediment particles, probably by slime excretion.

The ultrastructure of *D. limicola* and *D. magnum* has been examined (Widdel et al., 1983). Ultrathin sections of both species exhibited intracytoplasmic membranes and a wavy outer membrane. The wavy structure was more regular in *D. magnum* (Fig. 23.96) than in *D. limicola*.

Desulfonema species are nutritionally versatile sulfate reducers oxidizing a range of fatty acids and dicarboxylic acids; also, hydrogen, lactate, benzoate or higher phenyl-substituted organic acids may be oxidized. Sulfate is used as an external electron acceptor; alternatively sulfite or thiosulfate may be reduced. Nitrate, fumarate or malate do not serve as electron acceptors. Sugars, pyruvate or fumarate are not fermented. Elemental sulfur inhibits growth, probably by increasing the redox potential. Filaments are damaged by oxygen.

Desulfonema species may be cultivated under strictly anoxic conditions in reduced synthetic media* with sulfate as the electron acceptor and acetate, propionate, higher fatty acids, succinate, lactate or benzoate as electron donors. Good growth may be obtained by combinations of organic substrates. Growth on acetate as sole organic substrate is very slow but can be stimulated by low concentrations (~50 mg/l) of additional electron donors, e.g. formate, fatty acids or succinate. Generally, addition of sterilized extracts from anaerobically digested complex organic matter (sludge extracts) promotes growth on any organic substrate. Ammonium ions are used as nitrogen source. *D. limicola* grows well with at least 13 g NaCl and 2 g MgCl₂·6H₂O/l medium and biotin as growth factor. For optimum growth of *D. magnum*, 20 g NaCl, 5 g MgCl₂·6H₂O and at least 0.8 g CaCl₂·2H₂O/l medium are necessary; biotin, 4-aminobenzoic acid and vitamin B₁₂ are required as growth factors. The high requirement for calcium ions has not been reported for any other sulfate-

---

*Defined medium has the following composition (in g/l distilled water): Na₂SO₄, 4.0; KH₂PO₄, 0.2; NH₄Cl, 0.25; NaCl, 20; KCl, 0.5; MgCl₂·6H₂O, 3.0 for *D. limicola* and 5.0 for *D. magnum*; and CaCl₂·2H₂O, 0.15 for *D. limicola* and 1.4 for *D. magnum*. The dissolved salts are autoclaved. For agar medium, 2 g of repeatedly washed, separately autoclaved molten agar in ~70 ml of distilled water are added per l (final volume) of the hot autoclaved medium and mixed immediately. After this is cooled under an anaerobic atmosphere, the following volumes from separately sterilized stock solutions are added per l medium while access of air is prevented by flushing with a mixture of N₂ + CO₂ (CO₂ content: 5–20%, depending on the desired pH): solution of 84 g NaHCO₃/l (autoclaved under CO₂ atmosphere), 30 ml; trace element solution (see below), 1 ml; solution of 3 mg Na₂SeO₃·5H₂O + 0.5 g NaOH/l, 1 ml; solution of 120 g Na₂S·9H₂O/l (autoclaved under N₂ atmosphere), 3 ml; and filter-sterilized solution of 10 mg biotin (to be dissolved in hot water) + 40 mg 4-aminobenzoic acid + 50 mg vitamin B₁₂/l, 1 ml. The pH of the mixed medium is adjusted with sterile HCl or Na₂CO₃ solution to 7.6 for *D. limicola* and to 7.0 for *D. magnum*. The medium may be dispensed into small culture bottles (50 or 100 ml); bottles are completely filled and tightly sealed with screw caps or are provided with an anaerobic gas phase and sealed with butyl rubber stoppers. The desired organic substrates are added from sterile stock solutions. For *D. limicola*, 5–10 ml from a solution of 280 g of sodium acetate trihydrate per l are added per l of medium. Growth on acetate is stimulated by the addition of 1 ml from a mixture of organic acids (see below) per l of culture medium. For *D. magnum*, 3–5 ml from a solution of 150 g of sodium benzoate per l are added per l of medium. Growth of both species may also be stimulated by the addition of 2—6% (v/v) of an autoclaved, particle-free supernatant from anaerobically digested rumen fluid, liquid animal manure or sewage sludge (dry weight content: 5–10%). In media prepared without agar, a sediment of aluminum phosphate per l of medium is precipitated before inoculation: 5 ml of an autoclaved solution of 48 g of AlCl₃·6H₂O per l are added, and the pH is readjusted with 1.6 ml from a solution of 106 g of Na₂CO₃ per l.

Trace element solution (without complexing agent) contains (per l): 25% HCl in H₂O, 10 ml; FeCl₂·4H₂O. 1.5 g; CoCl₂·6H₂O, 190 mg; MnCl₂·4H₂O, 100 mg; ZnCl₂, 70 mg; H₃BO₃, 6 mg; Na₂MoO₄·2H₂O, 36 mg; NiCl₂·6H₂O, 24 mg; and CuCl₂·2H₂O, 2 mg. The FeCl₂ is initially dissolved in the HCl solution, and then distilled water and the other components are added.

Mixture of organic acids (modified after Bryant, 1973) contains (per l): isobutyric acid, 5 g; valeric acid, 5 g; isovaleric acid, 5 g; 2-methylbutyric acid, 5 g; caproic acid, 2 g; heptanoic acid, 2 g; octanoic acid, 2 g; and succinic acid, 45 g. The acids are neutralized with NaOH.

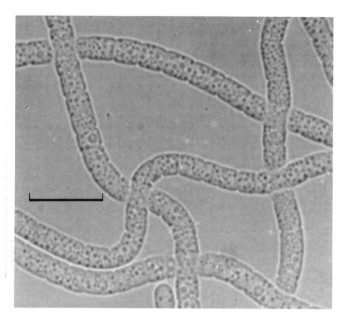

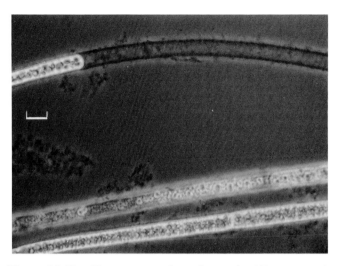

Figure 23.95. Phase-contrast photomicrograph of *D. magnum*. A trail of the gliding movement is visible in the synthetic sediment of aluminum phosphate precipitated in the medium. *Bar*, 10 μm.

Figure 23.93. Brightfield photomicrograph of *Desulfonema limicola* isolated from marine mud and grown on acetate as electron donor. *Bar*, 10 μm.

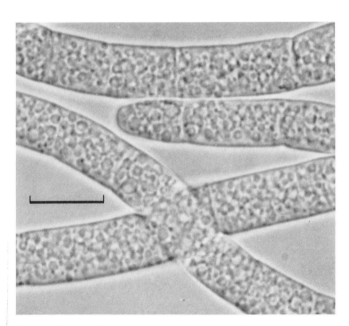

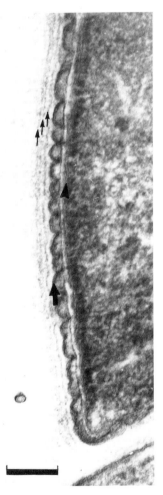

Figure 23.94. Brightfield photomicrograph of *D. magnum* isolated from marine mud and grown on benzoate as electron donor. *Bar*, 10 μm.

reducing bacterium. Gliding movement and growth are supported by addition of artificial sediments such as precipitated aluminum phosphate or sloppy agar (0.2%).

Desulfonema species occur in anoxic sediments, especially if they are rich in decomposing algal material. In samples taken from such habitats, the filaments may be observed under the microscope without a preceding enrichment in the laboratory. Only marine, salt-requiring *Desulfonema* species have been isolated so far in pure culture. However, observation of morphologically similar, sometimes thinner filaments grown in anaerobic enrichments from pond and ditch sediments suggests that freshwater forms may also occur. None of the electron donors known to be oxidized by *Desulfonema* species allows a reliable selective enrichment. Since the

Figure 23.96. Electron micrograph of ultrathin section of *D. magnum*. Block staining with uranyl acetate, poststaining with lead citrate. *Large arrowhead*, cytoplasmic membrane; *large arrow*, waved outer membrane; *small arrows*, outer wall layers; *bar*, 0.1 μm. (Reproduced with permission from F. Widdel, G.-W. Kohring and F. Mayer, Archives of Microbiology *134:* 286–294, 1983, © Springer-Verlag.)

filamentous gliding sulfate reducers grow relatively slowly (doubling times around 30 h or longer), they are often outcompeted in enrichments by unicellular sulfate reducers after some transfers. A selective advantage of *Desulfonema* in nature is probably the ability for gliding movement that allows the filaments to spread in sediments and to exploit favorable growth conditions. Moreover, the long filaments resist grazing by protozoa (Widdel, 1983).

Enrichment and Isolation Procedures

Filamentous gliding sulfate-reducing bacteria can be enriched in raw cultures if anoxic sediment samples from sulfate-rich freshwater or marine habitats are mixed with algal material or cellulose powder. In case of low sulfate concentrations, $CaSO_4$ should be added. Enrichments are incubated under an anoxic gas phase in a sealed bottle in the dark at room temperature. After 1–2 weeks, cell filaments may form dense silky layers covering the sediment and the glass wall.

Of the defined substrates known for *D. limicola* and *D. magnum*, isobutyrate (5 mmol/l) and benzoate (3 mmol/l), respectively, are most suitable to favor enrichment of the filaments in synthetic media. An inoculum of 2–5% (v/v) of black marine mud should be used. No artificial substrata for gliding movement should be added to the enrichment subcultures, so that filaments are forced to grow at the glass wall. If possible, transfers should be made from the glass wall. Parts of the layers may be sucked into a Pasteur pipette. However, despite these precautions, unicellular sulfate reducers often become dominant. *Desulfonema* may be obtained in pure culture only if the number of these competitors is not significantly higher than the number of filaments. Before the enrichment medium becomes turbid due to spreading of unicellular competitors, tufts of filaments are taken from the glass wall into Pasteur pipettes and washed anaerobically to remove the bulk of other cells. For washing, a fine-mesh copper grid (as used in electron microscopy) fixed in a conically drawn glass tube by means of a thin resin layer is used as a sieve (Widdel, 1980, 1983). Anoxic medium is kept above the grid by the level of an elevated, bent outlet tubing. After addition of filament tufts, sterile medium passes through the grid; *Desulfonema* filaments are retained, whereas unicellular competitors and commensals pass through.

In the case of *D. magnum*, a pure culture was finally obtained from the washed filaments by transferring one of the relatively thick, visible filaments through a series of small portions of sterile anoxic medium.

D. limicola may be isolated from washed filaments in agar dilution series. The following soft agar medium (0.8%) may be used. A 3.3% (w/v) agar is prepared in distilled water; the agar should be washed several times in distilled water before it becomes molten. The same concentrations of NaCl, $MgCl_2$ and $CaCl_2$ as in the enrichment medium are added to the agar. The molten agar is dispensed in 3-ml amounts into test tubes (20 ml) which are sealed with aluminum caps (or cotton) and autoclaved. The agar is kept molten in a water bath at ~60°C. Reduced culture medium containing a suitable organic substrate and growth-promoting supplements is prewarmed to 41°C, and 9-ml amounts are added to each tube of liquified agar; exposure to air is minimized by dipping the tip of the pipette into the agar. For one dilution series, about six tubes are prepared and kept at 41°C. The aluminum caps are replaced by sterile butyl rubber stoppers. Starting with an inoculum of 0.5 ml containing *Desulfonema* filaments, serial dilutions are made. Before the agar solidifies, 5–7 µl from a 5% (w/v) sodium dithionite solution are aseptically added to each tube by means of a 0.1-ml pipette, starting at the highest dilution; the pipette is dipped into the agar and used at the same time for gentle

mixing. The dithionite solution is prepared by dissolving $Na_2S_2O_4$ powder in sterile water under an atmosphere of N_2. The agar in the tubes is then hardened in cold water. The tubes are immediately gassed with a N_2-CO_2 mixture (5–20% CO_2, depending on desired pH) and sealed with rubber stoppers. The tubes are incubated in the dark at 25–30°C for 2–5 weeks.

Filamentous sulfate reducers may form fluffy colonies. If, however, the gilding filaments (as in *D. magnum*) migrate through the agar, the described method is not useful for isolation, since separate colonies are not obtained. Colonies of filaments are picked with medium-containing Pasteur pipettes. These may previously be drawn in a flame to an appropriate diameter. If the filaments cannot be reached without touching colonies of other bacteria, a part of the soft agar is carefully sucked off with a Pasteur pipette connected to a vacuum pump; however, a minimum distance of 8 mm should be kept between filaments and agar surface. In order to prevent contamination by bacteria liberated from disrupted colonies, the agar surface is sterilized, e.g. by addition of bromine vapor to the head space of the agar tube. The slow penetration of bromine into the agar is visible by a yellow zone. After 1 min, the bromine is removed with a gas stream of N_2. The bromine dissolved in the upper agar zone is reduced by injection of ~0.5 ml SO_2 gas (e.g. made from sodium bisulfite plus acid in a serum bottle) into the head space. Immediately after decolorization of the bromine zone, the SO_2 is removed with N_2.

A few isolated filaments often do not start to grow if transferred into large volumes (>20 ml) of liquid medium in common tubes or bottles. Such filaments should be transferred into media in special anaerobic glass tubes (15 ml) with pointed, conical bottoms. The filaments sink to this narrow part of the tube where they can establish a growth-favoring microenvironment and where growth can be observed under the dissecting microscope. Initiation of growth may be promoted by addition of sludge extract and dithionite as strong reductant. In the beginning, tubes are incubated without shaking. If growth is visible by increasing numbers of filaments attached to the glass wall, the culture may be shaken twice a day.

Freshly isolated filamentous sulfate reducers usually spread on surfaces and form silky layers that may cover the whole inner wall of the culture vessel. After a number of subcultures, however, *Desulfonema* filaments tend to creep together and form irregular clumps; such cultures grow only poorly, and filaments in clumps may soon die off. Clump formation is avoided by providing an insoluble substratum (aluminum phosphate or sloppy agar) for gliding movement and by shaking the culture once or twice a day.

Maintenance Procedures

Pure cultures are maintained in liquid medium with an added sediment in completely filled screw-capped bottles or, under an anaerobic gas phase, in bottles sealed with butyl rubber stoppers. Filaments remain viable longest with substrates on which growth is relatively slow. The enrichment substrate isobutyrate may affect *D. limicola* after a number of transfers. Stock cultures of *D. limicola* may be kept on acetate plus low concentrations of other fatty acids, and those of *D. magnum* may be kept on benzoate. *D. limicola* is stored at 2–5°C. *D. magnum* is damaged at such low temperatures and, therefore, is stored at ~20°C. Stock cultures are transferred every 2–4 months. Strains may also be preserved indefinitely by suspending the filaments in anaerobic medium containing 5% (v/v) dimethyl sulfoxide and storing in liquid nitrogen.

Differentiation of the genus **Desulfonema** from other genera

Desulfonema species are differentiated from all other genera of sulfate-reducing bacteria by their striking filamentous morphology. The filaments consist of regularly arranged, nearly cylindrical cells. Single cells are usually not observed but may be liberated by shearing forces. *Desulfonema* species do not live suspended in liquid medium; the filaments are always attached to a surface which they need for gliding movement.

Desulfonema is distinguished from *Beggiatoa* species that may be

abundant at the oxic-anoxic interface in sediments by the absence of highly refractile sulfur globules. Granules of poly-β-hydroxybutyric acid that are often present in *Desulfonema* are less refractile than sulfur globules. In sediment samples kept under completely anaerobic conditions, *Desulfonema* continues to move and to multiply, whereas *Beggiatoa* becomes nonmotile, loses the sulfur droplets, and dies off after some days.

Desulfonema can be differentiated from filamentous gliding cyanobacteria and green bacteria by the absence of pigments. Layers of *Desulfonema* are whitish, and filaments appear colorless in the brightfield microscope.

D. limicola and *D. magnum* are morphologically similar to filamentous organisms described by Skuja (1956) as "*Achroonema splendens*" and "*Achroonema macromeres*" that were classified in the family "Pelonemataceae" (this volume). "*Achroonema*" species have not been isolated so far, and their metabolism is unknown. "*Achroonema*" types may have an anaerobic metabolism, since they have been observed in anoxic hypoliminia containing H_2S. The purely morphological descriptions of "*Achroonema*" species do not allow identification with *Desulfonema* or other filamentous organisms studied in pure culture.

Natural Relationships

The genealogical relationship of *D. limicola* has been investigated by cataloging of oligonucleotides from 16S ribosomal RNA (Fowler et al., 1986). Of the species studied, *Desulfosarcina variabilis* (Widdel and Pfennig, 1984) is the closest relative to *D. limicola*, with the S_{AB} value being 0.53. The next relatives are *Desulfococcus niacini* and the sulfur-reducing, nonsulfate-reducing *Desulfuromonas* species with S_{AB} values of about 0.37. The similarity of *D. limicola* to *Desulfobulbus*, *Desulfobacter* and *Desulfovibrio* species was 0.32 or less.

Further Reading

Widdel F. 1983. Methods for enrichment and pure culture isolation of filamentous gliding sulfate-reducing bacteria. Arch. Microbiol. *134:* 282–285.
Widdel, F., G.-W. Kohring and F. Mayer. 1983. Studies on dissimilatory sulfate-reducing bacteria that decompose fatty acids. III. Characterization of the filamentous gliding *Desulfonema limicola* gen. nov. sp. nov., and *Desulfonema magnum* sp. nov. Arch. Microiol. *134:* 286–294.

List of species of the genus **Desulfonema**

1. **Desulfonema limicola** Widdel 1981, 382.[VP] (Effective publication: Widdel 1980, 379.)

li.mi′co.la. L. n. *limus* mud; L. suff., verbal n. *cola* dweller; M.L. masc. n. *limicola* mud dweller.

Multicellular gliding filaments, 3 μm in diameter and 0.05–1 mm in length; individual cells are 2.5–3.5 μm long.

Hydrogen plus carbon dioxide, formate, acetate, propionate, butyrate, isobutyrate, valerate, isovalerate, 2-methylbutyrate, higher fatty acids up to myristate (C_{14}), lactate, pyruvate, succinate or fumarate may serve as electron donor and carbon source. Growth on hydrogen plus carbon dioxide or formate does not require an additional carbon source (chemoautotrophic growth) but is stimulated by acetate. Alcohols and benzoate are not utilized. Sulfate, sulfite or thiosulfate serve as electron acceptors. Biotin is required as growth factor.

pH range: 6.5–8.8; optimum: 7.6. Temperature range: 10–36°C; optimum: 30°C.

The type strain requires a saline medium with at least 13 g NaCl and 2 g $MgCl_2 \cdot 6H_2O/l$ medium for optimum growth. However, morphologically similar filaments have been also observed in freshwater sediments.

Cytochrome *c* is present in the membrane and cytoplasmic fraction; cytochrome *b* is also present in the membranes but only in small amounts. The sulfite reductase, desulfoviridin, is present in the cytoplasm.

The mol% G + C of the DNA is 34.5 (T_m).

Type strain: DSM 2076 (strain 5ac10 of Widdel et al., 1983).

2. **Desulfonema magnum** Widdel 1981, 382.[VP] (Effective publication: Widdel 1980, 381.)

mag′num. L. adj. *magnus* large, big.

Multicellular gliding filaments 6–8 μm in diameter and 0.1–2 mm in length; individual cells are 9–13 μm long.

Acetate, propionate, butyrate, isobutyrate, valerate, isovalerate, 2-methylbutyrate, higher fatty acids up to decanoate (C_{10}), succinate, fumarate, malate, benzoate, phenylacetate, 3-phenylpropionate, hippurate or 4-hydroxybenzoate may serve as electron donor and carbon source. Formate is used in the presence of acetate. Not utilized are hydrogen alcohols, lactate, pyruvate, 2-hydroxybenzoate, 3-hydroxybenzoate and cyclohexanecarboxylate. No other compounds instead of sulfate are known to serve as electron acceptors. Biotin, 4-aminobenzoic acid and vitamin B_{12} are required as growth factors.

pH range: 6.6–7.5; optimum: 7.0. Temperature range: 15–37°C; optimum: 32°C. Isolated cultures in the laboratory die off within some days at temperatures below 10°C.

Optimum growth of the type strain requires 20 g NaCl, 5 g $MgCl_2 \cdot 6H_2O$ and at least 0.8 g $CaCl_2 \cdot 2H_2O/l$ culture medium.

The membrane fraction contains cytochromes *b* and *c*; the cytoplasmic fraction contains only traces of cytochromes. Desulfoviridin is not present.

The mol% G + C of the DNA is 41.6 (T_m).

Type strain: DSM 2077 (strain 4be13 of Widdel et al., 1983).

Genus **Achromatium** Schewiakoff 1893, 1[AL]

J. W. M. LA RIVIÈRE AND K. SCHMIDT

A.chro.ma′ti.um. Gr. pref. *a* not; Gr. n. *chromatium* color, paint; M.L. neut. n. *Achromatium* that which is not colored.

Spherical to ovoid or cylindrical with hemispherical ends, 5–33 × 15–100 μm. Division by constriction in the middle. **Movement, if any, of a slow rolling jerky type on solid surfaces.** (Photosynthetic) pigments absent. **Sulfur droplets and large spherules of calcium carbonate are typical inclusions.** No resting stages are known. **Aerobic,** apparently requires H_2S. Gram- and catalase-negative. Pure cultures are not available.

Type species: *Achromatium oxaliferum* Schewiakoff 1893, 1.

Further Descriptive Information

Cells are spherical, ovoid or cylindrical, depending on the stage of the life cycle. The size of *A. oxaliferum* varies between a minimum width of the short axis of 5 μm and a maximum length of the long axis of 100 μm. "*A. volutans*" is smaller, ranging from spheres with a diameter of 5 μm, when young, to ovals of up to about 40 μm in length before division.

Cell walls of *A. oxaliferum* could easily be lysed by lysozyme.

The $CaCO_3$ inclusions in *A. oxaliferum* are highly refractile and can be easily removed by treating the cells with 0.05 M acetic acid.

Locomotion of *A. oxaliferum* may be caused by peritrichous filaments within the slime layer which surround the cells (de Boer et al., 1971).

Ultrathin sections gave little information about the fine structure of *A. oxaliferum* but revealed typical Gram-negative membranes, sulfur and calcium carbonate inclusions, and probably ribosomes (de Boer et al., 1971).

Cells divide by constriction in the middle. Before constriction takes place, spherical cells elongate to a definite size (80–100 μm for *A. oxaliferum*; 40 μm for "*A. volutans*") then divide in two. In the case of *A. oxaliferum*, daughter cells are connected by a hyaline "bridge" before they are completely separated (Fig. 23.97). This phenomenon has not been observed with "*A. volutans*" (Fig. 23.98). Daughter cells of "*A. volutans*" are flat at one side immediately after separation, thus suggesting a slightly different mechanism of division.

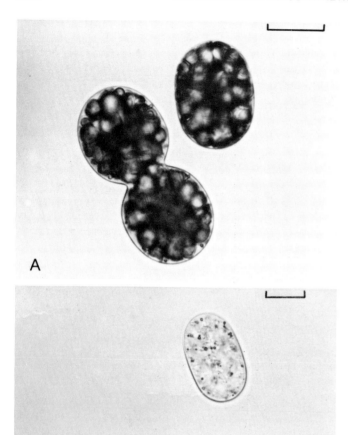

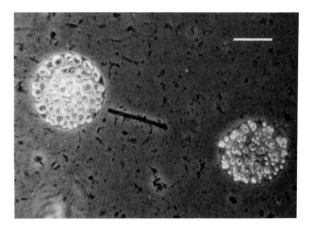

Figure 23.98. "*A. volutans*" cells. *Bar*, 20 μm. (Reproduced with permission from J. W. M. la Rivière and K. Schmidt. 1981. Morphologically conspicuous sulfur-oxidizing eubacteria. *In* Starr, Stolp, Trüper, Balows and Schlegel (Editors), The Prokaryotes. A Handbook on Habitats, Isolation, and Identification of Bacteria. Springer-Verlag, Berlin.)

Enrichment and Isolation Procedures

No enrichment procedure is available. "Isolation" of *A. oxaliferum* is based on concentration of cells from natural habitats rather than on growing them under selective growth conditions. This can best be done by slowly rotating mud particles in a tilted beaker until a white band becomes visible right above the mud particles (Fig. 23.99). The white band contains heavy CaCO$_3$-laden *A. oxaliferum* cells. The cells are pipetted off with a Pasteur pipette and transferred to another beaker. This procedure can be repeated several times until the *Achromatium* cells are washed free of contaminants. During this treatment the pH of the liquid medium should be kept slightly alkaline, as the CaCO$_3$ crystals are dis-

Figure 23.97. *A. oxaliferum* cells. *A*, untreated. *B*, after treatment with 0.05 M acetic acid. *Bar*, 20 μm. (Reproduced with permission from J. W. M. la Rivière and K. Schmidt. 1981. Morphologically conspicuous sulfur-oxidizing eubacteria. *In* Starr, Stolp, Trüper, Balows and Schlegel (Editors), The Prokaryotes. A Handbook on Habitats, Isolation, and Identification of Bacteria. Springer-Verlag, Berlin.)

Nutritional requirements are not yet known. Observation in natural habitats and some experiments in the laboratory have shown that growth of *Achromatium* is dependent on the presence of a well-balanced concentration of H$_2$S, O$_2$ and CO$_2$. Organic substrates, such as organic acids and casamino acids, promote growth (la Rivière and Schmidt, 1981).

Achromatium has been found in or on mud of fresh or saline waters, consisting mainly of decaying organic material where H$_2$S is produced and O$_2$ is present in suitable concentrations. The presence of sulfate reducers, algae and cyanobacteria is possibly required for optimal growth (la Rivière and Schmidt, 1981). *A. oxaliferum* is found in Ca^{2+}- and CO$_2$-containing fresh and marine waters (Bersa, 1920; Gicklhorn, 1920; Bavendamm, 1924; Skuja, 1948; Starr and Skerman, 1965; la Rivière and Schmidt, 1981). "*A. volutans*" was observed in saline waters only (Hinze, 1903, 1913, Kolkwitz, 1918; Lackey and Lackey, 1961). It normally contains sulfur inclusions but lacks calcium carbonate inclusions.

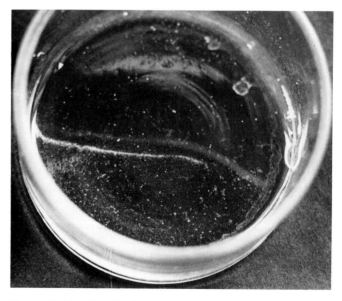

Figure 23.99. Topside view of a beaker in which *A. oxaliferum* cells have been concentrated in a white band by gentle swirling. (Reproduced with permission from J. W. M. la Rivière and K. Schmidt. 1981. Morphologically conspicuous sulfur-oxidizing eubacteria. *In* Starr, Stolp, Trüper, Balows and Schlegel (Editors), The Prokaryotes. A Handbook on Habitats, Isolation, and Identification of Bacteria. Springer-Verlag, Berlin.)

solved under acidic conditions (de Boer et al., 1971; la Rivière and Schmidt, 1981).

Maintenance Procedures

Achromatium can be maintained in natural populations only. Cells survived for about 10 months when loosely packed mud was stored at 5°C in bottles in which the overlaying water column was about 4 times as high as the mud layer (la Rivière and Schmidt, 1981). Stirring the mud from time to time was recommended by West and Griffiths (1913) when it was placed in small cylinders (15 cm wide, 5 cm high) and covered with tap water.

Differentiation of the species of the genus **Achromatium**

Although one of the two species ("*A. volutans*") does not appear on the Approved Lists, it is retained in the present description because of its marked differences from the type species. Thus the genus contains (a) the forms which contain the characteristic calcium carbonate inclusions, as are found in fresh and brackish waters, and (b) those lacking these inclusions, as are usually found in marine environments (Table 23.29).

Further Reading

de Boer, W.E., J.W.M. la Rivière, and K. Schmidt. 1971. Some properties of *Achromatium oxaliferum*. Antonie van Leeuwenhoek J. Microbiol. Serol. *37:* 553–563.

Kolkwitz, R. 1918. Über die Schwefelbakterien des Solgrabens von Artern. Berl. Deut. Bot. Ges. *36:* 218–224.

la Rivière, J.W.M. and K. Schmidt. 1981. Morphologically conspicuous sulfuroxidizing eubacteria. *In* Starr, Stolp, Trüper, Balows and Schlegel (Editors), The

Taxonomic Comments

Pending pure culture studies, any classification can only be provisional. The present classification is based on the absence of pigment and the gliding type of movement seen on solid surfaces with no "apparent" means of locomotion.

However, the finding of peritrichous filaments (de Boer et al., 1971) would remove *Achromatium* from the gliding bacteria if further study were to assign a locomotor role to these filaments. Pending such studies, *Achromatium* is left in the category of the gliding bacteria but as a *genus incertae sedis.*

Table 23.29.
Differential characteristics of the species of the genus **Achromatium**[a]

Characteristic	A. oxaliferum	"A. volutans"
Calcium carbonate inclusions	+	−
Sulfur inclusions	+	+
Found in freshwaters	+	−
Found in saline waters	+	+

[a]Symbols: +, positive; and −, negative.

Prokaryotes. A Handbook on Habitats, Isolation, and Identification of Bacteria. Springer-Verlag, Berlin, pp. 1037–1048.

List of species of the genus **Achromatium**

1. **Achromatium oxaliferum** Schewiakoff 1893, 1.[AL]
   ox.al.if′er.um. M.L. n. *oxalatum* oxalate; Gr. n. *oxalis* sorrel, a sour plant; L. v. *fero* to carry; M.L. adj. *oxaliferum* oxalate-containing.
   See generic description and Table 23.29.

2. **"Achromatium volutans"** (Hinze) van Niel 1948, 999. (*Thiophysa volutans* Hinze 1903, 310.)
   vol′u.tans. L. part. adj. *volutans* rolling.
   See generic description and Table 23.29.

Genus **Agitococcus** *Franzmann and Skerman 1981, 177* [VP]

P. D. Franzmann and V. B. D. Skerman

A. gi′to.coc′cus. L. v. *agito* to shake; Gr. n. *coccus* a grain or berry; M.L. masc. n. *Agitococcus* shaking coccus.

Cocci, 1–2 μm in diameter, which distend with sudanophilic granules in old cultures. **Twitching, gliding motility. No flagella or fimbriae present.** Capsules are produced. **Aerobic. Gram-negative** by staining and cell wall structure.

Growth occurs between 15 and 37°C and between pH 6 and 10. No growth occurs at 4 or 41°C or at pH 5. **Chemoorganotrophic. Do not oxidize or ferment glucose. Tween compounds are actively metabolized.**

The mol% G + C of the DNA is 40–43.

Type species: *Agitococcus lubricus* Franzmann and Skerman 1981, 177.

Further Descriptive Information

Cells of the genus *Agitococcus* are coccoid, but when they are filled with sudanophilic inclusions, larger distended forms occur. These inclusions occur more frequently in aging cells on a nutritious medium such as Tween 80 agar* than on lake water agar.†

Thin sections show a cell wall characteristic of Gram-negative bacteria and large white areas once occupied by sudanophilic inclusions. Critical-point-dried preparations (Fig. 23.100) show strands of extracellular polysaccharide. No fimbriae are present.

Colonies on casitone-yeast extract agar (CYEA‡) grow to 2–3 mm in diameter and are erose, flat, transparent and glistening, smooth and butyrous. Colonies on Tween 80 agar are 2–3 mm in diameter, entire, low convex to umbonate, opaque, glistening, smooth and butyrous. One strain was mucoid.

Other characteristics of the genus are given in Table 23.30 for the type species, *Agitococcus lubricus*. The methods used for the biochemical and physiological characterization are given by Franzmann and Skerman (1981).

Isolation, Maintenance and Preservation Procedures

Strains of this genus are recognized by their morphologically distinct microcolonies (Fig. 23.101) after growth on lake water agar. Single drops of water samples are allowed to flow across the surface of a lake water agar plate. Excess moisture is evaporated from the surface of the agar at 22°C in a sterile atmosphere. Plates are incubated and examined periodically with a Leitz PHACO × 32 phase-contrast objective. Typical microcolonies will often appear within 14 h, and single cells are selected by micromanipulation as described by Skerman (1968). Microcolonies grown from the isolated cells are transferred to a fresh medium.

Active growth is best maintained on Tween 80 agar at 28°C. Strains

*Tween 80 agar contains: Tween 80, 10.0 g; and casitone-yeast extract (Difco) agar (CYEA), 1 l.
†Lake water agar contains: lake water (filtered through a 0.2-μm membrane filter), 1 l; and agar (Difco), 15.0 g.
‡CYEA (in g/l) contains: casitone (Difco), 5.0; yeast extract (Difco), 3.0; $MgSO_4 \cdot 7H_2O$, 2.0; and agar (Difco), 15.0; at pH 7.2.

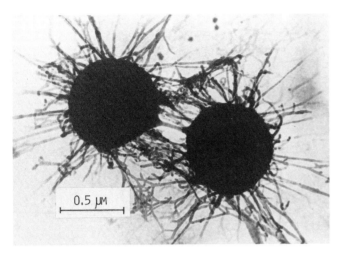

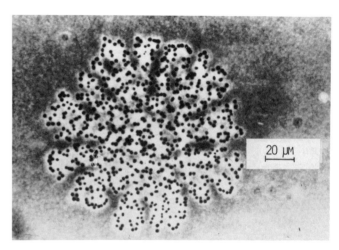

Figure 23.100. Critical point-dried preparation of *Agitococcus lubricus* strain UQM 1982 grown for 24 h on lake water agar at 28°C. (Reproduced with permission from P. D. Franzmann and V. B. D. Skerman, International Journal of Systematic Bacteriology *31:* 177–183 (Fig. 4), 1981, ©International Union of Microbiological Societies.)

Figure 23.101. *A. lubricus* strain on an isolation plate of lake water agar after incubation for 21 h at 22°C. (Reproduced with permission from P. D. Franzmann and V. B. D. Skerman, International Journal of Systematic Bacteriology *31:* 177–183 (Fig. 1), 1981, ©International Union of Microbiological Societies.)

Table 23.30.

Morphological, biochemical and physiological characteristics of **A. lubricus**[a]

Characteristic/test	Reaction	Characteristic/test	Reaction
Cell shape	Coccus	Growth at pH	
Cell diameter (μm)	1.0–2.0	5.0	−
Capsule present	+	6.0	+
Sudanophilic inclusions	+	10.0	+
Twitching motility	+	Growth on NaCl	
Mol% G + C of DNA (T_m)	42–43	0.1%	+
Oxidase	+	0.5%	+
Catalase	−	1.0%	−
Benzidine	+	Growth in nitrogen-free medium	−
Acid from glucose (O/F)[b]	−	Growth on *Nitrosomonas* sp. medium	−
Anaerobic growth	−	Gelatin hydrolysis	−
Acid in TSI[c]	−	Proteolysis of skim milk	+
H₂S production (lead-acetate strip test)	−	Serum liquefaction	−
H₂S in TSIA[d]	−	Hemolysis	−
Deamination of phenylalanine	−	Decolorization of chocolate agar	−
Indole production	−	Deposition of iron	−
Nitrate reduction	−	Tween 80 hydrolysis	+
Urease	−	Tween 40 hydrolysis	+
Lecithinase	+	Tween 20 hydrolysis	+
Tributyrin hydrolysis	−	Susceptibility to[e]	
Starch hydrolysis	−	Penicillin G (4 U)	+
Cellulose hydrolysis	−	Chloramphenicol (25 μg)	+
Alginate hydrolysis	−	Tetracycline (10 μg)	+
Growth at		Erythromycin (5 μg)	+
4°C	−	Streptomycin (10 μg)	+
15°C	+	Kanamycin (30 μg)	+
37°C	+	Neomycin (10 μg)	+
41°C	−	Utilization of	
Growth on 0.1% sodium lauryl sulfate	+	Acetate	−
		Propionate	−
		Glycerol	−

[a]Symbols: +, 90% or more of strains are positive; and −, 90% or more of strains are negative.

[b]O/F, oxidation/fermentation.

[c]TSI, triple sugar iron.

[d]TSIA, triple sugar iron agar.

[e]Antibiotics were supplied in disks from Mast Laboratories, U.K.

should be subcultured every 7 days. Cultures suspended in casitone-yeast extract broth containing 1% Tween 80 and 10% glycerol have been preserved successfully in liquid nitrogen when they have been frozen at a rate of 1°C/min to −100°C. Strains have not been successfully lyophilized.

Differentiation of the genus **Agitococcus** from other taxa

The genus *Agitococcus* bears little resemblance to other Gram-negative cocci. Optically they show some resemblance to the published illustrations of *Nitrosococcus*, but *Agitococcus* is heterotrophic and has a predilection for Tween compounds. The cells are larger than those of the *Moraxella-Acinetobacter* group with which they show little affinity.

Taxonomic Comments

Eighteen strains of *Agitococcus* showed virtually no phenotypic variation (Franzmann, 1983). Twelve strains were examined for the mol% G + C of their DNA. Nine strains had a mol% G + C of the DNA in the range of 40.7–42.7. Of the other three strains, two had a mol% G + C in the range of 52.1–53.1, and the remaining strain had a mol% G + C of 62.4. Three strains with similar mol% G + C of their DNA (UQM 1981, UQM 1982, UQM 1983: 42.7, 42.7 and 42.1, respectively) (Franzmann and Skerman, 1981) were selected for the description of the single species, *Agitococcus lubricus*. The divergency of other strains suggests that other species may need to be defined.

Further Comments

Agitococci have been found in the majority of freshwater samples examined. They have formed a minority of most populations. Initially the cocci form a compact monolayer on the surface of an unsupplemented lake water agar, but within a few days, groups of cells begin to migrate from the edge of the colony, leaving a broad "slime trail" in their wake (Fig. 23.101). When observed microscopically, these groups of cells show alternate periods of migratory and stationary behavior. Movement, when it occurs, is abrupt. When colonies are covered with a drop of water and a coverslip, the cells exhibit an intense twitching activity.

The tendency to migrate appears to be related to the availability of food. Cells grown on lake water agar supplemented with Tween compounds produce more regular heaped up colonies with little tendency to migrate. In this, they mimic the behavior of some other gliding bacteria.

Cells in microcolonies are usually well separated by slime (Fig. 23.102).

List of species of the genus **Agitococcus**

At this stage only one species has been proposed for the genus.

1. **Agitococcus lubricus** Franzmann and Skerman 1981, 177.[VP]
lu'bri.cus. L. adj. *lubricus* slippery.

The characters of the species are given in Table 23.30.
Type strain: UQM 1981.

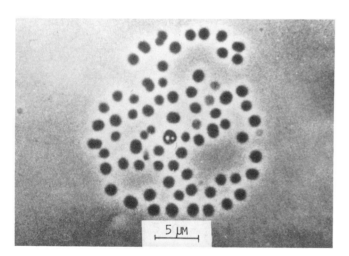

5 µM

Figure 23.102. *A. lubricus* strain UQM 1981 grown for 19 h on lake water Noble agar at 28°C. (Reproduced with permission from P. D. Franzmann and V. B. D. Skerman, International Journal of Systematic Bacteriology *31:* 177–183 (Fig. 2), 1981, ©International Union of Microbiological Societies.)

Genus **Herpetosiphon** Holt and Lewin 1965, 2408[AL]

J. G. HOLT

Her.pe.to.si′phon. Gr. n. *herpeton* gliding animal, reptile; Gr. masc. n. *siphon* tube or cylinder; M.L. masc. n. *Herpetosiphon* gliding tube.

Unbranched, flexible rods or filaments 0.5–1.5 × 5–150 µm or more (to several millimeters), consisting of individual cells 2–3 µm long. Often ensheathed, although sheaths may be difficult to visualize. Filament breakage or cell lysis results in empty ends or spaces (necridia). Resting stages not known. **Motile by gliding.** Gram-negative.

Chemoorganotrophs. **Metabolism is respiratory, with molecular oxygen used as the terminal electron acceptor.** Cellulose and chitin may be degraded, carboxymethyl cellulose may be depolymerized, or starch may be hydrolyzed. Gelatin is liquified. Indole, ammonia or H_2S is not produced. Produce yellow, red or orange carotenoid pigments.

Strict aerobes.

Marine forms require seawater for growth.

The mol% G + C of the DNA is 44.9–53.1 (Bd) (Mandel and Lewin, 1969).

Type species: *Herpetosiphon aurantiacus* Holt and Lewin 1968, 2408.

Further Descriptive Information

In their original description of the genus *Herpetosiphon*, Holt and Lewin (1968) noted the existence of a sheath surrounding the filaments of *H. aurantiacus*, the type species (Fig. 23.103). Lewin (1970b) later described four new species, all being ensheathed. A controversy over the presence of sheaths in *Herpetosiphon* ensued with the publication of a paper by Reichenbach and Golecki (1975) who were unable to find such a

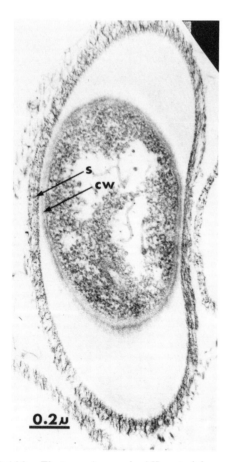

Figure 23.103. Electron micrograph of *Herpetosiphon aurantiacus* ATCC 23779 stained with uranyl acetate and showing a sheath (*S*) and the cell wall (*CW*). (Electron micrograph taken by J. A. Lauritis.)

structure. Unfortunately, they did not study any of the cultures of *H. aurantiacus* deposited by Holt and Lewin; instead, they used a new strain, Hp a2, which they named "*H. giganteus*," and reported that they were unable to find evidence for a sheath. The observations of Reichenbach and Golecki were refuted by Skerman et al. (1977). The latter investigators studied strains of *Herpetosiphon* isolated locally and strain Hp a2 of Reichenbach and Golecki. Skerman et al. claim that their local isolates are similar to the type strain of *H. aurantiacus* obtained from the ATCC, but it is unclear in the paper whether they found sheaths in the type strain which they presumably examined. Shortly after the genus was described, ultrathin sections of the type strain, ATCC 23779, were examined in the electron microscope (J. Lauritis, personal communication), and evidence for a sheath was found (Fig. 23.103). It is probable that the empty spaces on the ends of filaments seen by Holt and Lewin (1968) were, in fact, necridia. However, thin sections of *H. aurantiacus* do show the presence of a thin sheath, and the evidence of Skerman et al. seems to corroborate the observation. Sheath formation in the remaining species of the genus has not been observed in the electron microscope. Further work is necessary to describe the presumed sheath, and as Reichenbach (1981) suggests, there is a need to determine the relationship of the thin sheaths seen by Skerman et al. and by us, to what he considers the outer membrane. It is still unclear whether these organisms produce a classic sheath or whether they have a unique cell surface.

Older cultures may give rise to the formation of large (2.5–3.5 µm) bulbs within the filaments (Reichenbach and Golecki, 1975), which appear to be the result of senescence.

Pure cultures exhibit the ability to lyse and digest living bacterial and yeast cells. Lewin (1970b) reported that *H. geysericola* could be grown on a lawn of "*Aerobacter*," and Brauss et al. (1969) isolated a presumed herpetosiphon from water that was lytic on yeast cells. Reichenbach and Dworkin (1981c) describe isolation techniques with baits of bacterial or yeast cells used. A controlled study of the phenomenon was reported by Quinn and Skerman (1980) who found that a number of strains of *H. aurantiacus* (including "*H. giganteus*") and *H. geysericola* were lytically active against a variety of Gram-positive and Gram-negative bacteria. They were ineffective against spores and encapsulated strains. Trick and Lingens (1984) isolated a herpetosiphon from bulking sewage sludge and reported their isolates to be lytic against Gram-negative bacteria.

On agar media such as 0.3% peptonized milk in 1.5% agar (Holt and Lewin, 1968) or on other dilute media (Reichenbach and Dworkin, 1981c), colonies show a rough swirled texture. Heavy growth may result in the formation of large fruiting body-like structures that do not contain resting stages. These protuberances may reach lengths of 1–5 mm. Brauss et al. (1969) described an organism isolated from water, which appears to be a herpetosiphon, that produced similar structures.

The main carotenoid pigments of *H. aurantiacus* ("*H. giganteus*" sensu Reichenbach and Golecki) were found to be a unique type, *x-O*-acyldiglucosyloxycarotenoids (Kleinig and Reichenbach, 1977; Reichenbach et al., 1978). Additionally, a monoglucosyloxycarotene and γ-carotene were found. These same authors reported that the primary isoprenoid quinone was MK-6 menaquinone, with a minor component of MK-7 menaquinone.

A unique restriction endonuclease of class II has been isolated from "*H. giganteus*" (Brown et al., 1980) and named *Hgi*AI. The enzyme has a digestion pattern different from those of other gliding bacteria (Mayer and Reichenbach, 1978).

Enrichment and Isolation Procedures

Herpetosiphon can be isolated from a wide variety of habitats, including freshwater, marine shores, soil, dung, decaying plant material and hot springs. Prior enrichment does not seem to be necessary, as most isolation techniques rely on the ability of the filaments to glide away from the point of inoculation. Any of a number of dilute agar media made with either freshwater or seawater can be used for isolation. In the original isolation of *H. aurantiacus* a medium of 0.3% peptonized milk in 1.5% agar was used (Holt and Lewin, 1968). Reichenbach and co-workers have used water agar containing cells of *Escherichia coli* or yeast (Reichenbach and Dworkin, 1981c). Often, a freshwater or seawater agar (1–1.5%) without added nutrients has been used (Lewin and Lounsbery, 1969; Skerman et al., 1977; Reichenbach and Dworkin, 1981c). Cycloheximide (0.0025%) can be added to the medium to suppress the growth of eucaryotic contaminants. Material from a natural habitat is placed in the center or in a single streak on the plate, and the herpetosiphons will glide away from the point of inoculation. Isolation of pure cultures is accomplished by picking material from the leading edge of a characteristic rough, swirled swarm, which is best viewed microscopically under low power.

Maintenance Procedures

Cultures of *Herpetosiphon* respond well to preservation by routine lyophilization or frozen storage at ultracold temperatures (−70C). Sanfilippo and Lewin (1970) found good survival of herpetosiphons in liquid nitrogen without additives.

Differentiation of the genus **Herpetosiphon** from other genera

For the differentiation of *Herpetosiphon* from other genera, please refer to the key to the groups of nonphotosynthetic, nonfruiting gliding bacteria (p. 2010).

Taxonomic Comments

Reichenbach and Golecki (1975) were unable to find sheaths in a strain of *Herpetosiphon* they isolated, strain Hp a2, and proposed that the genus be redefined as sheathless. They named their strain *Herpetosiphon giganteus* (basionym: *Flexibacter giganteus* Soriano 1945, 93) and proposed that the genus be redefined with "*H. giganteus*" replacing the type species, *H. aurantiacus*. Their study did not include the type strain of *H. aurantiacus* (ATCC 23779), and therefore proper nomenclatural procedures for comparing type strains were not followed. *H. aurantiacus* has priority and has been retained as the type species in the Approved Lists of Bacterial Names (Skerman et al., 1980). "*H. giganteus*" is presumably an illegitimate subjective synonym of *H. aurantiacus* and is not included in this treatment.

Lewin (1970b) described three new species from beach sand, *H. persicus*, *H. cohaerens* and *H. nigricans*, and one from a hot spring in Baja California, *H. geysericola* (basionym: *Phormidium geysericola* Copeland 1936, 186). All of these species have been grown in pure culture, and type strains are on deposit in the ATCC. They have not been studied very much since Lewin's original description. These four species along with the type species, *H. aurantiacus*, were included in the eighth edition of the *Manual* (Lewin and Leadbetter, 1974) and are retained here. The marine species were included in a numerical taxonomic study of a large collection of gliding bacteria (Colwell, 1969), with data used from Lewin and Lounsbery (1969) and Fager (1969). Fager had analyzed the phenotypic data of Lewin and Lounsbery and concluded that the three species formed a group separate from the other gliders. Colwell's analysis, using a different program, showed that the three species did not cluster together. None of these studies included the type species of the genus, and as Colwell points out, there were a very small number of features used.

The phylogenetic position of *Herpetosiphon* has been speculated upon since its description. Using phenotypic criteria and DNA base ratios, early workers speculated that these organisms were apochlorotic counterparts of cyanobacteria such as *Lyngbya* (Holt and Lewin, 1968; Mandel and Lewin, 1969; Lewin, 1970b; Reichenbach and Golecki, 1975). Lewin (1969) considered *Herpetosiphon* to be a member of the family *Cytophagaceae*. Analyses of the lipids of the genus (Kleinig and Reichenbach, 1977; Reichenbach et al., 1978) show that the carotenoids are similar to those found in the *Myxobacterales* but not the *Cytophagales*. The menaquinone pattern of *Herpetosiphon* (mainly MK-6) is unlike other gliders studied. Godchaux and Leadbetter (1983) reported the absence of certain sulfonolipids (capnoids) in *Herpetosiphon*, while they are present in those species of the *Cytophagales* which they studied.

The application of 16S rRNA cataloging to define phylogenetic groupings among the procaryotes has given good insights into the place of *Herpetosiphon* in the evolution of the bacteria. Prior to these studies, gliding motility was the thread that bound many diverse groups together, and as Reichenbach et al. (1986) have pointed out, there are gliding bacteria in at least six of the (then) nine major phylogenetic groups of eubacteria. As explained above, the phenotypic and chemotaxonomic data did not give clear evidence for phylogenetic placement, and all statements about evolutionary relationships were speculative. Reichenbach (1981), in his excellent review of the taxonomy of the gliding bacteria, suggested a close relationship of *Herpetosiphon* to the family *Chloroflexaceae* on the basis of morphology and closeness of DNA base ratios (mol% G + C of 45–53 vs. 53–55). This observation has been substantiated by studies in which the 16S rRNA of *Herpetosiphon* was compared with that of green phototrophic bacteria (Gibson et al., 1985). They compared the 16S rRNA of *Chloroflexus*, *Chlorobium*, *Prosthecochloris*, *Chloroherpeton*, *Thermomicrobium roseum*, and two herpetosiphons, *H. aurantiacus* ATCC 23779 and strain Wie 2 of E. Senghas. When these were analyzed by signature analysis, evidence suggested that *Chloroflexus* and *Herpetosiphon* formed a phylogenetic grouping very distant from the *Chlorobium* group. Reichenbach et al. (1986) showed by S_{AB} analysis that the gliding bacteria were not related phylogenetically to the cyanobacteria, and using the data of Gibson et al. (1985), they argued that *Herpetosiphon* is related to *Chloroflexus* and not to any other gliders. Finally, in a more recent study, Oyaizu et al. (1987) using sequence data of the 16S rRNA of *Herpetosiphon* and relatives refined the results of the earlier work and have shown that *Herpetosiphon*, the *Chloroflexaceae* and *Thermomicrobium* all belong to a separate phylogenetic "phylum" of the eubacteria. The authors conclude that *Herpetosiphon* is the most rapidly evolving line in the group, while *Thermomicrobium* is the slowest. In their study, data from only one strain of *H. aurantiacus*, fortunately the type strain, were used; it is hoped future studies will be expanded to include more strains and species from the genus. It is noteworthy that Gibson et al. (1985) using two strains of *H. aurantiacus*, ATCC 23779 and Wie 2, found that 10 of 35 signature sequences differed between the two. One wonders how the phylogenetic tree of Oyaizu et al. would have appeared with data from other strains of *Herpetosiphon*.

Further Reading

Oyaizu, H., B. Debrunner-Vossbrinck, L. Mandelco, J.A. Studier and C.R. Woese, 1987. The green non-sulfur bacteria: a deep branching in the eubacterial line of descent. Syst. Appl. Microbiol. *9:* 47–53.

Reichenbach, H. 1981. Taxonomy of the gliding bacteria. Annu. Rev. Microbiol. *35:* 339–364.

Reichenbach, H. and M. Dworkin. 1981. The order *Cytophagales* (with addenda on the genera *Herpetosiphon*, *Saprospira* and *Flexithrix*). *In* Starr, Stolp, Trüper, Balows and Schlegel (Editors), The Prokaryotes. A Handbook on Habitats, Isolation, and Identification of Bacteria. Springer-Verlag, Berlin, pp. 356–379.

Differentiation of the species of the genus **Herpetosiphon**

The differential characteristics of the species of the genus *Herpetosiphon* are listed in Table 23.31 which is reproduced from the eighth edition of the *Manual* (Lewin and Leadbetter, 1974).

Table 23.31.
Differential characteristics of the species of the genus **Herpetosiphon**[a]

	Color of cell mass	Cellulose hydrolyzed	Starch hydrolyzed	Tyrosine degraded	Catalase	Seawater required	Thermophilic	Nitrate as sole nitrogen source	Mol% G + C of DNA
1. *H. aurantiacus*	Orange	−	+	+	+	−	−		48.1
2. *H. geysericola*	Orange	+	+		+	−	+		48.5
3. *H. cohaerens*	Orange	−	−	−	−	+	−	−	44.9
4. *H. persicus*	Orange	−	−	−	−	+	−	+	52.6
5. *H. nigricans*	Yellow	−	−	+	−	+	−	+	53.1

[a] Symbols: −, 90% or more of strains are negative; and +, 90% or more of strains are positive.

List of species of the genus **Herpetosiphon**

1. Herpetosiphon aurantiacus Holt and Lewin 1968, 2408.[AL]

au.ran.ti′a.cus. M.L. neut. n. *aurantium* specific name of the orange; M.L. adj. *aurantiacus* orange-colored.

Cells, 1.0–1.5 × 5–10 μm, in unbranched, flexible and usually sheathed filaments, which may exceed 500 μm in length.

Cellulose is not hydrolyzed. Starch is hydrolyzed. A crystalline suspension of tyrosine is degraded, with formation of a reddish brown pigment. Growth has been reported only in complex media; minimal nutritional requirements are unknown.

The mol% G + C of the DNA is 48.1 (Bd).

Type strain: ATCC 23779.

2. Herpetosiphon geysericola (Copeland) Lewin 1970, 517.[AL]
(*Phormidium geysericola* Copeland, 1936, 186.)

gey.ser.i′cola. Icelandic n. *geysir* gusher, name of a hot spring; L. n. *cola* dweller; M.L. n. *geysericola* hot springs dweller.

Flexible, sheathed rods or filaments 0.5 × 10–150 μm or more.

Cellulose is digested. Carboxymethyl cellulose is depolymerized. Starch is hydrolyzed.

High temperatures tolerated; recorded from hot springs at 60–80°C. pH tolerated (in nature): 8–9.

The mol% G + C of the DNA of the single strain (suggested neotype) examined is 48.5 (Bd).

3. Herpetosiphon cohaerens Lewin 1970, 518.[AL]

co.hae′rens. L. part. adj. *cohaerens* cohering, uniting together.

Unbranched, flexible, sheathed rods or filaments 0.7 μm (1.0 μm if sheath is included) × 60–150 μm longer.

Cellulose and starch are not attacked; carboxymethyl cellulose is not depolymerized. Glucose and sucrose promote growth, while acetate, galactose, glycerol and lactate do not. Tryptone or glutamate, but not nitrate, can serve as sole nitrogen source. No acid is produced in litmus milk, although coagulation occurs; the resultant curd is not digested, but the litmus is reduced. A crystalline suspension of tyrosine or dihydroxyphenylalanine is not degraded. There are no known growth factor requirements.

Cell masses orange. Extracts, in hexane, have an absorption maximum at 471 nm, attributable to the carotenoid saproxanthin.

Seawater ranging from one-half to double strength is required for growth.

The mol% G + C of the DNA of the type strain is 44.9 (Bd).

Type strain: II-2; ATCC 23123.

4. Herpetosiphon persicus Lewin 1970, 518.[AL]

per′si.cus. L. adj. *persicus* Persian (of fruit = peach), i.e. peach-colored.

Unbranched, flexible, sheathed rods or filaments 0.7 μm (1.0 μm if sheath is included) × 30–150 μm or longer.

Cellulose and starch are not attacked; carboxymethyl cellulose is not depolymerized. Glucose is a suitable carbon source; galactose and sucrose also promote growth, but acetate, glycerol and lactate do not. Tryptone, glutamate or nitrate can serve as sole nitrogen source. Acid is not produced from litmus milk, although coagulation occurs; the curd is not digested, but the litmus is reduced. A crystalline suspension of tyrosine or dihydroxyphenylalanine is not degraded. There are no known growth factor requirements.

Cell masses orange; extracts, in hexane, have an absorption maximum at 471 nm, attributable to the carotenoid saproxanthin.

Seawater ranging from one-half to double strength is required for growth.

The mol% G + C of the DNA of the type strain is 52.6.

Type strain: T-3; ATCC 23167.

5. Herpetosiphon nigricans Lewin 1970, 518.[AL]

ni′gri.cans. L. part. adj. *nigricans* blackening.

Unbranched, flexible sheathed rods or filaments 0.5 μm (1.0 μm if sheath is included) × 5–50 μm.

Cellulose and starch are not attacked; carboxymethyl cellulose is not depolymerized. Glucose is a suitable carbon source; galactose and sucrose also promote growth, but acetate, glycerol and lactate do not. Casamino acids, tryptone, glutamate or nitrate can serve as sole nitrogen source. Acid is not produced from litmus milk, although coagulation occurs; the curd is digested, and the litmus is reduced. A crystalline suspension of tyrosine is degraded, with the formation of a pigmented product, but dihydroxyphenylalanine is not degraded. There are no known growth factor requirements.

Cell masses yellow; extracts, in hexane, have an absorption maximum at 450 nm, attributable to the carotenoid zeaxanthin.

Seawater ranging from one-half to double strength is required for growth.

The mol% G + C of the DNA of the type strain is 53.1 (Bd).

Type strain: SS-2; ATCC 23147.

SECTION 24

Fruiting Gliding Bacteria: The Myxobacteria

ORDER **MYXOCOCCALES** TCHAN, POCHON AND PRÉVOT 1948, 398[AL]*

HOWARD D. McCURDY

Myx.o.coc.ca′les. N.L. masc. n. *Myxococcaceae* type family of order; *-ales* ending to denote order; N.L. fem. pl. n. *Myxococcales* the *Myxococcaceae* order

Unicellular rods of <1.5 μm in diameter, which may be slender, flexible and tapered at the ends (cell type I) or may be cylindrical and more rigid with blunt, rounded ends (cell type II). Capable of slow **gliding movement** when in contact with a solid surface or air-water interface (but not when in suspension) at a rate of up to 10 μm/min but lacking detectable locomotor organelles. This organism typically produces an extracellular polysaccharide slime in which the cells are embedded or which is deposited as a trail behind gliding cells. Gram-negative.

Under conditions of nutrient deprivation, **cells aggregate to form fruiting bodies** composed of modified slime and cells, which are often brightly colored and of macroscopic dimensions. **Fruiting bodies vary** in complexity, **from simple mounds to complex structures** consisting of sporangia of characteristic shape and dimensions which may be sessile or borne singly or in groups on simple or branched stalks.

Within the fruiting bodies, the cells are converted to resting cells called either myxospores or microcysts. The myxospores of species of cell type II (the *Polyangiaceae*) differ little from vegetative cells and are always contained within sporangia. In all other species (cell type I), the myxospores are much shortened rods or spheres surrounded by a spore coat that confers some degree of individual resistance to heat, ultraviolet light and desiccation. Myxospores of this kind are also termed microcysts. In the *Polyangiaceae*, the unit of resistance appears to be the entire sporangium.

Chemoorganotrophs. Strictly aerobic; energy-yielding metabolism is **respiratory,** never fermentative. Typically **produce extracellular enzymes hydrolyzing** such macromolecules as **proteins, nucleic acids, fatty acid esters and various polysaccharides** including, in some *Polyangiaceae*, cellulose. Most are capable of lysing other eucaryotic and procaryotic microorganisms. Photosynthetic pigments are lacking, but carotenoid pigments, typically of the tertiary glycoside class (Kleinig et al., 1970, 1971; Reichenbach and Kleinig, 1971), melanin, and protoporphyrin pigments (Burchard and Dworkin, 1966a) are often produced. Hence the **myxobacters are generally brightly colored.**

The mol% G + C of the DNA is 67–71 (T_m, Bd) (Mandel and Leadbetter, 1965; McCurdy and Wolf, 1967).

Further Comments

The cells of myxobacters stain poorly by routine bacteriological techniques and are best observed by phase-contrast microscopy. They are never in chains or pairs. There is a tendency for cells to autolyze and to form spheroplasts under a variety of conditions (anaerobiosis, refrigeration temperatures, in the presence of certain cations, in old cultures).

In addition to their gliding motility and flexibility, the myxobacters are distinguished from other Gram-negative bacteria by their content of 2- and 3-hydroxy fatty acids and the exclusive presence of menaquinones in their respiratory chains (Fautz et al., 1981). Their vegetative cells are of typical Gram-negative structure, although on examination the diaminopimelic acid-containing peptidoglycan has been found to be present in relatively low amounts (0.6% (dry weight)) and organized in patches (White et al., 1968). The outer membrane lipopolysaccharide is similar to that of other Gram-negative bacteria but differs in lacking heptose and in containing odd-numbered and isobranched fatty acids of 16 rather than 14 carbon length (Sutherland and Smith, 1973; Rosenfelder et al., 1974). Some contain the unusual sugar 3-*o*-methyl-D-xylose (Weckesser et al., 1971). The cell membrane is marked by a predominance of branched, and the presence of diunsaturated, fatty acids (Ware and Dworkin, 1973).

As for other gliding bacteria, the myxobacteria are more sensitive to actinomycin than are other Gram-negative bacteria (Dworkin, 1969).

All examined myxobacters except *Nannocystis* possess unipolar tufts of fimbriae (MacRae et al., 1977) which function as organelles of swarming or social motility but which are not motility organelles as such (Dobson et al., 1979.)

The vegetative colony of the myxobacters (Fig. 24.1), termed a swarm, has a characteristic appearance as a result of slime production and the tendency of cells to glide in more or less organized groups. The swarm is typically flat and thin with many concentric ridges or dense waves and with radiating lines or folds. It spreads extensively, sometimes rapidly, over the agar surface as a result of the outward movement of cells at the periphery. Frequently, the latter advance as groups forming tonguelike extensions or isolated clumps and streams. In the *Polyangiaceae* especially, the underlying agar may be etched, eroded and penetrated. Some members of this family may display prominent peripheral ridges, especially in contact with eubacterial colonies; others may separate into large clumps of migrating cells which furrow and penetrate deeply into the agar (Fig. 24.2).

Continued cultivation on rich media yields mucoid, nonspreading, nonfruiting or poorly fruiting colonies which resemble those of the nongliding bacterial colonies. Such variants usually grow dispersely in

---

* *AL* denotes inclusion of this name on the Approved Lists of Bacterial Names (1980).

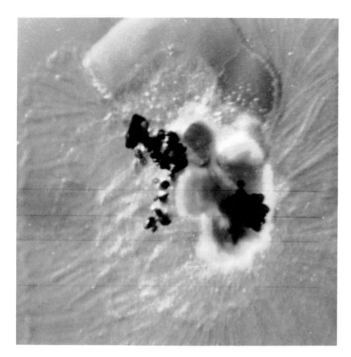

Figure 24.1. *Stigmatella brunnea* vegetative colony. Light photomicrograph (× 10).

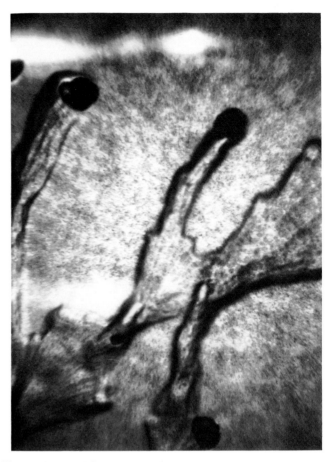

Figure 24.2. *Polyangium cellulosum* migrating cell mass on agar. Light photomicrograph (× 90).

liquid media. In some instances, these changes are associated with changes in the character of the slime (Grimm and Kühlwein, 1973b). In other, perhaps most, instances, dispersed growth and loss of swarming is associated with the loss of fimbriae (Dobson et al., 1979).

Fruiting body formation is initiated as a result of nutrient depletion. In *Myxococcus xanthus*, the omission of any one of the essential or strongly growth-limiting amino acids or starvation for carbon-energy or inorganic phosphate results in fruiting-body induction (Bretscher and Kaiser, 1978).

The process consists of a number of stages. After induction, the cells aggregate into mounds which, in some species (e.g. *Myxococcus)*, may end the process, or further morphogenetic movements may result in the formation of such structural elements as stalks and sporangia. In the final stages, the surviving cells differentiate into myxospores. It has been suggested that in certain species, sacrificial autolysis of some cells may be a necessary part of the process (Wireman and Dworkin, 1975). In two species at least (Qualls et al., 1978; Reichenbach, 1974a and b), light is required for fruiting.

Although it is clear that the fruiting bodies of myxobacters are the resistant or resting stage, they have another function as well: to ensure a multicellular and, therefore, an adequately functional inoculum for the initiation of growth on a fresh substrate by organisms possessing a cooperative ("wolf pack") feeding habit (Dworkin, 1972).

In those myxobacters in which the myxospore is a microcyst, the hard slime coat surrounding the cell confers considerably more resistance to heat, desiccation, mechanical disruption and ultraviolet light than is possessed by vegetative cells. The conversion of vegetative cells into microcysts without fruiting body formation can be induced in all species examined by the addition of 0.5 M glycerol to liquid cultures (Dworkin and Gibson, 1964; McCurdy and Khouw, 1969; Reichenbach and Dworkin, 1970; Gerth and Reichenbach, 1978; H. D. McCurdy, unpublished observations). Other inducers include DMSO, indole, certain amino acids, *t*-butanol, phenethyl alcohol and certain monovalent cations (Gerth and Reichenbach, 1978; H. D. McCurdy, unpublished observations). However, such microcysts may differ from fruiting body microcysts in several physiological and structural properties (Kaiser et al., 1979).

Some students of the myxobacters disagree on terminology. Reichenbach and Dworkin (1981) have suggested use of the term "sporangiole" in lieu of the older term "sporangium" for spore-containing structures, since these investigators associate the suggestion of sexuality with the latter.

However, no accepted definition of "sporangium" is conditional upon sexuality; it is defined merely as a saclike structure containing an indefinite number of spores (see, for example, Alexopoulos, 1962; Bold and Wynne, 1978). Indeed, in the *Mucorales* cited by Reichenbach and Dworkin, sporangia are the products of asexual reproduction by haploid thalli. Sporangioles, which are similarly derived, are defined as *small* sporangia containing *few* spores. Thus it is difficult to use the argument of Reichenbach and Dworkin as a basis for changing accepted terminology.

These same authors also suggest, in the interest of uniform terminology, that in spite of its long use the term "microcyst" be abandoned in favor of the term "myxospore" in application to all myxobacter resting cells. They would have conformity with this view in spite of their own observation (Reichenbach and Dworkin, 1981, p. 370) that the term "cyst" is best applied to "dormant, encapsulated single cells" which microcysts are and in spite of the clear physiological differences between these cells and other myxospores.

Most myxobacters grow poorly or not at all on conventional bacteriological media (nutrient broth, etc.). They may be divided conveniently into two physiological groups: the bacteriolytic, which includes all *Myxococcaceae*, *Archangiaceae*, *Cystobacteraceae* and most *Polyangiaceae*; and the cellulolytic, all of which are members of the genus *Polyangium*. The cellulolytic myxobacters have very simple requirements. Nitrogen is supplied by NH_4^+ or NO_3^-, while carbon and energy are derived from cellulose, cellobiose or glucose. Most also yield good growth in casitone (Difco) media and lyse dead bacterial cells.

The bacteriolytic myxobacteria may be cultivated on agar media containing living or killed bacteria or yeast which they lyse. Their frequent observation on herbivorous dungs probably reflects the abundance therein of bacteria and other organic materials as sources of food. Most will also grow well on agar media containing enzymatically hydrolyzed protein and salts including relatively high concentrations of Mg^{2+} or Ca^{2+}. However, cultivation on liquid media may present special problems, and a solid medium which supported good growth may fail to do so if agar is omitted.

Myxobacter cultures emit characteristic musty odors which the trained observer will associate with different groups. For example, the bacteriolytic types often have a beetlike odor in fresh cultures, whereas the odor of many polyangia is streptomycetous (geosmin production has been confirmed in *Nannocystis exedens* (Trowitzsch et al., 1981)).

The minimal nutritional requirements of most bacteriolytic myxobacters are still poorly known. Defined media originally reported for three species contained complex amino acid mixtures meeting both carbon-energy and nitrogen requirements (Dworkin, 1962; Mayer, 1967; Hemphill and Zahler, 1968; McCurdy and Khouw, 1969). Bretscher and Kaiser (1978) demonstrated, however, that *Myxococcus xanthus* could be cultivated on a medium in which pyruvate and aspartate were the predominant carbon-energy sources and which contained the required amino acids leucine, isoleucine, valine and methionine (with the latter replaceable by vitamin B_{12}). No definite obligate vitamin requirements have been demonstrated for most species, but some bacteriolytic *Polyangiaceae* appear to require, or are stimulated by, vitamin B_{12} and perhaps other factors as well (McCurdy, 1964, 1969b; Reichenbach, 1970). None appear able to use sugars for carbon-energy, although some strains of *Stigmatella aurantiaca* do produce detectable acid from glucose (Gerth and Reichenbach, 1978), and the incorporation of several sugars into casitone media has been found to stimulate the growth of some fresh isolates (J. Peterson, University of Missouri, personal communication; H. D. McCurdy, unpublished observation). Furthermore, the addition of a polysaccharide such as starch (which is rapidly hydrolyzed), glycogen, agar or carboxymethyl cellulose (Dworkin, 1962; Schürmann, 1967; McCurdy, 1969b) as well as certain other soluble polymers will often permit growth in liquid media that will not otherwise support growth.

The strictly aerobic, respiratory metabolism of the bacteriolytic myxobacters and their use of pyruvate and/or amino acids but not sugars as carbon-energy sources suggest that the tricarboxylic acid cycle is the main pathway of energy metabolism. Enzymes of the tricarboxylic acid cycle as well as typical aerobic bacterial electron transport systems have been detected in *Myxococcus xanthus* (Dworkin and Niederpruem, 1964), *Stigmatella erecta* (McCurdy and Khouw, 1969) and *Polyangium cellulosum* (Sarao et al., 1985). Some Embden-Meyerhof enzymes were detected in both organisms, although hexokinase was evidenced only in *S. erecta* and *P. cellulosum*. This may explain why acid from glucose has been detected in some *Stigmatella* organisms but not in *Myxococcus*. The intermediary metabolism of the cellulolytic myxobacters has not been studied at all but can be expected to differ from the bacteriolytic group.

The mol% G + C of the DNA (Mandel and Leadbetter, 1965; McCurdy and Wolf, 1967) of all myxobacters is 67–70 which differentiates them from the *Cytophagales* generally, although certain nonfruiting gliders seemingly unrelated to the *Myxococcales* have a mol% G + C of 70 (Shilo, 1970; Stewart and Brown, 1971). Although the genome of *M. xanthus* (and *S. aurantiaca*) was initially estimated to be 3 or 4 times larger than that of *Escherichia coli* (Zusman et al., 1978), it is probably in the range of $3.1–3.8 \times 10^9$ daltons or about 24–53% larger than the *E. coli* genome (Yee and Inouye, 1981).

Genetic studies of the *Myxococcales* have been limited largely to *Myxococcus xanthus* for which auxotrophic mutants, motility mutants and morphogenetic mutants have been isolated, resulting from spontaneous mutations or mutagenesis by ultraviolet light, nitrosoguani-

dine, ethyl methanesulfonate and ICR 191 (Burchard and Parish, 1975; MacRae and McCurdy, 1976; Hodgkin and Kaiser, 1977; Grimm, 1978).

The extreme instability of fruiting body formation in many species of myxobacters might suggest that significant parts of the morphogenetic program are subject to phase variation, as has been described for colonial morphology in *M. xanthus* (Burchard and Dworkin, 1966a; Wireman and Dworkin, 1975; Burchard et al., 1977) and *Archangium violaceum* (Grimm and Kühlwein, 1973a, b), or are plasmid-determined.

Evidence has been obtained for endogenous cryptic plasmids in strains of *Myxococcus fulvus* and *M. xanthus* $MxFb_t$ (Brown and Parish, 1976). Moreover, chloramphenicol resistance in $MxFb_t$ was correlated with the appearance of a peak of extrachromosomal, covalently closed DNA molecules.

Chloramphenicol resistance as well as resistance to other antibiotics has been transferred to *Myxococcus xanthus* and *M. virescens* from R^+ strains of *Pseudomonas fluorescens* and *E. coli* (Brown and Parish, 1976). Chloramphenicol resistance may also be transduced into *M. virescens* by the specialized transducing phage P1CM, with the accompanying appearance of plasmids not observed in the parental strain. DNA from the transduced myxococci could then be employed to clone certain genes in *E. coli* (Morris et al., 1978).

More recently, the transposon Tn5, carrying kanamycin resistance, has been introduced into *M. xanthus* from *E. coli* by use of P1:Tn5. Only the Tn5 sequences were found in the transductants (Kuner and Kaiser, 1981). Tn5 provides a good selectable marker for isolating and mapping mutants and for cloning *M. xanthus* genes in *E. coli* (see also O'Connor and Zusman, 1983).

Bacteriophages have so far been reported only for *Myxococcus* species. These were isolated from soil, dung and carrier strains. All belong to four major groups, the prototypes of which are Mx1 (Burchard and Dworkin, 1966b), Mx4 (Campos et al., 1978), Mx8 and Mx9 (Martin et al., 1978). All, with the possible exception of the Mx1 group (Ov, Om, Oa, Ob and O2) (Brown et al., 1976), are generalized transducers. Most are morphologically similar to the T-even bacteriophages of *E. coli*.

Bacteriocins and bacteriocinlike activities have also been detected in various *Myxococcus* species (McCurdy and MacRae, 1974; Brown et al., 1976; Hirsch, 1977).

Most known myxobacters occur in soil of neutral or alkaline pH, although *Angiococcus disciformis* (*Cystobacter disciformis*) and *Polyangium sorediatum* have been reported to prefer acid soils (Krzemieniewska and Krzemieniewski, 1927). Myxobacters develop especially abundantly on decaying plant material, the bark of living or dead trees and the dung of herbivorous animals, on all of which they are detected by the appearance of fruiting bodies. Only one species has been described as aquatic (Geitler, 1924), but a number have been isolated from freshwater environments (Jeffers, 1964; Brauss et al., 1968; Shilo, 1970; Hook, 1977), and it appears that many are capable of growth on the surfaces of natural waters with high organic content (H. D. McCurdy, unpublished observation).

The distribution of myxobacters is worldwide. They have been obtained in Europe, Asia, Australia, the Americas, Iceland and Africa. Although their numbers appear highest in temperate, cultivated soils, they have also been recovered from forest soils, marine and freshwater beaches and dunes, mountain soils, tropical soils and arctic tundra.

No completely satisfactory method has been devised to estimate soil populations, but it is evident that their numbers may be considerable. For example, Singh (1947) obtained estimates of 2,000–76,000/g in soils. McCurdy (1969b), using a direct plating technique on myxococcal populations alone in soil, found a range of 1,000–450,000/g. Numbers in sludge compost were found to exceed 500,000/g (Singh, 1947). The ecological role of the *Myxococcales* is as scavengers, and often too as predators, in the aerobic decomposition of various biological macromolecules. However, there has not yet been a systematic ecological study which would permit a definitive analysis of the specific niches of the various species.

In addition to various lytic enzymes, the production of antibiotic substances is probably common among myxobacters. For example, antibacterial antibiotics have been characterized from *Myxococcus coralloides* (Arias et al., 1979), *M. xanthus* (Rosenberg et al., 1973; Vaks et al., 1974; Gerth et al., 1982), *M. fulvus* (Irschik et al., 1983), *Cystobacter fuscus* (Kunze et al., 1982) and *M. virescens* (Gerth et al., 1982). Antifungal antibiotics have been described from *Polyangium cellulosum* (Connor et al., 1977; Ringel et al., 1977) and *M. fulvus* (Gerth et al., 1980).

Enrichment of Bacteriolytic Myxobacters

Incubation of Natural Materials

Bits of decaying plant material, herbivorous dung or the bark from living or dead trees are placed in Petri dishes on two or three layers of filter paper and soaked for several hours in distilled water containing 30–50 mg Acti-Dione per l. After the water is poured off, the material is incubated.

Soil Baiting

Petri dishes are half-filled with soil which has been moistened to a muddy consistency with Acti-Dione-containing distilled water (30–50 μg/ml). About a dozen autoclaved, urine-free dung pellets from rabbits on an antibiotic-free diet are pressed partially into the soil in each dish.

Singh Plates

A thick paste of living or killed *Escherichia coli, Micrococcus luteus, Enterobacter aerogenes* or baker's yeast is spread as cross-streaks on 2% water agar (pH 7.0) containing 30 μg each of Acti-Dione and nystatin per ml. Small bits of soil or other inoculum are placed on the streaks, and the plates are incubated (Singh, 1947).

Water Samples

Water from natural sources is drawn through 0.45-μm membrane filters previously coated with bacteria or yeast from approximately 10 ml of broth culture. The filter is then placed on 1.5% water agar containing 30 mg Acti-Dione per l and 100 mg $CaCl_2 \cdot 2H_2O$ per l and sometimes supplemented with 0.01% peptone.

All of these preparations are incubated at about 27°C in freezer boxes to maintain relatively humid conditions. Myxobacters are usually detected by means of a dissecting microscope, with reflected illumination used for sighting fruiting bodies and transmitted light used for sighting swarms. On agar enrichments, swarms are frequently detected even in the absence of fruiting body formation. The first organisms detected after 3–4 days are usually myxococci. These are followed by species of the *Archangiaceae, Cystobacteraceae* and, finally, *Polyangiaceae*. Generally, no new development occurs after 3 weeks. As soon as possible, fruiting bodies or swarm edges as free as possible from eubacterial contamination are transferred to one or more of the following media. A useful tool for transfers is a stainless steel needle rubbed to a very fine, flattened tip. Individual sporangia may be easily picked up by means of this tool. Fine glass needles are preferred by some workers (Reichenbach and Dworkin, 1981).

Media

All of the following media are prepared with distilled water:

1. (*Escherichia coli* medium (ECM) agar (modified): *E. coli*, 100 mg (dry weight); $MgSO_4 \cdot 7H_2O$, 0.05 g; $CaCl_2 \cdot 2H_2O$, 0.05 g; agar, 1.5 g; and water, 100 ml.
2. Yeast-calcium agar: baker's yeast, 0.5%; $CaCl_2 \cdot 2H_2O$, 0.1%; vitamin B_{12}, 0.5 μg/ml; and agar, 1.5%, pH 7.2. (H. Reichenbach, personal communication).
3. Dung pellet agar: 5–6 rabbit dung pellets are placed in a Petri dish and partially covered with 1.5% agar containing 0.1% $CaCl_2 \cdot 2H_2O$, pH 7.2.
4. Sp agar: raffinose, 1g; sucrose, 1g; galactose, 1g; soluble starch, 5g; casitone, 2.5 g; K_2HPO_4, 0.25 g; $MgSO_4 \cdot 7H_2O$, 0.5 g; and agar, 15 g. For the growth of *Chondromyces* species, this medium is supple-

mented with *E. coli* extract (for details, see McCurdy, 1964). For routine cultivation of most bacteriolytic forms, the sugars are omitted.
5. Casitone-yeast extract agar: casitone, 2.5 g; $MgSO_4 \cdot 7H_2O$, 0.05 g; $CaCl_2 \cdot 2H_2O$, 0.05 g; yeast extract, 1 g; soluble starch, 0.5 g; and agar, 15 g, pH 7.2–7.4.

Enrichment of Cellulolytic Species

Each of the following media has proved useful for the isolation of cellulolytic polyangia:

6. Stanier's mineral salts agar (Stanier, 1942): KNO_3, 0.75 g; K_2HPO_4, 0.75 g; $MgSO_4 \cdot 7H_2O$, 0.2 g; $CaCl_2 \cdot 2H_2O$, 0.1 g; $FeCl_2$, 0.2 g; agar, 15 g; and H_2O, 1 l. My colleagues and I employ this medium adjusted to pH 6.0 and 7.4 for each sample. For inhibition of fungi, 3 μg Acti-Dione per ml are added.
7. Isolation medium 1 (IM-1) (McCurdy, 1969b): same as Stanier's medium but supplemented with 0.3 g cellobiose and 0.3 g casitone per l.

Each of these media is overlaid with filter paper or a thin agar overlay containing 0.5% cellulose powder and inoculated with finely crumbled soil or plant material. Cellulolytic polyangia appear as yellow, orange, brown or even black areas in which cellulolytic activity becomes obvious after 2–3 weeks. Transfer for purification purposes is best done from the swarm stage. IM-1 also permits isolation of some noncellulolytic species such as *Polyangium fumosum*, which are difficult to observe on other enrichments.

Isolation of Pure Cultures

Often, it is possible to obtain pure cultures by serial transfer of swarm edges which move ahead of contaminant bacterial growth. Frequent examination may be necessary to choose the best times for transfer.

When serial transfer fails, pure cultures may be obtained by plating dispersed vegetative cells. Portions of a swarm as free as possible from contaminating organisms are dispersed in DM (soluble starch, 0.5%; $MgSO_4 \cdot 7H_2O$, 0.05%; and K_2HPO_4, 0.025%, in distilled water) (McCurdy, 1963) in an Omnimixer or similar device with 200-μm glass beads. The suspension is serially diluted in DM and is surface- or pourplated by use of the previously described medium 1, 4 or 5.

Myxobacter colonies may take as long as a month to appear; thus plates should be incubated in adequate humidity. The colonies may also be difficult to detect. It is convenient to use a 60× dissecting microscope equipped with a mirror permitting "semi-darkfield" illumination to detect the thin surface and ephemeral subsurface colonies.

The cellulolytic polyangia are difficult to isolate. They are slow growing, and primary enrichments are rapidly overgrown with contaminants. Swarms should be transferred as soon as they are observed after dispersal and dilution. Suspensions should be spread on the surfaces of both filter paper and cellulose agar overlay plates as well as Stanier's medium containing 1% cellobiose or glucose, and the transfer is repeated as soon as colonies appear. The swarms of polyangia often penetrate deep into the agar, and this may be exploited by inverting the agar and transferring the penetrating growth.

Recently, Reichenbach (1983) described a new method for the purification of myxobacters in which antibiotics are used in high concentrations.

The purity of isolates may be confirmed by inoculation into trypticase broth, brain heart infusion and nutrient broth in which most myxobacters grow poorly or not at all.

Almost all myxobacters capable of fruiting may be preserved as fruiting bodies dried on agar over filter paper in a vacuum evaporator. However, the most convenient method is simply to grow them on slants of an appropriate medium in 5–10-ml screw-capped vials and store them at −70°C. By use of this method, cultures have been maintained for as long as 8 years. Myxobacters die out rapidly at temperatures of −18 to 4°C.

Procedures for Testing Special Characters

The identification of myxobacters is based primarily upon the morphology of their fruiting bodies, myxospores, swarms and vegetative cells. Differences in slime composition are detected by flooding vegetative colonies with 0.01% Congo red. Other tests are applied to the myxobacters according to conventional methods (McCurdy, 1969b), except where dispersed inocula are required (e.g. antibiotic sensitivity), in which case the swarms are dispersed by homogenization in the presence of 200-μm glass beads. Liquid cultivation of any of the myxobacters obtained in pure culture may be carried out in the previously described medium 4 or 5 with the agar omitted.

To induce fruiting body formation, media of low nutrient content are best. Among the media on which growth yields fruiting bodies are the previously described media 1 and 3. Medium 4, from which the sugars are omitted and in which the casitone concentration is reduced to 0.5 g/l, will also support fruiting. Transferring swarms from growth media to water agar ($CaCl_2 \cdot 2H_2O$, 0.17%; $MgSO_4 \cdot 7H_2O$, 0.05%; and agar, 1.5%) or to bacterial streaks on this medium is perhaps the best general method for fruiting body induction.

For further, more detailed consideration of methods for the isolation, cultivation and characterization of myxobacters, see Reichenbach and Dworkin, 1981; McCurdy, 1969b; Peterson, 1969; and Reichenbach, 1983.

Taxonomic Comments

The classification used here is the same as that used in the eighth edition of the *Manual* and is based upon the formal revisions proposed by McCurdy (1969b, 1970, and 1971a and b). Organisms of cell type I (the *Myxococcaceae*, *Cystobacteraceae* and *Archangiaceae*) were originally separated from those of cell type II (*Polyangiaceae*) on the basis of correlated differences in myxospore structure, adsorption of Congo red, and other cultural characteristics. Recent studies have confirmed the validity of the revised classification. Using ribosomal oligonucleotide cataloging, Ludwig et al. (1983) found the cell type I families to be closely related to one another but clearly separate from *Polyangium cellulosum* and *Nannocystis exedens* (cell type II, *Polyangiaceae*). Furthermore, Fautz et al. (1981) reported significant differences between these two groups in hydroxy fatty acid content: The *Polyangiaceae* contained none; members of the remaining families contained them in abundance.

Although no other classification has been formally published, Reichenbach (1974a) and Reichenbach and Dworkin (1981) have suggested a somewhat different classification (summarized in Table 24.1) from that used here. In it, the family *Polyangiaceae* is designated the "*Sorangiaceae*," and the order is divided into two suborders, the "*Cystobacterineae*" and "*Sorangineae*" (sic), based on the same cellular morphological differences previously noted. This classification, however, poses nomenclatural problems. As noted by McCurdy (1970), *Polyangium vitellinum* is the oldest myxobacter in the literature and must, therefore, be the nomenclatural type not only of the genus but also of the family, any proposed suborder and, indeed, the entire order.

Reichenbach and Dworkin have also proposed that the genus *Sorangium* be redefined to include only cellulolytic polyangia. However, Jahn's (1924) *Sorangium schroeteri*, considered by Peterson (1974) to be the same as *Polyangium sorediatum* (Thaxter, 1904), was not described as cellulolytic and, indeed, is too incompletely characterized for reidentification (i.e. no pure cultures; vegetative cells not described). If a type is designated for cellulolytic myxobacters, apparently it would have to be *Polyangium cellulosum* (Imshenetski and Solntzeva, 1936; McCurdy, 1970), although *Polyangium spumosum* (Krzemieniewska and Krzemieniewski, 1937b; McCurdy, 1970), if proved to be cellulolytic, could be an alternative candidate.

Since very few genera of the *Polyangiaceae* have been studied in any detail, it seems premature to erect additional genera such as *Sorangium*

or "*Haploangium*." The latter was suggested for polyangia with solitary sporangia in spite of their occurrence in other species (e.g. *Polyangium vitellinum*!). On the other hand, *Nannocystis* (sic) is so distinctive that its placement in a family separate from the *Polyangiaceae* might be justified (see the description of *Nannocystis exedens*).

The "*Cystobacterineae*" exhibit such a high degree of similarity in their 16S rRNA oligonucleotide catalogs, that a case might be made for making them a single family but, given their considerable morphological diversity, not for making them a single genus, as was suggested by Ludwig et al. (1983). In that case, the erection of a new suborder would then be superfluous rather than merely unnecessary.

The taxonomy of many of the *Myxococcales* is still largely based on the characteristics of the fruiting bodies, even though these structures are known to vary greatly in response to environmental influences and either may not be formed or are arrested in their development as a result of mutation or unfavorable conditions. Imperfectly formed fruiting bodies of certain species simulate the mature fruiting bodies of other members of the group. Accordingly, in identifying these organisms, it is essential to study fruiting body formation, preferably with pure cultures, under a wide range of defined nutritional and environmental conditions and over a considerable period of time. This principle has not always been followed in the taxonomy of the myxobacters, and the biochemical data conventionally used in bacterial taxonomy are often lacking.

It should be noted that the *Myxococcales* are unique among bacteria, in that in most cases the type materials are represented by herbarium specimens, not by type cultures. Such specimens, although often giving a good impression of fruiting body structure, offer little or no information about vegetative cell morphology and other phenotypic properties. Since future work with these organisms will undoubtedly be based on the comparative study of pure cultures, it would be desirable, insofar as possible, to designate type or neotype strains of each species. However, since the Code of Nomenclature of Bacteria does not cover this point and in the absence of a ruling by the Judicial Commission, after mention of the location of the type specimens the location of representative strains for all those species for which cultures are now available have been noted.

The following reviews may be consulted for further information about the general biology of the *Myxococcales*: Parish, 1979; White, 1981; Kaiser et al., 1979; and Rosenberg, 1984.

Table 24.1.
Taxonomy of the myxobacteria

Reichenbach and Dworkin (1981)	The *Manual*
Order "*Myxobacterales*"	Order *Myxococcales*
Suborder "*Cystobacterineae*"	Family I. *Myxococcaceae*
Family I. *Myxococcaceae*	Genus *Myxococcus*
Genus *Myxococcus*	Family II. *Archangiaceae*
Genus *Corallococcus*	Genus *Archangium*
Genus *Angiococcus*	Family III. *Cystobacteraceae*
Family II. *Archangiaceae*	Genus I. *Cystobacter*
Genus *Archangium*	Genus II. *Melittangium*
Family III. *Cystobacteraceae*	Genus III. *Stigmatella*
Genus *Cystobacter*	Family IV. *Polyangiaceae*
Genus *Melittangium*	Genus I. *Polyangium*
Genus *Stigmatella*	Genus II. *Nannocystis*
Suborder "*Sorangineae*"	Genus III. *Chondromyces*
Family "*Sorangiaceae*"	
Genus *Sorangium*	
Genus *Polyangium*	
Genus "*Haploangium*"	
Genus *Chondromyces*	
Genus *Nannocystis*	

Key to the families of the order **Myxococcales**

I. Vegetative cells tapered, microcysts produced
   A. Microcysts spherical or oval

   Family I. *Myxococcaceae*, p. 2144

   B. Microcysts rod-shaped
      1. Microcysts not in sporangia

   Family II. *Archangiaceae*, p. 2148

      2. Microcysts in sporangia

   Family III. *Cystobacteraceae*, p. 2149

II. Vegetative cells of uniform diameter with blunt, rounded ends; myxospores resemble vegetative cells

   Family IV. *Polyangiaceae*, p. 2158

FAMILY I. **MYXOCOCCACEAE** JAHN 1924, 84[AL]

E. R. BROCKMAN

Myx.o.coc.ca′ce.ae. M.L. masc. n. *Myxococcus* type genus of the family; -*aceae* ending to denote a family; M.L. fem. pl. n. *Myxococcaceae* the *Myxococcus* family.

Vegetative cells slender, straight to slightly tapered, flexible rods. **Refractile microcysts spherical or ellipsoidal.**

Type genus: *Myxococcus* Thaxter 1892, 403.

Genus **Myxococcus** *Thaxter 1892, 403*[AL]

E. R. BROCKMAN

Myx.o.coc′cus. Gr. fem. n. *myxa* mucus, slime; Gr. n. *coccus* berry; M.L. masc. n. *Myxococcus* slime coccus.

Vegetative cells are slender rods with tapering ends, 0.4–0.7 × 2.0–10.0 μm. Motile by gliding motility. Fruiting bodies contain **refractile, spherical or ellipsoidal microcysts** up to 2.3 μm in the largest dimension. The **microcysts are not enclosed in a sporangium.**

Chemoorganotrophs. Metabolism respiratory. Those which have been studied require several amino acids and are capable of hydrolyzing protein, starch, nucleic acids and various fatty acid esters. **Known to lyse bacteria, yeast and certain filamentous fungi.** Noncellulolytic. Strict aerobes. Fail to grow at 40°C or above. **Colonies adsorb Congo red.**

Resistant to 10-unit disks of penicillin. Sensitive to 10-μg disks of neomycin and tetracycline and to 5-μg disks of erythromycin.

The mol% G + C of the DNA of the examined species is in the range of 68–71 (Mandel and Leadbetter, 1965).

Type species: *Myxococcus fulvus* (Cohn) Jahn 1911, 198.

Further Comments

The species of this genus are free-living, may be isolated from soil and freshwater, and are common inhabitants on tree bark, dung of herbivorous animals, and decomposing vegetation. Fruiting body morphology, pigmentation and microcyst shape and size remain the major characteristics by which the species of this genus are identified.

In the following species descriptions, only those species that have been studied in pure culture have been accepted as valid species. In the eighth edition of the *Manual*, eight previously identified *Myxococcus* species were given *species incertae sedis* status, and it is possible that some of these organisms will, given future study, prove to be valid

species. In fact, one of these, *Myxococcus disciformis*, has now been examined (Hook et al., 1980) in sufficient detail to reclassify the organism; it is now placed in the genus *Cystobacter* on the basis that it forms myxospores within a definite sporangium.

Enrichment and Isolation Procedures

The details of the enrichment and isolation procedures for myxobacteria are well-described in the introductory remarks to the order and in the literature and will not be duplicated here. Myxobacteria have generally been isolated from tree bark, soils and dung of various animals and, on occasion, water. The moist chamber method (Gilbert and Martin, 1933) is generally used for tree bark samples. To obtain myxobacteria from soil and dung, the methods described by Dawid (1981), Kühlwein (1950), Kühlwein and Reichenbach (1965), McCurdy (1963, 1969b), Peterson (1969), Reichenbach and Dworkin (1981), Singh and Singh (1971), and Solntseve (1939) may be followed. Myxobacteria may be obtained from water by using the methods of Bernátová et al. (1980), Brauss et al. (1968), Brockman (1977), Gräf (1975), Raverdy (1973), and Roper and Marshall (1977). If a freshwater or distilled water medium is used, myxobacteria may also be isolated from seawater, especially coastal and estuarine waters (Brockman, 1973).

Maintenance Procedures

The methods described in the introductory remarks to the order and those described by Reichenbach and Dworkin (1981) may be used for the maintenance of myxobacterial cultures.

Differentiation of the genus **Myxococcus** *from other genera*

The genus *Myxococcus* is differentiated from other genera of the fruiting body-forming gliding bacteria in that its species have slender vegetative cells with slightly tapered ends and refractile, spherical or ellipsoidal microcysts produced within a fruiting body that is not bounded by a wall.

An abnormal fruiting body of *Archangium gephyra* could be confused with a fruiting body of a *Myxococcus* species. The *Archangium* species fruiting body, when placed in a wet mount and broken apart by pressure

applied to the coverslip, will fracture into irregular masses. Also, the microcysts of the *Archangium* species will normally be seen as very short rods, not spheres or ellipsoids.

Taxonomic Comments

There are several unsolved problems concerning the taxonomy of *Myxococcus* species, and future studies are required to clarify the present status of these species. Such studies might include a better understanding of the various morphological forms of fruiting bodies observed with *M. coralloides*: Is *M. blasticus* a true variant of *M. coralloides*? Which is most important to taxonomy, the size or the shape of the mycrocyst? Is the only difference between *M. xanthus* and *M. virescens* a single pigment? How stable is stalk formation, and is this a justification for a species status? These problems, and many others, require solutions before investigators will be satisfied with the taxonomy of this genus.

Although current and future methods that explore the molecular nature of these species will undoubtedly unravel distinct differences between them, the student who does not have access to such methods will require, on the other hand, clear, easy-to-use tests for the identification of an isolate. Tests with an emphasis on the physiology of the species are needed.

Further Reading

Beebe, J.M. 1941. Studies on myxobacteria. Iowa State Coll. J. Sci. *15:* 307–337.
Dawid, W. 1976. Fruchtkörperbildende Myxobakterien. I. Die *Myxococcus*—Arten. *M. fulvus, M. virescens, M. xanthus, M. stipitatus.* Mikrokosmos *65:* 72–79.
Krzemieniewska, H. and S. Krzemieniewski. 1926. Miksobakterje Polski (Die Myxobakterien von Polen). Acta Soc. Bot. Pol. *4:* 1–54.
Kühlwein, H. 1960. Zur Systematik und Verbreitung der Myxobakterien. Zentralbl. Bakteriol. Parasitenkd. Infektionskr. Hyg. Abt. II *113:* 480–490.
Solntseva, L.I. 1940. Biology of the myxobacteria. I. *Myxococcus* (in Russian with English summary). Mikrobiologiya *9:* 217–231.

Differentiation of the species of the genus **Myxococcus**

The differential characteristics of the species of the genus *Myxococcus* are indicated in Table 24.2.

List of species of the genus **Myxococcus**

1. **Myxococcus fulvus** (Cohn) Jahn 1911, 198.[AL] (*Micrococcus fulvus* Cohn 1875, 181.)*

ful'vus. L. adj. *fulvus* reddish-yellow.

Vegetative cells are slender, only slightly tapering with rounded ends, 0.4–0.8 (average: 0.6) $\times$ 5–9 (average: 6) μm (Fig. 24.3).

Fruiting bodies are spherical, elongated or pear-shaped and constricted below, may have a definite slimy stalk which usually does not persist, and at first are coherent but later are deliquescent. When moist, the fruiting bodies are white, pink, flesh-red, reddish orange or brownish red; when dry, they are deep red to brown; 150–400 μm (Fig. 24.4).

Microcysts are spherical to slightly oval, refractile and 1.4–1.5 μm (Fig. 24.5).

Colonies on casitone-Mg^{2+} agar are thin with a filamentous margin; at first, they are translucent, gray-white to light pink, and often yellow (particularly when grown in the dark), becoming more opaque, light flesh-colored to reddish orange to pink and even purple (when grown in the light). Growth is similar on *Escherichia coli* medium but less pigmented and with moderate lysis; concentric zones of fruiting bodies are formed in the central portion of the colony (Fig. 24.6).

Vegetative cell pigment is extracted with methyl alcohol (Reichenbach and Kleinig, 1971; Meckel and Kester, 1980).

Sporopollenin is found in both vegetative cells and microcysts (Strohl et al., 1977).

Optimum pH: 6.5–7.0. Temperature range: 18–37°C; optimum: 26–30°C.

Table 24.2.

Differential characteristics of the species of the genus **Myxococcus**[a]

Characteristic	1. *M. fulvus*	2. *M. virescens*	3. *M. xanthus*	4. *M. stipitatus*	5. *M. coralloides*	6. *M. macrosporus*
Fruiting bodies deliquescent	+	+	+	+	−	−
Fruiting bodies raised on a well-defined, persistent stalk	±	−	−	+	−	−
Fruiting bodies fluoresce under ultraviolet light[b]	−	−	−	+	−	−
Microcysts 2.5 μm or more in diameter	−	+	+	−	−	+
Color of vegetative cell masses						
Yellow	−	+	+	+	−	−
Buff to tan	−	−	−	−	d	d
Flesh-colored to reddish-orange	+	−	−	−	d	d
Greenish diffusible pigment on agar	−	+	−	−	−	−
Hydrolyzes starch in 3 days or less	−	−	−	−	+	+[c]
Hydrolyzes esculin	−	−	−	−	±	−
Oxidase	−	−	−	+	−	−

[a] Characteristics determined on casitone-Mg^{2+} (McCurdy, 1969). Symbols: +, 90% or more of strains are positive; −, 90% or more of the strains are negative; ±, indefinite; and d, substantial portions of the species differ.
[b] Lampky and Brockman, 1977.
[c] Only one strain tested.

---

* **Editorial note:** Jahn (1924, 85) noted two varieties: var. *albus*, which is white and has small fruiting bodies, and var. *minatus*, which is cinnabarred or red-lead in color and has large fruiting bodies.

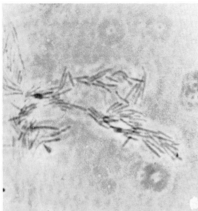

Figure 24.3.   *M. fulvus* vegetative cells. Phase-contrast micrograph (× 1000). (Reproduced with permission from W. Dawid, Mikrokosmos *65:* 74, 1976, ©Franckh'sche Verlagshandlung, Stuttgart.)

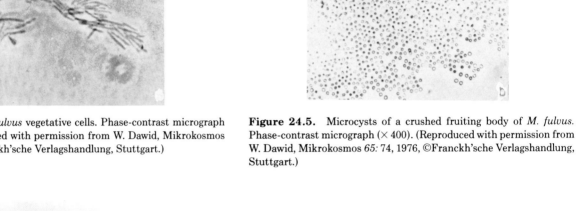

Figure 24.5.   Microcysts of a crushed fruiting body of *M. fulvus.* Phase-contrast micrograph (× 400). (Reproduced with permission from W. Dawid, Mikrokosmos *65:* 74, 1976, ©Franckh'sche Verlagshandlung, Stuttgart.)

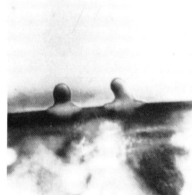

Figure 24.4.   Mature fruiting bodies of *M. fulvus.* Light micrograph (× 100). (Reproduced with permission from W. Dawid, Mikrokosmos *65:* 75, 1976, ©Franckh'sche Verlagshandlung, Stuttgart.)

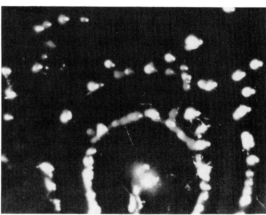

Figure 24.6.   Concentric ring formation of fruiting bodies of *M. fulvus* that formed after 7 days of incubation on *E. coli* agar. Light micrograph (× 25). (Reproduced with permission from W. Dawid, Mikrokosmos *65:* 75, 1976, ©Franckh'sche Verlagshandlung, Stuttgart.)

Gelatin is liquefied, casein is digested, starch is hydrolyzed, and growth occurs with a variety of filter sterilized carbohydrates.

This organism is resistant to 5-μg streptomycin disks. Sensitive to 10-μg chloramphenicol and kanamycin disks. Growth is inhibited by sulfadiazine (1.2 μg/ml), aureomycin (5.0 μg/ml), chloramphenicol (10 μg/ml), penicillin (20 μg/ml) and streptomycin (500 μg/ml) (Henis and Kletter, 1963).

Very common on dung-soil plates and on bacterial streaks inoculated with soil; also observed frequently on decaying plant material, the dung of various animals, and lichens. Found in freshwater and even littoral seawater.

The mol% G + C of the DNA is 69–71 (Bd) (Mandel and Leadbetter, 1965).

Reference strain: University of Windsor M17, ATCC 25199.

Other typical strains: University of Windsor M7 and M16.

Illustrations

Cohn, 1875, Plate b, Fig. 18; Baur, 1905, Figs. 1–3, and Plate 4, Figs. 1–13 and 16; Jahn, 1924, Figs. L–N, p. 43, and Fig. R, p. 47; Krzemieniewska and Krzemieniewski, 1928, Plate 1, Fig. 3, Plate 2, Fig. 14, and Plate 3, Figs. 38 and 40; Kühlwein, 1950, Figs. 2, 3, 5 and 6; Oetker, 1953, Figs. 2–5, 7, 8 and 12; Nolte, 1957, Figs. 1, 2, 4*b* and 5*a*; Reichenbach, 1966, Fig. 4; McCurdy, 1969b, Fig. 3; Peterson, 1969, Figs. 3 and 4; Smit and Clark, 1971, Plate 1 (*e, f*) and Plate 2 (*a*,

b); McNeil and Skerman, 1972, Figs. 21–24; Rückert, 1972, Fig. 7; Brockman and Todd, 1974, Fig. 1; Bisset, 1974, Figs. 1–4, and 1975, Figs. 1–10; Dawid, 1976a, Figs. 1–6.

2. **Myxococcus virescens** Thaxter 1892, 404.[AL]

vi.res′cens. L. part. adj. *virescens* green.

Vegetative cells are slender, tapered rods 0.4–0.8 (0.7) × 5–9 (7) μm.

Fruiting bodies are spherical to elongated, yellow to greenish yellow (in culture on artificial media, they easily become white; they become deliquescent in continued moisture), and 150–500 μm.

Microcysts are refractile, spherical and 1.7–2.3 μm in diameter.

Vegetative colonies grown on casitone-Mg^{2+} agar are thin, with many fine intertwining radiating lines and an indefinite edge, are yellowish white to yellow, and are clear in the central portion with formation of fruiting bodies. A diffusible green pigment develops on continued incubation. Colonies on *E. coli* medium are thinner and less pigmented with numerous fruiting bodies in concentric zones; lysis is moderate.

Sporopollenin is found in both vegetative cells and myxospores (Strohl et al., 1977).

This organism utilizes starch, inulin and sucrose (Beebe, 1943).

Optimum pH: 6.5–7.0. Temperature range: 18–37°C; optimum: 28°C.

Resistant to 5-μg streptomycin disks. Sensitive to 10-μg chloramphenicol and kanamycin disks.

Originally obtained on decaying matter from soil and dung of various animals. One of the earliest and most frequently encountered myxobacters on dung in contact with soil. Also isolated from river water (Raverdy, 1973).

The mol% G + C of the DNA is 68–70 (Bd) (Mandel and Leadbetter, 1965).

Type material: Farlow Herbarium, Harvard University, Cambridge, Massachusetts (U.S.A.).

Reference strain: University of Windsor M22, ATCC 25203.

Another typical strain: University of Windsor M100.

Illustrations

Krzemieniewska and Krzemieniewski, 1926, Plate I, Figs. 6 and 9; Krzemieniewska and Krzemieniewski, 1927, Plate 1, Figs. 1 and 6, Plate 2, Fig. 26, and Plate 3, Figs. 32–34; Badian, 1930, Plate 8; Oetker, 1953, Fig. 9; Reichenbach, 1966, Fig. 1; McCurdy, 1969b, Fig. 1; McNeil and Skerman, 1972, Figs. 19 and 20; Rückert, 1972, Fig. 10; Ståhl, 1972, Figs. 1 and 2; Dawid, 1974, Figs. 1, 5 and 7–13; Rückert, 1975, Fig. 2 (*right*); Dawid, 1976a, Figs. 11–15.

3. Myxococcus xanthus Beebe 1941, 195.[AL]

xan′thus. Gr. adj. *xanthus* orange, golden.

Vegetative cells are slender, flexible rods 0.5–1.0 (average: 0.75) × 4.0–10 (average: 5) μm.

Fruiting bodies are spherical to subspherical, constricted at the base, occasionally irregular from fusion of adjacent masses; up to 300–400 μm in diameter; and color constant, light yellowish orange to bright orange, yellow and tan but never greenish yellow (pigmentation varies with the medium).

Microcysts are refractile, spherical and 1.7–2.2 (2.0) μm in diameter.

Vegetative colonies resemble those of *M. virescens*, but no diffusible green pigment is produced.

Sporopollenin is found in both vegetative cells and microcysts (Strohl et al., 1977).

This organism may be cultured on a variety of synthetic media (Reichenbach and Dworkin, 1981).

Optimum pH: 7.2–8.2. Optimum temperature: 30°C; maximum growth range: 34–36°C (Janssen et al., 1977).

Resistant to 5-μg streptomycin disks. Sensitive to 10-μg chloramphenicol and kanamycin disks.

Originally obtained on dried cow dung. Common on sterile dung in contact with soil or soil inoculated bacterial streaks on water agar. Also found in surface freshwater and even coastal seawater (Brockman, 1973).

The mol% G + C of the DNA is 69.3–71.2 (Mandel and Leadbetter, 1965) and 67.1 (McCurdy and Wolf, 1967).

Reference strain: Dworkin (1962) strain FB, NCIB 9412 ATCC 19368.

Illustrations

Beebe, 1941, Figs. 1–28; Voelz and Dworkin, 1962, Figs. 1–11; Reichenbach, 1966, Figs. 5 and 8; Voelz, 1966, Figs. 1–4; Bacon and Eiserling, 1968, Figs. 1 and 2; Kühlwein, 1969, Figs. 3, *a* and *b*; McCurdy, 1969b, Fig. 2; Brockman and Todd, 1974, Fig. 2; Shimkets and Seale, 1975, Figs. 2–20; Dawid, 1976a, Figs. 7–10; MacRae and McCurdy, 1976, Figs. 1, *c* and *d*, 2, *a–d*, and 3, *a–d*.

4. Myxococcus stipitatus Thaxter 1897, 408.[AL]

sti.pi.ta′tus. L. masc. n. *stipes, stipitis* trunk, stalk; M.L. adj. *stipitatus* stalked.

Vegetative rods are slender, occasionally slightly tapering, flexible and 0.5–0.7 × 2.0–7.0 μm.

Fruiting bodies have a spore mass which is nearly spherical, milky or yellowish white to slightly pink and are up to 200 μm in diameter; they are raised on a stalk which may be as long as 200 μm and 30–50 μm in diameter. On artificial media, fruiting bodies are variable; stalks may be poorly developed, and adjacent fruiting bodies may fuse to form irregular rounded masses. When exposed to long wave ultraviolet light (320–380 nm), the fruiting bodies fluoresce yellowish green (Lampky and Brockman, 1977).

Microcysts are spherical (1.8 μm) to ellipsoidal (1.1–1.4 × 1.3–1.8 μm), optically dense or slightly refractile.

Vegetative colonies on casitone-Mg²⁺ agar (McCurdy, 1963) are grayish or yellowish white, flat, myceloid and almost moldlike. Fruiting body formation is seldom observed on *E. coli* medium or casitone-Mg²⁺ agar. Vegetative growth has yellowish-green fluorescence when it is exposed to long-wave ultraviolet light.

In liquid media, growth is luxuriant in the form of distinctive cottony, moldlike spheres. This organism is capable of growth in ordinary bacteriological media, e.g. nutrient broth or trypticase broth.

Sporopollenin is found in both vegetative cells and microcysts (Strohl et al., 1977).

Temperature range: 18–37°C.

Resistant to 5-μg streptomycin disks. Sensitive to 10-μg chloramphenicol and kanamycin disks.

Originally isolated on dung in laboratory cultures from Maine and Tennessee (U.S.A.). Has been isolated from various soils, tree bark, surface water and coastal seawater.

Type material: Farlow Herbarium, Harvard University, Cambridge, Massachusetts.

Reference strain: University of Windsor M78.

Illustrations

Thaxter, 1897, Plate 31, Figs. 30–33; Krzemieniewska and Krzemieniewski, 1926, Plate I, Figs. 10–12, and Plate II, Figs. 13 and 14; McCurdy, 1969b, Fig. 4; Smit and Clark, 1971, Plate 2, Fig. e; McNeil and Skerman, 1972, Figs. 19 and 20; Brockman and Todd, 1974, Figs. 3 and 4; Rückert, 1975, Fig. 2 (*middle*); Dawid, 1976a, Figs. 16 and 17.

5. Myxococcus coralloides Thaxter 1892, 404.[AL]

co.ral.lo.i′des or co.ral.loi′des. Gr. neut. n. *corallium* coral; Gr. n. *eidus* shape; M.L. adj. *coralloides* corallike.

Vegetative cells are slightly tapered rods 0.5–0.8 (average: 0.6) × 4–8 (average: 6) μm.

Fruiting bodies are firm, not deliquescent, and are extremely variable in shape, size and color, ranging from simple, barely visible papillae (<25 μm) or straight or branched tubules recumbent on the substrate, to erect, simple or branched columnar structures (20–30 × 50–250 μm). Or they may be flattened, cushionlike and constricted below, forming a short stalk (25–40 μm), while in other instances, they consist of irregular corallike masses up to 300 μm in size with constricted lobes and fingerlike outgrowths. Fruiting bodies may be flesh-colored, pink, reddish orange, orange or buff in different strains. When formed on agar media, the fruiting bodies often extend taprootlike into the underlying agar.

Microcysts are spherical, optically dense or refractile, 1.0–1.5 μm in diameter.

Colonies on casitone-Mg²⁺ agar are flat and thin with densely radiating lines. The color corresponds to that of the fruiting bodies, which are densely arranged in concentric rings and various other patterns in the central portion of the colony. Growth on *E. coli* medium is similar but less pigmented; lysis is moderate, and the underlying agar may be eroded. A brownish diffusible pigment is produced by some strains in old cultures.

Optimum pH: 7.0–7.5. Temperature range: 18–37°C; optimum: 25–30°C.

This organism is sensitive to 5-μg streptomycin disks and to 10-μg chloramphenicol and kanamycin disks.

Originally reported on lichens but very common on sterile dung in contact with soil, on moist bark and on bacterial streaks over agar inoculated with soil. Also frequently isolated from surface waters and coastal seawater.

The mol% G + C of the DNA is 67.6–68.1 (McCurdy and Wolfe, 1967).

Type material: Farlow Herbarium, Harvard University, Cambridge, Massachusetts.

Reference strain: University of Windsor M2, ATCC 25202.
Other typical strains: University of Windsor M1 and M25.

Illustrations

Thaxter, 1892, Plate 24, Figs. 29–33;Quehl, 1906, Plate 1, Figs. 1 and 9; Kofler, 1913, Figs. 4, 9 and 11; Jahn, 1924, Fig. Y, *a–h*; Krzemieniewska and Krzemieniewski, 1926, Table II, Fig. 20; Mishustin, 1942, Figs. 1–7; Reichenbach, 1962, Figs. 1–8, and 1966, Figs. 6,7 and 9; McCurdy, 1969b, Figs. 5–7; McNeil and Skerman, 1972, Figs. 17 and 18; Rückert, 1972, Fig. 8; Brockman and Todd, 1974, Figs. 5 and 6; Dawid, 1975, Figs. 1–22; Rückert, 1975, Fig. 2 (*left*).

6. **Myxococcus macrosporus** (Krzemieniewska and Krzemieniewski) Zahler and McCurdy 1974, 82.[AL] (*Chondrococcus macrosporus* Krzemieniewska and Krzemieniewski 1926, 16.)

ma.cro.spor′us. Gr. adj. *macros* long, large; Gr. n. *spora* seed; M.L. adj. *macrosporus* large-spored.

Vegetative cells are slender rods 0.4–0.5 × 7–8 μm.

Fruiting bodies are similar to those of *M. coralloides*, with or without projections of varying length, and yellow or light brown.

Microcysts are 1.6–2.0 μm in diameter.

Vegetative growth resembles that of *M. coralloides.*

The organism is resistant to 5-μg streptomycin disks and 10-μg chloramphenicol and kanamycin disks.

Originally obtained on leaves but also cultivated from soil with sterile rabbit dung. Not common.

Reference strain: University of Windsor M271.

Illustrations

Krzemieniewska and Krzemieniewski, 1926, Plate II, Fig. 19; Singh and Singh, 1971, Figs. 21–24.

FAMILY II. **ARCHANGIACEAE** JAHN 1924, 66[AL]

HOWARD D. MCCURDY

Ar.chan.gi.a′ce.ae. M.L. neut. n. *Archangium* type genus of the family; -*aceae* ending to denote a family; M.L. fem. pl. n. *Archangiaceae* the *Archangium* family.

The vegetative rods are slender with **tapered** ends. The **microcysts** are **very short rods, ellipsoids or spheres** which are never enclosed in sporangia; the **fruiting bodies consist of irregular masses** or projections of variable dimensions.

Type genus: *Archangium* Jahn 1924, 66.

Further Comments

Only one species, *Archangium gephyra,* is sufficiently well-characterized and distinguished from other myxobacter species to warrant rec-

ognition. It shows clear affinities to the *Myxococcaceae* and might well be included in that family. Several species described in the literature and included in the eighth edition of the *Manual* as *species incertae sedis* are now omitted. Because of the lack of pure culture data, generally inadequate descriptions and the absence of striking morphological features, they would be impossible to differentiate from immature variant fruiting bodies which are frequently observed in other, well-characterized species. Such variants are especially common in *Stigmatella, Cystobacter* and *Polyangium.*

Genus **Archangium** *Jahn 1924, 66*[AL]

HOWARD D. MCCURDY

Ar.chan′gi.um. Gr. fem. n. *arche* beginning, primitive; Gr. neut. n. *angium* vessel, receptacle; *Archangium* primitive vessel.

Vegetative cells are slender, **tapered,** flexible **rods.**

Sporangia are lacking; and fruiting bodies are irregular in form, swollen or brainlike, consisting internally of intestinelike twisted or intertwined masses with **no definite slime wall.**

Microcysts are **very short rods, ellipsoids or spheres** and are refractile or optically dense.

Vegetative colonies do not etch or erode agar media. Congo red is adsorbed.

Type species: *Archangium gephyra* Jahn 1924, 67.

List of species of the genus **Archangium**

1. **Archangium gephyra** Jahn 1924, 67.[AL]
ge′phy.ra. Gr. n. *gephyra* bridge.

Vegetative cells resemble those of *Cystobacter minus* and are slightly tapered with slightly swollen rounded ends 0.4–0.7 × 6–15 μm (Fig. 24.7).

The fruiting bodies (Fig. 24.8) are very variable in size and shape. They usually consist of an irregular, brainlike or elongated mass with a padded or swollen surface; this mass is firm in consistency. By reflected light, the color of these fruiting bodies is variable, light rose or reddish flesh-colored to orange. Later, when these bodies are observed on a dark background, they appear bluish violet. By transmitted light, the fruiting bodies appear yellowish to light red. When they are dry, they appear orange to red.

Internally, the fruiting body consists of a mesenteric mass of tubules which are periodically interrupted by cross-walls that may not entirely cut through the microcyst masses from one side to the other. The tubules, when pressed between slide and coverslip, break up into a number of irregularly rounded or polygonal masses 15–30 μm in diameter. Within these, the microcysts lie parallel in bundles.

Microcysts (Fig. 24.9) are spherical, oval or short, often bean-shaped, rods, optically dense or refractile, and 1.0–2.0 × 1.5–2.8 μm.

Vegetative colonies on agar media are thin, with many radiating ridges and concentric folds. The edge is thin, with tonguelike extensions. The colonies are orange in areas of cell accumulations. Slime production is moderate; colonies may be cut easily but readily adhere to a needle.

Growth on casitone-Mg²⁺ broth (McCurdy, 1969b) is slight and in the form of tight orange globules or rounded masses in shake culture. Growth is substantially improved by the addition of 0.1–0.2% agar.

This organism is easily cultivated on the usual complex media used for noncellulolytic myxobacters. Nitrate is not reduced, catalase and oxidase are produced. Esculin, starch (3 days), casein, gelatin, Tween 80, indoxyl acetate, RNA and DNA are hydrolyzed. It is noncellulolytic.

Aerobic. Optimum pH: 7.5. Temperature range: 18–40°C; optimum: 18–32°C.

Antibiotic sensitivity (disks): resistant to penicillin (10 units); sensitive to neomycin (10 μg), streptomycin (5 μg), tetracycline (10 μg), chloramphenicol (10 μg), kanamycin (10 μg) and erythromycin (5 μg).

Figure 24.7. *A. gephyra* vegetative cells. Light micrograph (× 3000).

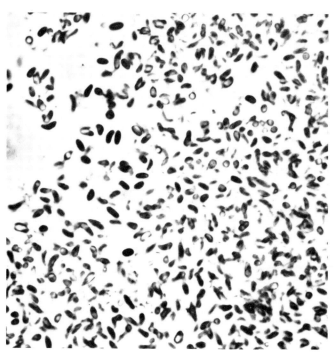

Figure 24.9. *A. gephyra* microcysts. Light micrograph (× 1000).

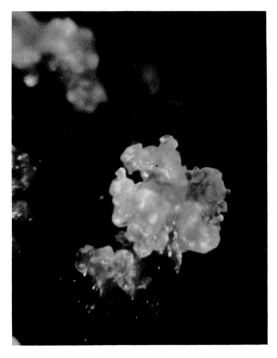

Figure 24.8. *A. gephyra* fruiting body on dung. Light micrograph (× 30).

Source and habitat: frequently observed on sterile rabbit dung in contact with soil and on *Escherichia coli* streaks over agar inoculated with soil.

The mol% G + C of the DNA is 67.8–68.3 (T_m).

Reference strain: Windsor M18, ATCC 25201.

Illustrations

Quehl, 1906, Plate 1, Fig. 7; Jahn, 1924, Plate 1, Fig. 5; Krzemieniewska and Krzemieniewski, 1936, Plate III, Figs. 25 and 26; McCurdy, 1969b, Fig. 8 (color); Dawid, 1976b, Fig. 3, and 1981, Plate II, Fig. 6, Plate III, Fig. 2, and Plate IV, Fig. 3.

FAMILY III. **CYSTOBACTERACEAE** McCURDY 1970, 286[AL]

HOWARD D. MCCURDY

Cys.to.bac.ter.a′ce.ae. M.L. *Cystobacter* type genus of the family; *-aceae* ending to denote a family; M.L. fem. pl. n. *Cystobacteraceae* the *Cystobacter* family.

Vegetative cells are tapered flexible **rods** which are converted to **refractile** or **phase-dense, rod-shaped microcysts** enclosed in **sporangia** of definite shape. The sporangia may be sessile, occurring singly or in groups and enclosed in a slime membrane or envelope, or may be borne on stalks (sporangiophores) which may be simple or branched. The sporangia may be solitary or in clusters at the tips of the stalks.

Vegetative colonies **do not etch or erode agar. Congo red is adsorbed** by the vegetative slime. All of the examined species grow well on media containing enzymatically hydrolyzed protein, starch and salts. **Bacteriolytic. Noncellulolytic.**

Key to the genera of the family **Cystobacteraceae**

I. Sporangia sessile
> Genus I. *Cystobacter*, p. 2150

II. Sporangia stalked
> A. Sporangia borne singly on an unbranched stalk
>> Genus II. *Melittangium*, p. 2153
> B. Sporangia borne singly or in clusters on branched or unbranched stalks
>> Genus III. *Stigmatella*, p. 2156

Genus I. **Cystobacter** *Schroeter 1886, 170*[AL]

HOWARD D. McCURDY

Cys.to.bac'ter. Gr. n. *cystis* bladder; M.L. n. *bacter* the masculine equivalent of the Gr. neut. n. *bakterion* a small rod; M.L. masc. n. *Cystobacter* bladder-forming rod.

Vegetative cells are slender, **tapered,** flexible rods.

Sporangia are usually sessile, occurring singly or in groups rounded, elongated or coiled and surrounded by a definite slime envelope or wall; they are either free or embedded in a second slimy layer.

Microcysts are rod-shaped, phase-dense or refractile, and rigid.

Vegetative colonies do not etch or erode agar media. **Congo red is adsorbed.**

The minimum nutritional requirements are now known, but all species are easily cultivated on media containing enzymatically hydrolyzed protein, salts and starch or glycogen. The latter is not utilized. **Cellulose is not digested.**

Type species: *Cystobacter fuscus* Schroeter 1886, 170.

Key to the species of the genus **Cystobacter**

I. Sporangia rounded, spherical to disk-shaped
> A. Sporangia rounded or spherical
>> a. Sporangia dark brown, 60 µm
>>> 1. *C. fuscus*
>> b. Sporangia pink to light brown, 60 µm
>>> 2. *C. minus*
> B. Sporangia disk-shaped, spheroidal or irregular; occasionally stipitate
>> 3. *C. disciformis*

II. Sporangia elongated or coiled
> 4. *C. ferrugineus*

List of species of the genus **Cystobacter**

1. **Cystobacter fuscus** Schroeter 1886, 170.[AL]

fus'cus. L. adj. *fuscus* dark, tawny.

Vegetative cells (Fig. 24.10) are distinctly tapered rods 0.6–0.8 × 3–20 µm (exponential cells are 0.65 × 8–10 µm).

Sporangia (Fig. 24.11) are smooth, flesh-colored when young, light to dark chestnut-brown when ripe, spherical, oval or elongated, and 50–130 µm in diameter with a definite wall, occurring singly or in groups of up to 100 or more (sori) and embedded in a glossy cohesive matrix. Sori are flat or heaped, occasionally with chains of sporangia raised in fingerlike projections. In some forms, the matrix is replaced by a folded outer membranelike layer.

Microcysts (Figs. 24.12 and 24.13) are rod-shaped, often fusiform, on the micrograph and bent, optically dense or definitely refractile, 0.4–1.5 × 2.5–5.0 µm.

Vegetative colonies on casitone-Mg^{2+} agar are rapid-growing, thick, and flat initially but with a definite edge later exhibiting prominent veins, ridges and accumulations with pointed extensions at the edge. When young, the colonies are yellow to yellowish-orange, becoming salmon or brownish orange with age. Older colonies are smooth, mucoid and translucent. A brownish pigment may diffuse into the medium. The vegetative slime is tenacious and difficult to cut; the colony is easily lifted intact from the agar surface. The colonies on *Escherichia coli* medium and dung pellet agar are similar but thinner and less pigmented. Clearing of *E. coli* medium is extensive. Fruiting bodies are produced on both media by freshly isolated strains.

Growth in casitone-Mg^{2+} broth is luxuriant, yellow to orange, and in the form of loose spheres or as a dense turbidity. The medium becomes viscous and turns brown with age.

This organism is easily cultivated on the usual complex media employed for the noncellulolytic myxobacteria. Nitrate is not reduced. Catalase-positive and oxidase-negative. Esculin, starch (3 days), casein, gelatin, Tween 80, indoxyl acetate, RNA and DNA are hydrolyzed. Urease is produced. Cellulose is not hydrolyzed.

Aerobic. Optimum pH: 6.9–8.2. Temperature range: 18–40°C.

Antibiotic sensitivity (disks): resistant to neomycin (10 µg) and penicillin (10 units); inhibited by tetracycline (10 µg), chloramphenicol (10 µg), kanamycin (10 µg), streptomycin (5 µg) and erythromycin (5 µg).

Source and habitat: originally obtained on rabbit dung from California (U.S.A.). Commonly obtained on moist bark and rabbit placed in contact with soil.

The mol% G + C of the DNA is 68.3 (T_m).

Reference strain: Windsor M31, ATCC 25194.

Illustrations

Thaxter, 1897, Plate 31, Figs. 37–39; Baur, 1905, Plate 4, Figs. 14, 15 and 17; Quehl, 1906, Plate 1, Figs. 8 and 16; Jahn, 1924, Plate 2, Fig. 12, and Fig. A, p. 9; Krzemieniewska and Krzemieniewski, 1926, Plate IV, Figs. 42 and 43; McCurdy, 1969b, Fig. 26 (color), and 1970, Figs. 4–6; Reichenbach and Dworkin, 1981, Plate II, Fig. b.

2. **Cystobacter minus** (Krzemieniewska and Krzemieniewski) McCurdy 1970, 288.[AL] (*Polyangium minus* Krzemieniewska and Krzemieniewski 1926, 33.)

mi'nus. L. neut. adj. *minus* less, smaller.

Vegetative cells are 0.6–0.8 × 3–11 µm and slightly tapered with somewhat swollen rounded ends as in *Archangium gephyra*.

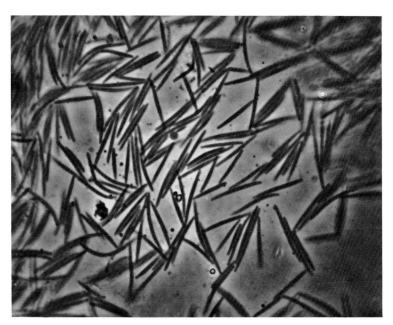

Figure 24.10. *C. fuscus* vegetative cells. Light micrograph (× 1350).

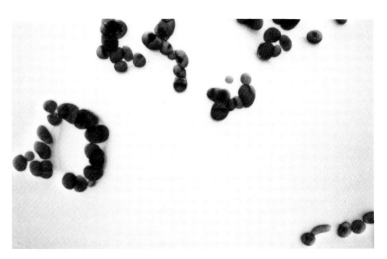

Figure 24.11. *C. fuscus* fruiting bodies. Light micrograph (× 45).

Sporangia (Fig. 24.14) are spherical or oval, 20–70 × 20–50 μm; pale pink at first, later becoming brownish; with definite walls 0.5–1.0 μm thick that are transparent, revealing contents. Sporangia are covered by a thin, transparent slime and occur in flat accumulations of up to 0.5 mm². A secondary sporangium may be formed within the first as a result of contraction of the contents and the formation of a new wall.

Microcysts are phase-dense or refractile, oval to short rod-shaped, and 0.8–1.2 × 1.3–2.7 μm.

Vegetative colonies on casitone-Mg²⁺ agar are at first grayish translucent or slightly pink with a definite edge. Later, the edge becomes thin and ill-defined. The surface is marked by many loosely spiralling lines. Colonies can be cultivated on casitone-Mg²⁺, *E. coli* medium and yeast-Ca²⁺ agars.

Nitrate is not reduced. Catalase is produced. This organism is oxidase-negative, hydrolyzes starch, esculin, RNA and DNA, is urease-negative, and does not digest cellulose.

Aerobic. Temperature range: 18–37°C; optimum: 28–30°C.

Antibiotic sensitivity (disks): inhibited by tetracycline (10 μg) and chloramphenicol (10 μg); resistant to neomycin (10 μg), kanamycin (10 μg), streptomycin (5 μg) and erythromycin (5 μg).

Source and habitat: first isolated from sterilized rabbit dung placed in contact with soil (Poland); may be obtained from soil placed on *Micrococcus luteus* streaks on water agar.

Relatively slow in appearing but not uncommon.

Reference strain: Windsor M307.

Illustrations

Krzemieniewska and Krzemieniewski, 1926, Plate IV, Figs. 47 and 48, and Plate V, Fig. 49; McCurdy, 1969b, Fig. 30, and 1970, Figs. 9–11.

3. **Cystobacter disciformis** (Thaxter) Brockman and McCurdy comb. nov. (*Myxococcus disciformis* Thaxter 1904, 412; *Angiococcus disciformis* (Thaxter) Jahn 1924, 89; *Angiococcus disciformis* (ex Jahn 1924) Hook, Larkin and Brockman 1980, 142.)

dis.ci.for′mis. Gr. n. *discus* a disk; L. n. *forma* form; M.L. adj. *disciformis* disk-shaped.

Vegetative cells are 0.5–0.7 × 5–10 μm.

Fruiting bodies: Sporangia are spheroidal, flattened, disk-shaped or irregular, 25–30 × 30–45 μm, solitary or in heaped groups with many attached directly to one another, interconnected by dried slime. Occasionally borne on slime sporangiophores. At first, they are yellowish, later becoming deep orange.

This organism grows in casitone-Mg^{2+} broth, but growth characteristics have not been described. Cultivated on dilute nutrient, casitone-Mg^{2+} and yeast-Ca^{2+} agars. The agar is not etched.

Catalase is produced. This organism hydrolyzes starch and casein but not urea, DNA or cellulose and is cytochrome oxidase-negative.

Temperature range: 19–34°C; optimum: 28–30°C.

Originally observed on muskrat and deer dung. Apparently common in forest and bog soils within the pH range of 3.6–6.4.

The mol% G + C of the DNA is 68.4 (Bd).

Reference strain: Central Michigan University strain CMU-1 (ATCC 33172).

Illustrations

Thaxter, 1904, Plate 27, Figs. 19–21; Krzemieniewska and Krzemieniewski, 1926, Plate II, Figs. 21 and 22; Hook et al., 1980, Figs. 1–5.

4. **Cystobacter ferrugineus** (Krzemieniewska and Krzemieniewski) McCurdy 1970, 288.[AL] (*Polyangium ferrugineum* Krzemieniewska and Krzemieniewski 1927, 89.)

fer.ru.gi′ne.us. L. adj. *ferrugineus* of the color of iron rust.

Vegetative cells are tapered with rounded ends, 0.6–0.8 × 4–15 μm.

Resting accumulations (Fig. 24.15) consist of irregular, branched and, occasionally, constricted coils. At first, these accumulations are grayish or flesh-colored, later becoming bright orange-yellow, orange-red or reddish brown. The enclosing membrane, when present, may be absent or difficult to observe, bearing the imprints of the enclosed microcysts. The external slime is colorless to yellow-orange.

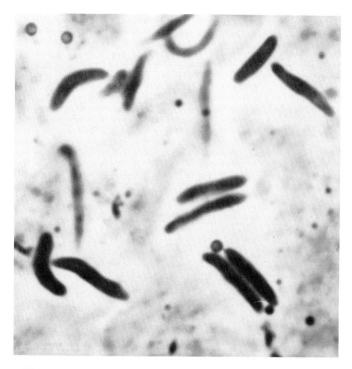

Figure 24.12. *C. fuscus* microcysts. Light micrograph (× 4000).

Figure 24.13. *C. fuscus* microcysts. Electron micrograph of thin section. *E*, envelope; *SC*, spore coat. *Bar,* 450 nm.

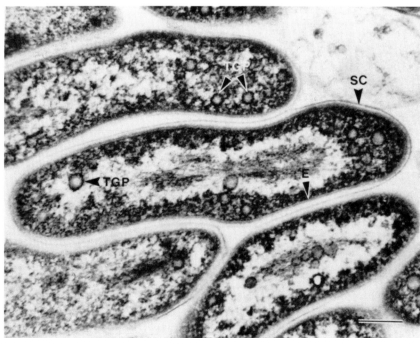

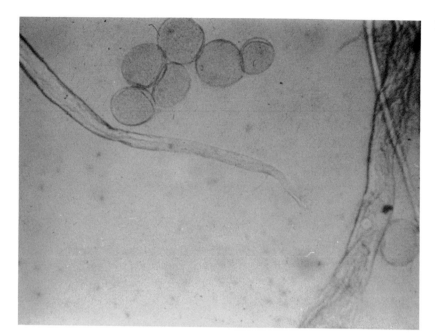

Figure 24.14. *C. minus* sporangia. × 270.

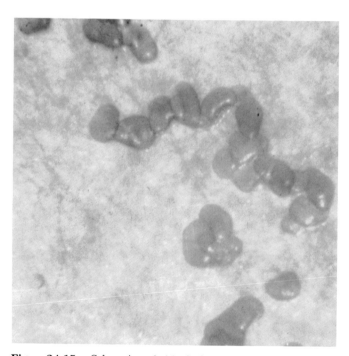

Microcysts are phase-dense or refractile, rigid, oval to short rod-shaped with rounded ends, 1.1–1.8 × 1.8–5 μm.

Vegetative colonies are grayish white to slightly salmon-colored with many fine radiating ridges and concentric ripples, later clearing in the center. The edge is slightly raised at first, later becoming thin with tonguelike extensions.

Cultivated easily on casitone-Mg^{2+}, *E. coli* medium and dung pellet agar. Oxidase- and urease-negative. Esculin is not hydrolyzed.

Aerobic. Maximum temperature: 37°C; optimum: 27–30°C.

Antibiotic sensitivity (disks): inhibited by tetracycline (10 μg), chloramphenicol (10 μg) and erythromycin (5 μg); resistant to neomycin (10 μg), streptomycin (5 μg) and penicillin (10 units). Its response to kanamycin (10 μg) is variable.

Originally obtained from Polish soil on rabbit dung, common on bacterial streaks over water agar inoculated with soil.

Reference strain: Windsor M203.

Illustrations

Krzemieniewska and Krzemieniewski, 1927, Plate V, Fig. 21; McCurdy, 1969b, Fig. 31 (color), and 1970, Figs. 1–3; Brockman and Todd, 1974, Fig. 10; Dawid, 1976c, Fig. 5; Reichenbach and Dworkin, 1981, Fig. 8*i*, Plate II*a* ("cellatus," color) and Plate II*b* (color); Dawid, 1981 Plate II, Figs. 7 and 8, Plate III, Fig. 3, and Plate IV, Fig. 4.

Figure 24.15. *C. ferrugineus* fruiting bodies. Light micrograph (× 120).

Genus II. **Melittangium** *Jahn 1924, 78*[AL]

HOWARD D. McCURDY

Me.lit.tan'gi.um. Gr. n. *melitta* bee; Gr. n. *angium* vessel; M.L. neut. n. *Melittangium* resembling a beehive.

Vegetative cells are tapered rods.
Sporangia are solitary, often on a stalk.
Microcysts are rod-shaped, optically dense or refractile.
Vegetative colonies do not etch or erode agar media. Congo red is adsorbed.

Minimum nutritional requirements are unknown, but this organism is cultivatable on media containing enzymatically hydrolyzed protein.

Type species: *Melittangium boletus* Jahn 1924, 78.

Key to the species of the genus **Melittangium**

I. Sporangia flattened like a mushroom cap

                                       1. *M. boletus*

II. Sporangia spherical or ellipsoidal
   A. Stalk short (<40 μm) or lacking

                                         2. *M. lichenicola*

   B. Stalk long (>40 μm) and bent

                                         3. *M. alboraceum*

List of species of the genus **Melittangium**

1. **Melittangium boletus** Jahn 1924, 78.[AL]

bo.le′tus. L. n. *boletus* a kind of mushroom.

Description is based on Jahn (1924), Krzemieniewska and Krzemieniewski (1928), and Solntseva (1941).

Vegetative rods are slightly tapered with rounded ends (Krzemieniewska and Krzemieniewski, 1928), 0.7–4.5 × 10.5 μm (Solntseva, 1941).

Sporangia (Fig. 24.16) are spherical or flattened, resembling a mushroom pileus, and 45–50 × 50–100 μm. At first, they are whitish, later becoming yellowish brown to nut-brown, and when dried, they are reddish brown. Sporangiophores are white or yellowish, 10–25 × up to 60 μm; occasionally, they are poorly developed or absent. The resting cells in the sporangia stand at right angles to the enclosing wall in several layers; the wall has a honeycomb structure because of the impingement of the resting cells against it. Myxospores are rod-shaped, 0.7–0.9 × 1.5–3.0 μm.

Vegetative colonies have not been described. Cultivated with good growth on 10% dung decoction agar and potato agar (Solntseva, 1941).

Starch is hydrolyzed. Cellulose is not digested (Solntseva, 1941).

Aerobic (Solntseva, 1941). pH range: 4.0–8.5 (Solntseva, 1941). Temperature range: 20–31°C (Solntseva, 1941).

Source and habitat: from dung of various herbivores and from wet bark (Solntseva, 1941).

Illustrations

Jahn, 1924, Plate 2, Figs. 17 and 18 and B, C–F, U–Q, T–U; Krzemieniewska and Krzemieniewski, 1926, Plate V, Figs. 55 and 56; McCurdy, 1970, Figs. 9 and 10; Dawid, 1981, Plate IV, Fig. 5.

2. **Melittangium lichenicola** (Thaxter) McCurdy 1971b, 53.[AL]
(*Chondromyces lichenicolus* Thaxter 1892, 402.)

li.che.ni′co.la. Gr. n. *lichen* lichen; L. n. *cola* dweller; M.L. n. *lichenicola* lichen dweller.

Vegetative rods are tapered, 0.6–0.9 × 7–12 μm. Cells in logarithmic growth phase are 0.6 × 6–8 μm.

Fruiting bodies are of two types: The first type (Figs. 24.17 and 24.18) consists of a single orange-red to bright red, spherical ellipsoidal or pear-shaped sporangium 15–35 × 25–35 μm, on a white to orange, rigid stalk 5–10 × 10–40 μm. When crowded, the sporangia may be confluent. Sporangiophores are occasionally lacking, but when they are well-developed, tapering at the tip, they are persistent, and the sporangia are caducous. The second type of fruiting body (Fig. 24.19) often accompanies the first, is more usual on artificial media, and consists of an orange to bright red irregular mass up to 1 mm in diameter with a swollen padded surface. Internally, the microcysts and slime are oriented to form numerous, closely appressed, intestinelike convoluted tubes of about 50–90 μm in diameter.

Microcysts (Fig. 24.20) are irregularly rod-shaped, often bent and narrowing at the ends, and are rigid, phase-dense or refractile with a slime capsule. Usually, they occur in sheaves and are difficult to separate.

Vegetative colonies grown on agar media spread very rapidly; they are very thin, nearly transparent, with occasional reddish-orange to bright red radial folds and accumulations. They characteristically extend onto the walls of the culture vessels and between agar-glass interfaces. Lysis on *Escherichia coli* medium is very extensive.

Growth in casitone-Mg^{2+} broth is poor, in the form of compact red spheres; the medium remains clear.

Cultivated on *E. coli* medium, dung pellet and casitone-Mg^{2+} agars but with only limited growth.

Figure 24.16. *M. boletus* fruiting bodies. × 90.

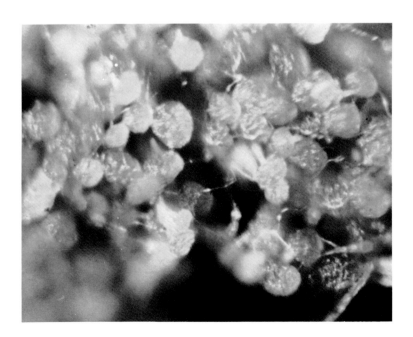

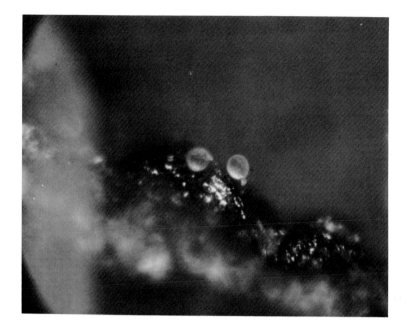

Figure 24.17. *M. lichenicola* fruiting bodies on bark. ×540.

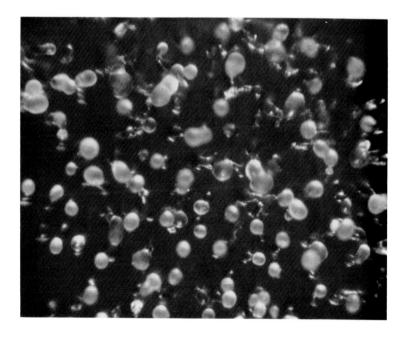

Figure 24.18. *M. lichenicola* fruiting bodies on agar. × 450.

Nitrate is not reduced. Catalase is produced. This organism is oxidase-negative; hydrolyzes starch, RNA, DNA and, usually, esculin; is urease-negative; and does not digest cellulose.

Temperature range: 18–37°C; optimum, 25–28°C.

Antibiotic sensitivity (disks): inhibited by 10 μg of tetracycline, chloramphenicol and kanamycin and by 5 μg of erythromycin. Response to neomycin (10 μg) and penicillin (10 units) is variable.

Originally observed on rabbit dung in contact with soil and on lichens. Very common on moist tree bark.

Type strain: Acc. nos. 4500 and 5170, Thaxter Collection, Farlow Herbarium, Harvard University, Cambridge, Massachusetts.

Reference strain: Windsor M201, ATCC 25946.

Illustrations

Thaxter, 1892, Plate 23, Figs. 20–23; Thaxter, 1897, Plate 31, Figs. 20–24; Quehl, 1906, Plate 1, Figs. 6 and 9; Jahn, 1924, Plate II, Figs. 19 and 20;

Krzemieniewska and Krzemieniewski, 1926, Plate V, Fig. 54; McCurdy 1970, Figs. 1–8; McNeil and Skerman, 1972, Fig. 15; Brockman and Todd, 1974, Fig. 9; Dawid, 1976c, Fig. 6, and 1981, Plate II, Figs. 9 and 10, Plate III, Fig. 4, and Plate IV, Fig. 9; Reichenbach and Dworkin, 1981, Plate 8h, Fig. 8f.

3. **Melittangium alboraceum** (Peterson) McCurdy 1971b, 54.[AL]
(*Podangium alboraceum* Peterson 1959, 167.)

al.bo.ra′ce.um. L. adj. *albus* white; L. masc. n. *racemus* the stalk of a cluster; M.L. adj. *alboraceum* implying a white stalk.

Vegetative cells are 0.8–1.0 × 4.5–5.0 μm, with no apparent tapering and with square ends.

Fruiting body consists of a single sporangium on a long, white, irregularly corkscrew-shaped sporangiophore 82–250 (average: 125) × 20 μm. The sporangium is an irregular globe, pale orange, crystalline, with a diameter of 35 μm and bounded by an elastic membrane which is difficult to see.

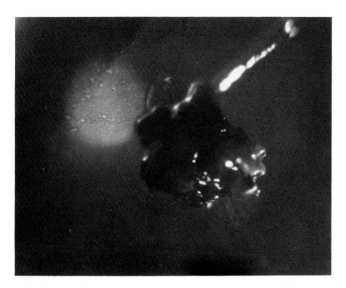

Figure 24.19. *M. lichenicola, Archangium*-like fruiting body on agar. × 30.

Figure 24.20. *M. lichenicola* microcysts. Electron micrograph of thin section. *CM*, cytoplasmic membrane; *ETR*, electron transparent region; *OM*, outer membrane; and *SC*, spore coat. *Bar*, 300 nm.

Myxospores are rod-shaped, 0.8 × 2.5 µm, slightly curved, and difficult to separate from the sporangium and one another.

This organism has not been cultivated.

Source and habitat: observed twice on elm bark.

Type strain: Three microscope slides, Peterson 72, University of Missouri Herbarium.

Illustrations

Peterson, 1959, Figs. 4–6.

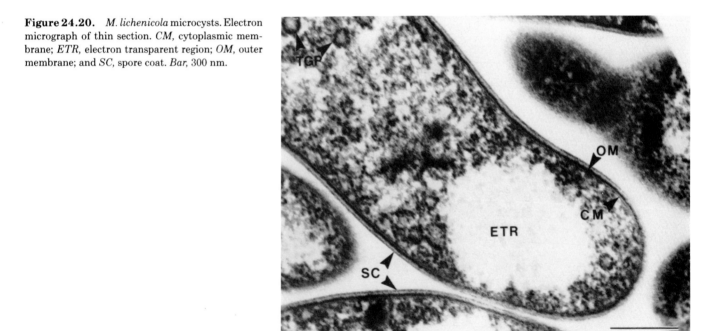

Genus III. **Stigmatella** *Berkeley and Curtis in Berkeley 1875, 97*[AL]

DAVID WHITE

Stig.ma.tel′la. L. neut. n. *stigma, stigmatis* brand or mark; M.L. fem. dim. ending *-ella*; M.L. fem. n. *Stigmatella* small brand or mark.

Vegetative cells are straight rods with tapered ends, 0.6–0.8 × 4–10 µm. **Myxospores are 0.9–1.2 × 2–4 µm,** phase-dense or refractile. **Sporangioles occur either singly or in clusters on stalks.** Vegetative swarms on agar are yellow-orange to red-brown, do not penetrate or etch agar, and adsorb Congo red.

This organism can be cultivated on media containing enzymatically hydrolyzed protein. Nitrate is not reduced. This organism is catalase-positive, is oxidase-negative, and hydrolyzes starch, Tween 80, indoxyl acetate, RNA, DNA, gelatin, casein and esculin. Urea is usually hydrolyzed (McCurdy, 1974).

Aerobic. Temperature range: 18–37°C; optimum: 30°C.

The mol% G + C of the DNA is 68.5–68.7 (T_m) (McCurdy and Wolf, 1967).

Type species: *Stigmatella aurantiaca* Berkeley and Curtis in Berkeley 1875, 97.

Further Descriptive Information

Detailed descriptions of both *S. aurantiaca* and *S. erecta* have been published (McCurdy and Khouw, 1969; Reichenbach and Dworkin, 1969). The carotenoid pigments and fatty acid composition of *S.*

aurantiaca have been analyzed (Kleinig and Reichenbach, 1969, 1970; Schröder and Reichenbach, 1970). A time lapse film showing the life cycle of *S. aurantiaca*, as well as a detailed scanning electron microscopic study of fruiting body formation with the orientations of the individual cells shown (Reichenbach et al., 1975–1976; Vásquez et al., 1985), has also been published. Techniques for culturing *S. aurantiaca* DW4 (ATCC 33878) and the induction of fruiting body formation were summarized by White (Appendix D in Rosenberg, 1984). These conditions include high cell densities and the presence of light (Qualls et al., 1978; White et al., 1980a). A lipoidal pheromone that stimulates aggregation is secreted into the medium during fruiting body formation (Stephens et al., 1982). Studies of *S. aurantiaca* DW4 under defined laboratory conditions have indicated that much of the reported variability in fruiting body morphology for *Stigmatella* may be due to the experimental conditions. For example, *Archangium*-like forms resembling intertwining ridges can form when the light is insufficient (Qualls et al., 1978). The presence or absence of stalks and the numbers of sporangia can be influenced by the cation composition if agarose is used as the solid medium (White et al., 1980b). Vegetative cells have polar fimbriae and an ultrastructure similar to that of other Gram-negative bacteria (Reichenbach et al., 1969; MacRae et al., 1977). Both peptidoglycan and lipopolysaccharide are present in the vegetative cells (Sutherland and Smith, 1973; D. White, unpublished observations). The myxospores differ from the vegetative cells in having an additional coat or capsule surrounding the wall (McCurdy and Khouw, 1969; Reichenbach et al., 1969; Voelz and Reichenbach, 1969). They are more resistant to heat, dessication and sonic oscillation than are vegetative cells (McCurdy and Khouw, 1969; Reichenbach and Dworkin, 1969). *Stigmatella* can be induced to form myxospores in suspension by the addition of any one of several inducers (e.g. glycerol, NA$^+$ (McCurdy and Khouw, 1969; Gerth and Reichenbach, 1978)). These myxospores are morphologically similar to myxospores found in fruiting bodies and share some of their resistant properties.

Vegetative swarms on agar frequently display a slightly raised radial pattern. The cells are distributed throughout the swarm. Significant amounts of slime are produced on agar plates. The slime is sufficiently cohesive as to make it often difficult to scrape cells from the agar surface. Freshly isolated strains usually grow as clumps in liquid media, but dispersed growing variants can be isolated during subculturing of the strains in broth. Even dispersed growing variants of *S. aurantiaca* may grow in clumps when calcium ion is added to the medium (Reichenbach and Dworkin, 1969). This may be due to the synthesis of an energy-dependent cohesive system (Gilmore and White, 1985). Strains will grow vegetatively and do not fruit when cultured on agar supplemented with amino acids or enzymatically hydrolyzed protein. Fruiting is induced by transferring the strains to nonnutrient agar,[*] although some strains will both grow and fruit on yeast agar.[†] When kept in the vegetative stage, some strains will fail to form fruiting bodies on nonnutrient agar even after a few subcultures in liquid media or on agar plates.

Cultures can be grown on enzymatically hydrolyzed protein, e.g.

Bacto casitone and Bacto tryptone (Difco) supplemented with magnesium sulfate.[‡] They are easily grown in liquid media in a reciprocating shaker or on agar plates. The generation time for *S. aurantiaca* DW4 grown on Bacto casitone and Bacto tryptone at 30°C is about 9–10 h. The generation time for *S. erecta* on complex media is 4.5 h (McCurdy and Khouw, 1969). A list of media has been published (Reichenbach and Dworkin, 1981). A defined medium has been published for *S. erecta* (McCurdy and Khouw, 1969).

Antibiotic sensitivity: resistant to penicillin (10 units); sensitive to streptomycin (5 µg), tetracycline (10 µg), chloramphenicol (10 µg), kanamycin (10 µg) and erythromycin (5 µg) (McCurdy, 1971a).

Found on rotting wood, dung, or soil in which organic material is being decomposed by other bacteria. *Stigmatella* probably makes use of other bacteria as the main nutrient source in nature.

Enrichment and Isolation Procedures

Stigmatella can be isolated from bark, rotting wood, dung pellets, or soil that has been placed in Petri dishes lined with 2–3 layers of filter paper and moistened with distilled or deionized water. When soil is being used, it is necessary also to use dung pellets as "bait." Bark and wood should be low in resins and tanning substances (Reichenbach and Dworkin, 1981). After several days of incubation at 30°C, fruiting bodies appear. These are then transferred to agar containing a suitable nutrient, e.g. autoclaved yeast or bacteria or enzymatically hydrolyzed protein. When swarms appear, a sample from the edge is transferred to fresh media. The details of the isolation and purification procedures were recently described (Reichenbach and Dworkin, 1981).

Maintenance Procedures

Cultures are routinely subcultured on agar plates or liquid media consisting of either enzymatically hydrolyzed protein or dead bacteria or yeast. Strains can be stored frozen in broth or on agar at −80°C or as dried fruits or myxospores (Reichenbach and Dworkin, 1969). It is important to freeze vegetative cells rapidly in dry ice and acetone or liquid nitrogen, as they may not survive slow freezing at −20°C or −80°C. Vegetative cells do not survive lyophilization well, nor can they be stored at −4°C or −20°C. Dried fruits are easily prepared by scraping vegetative cells from growth plates and transferring them in large masses to strips of sterile filter paper on nonnutrient agar. The plates are incubated at 30°C. Fruits will appear in a few days, and once the fruits are mature, the filter paper strips can be transferred to sterile screw-capped tubes and desiccated in a vacuum desiccator. When they are dried, they can be stored at 4°C or at room temperature. It is possible to revive strains stored at 4°C as dried fruiting bodies after several years. Details for strain preservation have recently been published (Reichenbach and Dworkin, 1981).

Further Reading

Reichenbach and Dworkin published a review of procedures for the isolation, characterization and culturing of myxobacteria (1981). There is also a detailed account of the developmental biology of the myxobacteria which includes an appendix of methods (Rosenberg, 1984).

List of species of the genus **Stigmatella**

1. **Stigmatella aurantiaca** Berkeley and Curtis in Berkeley 1875, 97.[AL]

au.ran.ti′a.ca. M.L. fem. adj. *aurantiaca* orange-colored.

Fruiting bodies on wood are yellowish orange or reddish brown, usually 50–100 µm tall, and consist of several sporangioles on a well-defined, usually unbranched stalk (Figs. 24.21 and 24.22). Sometimes, the sporangioles are attached to the stalk by tiny pedicels. In culture

on agar, the fruiting body morphology can be variable if the experimental procedures and culture conditions are not strictly controlled. For example, stalks may be absent, and the sporangioles may exist singly or in clumps of approximately 50–100 on a mound of slime or directly on the agar. The cells may aggregate into intertwining ridges resembling fruiting bodies of *Archangium*, rather than form discrete aggregates. When this occurs, the ridges do not develop morphologi-

---

[*] Nonnutrient agar (water agar) contains: 0.1% CaCl$_2$·2H$_2$O and 1.5% agar, autoclaved. Also used are: 3.4 mM CaCl$_2$·2H$_2$P, 10 mM *N*-2-hydroxyethylpiperazine-*N*′-2-ethanesulfonic acid (HEPES) buffer (pH 7.2), and 1.5% agar.

[‡] Bacto casitone or Bacto tryptone medium contains: 1% Bacto casitone or Bacto tryptone and 8 mM MgSO$_4$, autoclaved.

[†] Yeast agar (Reichenbach and Dworkin, 1981) contains: baker's yeast, 0.5% (by fresh weight of yeast cake); CaCl$_2$·2H$_2$O, 0.1%; cyanocobalamin, 0.5 µg/ml; and agar, 1.5%, autoclaved. For most myxobacteria, the cyanocobalamin is not necessary.

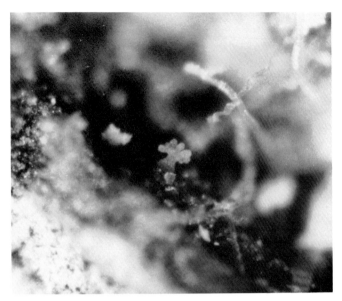

Figure 24.21. *S. aurantiaca* fruiting body on wood. Light micrograph (× 122).

cally, although myxospores can form (Inouye et al. 1980). However, under controlled laboratory conditions and with use of experimental procedures specifically designed to ensure consistent and reliable development, *S. aurantiaca* DW4 fruiting bodies that resemble those shown in Figures 24.21 and 24.22 develop with very little variability (Qualls et al. 1978). Cultures produce an antibiotic that inhibits electron transport in bovine heart mitochondria and in the photosynthetic electron transport chain of chloroplasts (Oettmeier et al., 1985).

The mol% G + C of the DNA is 68.5–68.7 (T_m) (McCurdy and Wolf, 1967).

Type strain: ATCC 25190.

Illustrations

Reichenbach and Dworkin, 1969, Figs. 1–9; Grilione and Pangborn, 1975, Fig. 4; Qualls et al., 1978, Fig. 2.

2. **Stigmatella erecta** (Schroeter 1886) McCurdy 1971a, 48.[AL] (*Cystobacter erectus* Schroeter 1886, 170.)

e.rec′ta. L. fem. adj. *erecta* erect.

S. erecta can be distinguished from *S. aurantiaca* in that *S. erecta* has a greater frequency of monosporangial fruiting bodies, darker (chestnut-brown or almost black) sporangioles in older fruiting bodies, and a tendency to "settle down" at maturity, i.e. the stalks wither and the sporangioles appear sessile in large masses of 50–100 (McCurdy, 1971a). The fruiting bodies of *S. erecta* can vary, depending upon conditions, in morphology. For example, on rabbit dung the fruiting bodies may be simply intertwining sausage-shaped masses similar to the fruit-

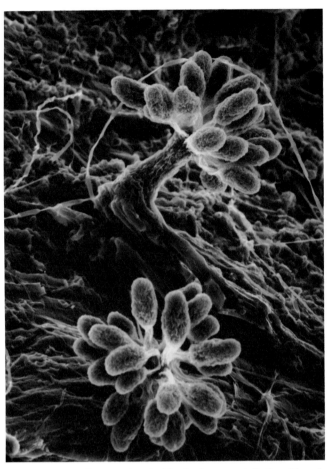

Figure 24.22. *S. aurantiaca* fruiting body on wood. Both a side and a top view are shown. Scanning electron micrograph (× 394).

ing bodies of *Archangium* or may be coralloid in morphology (McCurdy and Khouw, 1969). When in culture, the fruiting bodies of both *S. erecta* and *S. aurantiaca* may have degenerate forms which appear similar in the two organisms. Under these conditions, the species may be difficult to distinguish. *S. erecta* is found most frequently on dung of herbivorous animals and soil, whereas *S. aurantiaca* is usually isolated from rotting wood and bark (Reichenbach and Dworkin, 1969; McCurdy, 1971a).

The mol% G + C of the DNA is 68.7 (T_m) (McCurdy and Wolf, 1967).

Type strain: Windsor M26 (ATCC 25191).

Illustrations

McCurdy and Khouw, 1969, Figs. 1–3; Reichenbach and Dworkin, 1981, Fig. 8e.

FAMILY IV. **POLYANGIACEAE** JAHN 1924, 75[AL]

E. R. BROCKMAN

Po.ly.an.gi.a′ce.ae. M.L. neut. n. *Polyangium* type genus of the family; -*aceae* ending to denote a family; M.L. fem. pl. n. Polyangiaceae the *Polyangium* family.

Cylindrical vegetative **bacilli** with **blunt, rounded ends. Myxospores are similar to vegetative cells,** not refractile or phase-dense, **lacking** a hard **slime coat** in the examined species (McCurdy, 1964; Peterson, 1969). **Sporangia** are normally **sessile, isolated or in sori** (clusters) bound by a common membrane, or they may develop singly or in groups on branched or unbranched stalks.

The swarm cells etch, erode and penetrate agar media. The **vegetative slime does not adsorb Congo red.**

Cellulose may or may not be utilized as carbon and energy sources.

Type genus: *Polyangium* Link 1809, 42.

Key to the genera of the family **Polyangiaceae**

I. Sporangia normally sessile
  A. Vegetative cells cylindrical bacilli
             Genus I. *Polyangium*, p. 2159
  B. Vegetative cells short, blunt-ended bacilli or cocci
             Genus II. *Nannocystis*, p. 2162
II. Sporangia borne on a stalk
             Genus III. *Chondromyces*, p. 2167

Genus I. **Polyangium** Link 1809, 42[AL]

E. R. BROCKMAN

Po.ly.an'gi.um. Gr. adj. *poly* many; Gr. neut. n. *angion* vessel; M.L. neut. n. *Polyangium* many vessels.

Vegetative cells are cylindrical, of uniform diameter, **with blunt rounded ends.**

Sporangia are usually **sessile, solitary or in sori**, often bounded by a common layer of slime.

Myxospores resemble vegetative cells, not refractile or phase-dense, **lacking a slime capsule** in the examined species.

Colonies of all examined species etch, erode and penetrate the agar. **Congo red is not adsorbed** by the vegetative slime.

Cellulose may or may not be hydrolyzed.

Type species: *Polyangium vitellinum* Link 1809, 42.

Further Comments

Some species of this genus are noted as being difficult to culture in the laboratory and for their slow growth. In fact, only four of the ten species, *P. cellulosum*, *P. fumosum*, *P. luteum* and *P. sorediatum*, have been grown in pure culture. The following key is based primarily on sorus and sporangium pigmentation and morphology and is a simple, mechanical means of separating the species. Once the nutritional requirements of these bacteria have been clarified, a better key will, no doubt, be forthcoming.

Enrichment and Isolation Procedures

The techniques described for the order and those of Reichenbach and Dworkin (1981) may be used for the enrichment and isolation of *Polyangium* species.

Maintenance Procedures

The methods described for the order and those of Reichenbach and Dworkin (1981) may be used for the maintenance of *Polyangium* species.

Differentiation of the genus **Polyangium** from other genera

The genus *Polyangium* is differentiated from other genera of fruiting body-forming gliding bacteria in that its species have cylindrical vegetative cells with blunt, rounded ends and that the myxospores formed resemble the vegetative cells. The fruiting bodies or sori contain the myxospores and are usually sessile; the sporangium of *P. rugiseptum* has been observed to be stipitate only on occasion. Immature sori of *Polyangium* species may resemble the fruiting bodies of *Archangium* species, so it is important that mature sori be observed for their distinctive myxospores. Species of the genera *Nannocystis* and *Cystobacter* might be confused with those of the genus *Polyangium* if only the sori are observed. The vegetative cells of *Nannocystis* species, however, are short, fat bacilli which may become coccoid in older cultures. The vegetative cells of *Cystobacter* species are slender, tapered, flexible bacilli. The myxospores of *Nannocystis* and *Cystobacter* species are phase-dense, while those of *Polyangium* species lack this property.

Further Reading

Dawid, W. 1977. Fruchtkörperbildende Myxobakterien. V. Die *Polyangium—* Arten: *P. cellulosum*, *P. fumosum*, *P. sorediatum*, *P. vitellinum*. Mikrokosmos *66:* 364–373.

Krzemieniewska, H. and S. Krzemieniewski. 1930. Miksobakterje Polski. Część trzecia (Die Myxobakterien von Polen. III Teil). Acta Soc. Bot. Pol. *7:* 250–273.

McCurdy, H.D. 1970. Studies on the taxonomy of the *Myxobacterales*. II. *Polyangium* and the demise of the *Sorangiaceae*. Int. J. Syst. Bacteriol. *20:* 283–296.

Key to the species of the genus **Polyangium**

I. Not parasitic on algae
  A. Sorus not white or gray
    1. Ripe sporangia not brownish but are yellow, reddish yellow, orange or light red
      a. Ripe sporangia not solitary
        b. Sporangia not polygonal when appressed in the sorus
          c. Slime envelope transparent, white and colorless
            1. *P. vitellinum*
          cc. Slime envelope bright yellow
            2. *P. luteum*
        bb. Sporangia often polygonal when appressed in the sorus
          c. Cellulolytic
            3. *P. cellulosum*
          cc. Noncellulolytic
            4. *P. sorediatum*
      aa. Ripe sporangium solitary and usually sessile
          5. *P. rugiseptum*

2. Ripe sporangia brownish
    a. Ripe sporangia dull orange-brown, usually solitary and without contact, sessile, and collapsed and wrinkled when dry
        6. *P. minor*
    aa. Ripe sporangia reddish brown, variable in number, and embedded in yellow slime envelope
        7. *P. aureum*
B. Sorus white or gray
  1. Slime envelope white and foamy in appearance
    8. *P. spumosum*
  2. Slime envelope smoke-gray in color
    9. *P. fumosum*
II. Parasitic on the alga, *Cladophora*
    10. *P. parasiticum*

List of species of the genus **Polyangium**

1. **Polyangium vitellinum** Link 1809, 42.[AL]

vi.tel.li′num. L. masc. n. *vitellus* egg yolk; M.L. neut. adj. *vitellinum* like an egg yolk.

Vegetative rods (Fig. 24.23) are cylindrical with blunt rounded ends, 0.9–1.2 × 4–10 μm.

Sporangia (Figs. 24.24 and 24.25) are golden yellow, reddish yellow or brownish orange; oval, spherical or cushionlike; 75–400 μm, with a sporangial wall 2.7 μm thick; and definite, showing imprints of enclosed rods. The sporangia occur singly or in groups of up to 20 and, when fresh, are surrounded by a white slimy envelope that measures up to 16 μm thick. The contents are flesh-colored when the sporangia are young.

Myxospores in young sporangia resemble vegetative cells, are 0.9 × 3–5 μm, and often adhere together in sheaves. In older sporangia, irregular shrunken rods (Fig. 24.23) are common, and in some instances, cells appear to be absent; the cells may be mixed with a yellowish oily substance.

Colonies, when rising to form fruiting bodies, are milky white to slightly pinkish and creamy in consistency.

This organism is cultivated only on original substrate. It has not been obtained in pure culture.

Most often observed on very wet wood on bark in swamps or moist ditches. Also obtained on bark kept in a moist chamber, from hay and on rabbit dung in contact with soil.

Neotype strain: Acc. no. 4564, Thaxter collection, Farlow Herbarium, Harvard University, Cambridge, Massachusetts (U.S.A.).

Illustrations

Link, 1809, Fig. 65; Ditmar, 1813, Figs. A–C; Thaxter, 1892, Plate 25, Figs. 34–36,; Zukal, 1897, Plate 27, Figs. 6–10; Jahn, 1911, Fig. 3, and 1924, p. 77 and Plate II, Fig. 13; Krzemieniewska and Krzemieniewski, 1930, Plate 16, Figs. 4 and 5, and Plate 18, Fig. 25; McCurdy, 1969b, Fig. 32, and 1970, Figs. 15–17; Peterson, 1969, Figs. 9–11; Brockman and Todd, 1974, Fig. 11; Dawid, 1977, Figs. 17–21.

2. **Polyangium luteum** (ex Krzemieniewska and Krzemieniewski 1927) nom. rev.

lu′te.um. L. adj. *luteum* saffron or golden-yellow.

Vegetative cells are 0.8–1.0 × 6.0–8.0 μm with blunt, rounded ends.

Sori are golden yellow, 85–170 × 100–180 μm (Kühlwein and Schlicke, 1971), containing one or two, rarely three or four, spherical, oval or irregular sporangia of variable size (39–90 × 37–115 μm) with thin, colorless walls. The slime envelope enclosing the sporangia is

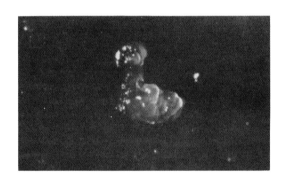

Figure 24.24. *P. vitellinum* 28-day-old sorus on an agar surface. Light micrograph (× 100). (Reproduced with permission from W. Dawid, *Mikrokosmos 66:* 372, 1977, ©Franckh'sche Verlagshandlung, Stuttgart.)

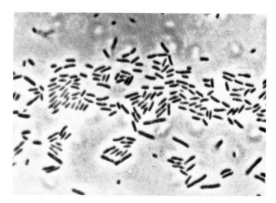

Figure 24.23. *P. vitellinum* vegetative swarm cells and shortened myxospores. Phase-contrast micrograph (× 1000). (Reproduced with permission from W. Dawid, *Mikrokosmos 66:* 373, 1977, ©Franckh'sche Verlagshandlung, Stuttgart.)

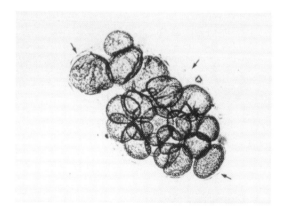

Figure 24.25. *P. vitellinum* sorus composed of numerous sporangia. The *arrows* point to the surrounding slime layer. Brightfield micrograph (× 250). (Reproduced with permission from W. Dawid, *Mikrokosmos 66:* 373, 1977, ©Franckh'sche Verlagshandlung, Stuttgart.)

bright yellow (Kühlwein and Schlicke, 1971, report the color in the cells, not in the slime envelope), double-contoured, up to 10 μm thick, and easily broken by slight pressure.

Myxospores are 0.7–0.8 × 3.8–5.8 μm.

Vegetative colonies are colorless to light yellow, depending on the culture media, with an irregularly fringed margin which penetrates the agar.

Cultivated on bacterial cells, rabbit dung and several artificial solid and liquid media.

Not observed to digest cellulose.

Obtained from rabbit dung in contact with soil from Radkowice (Kielce County), Poland; moist, acid, meadow bog soil from Germany (Rückert, 1972); and soil from Essex County, Ontario, Canada (McCurdy, 1969b).

Illustrations

Krzemieniewska and Krzemieniewski, 1927, Plate V, Figs. 22 and 23; Kühlwein and Schlicke, 1971, Plates 1–4.

3. **Polyangium cellulosum** (ex Imshenetski and Solntseva 1936) nom. rev.

cel.lu.lo′sum. M.L. n. *cellulosum* cellulose.

Vegetative rods are 0.8–1.2 × 3.0–10 μm.

Sporangia are 20–30 μm in diameter and, depending upon pressure from the mass, rounded to polygonal. From four to several hundred sporangia (usually several dozen) are clustered in sori which may or may not have discernible slime envelopes. The sori vary from slightly knobby rounded cushions, when formed free of constraints, to simple rows of sporangia, when formed within cellulose fibers; the color varies from pale yellow through shades of pink, orange, rusty-red and brown to shades of gray and black.

Myxospores are similar to vegetative cells, 1.0–3.0 μm in length.

Growth on filter paper overlaid on mineral salts medium is slow, appearing in 3–14 days. The advancing periphery of the colony is lightly pigmented in shades of yellow, pink or orange; with the formation of sori (2–4 weeks), the central portion becomes more deeply pigmented.

This organism is strongly cellulolytic; there is marked decomposition of filter paper under the colony.

Most isolates may be grown on agar or in liquid media containing cellobiose, nitrate and salts. Ammonium salts, organic nitrogen and simpler carbon sources may or may not be utilized. Starch is hydrolyzed (Pronina, 1962).

Temperature range: 20–37°C; optimum 28–32°C. Optimum pH: 6.8–7.2.

First isolated from Russian and Polish soils, this organism has now been found elsewhere in Continental Europe and in North America. Closely associated with agricultural soils as well as arid and semiarid soils in the United States and Mexico.

The mol% G + C of the DNA is 69 (Bd).

Reference strains: ATCC 15384, ATCC 25531, ATCC 25532, ATCC 25569.

Four subspecies have been described.

a. *"Polyangium cellulosum* subsp. *ferrugineum"* Mishustin 1938, 433.

b. *"Polyangium cellulosae* (sic) subsp. *fuscum"* Mishustin 1938, 435.

c. *"Polyangium cellulosae* (sic) subsp. *fulvum"* Mishustin 1938, 437.

d. *"Polyangium cellulosae* (sic) subsp. *luteum"* Mishustin 1938, 438.

Illustrations

Imshenetski and Solntseva, 1936, Figs. 1–5, and Table II, Fig. 2, and 1937, Figs. 1–8; Krzemieniewska and Krzemieniewski, 1937a, Plate III, Figs. 17–21, and Plate IV, Figs. 22–26; Mishustin, 1938, Figs. 4–14; McCurdy, 1969b, Figs. 33–38; Peterson, 1969, Figs. 7 and 8; Brockman and Todd, 1974, Fig. 12; Lampky, 1976, Figs. 1–15; Dawid, 1977, Figs. 1–7.

4. **Polyangium sorediatum** (ex Thaxter 1904) nom. rev.

so.re.di.a′tum. Gr. n. *sorus* a heap; M.L. dim. n. *soredium* a little heap; M.L. neut. adj. *sorediatum* having little heaps.

Vegetative rods are 0.8–1.2 × 3.0–6.0 μm.

Sori are yellow-orange, up to 0.5 mm in diameter, and flat or cushion-shaped, consisting of up to hundreds of sporangia. The latter are often contained in slime-delimited groups of several sporangia each. Sporangia are polygonal when appressed within the sorus but are nearly spherical when free and are 5–15 μm in diameter.

Myxospores are shorter than vegetative cells but similar, 0.8 × 3–4 μm.

Vegetative growth has not been described.

Pure culture (Dawid, 1981) has been obtained on *Escherichia coli*-smeared Ca²⁺-water agar. This organism is noncellulolytic.

Obtained from animal dung, decomposing plant material, tree bark, and soils rich in organic matter.

Illustrations

Thaxter, 1904, Plate 27, Figs. 22–30; Quehl, 1906, Plate 1, Figs. 2 and 3; Jahn, 1911, Figs. 1 and 2, p. 202; Jahn, 1924, Plate I, Fig. 6, and Plate II, Fig. 22; Krzemieniewska and Krzemieniewski, 1926, Plate III, Figs. 28–36, and Plate IV, Figs. 37–41, and 1927, Plate IV, Figs. 7–12, Plate V, Figs. 13–18, and Plate VI, Fig. 36; McCurdy, 1969b, Fig. 38; Dawid, 1977, Figs. 11–16, and 1981, Table II, Fig. 11, and Table IV, Fig. 7.

5. **Polyangium rugiseptum** (Peterson) McCurdy 1970, 295.[AL]

ru.gi.sep′tum. L. fem. n. *ruga* wrinkle; L. neut. n. *septum* enclosure; M.L. neut. n. *rugiseptum* wrinkled enclosure.

Vegetative cells have not been described.

Sporangia are solitary, usually sessile (Hu et al., 1985), globose or oval, glistening orange-red, wrinkled and, when dry, redder, and up to 200 μm (average: 85 μm). The sporangial wall is of two distinct layers: the inner, which is smooth, bright yellow and fairly strong, and the outer, which is irregular, flaky and dark orange-red. Sporangia may or may not contain fatty globules and amorphous material dispersed among the myxospores.

Myxospores are cylindrical with blunt ends, 0.8 × 4–6 μm, often becoming shrunken and irregular in shape (McCurdy, 1970) and lacking a definite arrangement in the sporangium.

This organism has not been cultivated.

Source and habitat: bark from various (ten species) living trees in Missouri (U.S.A.).

Type specimen: Peterson 51, University of Missouri Herbarium.

Illustrations

McCurdy, 1970, Fig. 8; Hu et al., 1985.

6. **Polyangium minor** (Peterson) McCurdy 1970, 294.[AL]

mi′nor. L. comp. adj. *minor* less, smaller.

Vegetative cells have more or less square ends and are 0.7 × 3–4.5 μm.

Sporangia are sessile, solitary or in groups of 4–10 but usually without contact, globose, oval or bean-shaped, 60–140 μm, and turgid, smooth and dull orange-brown when fresh, but collapsed, wrinkled, more glistening and orange when dry. Myxospores are not visible through the wall. The wall is bright yellow-orange by transmitted light and about 2 μm thick. An unknown amorphous material is observed inside the sporangium.

Myxospores are 0.7 × 2.5–3.5 μm and cylindrical with blunt ends, becoming irregular in old sporangia, and are arranged in distinct spherical groups which are difficult to separate.

Impure colonies on rabbit dung pellet agar and homogenized-bark agar are grayish yellow.

Source and habitat: obtained on numerous pieces of bark from four species of living tress in Missouri.

Type specimen: Peterson 41, University of Missouri Herbarium, Columbia, Missouri.

7. **Polyangium aureum** (ex Krzemieniewska and Krzemieniewski 1930) nom. rev.*

au're.um. L. neut. adj. *aureum* golden.

Vegetative cells are straight rods with curved ends; dimensions have not been given.

Sori are usually composed of 2–12 spherical or oval, light brown to reddish brown sporangia. Sporangia measure 15–50 × 20–60 μm (average: 32 × 37 μm). Each sporangium has an orange-yellow wall 3.5 μm thick. Sori are covered with a transparent, colorless, stretched membrane, but the sporangia are not appressed. Contents of older sporangia consist of either a colorless, granular mass or a light yellow oily liquid with few myxospores.

Myxospores resemble vegetative cells, are straight with rounded ends, and are 0.7–0.9 × 2.8–5.3 μm.

Vegetative colonies are indefinite and colorless; underlying agar is etched and penetrated.

Growth is very slow on *Micrococcus luteus*. Pure cultures have not been obtained.

Originally obtained on rabbit dung in contact with soil. Also on *Micrococcus luteus* streaks inoculated with soil.

Illustrations

Krzemieniewska and Krzemieniewski, 1930, Plate XVII, Figs. 14–17, and Plate XVIII, Fig. 29; McCurdy, 1969b, Fig. 31, and 1970, Fig. 7.

8. **Polyangium spumosum** (ex Krzemieniewska and Krzemieniewski 1930) nom. rev.†

spu.mo'sum. L. adj. *spumosum* foamy or frothy.

Vegetative cells are thick rods with blunt, rounded ends, 1.1–1.5 × 2.7–5.5 μm (Krzemieniewska and Krzemieniewski, 1937a).

Sori consist of numerous ellipsoidal sporangia, 7–24 × 9–34 μm, loosely arranged into spherical, oval, irregular to elongated accumulations not surrounded by a common membrane but covered by a weak layer of colorless slime. Sporangial walls are colorless to slightly brownish and transparent.

Myxospores from mature sporangia are cylindrical with blunt ends and 0.4–0.5 × 2–3 μm.

This organism can be cultivated in manure cultures and on filter paper which is digested, but it has not been obtained in pure culture. Vegetative growth is flesh-red (Krzemieniewska and Krzemieniewski, 1938a).

Obtained from Polish soils and decaying plant debris, peat and leaf mold; most often observed on damp blotting paper inoculated with these materials.

Illustrations

Krzemieniewska and Krzemieniewski, 1927, Plate V, Fig. 19, and 1937a, Plate 3, Figs. 12–16.

9. **Polyangium fumosum** Krzemieniewska and Krzemieniewski 1930, 253.[AL]

fu.mo'sum. L. neut. adj. *fumosum* smoky.

Vegetative cells are 0.6–0.9 × 3.7–7.3 μm with blunt to rounded ends.

Sori are usually flat, rounded or irregular in outline, consisting of 2–50 or more sporangia, at first milky white to pale pink, later developing a transparent brownish or smoky-gray pigment outlining the sporangia. The sporangial wall is definite, often double-contoured, slightly elongated to almost spherical, colorless and 17–72 × 13–60 μm (average: 35 × 45 μm). The dark slime enclosure of the sorus is 2.4–3.5 μm thick in the thinnest regions.

Myxospores are 0.7–0.9 × 2.5–5.7 μm with conspicuous terminal granules. In old sporangia, lysis may result in conversion of contents to a colorless, oily liquid and few or no cells.

Vegetative colonies light pink, delicate, becoming divided into migrating masses (200–500 μm) which leave radiating furrows and tunnels in the agar.

Growth is slow in pure culture on yeast-Ca²⁺ agar and *Micrococcus luteus* streaks over water agar.

Originally described on dung placed in contact with pine forest soil from Ciemianowka, Poland. Commonly encountered on *M. luteus* streaks on water agar inoculated with soil.

Reference strain: Windsor M257.

Illustrations

Krzemieniewska and Krzemieniewski, 1930, Plate XVI, Figs. 6–9 and 26; McCurdy, 1969b. Figs. 28 and 29, and 1970, Figs. 12–14; Dawid, 1977, Figs. 8–10.

10. **Polyangium parasiticum** (ex Geitler 1924) nom. rev.

pa.ra.si'ti.cum. Gr. adj. *parasiticum* parasitic.

Vegetative rods are 0.5–0.7 × 4–7 μm with rounded ends.

Sporangia are spherical or elongated, 15–50 μm but usually 25–40 μm, red-brown with distinct double-contoured walls, usually occurring in groups of 2–8, appressed and enclosed by a colorless, distinct slime.

Myxospores resemble vegetative cells but are slightly shorter.

Growth occurs only on the alga *Cladophora* in water and in dilute Benecke's solution at approximately 10°C; at first, this organism grows externally as a saprophyte, later entering and destroying the algal cells. This organism has not been cultivated on artificial media.

Reported only once on *Cladophora* (*fracta*?) obtained from a weakly salty pool in an unused clay pit in the town of Vösendorf (now in Liesing District, Vienna), Austria.

Illustrations

Geitler, 1924, Figs. A–H, J and K.

Genus II. **Nannocystis** *Reichenbach 1970, 137*[AL]

H. REICHENBACH

Nan.no.cys'tis. Gr. masc. n. *nannos* dwarf; Gr. fem. n. *cystis* bladder; M.L. fem. n. *Nannocystis* tiny bag.

Vegetative cells are stout rods with blunt ends and move by gliding. Myxospores are ovoid or nearly spherical. Fruiting bodies are solitary sporangia. Swarm colony deeply corrodes the agar surface. Aerobic organotrophic organisms.

The mol% G + C of the DNA is 70–72 (Bd, T_m).

Type species: *Nannocystis exedens* Reichenbach 1970, 137.

Enrichment and Isolation Procedures

Nannocystis lives in soil, decaying plant material, and dung of herbivorous animals in warm and temperate climate zones all over the world. It is a very common myxobacterium and, in the upper well-aerated layers, is present in virtually every pinch of soil, at least in environments in the normal pH range.

Nannocystis may be enriched and isolated by inoculating streaks of living *Escherichia coli* on water agar containing cycloheximide with small amounts of suitable material collected in nature, such as soil, rotting plant material, dust and particles from dung, etc. The crude cultures are incubated at 28–30°C for 4–14 days. Small clumps and ridges of cells will then emerge from the inoculum and migrate along the streaks and over the agar surface. The strains may be purified by

---

*Editorial note: This species was described by Krzemieniewska and Krzemieniewski in 1930 as being very similar to the "*P. morula*" that was described by Jahn in 1911.

† Editorial note: Two forms, differing in sporangial size, are known (Krzemieniewska and Krzemieniewski, 1937a): One has smaller sporangia, 7–18 × 9–23 μm; the other has sporangia 13–24 × 16–34 μm. The size difference remains constant after subculture.

serial transfers to living and, later, to autoclaved *E. coli* on water agar. Soil amoebae, which often are a very serious problem in crude cultures, may be eliminated by exposing the culture plate to the vapors of a 5% NH₃ solution for 30–120 s and then transferring the myxobacterium to a fresh plate. Molds, which occasionally grow in spite of the cycloheximide, may be suppressed by dusting the inoculum with nystatin. Pure strains grow well on streaks of autoclaved *E. coli* on water agar or on agar containing 0.5% baker's yeast (vy/2-agar). Fruiting bodies are best obtained by growing the organism on streaks of living *E. coli* on water agar but often are also observed on autoclaved *E. coli* or vy/2-agar. After a few transfers, however, the ability of a strain to form fruiting bodies is usually irrevocably lost. *Nannocystis* grows well in the form of tiny flakes in liquid media containing 0.3% casein peptone (e.g. MD1 liquid medium) and grows particularly vigorously in media with single-cell protein (Kohl et al., 1983). For details on media, isolation and cultivation, see Reichenbach, 1970; Reichenbach and Dworkin, 1981; and Reichenbach, 1983.

Maintenance Procedures

Vegetative cells from plates or liquid cultures may be stored in MD1 liquid medium at −80°C or in liquid nitrogen but cannot be lyophilized. Small squares (1 × 1 cm) of agar can be cut out from cultures with fruiting bodies, placed on pieces of sterile filter paper in empty Petri dishes, and dried in a desiccator under vacuum. When stored at room temperature, the dry fruiting bodies will germinate for at least 6 years as soon as they are transferred to a suitable growth medium.

Differentiation of the genus **Nannocystis** from other genera

The genera most related to *Nannocystis* are *Polyangium* and "*Sorangium*." The vegetative cells of the latter two genera are decidedly cylindrical and more regular in outline; their myxospores are rod-shaped; their fruiting bodies, at least in their typical form, are always composed of several to many sporangia which are closely packed and flattened against each other; the pattern of channels and paths etched into the agar surface by their swarm colonies is, in general, more coarse and less densely interwoven than that of *Nannocystis*. The "*Sorangium*" species are cellulose degraders. The pigments of *Nannocystis* are different from those of all other myxobacteria (Reichenbach and Kleinig, 1984).

Taxonomic Comments

A recent study on the oligonucleotide pattern of the 16S rRNA of several myxobacteria has shown that *Nannocystis* clearly belongs to the myxobacteria but that it forms a branch of its own within the *Polyangium*/"*Sorangium*" group (Ludwig et al., 1983). That *Nannocystis* is a member of the *Polyangium*/"*Sorangium*" group is further supported by the fatty acid patterns of myxobacteria. Although organisms of the *Cystobacter* group contain appreciable amounts of 3- hydroxy and, particularly, 2-hydroxy fatty acids, mainly with branched chains, there are no hydroxy acids at all in the overall fatty acid patterns of members of the *Polyangium*/"*Sorangium*" group including *Nannocystis* (Fautz et al., 1979, 1981). The 16S rRNA data also suggest a relatively distant relationship between *Nannocystis* and *Polyangium*/ "*Sorangium*," and this is again supported by chemosystematic data. Although the main pigments of all myxobacteria, including *Polyangium*/"*Sorangium*" and *Chondromyces*, are carotenoid glycosides and the fatty acid esters of those, *Nannocystis* has no carotenoid glycosides at all but contains unusual monocyclic aromatic carotenoids not found in any other myxobacterium (Reichenbach and Kleinig, 1984). Furthermore, *Nannocystis* appears to be the only myxobacterium, and one of the very few procaryotes, that synthesizes and contains considerable amounts of sterols and squalene (Kohl et al., 1983). The taxonomic conclusions that could perhaps be drawn from all these data are that *Nannocystis* should be placed into a family of its own within a suborder of the *Myxococcales*.

Only one species, *N. exedens*, is distinguished within the genus. However, quite often organisms are isolated from soil that clearly resemble *N. exedens* but show different swarm patterns and growth behavior on the standard media. No fruiting bodies have been observed so far with these atypical strains. Such isolates may represent other species or even genera and have to be studied more intensely.

List of species of the genus **Nannocystis**

1. **Nannocystis exedens** Reichenbach 1970, 137.[AL]

ex.e′dens. L. v. *exedere* to eat away; L. part. adj. *exedens* eating away, corroding (the agar).

Vegetative cells are short stout rods with blunt ends, 1.5–5 µm long and 1.1–2 µm wide (Fig. 24.26). Although the cells of *N. exedens* are clearly of the *Polyangium*/"*Sorangium*" type, they tend to be less regular in outline than the cells of the former, often being somewhat fatter near one end and becoming shorter in old cultures until they are ovoid or almost cube-shaped. The cells move slowly by gliding, leaving conspicuous slime tracks on the surface of the substrate (Fig. 24.27). On agar plates, the cells usually migrate in small groups or packs which penetrate deeply into the agar and produce holes and tunnels within the agar.

The fruiting bodies of *N. exedens* are solitary sporangia (Figs. 24.28 and 24.30). Usually they are embedded within the agar, but they may also be found on the surface of the substrate. In the latter case, they may be somewhat raised above the surface, forming tiny knobs or heads. The shape and the size of the fruiting bodies are quite variable. The sporangia within the agar are usually slender and ovoid to spherical and may be as small as 6 × 3.5 µm (these contain only 4–5 myxospores); the larger ones are about 30 × 15 µm. Sporangia on the surface may become much larger, 110 × 40 µm and more, are bean- or sausage-shaped, often bent and sometimes quite irregular, and may even be branched. The sporangia have a tough wall. A fine and regular striation may occasionally be seen on their surface (Fig. 24.28), but sporangia from one and the same culture may differ in this respect. The fruit-ing bodies may be colorless or pale yellow-brown to dark red-brown.

The myxospores are ovoid to almost spherical, are optically dark to refractile in phase contrast, and measure between 0.75 and 1.5 µm in diameter (Fig. 24.29). They are not surrounded by a capsule and, on electron micrographs of a freeze fracture specimen, show a striking pattern of infoldings of the surface membranes (Fig. 24.30).

On water agar with streaks of living or autoclaved *E. coli*, the swarm colonies of *N. exedens* produce a typical, more or less deep corrosion of the agar plate in the form of radiating furrows, channels, tunnels, bubbles and holes (Fig. 24.31). The pattern is highly variable, sometimes differing even in different sections of the same swarm. Most cells are found in ridges and tiny spherical clusters or masses in and on the agar in the outer fringe of the swarm. On yeast (vy-2)-agar, the swarm colonies form shallow craters which gradually enlarge until, in the course of 2–3 weeks, they reach the edge of the dish. The agar surface is only slightly corroded in this case. On media with low (0.05–0.3%) peptone concentrations, the swarms consist of round or irregular flat sheets or mounds, and agar corrosion is usually moderate or absent. The sheets are bright orange, red or purple. Also, on autoclaved *E. coli* the swarms are always brightly colored, from yellow-orange to brick-red, purple, and brown to almost black, depending on the strain and somewhat on the age of the culture.

As mentioned previously, the organism also grows well in liquid media, initially as relatively coarse flakes which become smaller with every transfer so that after some time a single cell suspension may be reached. In liquid culture, too, particularly when grown on single-cell

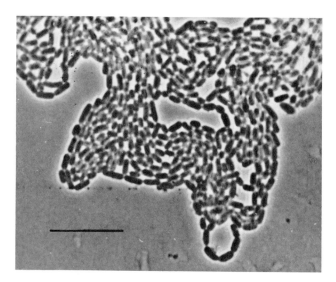

Figure 24.26. *N. exedens* vegetative cells in situ on agar surface in a chamber culture. Phase-contrast micrograph. *Bar,* 13 μm.

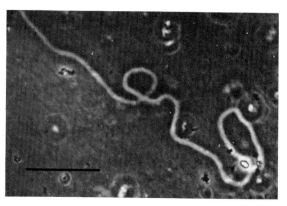

Figure 24.27. *N. exedens* slime track produced by a pack of a few cells migrating over a thin film of peptone agar in a chamber culture. Phase-contrast micrograph. *Bar,* 28 μm.

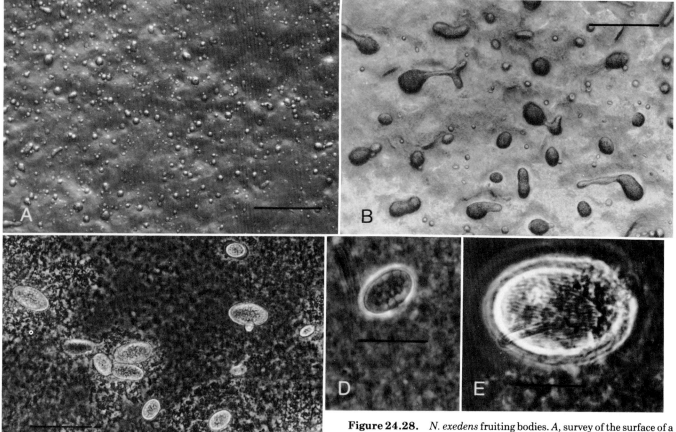

Figure 24.28. *N. exedens* fruiting bodies. *A,* survey of the surface of a culture plate with numerous sporangia on and within the agar. Oblique illumination. *Bar,* 310 μm. *B,* surface of a culture plate (at higher magnification) on which large irregularly shaped sporangia are seen on top of the agar and small ovoid ones are seen within it. Oblique illumination. *Bar,* 30 μm. *C,* slide mount showing ovoid sporangia from within the agar. Phase-contrast micrograph. *Bar,* 50 μm. *D,* small sporangium at high magnification. The myxospores within it are clearly recognizable. Phase-contrast micrograph. *Bar,* 13 μm. *E,* ovoid sporangium from within the agar. A fine striation on its surface is shown. Phase-contrast micrograph. *Bar,* 12 μm.

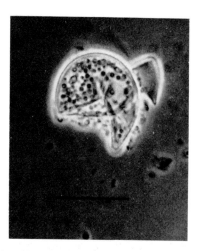

Figure 24.29. *N. exedens* crushed sporangium with spherical myxospores. Phase-contrast micrograph. *Bar*, 16 μm.

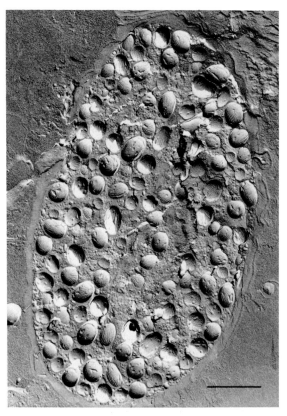

Figure 24.30. *N. exedens* sporangium with myxospores. The sporangium is surrounded by a thick wall. The surface membranes of the ovoid myxospores show a pattern of folds. Zeiss EM 10 B electron micrograph of a freeze fracture specimen. *Bar*, 3.2 μm. (Courtesy of I. Geffers.)

protein, *N. exedens* is brightly colored, usually orange to tomato-red.

All strains grow well on agar containing whole yeast cells (vy/2-agar). The yeast cell is clearly attacked but is not completely decomposed. In particular, the walls remain, and in contrast to most other myxobacteria, no clear lysis zones arise. All strains grow well on streaks of living or autoclaved *E. coli* or other food bacteria; the bacteria are degraded in the process. But not all bacteria are equally suitable. For example, on *Micrococcus luteus*, growth drastically declines with many strains after a few transfers, and the bacteria finally starve to death. This never happens on *E. coli*. Peptone from casein is a good substrate but is tolerated only at relatively low concentrations (0.05–0.1%); in agar media, 0.3% is strongly inhibitory for most strains, although this concentration is suitable in liquid media (e.g. MD1 liquid medium). *N. exedens* seems to utilize only complex nitrogen sources; inorganic nitrogen, aspartic and glutamic acid do not stimulate growth. Neither do various sugars. Vitamin B_{12} enhances the growth of many strains but is not strictly required. Cellulose and starch are not decomposed. Agar is obviously broken down but is not required for growth. It has not been possible to demonstrate an unequivocal growth stimulation by agar. When agar is added to a liquid medium at low concentration, the tiny agar flakes arising under this condition become indented at their edges after the medium is inoculated. It seems that the agar is attacked only in direct contact with cells. As agar is not a usual substrate in soil, the natural substrate for the agarolytic enzymes of *N. exedens* is likely to be some other polysaccharide. Gelatin is liquefied and casein is hydrolyzed. Optimum temperature: 30–36°C; optimum pH: around 7. The organism is strictly aerobic and catalase-positive. The cultures often have an earthly smell which is due in part to geosmin (Trowitzsch et al., 1981). The main pigments of *N. exedens* are monocyclic aromatic carotenols and carotenones (Reichenbach and Kleinig, 1984). The dark brown to black pigments appear to be extracellular and melaninlike. The organism contains quantities of squalene and sterols (about 0.4% each), such as cholest-8(9)-en-3β-ol which it synthesizes de novo (Kohl et al., 1983).

N. exedens is an ubiquitous soil organism, having been isolated from samples obtained worldwide. The bacterium seems not to thrive in cold climate zones, including mountains at high altitudes, and in soils with extreme pH values.

In general, *N. exedens* appears remarkably uniform in its characteristics, although there is a certain variability between strains. Some strains grow very well on agar containing 0.3% casein peptone (e.g. cy-agar), while most do not; some tolerate 0.8% NaCl in the agar medium fairly well; a few produce clear lysis zones in yeast-agar by almost totally decomposing the yeast cells; the color of the swarm colonies may vary considerably. The taxonomic importance of all this has not yet been established, and a subdivision of the species, based on these characteristics, would not be justified.

The mol% G + C of the DNA is 70–71 (Bd) and 71–72 (T_m), respectively (Behrens et al., 1976).

Type strain: DSM 71, ATCC 25963 (equals Na e1 or *N. exedens* HR1).

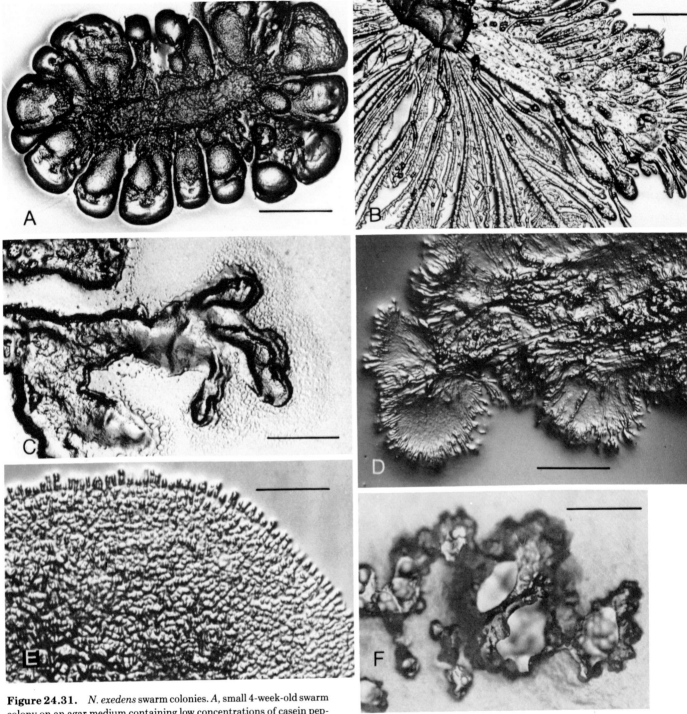

Figure 24.31. *N. exedens* swarm colonies. *A*, small 4-week-old swarm colony on an agar medium containing low concentrations of casein peptone. The organism produced a series of deep bubblelike caverns within the agar plate. *Bar*, 6 mm. *B*, swarm on a streak of autoclaved yeast on water agar. The organism etched a system of feathery branched trenches into the agar surface. *Bar*, 6 mm. *C*, tip of a trench. At the very edge of the colony, the bacteria form a delicate veillike swarm which later tends to contract somewhat and to sink into the agar. *Bar*, 1300 μm. *D*, typical swarm pattern on water agar with streaks of living *E. coli*. The organism has decomposed the food bacteria, and the swarm is now expanding to the plain agar surface. *Bar*, 2.5 mm. *E*, on water agar with autoclaved *E. coli*, a delicate and uniform corrosion pattern may arise. *Bar*, 830 μm. *F*, deep agar corrosion on yeast agar. *Bar*, 470 μm.

Genus III. **Chondromyces** *Berkeley and Curtis in Berkeley 1874, 64*[AL]

HOWARD D. MCCURDY

Chon.dro′my.ces or Chon.dro.my′ces. Gr. n. *chondrus* cartilage, gristle; Gr. n. *myces* fungus; M.L. masc. n. *Chondromyces* cartilaginous fungus.

Vegetative cells are **cylindrical, untapered rods** with blunt rounded ends.

Sporangia are borne singly or in clusters **on simple or branched stalks**.

Myxospores lack capsules and **resemble vegetative rods**.

Vegetative swarms etch, erode and penetrate agar media. Vegetative slime **does not adsorb Congo red dye**.

Aerobic. Temperature range: 18–37°C; optimum: 28–30°C.

The mol% G + C of the DNA is 69–70 (T_m).

Key to the species of the genus **Chondromyces**

I. Sporangium in spherical clusters, not in chains
  A. Sporangia on branched stalks
          1. *C. crocatus*
  B. Sporangia on unbranched stalks
    AA. Sporangia with apical appendages
      a. Sporangia fused on their bases
          2. *C. lanuginosus*
      b. Sporangia not fused
          3. *C. apiculatus*
    BB. Sporangia without apical appendages, borne on conspicuous pedicels
          4. *C. pediculatus*
II. Sporangia in chains
          5. *C. catenulatus*

List of species of the genus **Chondromyces**

1. **Chondromyces crocatus** Berkeley and Curtis in Berkeley 1874, 64.[AL]

cro.ca′tus. L. adj. *crocatus* saffron-yellow.

Vegetative cells (Fig. 24.32) are 1.1–1.4 × 3–12 μm.

Sporangia are broadly spindle-shaped, conical or nearly spherical, 10–25 × 15–30 μm, straw-colored initially, finally becoming golden yellow or orange. Sporangia are borne in spherical clusters on usually branched stalks up to 700 μm or more in height (Figs. 24.33–24.35). Stalks are orange to brown, striated, and often spirally twisted, with several hollow ducts, containing few cells. Irregular forms with ramifying branches and few sporangia or with secondary fruiting structures arising from sporangia germinating in situ may be observed in culture.

Myxospores lack capsules (Figs. 24.36 and 24.37), differ little from vegetative cells except for the presence of conspicuous granules at one or both ends, and are 1.0–1.3 × 3–6 μm.

Vegetative colonies on most media are initially translucent and almost colorless, later becoming yellowish orange and heaped at the periphery to form a "front" which is particularly conspicuous in contact with masses of other living bacteria. The underlying agar is pitted, eroded and penetrated by columns of vegetative cells.

Growth on *Escherichia coli* agar is poor, with lysis generally limited to the immediate area of the colony. Lysis of living bacteria requires direct contact. This organism is cultivated in pure culture on complex media containing enzymatically hydrolyzed protein and Mg^{2+}. Growth is

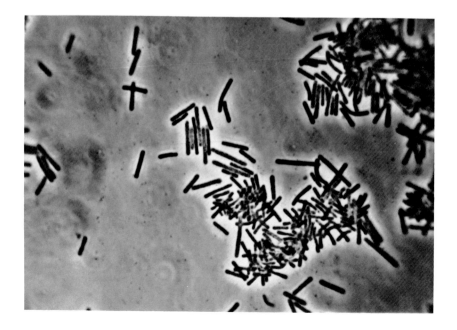

Figure 24.32. *C. crocatus* vegetative cells. Light micrograph (× 900).

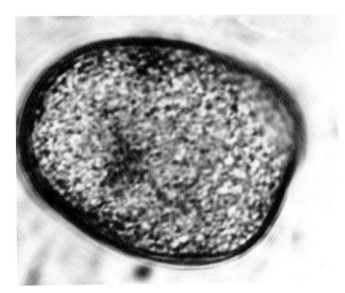

Figure 24.33. *C. crocatus* sporangium. Light micrograph.

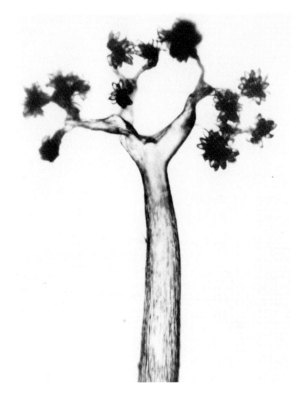

Figure 24.35. *C. crocatus* fruiting body. Light micrograph (× 130).

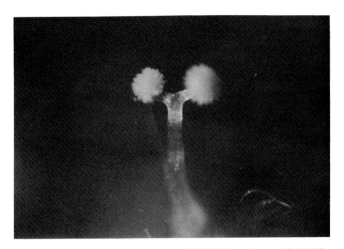

Figure 24.34. *C. crocatus* fruiting body. Light micrograph (× 90).

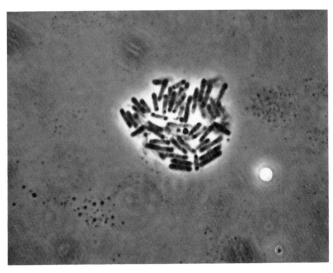

Figure 24.36. *C. crocatus* myxospores. Light micrograph (× 1000).

stimulated by, and initially requires, an extract from bacterial cells.

Nitrate is not reduced. Catalase and oxidase are not produced. This organism hydrolyzes starch, Tween 80, indoxyl acetate, RNA, DNA, gelatin and casein and does not hydrolyze urea, esculin or cellulose. Agar digestion has not been detected.

Temperature range: 18–37°C; minimum: 18°C; optimum: 28–30°C.

Antibiotic sensitivity (disks): resistant to neomycin (10 μg), kanamycin (10 μg) and penicillin (10 units) and inhibited by streptomycin (5 μg), tetracycline (10 μg), chloramphenicol (10 μg) and erythromycin (5 μg).

The streptomycetelike odor produced differs from that of myxobacters with tapered cells.

First observed on decayed melons from South Carolina (U.S.A.). Later found by Thaxter (1892) on old straw from Ceylon. Commonly found on dung in contact with soil, on bacterial streaks inoculated with soil, or on bark.

Neotype specimen: Acc. no. 601, Thaxter Collection, Farlow Herbarium, Harvard University, Cambridge, Massachusetts.

Reference strain: Windsor M38, ATCC 25193.

Illustrations

Berkeley, 1857, p. 313; Thaxter, 1892, Plates 22 and 23, Figs. 1–11; Quehl, 1906, Plate 1, Fig. 10; Jahn, 1924, Plate 2; Emoto 1934, Figs. 1–5; McCurdy, 1969a, Figs. 1–13, 1969b, Fig. 22 (color), and 1971a, Figs. 1–3; McNeil and Skerman, 1972, Figs. 1–4; Brockman and Todd, 1974, Figs. 15–18; Grilione and Pangborn, 1975, Figs. 1 and 2; MacRae and McCurdy, 1975, Figs. 1–13.

2. **Chondromyces apiculatus** Thaxter 1897, 405.[AL]

a.pi.cu.la′tus. L. n. *apex, apicis* point; M.L. adj. *apiculatus* having a small point.

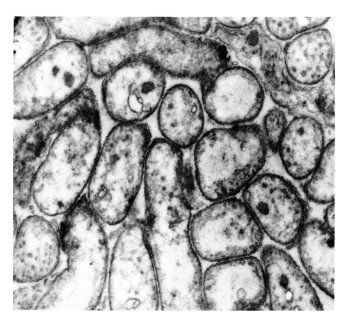

Figure 24.37. *C. crocatus.* Electron micrograph (× 20,700).

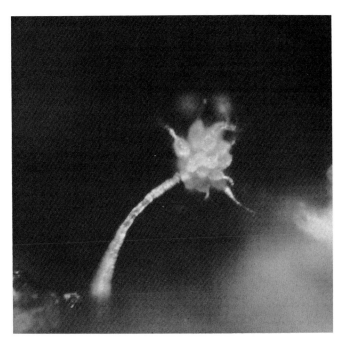

Figure 24.38. *C. apiculatus* fruiting body. Light micrograph (× 200).

Vegetative rods are 1.1–1.4 × 3–14 μm.

Sporangia (Fig. 24.38) are straw-colored to bright orange to brownish orange, variable in form and size, cylindrical to broadly turnip-shaped, and 25–40 × 35–50 μm, with colorless, pointed, frequently branched, apical appendages up to 35 μm long. Pedicels are absent or up to 30 μm long and colorless. Sporangia are borne in spherical clusters of up to 60 or more, although they are usually fewer in number than in *C. crocatus*. The stalk is seldom branched, is up to 700 μm in height, has a diameter of 15–40 μm, is longitudinally striated, and is tunneled and without cells internally. Forms without stalks, with basally fused sporangia, or with large, irregular, solitary sporangia are common. Secondary fruiting body formation as in *C. crocatus* or sporangium formation at tips of appendages is often observed.

Myxospores are similar to vegetative cells, 1.0–1.3 × 3–6 μm. In all other characteristics, this organism is similar to *C. crocatus*.

Originally isolated from antelope dung from Liberia. Commonly observed on rabbit dung placed in contact with soil.

The mol% G + C of the DNA is 69.3 (T_m).

Type specimen: Acc. no. 4481, Thaxter Collection, Farlow Herbarium, Harvard University, Cambridge, Massachusetts.

Reference strain: Windsor M6.

Illustrations

Thaxter, 1897, Plate 30, Figs. 1–15; Quehl, 1906, Plate 1, Figs. 13 and 14; Jahn, 1924, Fig. 5; Kühlwein, 1952, p. 403; McCurdy, 1969b, Fig. 23 (color), and 1971a, Figs. 6 and 7; McNeil and Skerman, 1972, Figs. 3–6; Dawid, 1981, Plate II, Fig. 12, and Plate III, Fig. 8; Reichenbach, 1974b, Figs. 1–5; Reichenbach and Dworkin, 1981, Plate IIg, Fig. 8, *j–m*.

3. **Chondromyces pediculatus** Thaxter 1904, 410.[AL]

pe.di.cu.la′tus. L. dim. n. *pediculus* a small foot (stalk); M.L. adj. *pediculatus* having a small foot or stalk.

Sporangia (Fig. 24.39) are pale yellow to orange and, when dry, orange-red, nearly spherical to long cylindrical, club-shaped or pyriform, usually broader and truncated at the distal end, rough-surfaced, and 25–40 × 35–60 μm. They are borne in groups of up to 60 in umbel-shaped heads on slender pedicels 20–40 μm long. The stalk is unbranched, up to 750 μm in height, striated, sometimes twisted, and colorless initially, becoming orange to brown when dry.

Myxospores are 1.0–1.2 × 3–7 μm.

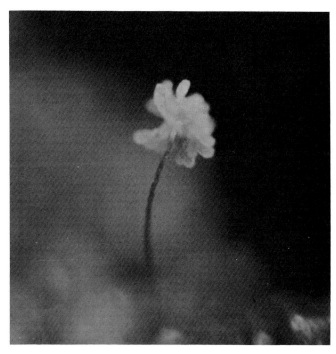

Figure 24.39. *C. pediculatus* fruiting body. Light micrograph (× 150).

Vegetative colonies are orange to reddish orange and resemble those of *C. crocatus*. Congo red is not adsorbed.

Cultivated on dung pellet agar and living bacteria. Growth is slow. This organism was obtained once in pure culture on *E. coli* extract-enriched casitone-Mg²⁺ agar.

Urease is not produced.

Originally isolated on goose dung from South Carolina (U.S.A.). Obtained on rabbit dung in contact with soil.

Type specimen: Acc. no. 4524, Thaxter Collection, Farlow Herbarium, Harvard University, Cambridge, Massachusetts.

Illustrations

Thaxter, 1904, Plate 26, Figs. 7–13; McCurdy, 1969b, Fig. 24 (color), and 1971a, Figs. 8 and 9; McNeil and Skerman, 1972, Figs. 7–10.

4. Chondromyces catenulatus Thaxter 1904, 410.[AL]

ca.te.nu.la′tus. L. n. *catena* chain; L. dim. n. *catenula* a small chain; M.L. adj. *catenulatus* having small chains.

Rods in "rising spore mass" are 1.0–1.3 × 4–6 μm. Cells in vegetative colonies have not been described.

Sporangia are light yellow to orange, fusiform, long elliptical or irregular in shape, 18 × 20–50 μm, and united in chains up to 300 μm long which may be once- or twice-branched (Fig. 24.40). They are separated by shriveled, membranous isthmuses. The stalk is simple, orange to rust-colored, up to 400 μm in height, and broad at the base, tapering above and several times cleft into swollen, tapering parts, with each bearing one or several sporangial chains (Thaxter, 1904, Plate 26, Fig. 5).

Myxospores are nonrefractile cylindrical rods with blunt rounded ends, 1.2–1.4 × 3–6 μm.

Cultivated only on decaying poplar wood from New Hampshire (U.S.A.), it has not been reported in pure culture.

Type specimen: Acc. no. 4517, Thaxter Collection, Farlow Herbarium, Harvard University, Cambridge, Massachusetts.

Illustrations

Thaxter, 1904, Plate 26, Figs. 1–5; McCurdy, 1969b, Fig. 41 (color), and 1971a, Figs. 4 and 5; McNeil and Skerman, 1972, Figs. 11 and 12.

5. Chondromyces lanuginosus Kofler 1913, 861.[AL]

la.nu.gin.os′us. L. adj. *lanuginosus* downy, wooly.

Vegetative cells are cylindrical with blunt rounded ends, 0.9–1.0 × 3–8 μm.

Sporangia (Fig. 24.41) are fused at their bases to form discoid or nearly spherical clusters containing up to 80 sporangia, each with an apical tuft of hairs. Diameter of clusters is variable (40–250 μm), as is the length of the apical hairs (7–30 μm). Stalks are simple or occasionally branched, bearing 1–30 clusters. Sporangia initially are white, changing to yellow, light pink and, lastly, orange. Stalks are at first colorless but become yellow. Sometimes, the sporangial clusters give rise to secondary stalks which are thinner than the primary ones and which are tipped with smaller clusters.

Myxospores do not differ from vegetative cells and are only slightly smaller, 0.6–1.0 × 2.6 μm.

Grown in laboratory culture on hay (Krzemieniewska and Krzemieniewski 1946, 27), pure cultures have not been obtained.

Found on the dung of herbivores in Canada (Faull, 1916) and Austria (Kofler, 1913) and from soil in Poland (Krzemieniewska and Krzemieniewski, 1946).

Neotype specimen: Acc. no. 4494 collected by J. H. Faull, Thaxter Collection, Farlow Herbarium, Harvard University, Cambridge, Massachusetts.

Illustrations

Kofler, 1913, Plate I, Figs. 1–3; Faull, 1916, Plates 5 and 6; Jahn, 1924, Fig. X; Krzemieniewska and Krzemieniewski, 1946, Plate 1, Figs. 1–3; McCurdy, 1969b, Fig. 25 (color), and 1971a, Fig. 10; Dawid, 1981, Plate IV, Fig. 11.

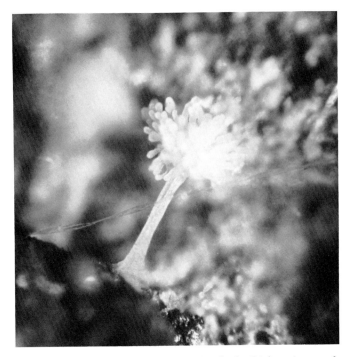

Figure 24.40. *C. catenulatus* fruiting body. Light micrograph (× 120).

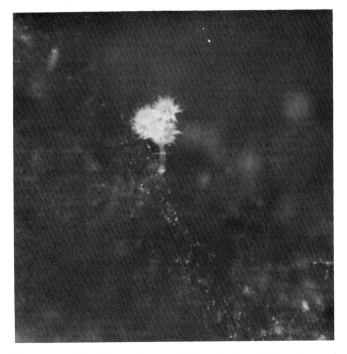

Figure 24.41. *C. lanuginosus* fruiting bodies. Light micrograph (× 100).

SECTION 25

Archaeobacteria

Helmut König and Karl O. Stetter

In addition to the normal procaryotes (eubacteria) and the eucaryotes, the archaeobacteria represent the third line of descent in the evolution of life. This definition is based mainly on sequence comparisons of the 16S rRNA by Woese. Some species of methanogenic and extremely halophilic archaeobacteria have been known for a long time, but their exceptional phylogenetic position had not previously been recognized.

The archaeobacteria are predominantly terrestrial and aquatic microbes, occurring in anaerobic or hypersaline or hydrothermally and geothermally heated environments; also, some occur as symbionts in animal digestive tracts. They consist of aerobes, anaerobes and facultative anaerobes which grow chemolithoautotrophically, organotrophically or facultatively organotrophically. Archaeobacteria may be mesophiles or thermophiles, with some species growing even above 100°C.

A unique biochemical feature of archaeobacteria is the presence of glycerol isopranyl ether lipids. The lack of murein in cell walls makes archaeobacteria insensitive to β-lactam antibiotics. The "common arm" of the tRNAs contains pseudouridine or 1-methylpseudouridine instead of ribothymidine. The sequences of 5S, 16S and 23S rRNAs are very different from the corresponding ones in eubacteria and eucaryotae.

Archaeobacteria share some molecular features with the eucaryotae: (a) the elongation factor 2 (EF-2) contains the amino acid diphthamide and is therefore ADP-ribosylable by diphtheria toxin, (b) amino acid sequences of the ribosomal "A" protein exhibit sequence homologies with the corresponding eucaryotic (L-7/L-12) protein, (c) the methionyl initiator tRNA is not formylated, (d) some tRNA genes contain introns, (e) the aminoacyl stem of the initiator tRNA terminates with the base pair "AU," (f) the DNA-dependent RNA polymerases are multicomponent enzymes and are insensitive to the antibiotics rifampicin and streptolydigin, (g) like the α-DNA polymerases of eucaryotae, the replicating, archaeobacterial DNA polymerases are not inhibited by aphidicolin or butylphenyl-dGTP, and (h) protein synthesis is inhibited by anisomycin but not by chloramphenicol.

Autotrophic archaeobacteria do not assimilate carbon dioxide via the Calvin cycle. In *Methanobacterium*, CO_2 is fixed via an acetyl-CoA pathway, whereas in *Acidianus* and *Thermoproteus*, autotrophic CO_2 fixation occurs via a reductive tricarboxylic acid pathway. Fixation of dinitrogen has been demonstrated by some methanogens.

Gram stain results may be positive or negative within the same order, due to very different types of cell envelopes. Gram-positive-staining species possess pseudomurein, methanochondroitin and heteropolysaccharide cell walls; Gram-negative-staining cells have (glyco-) protein surface layers. The cells may have a diversity of shapes, including spherical, lobed, spiral, plate- or rod-shaped; unicellular and multicellular forms in filaments or aggregates also occur. The diameter of an individual cell may be from 0.1 to >15 μm, and the length of the filaments can be up to 200 μm. Multiplication is by binary fission, budding, constriction, fragmentation or unknown mechanisms. Colors of cell masses may be red, purple, pink, orange-brown, yellow, green, greenish-black, gray and white.

The phylogeny of the archaeobacteria has been explored mainly by Woese by comparison of 16S rRNA catalog and sequences. Two main phylogenetic branches are evident (Fig. 25.1): I. The *"methanogen"* branch which comprises the methanogens, the extremely halophilic bacteria, *Thermoplasmales, Thermococcales* and the recently discovered archaeobacterial sulfate reducers (tentatively named *"Archaeoglobales,"* not shown); and II. The *thermophilic S⁰-metabolizer's* branch, comprising *Sulfolobales, Thermoproteales* and *Pyrodictium.* The phylogenetic tree shows highly divergent groups, indicating that each represents a different order. Some of these groups, however, have only been described at the genus level because very few members are known (e.g. *Thermoplasma*). On the other hand, members of some genera (e.g. *Sulfolobus acidocaldarius* and *Sulfolobus solfataricus; Acidianus infernus* and *Acidianus brierleyi,* not shown) exhibit very divergent 16S rRNA sequences, indicating that they may represent different genera or even families. However, too few distinguishing physiological or morphological features are known; thus, higher taxa for these species are often not described. The 16S rRNAs show evidence for a faster evolution in some bacteria than in other organisms. For further elucidation of the natural system of archaeobacteria, it will be important to compare also other semantophoretic features (e.g. protein sequences) and to correlate these results with those of 16S rRNA cataloging or sequencing.

In the following determinative key of the archaeobacteria, higher taxa are evident from the 16S rRNA analyses, but they have not been validly published (identified by quotation marks); these are shown in order to present the new phylogenetic data.

Key to the groups and taxa of the **Archaeobacteria**

Cytoplasmic membranes of cells contain phytanyl ether lipids. The RNA polymerases are multisubunit enzymes of the AB′B″C, (A+C)B′B″ or BAC type. EF-2 is ADP-ribosylated by diphtheria toxin. Cell walls lack muramic acid. The 16S rRNA sequence is different from eubacteria and eucaryotae.

    I. Cells are able to form methane as the dominating metabolic end product. H_2-CO_2, formate, acetate, methanol, methylamines or H_2-methanol can serve as substrates. S⁰ may be reduced to H_2S without gain of en-

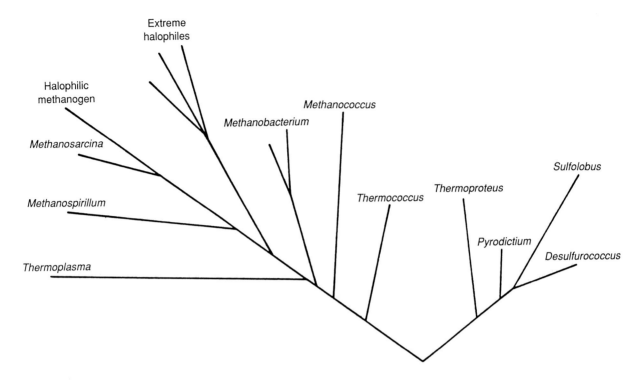

Figure 25.1. Archaeobacterial phylogenetic tree based upon 16S rRNA sequence comparisons. (Reproduced with permission from C. R. Woese, Microbiological Reviews *51:* 221–271, 1987, ©American Society for Microbiology, Washington, D.C.

ergy. Strictly anaerobic. Blue-green epifluorescence when excited at 420 nm. Cells possess coenzyme M, factor 420, factor 430, and methanopterin. RNA polymerase is of the AB'B''C type.

Group I: Methanogenic Archaeobacteria, p. 2173

II. Cells are able to form H_2S from sulfate by dissimilatory sulfate reduction. Traces of methane formed in addition. Extremely thermophilic (growth up to 92°C). Strictly anaerobic. Blue-green fluorescence at 420 nm under the UV microscope. Cells possess factor 420 and methanopterin, but no coenzyme M and no factor 430. RNA polymerase is of the (A+C)B'B'' type.

Group II: Archaeobacterial Sulfate Reducers, p. 2216

III. Cells are Gram-negative or Gram-positive, aerobic or facultatively anaerobic chemoorganotrophs. Rods and regular to highly irregular cells. Requirement for high concentrations of sodium chloride (1.5 M or above). Neutrophilic or alkalophilic. Mesophilic or slightly thermophilic (up to 55°C). RNA polymerase of the AB'B''C type. Some species contain bacteriorhodopsin and are able to use light for ATP synthesis.

Group III: Extremely Halophilic Archaeobacteria, p. 2216

IV. Thermoacidophilic coccoid cells lacking a cell envelope. Cytoplasmic membrane contains a mannose-rich glycoprotein and a lipoglycan. Aerobic. RNA polymerase of the BAC type.

Group IV: Cell Wall-less Archaeobacteria, p. 2233

V. Obligately thermophilic aerobic, facultatively aerobic or strictly anaerobic bacteria. Gram-negative rods, filaments or cocci. Optimal growth temperature: between 70 and 105°C. Acidophiles and neutrophiles. Autotrophic or heterotrophic growth. Most species are sulfur metabolizers. RNA polymerase of the BAC type.

Group V: Extremely Thermophilic S⁰-Metabolizers, p. 2236

Further Reading

Balch, W.E., C.E. Fox, L.J. Magrum, C.R. Woese and R.S. Wolfe. 1979. Methanogens: reevaluation of a unique biological group. Microbiol. Rev. *43:* 260–296.

Brock, T.D. 1978. The genus *Thermoplasma. In* Starr (Editor), Thermophilic Microorganisms and Life at High Temperatures. Springer-Verlag, Heidelberg, pp. 92–116.

Grant, W.D. and H.N.M. Ross. 1986. The ecology and taxonomy of halobacteria. F.E.M.S. Microbiol. Rev. *39:* 9–15.

Kushner, D.J. 1985. The *Halobacteriaceae. In* Woese and Wolfe (Editors), The Bacteria. A Treatise on Structure and Function, Vol. VIII: Archaebacteria. Academic Press, New York, pp. 171–214.

Larsen, H. 1981. The family *Halobacteriaceae. In* Starr, Stolp, Trüper, Balows and Schlegel (Editors), The Prokaryotes. A Handbook on Habitats, Isolation, and Identification of Bacteria. Springer-Verlag, Berlin, pp. 985–994.

Mah, R.A. and M.R. Smith. 1981. The methanogenic bacteria. *In* Starr, Stolp, Trüper, Balows and Schlegel (Editors), The Prokaryotes. A Handbook on Habitats, Isolation, and Identification of Bacteria. Springer-Verlag, Berlin, pp. 948–977.

Stetter, K.O. 1986. Diversity of extremely thermophilic archaebacteria. *In* Brock (Editor), Thermophiles: General, Molecular and Applied Microbiology. John Wiley and Sons, New York, pp. 39–74.

Stetter, K.O. and W. Zillig. 1985. *Thermoplasma* and thermophilic sulfur-dependent archaebacteria. *In* Woese and Wolfe (Editors), The Bacteria. A Treatise on Structure and Function, Vol. VIII: Archaebacteria. Academic Press, New York, pp. 85–170.

Stetter, K.O., G. Lauerer, M. Thomm and A. Neuner. 1987. Isolation of extremely thermophilic sulfate reducers: evidence for a novel branch of archaebacteria. Science *236:* 822–824.

Torreblanca, M., F. Rodriguez-Valera, G. Juez, A. Ventosa, M. Kamekura and M. Kates. 1986. Classification of non-alkaliphilic halobacteria based on numerical taxonomy and polar lipid composition, and description of *Haloarcula* gen. nov. and *Haloferax* gen. nov. Syst. Appl. Microbiol. *8:* 89–99.

Whitman, W.B. 1985. Methanogenic bacteria. *In* Woese and Wolfe (Editors), The Bacteria, A Treatise on Structure and Function, Vol. VIII: Archaebacteria. Academic Press, New York, pp. 3–84.

Woese, C. R. 1987. Bacterial evolution. Microbiol. Rev. *51:* 221–271.

GROUP I. **METHANOGENIC ARCHAEOBACTERIA**

David R. Boone and Robert A. Mah

The methanogenic archaeobacteria have long been distinguished from other microorganisms because they alone produce a hydrocarbon (CH_4) as the major catabolic product. Barker (1956) pointed out that "those investigators who have had personal experience with the methane bacteria have been impressed by the striking physiological characteristics of all members of the group and have preferred to think of them as belonging to a physiological family. . . ." In 1974, Bryant, as one of "those investigators," placed the methanogens as a separate group in the eighth edition of the *Manual* (Bryant, 1974). Since that time, a multitude of data has confirmed Barker's and Bryant's judgment. Woese and Fox (1977) analyzed 16S rRNA oligonucleotides and showed that rRNA changes only very slowly. Thus, cataloging 16S rRNA reveals details in the ancient evolution of cell lines and indicates that methanogens belong to a new kingdom, archaeobacteria, distinct from eubacteria and eucaryotes.

This finding of an ancient divergence of archaeobacteria from other organisms stimulated interest in methanogens. Many unique features were found, confirming that the methanogens are fundamentally different. They have unusual coenzymes such as coenzyme M (Bryant et al., 1971; Taylor et al., 1974), F_{420} (Cheeseman et al., 1972; Eirich et al., 1979), F_{430} (Gunsalus and Wolfe, 1978b), methanopterin (Vogels et al., 1982) and methanofuran (Leigh and Wolfe, 1983); their membranes are composed mainly of ether-linked isoprenoids rather than ester-linked phospholipids (Tornabene et al., 1978; Tornabene and Langworthy, 1979; Langworthy, 1985), and they contain no peptidoglycan (Kandler and Hippe, 1977; Kandler and König, 1985). Further, their ribosomal structure confirms their ancient divergence and provides a phylogenetic structure which is consistent with the physiological and morphological characteristics of the organisms (Balch et al., 1979; Fox, 1985).

Prior to 1977, division of methanogens into taxa depended on standard physiological and morphological characteristics used in examining other organisms. Since that time, various methods have been used for determining the phylogeny of these organisms. They include DNA/DNA homology for distinguishing between species and rRNA homology for higher phylogenetic distinction. rRNA homologies may be determined by directly comparing RNA sequences or by cataloging oligonucleotides from digests or by determining DNA/RNA homology (Fox, 1985). Data from these methods have been used to construct a taxonomy based on phylogeny, and the methanogens may be the first microbial group having its taxonomy based on phylogeny (Whitman, 1985). The phylogenetic data indicate at least three major divisions of methanogenic bacteria, *Methanobacteriales*, *Methanococcales* and *Methanomicrobiales*.

Key to the **Methanogenic Archaeobacteria**

A. Rod-shaped or lancet-shaped methanogens which catabolize H_2-CO_2 or formate; cell walls contain pseudomurein.

Order I. *Methanobacteriales*, p. 2174

B. Coccoid organisms from marine environments; protein cell walls; C_{40} isopranyl ethers are generally absent, and cells grow autotrophically by catabolizing H_2-CO_2 or formate.

Order II. *Methanococcales*, p. 2185

C. Pseudosarcinal, coccoid or sheathed rod-shaped methanogens which catabolize methyl groups; H_2-CO_2 and, sometimes, formate may also be used.

Order III. *Methanomicrobiales*, p. 2191

D. Other taxa

Two additional representatives of the methanogenic bacteria have been described, but they have not yet been assigned to any of the above orders.

1. Methane produced from H_2-CO_2 or formate, but not methanol.

Family *Methanoplanaceae*, p. 2211

2. Methane produced from methanol-H_2, but not H_2 and CO_2 or formate.

Genus *Methanosphaera*, p. 2214*

Acknowledgments

We thank Tatjana N. Zhilina (Institute of Microbiology, Academy of Sciences, Moscow, U.S.S.R.), Indra M. Mathrani, J. Gregory Ferry (Department of Anaerobic Microbiology, Virginia Polytechnic Institute and State University, Blacksburg), Paul H. Smith (Department of Microbiology and Cell Science, University of Florida, Gainesville), Kevin Sowers (Department of Microbiology, University of California, Los Angeles) and Daisy A. Kuhn (Department of Biology, California State University, Northridge) for discussions concerning this chapter and others we prepared in this volume. We also thank Thomas O. MacAdoo (Department of Foreign Languages and Literatures, Virginia Polytechnic Institute and State University, Blacksburg) for discussions and suggestions on taxonomic names.

The preparation of these chapters was supported by Department of Energy grant DE-AT03-80ER10684 and by Gas Research Institute contract CN5080-323-0423(D).

---

*Editorial note: Methanosphaera contains pseudomurein and has phylogenetic links to *Methanobacteriales* (Miller and Wolin, 1985a).

ORDER I. **METHANOBACTERIALES** BALCH AND WOLFE 1981, 216[VP†] (EFFECTIVE PUBLICATION: BALCH AND WOLFE *IN* BALCH, FOX, MAGRUM, WOESE AND WOLFE 1979, 268)

DAVID R. BOONE AND ROBERT A. MAH

Me.tha.no.bac.ter.i.al'es. N.L. fem. pl. n. *Methanobacteriaceae* type family of the order; *-ales* ending to denote an order; N.L. fem. pl. n. *Methanobacteriales* the order of *Methanobacteriaceae*.

Cells are short, lancet-shaped cocci to long, filamentous **rods. Non-motile.** Cells are typically Gram-positive, although some strains are reported to be Gram-variable. Cell wall structure may appear to be typically Gram-positive when viewed by electron microscopy of thin sections, but the wall does not contain muramic acid. **Pseudomurein is the predominant peptidoglycan polymer. Cell membranes are composed mainly of polyisoprenoid hydrocarbons ether-linked to glycerol.** The *Methanobacteriales* are **very strict anaerobes,** and they all **grow by oxidizing H$_2$.** Formate or CO may also be oxidized. CO$_2$ is the normal electron acceptor; sulfur may also be reduced to sulfide, but sulfide production does not lead to growth. Cells contain coenzyme M, F$_{420}$, F$_{430}$ and methanopterin. They form a highly specialized physiological group which **does not catabolize carbohydrates, proteinaceous material or organic compounds other than formate or CO.** They are widely distributed in nature, being found in anaerobic habitats, such as aquatic sediments, soil, anaerobic sewage digesters, and the gastrointestinal tracts of animals, and in ecosystems where geothermally produced H$_2$ accumulates.

The mol% G + C of the DNA is 27–61.

Type family: *Methanobacteriaceae* Barker 1956, 15, emend. Balch, Fox, Magrum, Woese and Wolfe 1979, 267.

Key to the families of the order **Methanobacteriales**

I. Little or no growth at 70°C or above

Family I. *Methanobacteriaceae*

II. No growth below 60°C; optimum temperature above 70°C

Family II. *Methanothermaceae*

Further Comments

Methanosphaera is a new and unassigned genus that may belong to the order *Methanobacteriales*. Cells of *Methanosphaera* contain pseudomurein and have moderately similar rRNA catalogs (S_{AB} = 0.45) to current members of *Methanobacteriales* (Miller and Wolin, 1985a). When more data are accumulated, the description of *Methanobacteriales* and its substituent families may be modified in order to include this genus in a new or existing family. *Methanosphaera* is treated under "Other Taxa" at the end of this section.

FAMILY I. **METHANOBACTERIACEAE** BARKER 1956, 15,[AL·] EMEND. BALCH AND WOLFE *IN* BALCH, FOX, MAGRUM, WOESE AND WOLFE 1979, 267

DAVID R. BOONE AND ROBERT A. MAH

Me.tha.no.bac.ter.i.a'ce.ae. N.L. neut. n. *Methanobacterium* type genus of the family; *-aceae* ending to denote a family; N.L. fem. pl. n. *Methanobacteriaceae* the *Methanobacterium* family.

Cells are short, lancet-shaped cocci to long, filamentous **rods.** Cells are typically Gram-positive, although some strains are reported to be Gram-variable. Cell wall structure may appear to be typically Gram-positive when viewed by electron microscopy of thin sections, but the wall does not contain muramic acid. **Pseudomurein is the predominant peptidoglycan polymer. Cell membranes are composed mainly of polyisoprenoid hydrocarbons ether-linked to glycerol.** The *Methanobacteriaceae* are **very strict anaerobes,** and they all **grow by oxidizing H$_2$.** Formate or CO may also be oxidized. **CO$_2$ is the normal electron acceptor; sulfur may also be reduced to sulfide,** but sulfide production does not lead to growth. Cells contain coenzyme M, F$_{420}$, F$_{430}$, and methanopterin. They form a highly specialized physiological group which **does not catabolize carbohydrates, proteinaceous material, or organic compounds other than formate or CO. Little or no growth occurs at 70°C or above.** They are widely distributed in nature, being found in anaerobic habitats, such as aquatic sediments, soil, anaerobic sewage digesters, and the gastrointestinal tracts of animals, and in ecosystems where geothermally produced H$_2$ accumulates.

The mol% G + C of the DNA is 27–61.

The type genus of this family is *Methanobacterium* Kluyver and van Niel 1936, 399, emend. Balch, Fox, Magrum, Woese and Wolfe 1979, 284.

Key to the genera of the family **Methanobacteriaceae**

I. Cells are short to long rods or filaments.

Genus I. *Methanobacterium*

II. Cells are short rods and lancet-shaped.

Genus II. *Methanobrevibacter*

---

†*VP* denotes that this name, although not on the Approved Lists of Bacterial Names, has been validly published in the official publication, *International Journal of Systematic Bacteriology.*

AL denotes the inclusion of this name on the Approved Lists of Bacterial Names (1980).

Genus I. *Methanobacterium* Kluyver and van Niel 1936, 399,[AL] emend. Balch and Wolfe in Balch, Fox, Magrum, Woese and Wolfe 1979, 284

DAVID R. BOONE AND ROBERT A. MAH

Me.tha.no.bac.ter'i.um. N.L. neut. n. *methanum* methane; Gr. masc. n. *bakterion* a small rod; N.L. neut. n. *Methanobacterium* methane (-producing) rod.

Curved, crooked to straight rods, long to filamentous, about 0.5–1.0 μm in width. **Endospores not formed. Gram stain results are variable. Nonmotile. Cells produce fimbriae. Very strictly anaerobic.** Optimum growth temperatures are 37–45°C for mesophilic species and 55°C or greater for thermophiles. Energy metabolism by reduction of CO_2 to CH_4; electron donors are limited to H_2, formate and CO (Kluyver and Schnellen, 1947). Ammonia is the sole nitrogen source, and sulfide may serve as sulfur source.

The mol% G + C of the DNA is between 32 and 61.

Type species: *Methanobacterium formicicum* Schnellen 1947, 85.

Further Descriptive Information

Rods are long and form chains or often filaments. *M. wolfei* cultures may also contain coccoid cells. The cell wall is a single, thick layer external to the cytoplasmic membrane and composed of pseudomurein (Kandler and König, 1978; König et al., 1982). The members of this genus generally stain Gram-positive, although results from *M. formicicum* and *M. bryantii* are variable. Intracytoplasmic membranous bodies are revealed by thin-section electron micrographs (Zeikus and Wolfe, 1972; Zeikus and Bowen, 1975a). Cells possess fimbriae (Doddema et al., 1979). Elemental sulfur may be reduced to sulfide, but this reaction does not support cell growth (Stetter and Gaag, 1983). Several species are autotrophic, but the mechanism of CO_2 fixation is not known; apparently, neither the reductive pentose cycle, the serine pathway, the hexose phosphate pathway nor the acetigenic pathway can be demonstrated (Daniels and Zeikus, 1978; Taylor et al., 1976; Stupperich and Fuchs, 1981; Ferry et al., 1976).

Agar colonies are tannish white or grayish white, round, diffuse and somewhat filamentous. Most strains are autotrophic, although some require growth factors present in rumen fluid, peptones or yeast extract. H_2 is used to reduce CO_2 to CH_4 for energy production by all strains; formate may replace H_2 as electron donor in *M. formicicum* or *M. thermoformicicum*. In either case the electrons enter metabolic pathways via factor 420-linked enzymes. CO_2 or formate may serve as carbon source; acetate is not required but is used when present.

Immunological analysis using polyclonal antibody probes and whole bacterial cells as antigens indicates the degree of antigenic relatedness among the species of *Methanobacterium* is not very strong. This indication of diversity is supported by the wide range of mol% G + C of the DNA within the species.

Members of the genus *Methanobacterium* may be present in methanogenic environments, such as anaerobic digesters, freshwater sediments, hot springs and marshy soils, or in the rumen of cattle or sheep. H_2-CO_2 or formate are methanogenic substrates; even though these substrates may be at concentrations so low that they are not detectable, they may be quantitatively important because of rapid turnover.

Enrichment and Isolation Procedures

Members of the genus *Methanobacterium* may be isolated directly from their methanogenic environments. The use of antibiotics such as penicillin may be helpful, especially if the numbers of methanogens are low. In enrichment cultures, H_2 concentration is usually high, and *Methanobacterium* species may be outcompeted by nonmethanogenic H_2 utilizers such as *Eubacterium limosum*. The methanogens' lower K_m values for H_2 may give them a selective advantage in nature when H_2 concentration is low, but the faster maximum growth rates of the nonmethanogens sometimes allow them to outcompete methanogens in enrichment cultures with excess H_2. In this case, incorporation of antibiotics such as penicillin or cycloserine may be necessary for isolation of methanogens. Formate may be used to enrich or isolate *M. formicicum* or *M. thermoformicicum*. Because species of *Methanobacterium* are autotrophic or have limited growth-factor requirements, media for isolation or enrichment need have little or no organic additions. Extracts from the natural habitat or rumen fluid additions to mineral media may meet all the nutritional requirements. Unusual metal ions such as nickel, cobalt, tungsten or molybdenum may be required. Ammonia is required as nitrogen source and sulfide as sulfur source. The most successful culture techniques involve the use of roll tubes, although plating methods may be used (Edwards and McBride, 1975; Balch et al., 1979). Agar plates are prepared and inoculated in an anaerobic chamber and then sealed in anaerobic jars for incubation.

Maintenance Procedures

Species of *Methanobacterium* may be stored after lyophilization or as liquid suspensions stored at liquid nitrogen temperatures, or cultures can be maintained by regular subculturing (Hippe, 1984).

Differentiation of the genus **Methanobacterium** from other genera

Members of the genus *Methanobacterium* can be distinguished from other genera of H_2-utilizing methanogens by their morphology and lack of motility. The only other rod-shaped, H_2-utilizing methanogens are in the genera *Methanospirillum*, *Methanomicrobium* and *Methanobrevibacter*. *Methanobrevibacter* rods are generally much shorter than those of *Methanobacterium*. *Methanospirillum* grows in long chains enclosed within a sheath, but the regularity of the gentle spiral curvature is easy to distinguish from the irregularly crooked *Methanobacterium* morphology. Also, *Methanospirillum* and *Methanomicrobium* are motile, whereas *Methanobacterium* is not.

Fimbriae occur and have not been found in other genera of methanogens (Doddema et al., 1979).

Further Comments

"*Methanobacterium thermaggregans*" (corrig.) was proposed as a new species of bacterium (Blotevogel and Fischer, 1985). However, the culture was obtained from cattle manure by inoculating medium with 50 mg penicillin G per liter and repeatedly growing and transferring the culture in the same medium until it appeared to be axenic. Because this culture is not a clone, the data from the reported tests are difficult to interpret, and "*M. thermaggregans*" is not listed as a species in this manual.

Differentiation of the species of the genus **Methanobacterium**

Table 25.1 provides information to distinguish among species of *Methanobacterium*.

Further Reading

Balch, W.E., G.E. Fox, L.J. Magrum, C.R. Woese and R.S. Wolfe. 1979. Methanogens: reevaluation of a unique biological group. Microbiol. Rev. *43*: 260–296.

Table 25.1.
Diagnostic and descriptive features of **Methanobacterium** *species[a]*

Characteristic	1. *M. formicicum*	2. *M. thermautotrophicum*	3. *M. wolfei*	4. *M. uliginosum*	5. *M. alcaliphilum*	6. *M. thermoformicicum*	7. *M. bryantii*	8. *M. thermalcaliphilum*
Substrates								
H_2-CO_2	+	+	+	+	+	+	+	+
Formate	+	−	−	−	−	+	−	−
Morphology								
Long rods	+	+	+	+	+	+	+	+
Filaments	+	+	−	−	+	+	+	+
Gram stain	var.	+	+	+	−	+	var.	−
Motility	−	−	−	−	−	−	−	−
Optimum growth chemoautotrophic	−	+	−	ND[a]	−	+	−	−
Optimum temperature (°C)	37–45	65–70	55–65	37–40	37	55–56	37–39	60
Optimum pH	6.6–7.8	7.2–7.6	7.0–7.5	6.0–8.5	8.1–9.1	7.0–8.0	6.9–7.2	7.5–8.0
Mol% G + C of DNA	38–42	50–52	61	29–34	57	43[b]	33–38	39

[a]Symbols and abbreviations: +, 90% or more of strains are positive; −, 90% or more of strains are negative; var., variable; and ND, not determined.
[b]From T. N. Zhilina, personal communication.
1. *M. formicicum*

List of species of the genus **Methanobacterium**

1. Methanobacterium formicicum Schnellen 1947, 85.[AL]

for.mi′ci.cum. N.L. n. *acidum formicum;* N.L. adj. *formicicum* pertaining to formic acid.

Original description supplemented by material from Mylroie and Hungate (1954, p. 58); Smith (1966, p. 159); Langenberg et al. (1968, p. 1124); Zeikus and Bowen (1975a, p. 373); and Bryant and Boone (1987b).

Cells are slender, crooked rods with blunt, rounded ends. Cells are long and often form chains or filaments. Cells are 0.4–0.8 μm wide and 2–15 μm long. Each strain has a relatively constant diameter, but its length may vary. Nonmotile. Endospores not formed. This organism has fimbriae (Doddema et al., 1979) and intracytoplasmic membranous elements.

Surface colonies are white to gray, flat and filamentous. Deep colonies are profusely filamented spheroids. In roll tubes with H_2-CO_2, colonies appear after 3–5 days, and complete growth occurs within 2 weeks, attaining a diameter up to 5 mm. Appearance of liquid cultures depends on the strain: medium may be uniformly turbid, or growth may occur as highly granular clumps which do not break up even with vigorous agitation (Langenberg et al., 1968).

Some strains may be autotrophic; acetate and cysteine may be stimulatory.

Habitat: may be numerous in anaerobic digesters or anaerobic freshwater sediments; may be present in low numbers in the rumen of cattle or as endosymbionts in anaerobic protozoa (van Bruggen et al., 1984).

The mol% G + C of the DNA is 41–42 (Bd).

Type strain (proposed): MF (DSM 1535), isolated from a sewage-sludge digester (Bryant and Boone, 1987b).

Reference strain: MS1 (van Bruggen et al., 1984).

2. Methanobacterium thermautotrophicum (corrig.) Zeikus and Wolfe 1972, 712.[AL]

therm.au.to.tro.phi′cum. Gr. adj. *thermos* hot; Gr. pref. *auto* self; Gr. adj. *trophikos* one who feeds; N.L. neut. adj. *thermautotrophicum* therm(ophilic) and autotrophic.

Cells are slender, cylindrical, irregularly crooked rods, 0.35–0.6 μm wide and 3–7 μm long, with frequent filaments 10–120 μm in length. Stains Gram-positive. Nonmotile. Endospores not formed. Cells contain intracytoplasmic membranous elements. Fibriae are present.

Deep colonies in roll tubes are tannish white, roughly spherical, diffuse and filamentous.

Growth is rapid in mineral medium with CO_2 as sole carbon source, NH_3 as sole nitrogen source, sulfide as sole sulfur source, and H_2-CO_2 as sole energy source. Not stimulated by organic additions, although acetate may be assimilated.

The mol% G + C of the DNA of the type strain is 50 (Balch et al., 1979) or 52 (Bd) (Zeikus and Wolfe, 1972) or 49 (T_m) (Brandis et al., 1981).

Habitat: thermophilic, anaerobic, sewage-sludge digesters.

Type strain: ΔH (DSM 1053, ATCC 29096), which was isolated from an anaerobic sewage-sludge digester.

Reference strains: YTB (DSM 1850) (Zeikus et al., 1980) and Marburg (DSM 2133) (Fuchs et al., 1980; Brandis et al., 1981).

3. Methanobacterium wolfei Winter and Lerp 1985, 223.[VP] (Effective publication: Winter and Lerp *in* Winter, Lerp, Zabel, Wildenauer, König and Schindler 1984, 460.)

wolf ′e.i. N.L. gen. n. *wolfei* of Wolfe; named for R. S. Wolfe for his pioneering research on the biochemistry of methanogenesis.

Cells are rods, 0.4 μm wide and 2.4–2.7 μm long, with rounded ends. Cells occur singly, in pairs, or in chains. Cell walls contain pseudomurein. Stains Gram-positive. Nonmotile.

Colonies on agar plates are 1–2 mm in diameter, convex with entire margins, and white to yellowish.

H_2-CO_2 is the sole catabolic substrate. Growth occurs in mineral medium; tungsten is required and cannot be replaced by nickel. Yeast extract may stimulate growth. Growth is not inhibited by 10 g NaCl per liter.

Habitat: Anaerobic digesters and anaerobic freshwater sediments.

The mol% G + C of the DNA is 61 (T_m).

Type strain: DSM 2970, isolated from a mixture of sewage-sludge and river sediment.

4. **Methanobacterium uliginosum** König 1985, 375.[VP] (Effective publication: König 1984, 1480.)

u.li.gi.nos'um. N.L. adj. *uliginosum* occurring wet, since it occurs in marshy soil.

Cells are rods 0.2-0.6 μm wide and 1.9-3.8 μm long; some spherical cells may be produced at the ends of the rods, and they may remain attached or be released. Cell walls are composed of pseudomurein, and a capsule may be present. Cells contain intracytoplasmic membrane systems. The organism stains Gram-positive. Nonmotile.

H_2-CO_2 is the sole catabolic substrate. Ammonia may be used as sole nitrogen source and sulfide as sole sulfur source, although this was not tested in the absence of L-cysteine.

Habitat: marshy soils.

The mol% G + C of the DNA is 29.4, as determined by its melting point, and 33.8, as determined by direct nucleotide analysis.

Type strain: P2St (DSM 2956), isolated by inoculation of enrichment cultures with marshy soil followed by treatment with antibiotics and purification by dilution in liquid medium.

5. **Methanobacterium alcaliphilum** Worakit, Boone, Mah, Abdel-Samie and El-Halwagi 1986, 381.[VP]

al.ca.li'phil.um. N.L. n. *alcali* (from Arabic *al* end; *qaliy* soda ash); Gr. adj. *philum* loving; N.L. adj. *alcaliphilum* liking alkaline media.

Original material supplemented by Boone et al. (1986).

Cells are long rods, 0.5-0.6 μm wide and 2-25 μm long, occurring individually or in pairs, more rarely in short chains or filaments. Organism stains Gram-negative. Nonmotile. Colonies grow to 1.0-1.5 mm in diameter. Endospores not formed.

Deep colonies in roll tubes are cream-colored, small (diameter, 0.2 mm), irregular spheroids. Surface colonies are yellowish to cream-colored, smooth, opaque, raised, convex and circular with entire margins.

H_2-CO_2 is the sole substrate for growth and methanogenesis. Growth factors present in peptone or yeast extract are required for growth. Acetate, when present, is assimilated.

Optimal growth occurs between pH 8.1 and 9.1 and near 37°C.

The mol% G + C of the DNA is 57 (Bd).

Habitat: alkaline lake sediments.

Type strain: WeN4 (DSM 3387), which was isolated from an alkaline lake of the Wadi el Natrun in Egypt (Boone et al., 1986; Worakit et al., 1986).

Reference strains: WeN1 (DSM 3457), WeN2 (DSM 3458), and WeN3 (DSM 3459) (Boone et al., 1986).

6. **Methanobacterium thermoformicicum** Zhilina and Ilarionov 1986, 489.[VP] (Effective publication: Zhilina and Ilarionov 1984, 785.)

ther.mo.for.mi'ci.cum. Gr. adj. *thermos* hot; N.L. n. *acidum formicum;* N.L. adj. *thermoformicicum* thermo(philic) and pertaining to formic acid.

Original description of the type culture described by Zhilina and Ilarionov (1984), supplemented with material of Zinder and Koch (1984) and Zhao et al. (1986).

Cells are slender, curved rods, 0.3-0.6 μm wide and 2-7 μm long, with frequent filaments 10-120 μm in length. Stains Gram-positive. Nonmotile. Endospores not formed.

Surface colonies in roll tubes are white to yellowish-gray, with a filamentous or entire margin. They are smooth, moist and translucent and reach a diameter of 0.5-1.0 mm after 5 days. Growth in liquid medium with formate may occur as a mat of interwoven cells.

Growth is rapid (specific growth rate, 0.56 h^{-1}) in mineral medium with CO_2 as sole carbon source, NH_3 as sole nitrogen source, sulfide as sole sulfur source and H_2-CO_2 as sole energy source. Growth on formate as sole organic carbon and energy source is just as rapid as on H_2-CO_2. Not stimulated by organic additions, although acetate may be assimilated. Growth is most rapid between pH 7.0 and 7.8 and at 50-60°C.

The mol% G + C of the DNA is 42.8 (T_m).

Habitat: mesophilic or thermophilic sewage-sludge digesters.

Type strain: Z-245 (DSM 3720) was isolated from a thermophilic manure fermentation.

Reference strains: CB12 (DSM 3664, ATCC 43574) (Zhao et al., 1986) and JF-1 (DSM 2639) (Schauer and Ferry, 1980).

7. **Methanobacterium bryantii** Boone 1987, 173* (ex Balch and Wolfe *in* Balch, Fox, Magrum, Woese and Wolfe 1979, 269).

bry.ant'i.i. N.L. gen. n. *bryantii* of Bryant; named for M. P. Bryant for his pioneering work on methanogens and for the separation and characterization of this organism from the "*Methanobacillus omelianskii*" syntrophic co-culture.

Original description of the type culture described by Bryant et al. (1967), supplemented with material of Bryant et al. (1971) and Langenberg et al. (1968).

Cells are slender rods with blunt, rounded ends, often forming chains and filaments which are irregularly crooked. Cells are 0.5-1.0 μm wide, and chains and filaments are 10-15 μm long. Gram stain results are variable. Nonmotile. Fimbriae are present.

Surface colonies, which can reach 1-5 mm in diameter, are flat with diffuse to filamentous edges and have a characteristic gray to light gray-green appearance. Deep colonies are rounded and filamentous. Cells tend to clump in liquid culture.

Ammonia is used as nitrogen source. Acetate, cysteine and B vitamins are highly stimulatory for growth.

Habitat: anaerobic digesters and sediments.

The mol% G + C of the DNA is 33-38 (Bd).

Type strain: (proposed): M.o.H. (DSM 863, ATCC 33272), isolated from the co-culture "*Methanobacillus omelianskii*," which was originally isolated from an anaerobic digester.

Reference strain: M.o.H.G. (DSM 863) (Balch et al., 1979).

8. **"Methanobacterium thermalcaliphilum"** Blotevogel, Fischer, Mocha and Jannsen 1985, 211.

ther.mal.ca.li'phi.lum Gr. adj. *thermos* hot; N.L. n. *alcali* (from Arabic *al* end; *qaliy* soda ash); Gr. adj. *philum* loving; N.L. adj. *thermalcaliphilum* liking hot, alkaline media.

Cells are slender rods, often forming chains and filaments. Cells are 0.3 μm wide and 3-4 μm long or with longer filaments. Gram stain results are negative. Nonmotile.

Surface colonies, which can reach 1-3 mm in diameter, are pale yellow and entire.

Ammonia is used as nitrogen source. Compounds present in yeast extract are highly stimulatory for growth.

Habitat: methanogenic digesters.

The mol% G + C of the DNA is 38 (T_m).

Type strain: AC60 (DSM 3267), isolated from an anaerobic digester.

*****Editorial note:** This is a request for an opinion to revive the name and assign strain M.o.H. (DSM 863) as the type strain.

Genus II. **Methanobrevibacter** *Balch and Wolfe 1981, 216* VP *(Effective publication: Balch and Wolfe in Balch, Fox, Magrum, Woese and Wolfe 1979, 284)*

Terry L. Miller

Me.tha.no.bre.vi.bac′ter. M.L. n. *methanum* methane; L. adj. *brevis* short; M.L. n. *bacter* masc. equivalent of Gr. neut. n. *bakterion* rod, staff; M.L. masc. n. *Methanobrevibacter* short methane (-producing) rod.

Oval rods or cocci to short rods, usually occurring in pairs or chains; about 0.5–0.7 μm in width and 0.8–1.4 μm in length. **Nonsporing, Gram-positive. Cell walls are composed of pseudomurein. Nonmotile.** Very strict anaerobes. Optimum temperature: 37–39°C; maximum: ~45°C; minimum: ~30°C.

Energy for growth is obtained by reduction of CO_2 to CH_4 by using H_2 and sometimes formate as the electron donor. Acetate, methanol, methylamines or other organic compounds are not used as electron donors for CH_4 formation. All use NH_4^+ as a major source of cell nitrogen. One or more B vitamins are required for growth. Acetate may be a major source of cell carbon.

The mol% G + C of the DNA is 27.5–31.6 (Bd).

Type species: *Methanobrevibacter ruminantium* (Smith and Hungate) Balch and Wolfe 1981, 216.

Further Descriptive Information

Cells are coccobacillary with tapered ends to short rods with rounded ends (Fig. 25.2). They occur singly but more often in pairs or short chains and may appear in long chains. Cell walls are composed of pseudomurein (König et al., 1982). Pseudomurein is composed of N-acetyl amino sugars, L-amino acids and neutral sugars. The glycan moiety of *M. ruminantium* and *M. smithii* contain D-glucosamine, D-galactosamine and L-talosaminuronic acid. *M. arboriphilicus* (strains DH1 and AZ) contain only D-galactosamine and D-talosaminuronic acid. The peptide moiety of all species contains L-alanine, L-glutamate and L-lysine; however, L-threonine can partially or completely replace L-alanine in the wall of *M. ruminantium. M. smithii* cell wall contains ornithine as an additional component of the peptide moiety. *M. ruminantium* and *M. arboriphilicus* (DH1) have high phosphate levels in their cell walls. The lipid composition of one strain of each species has been examined (Tornabene et al., 1979; Tornabene and Langworthy, 1979). The lipids of the species differ primarily in the composition of the isoprenoid hydrocarbon neutral lipid.

Ultrastructural features of the type strains of each species are shown in Figure 25.3.

M. ruminantium and *M. smithii* require acetate as a major source of cell carbon. Acetate is a precursor of 60% of the cell carbon of *M. ruminantium* (Bryant et al., 1971). CO_2 can serve as the sole carbon source of *M. arboriphilicus,* but one or more B vitamins are required for growth. *M. ruminantium* is more nutritionally fastidious than the other species. It requires 2-methylbutyrate, 2-mercaptoethanesulfonic acid (coenzyme M) and a mixture of amino acids (Bryant et al., 1971; Taylor et al., 1974). Trace metal requirements have not been determined, although *M. smithii* was shown to require nickel (Diekert et al., 1981). All of the species grow well with H_2 and CO_2 as the energy source. *M. ruminantium* and *M. smithii* can use formate as an energy source, but growth is usually slow and cultures do not grow to the extent observed with H_2 and CO_2. *M. arboriphilicus* does not usually grow with formate, although a recent sewage-sludge isolate that is morphologically and immunologically similar to *M. arboriphilicus* strain DC grows with formate as the sole energy source (Morii et al., 1983).

M. smithii and *M. arboriphilicus* are resistant to many antibiotics that inhibit eubacterial membrane function or cell wall, RNA or protein synthesis (Hilpert et al., 1981; Pecher and Böck, 1981).

Methanobrevibacter species occur in ruminants, human and other animal gastrointestinal tracts, municipal sewage sludges and decaying woody tissues.

Enrichment and Isolation Procedures

All enrichments and isolations must be carried out under strictly anaerobic conditions. Isolation and cultivation procedures are based on the techniques developed by Hungate (1969). Serum bottle modifications of the Hungate technique have been developed (Miller and Wolin, 1974; Balch and Wolfe, 1976) that allow the use of syringes for additions and incubation under elevated gas pressures to increase the availability of the energy sources, H_2 and CO_2. Liquid cultures with H_2 and CO_2 are incubated with rotation or shaking. The development of anaerobic glove boxes based on the design of Aranki and Freter (1972) have helped to facilitate the isolation and handling of pure cultures.

M. smithii can be enumerated and isolated semiselectively from human fecal samples by plating on medium 1 of Balch et al. (1979), supplemented with 0.1% additional NH_4Cl, 10% rumen fluid, 2% agar (modified medium 1) and clindamycin and cephalothin (Miller and Wolin, 1982). Many eubacteria are inhibited by these antibiotics. Methanogens are insensitive due to their unique macromolecular properties. The roll tubes are incubated statically at 37°C under 80% H_2 and 20% CO_2 gas phase. The presence of methanogens is confirmed by gas chromatographic analysis for CH_4 in the head space of the roll tubes. A single methanogenic colony can produce detectable CH_4. Colonies are picked from the most dilute inoculum having roll tube methane and are subcultured in liquid medium. Purity of cultures is established by noting that all cells show factor 420 fluorescence, when viewed with epifluorescent microscopy, and lack of growth in complex media with energy sources other than H_2 and CO_2 or formate. The above antibiotic medium may also be used to enrich or enumerate *Methanobrevibacter* species in rumen contents and animal feces (Miller et al., 1986a, b). The antibiotic medium is not specific for *Methanobrevibacter* and may be useful for enriching and/or enumerating other methanogens in other ecosystems.

Maintenance Procedures

M. ruminantium, M. smithii and *M. arboriphilicus* can be maintained for short periods (weeks) on agar slants of modified medium 1 without antibiotics (see above). A broth culture (24–48 h, 0.1–0.3 ml) is inoculated into a tube containing 10 ml of reduced agar medium and 1 ml of reduced liquid medium. Inoculated tubes are regassed and pressurized to 2 atm with 80% H_2 and 20% CO_2 and incubated statically and horizontally at 37°C. After growth, the head space is regassed with H_2-CO_2, and the culture is stored at 4°C. Cultures are directly transferred to fresh slant tubes every 2 weeks.

M. ruminantium, M. smithii and *M. arboriphilicus* have been preserved for longer periods (months) by preparing agar-liquid cultures on the basis of biphasic culture techniques (Krieg and Gerhardt, 1981; Miller and Wolin, 1985a; Miller et al., 1986a). Double-strength modified medium 1 without antibiotics, containing 3% Difco agar, is prepared and dispensed into serum bottles under an atmosphere of 80% N_2 and 20% CO_2. After autoclaving, double-strength reducing agent is added, the head space of the bottle is replaced with 80% H_2 and 20% CO_2, and the bottle is laid on its side. When the agar solidifies, an amount of reduced single-strength broth medium is added in the ratio of 1 volume of liquid medium to 3 volumes of solid medium. An inoculum equivalent to 10% of the liquid volume is added, and the bottles are pressurized to 2 atm with 80% H_2 and 20% CO_2. Cultures are incubated at 37°C with gentle rocking and regassed and pressurized 1–2 times daily until an A_{660} of >2.0 (1-cm cuvette) is obtained. After outgrowth, biphasic culture bottles are regassed and repressurized with 80% H_2 and 20% CO_2, precooled for 1 h at 4°C and stored at −76°C.

Cultures are removed every 6 months, rapidly thawed under warm running water, and transferred by using a 10% inoculum into reduced single-strength broth medium. Cells of *M. smithii* remain viable after 1 year of storage at −76°C. Addition of sterile glycerol (20%, v/v) to biphasic cultures of *Methanobrevibacter* species did not enhance viability and resulted in growth lags of 1–2 days when transfers were made into a liquid

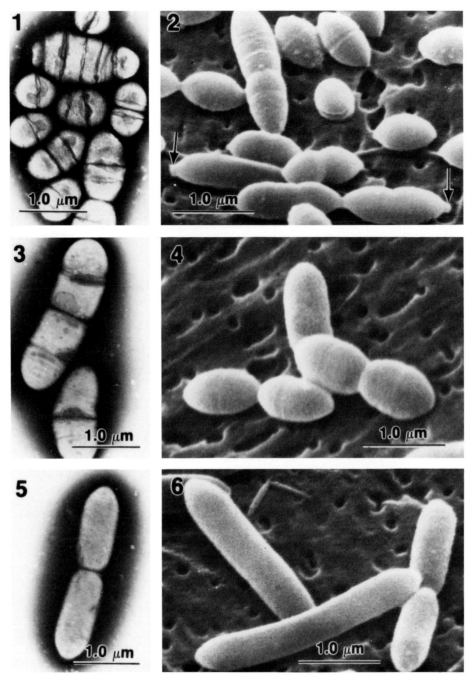

Figure 25.2. Morphology of *Methanobrevibacter* species. The three species were grown in liquid modified medium 1 (see text) with 2 atm 80% H_2 and 20% CO_2 at 37°C. Cultures were regassed and repressurized 1–2 times daily for 2–4 days. Final A_{660} ($d = 1$ cm) were: *M. ruminantium*, 1.3 (72 h); *M. smithii*, 3.6 (96 h); and *M. arboriphilicus*, 1.2 (48 h). *Part 1, M. ruminantium* strain M1. Negative stain preparation, 2% sodium phosphotungstate (2% NaPTA), pH 7.0. The multiple septa of the cells are penetrated by the stain. *Part 2*, scanning electron micrograph (*SEM*) of *M. ruminantium* strain M1. Cells from culture fluid were collected on a filter with mild vacuum and fixed in situ with 2% glutaraldehyde in 0.09 N sodium cacodylate, pH 7.2, for 30 min followed by rinsing with the same buffer and fixing in 1% osmium in veronal acetate buffer (Kellenberger et al., 1958) for 1 h. After rinsing in double-distilled water and dehydration in a graded ethanol series the material was critical point-dried from liquid CO_2 and sputter-coated with gold. The division septa are apparent; cell ends appear more tapered than that seen by negative staining (*Part 1*), and remnants of wall material from a recent cell division are observed (*arrows*). *Part 3, M. smithii* strain PS. Negative stain (2% NaPTA). Multiple septa are penetrated by the stain. *Part 4*, SEM of *M. smithii* strain PS (prepared as in *Part 2*). Some cell septa are visible, and the cell ends are rounder than *M. ruminantium* (*Part 2*). *Part 5, M. arboriphilicus* strain DH1. Negative stain (2% NaPTA). The cell surface is smooth. *Part 6*, SEM of *M. arboriphilicus* strain DH1. Septa are not present. The ends of the cells are slightly truncated.

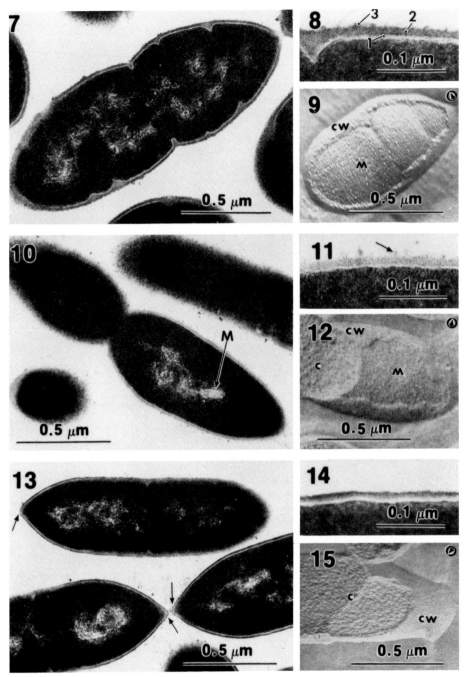

Figure 25.3. Ultrastructure features of *Methanobrevibacter* species. Cultures were grown as described in Figure 25.2. *Part 7,* thin section of *M. ruminantium* strain M1, prepared as described by Samsonoff et al. (1970). The thick cell wall is invaginated at multiple septa sites. *Part 8,* thin section through the cell wall of *M. ruminantium* strain M1. The cell wall is composed of three layers, as previously reported by Zeikus and Bowen (1975): a thin electron-dense inner layer (*1*), a thicker less-electron-dense middle layer (*2*), and a rough irregular outer layer (*3*). *Part 9,* freezed-etched preparation of *M. ruminantium* strain M1. Cells were harvested by centrifugation, frozen in Freon-22, stored in liquid N₂ and fractured in a Balyers 360M freeze-fracture device. After 1 min of etching at −110°C, the samples were shadowed with carbon-platinum. No organized structural patterns can be seen in the cell wall (*cw*). Fractures through the cytoplasmic membrane (*m*) revealing the protoplasmic face (Branton et al., 1975) are frequent. *Encircled arrow* indicates the direction of shadow. *Part 10,* thin section of *M. smithii* strain PS (prepared as in *Part 7*). Membranous structures (*M*) are frequently seen near the nucleoid and in some instances extend to the cytoplasmic membrane (not shown). *Part 11,* thin section through the cell wall of *M. smithii* strain PS. The wall appears as a single electron-dense thick layer with a rough irregular outer surface (*arrow*). *Part 12,* freeze-etched preparation of *M. smithii* strain PS (prepared as in *Part 9*). No organized structural pattern is seen in the cell wall (*cw*). Most fractures are through the cytoplasm (*c*) and only occasionally occur through the cytoplasmic membrane (*m*), revealing the protoplasmic face. *Encircled arrow* indicates the direction of shadow. *Part 13,* thin section of *M. arboriphilicus* strain DH1 (prepared as in *Part 7*). The cell ends are slightly truncated (*arrows*). *Part 14,* thin section through the cell wall of *M. arboriphilicus* strain DH1. The cell wall appears as a single layer which is more electron dense toward the outer surface. *Part 15,* freeze-etched preparation of *M. arboriphilicus* strain DH1 (prepared as in *Part 9*). The cell wall (*cw*) has no apparent organized structural pattern. Fractures occur frequently through the cytoplasm (*c*) but not through the cytoplasmic membrane. *Encircled arrow* indicates the direction of shadow.

medium. This method of culture storage is routinely used in my laboratory to stock a wide variety of other genera and species of methanogens, including thermophilic species. Biphasic cultures have also been used to

obtain sufficient cells for cell wall and DNA analyses (Miller and Wolin, 1985a; König, 1986; Miller et al., 1986a).

Differentiation of the genus **Methanobrevibacter** from other genera

The genus *Methanobrevibacter* is phylogenetically differentiated from other genera by the oligonucleotide codon sequences of its 16S rRNA (Balch et al., 1979). *Methanobrevibacter* is Gram-positive, and all other genera except *Methanosarcina* and *Methanobacterium* are Gram-negative. *Methanobrevibacter* is distinguished from *Methanosarcina* on the basis of morphology, energy sources for growth and the presence of pseudomurein in *Methanobrevibacter* cell walls. *Methanobrevibacter* is differentiated from *Methanobacterium* on the basis of morphology.

Acknowledgments

I thank W. A. Samsonoff for electron microscopic analyses and the electron micrographs presented in this description and E. Currenti and E. Kusel for technical assistance.

Further Reading

Balch, W.E., G.E. Fox, L.J. Magrum, C.R. Woese and R.S. Wolfe. 1979. Methanogens: reevaluation of a unique biological group. Microbiol. Rev. *43:* 260–296.
Kanler, O. (Editor). 1982. *Archaebacteria.* Gustav Fisher Verlag, Stuttgart.
Kandler, O. and W. Zillig (Editors). 1986. *Archaebacteria '85.* Gustav Fischer Verlag, Stuttgart.
Mah, R.A. and M.R. Smith. 1981. The methanogenic bacteria. *In* Starr, Stolp, Trüper, Balows and Schlegel (Editors), The Procaryotes. A Handbook on Habitats, Isolation, and Identification of Bacteria. Springer-Verlag, Berlin, pp. 948–977.
Woese, C.R. and R.S. Wolfe (Editors). 1985. The Bacteria: A Treatise on Structure and Function, Vol. VIII: Archaebacteria. Academic Press, New York.

Differentiation of the species of genus **Methanobrevibacter**

Some characteristics of the type species of *Methanobrevibacter* are summarized in Table 25.2.

List of species of the genus **Methanobrevibacter**

1. **Methanobrevibacter ruminantium** (Smith and Hungate 1958) Balch and Wolfe 1981, 216.[VP] (Effective publication: Balch and Wolfe *in* Balch, Fox, Magrum, Woese and Wolfe 1979, 284.) (*Methanobacterium ruminantium* Smith and Hungate 1958, 717.[AL])

ru.mi.nan'ti.um. L. part. adj. *ruminans, ruminantis* ruminating; M.L. neut. pl. n. *ruminantia* ruminants; M.L. pl. gen. *ruminantium* of ruminants.

Only one strain of the species (M1 or DSM 1093), isolated from bovine rumen contents by Bryant (1965), has been phylogenetically characterized. The following features are based on studies of this strain.

Short oval rod or coccobacillus with tapered ends 0.7 μm in width and 0.8–1.7 μm in length. Cells occur predominantly in pairs in young cultures and in chains in older cultures. Strong Gram-positive reaction, even in relatively old cultures. Nonmotile. Flagella appear to be absent by negative staining or freeze-fracture procedures (W. A. Samsonoff, personal communication). Langenberg et al. (1968) first described the coccoid appearance and the presence of large numbers of cross-walls, presumably because the cells are constantly dividing (Fig. 25.2, *Parts 1 and 2*).

Surface colonies on organically complex agar medium in roll tube cultures with H_2-CO_2 gas phase are translucent, convex and circular with entire margins and frequently light yellow in appearance. They may be visible after ~3 days incubation at 37°C and can reach a diameter of 3–4 mm, depending on the number of colonies and the availability of the energy source. Colonies in deep agar are lenticular.

M. ruminantium requires acetate as a major source (60%) of cell carbon (Bryant et al., 1971). In addition to one or more B vitamins, it requires 2-mercaptoethanesulfonic acid (coenzyme M), 2-methylbutyric acid and a mixture of amino acids (Bryant, 1965; Bryant et al., 1971; Taylor et al., 1974). Coenzyme M transport is energy-dependent and is inhibited by 2-bromoethanesulfonic acid (Balch and Wolfe, 1979b). Radioisotopic studies indicate that 2-methylbutyric acid is a precursor of isoleucine via a reductive carboxylation pathway (Robinson and Allison, 1969). The amino acids cannot replace the requirement for NH_4^+ as the major source of cell nitrogen. Growth is inhibited in modified medium 1 containing 2% oxgall and 0.1% sodium deoxycholate (T. L. Miller, unpublished data). H_2 and CO_2 serve as energy sources. Growth with formate as an energy source is slow, and cultures do not grow to the same optical density as with H_2 and CO_2. Formate is probably first converted to H_2 and CO_2 via a formate dehydrogenase coupled to a hydrogenase. A mag-

nesium and ATP-dependent methyl-coenzyme M methylreductase system has been demonstrated in cell-free extracts (Gunsalus and Wolfe, 1978a; Romesser and Wolfe, 1982).

Rabbit antisera and the corresponding antigen preparations of strain M1 do not cross-react with antigens and antisera, respectively, of other species of the genus or other members of the family (Conway de Macario et al., 1982b).

Table 25.2.

Characteristics of the type strains of the species of the genus **Methanobrevibacter**[a]

Characteristic	1. *M. ruminantium*, M1	2. *M. smithii*, PS	3. *M. arboriphilicus*, DH1
Morphology	Oval rod or cocus	Oval rod or cocus	Short rod
Nutritional requirement			
Acetate	+	+	−
B vitamins	+	+	+
Coenzyme M	+	−	−
2-Methylbutyrate	+	−	−
Amino acids	+	−	?
NH_4^+	+	+	+
Energy sources			
H_2-CO_2	+	+	+
Formate	+	+	−
Bile inhibition	+	−	+
Mol% G + C of DNA (Bd)	30.6	31.0	27.5
Serology[b]			
M1 antiserum	4+	−	−
PS antiserum	−	4+	−
DH1 antiserum	−	−	4+

[a]Symbols: +, positive; −, negative; and ?, not known.
[b]Rabbit antisera tested at the highest dilution that produces the maximal reaction with the homologous antigen in an indirect immunofluorescence test. (See Conway de Macario et al. (1982b).)

There is limited information on the antibiotic sensitivity of the strain. Clindamycin (2 µg/ml) and cephalothin (8 µg/ml) are not lethal in liquid or solid media. Bacitracin (100 µg/ml) inhibits growth in liquid medium (T. L. Miller, unpublished data). Growth and CH_4 production are inhibited by 2-bromoethanesufonate until the coenzyme M concentration exceeds a 1:1 molar ratio with bromoethanesulfonate (Balch and Wolfe, 1979a).

The strain isolated by Smith and Hungate (1958) was present in rumen contents in concentrations of 10^6-10^8/ml in grass and/or alfalfa-fed steers. It is no longer in extant culture. Both coenzyme M-requiring and nonrequiring *Methanobrevibacter* strains are present in high concentrations in bovine rumen contents (Lovley et al., 1984; Miller et al., 1986b). The taxonomic relationship of the *Methanobrevibacter* species isolated in the latter studies to the *M. ruminantium* type strain or to each other has not yet been clearly established (Miller et al., 1986b).

The mol% G + C of the DNA is 30.6 (Bd) (Balch et al., 1979).

Type strain: Ml (DSM 1093).

2. Methanobrevibacter smithii Balch and Wolfe 1981, 216.[VP] (Effective publication: Balch and Wolfe *in* Balch, Fox, Magrum, Woese and Wolfe 1979, 284.)

smith'i.i. M.L. gen. n. *smithii* of Smith; named after P. H. Smith who isolated the type strain.

Cells are short oval rods or coccobacilli with tapered ends, 0.6-0.7 µm in width and ~1.0 µm in length. Cells occur most frequently in pairs or in chains of 4-6 cells. Gram-positive. Nonmotile. A strain cited as "PS1," but recently confirmed to have been strain PS, was reported to have a single polar flagellum (Doddema et al., 1979; H. D. Doddema and G. D. Vogels, personal communication). Other investigators have found that flagella are absent from cells of strain PS or human fecal strains that are morphologically, physiologically and immunologically indistinguishable from strain PS (Miller et al., 1982; M. Edwards and W. A. Samsonoff, personal communication). Multiple septa are frequently observed on the cell surface (Fig. 25.2, *Parts 3* and *4*), but septa formation is not as extensive as that observed with *M. ruminantium* cells.

Surface colonies in roll tube cultures on complex rumen fluid-containing medium are translucent, effuse to low convex, usually circular or elliptical with entire margins and light to dark tan, often with a tiny brown center. They can reach a diameter of 2-3 mm in roll tubes with few colonies and excess energy source.

One or more B vitamins are required or stimulatory to growth, and acetate is required as a major source of cell carbon (Bryant et al., 1971). Nickel is required (Diekert et al., 1981). Other trace metal requirements have not been investigated. Growth of the type strain or human fecal strains is not inhibited in modified medium 1 containing 2% oxgall and 0.1% sodium deoxycholate and H_2 and CO_2 as energy sources (Miller et al., 1982). NH_4^+ is the sole source of cell nitrogen, and H_2S may serve as the sole source of cell sulfur (Bryant et al., 1971). H_2 and CO_2 are the preferred energy sources. Growth on formate is poor. In the presence of H_2 and CO_2, CO is removed from the gas phase (Daniels et al., 1977); however, CO has not been shown to support growth and methane production. A factor 420-dependent formate dehydrogenase oxidizes formate to CO_2 and reduced factor 420 (Tzeng et al., 1975a). A hydrogenase is factor 420-linked, and biosynthetic reducing power may be generated via factor 420:NADPH oxidoreductase (Tzeng et al., 1975b). These enzymatic reactions were the first demonstration of the function of factor 420 in electron transfer reactions in methanogens. *M. smithii* also contains the cofactors 2-mercaptoethanesulfonic acid (Balch and Wolfe, 1979a) and factor 430 (Diekert et al., 1981). Cells also have corrinoids (Krzyck and Zeikus, 1980). The polyamine content is low (Scherer and Kneifel, 1983).

Antisera and the corresponding antigen preparations of strain PS do not cross-react with antigens and antisera, respectively, of other species in the genus (Conway de Macario et al., 1982b). PS antisera strongly cross-reacts with human fecal strains (Conway de Macario et al., 1982a; Miller and Wolin, 1982; Miller et al., 1982).

The following antibiotics produce zones of inhibition (20-40 mm): bacitracin, gardimycin, enduracidin, chloramphenicol and lasalocid

(Hilpert et al., 1981). In rumen fluid medium, monensin causes a delayed growth response (Chen and Wolin, 1979). Bacitracin (10 µg/ml) completely inhibits growth in liquid modified medium 1 (T. L. Miller, unpublished data).

The type strain PS was isolated from an anaerobic sewage-sludge enrichment with formate as the exogenously added energy source (Smith, P.H. 1961. Bacteriol. Proc. Abstr. A 40, p. 60). *M. smithii* is the dominant methanogen in feces of humans who harbor methanogens in their large bowel (Nottingham and Hungate, 1968; Miller and Wolin, 1982). Their concentrations range from extremely low numbers (a few cells per gram dry weight feces) to as high as 10^{10}/g dry fecal weight and in some individuals can be equal to 10% of the total concentration of viable anaerobic bacteria (Weaver et al., 1986). *Methanobrevibacter* species have been isolated from feces of several different animals, but, to date, *M. smithii* appears to be unique to the human large bowel ecosystem (Miller et al., 1986a; Miller and Wolin, 1986; Weaver et al., 1986).

The mol% G + C of the DNA of the type strain is 31.0 (Bd) (Balch et al., 1979) or 30.0 (T_m) (T. L. Miller, unpublished data). The range of mol% G + C of three human fecal isolates is 28.8-29.5 (T_m) (T. L. Miller, unpublished data).

Type strain: PS (DSM 861).

3. Methanobrevibacter arboriphilicus (Zeikus and Henning 1975) Balch and Wolfe 1981, 216.[VP] (Effective publication: Balch and Wolfe *in* Balch, Fox, Magrum, Woese and Wolfe 1979, 284.) (*Methanobacterium arbophilicum* Zeikus and Henning 1975, 550.[AL])

ar.bor.i.phil'i.cus. L. gen. n. *arbor* tree; M.L. adj. *philicus* equivalent of Gr. adj. *philus* loving; M.L. adj. *arboriphilicus* tree-loving.

Four strains of *M. arboriphilicus* are presently in pure culture (strains DH1 (DSM 1125), DC (DSM 1536), AZ (DSM 744) and A2 (DSM 2462)). Strains DH1 and DC were found to have identical 16S rRNA oligonucleotide codon catalogs (Balch et al., 1979). The codon catalog of strain AZ has a similarity index value of 0.84 with strains DH1 and DC. The lack of detectable immunologic cross-reactivity between reciprocal rabbit antisera and antigens between strains DH1, DC and AZ and the existence of distinct immunovars indicate strain differences (Conway de Macario et al., 1982a). Strain A2 weakly cross-reacts with strain DC antiserum but not with strain AZ or DH1 antisera (Morii et al., 1983). Some physiological features of the strains are summarized in Table 25.3.

Cells of DH1 grown in liquid culture are short rods with rounded ends, 0.5 µm in width and 1.2-1.4 µm in length. Some cells may have a slightly truncated end (Fig. 25.3, *Part 13*). They occur singly or in pairs. In agar medium, cells are elongated, often as much as 12 times the length of cells grown in liquid medium (Zeikus and Henning, 1975). Cells in liquid culture tend to clump together and are not easily dispersed by vigorous

Table 25.3.
Physiological features of **M. arboriphilicus**[a]

Characteristic	Strain			
	DH1	DC	AZ	A2
Mol% G + C of DNA (Bd)	27.5	27.7	31.6	29.6
Serology[b]				
DH1 antiserum	4+	—	—	—
DC antiserum	—	4+	—	1+
AZ antiserum	—	—	4+	—
16S rRNA codon catalog S_{AB}[c]	1.0	1.0	0.84	ND
Energy source				
H_2-CO_2	Yes	Yes	Yes	Yes
Formate	No	No	No	Yes

[a]Symbols: —, no reaction; and ND, not determined.
[b]Rabbit antisera tested at the highest dilution that produces the maximal reaction with the homologous antigen in an indirect immunofluorescence test. (See Conway de Macario et al. (1982a).)
[c]Relative to DH1. (See Balch et al. (1979).)

shaking or vortexing. Gram-positive. Nonmotile. Cells of strain AZ were reported to have a single polar flagellum (Doddema et al., 1979). Flagella appear to be absent from cells of strain DH1 by negative stain or freeze-fracture procedures (W. A. Samsonoff, personal communication). Multiple division septa are not usually present (Fig. 25.2, *Parts 5* and *6*).

Surface colonies in organically complex agar medium in roll tubes with H_2 and CO_2 gas phase are roughly round, diffuse or filamentous and creamy white to yellow or dark brown. Mature colonies do not exceed 5 mm in diameter.

Carbon dioxide is the major and possibly sole source of cell carbon; however, one or more B vitamins are required. Growth is stimulated by trypticase, yeast extract and rumen fluid. Growth is inhibited in modified medium 1 containing 2% oxgall and 0.1% sodium deoxycholate (T. L. Miller, unpublished data). H_2 and CO_2 may be the sole or preferred energy sources. Methane formation from H_2 and CO_2 by cell suspensions of strain AZ is dependent on sodium ion (Perski et al., 1982). Growth with formate as sole energy source has been reported for strain A2 (Morii et al., 1983). The other strains do not use formate as an energy source. Ex-

tracts of DH1 oxidize CO with reduction of benzyl viologen, but CO cannot substitute for H_2 as the electron donor for CO_2 reduction to CH_4 (Daniels et al., 1977). Strains DH1 and AZ synthesize coenzyme M (Balch and Wolfe, 1979a). Strain DH1 contains corrinoids (Krzycki and Zeikus, 1980). Strain AZ has a low polyamine content (Scherer and Kneifel, 1983).

Strain DH1 is inhibited (2 µg/ml) by chloramphenicol and ansiomycin (Pecher and Böck, 1981). The following antibiotics produce zones of inhibition (13-23 mm) with strain AZ: bacitracin, gardimycin, enduracidin, chloramphenicol, gentamicin and lasalocid (Hilpert et al., 1981).

The mol% G + C of the DNA is 27.5-31.6 (Bd or T_m).

The type strain, DH1, was isolated from enrichments of decaying cottonwood tissue (Zeikus and Henning, 1975). Strains AZ and A2 were isolated from enrichments of anaerobic sewage sludge (Zehnder and Wuhrmann, 1977; Morii et al., 1983). Strain DC was isolated in the laboratory of R. S. Wolfe from an anaerobic sewage-sludge enrichment provided by D. Castignetti (D. Castignetti, personal communication).

Type strain: DH1 (DSM 1125).

FAMILY II. **METHANOTHERMACEAE** STETTER 1982, 266^{VP} (EFFECTIVE PUBLICATION: STETTER *IN* STETTER, THOMM, WINTER, WILDGRUBER, HUBER, ZILLIG, JANEKOVIC, KÖNIG, PALM AND WUNDERL 1981, 176)

K. O. STETTER

Me.tha.no.ther.ma′ce.ae. M.L. neut. n. *Methanothermus* type genus of the family; -*aceae* ending to denote a family; M.L. fem. pl. n. *Methanothermaceae* the *Methanothermus* family.

Rod-shaped cells, 0.3-0.4 µm in diameter and 1-3 µm in length, occurring singly and in short chains. Gram-positive. The cell envelope contains pseudomurein and an outer S-layer. Two tufts of polar flagella. Strictly anaerobic. Chemolithotrophic. Utilize H_2 and CO_2 to form methane. Molecular sulfur is reduced to H_2S (Stetter and Gaag, 1983). No growth below 60°C.

Free-living in hot anaerobic environments within solfatara fields.

The mol% G + C of the DNA is 33. Two species (Stetter et al., 1981; Lauerer et al., 1986a). Comparison with members of the *Methanobacteriaceae* by means of 16S rRNA cataloging revealed that they are phylogenetically distant ($S_{AB} = 0.38$; E. Stackebrandt, personal communication).

Type genus: *Methanothermus* Stetter, Thomm, Winter, Wildgruber, Huber, Zillig, Janekovic, König, Palm and Wunderl 1982, 267.

Genus **Methanothermus** *Stetter 1982, 267^{VP} (Effective publication: Stetter in Stetter, Thomm, Winter, Wildgruber, Huber, Zillig, Janekovic, König, Palm and Wunderl 1981, 177)*

K. O. STETTER

Me.tha.no.ther′mus. M.L. n. *methanum* methane; Gr. fem. n. *therme* heat; M.L. masc. n. *Methanothermus* methane (-producing) thermophile.

Straight to slightly curved rods, usually 0.3-0.4 × 1-3 µm, **occurring singly and in short chains. The cell envelope consists of** a double layer, an inner of **pseudomurein and an outer S-layer** (Sleytr and Messner, 1983) **of protein** subunits (Fig. 25.4). At the poles, channels are visible, leading radially through the pseudomurein. Gram-positive. Strictly anaerobic. **Optimum temperature: 80-85°C;** maximum: ~97°C; minimum: 55-60°C.

Chemolithotrophic, growing on hydrogen and CO_2. The end product is methane. Formate, acetate, methanol and methylamines can not serve as substrates (Stetter et al., 1981). In the presence of molecular sulfur and hydrogen and CO_2, large amounts of H_2S are formed, and sulfur granules attached to the cells are visible (Stetter and Gaag, 1983).

The mol% G + C of the DNA is 33.

Type species: *Methanothermus fervidus* Stetter 1982, 267.

Further Descriptive Information

Cells are rigid. They occur singly, in pairs and in short chains. At 97°C, irregular giant cells with large diameter (up to ~2 µm) appear. At 65°C and below, the rods become curly and occur in clumps. Cells divide by binary fission.

The S-layer of the envelope can be removed by pronase or sodium dodecyl sulfate. The pseudomurein sacculus consists of *N*-acetylglucosamine, *N*-acetylgalactosamine, *N*-acetyltalosaminuronic acid, glutamic acid, alanine and lysine (Stetter et al., 1981). Cells of *Methanobacterium*

formicicum show a slight serological cross-reaction with *Methanothermus fervidus* cells (Macario and Macario, 1983). The RNA polymerase shows a subunit pattern with a spacing similar to the enzyme of *Methanobacterium thermoautotrophicum* (strains ΔH and Winter, Madon, Thomm and Stetter, unpublished observation; Stetter et al., 1980). However, no serological cross-reaction could be observed in the Ouchterlony immunodiffusion test (Stetter et al., 1981).

Methanothermus fervidus was isolated from samples of Icelandic solfatara fields with a pH of 6.5 and 85°C.

Enrichment and Isolation Procedures

Methanothermus fervidus can be enriched anaerobically in medium 1 (Balch et al., 1979) at pH 6.5 in stoppered serum bottles made of "type III" glass with a gas phase of H_2 and CO_2 (80:20) at ~70°C. No growth occurs above pH 7. *Methanothermus fervidus* can be isolated by plating on medium 1 solidified by polysilicate and by incubation with H_2 and CO_2 in a pressure cylinder (Balch et al., 1979) at 85°C. After 3 days, round, smooth, opaque, slightly grayish colonies, 1-3 mm in diameter appeared. No growth on agar (Stetter et al., 1981).

Maintenance Procedure

Stock cultures of *Methanothermus*, stable at least 4 months without transfer, were obtained by 6 h growth (5% inoculation) followed by renewing the gas phase of 200 kPa of $H_2 + CO_2$ (80:20) and storage at 4°C.

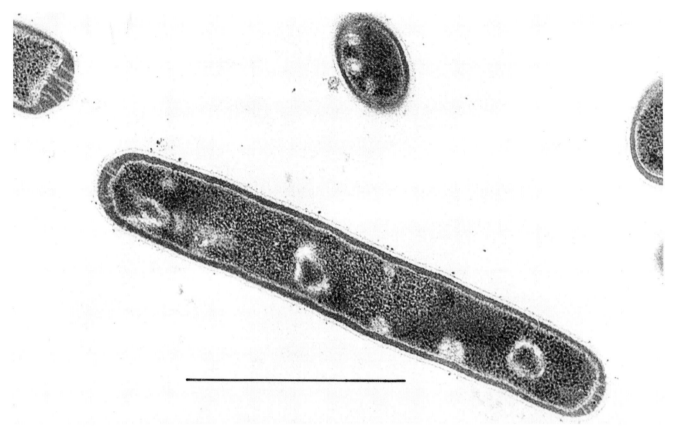

Figure 25.4. Thin section of *Methanothermus fervidus.* Contrasted with lead citrate and uranyl acetate. Electron micrograph. *Bar,* 1 μm. (Reproduced with permission from K.O. Stetter, 1984. Microbial growth on C₁ compounds. *In* Proceedings of the 4th International Symposium, ©American Society for Microbiology, Washington, D.C., p. 178.)

Differentiation of the genus **Methanothermus** *from other genera*

The genus *Methanothermus* belongs to the order *Methanobacteriales* due to its positive Gram reaction, the presence of a pseudomurein cell wall and its rod shape. From the genera *Methanobacterium* and *Methanobrevibacter* it differs by the lack of serological cross-reaction of its RNA polymerases, the high temperature optimum, and the existence of an S-layer (Sleytr and Messner, 1983) outside of the cell wall.

Taxonomic Comments

The phylogenetic relationship of the genus *Methanothermus* studied by 16S rRNA cataloging yielded a S_{AB} value of 0.38 with the other members of the *Methanobacteriales* (E. Stackebrandt, personal communica-

tion). This indicates again that *Methanothermus* belongs to the new family *Methanothermaceae* separate from the *Methanobacteriaceae* but within the *Methanobacteriales.*

Further Reading

Stetter, K.O., M. Thomm, J. Winter, G. Wildgruber, H. Huber, W. Zillig, D. Janekovic, H. König, P. Palm and S. Wunderl. 1981. *Methanothermus fervidus,* sp. nov., a novel extremely thremophilic methanogen isolated from an Icelandic hot spring. Zentralbl. Bakteriol Mikrobiol. Hyg. I. Abt. Orig. *C2:* 166–178.

Lauerer, G., J.K. Kristjansson, T.A. Langworthy, H. König and K.O. Stetter. 1986. *Methanothermus sociabilis* sp. nov., a second species within the *Methanothermaceae* growing at 97°C. Syst. Appl. Microbiol. *8:* 100–105.

Differentiation of the species of the genus **Methanothermus**

Only two species of *Methanothermus* are presently known.

List of species of the genus **Methanothermus**

1. **Methanothermus fervidus** Stetter 1982, 267.^VP (Effective publication: Stetter *in* Stetter, Thomm, Winter, Wildgruber, Huber, Zillig, Janekovic, König, Palm and Wunderl 1981, 177.)

fer′vid.us. L. masc. adj. *fervidus* fervent; on account of its growth in almost boiling water.

See the generic description for the features.

The mol% G + C of the DNA is 33 (T_m).

Type strain: DSM 2088.

2. **Methanothermus sociabilis** Lauerer, Kristjansson, Langworthy,

König and Stetter 1986b, 573.^VP (Effective publication: Lauerer, Kristjansson, Langworthy, König and Stetter 1986a, 100.)

so.ci.a′bi.lis. L. masc. adj. *sociabilis* social; on account of its growth in large aggregates.

See the generic description for the features. Cells grow in large clusters. Optimal growth: ~88°C.

The mol% G + C of the DNA is 33. The DNA homology with *M. fervidus* is ~63%. The lipid pattern is different from *M. fervidus.*

Type strain: DSM 3496.

ORDER II. **METHANOCOCCALES** BALCH AND WOLFE 1981, 216^{VP} (EFFECTIVE PUBLICATION: BALCH AND WOLFE *IN* BALCH, FOX, MAGRUM, WOESE AND WOLFE 1979, 285)

WILLIAM B. WHITMAN

Me.tha.no.coc.cal′es. M.L. fem. pl. n. *Methanococcaceae* type family of order; *-ales* to denote order; M.L. fem. pl. n. *Methanococcales* the *Methanococcaceae* order.

Strictly anaerobic methane-producing bacterium. Hydrogen or formate may be electron donors. The cell wall is composed of protein.

The order includes one family, *Methanococcaceae* Balch and Wolfe 1981, 216.

FAMILY **METHANOCOCCACEAE** BALCH AND WOLFE 1981, 216^{VP} *(EFFECTIVE PUBLICATION: BALCH AND WOLFE* IN *BALCH, FOX, MAGRUM, WOESE AND WOLFE 1979, 285)*

Me.tha.no.coc.ca′ce.ae. M.L. neut. n. *Methanococcus* (Kluyver and van Niel) Barker 1936 type genus of the family; *-aceae* ending to denote family; M.L. fem. pl. n. *Methanococcaceae* the *Methanococcus* family.

Irregular coccus with a protein cell wall. Motile by means of flagella. Obligately anaerobic methane-producing bacterium which uses carbon dioxide as an electron acceptor. Hydrogen or formate may be electron donors. Temperature range varies from mesophilic to extremely thermophilic.

The type and only genus is *Methanococcus* (Kluyver and van Niel 1936, 400, emend. Barker 1936, 430) Mah and Kuhn 1984, 264.

Genus **Methanococcus** *(Kluyver and van Niel 1936, 400, emend. Barker 1936, 430; Mah and Kuhn 1984, 264)*^{AL} *(Nom. Cons. Opin. 62 Jud. Comm. 1986a, 491)*

Me.tha.no.coc′cus. M.L. n. *methanum* methane; M.L. n. *coccus* a spherical cell; M.L. masc. n. *Methanococcus* methane coccus.

Irregular coccus, 1.0–2.0 µm in diameter during balanced growth. Cells from older cultures or colonies are extremely irregular. Cells lose integrity during Gram staining and lyse completely within 10 s when suspended in either distilled water or 0.01% sodium dodecyl sulfate. **Motile, by means of polar tufts of flagella. Obligate anaerobic.** Either mesophilic (temperature optima: 35–40°C), thermophilic (temperature optimum: 65°C) or extremely thermophilic (temperature optimum: 85°C); pH optima between 6 and 8. NaCl required for growth, optimal concentrations 0.5–4% (w/v). **Obligate methanogenic; H$_2$ and, in most cases, formate serve as electron donors. Acetate, methanol and methylamines are not substrates for methanogenesis.** With one exception, all species grow autotrophically in mineral medium. Amino acids and acetate are stimulatory for some species. Nitrogen sources include ammonium, N$_2$ gas and alanine. Storage materials include glycogen. Organism is found in **salt marsh, marine** and **estuarine sediments.**

The mol% G + C of the DNA is 29–34 (liquid chromatography and Bd).

Type species: *Methanococcus vannielii* Stadtman and Barker 1951, 269 (Judicial Commission, Opinion 62, 1986a, 491).

Further Descriptive Information

Cell morphology. In growing cultures, cells are slightly irregular and uniform in size, between 1 and 2 µm in diameter (Fig. 25.5A). Pairs of cells are common. In stationary cultures, colonies or enrichment cultures, cell shape is very irregular, and large cells up to 10 µm in diameter are observed (Jones et al., 1977). In wet mounts, a few cells in a preparation may slowly swell and burst (Ward, 1970). Cells on the edge of a slide where drying may occur are much larger, less irregular, and more transparent than cells from the center of the slide (Fig. 25.5). Cells from older cultures are mechanically fragile and rupture during vigorous stirring or upon harvesting by some continuous centrifugation devices. Cells are also osmotically fragile, and they lyse rapidly in distilled water. Cell integrity is maintained in 2% NaCl (w/v). All species lyse rapidly in 0.01% sodium dodecyl sulfate, and species which have been investigated contain a protein cell wall. In *M. vannielii* and *M. jannaschii,* the outer cell surface is composed of tetragonally and hexagonally ordered structures, respectively (Jones et al., 1977, 1983c).

The pattern of flagellation has been described in three species. *M. vannielii* and *M. jannaschii* both contain two tufts or bundles of flagella at the same pole. *M. thermolithotrophicus* contains a single polar tuft of about 20 flagella. In *M. jannaschii* and *M. thermolithotrophicus,* the flagella are up to 5 and 3 µm in length, respectively.

Colonial morphology. Colonies are round, entire and slightly convex. Their surface is smooth or shiny. Their color varies from pale green to yellow, depending on the species and the growth conditions. Colony size is 1–2 mm after 5 days, except for *M. thermolithotrophicus,* which is larger. However, colony size depends greatly on the culture conditions (Jones et al., 1983b). With transmitted light, colonies are translucent with either irregular or circular dark centers.

Growth conditions. All species grow rapidly on H$_2$ + CO$_2$ in pressurized culture tubes (Balch and Wolfe, 1976). Under optimal conditions, generation times vary from <1 h for the thermophilic species to <3 h for the mesophilic species. All species grow with formate except *M. jannaschii,* although it contains a formate dehydrogenase (Jones et al., 1983c). Acetate, methanol and methylamines are not substrates for methanogenesis. Other growth conditions are described in Table 25.4.

Mineral requirements. In addition to NaCl, high concentrations of magnesium salts are stimulatory or required by the methanococci (Whitman et al., 1982, 1986; Corder et al., 1983; Jones et al., 1983a). Calcium is required by *M. voltae* (Whitman et al., 1982). Selenium is stimulatory to all species which have been tested (Jones and Stadtman, 1977; Whitman et al., 1982; Jones et al., 1983a, c). Iron, nickel and cobalt are required or stimulatory for *M. voltae* (Whitman et al., 1982), and tungsten and nickel are required or stimulatory for *M. vannielii* (Jones and Stadtman, 1977; Diekert et al., 1981). Requirements for iron, nickel, cobalt and tungsten have not been investigated in other methanococci.

Carbon sources. Except for *M. voltae,* the methanococci will grow in mineral medium with sulfide as the sole reducing agent and carbon dioxide as the sole carbon source (Whitman et al., 1986). Under these conditions, acetate is stimulatory to *M. maripaludis* but not to *M. vannielii* and *M. thermolithotrophicus. M. voltae* requires acetate, isoleucine and leucine for growth (Whitman et al., 1982). Isovalerate and 2-methylbutyrate can substitute for leucine and isoleucine, respectively. Pantoyllactone and pantoic acid, which are formed from pantothenate during autoclaving, are also stimulatory to growth (Whitman, unpublished

Figure 25.5. Phase-contrast photomicrograph of *M. thermolithotrophicus*. Effect of drying on the apparent cell morphology. Photomicrographs from the same slide: *A*, center; *B*, between *A* and *C*; *C*, edge of coverslip. *Bar*, 10 µm.

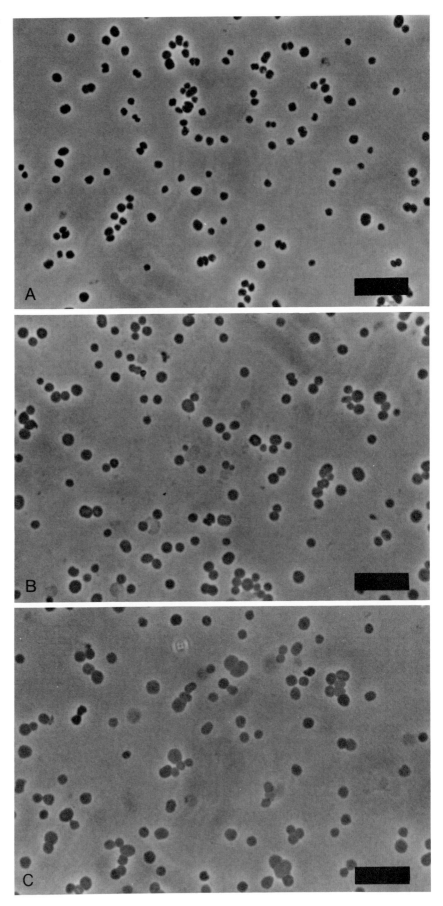

Table 25.4.
Differential characteristics of the species of the genus
Methanococcus[a]

Characteristic	1. *M. vannielii*	2. *M. voltae*	3. *M. maripaludis*	4. *M. thermolithotrophicus*	5. *M. jannaschii*
Optimum temperature					
35–40°C	+	+	+	−	−
65°C	−	−	−	+	−
85°C	−	−	−	−	+
Nitrogen source					
N$_2$	−	−	+	+	
Alanine	−	−	+		
Autotrophic growth	+	−	+	+	+
Mol% G + C of DNA	33	30	33	34	31

[a]Symbols: +, property of the species; −, not a property of the species; and ( ), not relevant or not tested. The properties of the species are based upon the description of a single strain.

data). Glycogen has been identified as a storage product in most methanococci (König et al., 1985).

Sulfur and nitrogen sources. Sulfide is sufficient as a sulfur source for all methanococci. Most species will also reduce elemental sulfur to sulfide (Stetter and Gaag, 1983; Whitman, unpublished data). Cysteine, dithiothreitol and sulfate do not substitute for sulfide for *M. voltae* and *M. jannaschii* (Whitman et al., 1982; Jones et al., 1983c). *M. thermolithotrophicus* is also reported to utilize sulfate, sulfite and thiosulfate as sole sulfur sources (Daniels et al., 1986).

Ammonium is sufficient as a nitrogen source for all methanococci and is required by *M. voltae* even during growth with amino acids (Whitman et al., 1982). N$_2$ gas and alanine are additional nitrogen sources for *M. maripaludis* (Whitman, unpublished data). *M. vannielii* cannot utilize N$_2$ gas or amino acids as nitrogen sources, but it will utilize purines (DeMoll and Tsai, 1986). *M. thermolithotrophicus* also utilizes N$_2$ gas (Belay et al., 1984).

Immunological data. Rabbit antisera to formalin-treated whole cells of methanococci cross-react weakly with other members of the genus but not other methane-producing bacteria (Conway de Macario et al., 1981). Antiserum to *M. voltae* cross-reacts with *M. vannielii* cells. Similarly, antiserum to *M. vannielii* cross-reacts with *M. maripaludis* (Jones et al., 1983a).

Antibiotic sensitivity and pathogenicity. Like other methanogens, methanococci are generally resistant to low concentrations of many common antibiotics (Jones et al., 1977). Some antibiotics which are inhibitory at low concentrations are: adriamycin, chloramphenicol, efrapeptin, leucinostatin, metronidazole, monensin, pleuromutilin, pyrollnitrin, and virginiamycin (Elhardt and Böck, 1982; Böck and Kandler, 1985).

The methanococci have not been reported to be associated with disease.

Habitats. To date, methanococci have only been isolated from marine environments. *M. vannielii* was isolated from the shore of the San Francisco Bay (Stadtman and Barker, 1951b). *M. voltae* was isolated from sediments from the mouth of the Waccasassa estuary in Florida (Ward, 1970). *M. maripaludis* was isolated from salt-marsh sediments near Pawley's Island, South Carolina (Jones et al., 1983a). *M. thermolithotrophicus* was isolated from geothermally heated sediment at Stufe di Nerone

near Naples, Italy (Huber et al., 1982). *M. jannaschii* was isolated from surface material collected at the base of a submarine hydrothermal vent on the East Pacific Rise (Jones et al., 1983c). In all cases, only a single strain of each species has been described. Therefore, the distribution is not well-known. All species were isolated from enrichments except *M. maripaludis*, which was the most abundant H$_2$-utilizing methanogen in the samples examined (Jones et al., 1983a).

Biochemistry. A number of enzymes from *M. vannielii* have been purified and characterized. Two forms of formate dehydrogenase have been described (Jones et al., 1979; Jones and Stadtman, 1980, 1981). The selenium-dependent formate dehydrogenase contains selenocysteine, molybdenum, iron and acid-labile sulfur. The selenium-independent form is lacking selenocysteine. Both enzymes reduce the deazaflavin coenzyme F$_{420}$. A selenium-containing hydrogenase which is deazaflavin-dependent has also been purified and shown to contain selenocysteine (Yamazaki, 1982). The 8-hydroxy-5-deazaflavin-dependent NADP$^+$ reductase has been purified and shown to be stereospecific with respect to NADP$^+$ as well as the deazaflavin (Yamazaki and Tsai, 1980; Yamazaki et al., 1980). At physiological pH, the reductase probably functions in the direction of NADP$^+$ reduction. In addition, the reductase is specific for the deazaflavin of coenzyme F$_{420}$, and riboflavin and dideazaflavin are inactive (Yamazaki et al., 1982).

Enrichment and Isolation Procedures

Methanococci may be easily isolated after enrichment under H$_2$ + CO$_2$ (80:20) in pressurized tubes or bottles (Miller and Wolin, 1974; Balch and Wolfe, 1976). Because of their rapid growth, methanococci frequently outgrow other H$_2$-utilizing methanogens in marine sediments. Therefore, this enrichment is somewhat specific. The enrichments are transferred to medium containing antibiotics (0.2 mg/ml penicillin G, erythromycin and streptomycin sulfate) before plating on agar plates or in roll tubes (Jones et al., 1983a, b; Godsy, 1980). In some cases, it is necessary to include antibiotics in the solid medium to prevent growth of spreading bacteria over colonies of methanococci. Isolated colonies are picked with a syringe needle and transferred to liquid medium. Purity may be demonstrated by microscopic examination, restreaking on agar medium and absence of growth in mineral medium supplemented with 1% yeast extract under N$_2$ + CO$_2$ (80:20).

Maintenance Procedures

A useful medium for rapid growth of methanococci consists of (in g/l): KCl, 0.34; NaCl, 22; MgSO$_4$·7H$_2$O, 3.5; MgCl$_2$·6H$_2$O, 2.8; NH$_4$Cl, 0.5; CaCl$_2$·2H$_2$O, 0.14; K$_2$HPO$_4$, 0.14; NaHCO$_3$, 5; Fe(NH$_4$)$_2$(SO$_4$)$_2$·6H$_2$O, 0.01; and 10 ml/l of trace metal solution (in g/l): (nitrilotriacetic acid, neutralized with KOH, 1.5; MnSO$_4$·2H$_2$O, 0.1; Fe(NH$_4$)$_2$(SO$_4$)$_2$·6H$_2$O, 0.2; CoCl$_2$·6H$_2$O, 0.1; ZnSO$_4$·7H$_2$O, 0.1; CuSO$_4$·5H$_2$O, 0.01; NiCl$_2$·6H$_2$O, 0.025; Na$_2$SeO$_3$, 0.2; Na$_2$MoO$_4$·2H$_2$O, 0.1; and Na$_2$WO$_4$·2H$_2$O, 0.1. An oxygen indicator, rezasurin (1 mg/l), may also be added prior to boiling the medium under N$_2$ + CO$_2$ (80:20). After boiling, 2-mercaptoethanesulfonate, 0.5 g/l, is added to reduce the medium. After dispensing the medium anaerobically and sterilizing, the medium may be stored for several months in an anaerobic chamber (Coy Laboratories, Ann Arbor, Michigan). Just prior to inoculation, one part of sterile 2.5% Na$_2$S·9H$_2$O (w/v) is added to 50 parts of medium. For *M. voltae*, the mineral medium must be supplemented with either yeast extract, 2 g/l, or NaCH$_3$COO·3H$_2$O, 0.14 g/l, L-isoleucine, 0.5 g/l, L-leucine, 0.5 g/l, and pantoyllactone, 1.3 mg/l (Whitman et al., 1986).

Because the methanococci lyse rapidly shortly after the cessation of growth in liquid media, stock cultures are grown below the temperature optimum (30°C for the mesophilic species) and stored at room temperature for up to 3 weeks. Strains of all the mesophilic methanococci have been stored with little loss in viability up to 3 years in 25% glycerol at −70°C (Whitman et al., 1986). Tube cultures are first concentrated by centrifugation and resuspended in a one-fifth volume of medium containing yeast extract and 25% glycerol (v/v). Portions of the cell suspension are transferred to sterile 1-ml screw-top vials in the anaerobic chamber. The vials are then stored at −70°C without anaerobic precautions. To revive the cultures, 0.2 ml of the cell suspension is allowed to thaw in the anaerobic chamber and transferred to fresh medium. Methanococci have also been stored in liquid nitrogen for at least 7 months

(Leigh, 1983) and in 10% glycerol in liquid nitrogen for 2 years (L. A. Hook, personal communication).

Differentiation of the genus **Methanococcus** from closely related genera

A number of morphologically and nutritionally similar species of *Methanogenium* and *Methanomicrobium* have also been obtained from marine environments (Romesser et al., 1979; Rivard and Smith, 1982; Ferguson and Mah, 1983; Rivard et al., 1983). The methanococci may be distinguished from these other species by their faster growth rate, requirement for NaCl, lack of organic growth requirements (except *M. voltae*) and lower mol% G + C of the DNA. However, until more species have been identified and more strains of known species characterized, identification of isolates based solely on morphology and growth characteristics is equivocal. Use of salt or mineral requirements is particularly deceptive (see below). Thus, antigenic cross-reactivity (Conway de Macario et al., 1981), RNA/DNA hybridization (Tu et al., 1982) and 16S rRNA partial sequencing (Balch et al., 1979) are helpful for final identification of new isolates.

Methanococci may also be readily distinguished by sodium dodecyl sulfate-polyacrylamide gel electrophoresis (SDS-PAGE) of cellular proteins (Whitman and Premachandran, unpublished data). Cultures are grown to an absorbance of 1.0 cm^{-1} at 600 nm, and 5-ml cultures are harvested by centrifugation. The cells are resuspended in 0.1 ml of mineral medium or a salt solution prepared without reducing agents. This cell suspension may be stored at $-20°$C prior to electrophoresis. After thawing, the suspension is vortexed to form an even suspension, and 15 µl are added to 60 µl of sample buffer containing sodium dodecyl sulfate and 2-mercaptoethanol (Laemmli, 1970). A portion, 35 µl, of this mixture is electrophoresed on a 12% polyacrylamide gel according to the procedure of Laemmli (1970). The protein profile on SDS-PAGE is sufficiently distinctive to readily distinguish species of mesophilic methanococci from each other (Fig. 25.6) or from other methanogenic bacteria like *Methanogenium* species (data not shown).

Taxonomic Comments

In the eighth edition of *Bergey's Manual*® (Bryant, 1974), the genus *Methanococcus* included methane-producing cocci which did not form regular packets (i.e. *Methanosarcina*) or chains (i.e. some species of *Methanobacterium*, now *Methanobrevibacter*). At that time, the type species, *Methanococcus mazei*, was not available in pure culture, and only one other species, *M. vannielii*, was known. Upon analysis of the partial sequence of the 16S rRNAs of methanogens (Balch et al., 1979) and isolation of a bacterium with the phenotype of *M. mazei* (Mah, 1980), it became apparent that *M. mazei* was related to the *Methanosarcinaceae* and that *M. vannielii* was related to a new species of methanococcus, *M. voltae*. Thus, it was proposed that *M. vannielii* become the new type species for the genus and *M. mazei* be reclassified as *Methanosarcina mazei* (Balch et al., 1979; Mah and Kuhn, 1984; Judicial Commission, 1986a). This proposal was adopted in the present work, and the genus *Methanococcus* now includes five phenotypically and phylogenetically related species.

Likewise, species which more closely resemble *M. mazei* should be placed in the *Methanosarcinaceae*. Thus, *Methanococcus halophilus* Zhilina 1984, 270, which utilizes methylamines for methane synthesis, has not been classified with the *Methanococcaceae* (Zhilina, 1983). Similarly, *Methanococcus frisius* Blotevogel, Fischer and Lüpkes 1986, 573 resembles *Methanosarcina mazei* by nutritional and morphological criteria (Blotevogel et al., 1986). It should also be classified with the *Methanosarcinaceae*.

The placement of the genus *Methanococcus* in a separate order, *Methanococcales*, is based largely on an analysis of the 16S rRNA (Balch et al., 1979). While significant phenotypic differences exist between the *Methanococcales* and members of other orders, the known phenotypic differences are probably not sufficient in themselves to justify creation of a new order. Thus, the present classification system anticipates the fur-

ther molecular and biochemical characterization of the *Methanococcales*.

The phylogeny of all species presently included in the genus has been analyzed by 16S rRNA homology (Jones et al., 1983c). Although these species are more closely related to each other than other methane-producing bacteria, they are not a closely knit group. In particular, the 16S rRNA of *M. jannaschii* is different enough from the other methanococci to justify creation of a new genus (Balch et al., 1979). Because the description of *M. jannaschii* is based on a single isolate and its phenotype is similar to other methanococci, creation of a new genus was not undertaken at this time. However, further characterization of *M. jannaschii* and isolation of additional species may make the addition of another genus to the family *Methanococcaceae* necessary.

The present description of the methanococci is based on the description of a single isolate for most species. Therefore, the phenotypic characteristics described may not be truly representative of the species. In addition, if additional species are discovered, they may not be distinguished from the known species by the limited number of characteristics which have been described. Thus far, new species have been determined principally by immunological comparisons, sequence data or nucleic acid hybridization. The importance of the phenotypic properties described thus far will have to await the isolation and characterization of additional strains of known species.

This difficulty is illustrated by a description of methanococci isolated

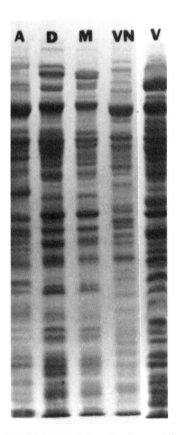

Figure 25.6. SDS-PAGE of whole cells of mesophilic methanococci. *Lanes (left to right) are "Methanococcus aeolicus," "M. deltae," M. maripaludis, M. vannielii and M. voltae.*

from sediments of salt marshes (Whitman et al., 1986). Thus, it was not possible to identify natural isolates by their sodium or magnesium requirements, which were somewhat variable. Although strains related to *M. voltae* were recognized by their requirement for isoleucine, leucine and acetate, the larger number of autotrophic isolates could not be identified by their nutritional properties or their mol% G + C of the DNA. Subsequent comparison of these isolates by SDS-PAGE proved very useful in identifying these isolates (Whitman and Premachandran, unpublished results). Moreover, these results indicate that *M. maripaludis* and "*Methanococcus deltae*," which has not been validly published, are more similar to each other than are other species in this genus (see below and Fig. 25.6). While the results are not sufficient to decide whether or not "*M. deltae*" (the latter of the two to be described) is a valid species, they clearly illustrate that caution must be exercised when species are compared on a limited number of nutritional characteristics (Corder et al. 1983).

In addition to the five validly published species of methanococci, an isolate has been described parenthetically in the literature, which appears to warrant species status (Schmid et al., 1984; Whitman et al., 1986; and Whitman, unpublished results). "*Methanococcus aeolicus*" is a mesophilic, coccal-shaped methane-producing bacterium which readily lyses in 0.01% sodium dodecyl sulfate or distilled water. Cells are 1.5–2.0 μM in diameter. Growth is autotrophic with hydrogen or formate as the electron donors. Ammonium and N_2 gas can serve as nitrogen sources. Sodium and magnesium salts are required for growth. "*M. aeolicus*" may be readily distinguished from other mesophilic methanococci by SDS-PAGE (Fig. 25.6).

Acknowledgments

I would like to thank W. J. Jones for providing cultures of *M. maripaludis, M. thermolithotrophicus* and *M. vannielii*, manuscripts prior to publication, and helpful discussions; L. A. Hook for providing a culture of "*M. deltae*" and helpful discussions; K. O. Stetter for providing a culture of "*M. aeolicus*"; and M. Rigler and J. Patton for assistance in preparation of the photomicrographs. This work was supported in part by National Science Foundation grants PCM-8214068 and PCM-8351355.

Further Reading

Balch, W.E., G.E. Fox, L.J. Magrum, C.R. Woese, and R.S. Wolfe. 1979. Methanogens: reevaluation of a unique biological group. Microbiol. Rev. *43:* 260–296.

Mah, R.A., and P.H. Smith. 1983. The methanogenic bacteria. *In* Starr, Stolp, Trüper, Balows and Schlegel (Editors), The Prokaryotes. A Handbook on Habitats, Isolation, and Identification of Bacteria. Springer-Verlag, Berlin, pp. 948–977.

Whitman, W.B. 1985. Methanogenic bacteria. *In* Woese and Wolfe (Editors), The Bacteria, Vol. VIII: Archaebacteria. Academic Press, Orlando, Fla., pp. 3–84.

List of species of the genus Methanococcus

1. Methanococcus vannielii Stadtman and Barker, 1951, 269.[AL]

van.niel'i.i. M.L. gen. n. *vannielii* of van Niel; named for C. B. van Niel, the bacteriologist who developed the carbon dioxide reduction theory of methane formation.

Cell morphology, nutrition and physiology are described in Tables 25.4 and 25.5 and in the generic description.

The mol% G + C of the DNA is 31–33 (Bd and liquid chromatography).

Type strain: SB (DSM 1224).

2. Methanococcus voltae Balch and Wolfe 1981, 216.[VP] (Effective publication: Balch and Wolfe *in* Balch, Fox, Magrum, Woese and Wolfe 1979, 285.)

vol'tae. M.L. gen. n. *voltae* of Volta; named for the Italian physicist A. Volta for discovery of the combustible nature of gas from anaerobic sediments.

Cell morphology, nutrition and physiology are described in Tables 25.4 and 25.5 and in the generic description.

The mol% G + C of the DNA is 30–31 (Bd and liquid chromatography).

Type strain: PS (DSM 1537).

3. Methanococcus maripaludis Jones, Paynter and Gupta 1984, 270.[VP] (Effective publication: Jones, Paynter and Gupta 1983, 91.)

ma.ri.pa.lu'dis. L. n. *mare* sea; L. n. *palus* marsh; M.L. pl. gen. n. *maripaludis* of the sea marsh.

Cell morphology, nutrition and physiology are described in Tables 25.4 and 25.5 and in the generic description.

The mol% G + C of the DNA is 33 (Bd and liquid chromatography).

Type strain: JJ (DSM 2067).

4. Methanococcus thermolithotrophicus Huber, Thomm and Stetter 1984, 270.[VP] (Effective publication: Huber, Thomm, König, Thies and Stetter 1982, 47.)

ther.mo.li.tho.tro'phi.cus. Gr. fem. n. *therme* heat; Gr. masc. n. *lithos* stone; Gr. masc. n. *trophos* one who feeds; M.L. masc. adj. *thermolithotrophicus* grows lithotrophically at elevated temperatures.

Cell morphology, nutrition and physiology are described in Tables 25.4 and 25.5 and in the generic description.

The mol% G + C of the DNA is 31–34 (Td and liquid chromatography).

Type strain: SN-1 (DSM 2095).

5. Methanococcus jannaschii Jones, Leigh, Mayer, Woese and Wolfe 1984, 503.[VP] (Effective publication: Jones, Leigh, Mayer, Woese and Wolfe 1983, 254.)

jan.nasch'i.i. M.L. gen. n. *jannaschii* of Jannasch; named for the marine microbiologist H. Jannasch.

Cell morphology, nutrition and physiology are described in Tables 25.4 and 25.5 and in the generic description.

The mol% G + C of the DNA is 31 (Bd).

Type strain: JAL-1 (DSM 2661).

Species Incertae Sedis

a. Methanococcus halophilus Zhilina 1984, 270.[VP] (Effective publication: Zhilina 1983, 290.)

Irregular coccus, 0.5–2 μm in diameter, which is nonmotile. Strict anaerobe which uses methylamines and methanol as substrates for methanogenesis. Hydrogen gas, formate and acetate are not utilized as substrates for methanogenesis. Best growth is found at 26–36°C, pH 6.5–7.4 and 7–9% NaCl.

This bacterium more closely resembles *Methanolobus tindarius* or "*Methanococcoides methylutens*" of the family *Methanosarcinaceae* than other species of *Methanococcus* (Mah and Kuhn, 1984). For this reason, it has not been included in the "List of Species of the Genus *Methanococcus*."

Type strain: Z-7982 (DSM 3094).

b. Methanococcus frisius Blotevogel, Fischer and Lüpkes 1986, 573.[VP] (Effective publication: Blotevogel, Fischer and Lüpkes 1986, 127.)

fri'si.us. L. masc. adj. *frisius* pertaining to Frisia, a region in the northwest of the Federal Republic of Germany.

Regular, nonmotile coccus, 0.9–1.6 μm in diameter. Strict anaerobe which uses hydrogen gas, methanol or methylamines as substrates for methanogenesis. Formate and acetate are not utilized as substrates for methanogenesis. Best growth is found at 36°C, pH 6.5–7.2 and 2% NaCl.

This bacterium more closely resembles species of the family *Methanosarcinaceae* than other species of *Methanococcus* (Mah and Kuhn, 1984). For this reason, it has not been included in the "List of Species of the Genus *Methanococcus*."

The mol% G + C of the DNA is 38.2 ± 1.0 (Td).

Type strain: C16 (DSM 3318).

Other Organisms

a. "*Methanococcus deltae*" Corder, Hook, Larkin and Frea 1983, 28.

del'tae. Gr. gen. n. *deltae* of the delta.

The cell morphology and nutrition closely resemble *M. maripaludis* strain JJ, except that *M. deltae* is slightly larger in diameter (1.2 μm). Otherwise, *M. deltae* uses H₂ or formate as electron donors and has a temperature optimum between 35 and 40°C. Growth is autotrophic. Acetate but not amino acids are stimulatory to growth. Nitrogen sources include ammonium, N₂ gas and alanine.

Isolated from sediments of the Mississippi River delta.

The mol% G + C of the DNA is 34 (liquid chromatography).

Type strain: ΔRC (ATCC 35294, DSM 2771).

b. "*Methanococcus aeolicus.*"

Mentioned parenthetically in Schmid et al., 1984, this bacterium has not been fully described; however, preliminary data suggest that it represents a new species of *Methanococcus*. The SDS-PAGE pattern is distinctive (Fig. 25.6). Nutritional properties closely resemble other autotrophic methanococci (Whitman et al., 1986). It is capable of autotrophic growth and is not stimulated by acetate or amino acids. Hydrogen gas and formate are substrates for methanogenesis; acetate, methylamines and methanol are not substrates. Nitrogen sources include ammonium and N₂ gas. The type strain has not been designed.

Table 25.5.

Descriptive characteristics of the species of the genus **Methanococcus**[a]

Characteristic	1. *M. vannielii*	2. *M. voltae*	3. *M. maripaludis*	4. *M. thermolithotrophicus*	5. *M. jannaschii*
Irregular coccus	+	+	+	+	+
Cell diameter					
1.0 μm	+	−	+	+	+
1.5 μm	−	+	−	−	−
Substrate for methane synthesis					
H₂ + CO₂	+	+	+	+	+
Formate	+	+	+	+	−
Growth requirement					
Acetate	−	+	−	−	−
Isoleucine	−	+	−	−	−
Leucine	−	+	−	−	−
Ca²⁺ (1 mM)	−	+	−	−	−
Growth stimulatory					
Selenium	+	+	+		+
Pantoyllactone	−	+	−		
Acetate	−		+	−	
Amino acids	−		+		
Sulfur source					
Sulfide	+	+	+	+	+
Elemental sulfur	+	+	+	+	+
Thiosulfate	−	−	−	+	
Sulfite	−	−	−	+	
Sulfate	−	−	−	+	
Nitrogen source					
NH₃	+	+	+	+	+
N₂	−	−	+	+	
Alanine	−	−	+		
Temperature range					
20–40°C	+	−	−	−	−
20–45°C	−	+	+	−	−
30–70°C	−	−	−	+	−
50–86°C	−	−	−	−	+
pH range					
5–7	−	−	−	−	+
6.5–8	−	+	+	+	−
7–9	+	−	−	−	−

[a]Symbols: +, property of the species; −, not a property of the species; and ( ), not relevant or not tested. The properties of the species are based upon the description of a single strain.

ORDER III. **METHANOMICROBIALES** BALCH AND WOLFE 1981, 216[VP] (EFFECTIVE PUBLICATION: BALCH AND WOLFE *IN* BALCH, FOX, MAGRUM, WOESE AND WOLFE 1979, 286)

DAVID R. BOONE AND ROBERT A. MAH

Me.tha.no.mi.cro.bi.al'es. N.L. fem. pl. n. *Methanomicrobiaceae* type family of the order; *-ales* ending to denote an order; N.L. fem. pl. n. *Methanomicrobiales* the *Methanomicrobiaceae* order.

A wide range of morphological types are contained in this order. **Cells are coccoid bodies, pseudosarcina or rods,** Gram-negative or Gram-positive, **nonmotile or motile. Cells do not contain muramic acid.** Lipids are predominantly isoprenoid hydrocarbons ether-linked to glycerol. Cells are very **strictly anaerobic. They grow by oxidation of H_2 or formate with the reduction of CO_2 to CH_4 or by fermentation of methylated amines, methanol or acetate to CH_4 and CO_2.** Some strains oxidize 1-propanol, 2-propanol, 2-butanol or ethanol to propionate, acetone, 2-butanone or acetate (respectively) and reduce

CO_2 to CH_4. Some strains reduce elemental sulfur, but this may not lead to growth. Cells contain coenzyme M and coenzyme F_{420}. The *Methanomicrobiales* form a highly specialized physiological group which does not utilize carbohydrate, proteinaceous materials or other organic compounds as energy sources other than those listed above. They are widely distributed in nature, being found in anaerobic habitats, such as aquatic sediments, anaerobic sewage-sludge digestors and the gastrointestinal tracts of animals.

Key to the families of the order **Methanomicrobiales**

I. Cells grow by oxidizing H_2, formate or various alcohols with two or more carbons and by reducing CO_2 to CH_4.
Family I. *Methanomicrobiaceae*, 2191
II. Cells grow by reducing CO_2 (or methylotrophic substrates) with H_2 or by fermenting methanol, methylamines or acetate.
Family II. *Methanosarcinaceae*, 2198

FAMILY I. **METHANOMICROBIACEAE** BALCH AND WOLFE 1981, 216[VP] (EFFECTIVE PUBLICATION: BALCH AND WOLFE *IN* BALCH, FOX, MAGRUM, WOESE AND WOLFE 1979, 286)

DAVID R. BOONE AND ROBERT A. MAH

Me.tha.no.mi.cro.bi.a'ce.ae. N.L. neut. n. *Methanomicrobium* type species of the family; *-aceae* ending to denote a family; N.L. fem. pl. n. *Methanomicrobiaceae* the *Methanomicrobium* family.

Cells are Gram-negative, cocci to straight or slightly curved rods. Cells oxidize H_2, formate, ethanol, 1-propanol, 2-propanol or 2-butanol to H^+, $H^+ + HCO_3^-$, acetate, propionate or 2-butanone, respectively. These oxidations are linked to CO_2 reduction to CH_4.

The mol% G + C of the DNA is 44–61.
Type genus: *Methanomicrobium* Balch and Wolfe 1981, 216.

Key to the genera of the family **Methanomicrobiaceae**

I. Rod-shaped cells, straight or slightly curved, but not helical
Genus I. *Methanomicrobium*
II. Sheathed, rod-shaped cells twisted into a gentle helix
Genus II. *Methanospirillum*
III. Coccoid organisms lysed by detergents or hypotonic solution
Genus III. *Methanogenium*

Genus I. **Methanomicrobium** Balch and Wolfe 1981, 216[VP] (Effective publication: Balch and Wolfe in Balch, Fox, Magrum, Woese and Wolfe 1979, 286)

M. J. B. PAYNTER

Me.tha.no.mi.cro'bi.um. M.L. n. *methanum* methane; Gr. adj. *micros* small; Gr. adj. *bios* life; M.L. neut. n. *Methanomicrobium* methane (-producing) small life (-form).

Short, straight to slightly curved, irregular rods, 0.6–0.7 μm wide and 1.5–2.5 μm long, with rounded ends. Morphology may be influenced by substrate availability, becoming coccoid (0.5–1.0 μm in diameter) under starvation conditions. **Cells occur singly, in pairs but not in chains.** Capsules are not formed. Endospores are not produced. **Gram stain results are negative. Species may be motile, with monotrichous polar flagellation, or nonmotile. Strictly anaerobic.** Growth between 25 and 45°C with an optimum at ~40°C. Growth and methanogenesis occur from pH 5.9 to 7.7 with an optimum between 6.1 and 7.0. **Hydrogen-carbon dioxide serves as substrate for methanogenesis and growth: One of the two known species also**

uses formate. Acetate is a required nutrient. Species may have no other requirements for organic nutrients or may have several.

The mol% G + C of the DNA is 44.9–48.8 (Bd).

Type species: *Methanomicrobium mobile* strain BP (Paynter and Hungate) Balch and Wolfe 1981, 216.

Further Descriptive Information

Cell morphology is dependent upon the nutritional status. In media with less than optimal concentrations of required nutrients, or when starvation occurs, cells become pleomorphic and have a tendency to lyse (Rivard et al., 1983; Tanner, R. S. 1982. Ph.D. thesis, University of Illinois). A rigid cell wall is lacking for *Methanomicrobium mobile;* muramic acid is absent, and the cell envelope appears to be a layer of regularly arranged protein subunits that is sensitive to sodium dodecyl sulfate (SDS) and trypsin (Kandler and König, 1978). The chemical nature of *Methanomicrobium paynteri* cell wall has not been determined. However, cells are also osmotically fragile and disintegrated by SDS, sodium desoxycholate or Triton X-100, suggesting a similar type wall structure (Rivard et al., 1983).

Motility of *M. mobile* may be difficult to observe. Brief exposure to air, or growth under less than optimal nutritional conditions (M. J. B. Paynter, unpublished data), results in very weak tumbling motility which is difficult to distinguish from Brownian motion.

Colonies of *M. mobile* grown on hydrogen-carbon dioxide in a medium containing clarified rumen fluid* are barely visible after 4 days of incubation at 39°C. Growth for 15 days results in surface colonies of 0.7–1.0 mm in diameter, with entire edges, translucent, colorless to pale yellow, smooth and convex. Deep colonies are lenticular. *M. paynteri,* grown for 14 days at 37°C on hydrogen-carbon dioxide, in medium no. 3[†] of Balch et al. (1979), produces colonies of 1.0–2.0 mm in diameter which are circular, with entire edges, and off-white. Initially, colonies are semitransparent but become more opaque with age.

Rabbit antiserum prepared against freeze-dried cells of *M. mobile* does not react in the indirect immunofluorescence assay with methanogens of other families or with *Methanospirillum hungatei.* There is a weak reaction with species of the genus *Methanogenium* (Conway de Macario et al., 1982a). Cells of *M. paynteri* have a weak positive reaction with the anti-*M. mobile* probe but not with antisera to methanogens belonging to other families (Rivard et al., 1983).

Methanomicrobium has been isolated from bovine rumen and marine sediment, environments with relatively high sodium ion concentrations.

Enrichment and Isolation Procedures

Because of the organisms' strict anaerobic nature, all manipulations must be adioxic. Cultivation requires that media be both adioxic and at a negative redox potential. This is achieved for tube and flask cultures by using reducing agents and the anaerobic procedures of Hungate (1950, 1969) with modifications (Balch et al., 1979). Anaerobiosis can also be achieved by using an anaerobic glove box. This allows cultivation on reduced agar media contained in Petri plates.

M. mobile is isolated by serial dilution of bovine rumen contents on a clarified rumen fluid medium (see Footnote *) with 80% H_2 and 20% CO_2 as the gas phase (Paynter and Hungate, 1968). *M. paynteri* is enriched when marine sediment is incubated with medium no. 3 (see Footnote †) of Balch et al. (1979) under an 80% H_2 and 20% CO_2 atmosphere (Rivard et al., 1983). Growth in closed vessels is improved if the atmosphere is pressurized to ~2 atm or if the gas phase is periodically flushed with the gas mixture.

Purification is accomplished by repeated serial dilution on the enrichment or isolation medium.

Maintenance Procedures

M. paynteri survives for several months at room temperature under nutrient starvation conditions (Rivard et al., 1983). *M. mobile* requires transfer every 2–3 weeks when grown in H_2–CO_2 rumen fluid broth. Colonies in rumen-fluid agar roll tubes survive for several months under dry-ice storage (M. J. B. Paynter, unpublished data). Cultures of both species are preserved in liquid nitrogen.

Differentiation of the genus **Methanomicrobium** from other genera in the family **Methanomicrobiaceae**

Distinctive features are presented in Table 25.6.

The mol% G + C for the DNA of *Methanomicrobium* is similar to that for *Methanospirillum.* However, immunological reactions suggest that these two genera are not very closely related.

Oligonucleotide catalogs of 16S rRNAs clearly delineate the different genera. Association coefficient (S_{AB}) values for binary couples of *M. mobile* to *M. hungatei* and *Methanogenium* species are 0.36 and 0.49–0.54, respectively (Balch et al., 1979).

Differentiation of the species of the genus **Methanomicrobium**

Characteristics are presented in Table 25.7.

List of species of the genus **Methanomicrobium**

1. **Methanomicrobium mobile** (Paynter and Hungate 1968) Balch and Wolfe 1981, 216.[VP] (Effective publication: Balch and Wolfe *in* Balch, Fox, Magrum, Woese and Wolfe 1979, 286. (*Methanobacterium mobilis* Paynter and Hungate, 1968, 1951).)

mo′bi.le. L. neut. adj. *mo′*bi.le motile, movable.

Characteristics are as described for the genus. Cells are 0.7×1.5–2.0 µm long. The polar flagellum is ~81 Å wide and up to 12.5 µm long. Lipophilic core components of polar lipids extracted from cells include diphytanylglycerol diether, bidiphytanyldiglycerol tetraether and several unidentified novel core lipids (Grant et al., 1985).

Substrate for growth and methanogenesis is H_2–CO_2 or formate. H_2 or formate can serve as electron donor for reduction of CO_2 to CH_4. Acetate, propionate, butyrate, isobutyrate, valerate, isovalerate, caproate, succinate, glucose, pyruvate, methanol, ethanol, propanol, isopropanol and butanol are not substrates.

Acetate isobutyrate, 2-methylbutyrate, isovalerate, tryptophan, pyridoxine, thiamine and biotin are required for growth; *p*-aminobenzoate is not required but is stimulatory.

An unidentified heat stable factor is required for growth and methanogenesis. It is present in bovine rumen fluid, mixed rumen bacteria and *M. thermoautotrophicum,* from which it has been partially purified (Tanner, R. S. 1982. Ph.D. thesis, University of Illinois).

---

*Clarified rumen fluid medium (final percentage composition (w/v): rumen contents centrifuged at $25,000 \times g$ for 15 min, 30 (v/v); KH_2PO_4, 0.05; K_2HPO_4, 0.05; NaCl, 0.1; $(NH_4)_2SO_4$, 0.05; $MgSO_4$, 0.01; $CaCl_2$, 0.01; resazurin, 0.0001; $NaHCO_3$, 0.5; cysteine·HCl, 0.03; Na_2S, 0.03; 80% H_2 and 20% CO_2 gas phase.

†Medium no. 3 of Balch et al. (1979) (g/l distilled water): KCl, 0.335; $MgCl_2\cdot2H_2O$, 2.75; $MgSO_4\cdot7H_2O$, 3.45; NH_4Cl, 0.25; $CaCl_2\cdot2H_2O$, 0.14; K_2HPO_4, 0.14; NaCl, 9.0; $Fe(NH_4)_2(SO_4)_2\cdot7H_2O$, 0.002; $NaHCO_3$, 5.0; sodium acetate, 1.0; yeast extract (Difco), 2.0; Trypticase (BBL), 2.0; L-cysteine·HCl·H_2O, 0.5; $Na_2S\cdot9H_2O$, 0.5; trace mineral solution, 10 ml/l; trace vitamins solution, 10 ml/l. Gas phase: 80% H_2 and 20% CO_2. The trace mineral solution contains (g/l distilled water): nitrilotriacetic acid, 1.5; $MgSO_4\cdot7H_2O$, 3.0; $MnSO_4\cdot2H_2O$, 0.5; NaCl, 1.0; $FeSO_4\cdot7H_2O$, 0.1; $CoSO_4$ or $CoCl_2$, 0.1; $CaCl_2\cdot2H_2O$, 0.1; $ZnSO_4$, 0.1; $CuSO_4\cdot5H_2O$, 0.01; $AlK(SO_4)_2$, 0.01; H_3BO_3, 0.01; $Na_2MoO_4\cdot2H_2O$, 0.01. Dissolve nitriloacetic acid with KOH to pH 6.5, add minerals, adjust pH to 7.0 with KOH. The trace vitamin solution contains (mg/l distilled water): biotin, 2; folic acid, 2; pyridoxine·HCl, 10; thiamine·HCl, 5; riboflavin, 5; nicotinic acid, 5; DL-calcium pantothenate, 5; vitamin B_{12}, 0.1; *p*-aminobenzoic acid, 5; lipoic acid, 5.

Table 25.6.

Differential characteristics of the genera **Methanomicrobium,** **Methanogenium** *and* **Methanospirillum**[a]

Characteristic	*Methanomicrobium*	*Methanogenium*	*Methanospirillum*
Cell morphology			
Short, straight to curved rods, no filaments, sometimes coccoid	+	+	−
Slender curved rods, form long spiral filaments	−	−	+
Presence of cell sheath	−	−	+
Mol% G + C of DNA	44.9–48.8	51.6–61.2	45.0–46.5
Immunological response of cells to *M. mobile* antiserum	+	Weak	−

[a]Symbols: +, property of the genus; and −, not a property of the genus.

Growth occurs from 30 to 45°C with an optimum at ~40°C; no growth at 28 or 50°C. The pH range is 5.9–7.7 with an optimum at 6.1–6.9, in bicarbonate or acetate buffers. Tris-hydrochloride (0.1 M) buffer is completely inhibitory, and phosphate (0.1 M) reduces methanogenesis by ~50%. The organism is isolated from the bovine rumen; ~10^8 organisms/ml of rumen contents.

The mol% G + C of the DNA is 48.8 (Bd).

Type strain: BP (DSM 1539).

2. **Methanomicrobium paynteri** Rivard, Henson, Thomas and Smith 1984, 91.[VP] (Effective publication: Rivard, Henson, Thomas and Smith 1983, 489.)

Table 25.7.

Differential characteristics of the species of the genus **Methanomicrobium**[a]

Characteristic	1. *M. mobile*	2. *M. paynteri*
Motility	+	−
Substrates for growth and methanogenesis		
$H_2 + CO_2$	+	+
Formate	+	−
Nutrient requirement		
Acetate	+	+
Unidentified growth factor present in rumen fluid and *M. thermoautotrophicum*	+	−
Growth and methanogenesis inhibited by Tris-HCl or phosphate buffers (0.1 M)	+	−

[a]Symbols: +, property of the species; and −, not a property of the species.

payn.ter′i. N.L. gen. n. *paynteri* of Paynter; named after M. J. B. Paynter who first isolated a species of the genus.

See genus description for general characteristics.

The only substrate for growth and methanogenesis is H_2-CO_2. Ethanol, methanol, methylamine, dimethylamine, trimethylamine, formate, acetate, pyruvate, propionate, glutamate and glucose are not used. Growth is stimulated by yeast extract and trypticase peptones, but the unidentified factor for *M. mobile* is not required. Optimum sodium ion concentration is 0.15 M, with growth occurring from 0 to 0.8 M. Optimal pH: 7.0, ranging from 6.6 to 7.3: limits are not known. Tris-HCl, phosphate and a variety of other buffers are not inhibitory. Temperature range: 25–42°C with an optimum at 40°C; no growth at 20 or 45°C.

Oligonucleotide catalogs of 16S rRNA support the placing of this organism in the family *Methanomicrobiaceae.*

Isolated from marine sediment collected from a mangrove swamp, Grand Cayman, British West Indies.

The mol% G + C of the DNA is 44.9 (Bd).

Type strain: G-2000 (ATCC 33997; DSM 2545).

Genus II. **Methanospirillum** *Ferry, Smith and Wolfe 1974, 469*[AL]

JAMES G. FERRY

Me.tha.no.spi.ril′lum. M.L. n. *methanum* methane; Gr. n. *speira* a spiral; M.L. neut. n. *Methanospirillum* methane (-producing) spiral.

Symmetrically curved rods 0.4–0.5 × 7.4–10 μm **that usually form wavy filaments** from 15 to several hundred μm in length. Gramnegative. **Progressively motile by means of polar, tufted flagella.** Organism is strictly **anaerobic.** Optimum temperature: 30–37°C. **Formate or H_2 are substrates** for growth and methanogenesis. Autotrophic to heterotrophic nutrition.

The mol% G + C of the DNA is 45 (Bd) and 46.5–49.5 (Td).

Type species: *Methanospirillum hungatei* Ferry, Smith and Wolfe 1974, 469.

Further Descriptive Information

The cellular morphology of *Methanospirillum hungatei* strain JF-1, taken from a culture in midgrowth phase, is shown in Fig. 25.7. Phasecontrast micrographs of lysed cells expose a continuous outer sheath which encases individual cells joined at the ends which form filaments (Ferry et al., 1974). Thin sections of filaments show a double-layered cell envelope comprised of the outer sheath and a cell wall sacculus contiguous with the outer membrane of individual cells that are joined by a "cell

spacer" structure (Zeikus and Bowen, 1975b). The rigid protein sheath contains a wide variety of amino acids, no amino sugars and only a trace of neutral sugars and exhibits a distinct fibrillar surface pattern (Kandler and König, 1978; Sprott and McKellar, 1980). Negatively stained cells of strain JF-1 show surface striations (Fig. 25.8) which result from the presence of circumferential rings likened to the hoops of a barrel (Sprott et al., 1987). The flexible cell wall sacculus is involved in septum formation (Sprott et al., 1979; Sprott and McKellar, 1980). Monoclonal antibodies against *M. hungatei* strain JF-1 do not bind pseudomurein components or their analogs (Conway de Macario et al., 1982b, c).

Surface colonies of *M. hungatei* strain JF-1 (1–3 mm in diameter) appear yellow, circular and convex with lobate margins (Ferry et al., 1974). Microscopic examination of agar surface colonies shows a unique optical pattern of regular light and dark striations approximately two cell lengths (16 μm) apart (Fig. 25.9). Light blue surface colonies with serrated edges are reported for *M. hungatei* strain GP1 (Patel et al., 1976).

Good growth of strain JF-1 occurs in a mineral salts medium and a H_2-

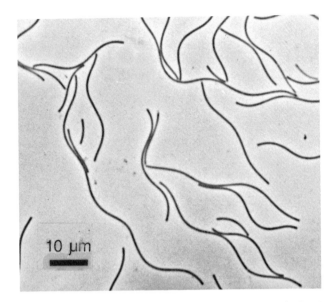

Figure 25.7. Phase-contrast micrograph of *M. hungatei,* showing single cells and filaments. Wet mounts of cultures were prepared on glass slides which had been coated with 2% washed Nobel agar (Difco).

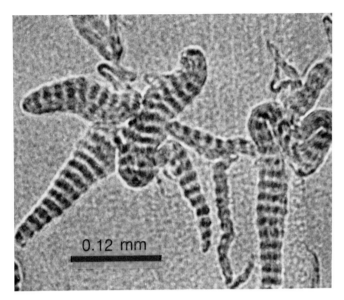

Figure 25.9. Colony of *M. hungatei* developing on the surface of an agar plate.

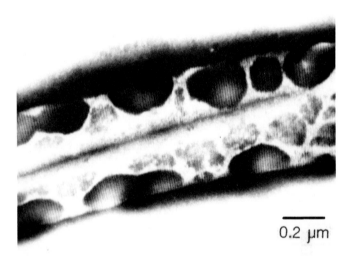

Figure 25.8. Negatively stained whole cells of *Methanospirillum hungatei* strain JF-1. An RCA EMU-3C electron microscope was used for observing cells stained with a 0.02% (w/v) aqueous solution of phosphotungstic acid adjusted to pH 7.0 with potassium hydroxide.

The energy-yielding metabolism (Ferry and Wolfe, 1977; Sprott et al., 1983) and biosynthetic pathways (Sprott et al., 1979; Ekiel et al., 1983) have received attention. Among 28 antibiotics tested, only enduracidin, chloramphenicol, gramicidin S and monesin inhibited growth (Hilpert et al., 1981). A decline in the growth rate and intracellular ATP concentration occurs when cultures are exposed to dicyclohexylcarbodiimide (Sprott and Jarrell, 1982).

Strains of *M. hungatei* have been isolated from sewage-sludge and pear waste digestors. A salt-tolerant strain has been isolated from marine sediments by K. R. Sowers in the author's laboratory. *M. hungatei* is the dominant H_2-utilizing organism associated with benzoate and fatty acid-oxiding organisms in enrichment cultures from nonmarine habitats (Ferry and Wolfe, 1976; Boone and Bryant, 1980; McInerney et al., 1981; Mountfort and Bryant, 1982). Formate is metabolized at low concentrations, which implies that this substrate may be directly utilized in some habitats (Schauer et al., 1982).

Enrichment and Isolation Procedures

All procedures for the preparation of culture media and transfer of cultures are done under an O_2-free atmosphere of H_2-CO_2 (80:20) (Balch et al., 1979). Media for enrichment of *M. hungatei* contains minerals, vitamins, sodium formate, sodium acetate and cysteine-sulfide reducing agent. A CO_2-bicarbonate buffer system is used to maintain the pH between 6.8 and 7.2 (Ferry et al., 1974; Patel et al., 1976). Additions of acetate and effluent from the habitat of the inoculum is recommended for enrichment and isolation of new strains. Isolation media may include additions of yeast extract and Trypticase. Colonies are most easily identified in deep agar roll tubes as diffuse light yellow colonies that develop in correlation with the formation of methane.

Maintenance Procedures

Methanospirillum strains are maintained in the author's laboratory by biweekly transfer on agar slants of isolation medium.

CO_2 (80:20) atmosphere (Ferry and Wolfe, 1977), but strain GP1 also requires acetate as a carbon source (Ekiel et al., 1983). The addition of amino acids and a B-vitamin mixture, or yeast extract and Trypticase, stimulate the growth of strain JF-1, but yeast extract and tryptone inhibit the growth rate of strain GP1 (Breuil and Patel, 1980). Other differences between strains JF-1 and GP1 include amino acid composition of the outer sheath and the DNA base composition (Patel et al., 1976).

Differentiation of the genus **Methanospirillum** from other genera

The genus *Methanospirillum* is distinguished from other genera of methanogenic bacteria primarily by its spiral shape, double-layered cell envelope and comparative cataloging of the 16S rRNA (Balch et al., 1979). Immunologic fingerprinting (Conway de Macario et al., 1982b, c) and 16S rRNA cataloging show the genus *Methanospirillum* most closely related to the genus *Methanogenium*. The protein sheath from *M. hungatei* and the protein cell walls of other genera contain a similar distribution of amino acids, but unlike the protein cell walls, the sheath is resistant to 2% SDS or 4 M urea at alkaline pH (Kandler, 1982).

The cellular lipid fraction of *M. hungatei* contains dibiphytanyl diglycerol tetraethers common to other genera of methanogenic bacteria, but the fraction is unique in that one of the free hydroxyl groups is esterified with glycerophosphoric acid and the other is glycosidically linked to a disaccharide (Kushwaha et al., 1981).

Further Reading

Conway de Macario, E., M.J. Wolin and A.J.L. Macario. 1981. Immunology of archaebacteria that produce methane gas. Science *214:* 74–74.
Patel, G.B., L.A. Roth and G.D. Sprott. 1979. Factors influencing filament length of *Methanospirillum hungatii.* J. Gen. Microbiol. *112:* 411–415.
Sprott, G.O. and K.F. Janell. 1981. K⁺, Na⁺ and Mg²⁺ content and permeability of *Methanospirillum hungatei* and *Methanobacterium thermoaustotrophicum.* Can. J. Microbiol. *27:* 444–451.
Zeikus, J.G. and V.G. Bowen. 1974. Comparative ultrastructure of methanogenic bacteria. Can. J. Microbiol. *21:* 121–129.

List of species of the genus **Methanospirillum**

1. **Methanospirillum hungatei** Ferry, Smith and Wolfe 1974, 469.[AL] (*Methanospirillum hungatii* [sic] Ferry, Smith and Wolfe 1974, 469.)

hun.gat′e.i. M.L. gen. n. *hungatei* of Hungate; named for R. E. Hungate who has made many contributions to the ecological study of methanogenic bacteria.

The description of the species is the same as that given for the genus. *Type strain:* ATCC 27890, DSM 864.

Genus III. **Methanogenium** Romesser, Wolfe, Mayer, Spiess and Walther-Mauruschat 1981, 216[VP] (Effective publication: Romesser, Wolfe, Mayer, Spiess and Walther-Mauruschat 1979, 152)

JAMES A. ROMESSER

Me.tha.no.gen′i.um. M.L. n. *methanum* methane; Gr. v. suff. *genium* producing; M.L. neut. n. *methanogenium* methane-producing.

Irregular cocci occurring singly or in pairs, usually 1.0–2.6 μm in diameter. **Gram-negative.** Non-sporeforming. No motility observed, although some strains flagellated. **Strictly anaerobic. Chemolithotrophic, utilizing hydrogen or sometimes formate as the electron donor, reducing carbon dioxide to methane. Growth factors required. NaCl generally required or stimulatory for growth.** Optimal temperatures range between 20 and 60°C, and optimal pH, between 6.2 and 7.3.

The mol% G + C of the DNA is 52–61 (Bd).

Type species: *Methanogenium cariaci* Romesser, Wolfe, Spiess and Walther-Mauruschat 1981, 216.

Further Descriptive Information

Cells are highly irregular (almost raisin-shaped) cocci. The cells can be made to round up into more regular cocci by lowering the salt concentration, but a reduction in cell growth rate is generally observed. Although the cells stain Gram-negative, micrographs of ultrathin sections of *M. cariaci* and *M. marisnigri* do not show an outer membrane (Romesser et al., 1979). The cell walls appear to be constructed of protein subunits and lack muramic acid or amino sugars (Kandler and König, 1978). Freeze-etched analysis has shown the cell walls to have a periodic surface pattern consisting of structural units about 14 nm in diameter (Romesser et al., 1979). *M. cariaci, M. marisnigri* and *M. tationis* have peritrichously arranged flagella but have not been observed to be motile. Some strains of *M. thermophilicum* have a single flagellum. *M. aggregans* appears to form capsules. *M. cariaci* and some strains of *M. thermophilicum* bear long, thin pili.

Colonies are shiny, yellow, beige or white, circular and have entire edges. Colonies of *M. marisnigri,* "*M. olentangyi,*" *M. aggregans* and *M. bourgense* are convex; those of *M. cariaci* are umbonate.

All strains require organic growth factors, and most either require or are stimulated by NaCl. All strains utilize hydrogen and CO₂ or formate for growth except for "*M. olentangyi*" which cannot use formate.

Both mesophilic and thermophilic strains have been described.

The cells occur in anaerobic marine or freshwater sediments, where they presumably function as hydrogen scavengers.

Enrichment and Isolation Procedures

The organisms may be cultivated in 125-ml serum vials in sterile growth medium prepared under strictly anaerobic growth atmosphere (80% H₂ and 20% CO₂) by a modification of the Hungate technique (1950), as described by Bryant and Robinson (1961) and revised by Balch and Wolfe (1976). Enrichment medium contains the following constituents in a mixture of 30% distilled water and 70% seawater at the indicated final concentration (w/v) in percent: ammonium acetate, 0.05; sodium formate, 0.1; Trypticase (BBL), 0.2; yeast extract, 0.1; Na₂CO₃, 0.1; NaHCO₃, 0.2; cysteine hydrochloride, 0.05; Na₂S + 9H₂O, 0.05; resazurin, 0.0001. The pH of the medium after equilibration with 80% H₂ and 20% CO₂ gas atmosphere at 137 kPa is 7.4. Enrichments for *M. cariaci* and *M. marisnigri* are incubated at 20°C, "*M. olentangyi,*" *M. tationis, M. aggregans* and *M. bourgense* at 37°C, and *M. thermophilicum* at 55°C. Methane formation is measured periodically by gas chromatography.

Isolation of these methanogens is achieved by streaking enrichment cultures on agar plates in a Freter type anaerobic hood (Aranki and Freter, 1972) as described by Romesser et al. (1979). Alternatively, agar roll tubes may be used. Colonies are yellow, beige or white and exhibit a dull greenish-blue fluorescence when illuminated with long wave UV light. Wet mounts of cells exhibit osmotic fragility.

Maintenance Procedures

Cultures are maintained by serial transfer in broth culture or on agar slants. Incubation at suboptimal growth temperatures is recommended so that transfers need not be made as frequently. Cells are very susceptible to freeze-thaw lysis, and storage procedures requiring freeze-thaw are not recommended.

Differentiation of the genus **Methanogenium** *from other genera*

Although similar to the genus *Methanococcus* in morphology and cell wall structures, the genus *Methanogenium* is distinct because of the higher mol% G + C of its DNA (52–61 vs. 31–41 for *Methanococcus*) and a lack of relatedness when 16S rRNA oligonucleotide catalogs are compared (Fox et al., 1977; Balch et al., 1979). Serological cross-reactions between *Methanogenium* and *Methanococcus* have not been detected by using the immunofluorescent techniques described by Conway de Macario et al. (1982b, d).

The genus *Methanogenium* differs from the genus *Methanococcoides* in that the latter has a low mol% G + C of its DNA (42%) and shows no serological cross-reactivity by immunofluorescence techniques. In addition, the genus *Methanococcoides* does not utilize H_2 and CO_2 or formate for growth but rather uses the methylotrophic substrates trimethylamine, methylamine or methanol.

Taxonomic Comments

Precise determination of phylogenetic relationships of the genus *Methanogenium* to other genera of methanogens will depend heavily on continued studies of relatedness of 16S and 5S rRNA oligonucleotide sequences and on other studies of its nucleic acids. Immunological comparative analysis of the cell envelopes of *Methanogenium* species (Conway de Macario et al., 1982b, d; Macario et al., 1987) has shown considerable antigenic diversity within the genus but that there is sufficient antigenic cohesiveness within the group for this technique to be used to distinguish *Methanogenium* from other genera.

Whitman (1985) has reported that S_{AB} data suggest that *Methanoplanus limicola* may, in fact, be a species of *Methanogenium*. Tu et al. (1982) originally assigned this species to the new genus *Methanoplanus*, based on DNA/RNA hybridization experiments and its novel morphology.

Further Reading

Balch, W.E., G.E. Fox, L.J. Magrum, C.R. Woese and R.S. Wolfe. 1979. Methanogens: reevaluation of a unique biological group. Microbiol. Rev. *43:* 260–296.

Whitman, W.B. 1985. Methanogenic bacteria. *In* Woese and Wolfe (Editors), The Bacteria: A Treatise on Structure and Function, Vol. VIII: The Archaebacteria. Academic Press, New York, pp. 3–84.

Differentiation of the species of the genus **Methanogenium**

The differential characteristics of the species of the genus *Methanogenium* are indicated in Table 25.8.

List of species of the genus **Methanogenium**

1. **Methanogenium cariaci** Romesser, Wolfe, Mayer, Spiess and Walther-Mauruschat 1981, 216.[VP] (Effective publication: Romesser, Wolfe, Mayer, Spiess and Walther-Mauruschat 1979, 152.)

car.i.a′ci. L. gen. n. *cariaci* of the Cariaco.

See Table 25.8 and Fig. 25.10, *A–C,* and the generic description for many characteristics.

Cells up to 2.6 µm in diameter. Yeast extract required for growth. Optimal growth in 0.46 M NaCl.

Colonies are circular, umbonate, greenish-yellow with entire edges and a shiny surface.

Type strain isolated from sediment from the Cariaco Trench.

The mol% G + C of the DNA is 52 (Bd).

Type strain: ATCC 35093 (DSM 1497).

2. **Methanogenium marisnigri** Romesser, Wolfe, Mayer, Spiess and Walther-Mauruschat 1981, 216.[VP] (Effective publication: Romesser, Wolfe, Mayer, Spiess and Walther-Mauruschat 1979, 152.)

mar.is.ni′gri. L. gen. n. *maris* of the sea; L. adj. *niger* black; M.L. neut. n. *marisnigri* Black Sea.

See Table 25.8 and the generic description for many characteristics.

Cells up to 1.3 µm in diameter. Trypticase (BBL) required for growth. Optimal growth in 0.1 M NaCl.

Colonies are circular, convex, yellow with entire edges and a shiny surface.

Type strain isolated from sediment from the Black Sea.

The mol% G + C of the DNA is 61 (Bd).

Type strain: ATCC 35101 (DSM 1498).

3. **Methanogenium thermophilicum** Rivard and Smith 1982, 436.[VP]

ther.mo.phil′i.cum. Gr. n. *therme* heat; Gr. adj. *philicum* loving; M.L. adj. *thermophilicum* heat-loving.

See Table 25.8 and the generic description for many characteristics.

Cells 1.0–1.3 µm in diameter. Trypticase (BBL) and vitamin solution required for growth. Optimal growth in 0.20 M NaCl.

Colonies are beige and circular with entire edges.

Type strain isolated from sediment underlying high temperature effluent channel from nuclear power plant.

The mol% G + C of the DNA is 59 (Bd).

Type strain: DSM 2373.

Two other strains of *M. thermophilicum* have been described. *M. thermophilicum* Los Angeles (Ferguson and Mah, 1983) has an optimal growth temperature of 60°C, is not flagellated, utilizes either formate or H_2 and CO_2 for growth, and requires Trypticase (BBL) and yeast extract for growth; the mol% G + C of the DNA is 60. *M. thermophilicum* Ratisbona (Zabel et al., 1985) has an optimal growth temperature of 58°C, has a single flagellum and several pili, and utilizes either formate or H_2 and CO_2 for growth; the mol% G + C of the DNA is 57.

4. **"Methanogenium olentangyi"** Corder, Hook, Larkin and Frea 1983, 32.

o.len.tan′gy.i. M.L. gen. n. *olentangyi* of the Olentangy.

See Table 25.8 and the generic description for many characteristics.

Table 25.8.

Characteristics differentiating the species of the genus **Methanogenium**[a]

Characteristic	1. *M. cariaci*	2. *M. marisnigri*	3. *M. thermophilicum*	4. *"M. olentangyi"*	5. *M. tationis*	6. *M. aggregans*	7. *M. bourgense*
Flagella	+	+	±	−	+	−	−
Capsule	−	−	−	−	−	+	−
Pili	+	−	±	−	−	−	−
Requires acetate	+	−	−	+	+	+	+
Growth on formate	+	+	+	−	+	+	+
Growth at 60°C	−	−	+	−	−	−	−
Growth at 15°C	+	+	−	−	−	−	−
Mol% G + C of DNA	52	61	59	54	54	52	59

[a]Symbols: +, 90% or more of strains are positive; −, 90% or more of strains are negative; and ±, some strains possess trait.

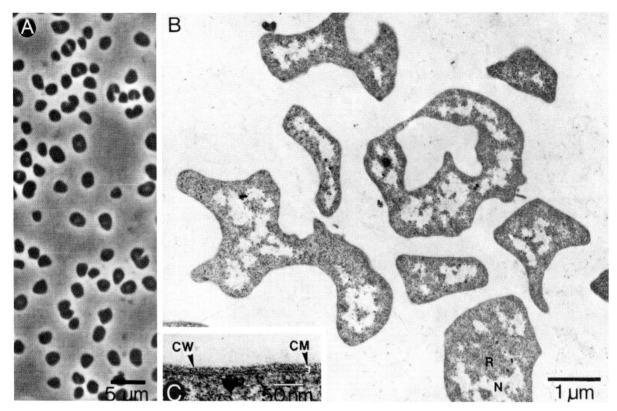

Figure 25.10. *M. cariaci. A,* phase-contrast photomicrograph of living cells. *Bar,* 5 μm. *B,* ultrathin section (× 14,000). *C,* section showing cell wall (*CW*) and cytoplasmic membrane (*CM*) (× 161,000). (Reproduced with permission from J. A. Romesser, R. S. Wolfe, F. Mayer, E. Spiess and A. Walther-Mauruschat, Archives of Microbiology *121:* 147–153, 1979, ©Springer-Verlag, Berlin).

Cells 1.0–1.5 μm in diameter. Optimal growth in 0.17 M NaCl.

Colonies are circular, mucoid, yellow, shiny and convex.

Type strain isolated from sediment from Olentangy River, Ohio.

The mol% G + C of the DNA is 54 (Bd).

Type strain: RC/ER.

5. **Methanogenium tationis** (corrig.) Zabel, König and Winter 1986, 355.[VP] (Effective publication as *M. tatii* [sic]: Zabel, König and Winter 1984, 313.)

ta′ti.o′nis. L. gen. n. *tationis* of the Tatio.

See Table 25.8 and the generic description for many characteristics.

Average cell diameter is 3 μm. Yeast extract, peptone and 0.1 M NaCl required for optimal growth.

Colonies are yellow.

Type strain isolated from mud from a small, moderately thermophilic sulfataric pool on Mount Tatio, Chile.

The mol% G + C of the DNA is 54 (Td).

Type strain: DSM 2702.

6. **Methanogenium aggregans** Ollivier, Mah, Garcia and Robinson 1985, 129.[VP]

ag′gre.gans. L. part. *aggregans* adding to, aggregating, forming clumps.

See Table 25.8 and the generic description for many characteristics.

Average cell diameter is 1 μm. Either yeast extract or Trypticase (BBL) required for growth. Less than 0.003 M NaCl required for optimal growth.

Colonies are white or yellow, circular and convex.

Type strain isolated from a sewage-sludge digester at Bourg-en-Bresse, France.

The mol% G + C of the DNA is 52.

Type strain: DSM 3027.

7. **Methanogenium bourgense** Ollivier, Mah, Garcia and Boone 1986, 300.[VP]

bourg.en′se. N.L. neut. adj. *bourgense* from Bourg-en-Bresse, France.

See Table 25.8 and the generic description for many characteristics.

Cells are 1–2 μm in diameter. Either yeast extract or Trypticase (BBL) stimulate growth. Optimal growth obtained in 0.017 M NaCl.

Colonies are white or yellow, circular and convex.

Type strain isolated from a digester fermenting tannery by-products, which was originally inoculated with digested sewage sludge from Bourg-en-Bresse, France.

The mol% G + C of the DNA is 59.

Type strain: DSM 3045.

FAMILY II. **METHANOSARCINACEAE** BALCH AND WOLFE 1981, 216, [VP] EMEND. SOWERS, JOHNSON AND FERRY 1984, 448 (EFFECTIVE PUBLICATION: BALCH AND WOLFE *IN* BALCH, FOX, MAGRUM, WOESE AND WOLFE 1979, 288)

DAVID R. BOONE AND ROBERT A. MAH

Me.tha.no.sar.cin.a′ce.ae. N.L. neut. n. *Methanosarcina* type genus of the family; -*aceae* the ending to denote a family; N.L. fem. pl. n. *Methanosarcinaceae* the *Methanosarcina* family.

Cells are irregular spheroid bodies occurring individually or typically in aggregates of cells or "cysts" or as sheathed rods. Spheroid cells are 0.8–2.5 μm in diameter and have a highly variable Gram reaction. Individual coccoid cells have a protein cell wall. Exterior to the wall, a heteropolysaccharide material may be present and may confer resistance to lysis by osmotic shock or sodium dodecyl sulfate. A second morphological state is pseudosarcina or an aggregate of cells; cell division planes are usually nonperpendicular. Most cells in this state have a heteropolysaccharide outer layer, but marine strains may not. These aggregates may be comprised of a few cells, or they may be very large, up to several millimeters in diameter, with an appearance similar to mulberries. A third morphological state has been termed a "cyst," which is apparently composed of an outer, cellular layer enclosing a central cavity filled with cells in the first morphological state. A single strain may occur in one or more of these three forms during different phases of growth. A fourth morphological state, sheathed rods, occurs only in the genus *Methanothrix*.

Cells are mesophilic or thermophilic. Methanol and methylated amines may be catabolized, but formate is not. Many strains also grow on H_2-CO_2 or acetate. Catabolic products are CH_4 and CO_2 (plus NH_4^+ from methylated amines). Molecular sulfur may be reduced to H_2S, but this reaction may not lead to growth.

Habitats: any anaerobic environment, especially where acetate or methyl amines are available, including aquatic sediments, anaerobic sewage digesters and gastrointestinal tracts, especially the rumen.

The mol% G + C of the DNA is 36–48.5.

Type genus: *Methanosarcina* Kluyver and van Niel 1936, 400.

Key to the genera of the family **Methanosarcinaceae**

I. Aggregates of cells are present during some phase of growth; other forms may include cocci or "cysts." Cells catabolize either H_2-CO_2 or acetate, in addition to methanol and methylamines.

Genus I. *Methanosarcina*

II. Irregular cocci with substrates limited to methylamines and methanol. Optimum NaCl concentration is near 0.5 M, and poor or no growth is obtained with 1.5 M NaCl. Organisms contain internal membrane structures and have no vitamin requirements. DNA/RNA homology high with *Methanolobus* species and low with *Methanococcoides* species.

Genus II. *Methanolobus*

III. Rod-shaped cells enclosed in a sheath; may occur in very long chains. Acetate is the sole substrate.

Genus III. *Methanothrix*

IV. Irregular cocci with substrates limited to methylamines and methanol. Optimum NaCl concentration is near 0.5 M, and poor or no growth is obtained with 1.5 M NaCl. Organisms contain no intramembranous structures; require vitamins for growth. DNA/RNA homology high with *Methanococcoides* species and low with *Methanolobus* species.

Genus IV. *Methanococcoides*

Taxonomic Comments

The taxonomic relationship between these groups is not entirely clear. *Methanothrix* is morphologically different and is the only genus which is unable to catabolize methanol or trimethylamine (however, some mixed cultures containing strongly epifluorescent cells with the morphology of *Methanothrix* as the sole methanogen grow by reducing trimethylamine with H_2 (D. R. Boone, unpublished data). This family contains all but one of the genera of methanogens able to catabolize methanol, methylated amines and acetate. *Methanosphaera*, currently unassigned to a family, requires both methanol and H_2 for growth. The *Methanosarcinaceae* can all grow on methanol and on trimethylamine as sole catabolic substrate.

A number of strains have been isolated which grow well only with high salt concentrations: *Methanococcus halophilus* Z-7982 (DSM 3094) (Zhilina, 1983), "*Halomethanococcus mahii*" SLP (ATCC 35705) (Paterek and Smith, 1985), strain SF1 (DSM 3243) (Mathrani and Boone, 1985), strain WeN5 (Boone et al., 1986) and the following five strains described by Zhilina (1986): strain Z-7301, strain Z-7302, strain Z-7303, strain Z-7305 and strain Z-7403. At the present time no formal taxonomic assignment has been proposed for most of these strains, but their physiological characteristics suggest that they may belong in a single genus. *M. halophilus* was proposed as a species with Z-7982 as type strain and appears on a validation list (Zhilina, 1984). However, the use of methylamines as catabolic substrate and inability of that species to use H_2-CO_2 (Zhilina, 1983) indicate it should be placed outside the genus *Methanococcus* (Mah and Kuhn, 1984a; Judicial Commission, 1986a). This species was not listed among the members of the genus *Methanococcus* in this manual because it appears that this species belongs, along with other halophilic, methylophagic methanogens, in a new, as yet undescribed, genus of bacteria within the family *Methanosarcinaceae*.

All *Methanosarcina* strains can use either acetate or H_2-CO_2 (or both) as catabolic substrate. The other two genera, *Methanococcoides* and *Methanolobus*, are more difficult to distinguish. Molecular analysis of DNA and RNA is the major basis for distinguishing these two genera (Sowers et al., 1984). Other differences (Sowers et al., 1984) include the presence of internal membranes and uniform inclusions in *Methanolobus* and vitamin requirements for *Methanococcoides*; *Methanolobus* also has a broader temperature range.

Genus I. *Methanosarcina* *Kluyver and van Niel 1936, 400,* [AL] *emend. Mah and Kuhn 1984a, 266*
(Nom. Cons. Opin. 63 Jud. Comm. 1986b, 492)

ROBERT A. MAH AND DAVID R. BOONE

Me.tha.no.sar.ci′na. N.L. n. *methanum* methane; M.L. n. *sarcina* a package, bundle; N.L. n. *Methanosarcina* methane sarcina.

Irregular spheroid bodies (1–1000 μm or more in diameter) **occurring alone or typically in aggregates of cells. Sometimes occur as large cysts** with a common outer wall surrounding individual coccoid cells. Refer to Figures 25.11–25.13 for typical morphologies. **Endospores not formed. Gram stain results are variable. Nonmotile. May contain gas vesicles (Fig. 25.14). Very strictly anaerobic.** Optimum growth temperatures are 30–40°C for mesophilic species and 50–55°C for thermophiles. **Energy metabolism via formation of methane from acetate, methanol, monomethylamine, dimethylamine, trimethylamine, H_2-CO_2, and possibly CO. Some strains do not use H_2-CO_2 as sole energy substrate.** N_2 may be fixed. The mol% G + C of the DNA is 36–43.

Type species: *Methanosarcina barkeri* Schnellen 1947, 73. (Judicial Commission, Opinion 63, 1986b, 492).

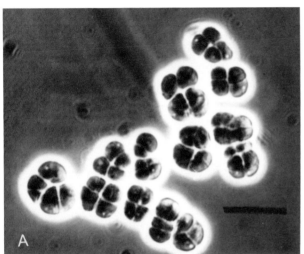

Figure 25.11. *Methanosarcina barkeri* 227. *A*, phase-contrast micrograph of typical pseudosarcinae. *Bar*, 10 μm. *B*, thin-section electron micrograph. *Bar*, 200 nm. (Courtesy of J. Pangborn, Facility for Advanced Instrumentation, University of California, Davis.)

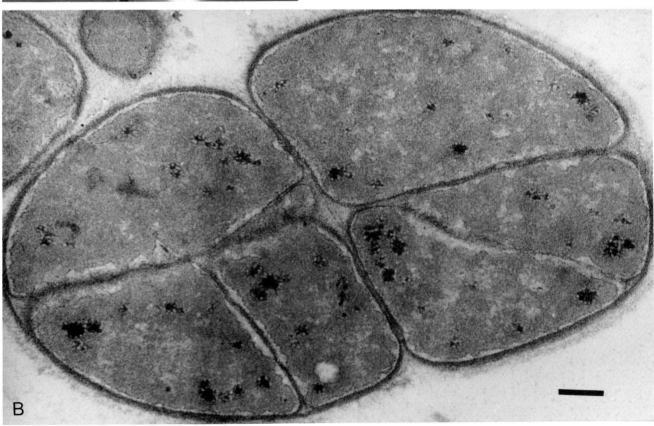

Further Descriptive Information

Aggregates are small to large spheroid bodies comprising many irregular subunits (Zhilina, 1971, 1976; Zeikus and Bowen, 1975a). The multilocular nature is visible only by transmission electron microscopy of thin sections, although phase-contrast microscopy reveals some surface indentations. The spheroid bodies may exist as: (a) small coccoid shapes 1–3 μm in diameter, with a tendency to irregularity; surface indentations are not visible in these bodies, but the bodies may be subdivided by irregular cross-walls which are apparent only when thin sections are examined by transmission electron microscopy; (b) larger coccoid bodies 5–10 μm in diameter, occurring in clusters of 5–10 or more; surface indentations are visible; and (c) large spheroid bodies 20–100 μm or more in diameter; surface indentations are visible, giving an appearance similar to mulberries (plant genus *Morus*). The larger clusters are always subdivided by irregular cross-walls, and surface indentations are always visible under phase-contrast microscopy. Occasionally, aggregates may form large rafts 1000 μm or more across. A cyst with a common outer layer may enclose myriads of smaller irregular coccoid elements. Such cysts may be ruptured by applying external pressure or may disaggregate enzymatically to release the coccoid elements. Some species undergo a life cycle involving these forms, or a single species may exist as only one of these forms.

The cell walls of *Methanosarcina* contain a protein layer adjacent to the cell membrane. External to this layer, there may often be an outer layer composed of heteropolysaccharide. This outer layer is absent in *Methanosarcina acetivorans*, which is sensitive to lysis by sodium dodecyl sulfate (SDS). The dissolution of the heteropolysaccharide outer layer of other *Methanosarcina* strains, which may occur during growth, gives rise to individual, SDS-sensitive, coccoid units. The heteropolysaccharide outer layer is comprised mainly of galactosamine, glucose, mannose and glucuronic or galacturonic acid. Sulfate is not a major component of this layer, but a small amount (5%) of protein is present. SDS-extracted cell wall material of *Methanosarcina mazei* contains five amino acids (molar amino acid concentrations relative to glycine are given in parenthesis): serine (1.8), glycine (1.0), lysine (0.9), ornithine (0.7), and alanine (0.2) (Robinson et al., 1985). These amino acids are apparently not contaminants from the inner, protein cell wall, since the concentrations of other detectable amino acids are less than one-tenth the molar amounts relative to glycine.

Immunological analysis using polyclonal antibody probes and whole bacterial cells as antigens indicates a close degree of antigenic relatedness among the species of *Methanosarcina* and no cross-reactivity with methanogens outside the family (Conway de Macario et al., 1982a; Macario and Conway de Macario, 1983). These findings augment the morphological and physiological factors which distinguish the species of *Methanosarcina* from other genera of methanogens. DNA and RNA interspecies hybridization and lack of intergeneric hybridization also support this generic composition (Sowers et al., 1984).

Gas vesicles may occur.

All species of *Methanosarcina* use methanol and methylamines as catabolic substrates. Most species can also use H_2-CO_2 and acetate. Stationary phase, H_2-CO_2-grown cells may require a period of adaptation for growth on acetate (Boone et al., 1987). However, if cells are grown with both H_2-CO_2 and acetate present, H_2-CO_2 is used first and then acetate is used without a long lag (Mah et al., 1981). Acetate is degraded by the aceticlastic reaction, with the methyl group reduced to CH_4 and the carboxyl group oxidized to CO_2 (Mah et al., 1978).

Members of the genus *Methanosarcina* may be isolated from freshwater and marine environments where acetate or methylamines are degraded. These include anaerobic digesters, freshwater and marine sediments, and the rumen of cattle or sheep. *Methanosarcina* species in pure culture also grow by using energy substrates other than acetate or methylamines, but these latter may be the major natural substrates. Existing *Methanosarcina* strains have a higher K_m for H_2 than other H_2-oxidizing methanogens and may not be competitive for H_2 in mixed-culture environments (Boone et al., 1987).

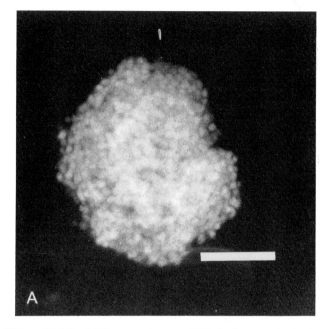

Figure 25.12. *Methanosarcina mazei* S-6. *A*, phase-contrast micrograph. *Bar*, 10 μm. *B*, scanning electron micrograph. *Bar*, 5 μm. (Courtesy of R. Robinson, Department of Microbiology, University of California, Los Angeles.) *C*, individual coccoid units viewed by Nomarski optics. *Bar*, 5 μm. (Courtesy of Ralph Robinson.)

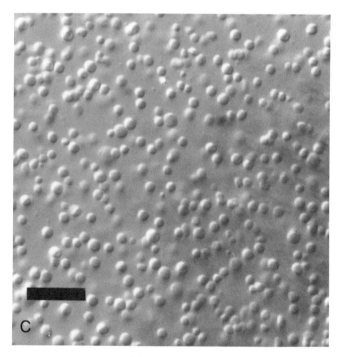

Figure 25.12C.

Enrichment and Isolation Procedures

Enrichment cultures of *Methanosarcina* may be initiated in media containing acetate, methanol or methylamines as substrate. NH_3 may serve as nitrogen source and sulfide as sulfur source. Some strains re-

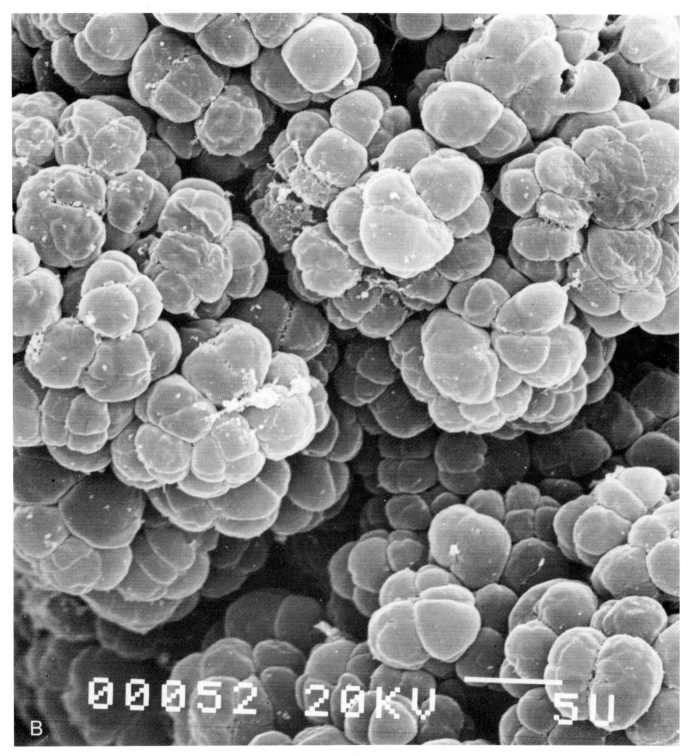

Figure 25.12B.

quire organic growth factors, and some may require unusual metal ions such as nickel or cobalt. Trimethylamine is the substrate of choice for rapid enrichment of *Methanosarcina*. Although *Methanolobus tindarius* (König and Stetter, 1982), *Methanococcoides methylutens* (Sowers and Ferry, 1983) and several halophilic isolates (Zhilina, 1983; Mathrani and Boone, 1985; Paterek and Smith, 1985; Zhilina, 1986; Zhilina and Zavar-zin, 1987) may also use trimethylamine (or methanol), *Methanosarcina* is morphologically distinctive and more commonly distributed. Methanol may also be used as an enrichment substrate, but nonmethanogens such as *Eubacterium limosum* may predominate (Sharak Genthner et al., 1981): growth of nonmethanogens may be inhibited by antibiotics such as penicillin, cycloserine or vancomycin. Acetate is perhaps the

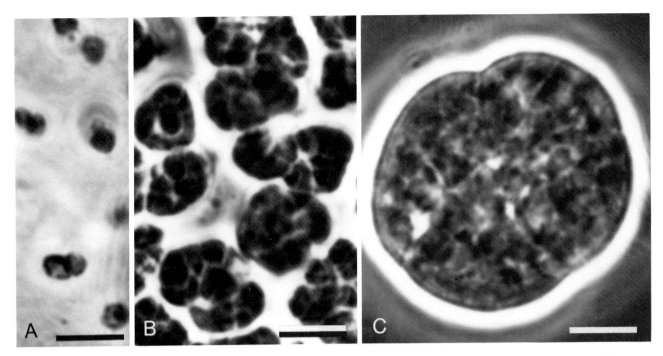

Figure 25.13. Phase-contrast photomicrographs of *Methanosarcina acetivorans* C2A. *Bars*, 5 μm. *A*, individual coccoid units. *B*, small aggregates of cells. *C*, a mature cyst. (Courtesy of K. Sowers, Department of Anaerobic Bacteriology, Virginia Polytechnic Institute and State University, Blacksburg.) (Reproduced with permission from K. R. Sowers, S. F. Baron and J. G. Ferry, Applied Environmental Microbiology 47: 972, 1984, ©American Society for Microbiology, Washington, D.C.)

most selective substrate for *Methanosarcina*, but growth is slower than with trimethylamine, and not all *Methanosarcina* species can use acetate. Also, at very long retention times (30 days), acetate enrichment cultures may yield *Methanothrix* instead of *Methanosarcina*, especially at pH values of 7.0 or above. Lowering the pH below 7.0 with frequent transfer of cultures (as soon as acetate is depleted) usually yields *Methanosarcina* in enrichment cultures.

Methanosarcina thermophila normally occurs only in large aggregates; in some media with high salt, it may form individual coccoid units (Sowers and Gunsalus, 1988). Because of its existence in large aggregates, the numbers of colony-forming units may be small compared with its metabolic importance in mixed-culture systems. Colonies of *M. ther-* *mophila* may occur in roll tubes inoculated with 100 μl or more of sample compared with an equivalent mass-density of *M. mazei* whose individual coccoid cells may form colonies when as little as 0.1 μl is inoculated. To isolate *M. thermophila* from roll tubes of low dilution, it may be necessary to incorporate antibiotics into the medium to inhibit nonmethanogenic species of bacteria (Zinder and Mah, 1979).

Maintenance Procedures

Species of *Methanosarcina* may be stored after lyophilization or, as liquid suspensions, at liquid nitrogen temperatures, or cultures can be maintained by regular subculturing (Hippe, 1984).

Differentiation of the genus **Methanosarcina** from other genera

Members of the genus *Methanosarcina* can be distinguished from most genera by morphology and by their ability to produce CH_4 as a metabolic product from most of the following substrates: H_2-CO_2, acetate, monomethylamine, dimethylamine, trimethylamine or methanol. Only three other genera of methanogens (*Methanolobus*, *Methanococcoides* and *Methanohalococcus*) use methylamines or methanol in the absence of added H_2; these organisms are unable to use H_2-CO_2 or acetate as sole catabolic substrate. *Methanosphaera stadtmanae* (Miller and Wolin, 1983; Miller and Wolin, 1985a) can use methanol only by reducing it with H_2 to methane. The only other genus which can dissimilate acetate, *Methanothrix*, can be distinguished easily by its square-ended rods occurring in long chains. It is easily differentiated from *Methanosarcina*, which typically grows in large, irregular, coccoid aggregates. The genus *Methanosarcina* may often be differentiated from other species of methanogens by its morphology alone. However, the life cycles of *Methanosarcina mazei* and *Methanosarcina acetivorans* include individual coccoid units which are difficult to distinguish from other coccus-shaped or coccoid methanogenic bacteria. By using epifluorescence microscopy, it is usually possible to identify the typical *Methanosarcina* morphology (large, irregular, coccoid, fluorescent aggregates) by microscopic examination alone.

Further Comments

The unusual morphologies exhibited by *Methanosarcina* species may be helpful in the recognition and classification of the species, but they have led to some confusion of terms. The term "sarcina" was used to describe methanosarcinae because of the superficial resemblance of these methanogens to true sarcinae. Methanosarcinae, however, exhibit nonperpendicular division planes, and numbers of cells or bodies within an aggregate are not usually a power of 2. Thus the term "pseudosarcina" ("pseudo-sarcine") was suggested by Mazé (1903) to describe the unordered appearance. Several other genera of microorganisms also exhibit this unusual pseudosarcina morphology, viz. *Geodermatophilus* (Ishiguro and Wolfe, 1970), blue-green bacteria (Stanier et al., 1971) and a sulfate reducer (Widdel, 1980).

The term "cyst" describes another unusual morphology exhibited by *Methanosarcina mazei* and *Methanosarcina acetivorans*. The methanosarcina cyst is a life-cycle stage in which a common wall surrounds a tightly packed mass of loose coccoid cells. This type of cyst differs from others because it is neither acellular, thick-walled, resistant to dessication nor connected to a fruiting structure. The cyst of *M. mazei* is a large body 100–1000 μm or more in diameter, containing tens of thousands of

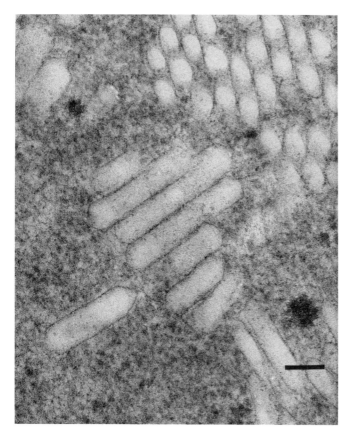

Figure 25.14. Thin-section electron micrograph of gas vesicles of *Methanosarcina vacuolata* W. *Bar*, 100 nm. (Courtesy of J. Pangborn.) (Reproduced with permission from R. A. Mah and M. R. Smith. 1981. *In* Starr, Stolp, Trüper, Balows and Schlegel (Editors), The Prokaryotes. A Handbook on Habitats, Isolation, and Identification of Bacteria. ©Springer-Verlag, Berlin, p. 974.)

coccoid units. In *M. acetivorans* the cysts may be smaller. Cysts of *Methanosarcina* may have a surface layer which appears to be composed of moribund cells surrounding myriads (or many, in the case of *M. acetivorans*) of coccoid elements. The cysts may be physically disrupted, releasing viable coccoid cells, or rupture of the cysts may occur spontaneously by the action of a disaggregating enzyme (Liu et al., 1985).

The separation of *Methanosarcina vacuolata* from other species of *Methanosarcina* is based on the characteristics of a single isolate (Zhilina and Zavarzin, 1979a). Although several other vacuolated strains of *Methanosarcina* have been described (Mah et al., 1977; Archer and King, 1983), it has not been demonstrated that these strains share the characteristics of the type strain of *M. vacuolata*, on which the species description was based, and these other strains may be *Methanosarcina barkeri* rather than *M. vacuolata*. Further, vacuolated *Methanosarcina* strains may lose their ability to form vacuoles for many months and regain them for no apparent reason (R. A. Mah, unpublished data). Thus, some strains currently classified as *M. barkeri* may in fact be phylogenetically closer to *M. vacuolata*. Answers to these questions require the characterization and comparison of additional strains.

Further Reading

Balch, W.E., G.E. Fox, L.J. Magrum, C.R. Woese and R.S. Wolfe. 1979. Methanogens: reevaluation of a unique biological group. Microbiol. Rev. *43*: 260–296.

Mah, R.A. 1980. Isolation and characterization of *Methanococcus mazei*. Curr. Microbiol. *3*: 321–326.

Mah, R.A. and D.A. Kuhn. 1984. Transfer of the type species of the genus *Methanococcus* to the genus *Methanosarcina*, naming it *Methanosarcina mazei* (Barker 1936) comb. nov. et emend. and conservation of the genus *Methanococcus* (Approved Lists 1980) with *Methanococcus vannielii* (Approved Lists 1980) as the type species. Int. J. Syst. Bacteriol. *34*: 263–265.

Mah, R.A. and D.A. Kuhn. 1984. Rejection of the type species *Methanosarcina methanica* (Approved Lists 1980), conservation of the genus *Methanosarcina* with *Methanosarcina barkeri* (Approved Lists 1980) as the type species, and emendation of the genus *Methanosarcina*. Int. J. Syst. Bacteriol. *34*: 266–267.

Robinson, R.W. 1986. Life cycles in the methanogenic archaebacterium *Methanosarcina mazei*. Appl. Environ. Microbiol. *52*: 17–27.

Sowers, K.R., S.F. Baron and J.G. Ferry. 1984. *Methanosarcina acetivorans* sp. nov., an acetotrophic methane-producing bacterium isolated from marine sediments. Appl. Environ. Microbiol. *47*: 971–978.

Zinder, S.H. and R.A. Mah. 1979. Isolation and characterization of a thermophilic strain of *Methanosarcina* unable to use H_2-CO_2 for methanogenesis. Appl. Environ. Microbiol. *38*: 996–1008.

Differentiation of the species of the genus **Methanosarcina**

Some differential characteristics of the species of the genus *Methanosarcina* are shown in Table 25.9.

List of species of the genus **Methanosarcina**

1. **Methanosarcina barkeri** Schnellen 1947, 73, emend. Bryant and Boone 1987a, 169.[AL]

bar′ker.i. N.L. gen. masc. n. *barkeri* of Barker; named for H. A. Barker, who made many definitive studies on this and other methanogenic bacteria.

Original material supplemented with material from Kluyver and Schnellen (1947), Stadtman and Barker (1951a), Mah et al. (1978), Weimer and Zeikus (1978), Hippe et al. (1979) and Murray and Zinder (1984).

Coccoid bodies, 1.5–2.0 µm in diameter, occurring mostly in irregular aggregates ranging from several to several hundred micrometers in size. Membranes contain C_{25} isoprenoids as major neutral lipid, but no C_{30} isoprenoids (Langworthy et al., 1982). Nonmotile. Stains Gram-positive. Not lysed by SDS.

Deep colonies in methanol agar with inorganic salts are whitish to light yellow and 0.5–1.0 mm in diameter. In liquid medium, growth may occur as a sediment with active gas formation.

Energy-yielding metabolism involves methane production. H_2-CO_2, methanol, monomethylamine, dimethylamine, and trimethylamine, acetate and CO may be used as substrate. The methyl group of methanol or

acetate is reduced to CH_4 without intermediate oxidation to CO_2. Carbohydrates, amino acids, formate, ethanol, propionate and butyrate are not fermented.

Ammonia serves as nitrogen source, and sulfide, as sulfur source. N_2 may be fixed. Growth and CH_4 formation are more rapid in medium with H_2-CO_2 or methanol than with acetate.

Optimum growth is obtained at pH 7.0 and at 30–40°C. Very strictly anaerobic.

The mol% G + C of the DNA is 39–44 (Bd).

Habitat: Freshwater and marine mud, rumens of ungulates, animal-waste lagoons and in sludge from anaerobic sewage-sludge digesters.

Type strain (proposed): MS (DSM 800; ATCC 43569) was isolated from a butyrate enrichment derived from an anaerobic sewage-sludge digester (Bryant and Boone, 1987a).

Reference strains: 227 (DSM 1538; ATCC 43567) (Mah et al., 1978); and UBS (DSM 1311) (Zeikus and Winfrey, 1976).

2. **Methanosarcina mazei** (Barker 1936) Mah and Kuhn 1984a, 263.[VP] (*Methanococcus mazei* Barker, 1936, 433.)

Table 25.9.
Diagnostic and descriptive features of **Methanosarcina** *species*[a]

Characteristic	*M. barkeri*	*M. mazei*	*M. acetivorans*	*M. thermophila*	*M. vacuolata*
Substrate					
H_2-CO_2	+	±	+	−[b]	+
Acetate	+	±	+	+	+
Methylamines	+	+	+	+	+
Methanol	+	+	+	+	+
Morphology					
Single cells or small aggregates	+	+	+	−	+
Large aggregates	−	+	+	+	−
Cysts	−	+	+	−	−
Life cycle	−	+	+	−	−
Gas vacuoles	−	+	+	−	+
Optimum temperature (°C)	30–50	30–40	35–40	50	40
Optimum NaCl (≥ 0.2 M)	−	−	+	−	−
Heteropolysaccharide outer layer	+	+	−	+	+
Lysis by SDS	−	+[c]	+	−	−

[a]Symbols: +, 90% or more strains are positive; ±, compounds may or may not be used; −, 90% or more strains are negative.
[b]Uses H_2-CO_2 very slowly.
[c]Only individual coccoid units, after release from cysts, are sensitive to lysis by SDS.

ma′ze.i. N.L. gen. masc. n. *mazei* of Mazé; named for P. Mazé, the French bacteriologist who first studied the organism.

Original description is supplemented with material from Mah (1980).

Individual, irregular coccoid cells 1.0–3.0 μm in diameter form irregular clumps 20–100 μm or more in diameter. These irregular clumps exhibit surface indentations and may cluster together in large rafts 1000 μm or more in diameter. The clumps later may become cysts, which can give rise to individual coccoid cells. A life cycle involving these morphological stages may occur (Zhilina and Zavarzin, 1979b; Liu et al., 1985; Robinson et al., 1985; Robinson, 1986). The organism is nonmotile. Stains Gram-negative. Isolated coccoid units, but not aggregates or cysts, are sensitive to lysis by SDS.

Colonies in roll tubes are buff white to tannish yellow, with a grainy appearance when young (<7 days). Older surface colonies are smooth, circular, transparent, glistening, mucoid and pulvinate with entire margins. Appearance of colonies in roll tubes may depend on whether cells are aggregated and on growth conditions which may cause strains to grow in a disaggregated state; colonies of disaggregated cells may appear transparent. Occasionally, gas is trapped in the mucoid colony surface, fulminating into clusters of bubbles.

Methanol, methylamine, dimethylamine and trimethylamine are converted to methane. Either acetate or H_2-CO_2 may be used. H_2-CO_2 may be used concurrently with trimethylamine or methanol. Butyrate, ethanol, butanol and acetone are not methanogenic substrates.

Methanogenic substrates are utilized as sole energy source in the presence of yeast extract and Trypticase peptone (BBL Microbiology Systems). The organism is stimulated by sludge supernatant fluid. Ammonia may serve as a nitrogen source.

Grows at 30–40° and pH 5.5–8.0; optimum growth is obtained at pH 7.0–7.2. Very strictly anaerobic.

During exponential methane formation, the generation times on the following substrates are: acetate, 17 h; methanol, methylamine or trimethylamine, 7–15 h; and H_2-CO_2, 9 h. Not all strains are capable of rapid growth on H_2-CO_2 or acetate.

The mol% G + C of the DNA is 42 (Bd).

Habitat: decaying leaves, garden soil, sewage-sludge digesters, black mud and feces of herbivorous animals; also isolated from urban solid waste and various sewage and animal-waste digesters and lagoons.

Type strain: S-6 (DSM 2053; ATCC 43572), which was isolated from an anaerobic sewage-sludge digester.

Reference strains: Z-558 (biotype 3; DSM 2244) (Zhilina and Zavarzin, 1979b); LYC (ATCC 43573) (Liu et al., 1985); and MC3 (DSM 2907) (Touzel and Albagnac, 1983).

3. **Methanosarcina acetivorans** Sowers, Johnson and Ferry 1984, 971.[VP]

a.ce.ti.vo′rans. L. n. *acetum* vinegar; L. part. adj. *vorans* consuming; N.L. adj. *acetivorans* consuming acetic acid.

Individual, irregular coccoid cells 1.5–2.5 μm in diameter. During growth on acetate, septate cell aggregates form. These small aggregates develop into cysts which contain individual coccoid elements within a common wall. Nonmotile. Stains Gram-negative. Cell walls are thin (10 nm), osmotically fragile and composed of protein. Cells lysed by SDS.

Colonies in roll tubes are pale yellow and are 0.5 mm in diameter after 14 days. Surface colonies are smooth, circular and convex with entire edges.

Acetate, methanol, monomethylamine, dimethylamine and trimethylamine are converted to methane. H_2-CO_2 and formate are not used. No organic growth factors are required. NaCl (optimum: 0.2 M and Mg^{2+} optimum: 50–100 mM) are required for growth.

Optimum growth is obtained at 35–40°C and pH 6.5–7.0. Very strictly anaerobic.

Minimum doubling time occurs with methanol as substrate (5.2 h). Monomethylamine, dimethylamine and trimethylamine give doubling times of 6.7, 7.8 and 7.3 h, respectively. Doubling time on acetate is 24.1 h.

The mol% G + C of the DNA is 41 (T_m).

Habitat: littoral marine sediments.

Type strain: C2A (ATCC 35395; DSM 2834), isolated from marine sediment.

4. **Methanosarcina thermophila** Zinder, Sowers and Ferry 1985, 522.[VP]

ther.mo.phi′la. Gr. adj. *thermos* hot; Gr. adj. *philos* loving; N.L. adj. *thermophila* heat-loving.

Irregular aggregates, 100 μm or more across, are comprised of coccoid bodies. These bodies appear to be individual cells; many nonperpendicular division planes are evident. Tetrads do not occur and individual cell bodies are rare. Nonmotile. Stains Gram-positive. Not lysed by SDS.

Surface colonies in agar roll tubes are yellow to brown and have a rough, granular appearance.

Growth occurs on acetate, methanol, monomethylamine, dimethylamine and trimethylamine. H_2-CO_2 and formate are not used, although H_2 may be used during growth on methanol. NH_3 serves as nitrogen source; N_2 is not fixed. Growth occurs in defined medium with *p*-aminobenzoate and methanol and acetate as catabolic substrate and sole carbon and energy source (Murray and Zinder, 1985).

Optimum growth temperature: 50°C; range: <35–55°C. Good growth occurs over a broad range of pH (5.5–8.0) with an optimum at 6.0. Very strictly anaerobic.

The mol% G + C of the DNA is 42 (Bd).

Habitat: thermophilic anaerobic digesters.

Type strain: TM-1 (DSM 1825; ATCC 43570), isolated from a 55°C anaerobic digester.

Reference strain: CHTI-55 (DSM 2906) (Touzel et al., 1985).

5. **Methanosarcina vacuolata** Zhilina and Zavarzin 1987, 283.[VP]

vac.u.o.la′ta. L. adj. *vacuus* empty; N.L. part. adj. *vacuolata* equipped with gas vacuoles.

Original material (Zhilina and Zavarzin, 1979a) supplemented with material from Zhilina (1971, 1976, 1978), Archer and King (1983, 1984), Lysenko and Zhilina (1985) and Zhilina and Zavarzin (1987).

Coccoid bodies, 1–2 μm in diameter, occurring sometimes as individual cells but mostly in irregular, rounded aggregates ranging from several to several hundred micrometers in size; individual cells within aggregates may not be distinguished by light microscopy. May contain gas vesicles. Membranes contain C_{30} isoprenoids (Osipov et al., 1985). Nonmotile. Stains Gram-positive. Not lysed by SDS.

Deep colonies in agar medium are light yellow, angular, granular and 0.5–1.0 mm in diameter. In liquid medium, growth may occur as a light yellow, easily dispersed sediment with clear supernatant medium.

Energy-yielding metabolism involves methane production. H_2-CO_2, methanol, methylamines and acetate may be used as substrate. Formate is not used. Growth on methanol faster than on acetate. Carbohydrates, amino acids, formate, ethanol, propionate and butyrate are not fermented.

Ammonia serves as nitrogen source, and sulfide, as sulfur source. Growth of some strains may be stimulated by addition of organic compounds, but all can grow autotrophically.

Optimum growth is obtained at pH 7.5 and 37–40°C. Very strictly anaerobic.

The mol% G + C of the DNA is 36.3 (T_m) (Lysenko and Zhilina, 1985).

Habitat: soil, freshwater mud, and sludge from anaerobic sewage-sludge digesters.

Type strain: Z-761 (Biotype-2 [Zhilina, 1976]; strain Z [Balch et al., 1979]; DSM 1232), isolated from a methanogenic digester.

Reference strains: FR-1 (DSM 2256) (Archer and King, 1983) and W (ATCC 43571) (Mah, R.A., M.R. Smith and L. Baresi. 1977. Abstr. Annu.

Meet. Am. Soc. Microbiol. *I32*: 160; Balch et al., 1979) are gas-vacuolated *Methanosarcina* strains which may belong to this species (see "Further Comments" below).

Further Comments

Physiologically, *M. vacuolata* is similar to *M. barkeri*; morphologically, these species are also similar except for the presence of gas vesicles in the former. These gas vesicles may be lost for extended periods of time (several years) and then reappear in cultures transferred monthly (R. A. Mah, personal communication). Thus, molecular data may be necessary to distinguish these species. DNA/DNA hybridization studies (Zhilina and Zavarzin, 1979a), membrane lipid analysis (Osipov et al., 1985), 16S rRNA cataloging (Balch et al., 1979), ribosomal protein analysis (Douglas et al., 1980) and immunological analysis (Zhilina and Zavarzin, 1987) indicate significant differences between *M. vacuolata* and *M. barkeri*.

Other gas-vacuolated strains may appear to be *M. vacuolata*, based on their physiologies and morphologies, but may be unrelated phylogenetically. For instance, it is not clear that strain W (Mah, R.A., M.R. Smith and L. Baresi. 1977. Abstr. Annu. Meet. Am. Soc. Microbiol. *I32*: 160) and strain FR-1, two other gas-vacuolated strains, are *M. vacuolata*. Strain W forms white colonies (unpublished data), whereas those of *M. vacuolata* are yellow.

The mol% G + C of the DNA of strain W and strain FR-1 is 40.5 (Balch et al., 1979) and 40.7 (Archer and King, 1983), respectively, compared with 36 for the type strain of *M. vacuolata*, strain Z-761.

Genus II. **Methanolobus** *König and Stetter 1983, 439ᵛᵖ (Effective publication: König and Stetter 1982, 488)*

K. O. STETTER

Me.tha.no.lob′us. M.L. neut. n. *methanum* methane; Gr. masc. n. *lobus* lobe; M.L. masc. n. *Methanolobus* methane (-producing) lobe.

Irregular cocci, 0.8–1.25 μm in diameter, sometimes forming loose aggregates (Fig. 25.15). Cells are surrounded by a protein subunit envelope (Fig. 25.16) covering the membrane. If flagellation present, monotrichous (Fig. 25.17). Gram-negative. Strictly anaerobic. Optimum temperature: 37°C; maximum: 40–45°C; minimum: 10–15°C. Growth occurs within a salt range of 0.3–7.5% with an optimum of ~3%. Chemoorganotrophic, growing on methanol and methylamines. No growth on H_2-CO_2, formate or acetate (König and Stetter, 1982). In the presence of molecular sulfur, H_2S, in addition to methane and CO_2, is formed from methanol (Stetter and Gaag, 1983).

The mol% G + C of the DNA is 38–42.

Type species: *Methanolobus tindarius* König and Stetter, 1983, 439.

Further Descriptive Information

Cells are fragile. They can be completely disintegrated by 1% SDS. The cell envelope (Sleytr and Messner, 1983) of *M. tindarius* contains a dominating protein with an apparent mol. wt. of 156,000 and which shows a positive periodate-Schiff staining and therefore is most likely a glycoprotein.

Grana of polyphosphate and glycogen granules (König et al., 1985) can be present. *M. tindarius* is able to fix dinitrogen (König et al., 1985). A plasmid with a mol. wt. of 4.6×10^6 is present in *Methanolobus vulcani* (Thomm et al. 1983). The RNA polymerase of *M. volcani* shows serological cross-reaction with that of *Methanosarcina barkeri* in the Ouchterlony immunodiffusion test (Thomm and Stetter, unpublished observation). Antibodies prepared against whole cells of *Methanosarcina* species show a slight cross-reaction with *M. tindarius*. On the other hand, there is no serological cross-reaction of antibodies prepared against *M. tindarius* with members of any other genera of methanogens except *Methanococcoides* (Macario and Macario, 1983; König and Stetter, unpublished observation). *Methanolobus* could be isolated from anaerobic samples taken from sea sediments with original temperatures

between 10 and 45°C and pH values between 5 and 8 in Sicily, Vulcano, Naples and Ischia, all situated in Italy. Therefore, this genus seems to be very common in sea sediments within the mesophilic temperature range.

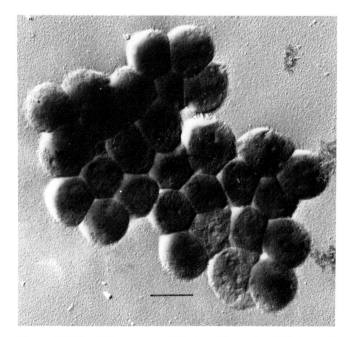

Figure 25.15. Cell aggregate of *Methanolobus vulcani*. Electron micrograph. Platinum shadowing. *Bar*, 1 μm.

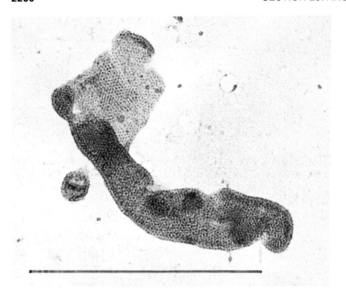

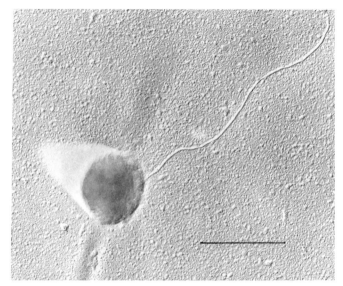

Figure 25.16. Isolated cell envelope of *Methanolobus tindarius*. Electron micrograph. Negative staining with uranyl formate. *Bar*, 1 μm. (Reproduced with permission from O. Kandler and H. König. 1985. The Bacteria: A Treatise on Structure and Function. ©Academic Press, New York.)

Figure 25.17. Cell of *Methanolobus tindarius* with flagellum. Electron micrograph. Platinum shadowing. *Bar*, 1 μm.

Enrichment and Isolation Procedures

Methanolobus can be enriched anaerobically in mineral medium (medium 3 of Balch et al., 1979; modified by omitting acetate, yeast extract and peptone) supplemented with methanol (0.5%) and a mixture of ampicillin, penicillin, kanamycin and tetracycline (each 100 μg/ml). Gas phase: N_2. Incubation at 37°C. Isolation on the same medium solidified by agar (1.5%). After 5 days, round, smooth, transparent, greenish-white to ocher-colored colonies, about 1–3 mm in diameter, become visible (König and Stetter, 1982).

Maintenance Procedures

Stock cultures of *Methanolobus* can be stored anaerobically at 4 and −20°C.

Differentiation of the genus **Methanolobus** *from other genera*

The genus *Methanolobus* is separated from the genus *Methanococcus* by its higher G + C content, its monotrichous flagellation and its inability to grow on H_2-CO_2 or formate. It is distinguished from the genus *Methanosarcina* by the existence of a protein S-layer (except *Methanosarcina acetivorans*; Sowers et al., 1984) instead of a rigid cell wall, the lack of galactosamine in its envelope, its negative Gram reaction, its motility and its inability to use acetate and CO_2-H_2 as energy source. It differs from the genus *Methanogenium* by its inability to grow on formate and H_2-CO_2 and by a different G + C content. The genus *Methanococcoides*, which was described later (Sowers and Ferry, 1983), is homologous in many features to *Methanolobus*. The type species *Methanococcoides methylutens* shows serological cross-reaction with antibodies prepared against *Methanolobus tindarius* (about ⅓ the intensity of the homologous reaction, König and Stetter, unpublished observation). Similar to *Methanolobus*, *Methanococcoides* is motile by monotrichous flagellation (König and Stetter, unpublished observation).

Taxonomic Comments

Phylogenetic relationship of *Methanolobus* to the *Methanosarcinaceae* is indicated by the serological cross-reaction between the RNA polymerase of *Methanolobus vulcani* and *Methanosarcina barkeri* and by the common property to utilize methanol and methylamines. This relationship was determined by 16S rRNA cataloging (E. Stackebrandt, personal communication) and DNA/RNA hybridization (Sowers et al., 1984).

Further Reading

König, H. and K.O. Stetter. 1982. Isolation and characterization of *Methanolobus tindarius* sp. nov., a coccoid methanogen growing only on methanol and methylamines. Zentralbl. Bakteriol. Mikrobiol. Hyg. I. Abt. Orig. *C3*: 478–490.

Sowers, K.R. and J.G. Ferry. 1983. Isolation and characterization of a methylotrophic marine methanogen, *Methanococcoides methyluteus* gen. nov., sp. nov. Appl. Environ. Microbiol. *45*: 684–690.

Sowers, K.R., J.L. Johnson and J.G. Ferry. 1984. Phylogenetic relationships among the methylotrophic methane-producing bacteria and emendation of the family *Methanosarcinaceae*. Int. J. Syst. Bacteriol. *34*: 444–450.

Differentiation of the species of the genus **Methanolobus**

Some differential features of the species *M. tindarius*, *M. siciliae* and *M. vulcani* are indicated in Table 25.10.

List of species of the genus **Methanolobus**

1. **Methanolobus tindarius** König and Stetter 1983, 439.^{VP} (Effective publication: König and Stetter 1982, 488.)

tin.da′ri.us. M.L. masc. adj. *tindarius* from Tindari, the place of isolation in Sicily, Italy.

See Table 25.10 and the generic description for features.

Type strain: T3 (DSM 2278).

2. **Methanolobus siciliae** sp. nov. Stetter and König.

si.ci′li.ae. L. n. gen. *siciliae* from Sicily, the place of isolation in Italy.

See Table 25.10 and the generic description for features. Flagella not observed.

Type strain: T4/M (DSM 3028).

3. **Methanolobus vulcani** sp. nov. Stetter, König and Thomm.

vul.ca′ni. L. gen. n. *vulcani* from Vulcan, the god after whom Vulcano Island was named (insula Vulcani).

See Table 25.10 and the generic description for features. Flagella rarely observed.

Type strain: PL-12/M (DSM 3029).

Table 25.10.

Characteristics differentiating **Methanolobus tindarius, M. siciliae** *and* **M. vulcani**

Characteristic	1. *M. tindarius*	2. *M. siciliae*	3. *M. vulcani*
Growth temperature (°C)			
Optimal	37	37	37
Maximal	40	48	45
Minimal	10	20	15
Mol% G + C of DNA	40	41.5	39
Serological cross-reaction with *M. tindarius* T3 (%)	100	31	14
DNA/DNA homology (%)			
M. tindarius^a	100	12	27
M. siciliae^a	ND^b	100	11
M. vulcani^a	40	11	100

^{a}Filter-bound unlabeled DNA.

^{b}ND, not determined.

Genus III. **Methanothrix** *Huser, Wuhrmann and Zehnder 1983, 439*^{VP} *(Effective publication: Huser, Wuhrmann and Zehnder 1982, 7)*

ALEXANDER J. B. ZEHNDER

Me.tha′no.thrix. M.L. n. *methanum* methane; Gr. n. *thrix* hair; M.L. fem. n. *Methanothrix* methane (-producing) hair.

Cells are rod-shaped with flat ends (Fig. 25.18*A*), usually 0.7–1.2 × 2.0–6.0 µm. Forms very long and **flexible filaments which tend to aggregate in characteristic bundles** (Fig. 25.18*B*). Resting stages are not known. One species produces gas vacuoles. Gram-negative. Nonmotile. **Strictly anaerobic.** Optimum temperature: 35–40°C; maximum, ∼50°C; minimum, 3°C, for the mesophilic strains; 35–75°C with an optimum at 65°C for the thermophilic strain. Optimum pH: 7.1–7.8; maximum, 8.3; minimum, 6.8. **Uses acetate exclusively as** energy source, which is split into methane and CO_2.

Acetate and CO_2 act as sole carbon sources.

The mol% G + C of the DNA is 52–61 (T_m, UV).

Type species: *Methanothrix soehngenii* Huser, Wuhrmann and Zehnder 1983, 439.

Further Descriptive Information

The individual cells in the filaments are held together by a sheathlike structure (Fig. 25.18*C*) which shows regular striation (Fig. 25.18*D*) similar to *Methanospirillum hungatei* (Zeikus and Bowen, 1975^b). This outer layer is composed of fibrilar glycoproteins (Kandler and König, 1985; Patel et al., 1986) forming a hollow tube composed of hoops piled on top of one another. The cells are separated by multilayered "cell-spacer" plugs. Their subunit arrangements resemble concentric rings (Zehnder et al., 1980; Patel et al., 1986). Sheath and plugs are extremely resilient to physical disruption. No rigid sacculus is present (Kandler and König, 1985; Beveridge et al., 1986b). All thermophilic *Methanothrix* so far observed contain gas vacuoles (Nozhevnikova and Yagodina, 1982; Zinder et al., 1984b). Mesophilic strains have not been reported to contain them. Polar lipids of the membrane are exclusively C_{20} di-*o*-phytanyl glycerol ether (Ekiel et al., 1985; Langworthy and Pond, 1986). Cells multiply by a type of septation which represents a new form of procaryotic division (Beveridge et al., 1986a).

Methanothrix grows chemoorganotrophically in a defined mineral salt medium that contains vitamins and acetate as sole organic compounds. Some strains require yeast extract. Methane is exclusively formed from the methyl group of acetate. H_2-CO_2, formate, methanol and methylamines cannot be used for growth and methane formation. Formate is split into hydrogen and carbon dioxide (Zehnder et al., 1980; Huser et al., 1982; Patel, 1984). This reaction does not sustain or stimulate growth or methane production; it inhibits them (Fathepure, 1983). Acetate and CO_2 are assimilated at a molar ratio of approximately 2:1. Reducing equivalents for biomass synthesis are produced from the oxidation of the methyl group of acetate (Zehnder et al., 1980; Patel, 1984). *M. concilii* requires carbon dioxide for the initiation of growth (Patel, 1984). Cell extracts show high carbon monoxide dehydrogenase (3 µmol min^{-1} mg^{-1} protein) and acetate thiokinase (5.3 µmol min^{-1} mg^{-1} protein) activities (Kohler and Zehnder, 1984). Coenzyme M (CoM), sarcinapterin and F_{420} with 4 or 5 glutamate residues are present. No methanopterin was found (Gorris and van der Drift, 1986). The F_{420} content is too low to cause visible autofluorescence under the UV microscope. In contrast to most other methanogens where F_{III} is the main corronoide, the predominant corronoide (∼70%) in *Methanothrix soehngenii* is 5α-methylbenzimiazolyl-β-cyanocobamide. F_{III} (5α-hydroxybenzimidazolyl-β-cyanocobamide) and vitamin B_{12} make up 10% each of the corronoide fraction (Kohler, 1986). Glycogen is formed from ADP-glucose via acetyl-CoA, pyruvate and glucose-6-P and is stored in the cell, composing ∼2% of the total dry weight of the bacteria. Besides acetate thiokinase, pyruvate synthase, phosphoenolpyruvate synthase and the enzymes of the gluconeogenesis, branching enzyme activity (1,4α-glucan-6-glucosyl transferase) was detected (Pellerin et al., 1987). The biosynthetic pathway of glucose-6-P resembles those of other methanogens (Jansen et al., 1982; Ekiel et al., 1985).

Evidence for a lytic bacteriophage for *Methanothrix* has been presented by Roustan et al. (1986). *M. soehngenii* strain FE and *M. concilii* are sensitive towards the virus.

Partial antigenic fingerprints of *M. concilii* with antisera S probes of a variety of methanogens revealed a weak reaction with anti-*Methanosarcina* TM1 but none with the others (Patel, 1984). Polyclonal antibodies against *M. soehngenii* strain FE were very strain-specific and reacted

Figure 25.18. *Methanothrix soehngenii. A*, scanning photomicrograph of filament fragments. *Bar*, 1.3 μm. *B*, phase-contrast photomicrograph showing the long filaments which form characteristic bundles. *Bar*, 45 μm. *C*, thin section through a filament showing common cross-wall and common outer layer. *Bar*, 0.4 μm. *D*, negative stain of the cell wall from lysed cells, illustrating laminar striation of the envelope and circular structure of the cross-wall. *Bar*, 0.4 μm.

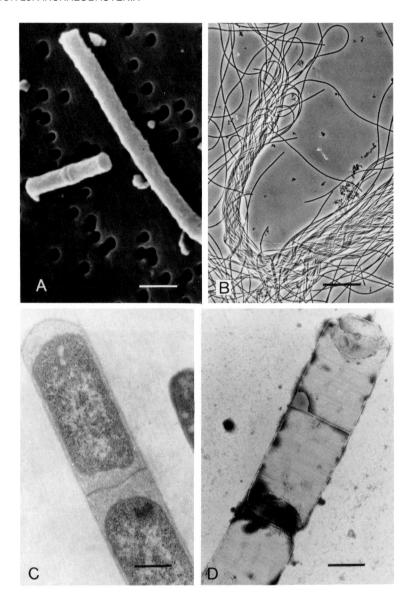

only weakly with *M. soehngenii* strain Opfikon and *M. concilii*. Some cross-reaction was also found with *Methanosarcina mazei* strain MC3. Anticomponent C of the methyl-CoM reductase of *M. mazei* strain MC3 recognized proteins from strain FE with a molecular weight comparable to the subunits of component C. These proteins are distributed randomly in the cytoplasm without any preferential localization in the vicinity of the cytoplasmic membrane (Thomas, 1986).

Growth and methane production of *Methanothrix* is almost completely inhibited with bromoethane sulfonic acid and dihydrostreptomycin at 0.01 mg/ml with penicillin G, ampicillin, D-cycloserin and novobiocin at 1 mg/ml and with vancomycin at 10 mg/ml (Huser et al., 1982; Patel, 1984).

Methanothrix can be isolated from sewage digesters, biogas fermenters, run with human and/or animal waste, and from sanitary landfills. This organism is one of the main microbial constituents of anaerobic contact reactors (Dubourguier et al., 1986) and of granular sludge grown in up-flow anaerobic sludge blanket (UASB) reactors (Hulshoff Pol et al., 1983; Dubourguier et al., 1985). No mesophilic strain has been found yet in unpolluted anoxic freshwater sediments. Thermophilic strains of *Methanothrix* were observed in sewage digesters (Zinder et al., 1984b) and were isolated from thermal lakes (Nozhevnikova and Chudina, 1984).

Enrichment and Isolation Procedures

Methanothrix can be isolated and enriched by using strict anaerobic procedures under an atmosphere of N_2-CO_2, on a mineral medium containing acetate as sole organic compound (Zehnder et al., 1980). The exact vitamin requirements are not known, but for *M. concilii*, some vitamins seem to be essential for growth (Patel, 1984). Sulfide of up to 100 mg/l can be used as sulfur source and reducing agent without negative effect on growth. Dithionite of 30 mg/l is slightly inhibitory. Some strains seem to require low concentrations of yeast extract (0.05%). Higher concentrations (>0.5%) have an inhibitory effect. Rumen fluid (20%) and manure extract (0.002%) can act stimulatory for growth or at least they reduce the lag phase. Higher yields are not reported with these additions. *Methanothrix* can be purified with the classical Hungate technique modified by Bryant (1972) and Balch and Wolfe (1976) from high dilutions. All attempts to isolate *Methanothrix* on solid medium have failed, with the exception of strain VNBF, which was obtained from roll tubes. *Methanothrix* is not very oxygen-sensitive under resting conditions.

Maintenance Procedure

Methanothrix strains can be lyophilized by common procedures used for anaerobes.

Taxonomic Comments

Methanothrix is probably identical with *Methanobacterium* species described by Söhngen (1906) and with "*Methanobacterium soehngenii*" from Barker (1936). All three organisms have common features, such as: formation of methane from acetate; growth on acetate and CO_2 as sole carbon source; similarity in size, with characteristic flat ends; and formation of long filaments, which are often associated in bundles.

The taxonomic relationship of *M. soehngenii* has been examined by means of 16S rRNA (Stackebrandt et al., 1982). The results revealed that *M. soehngenii* is related only distantly to members of the family *Methanobacteriales* ($S_{AB} = 0.27$). Its highest degree of relatedness was found with *Methanosarcina barkeri* ($S_{AB} = 0.44$). This S_{AB} value is just about at the lower limit for a new genus and at the upper limit for a new family.

These results and the common characteristics of *M. barkeri* to use acetate and to contain cytochrome *b* (Kühn et al., 1979) were the reasons not to create a new family but to assign *M. soehngenii* to the family *Methanosarcinae*. Numerical analysis of whole-cell protein patterns of methanogens supported these views (Thomas et al., 1986).

The only significant characteristic which distinguishes *M. soehngenii* from *M. concilii* is a difference in the G + C of the DNA of <10%. Therefore, it is questionable whether *M. concilii*, based only on this difference, should be treated as a separate species (Thomas, 1986).

Acknowledgments

I am grateful to H. C. Dubourguier for generously providing unpublished data from his laboratory and for stimulating discussions concerning the taxonomy of methanogens, especially *Methanothrix*.

Differentiation of the species of the genus **Methanothrix**

Some differential features of the species *M. soehngenii*, *M. concilii* and "*M. thermoacetophila*" are indicated in Table 25.11.

List of species of genus **Methanothrix**

1. **Methanothrix soehngenii** Huser, Wuhrmann and Zehnder, 1983, 439.[VP] (Effective publication: Huser, Wuhrmann and Zehnder 1982, 7.)

soehn'gen.i.i. M.L. gen. n. *soehngenii* of Söhngen; named after N. L. Söhngen, who first described this organism in his thesis (1906).

So far, three different strains have been isolated. They are strain Opfikon (Huser et al., 1982), strain VNBF (Fathepure, 1983) and strain FE (Touzel and Albagnac, 1985). Strain FE and Opfikon are very similar; they differ in their response toward a lytic bacteriophage (Roustan et al., 1986). The kinetic parameters of strain Opfikon for growth and methane formation are: half-saturation constant (K_s), 0.7 ± 0.05 mmol/l; yield (Y), 1.4 g cells/mol acetate; and a doubling time for growth of 84–144 h. Strain VNBF had a generation time of 23–29 h. Hydrogen or formate inhibit methane formation from acetate in strain VNBF but not in strain FE and Opfikon. Methane production of strain Opfikon was completely suppressed by methylviologen (5 μmol/l), benzylviologen (5 μmol/l), chloroform (20 μmol/l), sodium arsenate (100 μmol/l), potassium cyanide (100 μmol/l) and iodopropane (100 μmol/l). Fluoroacetate (100 μmol/l) inhibited the methane production rate by 50%; sodium nitrate (5 mmol/l) by 80%; and 2-bromoethane sulfonic acid (10 μmol/l), by 95%. In batch experiments, the acetate uptake rate at the beginning of the growth phase was much faster than the concomitant methane production rate (Huser et al., 1982). The reason for this uncoupling is not known.

The mol% G + C of the DNA is 52 (T_m).

Type strain: DSM 2139.

2. **Methanothrix concilii** Patel 1985, 223.[VP] (Effective publication: Patel 1984, 1394.)

con.ci'li.i. L. gen. n. *concilii* of a council; named after the National Research Council of Canada.

The characteristics of this species, of which the type strain is GP6, closely resembles those of *M. soehngenii*. The kinetic parameters of strain GP6 for growth and methane formation are: $K_s = 1.2 ± 0.1$ mmol/l; $Y = 1.13$–1.16 g cells mol acetate; and a doubling time calculated from methane production of 24 h. Some hydrogenase activity (0.02 μl H_2 min^{-1} ml culture) was found. Hydrogen, formate and penicillin G (0.1 mg/ml) had no negative effect on growth and methane production. Viologen dyes, potassium cyanide and D-cycloserine were potent inhibitors of growth. 2-Bromoethanesulfonic acid (10 μmol/l) reduced the growth rate by 89%, and yeast extract (5–6 g/l), by 87%.

The mol% G + C of the DNA is 61% (UV).

Type strain: NRC 2989.

3. "**Methanothrix thermoacetophila**" Nozhevnikova and Chudina 1984, 623.

ther.mo.a.ce.to.phi'la. Gr. n. *thermos* heat; L. n. *acetum* vinegar; Gr. n. *philos* lover; M.L. fem. adj. *thermoacetophila* thermophilic acetate-loving.

Several thermophilic monocultures have been obtained (Nozhevnikova and Yagodina, 1982), and strain Z-517 is characterized in more detail. This strain has a temperature optimum of 65°C and a generation time of about 24–32 h. Penicillin suppresses culture growth. All thermophilic strains observed up to now contain gas vacuoles (Zinder et al., 1984a). A pure culture is not available.

Table 25.11.
Differential characteristics of the species of the genus **Methanothrix**[a]

Characteristic	1. *M. soehngenii*[b]	2. *M. concilii*	3. "*M. thermoacetophila*"
Habitat			
Digester	+	+	+
Thermal lakes	−	−	−
Gas vacuoles	−	−	+
Inhibition of methane formation by hydrogen	D	−	+
Optimum temperature (°C)	35–40	37–40	65
Mol% G + C of DNA	52 (T_m)	61 (UV)	NR[b]

[a]Symbols: +, 90% or more of strains are positive; −, 90% or more of strains are negative; D, different reactions in different taxa; and NR, not reported.

[b]Includes the strains Opfikon, VNBF and FE.

Genus IV. **Methanococcoides** *Sowers and Ferry 1985, 223*[VP] *(Effective publication: Sowers and Ferry 1983, 688)*

K. R. SOWERS

Me.tha′no.coc.coi′des. *Methanococcus* established genus; Gr. adj. suff. *-ides* similar to; M.L. neut. n. *Methanococcoides* organism similar to *Methanococcus*.

Extremely irregular cocci, 1 ± 0.2 µm in diameter; occur singly or in pairs. Gram-negative. Nonmotile. **Strictly anaerobic**. Temperature range: 15–35°C; optimum: 30–35°C. NaCl and Mg^{2+} are required for growth; optimum NaCl concentration: 0.2–0.6 M; optimum Mg^{2+} concentration as $MgSO_4$: 0.025–0.2 M. **Trimethylamine, dimethylamine, methylamine and methanol are substrates** for growth and methanogenesis; **acetate, formate and H_2 are not**.

The mol% G + C of the DNA from the only described strain, TMA-10, is 42. (T_m).

Type species: *Methanococcoides methylutens* Sowers and Ferry 1983, 688.

Further Descriptive Information

The irregularly shaped cells (Fig. 25.19) become spherical, as the NaCl or Mg^{2+} concentrations (as $MgSO_4$) are decreased, and lyse when either is eliminated (Sowers and Ferry, 1983). Cultures will not grow if NaCl is substituted with KCl or $NaSO_4$, or if divalent cations such as Mn^{2+} are substituted for Mg^{2+} cations. Whole cells are immediately lysed by 0.01% sodium dodecyl sulfate or 0.001% Triton X-100. Electron microscopy of thin sections shows a monolayered cell wall approximately 10 nm thick. Acid hydrolysates of isolated cell walls yield a variety of amino acids, which indicates that the walls are protein. Aspartic and glutamic acids are predominant. Amino sugars are not detected. The membrane polar lipid fraction consists of 2,3-diphytanyl glycerol ethers; dibiphytanyl diglycerol tetraethers are not detected. Structures such as storage granules or internal membranes are not observed in the cytoplasm. Fimbrialike structures are occasionally observed in electron micrographs.

Surface colonies (0.5–1.5 mm) are yellow, circular and convex with entire edges. Colonies fluoresce blue-green under UV light.

Medium that contains seawater, mineral salts, biotin and substrate with an N_2 or N_2-CO_2 (80:20) atmosphere is required for growth of *M. methylutens* strain TMA-10 (Sowers and Ferry, 1985). A mixture of NaCl, $MgSO_4$, KCl and $CaCl_2$ may be substituted for seawater. Yeast extract, Trypticase or rumen fluid may be substituted as sources of biotin. Essential trace metals include nickel, iron and cobalt. Strains of *M. methylutens* will grow in the presence of vancomycin (100 mg/l).

Strains of *M. methylutens* have been isolated from a marine trench that contained large deposits of organic material.

Enrichment and Isolation Procedures

Culture media are prepared under an O_2-free atmosphere of N_2-CO_2 (80:20) (Balch et al., 1979). Enrichment medium contains a solution of 80% artificial seawater diluted with demineralized water plus minerals, vitamins, cysteine–sulfide-reducing agent and trimethylamine-HCl (Sowers and Ferry, 1983). Resazurin is added as an E_h indicator. The pH is

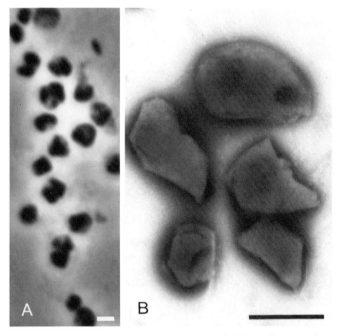

Figure 25.19. Phase-contrast micrograph (*A*) and ammonium molybdate-stained electron micrograph (*B*) of *M. methylutens* strain TMA-10 grown on trimethylamine. *Bars*, 1 µm.

maintained at 7.2 by a CO_2-bicarbonate buffer system. Alternatively, medium 3 of Balch et al. (1979) may be used with the addition of suitable substrate. Enrichment cultures are incubated at 20–30°C and assayed for turbidity and methane production. Isolation medium is the same as enrichment medium, with the addition of 2% purified agar (BBL Microbiology Systems) or Noble agar (Difco). Inocula are streaked onto agar roll tubes, or serial dilutions are added to molten agar and rolled (Hungate, 1969). Isolates are identified as yellow colonies that fluoresce blue-green in long wave UV light (Mink and Dugan, 1977).

Maintenance Procedures

M. methylutens is maintained by biweekly transfer on agar slants that contain isolation medium or a modification with salts substituted for seawater (Sowers and Ferry, 1983). Cultures may also be maintained by freezing in serum vials that contain enrichment medium and glycerol (1:1).

Differentiation of the genus **Methanococcoides** from other genera

The genus *Methanococcoides* is separated from *Methanosarcina* based on its inability to use acetate, comparative cataloging of the 16S rRNA (C. Woese, personal communication) and DNA/RNA homology values (Sowers et al., 1984). In addition, *Methanococcoides* lacks the thick (400 nm) heteropolysaccharide cell wall layer which is found among the *Methanosarcina* (Kandler, 1982), although one species of *Methanosarcina* also lacks a heteropolysaccharide layer (Sowers et al., 1984).

Unlike *Methanolobus*, *Methanococcoides* has no membranous internal structures or apparent storage granules (König and Stetter, 1982). The genera show no DNA/DNA homology and only 67% DNA/RNA homology. Immunological fingerprinting by indirect immunofluorescence

(S probe) shows only slight cross-reactivity between *M. methylutens* strain TMA-10 and *M. tindarius* strain T3 (E. Conway de Macario, personal communication).

Taxonomic Comments

The most comprehensive phylogenetic study of the *Methanosarcinaceae* is based on DNA/RNA and DNA/DNA homology values of only seven strains (Sowers et al., 1984). The division of genera in this family is supported by rRNA hybridization values obtained by Tu et al. (1982) for division of genera in the archaeobacteria. Although the phylogenetic divisions appear distinct at this time, the current divisions may become less distinct and warrant the merging of some genera as more methylotrophic strains become available and their phylogenies are determined. The maintenance of separate genera may also be impractical for identification purposes if more distinguishing phenotypic characteristics are not found among other strains.

Further Reading

Conway de Macario, E., M.J. Wolin and A.J.L. Macario. 1982. Antibody analysis of relationships among methanogenic bacteria. J. Bacteriol. *149*: 316–219.

List of species of the genus **Methanococcoides**

1. **Methanococcoides methylutens** Sowers and Ferry 1985, 223.[VP] (Effective publication: Sowers and Ferry 1983, 688.)
  meth.y.lu'tens. mod. chem. word *methyl-*; L. part. adj. *utens* using; *methylutens* using methyl.

The description of the species is the same as that given for the genus. *Type strain:* ATCC 33938; DSM 2657.

OTHER TAXA

FAMILY **METHANOPLANACEAE** WILDGRUBER, THOMM AND STETTER, 1984, 270[VP] (EFFECTIVE PUBLICATION: WILDGRUBER, THOMM AND STETTER *IN* WILDGRUBER, THOMM, KÖNIG, OBER, RICCHIUTO AND STETTER 1982, 36)

K. O. STETTER

Me.tha.no.pla.na'ce.ae. M.L. neut. n. *Methanoplanaceae* the *Methanoplanus* family.

Plate-shaped cells occurring as thin plates with sharp edges (Figs. 25.20 and 25.21). Gram-negative. The cell envelope shows a hexagonal surface pattern (Fig. 25.21). Strictly anaerobic. Chemolithotrophic. **H_2 and CO_2 or formate serve as energy source** for growth and methane formation. On hydrogen in the presence of molecular sulfur; H_2S is formed in addition to methane. The organism is mesophilic.

Habitat: free-living in anaerobic environments within swamps or as endosymbionts in marine ciliates.

The mol% G + C of the DNA is 38.7–47.5.

Comparison by DNA/RNA hybridization (Tu et al., 1982) with members of the genera *Methanosarcina* and *Methanogenium* showed a lower fractional stability (fs) between *Methanoplanus* and *Methanogenium* (fs = 0.59) than between *Methanogenium* and *Methanosarcina* (fs = 0.62), indicating phylogenetical distance.

Type genus: *Methanoplanus* Wildgruber, Thomm and Stetter 1984, 270.

Further Descriptive Information

Cells are fragile. They can be easily broken by detergents, e.g., SDS (2%) or by the French press. Cell division, possibly by constriction or budding, is indicated by the existence of Y-shaped cells. No septa formation visible. Grana of polyphosphate are visible within the cells (Wildgruber et al., 1982). Two species: *Methanoplanus limicola* was isolated from an anaerobic sample taken from a swamp composed of waste and water from steam drilling (pH 7; 19°C), and *Methanoplanus endosymbiosus* was isolated from homogenized cells of the marine ciliate *Metopus contortus*.

Enrichment and Isolation Procedures

Methanoplanus limicola can be enriched anaerobically in medium 3 (Balch et al., 1979) in pressurized (200 kPa H_2-CO_2 (80:20)) serum bottles at 30°C in the presence of vancomycin, penicillin and kanamycin with each at 150 µg/ml, and tetracycline at 100 µg/mg. It can be isolated by streaking onto polysilicate plates containing medium 3 (Balch et al., 1979). Round, smooth, bright ocher-colored colonies about 2 mm in diameter were visible after 3 months at 30°C. No growth on agar (Wildgruber et al., 1982). *Methanoplanus endosymbiosus* can be isolated from homogenized cells of *Metopus contortus* by plating the homogenate on solid media (van Bruggen et al., 1986a) containing penicillin (10³ IU/ml) or lysozyme (1 mg/ml). Incubation at 30°C for 3 weeks. Colonies about 2 mm in diameter were whitish yellow, convex and circular with entire margin.

Key to the genera of the family **Methanoplanaceae**

Only one genus exists: *Methanoplanus*.

Genus **Methanoplanus** Wildgruber, Thomm and Stetter 1984, 270[VP] (Effective publication: Wildgruber, Thomm and Stetter in Wildgruber, Thomm, König, Ober, Ricchiuto and Stetter 1982, 36)

K.O. STETTER

Me.tha.no.pla'nus. M.L. n. *methanum* methane; M.L. adj. *planus* flat; M.L. masc. n. *Methanoplanus* the methane (-producing) plate.

Cells are angular, crystallike plates 0.07–0.30 µm thick, 1.6–3.4 µm long and 1.5 µm wide and occur singly (Figs. 25.20 and 25.21). The **cells are sometimes branched**, without septa. The cell envelope shows a hexagonal surface pattern (Fig. 25.21). No sacculus is present. **Flagellate.** Strictly anaerobic. Optimum temperature: 32–40°C; maximum: 41°C; minimum: 16°C. Growth occurs in 0.4 and 6% NaCl.

Chemolithotrophic, growing on H_2 and CO_2 or formate. No growth occurs on methanol or methylamines. The **end product is methane** (Wildgruber et al., 1982). In the presence of molecular sulfur, H_2S is formed, in addition to H_2 and CO_2 (Stetter and Gaag, 1983). Cells are resistant to vancomycin, penicillin, kanamycin and tetracycline.

The mol% G + C of the DNA is 38.7–47.5.

Type species: *Methanoplanus limicola* Wildgruber, Thomm and Stetter 1984, 270.

Maintenance Procedures

Stock cultures of *Methanoplanus limicola* can be stored anaerobically at −20°C for several months after renewing the gas phase.

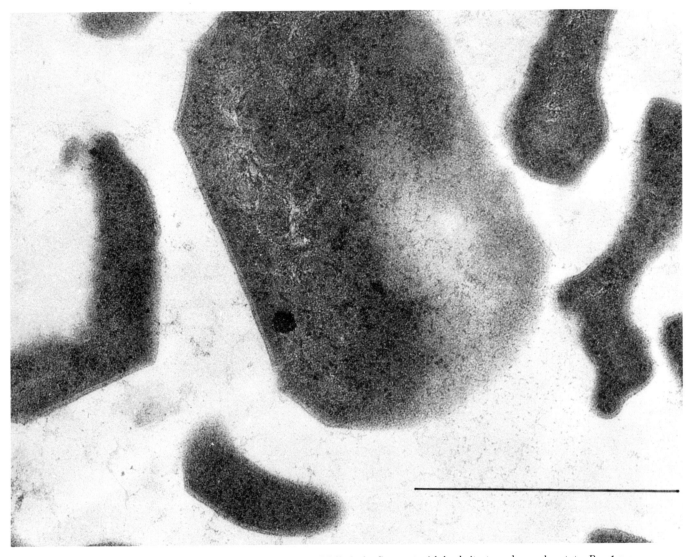

Figure 25.20.   Electron micrograph of thin section of *M. limicola*. Contrast with lead citrate and uranyl acetate. *Bar*, 1 μm.

Differentiation of the genus **Methanoplanus** *from other genera*

The genus *Methanoplanus* belongs to the order *Methanomicrobiales* due to its DNA/RNA hybridization and its relatively high G + C of the DNA. It differs from *Methanosarcina* by the lack of a rigid cell wall (except *M. acetivorans*; Sowers et al., 1984), the existence of flagella and the inability to use acetate, methanol and methylamines as energy sources. It differs from *Methanomicrobium* and *Methanogenium* by its flat shape and weak DNA/RNA hybridization.

Taxonomic Comments

The 16S rRNA/DNA hybridization between *Methanoplanus* and *Methanogenium* (Tu et al., 1982) yielded a lower thermostability of the hybrid (fs = 0.59) than that between *Methanogenium* and *Methanosarcina* (fs = 0.62). These results indicated that the genus *Methanoplanus* represents a new family, the *Methanoplanaceae*. However, very recent results of 16S rRNA cataloging show relationship to the *Methanomicro-*

biaceae (C.R. Woese, unpublished observation). Studies have yet to show the definitive phylogenetic status of the *Methanoplanaceae*.

Further Reading

Balch, W.E., G.E. Fox, L.J. Magrum, C.R. Woese and R.S. Wolfe. 1979. Methanogens: reevaluation of a unique biological group. Microbiol. Rev. *43*: 260–296.

Tu, J., D. Prangishvilli, H. Huber, G. Wildgruber, W. Zillig and K.O. Stetter. 1982. Taxonomic relations between archaebacteria including 6 novel genera examined by cross hybridization of DNA's and 16 S rRNA's. J. Mol. Evol. *18*: 109–114.

Van Bruggen, J.J.A., K.B. Zwart, J.G.F. Herman, E.M. van Hove, C.K. Stumm and G.D. Vogels. 1986. Isolation and characterization of *Methanoplanus endosymbiosus* sp. nov., an endosymbiont of the marine sapropelic ciliate *Metopus contortus* Quennerstedt. Arch. Microbiol. *144*: 367–374.

Wildgruber, G., M. Thomm, H. König, K. Ober, T. Ricchiuto and K.O. Stetter. 1982. *Methanoplanus limicola*, a plate-shaped methanogen representing a novel family, the *Methanoplanaceae*. Arch. Microbiol. *132*: 31–36.

Differentiation of the species of the genus **Methanoplanus**

1. Optimal growth temperature: 40°C. Mol% G + C of the DNA is 47.5. Acetate required.
            1. *M. limicola*

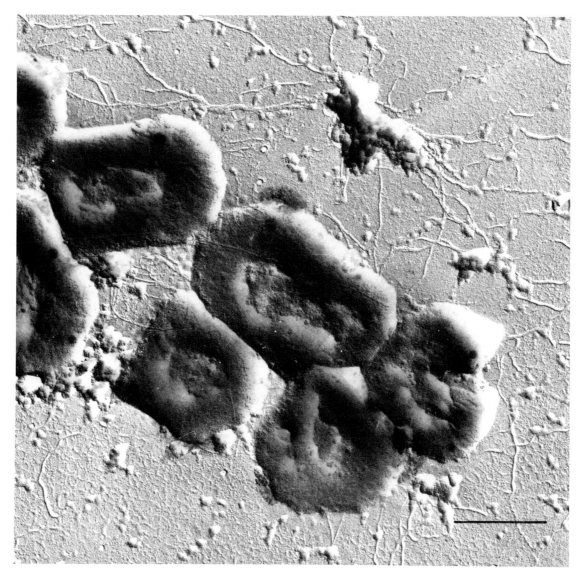

Figure 25.21. Electron micrograph of *M. limicola*. Platinum-shadowed. *Bar*, 1 μm.

2. Optimal growth temperature: 32°C. Mol% G + C of the DNA is 38.7. Acetate not required,.

2. *M. endosymbiosus*

List of species of the genus **Methanoplanus**

1. **Methanoplanus limicola** Wildgruber, Thomm and Stetter 1984, 270.[VP] (Effective publication: Wildgruber, Thomm and Stetter *in* Wildgruber, Thomm, König, Ober, Ricchiuto and Stetter 1982, 36.)

li.mi′co.la. L. masc. n. *limicola* inhabitant of a swamp.

Occurring in swamps. Tuft of flagella. Acetate required. Optimal growth temperature: 40°C. Cell envelope contains most likely a glycoprotein with a mol. wt. of 143,000.

The mol% G + C of the DNA is 47.5 (T_m).

Type strain: DSM 2279.

2. **Methanoplanus endosymbiosus** van Bruggen, Zwart, Herman, van Hove, Stumm and Vogels 1986b, 573.[VP] (Effective publication: van Bruggen, Zwart, Herman, van Hove, Stumm and Vogels 1986a, 373.)

en.do.sym.bi.o′sus. Gr. adj. *endo* inside; Gr. masc. adj. *symbiosus* living together; Gr. masc. adj. *endosymbiosus* living symbiotically inside of another organism.

Endosymbiont of the sapropelic marine ciliate *Metopus contortus*. Peritrichous flagellation. Acetate not required. Optimum growth temperature: 32°C. Tungsten (0.1 M) required. Cell envelope consists most likely of a glycoprotein with a mol. wt. of 110,000.

The mol% G + C of the DNA is 38.7.

Type strain: DSM 3599.

Genus **Methanosphaera** Miller and Wolin 1985b, 535[VP]
(Effective publication: Miller and Wolin 1985a, 121)

TERRY L. MILLER

Me.tha.no.sphae′ra. M. L. n. *methanum* methane; Gr. fem. n. *spaira* a sphere; N.L. fem. n. *Methanosphaera* methane-producing sphere.

Round cells, usually occurring **in pairs, tetrads and clusters,** about 1.0 μm in diameter. Resting cells, such as spores, are not known. Gram-positive. Nonmotile. **Very strict anaerobe. Cell walls are composed of pseudomurein.** Optimum temperature: near 37°C. Optimum pH: 6.5–6.9. **Chemoorganotrophic.**

Energy for growth is obtained by using 1 mol of H₂ to reduce 1 mol of methanol to 1 mol of CH₄. Methane is not produced from methanol in the absence of H₂. Carbon dioxide, carbon monoxide, sulfate, fumarate, choline or nitrate do not substitute for methanol. Methane is not produced from acetate, methylamines or formate with or without H₂. No growth or methane is obtained with ethanol and H₂. **Easily visible pigments are not produced, and cytochromes are absent.**

Carbon dioxide and acetate are required for growth. NH₄⁺ and one or more amino acids may be major sources of cell nitrogen. One or more B vitamins may be required for, or stimulatory to, growth.

The mol% G + C of the DNA is 26 (T_m).

Type species: *Methanosphaera stadtmanae* Miller and Wolin 1985b, 535.

Further Descriptive Information

The genus presently is represented by one species, *M. stadtmanae.* Specific information regarding the species is given in the species description.

Isolation and Enrichment Procedures

All enrichments and isolations require stringent anaerobic conditions. Selective enrichment procedures have not yet been developed. The type species was present in enrichments of human fecal material with methanol as the exogenously added methanogenic substrate and an initial 80% N₂ and 20% CO₂ gas phase and was subsequently isolated from subcultures of the enrichment with methanol and 80% H₂ and 20% CO₂ (Miller and Wolin, 1985a). *Methanosphaera* was isolated from an individual who harbored *Methanobrevibacter smithii* as the numerically dominant methanogen morphotype (Miller and Wolin, 1983, 1985a). *Methanosphaera* probably uses methanol produced by other organisms that degrade pectin in the intestinal habitat.

Maintenance Procedures

M. stadtmanae is maintained in anaerobic biphasic culture in phosphate-buffered, complex rumen fluid medium as described by Miller and Wolin (1985a) with a ratio of 1 volume of single-strength liquid medium to 4 volumes of double-strength agar medium. The methanol concentration is 1.2% in the agar phase and 0.6% in the liquid phase with a gas phase of 203 kPa H₂-CO₂ (80:20). An inoculum ($A_{660} \geq 0.7$, $d = 1.8$ cm) equivalent to 10% of the liquid phase is added, and the bottle is incubated at 37°C with gentle shaking. After outgrowth, the biphasic cultures are regassed and pressurized to 203 kPa with H₂-CO₂, precooled for 1 h at 4°C and frozen at −76°C. Biphasic cultures preserved with this method remain viable for up to 1 year of storage in the frozen state.

Differentiation of the genus **Methanosphaera** from other genera

Methanosphaera is presently the only described methanogen that is restricted to methanol and H₂ as its sole source of methanogenic substrates (Miller and Wolin, 1983, 1985a). *Methanosarcina barkeri* (strain Fusaro, DSM 804) was recently shown to grow and produce methane by direct reduction of 1 mol of methanol with 1 mol of H₂ (Müller et al., 1986). However, *Methanosarcina* is not restricted to this mechanism of methanogenesis and can use a variety of substrates for methanogenesis and growth, including methanol without H₂, methylamines, acetate and H₂ and CO₂.

Methanosphaera is phylogenetically differentiated from *Methanosarcina* and other genera of methanogens by the oligonucleotide codon sequence of its 16S rRNA (Miller and Wolin, 1985a; C. Woese, personal communication). Several characteristics indicate *M. stadtmanae* is closely related to the family *Methanobacteriaceae.* The 16S rRNA codon catalog relationships show a familial relationship to the *Methanobacteriaceae,* although the SAB index (0.45) indicates that it should not be included with either of the recognized genera of the family, *Methanobacterium* or *Methanobrevibacter.* The cell envelope of *M. stadtmanae* contains pseudomurein, the major polymer of the cell envelopes of the family (König et al., 1982; König, 1986). Cell envelopes of other families of methanogens do not contain pseudomurein. The amino acid composition of the pseudomurein of *M. stadtmanae* is distinguished from that of other members of the family by the presence of serine (König, 1986). Immunological fingerprinting showed a relationship between *M. stadtmanae* and *Methanobacterium thermoautotrophicum* and no relationship to any other member of the *Methanobacteriaceae* or any member of the other families of methanogens (Conway de Macario and Macario, 1986). Regardless of the characteristics that suggest *M. stadtmanae* is phylogenetically related to the *Methanobacteriaceae,* the present accepted description of the family excludes cocci and accepts only hydrogen and carbon dioxide and formate as substrates for methanogenesis by members of the family. Future studies of the nucleotide sequences of 16S rRNA may clarify the relationship of *M. stadtmanae* to the *Methanobacteriaceae.*

Further Reading

Kandler, O. and W. Zillig (Editors). 1986. Archaebacteria '85. Gustav Fischer Verlag, Stuttgart.

Miller, T.L. and M.J. Wolin. 1983. Oxidation of hydrogen and reduction of methanol to methane is the sole energy source for a methanogen isolated from human feces. J. Bacteriol. *101*: 1038–1045.

Miller, T.L. and M.J. Wolin. 1985. *Methanosphaera stadtmaniae* gen. nov., sp. nov.; a species that forms methane by reducing methanol with hydrogen. Arch. Microbiol. *141*: 116–122.

Whitman, W.R. 1985. Methanogenic bacteria. *In* Woese and Wolfe (Editors), The Bacteria. A Treatise on Structure and Function, Vol. VIII: Archaebacteria. Academic Press, New York.

Description of the species of the genus **Methanosphaera**

1. **Methanosphaera stadtmanae** Miller and Wolin 1985, 535.[VP] (Effective publication: Miller and Wolin 1985a, 121.) (*Methanosphaera stadtmaniae* [sic] Miller and Wolin 1985a, 121.)

stadt.man′ae. N.L. gen. n. *stadtmanae* of Stadtman; named in honor of T. C. Stadtman for her important contributions to the microbiology and biochemistry of methanogenesis.

Morphological characteristics are shown in Figure 25.22. A distinctive cleavage furrow is observed in dividing cells. Numerous electron-dense inclusions that are stable in the electron beam are usually, but not always, located near the cell wall (Fig. 25.22, *c–e*). The cell envelope consists of a single (18–20 nm thick) electron-dense layer (Fig. 25.22, *c* and *e*); its surface is smooth and lacks any organized structure. The peptide moiety of

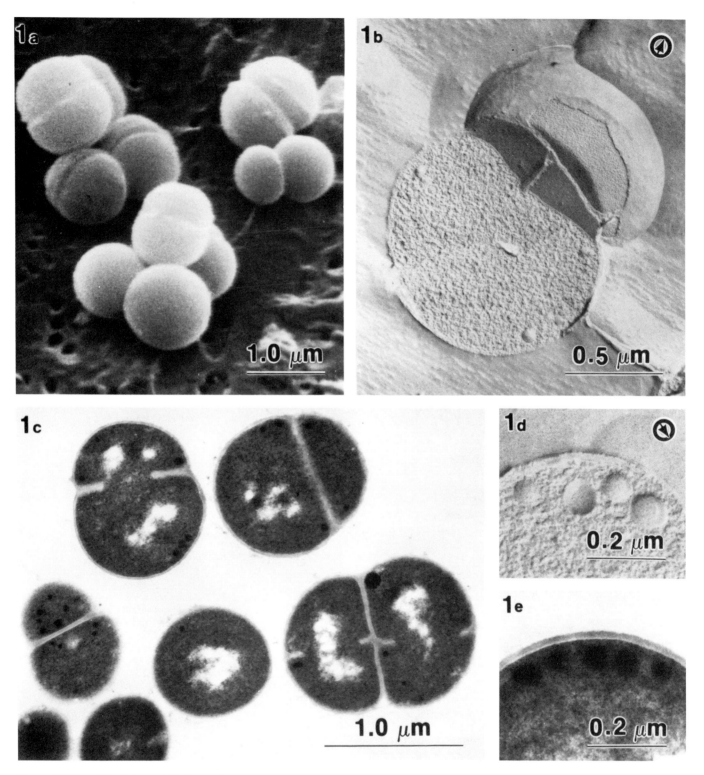

Figure 25.22. Morphology of *Methanosphaera stadtmanae*. The organism was grown in a liquid semidefined medium with 1.0% methanol and 203 kPa H_2-CO_2 (80:20) and cells were prepared for electron microscopy as described by Miller and Wolin, 1985a. *a*, scanning electron micrograph, illustrating the spherical cellular morphology and the cleavage furrow seen in rapidly dividing cells. *b*, freeze-fracture through dividing cells; the outer surface of the wall appears smooth; *encircled arrow* indicates the direction of the shadow. *c*, thin section through dividing cells re-

veals multiple septa and numerous electron-dense bodies. *d*, high magnification freeze-fracture through inclusion bodies, illustrating their presence in unfixed material. *e*, high magnification thin section through the electron-dense inclusion bodies near the cell wall, which consists of a single electron-dense layer. (Reproduced with permission from T. L. Miller and M. J. Wolin, *Archives of Microbiology 141*: 116–122, 1985, ©Springer-Verlag, Berlin).

the pseudomurein contains L-glutamate, L-lysine and L-serine. Flagella appear to be absent from cells treated by negative stains or by freeze-fracture procedures (W. A. Samsonoff, personal communication).

Surface colonies in complex rumen fluid medium are opaque to transluscent, effuse, circular or elliptical with entire margins and are light tan. Colonies in uncrowded roll tubes with excess methanol and hydrogen may reach a diameter of 2 mm.

Methanol and hydrogen are stoichiometrically converted to methane. Growth in a complex medium, with H_2 in excess, increases as the methanol concentration is increased, up to ~0.45 M (1.4%.). Higher concentrations of methanol are inhibitory. The growth yield is 4 g dry weight of cells/mol of methane.

Thiamine is required for growth, and biotin is stimulatory. Coenzyme M, vitamin B_{12} or other B vitamins are not required for growth. Radio-isotopic incorporation studies indicate ~50% of the cell carbon is derived from CO_2 and about 50% is derived from acetate (Miller and Wolin, 1983; T. L. Miller, unpublished data). Methanol or formate are not significant sources of cell carbon. Growth is not inhibited in a complex rumen fluid medium containing 2% oxgall and 0.1% sodium deoxycholate. NH_4^+ and isoleucine are essential for growth, and leucine is stimulatory to growth. 2-Methybutyric and isovaleric acids do not substitute for isoleucine and leucine, respectively. Sulfur and trace metal requirements have not been determined.

The following antibiotics do not inhibit growth in liquid culture medium (μg/ml): trimethoprim (10), methotrexate (10), sufanilamide (500), cephalothin (1.7) or clindamycin (6.7). Metronidazole (1 μg/ml) and bacitracin (10 μg/ml) completely inhibit growth. Monensin (10 μg/ml) and bromoethanesulfonate (1 mM) cause growth lags of ~5 days, after which cultures grow to turbidities similar to those obtained in controls without added inhibitors (see Miller and Wolin, 1985a).

The type strain MCB3 was isolated from enrichments of human feces (Miller and Wolin, 1983, 1985a). Similar morphotypes have been observed in human and some animal feces, but are usually far outnumbered by the numerically dominant H_2-CO_2-using *Methanobrevibacter* morphotype (Miller and Wolin, 1986; Miller et al., 1986a; T.L. Miller, unpublished data). In the intestinal habitat, the organism probably uses methanol produced by other intestinal organisms that degrade pectin.

The mol% G + C of the DNA of the type strain is 25.8 (T_m).

Type strain: MCB3 (DSM 3091).

Acknowledgments

I thank Dr. W. A. Samsonoff of the Wadsworth Center for providing the electron microscopic analysis.

GROUP II. **ARCHAEOBACTERIAL SULFATE REDUCERS**

ORDER **"ARCHAEOGLOBALES"**

Karl O. Stetter

Gram-negative cocci occurring singly and in pairs. Cell envelope consisting of glycoprotein subunits. H_2, formate, D(−)-lactate, D(+)-lactate, glucose and yeast extract are used as electron donors. As electron acceptors, sulfate, sulfite and thiosulfate, but no S^0, are used. DNA base composition is 46 mol% G + C. Only one group is presently known.

FAMILY **"ARCHAEOGLOBACEAE"**

Description of the family is the same as that for the order.

Genus **Archaeoglobus** Stetter 1988b, 328[VP] (Effective publication: Stetter 1988a, 172)

Description of the genus is the same as that for the order. A more complete description of the genus and its type species, *A. fulgidus*, was published while this volume was in proof stage (Stetter, 1988a).

GROUP III. **EXTREMELY HALOPHILIC ARCHAEOBACTERIA**

ORDER **HALOBACTERIALES** ORD. NOV.

William D. Grant and Helge Larsen

Hal.o.bac.ter.i.al'es. M.L. n. *Halobacterium* type genus of the family *Halobacteriaceae*: *-ales* ending to denote an order; M.L. fem. pl. n. *Halobacteriales* the *Halobacterium* order.

Rods, cocci, a multitude of **involution forms from disks to triangles.** Resting stages are not known. **Nonmotile or motile by tufts of polar flagella.** Gram-negative or Gram-positive (after fixation in 2% (w/v) acetic acid). **Aerobic or facultatively anaerobic** with or without nitrate. **Require** at least **1.5 M NaCl for growth.** Most strains grow best at 3.5–4.5 M NaCl. **Colonies are various shades of red due to** the presence of C_{50} **carotenoids** (bacterioruberins) that impart red coloration to mass developments in the natural environment. Retinal-based pigments capable of producing movements of ions across the cell membrane are probably also universally present. One of these pigments, bacteriorhodopsin, acts as a proton pump driven by light energy. Those organisms that contain this particular pigment are able to harness the proton gradient so produced for ATP synthesis. Optimum temperature for growth: 35–50°C. Chemoorganotrophic, using amino acids or carbohydrates as carbon source. Have an RNA polymerase of the ABB″C type. Osmoregulation is achieved by the intracellular accumulation of a large concentration of KCl.

Occur ubiquitously **in nature where the salt concentration is high, i.e. in salt lakes, soda lakes and salterns.** Are common in crude solar salts and proteinaceous products (fish and hides) heavily salted with solar salt.

The DNA is commonly comprised of a major component and a minor component, with the minor component making up to 10–30% of the total DNA. Strains with a minor DNA component usually harbor large plasmids (>100 kilobases (kb)). The mol% G + C of the major DNA component is 61–71, and that of the minor DNA component is 51–59 (Bd).

Further Descriptive Information

The archaeobacterial halophiles (halobacteria) can be unequivocally distinguished from other halophilic procaryotes by their archaeobacterial characteristics, particularly the possession of ether-linked phosphoglycerides readily detectable by the procedures of Ross et al. (1985) and Torreblanca et al. (1986a) and by their insensitivity to eubacterial inhibitors such as penicillin and chloramphenicol.

All halobacteria have diphytanyl (C_{20},C_{20}) glycerol ether core lipids, but certain strains have additional sesterterpanyl-phytanyl (C_{25},C_{20}) glycerol ether core lipids (De Rosa et al., 1982), and at least one strain has disesterterpanyl (C_{25},C_{25}) glycerol ether lipids (De Rosa et al., 1983). Bi-diphytanyl tetraethers (C_{40},C_{40}) have not been detected in any halobacteria to date.

The most striking feature of the halobacteria is their absolute requirement for high concentrations of NaCl. Although some strains may grow at salt concentrations as low as 1.5 M, most of the strains grow best at concentrations of 3.5–4.5 M and grow well in saturated NaCl (5.2 M).

Many isolates have been cultured only in nutrient-rich yeast extract or peptone-based media, but examples are known that grow in defined media (Rodriguez-Valera et al., 1980). Anaerobic growth occurs either by an uncharacterized fermentative mode (Gonzalez et al., 1978; Javor, 1984), by a fermentative mode linked to arginine utilization (Hartmann et al., 1980) or by dissimilatory nitrate reduction (Tomlinson et al., 1986).

Halobacteria may cause the spoilage of heavily salted proteinaceous products, being responsible for the "pink" in salted fish and the "red heat" of salted hides. Without further processing, solar salt may contain 10^5–10^6 viable halobacteria g^{-1}, surviving for many years under practical storage conditions. Salt lakes may contain 10^7–10^8 cells ml^{-1} (Nissenbaum, 1975; Post, 1977).

The characteristic red bacterioruberins possessed by all naturally occurring isolates seem to play a protective role against the strong sunlight where these organisms are found. Colorless strains are rare (Onishi et al., 1985) and usually only readily found as mutants produced in the laboratory. Isoprenoid quinones are of the menaquinone type (MK8 and MK8H$_2$) (Collins et al., 1981), not the ubiquinone type. Halobacteria contain small amounts of polyamines (Carteni-Farina et al., 1985), far less than most eubacteria and most other archaeobacteria.

To compensate for the high salt concentrations in the environment, the organisms accumulate mainly KCl (up to 5 M) and may be growth-limited by the amount of KCl in media. NMR studies indicate that most of the KCl is in the free state (Shporer and Civan, 1977). The functional and structural units of the cells are adapted to these high salt concentrations. Most intracellular enzymes have a requirement for high levels of KCl (Kushner, 1985) although normally NaCl will substitute. The molecular basis of the salt requirement is not fully understood, although halobacterial proteins are considerably more acidic overall than nonhalophilic counterparts. Detailed structural investigations of a few highly purified halobacterial proteins (malate dihydrogenase, glutamate dehydrogenase and ferredoxin) indicate that the high concentrations of negative charges in such proteins is associated with separate and distinct domains within these proteins. Denatured halophilic proteins lose the ability to retain large amounts of water and salt (Werber et al., 1986) and undergo a remarkable loss of secondary and tertiary structure.

The cell envelope of the noncoccoid isolates maintains its integrity only in the presence of NaCl or KCl. Upon gradual dilution of the growth medium with water, the cells change their shape, through irregular forms to spheres which undergo lysis. The composition of the growth medium affects the point at which lysis occurs. Gram staining procedures require modification to overcome the osmotic fragility of such cells. Fixation of air-dried smears with 2% (w/v) acetic acid for 5 min (Dussault, 1955), before the staining procedure is followed, gives good results.

Taxonomic Comments

In the eighth edition of the *Manual*, the family *Halobacteriaceae* was created for these organisms, a taxonomic status retained in the first volume of *Bergey's Manual® of Systematic Bacteriology*. However, it is clear from a comparison of oligonucleotide catalogs of archaeobacteria that the halobacteria comprise a taxonomic ranking equal in depth to any of the three orders of methanogens (Fox et al., 1980; Stackebrandt and Woese, 1981). 16S rRNA/DNA hybridization studies have produced similar results (Tu et al., 1982), leading many authors to ascribe ordinal status to the halobacteria, most recently Grant and Ross (1986) who suggested that the halobacteria might comprise an order with two families on the basis of 16S rRNA/DNA hybridization studies (see Fig. 25.23).

More recent complete sequence comparisons of archaeobacterial 16S rRNA (Jarsch and Böck, 1985; Lechner et al., 1985; Leinfelder et al., 1985; Yang et al., 1985; Kjems et al., 1987) have substantiated the ordinal status of these bacteria. Complete 16S rRNA sequences are now available for *Halobacterium salinarium* (Hui and Dennis, 1985; Mankin et al., 1985) *Haloferax volcanii* (Gupta et al., 1983), *Halococcus morrhuae* (Leffers and Garrett, 1984) and *Natronobacterium magadii* (H. N. M. Ross and W. D. Grant, unpublished results). Comparisons between these sequences, however, provide no evidence for any suprageneric groupings within the order, since each sequence is approximately 88% homologous with all of the others. The halobacteria are most closely related to the methanogenic archaeobacteria *(Methanomicrobiales)* as determined by such sequence comparisons (Yang et al., 1986).

Few numerical taxonomic studies of halobacteria have been carried out, and these have either contained few reference strains (Colwell et al., 1979) or have only been moderately successful in defining or redefining certain groups (Torreblanca et al., 1986a), such as the genera *Haloferax* and *Haloarcula* (both of which have type species originally classified in the genus *Halobacterium*). The discovery of the haloalkaliphilic phenotype (Tindall et al., 1984a) prompted a reappraisal of the taxonomy of the halobacteria on the basis of chemotaxonomic markers rather than standard biochemical tests (Ross and Grant, 1985).

The polar lipid composition of isolates has proved particularly useful in this respect (Ross et al., 1985; Kates, 1986). The lipids of halobacteria examined to date contain phytanyl or sesterterpanyl ether analogs of phosphatidylglycerol (PG) and phosphatidylglycerol phosphate (PGP). Most strains also contain phosphatidylglycerol sulfate (PGS). A family of glycolipids and sulfated glycolipids is also present with the exception of strains in one group. These glycolipids are derived from a basic mannosyl-glycosyl-diphytanyl glycerol by substitution of sugar or sulfate groups at the three or six positions of the mannose residue (Kates, 1978) (Fig. 25.24). Glycolipids include a sulfated tetraglycosyl diether (S-TeGD), triglycosyl diethers (TGD-1 and TGD-2) and diglycosyl diethers (DGD-1 and the uncharacterized DGD-2) as well as certain corresponding sulfated forms. The presence or absence of examples of these (and other minor unidentified lipids) can be used to rapidly assign an isolate to a particular group (Ross and Grant, 1985; Torreblanca et al., 1986a). The chromatographic procedure of Torreblanca et al. (1986) is particularly useful in distinguishing diglycosyl, triglycosyl, and tetraglycosyl glycolipids and their sulfated derivatives.

Polar lipid analyses and 16S rRNA/DNA hybridization studies not only generate groupings corresponding to the genera *Halococcus, Haloarcula, Haloferax, Natronococcus* and *Natronobacterium* but also indicate that a further redefinition of certain isolates currently classified in the genus *Halobacterium* may be necessary in the future with four extra putative generic groupings (Fig. 25.23). A recent immunological analysis of a more restricted range of isolates has produced similar groupings (Conway de Macario et al., 1986). It will be noted (Fig. 25.23) that certain isolates with identical specific epithets appear largely unrelated, highlighting a real historical problem, both for the future taxonomy of the group and for comparative biochemical studies between different laboratories.

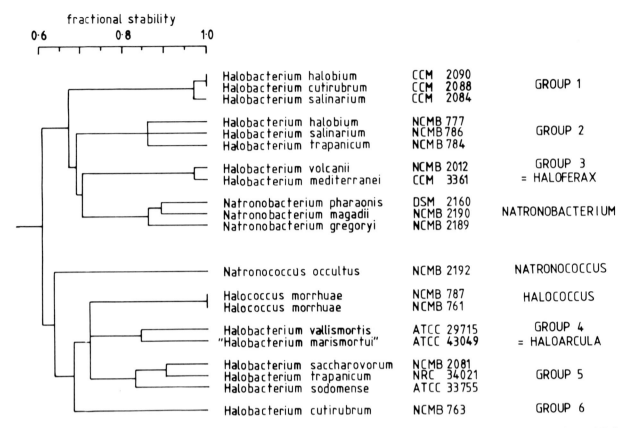

Figure 25.23. Relationships among halobacteria based on the thermal stability of 16S rRNA/DNA hybrids. *ATCC*, American Type Culture Collection; *CCM*, Czechoslovak Collection of Microorganisms; *DSM*, Deutsche Sammlung vor Mikroorganismen; *NCMB*, National Collection of Marine Bacteria, U.K. (Modified from H. N. M. Ross and W. D. Grant, Journal of General Microbiology *131:* 165–173, 1985.)

FAMILY **HALOBACTERIACEAE** GIBBONS 1974, 269[AL]

Hal.o.bac.ter.i.a′ce.ae. M.L. n. *Halobacterium* type genus of the family; *-aceae* ending to denote a family; M.L. pl. fem. n. *Halobacteriaceae* the *Halobacterium* family.

Description of the family the same as for the order.
Type genus: **Halobacterium** Elazari-Volcani 1957, 207.

Key to the groups and genera of the **Halobacteriaceae**

Current isolates comprise essentially two groups:

    I. Isolates that grow at neutrality or close to neutrality (pH 5–8) with a Mg^{2+} requirement of at least 5 mM.
    II. Haloalkaliphilic isolates that grow only at high pH (pH 8.5–11.0) with a very low Mg^{2+} requirement (<1 mM).

    I. Optimum pH for growth: 5–8.
        A. Cells are rods of varying length under optimal conditions in young liquid culture. Pleomorphic and coccoid forms may be present in old liquid culture and in agar-grown cultures. Cells lyse in distilled water. Cells are motile and uniformly stain Gram-negative. Mg^{2+} requirement moderate (5–50 mM). Amino acids are required for growth. Optimum concentration: 3.5–4.5 M NaCl. Characteristic sulfated triglycosyl and tetraglycosyl diethers present.
                Genus I. *Halobacterium,* p. 2219
        B. Cells are extremely pleomorphic. Under optimal conditions in liquid media, triangles, rectangles and irregular disks are commonly observed. Cells lyse in distilled water. Motile or nonmotile and uniformly stain Gram-negative. Mg^{2+} requirement moderate (5–50 mM). Amino acids not required for growth. Optimum concentration: 2–3 M NaCl. Characteristic triglycosyl diether lipid present.
                Genus II. *Haloarcula,* p. 2224
        C. Cells are extremely pleomorphic under optimal conditions in liquid media, pleomorphic rods and flat disks most commonly present. Cells lyse in distilled water. Cells are motile or nonmotile and uniformly stain Gram-negative. Mg^{2+} requirement high (20–50 mM). Amino acids are not required for growth. Opti-

mum concentration: 2–3 M NaCl. Characteristic sulfated diglycosyl diether lipid present. Phosphatidylglycerol sulfate absent.

Genus III. *Haloferax*, p. 2226

D. Cells are invariably coccoid. Under all conditions of growth, occurring in pairs, tetrads, sarcinae or irregular clusters. Cells are nonmotile and do not lyse in distilled water, and some cells at least stain Gram-positive. Optimum concentration: 3.5–4.5 M NaCl.

Genus IV. *Halococcus*, p. 2228

II. Optimum pH for growth: 8.5–11. Mg^{2+} requirement low (<1 mM).

E. Cells are rods of varying lengths in young liquid cultures but become coccoid as they age. Cells from agar cultures are coccoid. Cells lyse in distilled water. Motile or nonmotile and uniformly stain Gram-negative. Optimum concentration: 3.5–4.5 M NaCl. Glycolipids absent.

Genus V. *Natronobacterium*, p. 2230

F. Cells are invariably coccoid under all conditions of growth, occurring singly or in pairs, tetrads and irregular clusters. Cells suspended in distilled water show some leakage of contents as judged by an increase in viscosity of the suspension, but they appear intact when examined microscopically. At least some cells stain Gram-positive. Nonmotile. Optimum concentration: 3.0–4.0 M NaCl. Glycolipids are absent.

Genus VI. *Natronococcus*, p. 2232

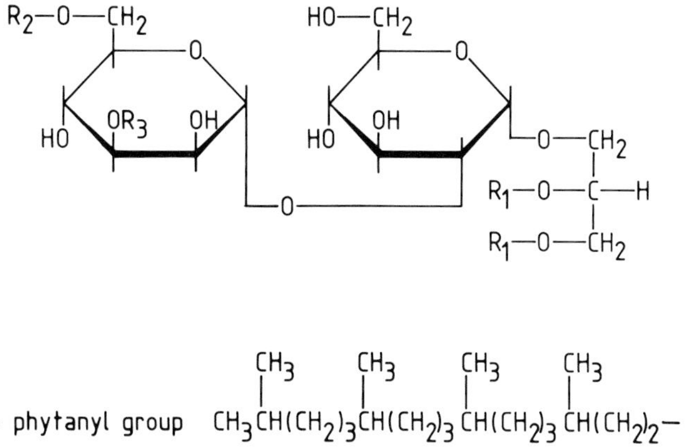

R_1 = phytanyl group

Fig. 25.24. Chemical structures of glycolipids in halobacteria. DGD-1 R_2 = H, R_3 = H; S-DGD-1 R_2 = $-SO_3^--OH$, R_3 = H; TGD-1 R_2 = β-gal*p*, R_3 = H; TGD-2 R_2 = β-glu*p*, R_3 = H; S-TGD-1 R_2 = $3SO_3^-$-β-gal*p*, R_3 = H; S-TeGD R_2 = $3SO_3^-$-β-gal*p*, R_3 = α-gal*f*. (Redrawn from M. Kates, FEMS Microbiology Reviews *39:* 95–101.)

Further Reading

Grant, W.D. and H.N.M. Ross. 1986. The ecology and taxonomy of the halobacteria. FEMS Microbiol. Rev. *39:* 9–15.

Kjems, J., R.A. Garrett and W. Ansorge. 1987. The sequence of the 16S RNA gene and its flanking region from the archaebacterium *Desulfurococcus mobilis*. Syst. Appl. Microbiol. *9:* 22–28.

Kushner, D.J. 1985. The *Halobacteriaceae. In* Woese and Wolfe (Editors), The Bacteria, Vol. VIII. Academic Press, London, pp. 171–214.

Larsen, H. 1982. The family *Halobacteriaceae. In* Starr, Stolp, Trüper, Balows and Schlegel (Editors), The Prokaryotes. A Handbook on Habitats, Isolation, and Identification of Bacteria. Springer-Verlag, Berlin, pp. 985–994.

Larsen, H. 1984. *Halobacteriaceae. In* Krieg and Holt (Editors), Bergey's Manual of Systematic Bacteriology, Vol. 1. The Williams & Wilkins Co., Baltimore, pp. 261–267.

Ross, H.N.M. and W.D. Grant. 1985. Nucleic acid studies on halophilic archaebacteria. J. Gen. Microbiol. *131:* 165–173.

Tindall, B.J., H.N.M. Ross and W.D. Grant. 1984. *Natronobacterium* gen. nov. and *Natronococcus* gen. nov., two new genera of haloalkaliphilic archaebacteria. Syst. Appl. Microbiol. *5:* 41–57.

Tindall, B.J. and H.G. Trüper. 1986. Ecophysiology of the aerobic halophilic archaebacteria. Syst. Appl. Microbiol. *7:* 202–212.

Torreblanca, M., F. Rodriguez-Valera, G. Juez, A. Ventosa, M. Kamekura and M. Kates. 1986. Classification of non-alkaliphilic halobacteria based on numerical taxonomy and polar lipid composition, and description of *Haloarcula* gen. nov. and *Haloferax* gen. nov. Syst. Appl. Microbiol. *8:* 89–99.

Yang, D., B.P. Kaine and C.R. Woese. 1986. The phylogeny of archaebacteria. Syst. Appl. Microbiol. *6:* 251–256.

Genus I. **Halobacterium** *Elazari-Volcani 1957, 207*[AL]

HELGE LARSEN AND WILLIAM D. GRANT

Hal.o.bac.te′ri.um. Gr. n. *halo, halos* the sea, salt; Gr. n. *bakterion* a small rod; M.L. neut. n. *Halobacterium* salt bacterium.

When grown under optimum conditions, the cells are **rod shaped** (0.5–1.2 × 1.0–6.0 μm) (Fig. 25.25). **Pleomorphic forms are common** (bent and swollen rods, clubs, spheres). **The cells divide by constriction** (Fig. 25.26). Resting stages are not known. Gram-negative. **Motile** by tufts of polar flagella. Some strains have gas vacuoles. **Most strains are strict aerobes,** but some strains exhibit facultatively anaerobic growth. Oxidase- and catalase-positive. **Extremely halophilic with growth occurring in media containing 3.0–5.2 M NaCl.** Most strains grow best at 3.5–4.5 M. Optimum temperature: 35–50°C; maximum: 55°C; minimum: 15–20°C. pH range for growth: 5.5–8.5. Chemoorganotrophic. **Amino acids are required for growth. Most strains are proteolytic.**

The DNA is usually composed of a major component and a minor component. The latter makes up 10–30% of the total DNA (Bd). Strains that have a minor component usually harbor a large plasmid (144 kb). The mol% G + C of the DNA of the major component is 67.1–71.2 (Bd, T_m), and that of the minor component, 57–60 (Bd).

Type species: *Halobacterium salinarium* (Harrison and Kennedy 1922) Elazari-Volcani 1957, 208.

Further Descriptive Information

Pleomorphism is a distinctive feature of the halobacteria including members of the genus *Halobacterium*. In some strains the cells are regular slender rods when grown at moderate temperature under optimal conditions, but they display a multitude of involution forms when in the stationary phase of growth, or grown at inappropriate temperature or NaCl concentrations. Upon gradual dilution of the medium with water, the cells change shape from rods through irregular transition forms to spheres, and the spheres undergo lysis. The composition of the growth medium may affect the point at which lysis occurs, since in media whose ion composition (with the exception of NaCl) is based on seawater (Torreblanca et al., 1986a), many strains are reported as being stable in 2% (w/v) total salts, whereas in other media lysis is widely reported to occur between 5 and 10% (w/v) NaCl (Kushner, 1985). The composition of the

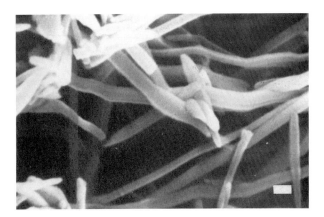

Figure 25.25. *Halobacterium salinarium* strain 1 (ATCC 19700; DSM 668), grown at 30°C in a medium in g/l of tap water: crude solar salt, 250.0; MgSO$_4$·7H$_2$O, 20.0; KCl, 5.0; CaCl$_2$·6H$_2$O, 0.2; yeast extract (Difco), 5.0; and tryptone (Difco), 5.0; at pH 6.8. This is a young culture, in which this strain tends to form long rods. *Bar,* 1 μm. (Prepared by G. Bentzen; photographed by the Laboratory of Clinical Electron Microscopy, University of Bergen.)

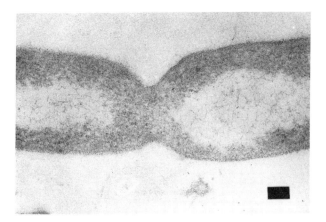

Figure 25.26. *Halobacterium salinarium* strain 1 (ATCC 19700; DSM 668), grown under the same conditions as given in the legend to Figure 25.25. Thin section of a cell in the process of division by constriction. *Bar,* 0.1 μm (Prepared by H. Steensland).

medium may also affect the minimum Mg^{2+} requirement for growth, originally considered to be 0.1–0.5 M in complex media (Larsen, 1984), but reported as much lower (0.005 M) in seawater-based medium (Torreblanca et al., 1986a).

The lysis phenomenon in hypotonic solutions is primarily not due to an osmotic effect but rather is due to the need for high concentrations of salt to maintain the cell envelope. The cell envelope of *Halobacterium* species has an outer layer visible in the electron microscope (Fig. 25.27) (Stoeckenius and Rowen, 1967; Steensland and Larsen, 1969) which is largely composed of a characteristic eucaryoticlike sulfated glycoprotein of high molecular weight (Wieland et al., 1982) responsible for maintaining the structural integrity of the cell wall. The surface of the cell envelope has a hexagonal surface pattern presumably due to the regular packing of glycoprotein subunits (Fig. 25.28). The proteinaceous subunits of the cell envelope are held together only in the presence of salt.

Some *Halobacterium* species (and other halobacteria), when grown under low oxygen tension, form patches in the cell membrane of a special chromophore, bacteriorhodopsin. The coloring principle is retinal; the membrane patches are referred to as the purple membrane. Bacteriorhodopsin acts as a proton pump driven by light energy absorbed by the pigment. Important energy-requiring phenomena in the cell utilize the energy made available by the proton gradient so produced. There is no doubt that the possession of bacteriorhodopsin confers survival value on illuminated cells otherwise starved of energy (Brock and Petersen, 1976; Hartmann et al., 1980; Rodriguez-Valera et al., 1982). Whether such cells behave as genuine autotrophs remains to be established, although there is evidence for an anaplerotic CO$_2$ fixation mechanism (Danon and Kaplan, 1977). The gene for the protein component of bacteriorhodopsin has now been sequenced and characterized (Dunn et al., 1981; DasSarma et al., 1984). Other retinal-based pigments are now known to be present in *Halobacterium* species, including halorhodopsin, an inwardly directed Cl$^-$ pump (Lanyi, 1986) similar in structure to bacteriorhodopsin. The gene for the protein component of this chromophore has also been sequenced (Hegemann et al., 1987). Other retinal pigments appear to function as signal transducers which mediate the phototactic responses of these cells (Stoeckenius and Bogomolni, 1982; Wolff et al., 1986). Halobacteria thus possess the only non-chlorophyll-mediated light energy transducing system.

Halobacterium species (and other halobacteria) have right-handed helical flagella which consist of bundles of several filaments (Alam and Oesterhelt, 1984). The constituting flagellins are glycoproteins carrying the same sulfated oligosaccharide moieties as the cell surface glycoprotein (Wieland et al., 1985).

Most strains grow well in complex media with yeast extract or casamino acids as carbon and energy sources. Many variations of complex media have been used over the years. Larsen (1982) details a number of these. Other complex media are described by Oren (1983), Tomlinson et al. (1986), and Torreblanca et al. (1986a). The most commonly used complex medium is based on the formulation of Gibbons and his collaborators.* Defined media have also been developed for certain isolates. (Rodriguez-Valera et al., 1980; Larsen, 1982). However, not all isolates grow in these media.

Halobacterium species have a requirement for amino acids. Rarely, carbohydrates and vitamins may stimulate the growth of some strains (Gochnauer and Kushner, 1969). Most isolates seem to have a complex organic nutrition and preferentially utilize amino acids as carbon and energy sources, but we do not have a general overview of the metabolic pathways in *Halobacterium* species. Most strains are strict aerobes, but some strains are facultative anaerobes growing fermentatively (Javor, 1984). In one instance, fermentative growth has been shown to be based on the conversion of arginine to ornithine (Hartmann et al., 1980). Even under aerobic conditions, growth is relatively slow; generation times of 3 h are the best that have been recorded, but a generation time of 6–7 h is more common.

Some strains contain gas vacuoles, forming pink or even white colonies on agar media. Upon cultivation in the laboratory, strains have a tendency to lose the ability to produce vacuoles at high frequency, and sectoring may occur in gas vacuolate colonies where reversion to non-gas vacuole forms has taken place. Observations such as this have led to the realization that certain strains of *H. salinarium* have considerable genetic instability due to the presence of multiple copies of different insertion elements which inactivate genes where they integrate into the major or minor DNA components. These insertion sequences are mainly clustered in the minor lower G + C component of the DNA which is covalently closed circular DNA. Mapping of integration sites has given insight into the complexity of bacteriorhodopsin gene expression and led to the isolation of a second gene whose product is involved. Other genes investigated in detail include genes encoding rRNAs, tRNAs, and a sta-

---

* The medium contains (in g/l): NaCl, 250.0; MgSO$_4$·7H$_2$O, 20.0; KCl, 2.0; trisodium citrate, 3.0; yeast extract, 10.0; and casamino acids, 7.5. Fe^{2+} and Mn^{2+} are added as trace elements at 10 and 0.1 ppm, respectively. The NaCl is sterilized separately from the rest of the components.

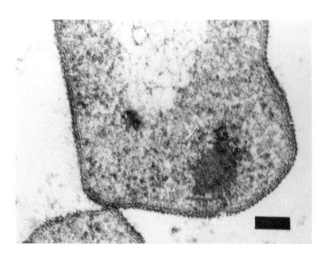

Figure 25.27. *Halobacterium* species strain 5, grown under the same conditions as given in the legend to Figure 25.25. Thin section. *Halobacterium* species have a gracilicute type envelope *Bar*, 0.1 µm. (Reproduced with permission from H. Steensland and H. Larsen, Journal of General Microbiology *55:* 325–326, 1969, ©Society for General Microbiology.)

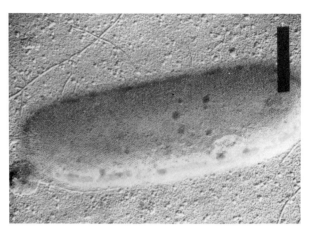

Figure 25.28. *Halobacterium salinarium* strain 1 (ATCC 19700; DSM 668), grown under the same conditions as given in the legend to Figure 25.25. Replica of the surface of a cell from a culture in late exponential phase. *Bar*, 0.5 µm. (Prepared by V. Mohr.)

ble 7S RNA whose function is unknown. A number of phages for *H. salinarium* strains have now been characterized (halophages). Most of these require high salt concentrations to maintain their viability. In some cases, lysogeny is established and insertional events also occur in phage DNA. The recent review of Pfeifer (1987) should be consulted for details of the genetics of *H. salinarium* and associated halophages.

The polar lipids of *Halobacterium* species are based on 2,3-di-*O*-phytanyl-*sn*-glycerol (C_{20},C_{20}) ethers. All strains have C_{20},C_{20} forms of PG, PGP, PGS and TGD-1. S-TGD-1 and S-TeGD are characteristic of the genus (Kates, 1986; Torreblanca et al. 1986a).

All isolates are insensitive to penicillin, chloramphenicol, streptomycin, erythromycin and tetracycline and sensitive to anisomycin, bacitracin, novobiocin and vibriostat reagent (0/129).

Halobacterium species make up a significant fraction of the microbial population of neutral salt lakes and salterns, particularly thallasohaline examples. Proteolytic organisms of this genus are largely responsible for the spoilage of proteinaceous products that have been heavily salted with such solar salt.

Enrichment and Isolation Procedures

Strong neutral brines, crude solar salt and salted products are potential sources of *Halobacterium* species. The material can be spread directly on the surface of agar media. The plates are wrapped in plastic bags to prevent drying and are incubated at 37–40°C. Red colonies appear after 4–21 days. Enrichments may be obtained in liquid media vigorously shaken to produce good aeration.

Members of the genus *Halobacterium* and other halobacteria may be obtained by these procedures. Selective procedures that are specific for particular genera or species have not been devised. However, thallasohaline brines and salted products might be expected to have very high numbers of *Halobacterium* species rather than other halobacteria (Marquez et al., 1987).

Maintenance Procedures

Growth on agar slants in screw-capped tubes can be kept in the refrigerator for 4 or 5 months. Lyophilization does not give reliable results. Preparations suspended in growth medium supplemented with 15% (w/v) glycerol may be stored at −70°C by using the bead procedure of Feltham et al. (1978). These preparations are viable for at least 10 years.

Differentiation of the genus **Halobacterium** from other genera

The key to the family *Halobacteriaceae* indicates characteristics useful in distinguishing *Halobacterium*, *Haloferax* and *Haloarcula*. The polar lipid composition of *Halobacterium* species is characterized by the lack of DGD-1, DGD-2 and TDG2 and the presence of TGD, S-TGD-1 and S-TeGD.

Taxonomic Comments

Klebahn (1919) was the first to describe distinctly the main morphological and physiological features of the group. He isolated from salt fish a salt-requiring red pleomorphic rod which he called *Bacillus halobius ruber*. Harrison and Kennedy (1922) isolated from salted cod a very similar organism which they named *Pseudomonas salinaria*. In Europe, Petter (1931) isolated several more strains of similar organisms but changed the name to *Bacterium halobium*. A number of Petter's strains are still available in culture collections today (e.g. NCMB). Lochhead (1934) had listed the organism of Harrison and Kennedy under the name *Serratia salinaria* and had isolated a closely related organism from salted buffalo hide, which he named *Serratia cutirubra*. Elazari-Volcani, when creating the genus *Halobacterium* in the seventh edition of the *Manual*, proposed that the Lochhead organism, the Petter organism and

the Harrison and Kennedy organism should be assigned to this genus as *H. cutirubrum*, *H. halobium* and *H. salinarium*, respectively. The genus also included an additional Dead Sea isolate, *H. marismortui*, and an organism isolated from Trapani salt, *H. trapanicum*.

The relationship of *H. halobium*, *H. salinarium* and *H. cutirubrum* has been the subject of considerable dispute over the years. In the eighth edition of the *Manual*, *H. cutirubrum* was considered a subjective synonym of *H. salinarium*. However, Colwell et al. (1979), on the basis of a numerical taxonomic analysis, came to the conclusion that *H. halobium* and *H. salinarium* were very similar, whereas *H. cutirubrum* was slightly different. Unfortunately, there are many different halobacteria residing in type collections with these specific epithets, and the relationship between the three species has been obscured by frequent failure to include the type strains in taxonomic analyses. Thus DNA/DNA base-pairing studies by Moore and McCarthy (1969) and Ross and Grant (1985) failed to include all of the type strains. The problem is compounded by the lack of any extant type strain of the original *H. halobium* (Tindall and Trüper, 1986), although a reference strain is available (NRC 34020). Oligonucleotide catalogs of strains of all three species are said to be identical (Fox et al., 1980), as are 16S rRNA gene sequences for *H. cutirubrum* (Hui and

Dennis, 1985) and *H. halobium* R[1] (Mankin et al., 1985), but the history of some of these strains is unclear, although the R$_1$ strain is a mutant of the suggested reference strain for *H. halobium* (NRC 34020) (Spudich and Stroeckenius, 1979).

Recently, Conway de Macario et al. (1986) have carried out an immunological analysis of different strains including the type strain of *H. cutirubrum* (NRC 34001), concluding that the strain was closely related to *H. halobium* R$_1$ and *H. salinarium* DSM 668. In Moore and McCarthy's study (1969), *H. salinarium* Larsen strain 1 (DSM 668), *H. halobium* strain Delft (CCM 2090) and *H. cutirubrum* CCNRLO9 (CCM 2088) were found to be closely related. In Ross and Grant's study (1985), *H. halobium* CCM 2090, *H. cutirubrum* (CCM 2088) and the type strain of *H. salinarium* NCMB 764 (NRC 34002) were compared; these authors found a close degree of relatedness (DNA/DNA homologies of >70%). Accordingly, although in no single study have all the type strains or reference strains of *H. halobium*, *H. salinarium* and *H. cutirubrum* been compared, the circumstantial evidence that they are extremely similar is overwhelming, and there is no reason to dissent from the view expounded in Volume 1 of *Bergey's Manual® of Systematic Bacteriology* that *H. cutirubrum* along with *H. halobium* should be subsumed into *H. salinarium*, the latter specific epithet having historical precedence. It should, however, be noted that in the analysis of Ross and Grant (1985) (Fig. 25.23) certain strains designated as *H. cutirubrum* (NCMB 763), *H. halobium* NCMB 777) and *H. salinarium* (NCMB 786) were shown to constitute a different polar lipid/16S rRNA group, and these organisms clearly should not be described as *H. salinarium* strains. It is of some concern that *H. halobium* NCMB 777 is supposedly the reference strain of *H. halobium* (NRC 34020).

H. marismortui, referred to in the seventh edition of the *Manual*, was considered to be *species incertae sedis* in the eighth edition, due to the lack of any extant type species or reference strain, and subsequently was deleted from Volume 1 of *Bergey's Manual® of Systematic Bacteriology*. However, a similar strain is now available, and this has been widely used in biochemical studies. This organism is clearly not a *Halobacterium* species and is considered *species incertae sedis* in the section devoted to the genus *Haloarcula*.

In Volume 1 of *Bergey's Manual® of Systematic Bacteriology*, *H. volcanii*, *H. vallismortis*, *H. saccharovorum* and *H. pharaonis* were added to the genus *Halobacterium*. Since then, *H. mediterranei* (Rodriguez-Valera et al., 1983), *H. sodomense* (Oren, 1983a) and *H. denitrificans* (Tomlinson et al., 1986) have been described.

H. volcanii and *H. mediterranei* were originally shown to constitute a new taxon by Ross and Grant (1985) (Fig. 25.23) on the basis of polar lipid analyses and nucleic acid hybridization studies, and both species have now been transferred to the new genus *Haloferax* (Torreblanca et al., 1986b). *Halobacterium vallismortis*, now transferred to the new genus *Haloarcula* (Torreblanca et al., 1986b) and *Halobacterium pharaonis*, transferred to the genus *Natronobacterium* (Tindall et al., 1984a, b) were also recognized by Ross and Grant (1985) as taxa separate from other *Halobacterium* species (Fig. 25.23).

The type strains of *H. saccharovorum* together with *H. sodomense* and *H. trapanicum* constitute an additional taxon distinct from other halabacteria (Ross and Grant, 1985) (Fig. 25.23). There is, however, some doubt over the polar lipid composition of these species. Ross and Grant (1985) describe the main polar lipids as C_{20},C_{20} derivatives of PG, PGP, PGS and a sulfated diglycosyl lipid. However, the structure of this glycolipid is uncertain, and Torreblanca et al. (1986a) consider the glycolipid of *H. sodomense* to be different from the others. It is thus not clear whether the lipids of all three species are identical. Torreblanca et al. (1986a) also report that their *H. saccharovorum* strain has a polar lipid composition identical with *H. salinarium* and thus completely different from that reported by Grant and Ross (1986), although both isolates are reputedly the type strain. A similar discrepancy is to be found with regard to *H. trapanicium*, and further lipid work with these organisms is clearly a priority.

That *H. saccharovorum*, *H. trapanicum* and *H. sodomense* constitute a distinct taxon is also supported by the observation that these halobacteria comprise the only group showing *dam* methylation of DNA (Lodwick et al., 1986). Immunological evidence does not support any close relationships between *H. salinarium* and *H. saccharovorum* (Conway de Macario et al., 1986), and these organisms also have different classes of fructose biphosphate aldolases (Dhar and Altekar, 1986). DNA/DNA homologies between *H. saccharovorum*, *H. sodomense* and *H. trapanicum* are between 45 and 52% (Ross and Grant, 1985). Until the structure(s) of the glycolipid(s) possessed by these strains are established and the discrepancies between the type strains of *H. saccharovorum* and *H. trapanicum* held by different culture collections are resolved, it is premature to activate the suggestion of Grant and Ross (1986) that these organisms merit reclassification as separate species within a new genus. Accordingly, they are treated as *species incertae sedis* in this volume of the *Manual*. An additional isolate named *H. trapanicum* (NCMB 784) is clearly not closely related to this group (Ross and Grant, 1985) (Fig. 25.23).

There is also some doubt over whether *H. denitrificans* is a member of the genus *Halobacterium* sensu stricto, and this, too, is treated here as *species incertae sedis*. Only limited chemotaxonomic analyses have been carried out on this isolate, and its relationship to other nitrate-reducing isolates remains to be unequivocably established. Carbon utilization at the expense of nitrate reduction may be characteristic of a wide range of halobacterial types (Javor, 1984). The nitrate-reducing halobacterium recently described by Tindall et al. (1987) also has a polar lipid pattern lacking PGS. The lack of PGS and the presence of sulfated diglycosyl diethers in both cases suggests an affinity with the genus *Haloferax*.

Further Reading

See references provided under "Further Reading" for the order *Halobacteriales*.

List of species of the genus **Halobacterium**

1. **Halobacterium salinarium** (Harrison and Kennedy 1922) Elazari-Volcani 1957, 208, [AL] emend. Larsen 1984, 262. (*Pseudomonas salinaria* Harrison and Kennedy 1922, 120; *Halobacterium halobium* (Petter 1931) Elazari-Volcani 1957, 210; *Halobacterium cutirubrum* (Lochhead 1934) Elazari-Volcani 1957, 209.)

sal.in.ar'i.um. L. adj. *salinarium* belonging or pertaining to salt works.

See the generic description for many features.

Rod-shaped (0.5–1.0 × 1.0–6.0 μm or more in length), but displays a multitude of involution forms, especially in deficient media or at elevated temperatures. Some strains contain gas vacuoles. Motile by tufts of polar flagella. Basically aerobic, but may grow anaerobically in the light, when bacteriorhodopsin is present, or fermentatively in the dark in the presence of arginine.

Best growth occurs at 3.5–4.5 M NaCl; good growth occurs in saturated NaCl (~5.2 M); no growth occurs below 3 M NaCl. Temperature range for growth: 20–55°C; optimum temperature: ~50°C. Mg^{2+} requirement: 0.005–0.05 M. pH range: 5.5–8.0.

Chemoorganotrophic. Amino acids are required for growth. Carbohydrates are not utilized, but stimulation of growth is observed in the presence of glycerol. Starch is not hydrolyzed. Indole-positive. Gelatin is hydrolyzed. Media become alkaline as a result of the deamination or decarboxylation of amino acids. Urease-negative. Arginine dehydrolase present.

Commonly found in proteinaceous products heavily salted with crude solar salt.

The DNA is composed of a major component and a minor component.

The mol% G + C of the major component of the DNA is 66–70.9, and that of the minor component, 57–60 (Bd).

Type strain: NRC 34002 (ATCC 33171; NCMB 764).

Further Comments

See "Taxonomic Comments" for the genus *Halobacterium*.

In view of the large numbers of uncharacterized halobacteria in culture collections with specific epithets of *halobium*, *salinarium* or *cutirubrum*, it is unwise to assume that an organism so named is *H. salinarium* sensu stricto. Only the organisms that have been characterized by chemotaxonomic procedures can definitely be ascribed to this species (Fig. 25.23 Group 1). They include: *H. cutirubrum* CCM 2088 (CCNRLO9); *H. cutirubrum* NRC 34001 (DSM 669); *H. halobium* CCM 2090 (strain Delft); *H. halobium* NCMB 736 (NRC 34007); *H. halobium* NRC 34020 (DSM 670); *H. halobium* NCMB 2080 (DSM 671); *H. salinarium* CCM 2148; *H. salinarium* CCM 2084 (CCNRLO 10); *H. salinarium* ATCC 19700 (DSM 668; Larsen strain 1).

The NRL and R₁ strains extensively used in genetic and biochemical studies are mutants of *H. halobium* NRC 34020. The R_1 strain is deposited as DSM 671 (NCMB 2080). *H. halobium* NRC 817 has also been extensively used in genetic studies (Pfeifer, 1987). This strain is not held by the NRC, the strain number is almost certainly a consequence of a misreading of the DSM catalog, and the strain is probably *H. halobium* NRC 34020 (DSM 670).

Species Incertae Sedis

The taxonomic position of the following species remains to be unequivocally established. See "Taxonomic Comments" for the genus *Halobacterium*.

i. **Halobacterium saccharovorum** Tomlinson and Hochstein 1977, 306.[AL] (Effective publication: Tomlinson and Hochstein 1976, 558.)

sacc.har.o′var.um. L. n. *saccharum* sugar; L. v. *voro* to devour; M.L. neut. n. *saccharovorum* sugar-devourer.

Rod-shaped cells (0.6–1.2 × 2.5 μm). Motile. Gas vacuoles are not present.

Strictly aerobic. Oxidase- and catalase-positive.

Growth occurs in media containing between 1.5 and 5.2 M NaCl; optimum concentration: 3.5–4.5 M NaCl. Mg^{2+} requirement: 0.005 M (Torreblanca et al., 1986b). Temperature range for growth: 30–56°C; optimum: ~50°C.

Chemoorganotrophic. Many sugars (glucose, galactose, mannose, fructose, ribose, maltose, lactose and sucrose) are utilized by a modified Entner-Doudoroff pathway (Tomlinson et al., 1974) with the production of acid. Amino acids are required for growth. Gelatin and starch are not hydrolyzed. Indole is not produced. Relatively insensitive to bacitracin (40 μg ml⁻¹) compared to other halobacteria.

The polar lipids are C_{20},C_{20} derivatives of PG, PGP, PGS and an uncharacterized glycolipid.

Isolated from marine salterns.

The mol% G + C of the DNA is 71.2 (Bd). A minor DNA component has not been detected, although large plasmids have been recorded (Gutierrez et al., 1986).

Type strain: ATCC 29252 (NCMB 2081; DSM 1137).

ii. **Halobacterium sodomense** Oren 1983a, 381.[VP]

so.do.men′se. M.L. adj. *sodomense* pertaining to Sodom, near the Dead Sea.

Rod-shaped cells (0.5 × 2.5–5 μm). Motile by a tuft of polar flagella. Gas vacuoles are not present.

Strictly aerobic. Oxidase- and catalase-positive.

Growth occurs in media containing between 0.5 (in the presence of 1.5–2 M Mg^{2+}) and 4.3 M NaCl; optimum concentration: 1.7–2.5 M NaCl in the presence of 0.6–1.2 M Mg^{2+}. Mg^{2+} requirement: 0.005 M (Torreblanca et al., 1986b), but best growth occurs in 0.6–1.2 M Mg^{2+}. Mg^{2+} can be partially replaced by Ca^{2+}. Temperature range for growth: 20–50°C; optimum temperature: ~40°C.

Chemoorganotrophic. Certain sugars (glucose, fructose, maltose, sucrose) and glycerol are utilized for growth with acid production. Galactose, mannose, ribose and lactose are not utilized. Amino acids are required for growth. The presence of starch or clay minerals (bentonite or kaolin) is necessary for growth. Starch is hydrolyzed. Gelatin is not hydrolyzed. Indole-negative.

The polar lipids are C_{20},C_{20} derivations of PG, PGP, PGS and an uncharacterized glycolipid.

Isolated from the Dead Sea.

The mol% G + C of the DNA is 68 (Bd). A minor DNA component has not been detected, although large plasmids have been reported (Gutierrez et al., 1986).

Type strain: ATCC 33755 (strain RD 26).

iii. **Halobacterium trapanicum** (Petter 1931) Elazari-Volcani 1957, 211,[AL] emend. Ross and Grant 1985, 165. (*Bacterium trapanicum* Petter 1931, 1419.)

tra.pa′ni.cum. M.L. adj. *trapanicum* obtained from salt of Trapani, Italy.

Description limited. Nonmotile, pleomorphic rods (0.7–1.0 × 1.5–3.0 μm). Cells contain low levels of carotenoid, and colonies are pale orange or almost colorless.

Strictly aerobic. Oxidase- and catalase-positive. Chemoorganotrophic. Glucose, fructose and sucrose are utilized with the production of acid. Indole-negative. Starch is not hydrolyzed. Gelatin-negative. Nitrate is reduced to nitrite.

The polar lipids are C_{20},C_{20} derivatives of PG, PGP, PGS and an uncharacterized glycolipid. Isolated from solar salt (Trapani, Sicily).

The mol% G + C of the DNA is 64.3 (Bd). A minor DNA component has not been detected, although large plasmids are present (Pfeifer et al., 1981). ("*H. capanicum*" is a typographical error.)

Type strain: NRC 34021 (NCMB 767).

iv. **Halobacterium denitrificans** Tomlinson, Jahnke and Hochstein 1986, 66.[VP]

de.ni.tri′fi.cans. M.L. part. adj. *denitrificans* denitrifying.

Highly pleomorphic and disk-shaped rods (0.8–1.5 × 2.0–3.0 μm). Nonmotile.

Facultatively anaerobic in the presence of nitrate and nitrite, producing nitrogen gas.

Growth occurs in media containing 1.5–4.5 M NaCl; optimum concentration: 2–3 M NaCl. Temperature range for growth: 30–55°C; optimum temperature: ~50°C.

Chemoorganotrophic, utilizing a wide range of carbon sources (glucose, galactose, fructose, maltose, sucrose, acetate, citrate, fumarate, glycerol, lactate, α-ketoglutarate, malate, succinate and pyruvate) with acid production from sugars. Starch is not hydrolyzed. Gelatin is liquefied. Lipolytic. H_2S is produced from thiosulfate. Urease- and indole-negative. Amino acids are not required for growth.

The polar lipids are described as C_{20},C_{20} derivatives of PG, PGP and a sulfated diglycosyl diether.

Isolated from San Francisco Bay salterns.

The mol% G + C of the DNA is not known.

Type strain: ATCC 35960 (strain S1).

Other Organisms

Halobacterium cutirubrum (NCMB 763).

This organism is clearly distinct from the *H. salinarium* taxon (Fig. 25.23).

The polar lipids are C_{20},C_{20} derivatives of PG, PGP, PGS, TGD-1 and S-DGD (Ross and Grant, 1985).

Originally deposited by J. M. Shewan and probably isolated from salted fish.

The DNA is composed of a major and a minor component. The mol% G + C of the major DNA component is 67.1, and that of the minor, 57.8 (Bd).

Halobacterium trapanicum (NCMB 784).
Halobacterium salinarium (NCMB 786).
Halobacterium halobium (NCMB 777).

These organisms together constitute a taxon distinct from other halobacteria (Fig. 25.23).

The polar lipids are C_{20},C_{20} and C_{25},C_{20} derivatives of PG, PGP, PGS and uncharacterized glycolipids (Ross and Grant, 1985).

Isolated from salted hides or salted fish.

The DNA of *H. salinarium* (NCMB 786) is comprised of a major and a minor component. The mol% G + C of the major DNA component is 69.9, and that of the minor, 60.0 (Bd).

It should be noted that NCMB 777 is listed as equivalent to NRC 34020. There is no doubt that NRC 34020 is a different organism.

Genus II. **Haloarcula** Torreblanca, Rodriguez-Valera, Juez, Ventosa, Kamekura and Kates 1986b, 573^{VP} (Effective publication: Torreblanca, Rodriguez-Valera, Juez, Ventosa, Kamekura and Kates 1986a, 98)

WILLIAM D. GRANT AND HELGE LARSEN

Hal.o.ar.cu'la. Gr. n. *halos* salt; L. fem. n. *arcula* small box; M.L. fem. n. *Haloarcula* salt (-requiring) small box.

Cells may be rods in liquid culture but are extremely pleomorphic, usually flat, 1–3 μm across with a range of shapes from triangles and squares to irregular disks. Resting stages are not known. Gram-negative. Some strains motile. **Aerobic or facultative anaerobic.** Oxidase and catalase-positive. **Extremely halophilic, with growth occurring in media containing 2.0–5.2 M NaCl;** optimum concentration; ~2.5 M NaCl. Temperature range for growth: 30–55°C; optimum temperature; 40–45°C. Mg^{2+} requirement for growth: 0.005 M. Chemoorganotrophic, utilizing many substrates as sources of carbon and energy. **Acids are produced from sugars. Amino acids are not required. The polar lipids are characterized by the presence of C_{20},C_{20} derivatives of TGD-2.**

The mol% G + C of the DNA is 61.9–64.7 (Bd). A minor DNA component may be present.

Type species: *Haloarcula vallismortis* Torreblanca, Rodriguez-Valera, Ventosa, Juez, Kamekura and Kates 1986b, 573.

Further Descriptive Information

In common with other noncoccoid halobacteria, a high molecular weight glycoprotein may be extracted from the cell envelopes of isolates. This glycoprotein is antigenically distinct from those produced by other groups (A. F. Dixon and W. D. Grant, unpublished results).

Cells contain bacterioruberins and, presumably, retinal pigments. The main polar lipids are C_{20},C_{20} derivatives of PG, PGP, PGS and TGD-2 (Evans et al., 1980; Ross and Grant, 1985). Torreblanca et al. (1986a) indicate that small amounts of DGD-2 are also present. It should be noted that Ross and Grant (1985) and Ross et al. (1985) misnamed TGD-1 as TGD-2 and TGD-2 as TGD-1, respectively.

All examples are insensitive to penicillin, chloramphenicol, streptomycin and tetracycline, and sensitive to anisomycin, bacitracin, novobiocin and vibriostat (0/129).

Organisms like these have been found in different thalassohaline and athalassohaline environments including the Dead Sea, salt pools in Death Valley and marine salterns.

Enrichment and Isolation Procedures

These organisms grow well on many of the standard media used for culturing halobacteria, including the one specified in the chapter on *Halobacterium.* There are no known ways of specifically enriching for organisms for this group.

Maintenance Procedures

See under *"Halobacterium."*

Differentiation of the genus **Haloarcula** from other genera

The key to the family *Halobacteriaceae* indicates those characteristics useful for distinguishing *Haloarcula* from other halobacterial genera. The pleomorphic nature of the cells, the use of a wide range of carbon sources and the relatively low Mg^{2+} requirement for growth are not in themselves sufficient to distinguish these organisms from other pleomorphic types, and they can be reliably separated from other halobacteria only by chemotaxonomic procedures. The polar lipids of these organisms characteristically contain TGD-2, and this is the simplest way of distinguishing the group.

Taxonomic Comments

The definition of the genus *Haloarcula* is based on the numerical taxonomic study of Torreblanca et al. (1986a), adopting the generic name first suggested by Javor et al. (1982) for a variety of pleomorphic isolates. The type species of the genus, *H. vallismortis,* was originally classified in the genus *Halobacterium* (Gonzalez et al., 1978; Larsen, 1984). Polar lipid analyses and 16S rRNA/DNA hybridization studies had indicated that this organism and the organism known as *"Halobacterium marismortui"* were closely related and should constitute a separate halobacterial taxon (Ross and Grant, 1985) (Fig. 25.23). Grant and Ross (1986) went on to suggest the generic name "Haloplanus" for these organisms, but they did not formally propose this in the absence of a significant number of phenotypic characteristics that would distinguish this taxon from other pleomorphic and nutritionally versatile halobacteria. Oligonucleotide catalog analyses have confirmed the close relationship of these organisms and a number of Javor's isolates (Nicholson and Fox, 1983).

Haloarcula encompasses phenons F, G, H, I and J of Torreblanca et al. (1986a). Phenon I corresponds to the polar lipid group/16S rRNA group of Grant and Ross (1986) that includes *"Halobacterium marismortui"* (Fig. 25.23). However, the other phenons are not obviously closely related, and they include *H. trapanicum* NCMB 767 (Phenon F). Torreblanca et al. (1986a) also include the organism *"Amoebobacter morrhuae"* considered to be *incertae sedis* in the eighth edition of the *Manual.* Both of these organisms have quite different polar lipid patterns and do not show any significant DNA/16S rRNA homology with *Haloarcula vallismortis* (H. N. M. Ross and W. D. Grant, unpublished observation), and there is no valid reason for including them in the genus *Haloarcula.* *Halobacterium trapanicum* NCMB 767 (NRC 34021) is considered as a *species incertae sedis* in the genus *Halobacterium* in this volume. It is also disturbing that the position of the two pleomorphic isolates of Javor et al. (1982) (*"Haloarcula californiae"* and *"Haloarcula sinaiiensis"*) in the numerical taxonomic study is not consistent with their relatedness as shown by chemotaxonomic studies such as polar lipid analyses (Torreblanca et al., 1986a; H. N. M. Ross and W. D. Grant, unpublished results) and 5S rRNA olignucleotide catalog comparisons (Nicholson and Fox, 1983).

Further Reading

See references provided under "Further Reading" for the order *Halobacteriales.*

Differentiation of the species of the genus **Haloarcula**

Some differential features of the species *H. vallismortis* and *H. hispanica* are given in Table 25.12.

List of species of the genus **Haloarcula**

1. **Haloarcula vallismortis** (Gonzalez et al., 1978) Torreblanca, Rodriguez-Valera, Juez, Ventosa, Kamekura and Kates 1986b, 573.[VP] (Effective publication: Torreblanca et al., 1986a, 98.) (*Halobacterium vallismortis* Gonzalez, Gutiérrez and Ramirez 1978, 710.)

val.lis.mor′tis. L. gen. n. *vallis* of the valley; L. gen. n. *mortis* of death; M.L. fem. n. *vallismortis* of the valley of death; named after Death Valley, California.

See Table 25.12 and the generic description for many features.

Cells are pleomorphic rods (0.6–1.0 × 3–5 µm). Motile.

Optimal growth in media containing 4.3 M NaCl; no growth below 2.5 M. Minimal Mg^{2+} concentration: 0.005 M (Torreblanca et al., 1986a). Temperature range for growth: 20–45°C; optimum temperature: 40°C.

Possibly facultatively anaerobic in the presence of nitrate. A variety of carbohydrates are utilized for growth (glucose, fructose, galatose, sucrose, maltose, trehalose, glycerol and gluconate). Acid is produced from sugars. Indole is produced. Nitrate is reduced, producing gas. Starch is hydrolyzed. H_2S is produced from cysteine.

Isolated from salt pools in Death Valley.

The mol% G + C of the DNA is 64.7 (Bd). A minor DNA component has not been detected, although large plasmids are present (Gutiérrez et al., 1986).

Type strain: ATCC 29715 (NCMB 2082) (strain J.F.54).

2. **Haloarcula hispanica** Juez, Rodriguez-Valera, Ventosa and Kushner 1986b, 573.[VP] (Effective publication: Juez, Rodriguez-Valera, Ventosa and Kushner 1986a, 75.)

his.pan′i.cus M.L. adj. *hispanicus* Spanish.

See Table 25.12 and generic description for many features.

Cells are small pleomorphic rods (0.5–1.0 × 0.3 µm). Motile by polar flagella.

Growth occurs in media containing 2–5.2 M NaCl. Minimal concentration is 0.005 M (Torreblanca et al., 1986a). Temperature range for growth: 25–50°C; optimum temperature: 35–40°C.

Possibly facultatively anaerobic in the presence of nitrate. Utilizes a range of compounds as sole carbon and energy sources (glucose, lactose, sucrose, glycerol, mannitol, sorbitol, acetate, citrate, lactate, malate, pyruvate, succinate, arginine, glutamine and lysine). Acids are produced from sugars. Starch is hydrolyzed. Some strains hydrolyze casein. Indole is variable. Nitrate is reduced with gas production. Susceptible to only high concentration of bacitracin (40 µg ml[−1]).

Isolated from marine salterns in Spain.

The mol% G + C of the DNA is 62.7 (T_m).

Type strain: ATCC 33960 (strain Y 27).

Other Organisms

The taxonomic status of the following organisms is uncertain because of a lack of detailed descriptive information.

See "Taxonomic Comments" for the genus *Haloarcula*.

i. *"Halobacterium marismortui"* Elazari-Volcani 1957, 210.

This organism was originally isolated from the Dead Sea as *"Flavobacterium marismortui"* (Elazari-Volcani, 1940). Its main distinguishing features were the production of acid from fructose, mannose, glucose and glycerol and the reduction of nitrate. In the eighth edition of the *Manual* the organism was relegated to *species incertae sedis* due to the lack of any extant type or reference species.

In 1970, Ginzburg et al. isolated a similar organism from the same source. This strain was originally referred to as *"Halobacterium* of the Dead Sea," but since 1978 it has become known as *"H. marismortui."* The original *"H. marismortui"* has some similarity to *Haloarcula vallismortis,* but the latter organism differs by virtue of its motility, the production of indole and its ability to hydrolyze starch (Gonzalez et al., 1978).

The Ginzburg strain has an identical polar lipid pattern to *H. vallismortis,* and the DNA/DNA homology between the two strains is 39% (Ross and Grant, 1985). Oligonucleotide catalog analysis of 5S rRNA has also shown considerable similarity between the two strains, but it has not shown complete identity (Nicholson and Fox, 1983). However, the Ginzburg strain does not completely fit the original description by Elazari-Volcani (A. Oren, personal communication) and is morphologically distinct, as a nonmotile extremely pleomorphic isolate (Fig. 25.29) that never produces rods, whereas *H. vallismortis* is usually rod-shaped and vigorously motile.

Further work is required to establish whether the two organisms can be considered different strains of the same genus, as suggested by Torreblanca et al. (1986a). The Ginzburg strain has been extensively used in biochemical analyses (e.g. Werber et al., 1986).

The polar lipids are C_{20},C_{20} derivatives of PG, PGP, PGS and TGD-2 (Evans et al., 1980; Ross and Grant, 1985).

The DNA is composed of a major and a minor component. The mol% G + C of the major component is 61.8, and that of the minor component, 54.7% (Ross and Grant, 1985).

Reference strain: ATCC 43049 (strain Ginzburg).

ii. *"Haloarcula californiae"* Javor, Requadt and Stoeckenius 1982, 1532.

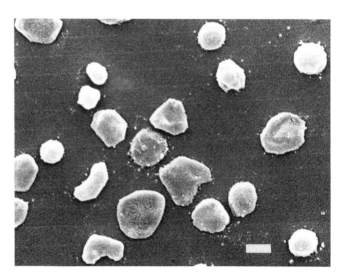

Figure 25.29. *"Halobacterium marismortui"* (ATCC 43049), grown at 37°C in the medium described under *"Halobacterium." Bar,* 1 µm. (Prepared and photographed by C. F. Norton.)

Table 25.12.
Characteristics differentiating **H. hispanica** *and* **H. vallismortis**[a]

Characteristic	H. hispanica	H. vallismortis
Tween hydrolysis	+	−
Gelatin hydrolysis	+	−
Urea hydrolysis	−	+
Sensitive to bacitracin (<40 µg ml[−1])	−	+

[a] Symbols: +, 90% or more of strains are positive; −, 90% or more of strains are negative.

Originally described largely on the basis of its unusual angular pleomorphic cells, with rectangular and square forms being common. Torreblanca et al. (1986a) described the organism as being nonproteolytic but lipolytic, producing H₂S from thiosulfate, reducing nitrates, and being amylase-negative. Amino acids are not required for growth, and acid is produced from sugars. The polar lipid composition is similar to that of *H. vallismortis,* and oligonucleotide catalog analysis of 5S rRNA indicates a close relationship with this organism and *"Halobacterium marismortui"* (Nicholson and Fox, 1983).

Isolated from a Californian saltern.

The mol% G + C of the DNA is stated as 68 (Javor et al., 1982).

Type strain: ATCC 33799.

iii. *"Haloarcula sinaiiensis"* Javor, Requadt and Stoeckenius 1982, 1532.

Stated as being different from *"H. californiae"* on the basis of restriction endonuclease digest patterns. Does not group with any other in the numerical taxonomic analysis of Torreblanca et al. (1986a). Oligonucleotide catalog analysis of 5S rRNA indicates a relationship with *"H. vallismortis,"* *"Halobacterium marismortui"* and *"Haloarcula californiae"* (Nicholson and Fox, 1983). Has the same polar lipid patterns as these organisms.

Isolated from a Red Sea sabkha.

Type strain: ATCC 33800.

iv. *"Amoebobacter morrhuae"* Penso 1947, 593.

Is referred to as *species incertae sedis* in the eighth edition of the *Manual.* Undoubtedly a halobacterium, although originally classified as a phototroph. The organism does not group with any other in the numerical taxonomic analysis of Torreblanca et al. (1986a). The polar lipid pattern is unusual (Torreblanca et al., 1986a), and 16S rRNA/DNA hybridization studies have failed to indicate any close relationship with any other halobacterium included in the study (H. N. M. Ross and W. D. Grant, unpublished results). However, the oligonucleotide catalog of the 16S rRNA is reported as only one base different from *H. salinarium* (Fox et al., 1980). Indole-positive. Amylase-, gelatinase- and sulfide-negative. Sugars are not utilized (H. N. M. Ross and W. D. Grant, unpublished results).

Isolated from salted cod.

The DNA has a major and a minor component. The mol% G + C of the major DNA component is 69.7, and that of the minor component, 57.3.

Type strain: NRC 51001.

v. Walsby's square bacterium Walsby 1980, 69.

Square bacteria were originally seen in brine from a sabkha in the Southern Sinai (Walsby, 1981), and since then they have been seen in a variety of other saline habitats in Israel, Calfornia and Senegal. The bacteria are characterized as flat, perfectly square boxes (Fig. 25.30) with

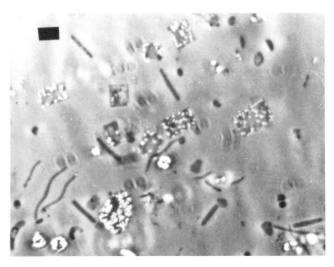

Figure 25.30. Phase-contrast light micrograph of a field of square bacteria. *Bar,* 10 μm. (Photograph supplied by A. E. Walsby.) (Reproduced with permission from A. E. Walsby, Nature (London) *283:* 69–71, 1980, ©Macmillan Magazines Ltd.)

sides 2–5 μm long and overall thickness 0.1–0.2 μm. The best analogy as to the shape and form of these organisms is that of the postage stamp, and sheets containing up to 64 have been described (Kessel and Cohen, 1982). The organisms are nonmotile and gas-vacuolate. To date, square bacteria have not been grown in culture, although other halobacteria can be readily isolated from such habitats. It is possible that the shape is determined by environmental factors. There is no doubt that these organisms are halobacteria, since they contain bacterioruberins and retinal pigments (Stoeckenius, 1981). They also have a hexagonal pattern of subunits on the cell surface similar to those found in other halobacteria (Kessel et al., 1985).

These organisms are difficult to see with the light microscope but are probably common in saline environments throughout the world. In the absence of any convincing laboratory cultures, it is not possible to tell whether more than one type exists. There is no a priori reason that these should be associated with the genus *Haloarcula* other than the observation that *Haloarcula* species do occasionally produce squares in culture, although the sheets of cells characteristic of Walsby's organisms have not been seen in any of the laboratory cultures of pleomorphic organisms.

Genus III. **Haloferax** *Torreblanca, Rodriguez-Valera, Juez, Ventosa, Kamekura and Kates 1986b, 573*[VP] *(Effective publication: Torreblanca, Rodriguez-Valera, Juez, Ventosa, Kamekura and Kates 1986a, 98)*

WILLIAM D. GRANT AND HELGE LARSEN

Hal.o.fe′rax. Gr. n. *halos* salt; L. adj. *ferax* fertile; M.L. neut. n. salt (-requiring) and fertile.

Cells extremely pleomorphic, most commonly flattened disks or cups (1–3 × 2–3 μm). Resting stages are not known. Gram-negative. **Motile, motility often difficult to observe.** One species is gas-vacuolate. Colonies have a mucoid appearance. **Strictly aerobic.** Oxidase- and catalase-positive. **Extremely halophilic, with growth occurring in media containing 1.5–4.5 M Na⁺**; optimum concentration: 2.5 M Na⁺. Temperature range for growth: 30–55°C; optimum temperature: ~35°C. Mg²⁺ requirement for growth: 0.02 M. Chemoorganotrophic utilizing many substrates as sources of carbon and energy. **Amino acids are not required. Acid is produced from sugars. Polyhydroxybutyrate is accumulated under certain conditions.**

The polar lipids are characterized by the presence of C₂₀,C₂₀ derivatives of S-DGD-1 and the absence of PGS.

The mol% of the G + C is 59.5–64.0 (Bd). A minor DNA component may be present.

Type species: Haloferax volcanii (Mullakhanbhai and Larsen 1975) Torreblance, Rodriguez-Valera, Juez, Ventosa, Kamekura and Kates 1986b, 573.

Further Descriptive Information

Rod-shaped cells are rare even under optimal conditions. In common with other halobacteria, a large glycoprotein can be extracted from cell envelopes (Rodriguez-Valera et al., 1983; Juez et al., 1986a). This is serologically distinct from the glycoproteins possessed by other taxa (A. F. Dixon and W. D. Grant, unpublished results). Cells lyse in hypotonic solutions but are more stable than other halobacterial cells, remaining intact in 0.5 M NaCl.

Cells contain bacterioruberins and retinal pigments but may not contain bacteriorhodopsin (Oren and Shilo, 1981; Oren, 1983b). The main polar lipids are C_{20},C_{20} derivatives of PG, PGP, DGD-1 and S-DGD-1 (Ross and Grant, 1985; Torreblanca et al., 1986a).

All examples are insensitive to penicillin, chloramphenicol, streptomycin and tetracycline and sensitive to anisomycin, bacitracin, novobiocin and vibriostat reagent (0/129).

Organisms like these probably make up a significant fraction of the microbial population of the Dead Sea and are presumably to be found in other high Mg^{2+} environments. However, they are also to be found in thallasohaline salterns.

Enrichment and Isolation Procedures

Organisms of this group have been isolated from the Dead Sea and from Spanish Mediterranean salterns. *H. volcanii* was originally enriched in a complex medium containing 0.2 M Mg^{2+} and 4 M NaCl (Mullakhanbhai and Larsen, 1975), but many other halobacteria will grow in this medium. No systematic attempts have been made to devise a suitable enrichment medium, but in view of the high Mg^{2+} tolerance (>1 M), relatively low NaCl requirement (<1 M), and utilization of carbohydrates, by the organisms, such an enrichment medium should not be difficult to construct. Rodriguez-Valera et al. (1980) have used media with simple carbon sources in a medium whose composition is based on seawater supplemented with NaCl. High Mg^{2+} brines may be directly spread on agar media, incubating plates in sealed plastic bags to prevent desiccation. Colonies appear after 3-14 days at 37°C.

Maintenance Procedures

See under "Halobacterium."

Differentiation of the genus **Haloferax** from other genera

The key to the family *Halobacteriaceae* indicates those characteristics useful for distinguishing *Haloferax* from other halobacterial genera. Although *Haloferax* species have a relatively high Mg^{2+} requirement, they can be reliably separated from other halobacteria only by chemotaxonomic procedures. The polar lipids of these organisms characteristically contain S-DGD-1 and its unsulfated derivative, lacking PGS, and this is the simplest way of distinguishing the group.

Taxonomic Comments

Two of the three species in the genus, *H. volcanii* and *H. mediterranei*, were previously classified in the genus *Halobacterium*. However, a comparison of oligonucleotide catalogs of halobacteria had indicated that *Haloferax volcanii (Halobacterium volcanii)* was likely to constitute a new taxon (Fox et al., 1980). Further 16S rRNA/DNA hybridization studies and polar lipid analyses (Tindall et al., 1984a; Ross and Grant, 1985) (Fig. 25.23) supported this view and confirmed the relationship between *H. volcanii* and *H. mediterranei*. The immunological analysis of Conway de Macario et al. (1986) and the fructose biphosphate aldolase study of Dhar and Altekar (1986) provide further supportive evidence. *H. volcanii* has 38% DNA/DNA homology with *H. mediterranei* (Ross and Grant, 1985). Another species, *H. gibbonsii*, has since been added to the genus (Juez et al., 1986a). Torreblanca et al. (1986a) have carried out an extensive numerical taxonomic study of halobacteria, and it is of some concern that *H. volcanii*, *H. mediterranei* and *H. gibbonsii* do not constitute a clearly circumscribed taxon on the basis of 102 phenotypic characteristics, although the chemotaxonomic evidence for such a taxon is very strong.

Further Reading

See references provided under "Further Reading" for the order *Halobacteriales*.

Differentiation of the species of the genus **Haloferax**

Some differential features of the species *H. volcanii*, *H. mediterranei* and *H. gibbonsii* are given in Table 25.13.

List of species of the genus **Haloferax**

1. **Haloferax volcanii** (Mullakhanbhai and Larsen 1975) Torreblanca, Rodriguez-Valera, Juez, Ventosa, Kamekura and Kates 1986b, 573.[VP] (Effective publication: Torreblanca et al. 1986a, 98.) [*Halobacterium volcanii* Mullakhanbhai and Larsen 1975, 213.]

vol.can'i.i. M.L. gen. n. *volcanii* of Volcani; named after Israel microbiologist B. E. Volcani, discoverer of life in the Dead Sea.

See Table 25.13 and the generic description for many features.

Cells are extremely pleomorphic, frequently disk- or cup-shaped even under optimal conditions (1-2 × 2-3 μm) (Fig. 25.31). In young cultures, many elongated disks occur, some of which may rotate around their long axis. Flagella have not been demonstrated, and the movement is different from that of the polarly flagellated strains of halobacteria.

Best growth occurs in media containing 1.5-2.5 M NaCl; 5 M NaCl is inhibitory. Minimal Mg^{2+} concentration: 0.02 M (Torreblanca et al., 1986a); tolerant to 1.5 M Mg^{2+}. Optimum growth temperature: 45°C.

Chemoorganotrophic. Growth occurs on sugars as the sole source of carbon (Larsen, 1984); acid is produced from glucose and, by implication, from a variety of sugars (Rodriguez-Valera et al., 1983). Indole is produced. H_2S is produced from thiosulfate. Nitrate is reduced to nitrite.

Found in the Dead Sea.

The DNA is composed of a major component and a minor compo-

Table 25.13.
Characteristics differentiating **Haloferax volcanii, H. mediterranei** *and* **H. gibbonsii**[a]

Characteristic	1. *H. volcanii*	2. *H. mediterranei*	3. *H. gibbonsii*
Exopolysaccharide production in liquid	−	+	−
Presence of gas vacuoles	−	+	−
Starch hydrolysis	−	+	−
Tween hydrolysis	−	+	+
Casein hydrolysis	−	+	+
Nitrate reduction	+	+	−
Gelatin hydrolysis	−	+	−

[a] Symbols: −, 90% or more of strains are negative; +, 90% or more of strains are positive.

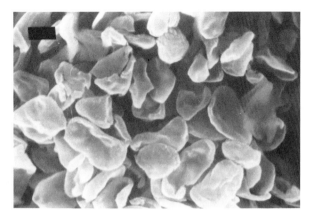

Figure 25.31. *Haloferax volcanii* strain DS2 (NCMB 2012), grown at 30°C in a medium consisting of (g/l of distilled water): NaCl, 125.0; MgCl$_2$·6H$_2$O, 50.0; K$_2$SO$_4$, 5.0; CaCl$_2$·6H$_2$O, 0.2; yeast extract (Difco), 5.0; and tryptone (Difco), 5.0; at pH 6.8. The culture was photographed at the end of the exponential growth phase. *Bar*, 1 μm. (Prepared by G. Bentzen; photographed by the Laboratory of Clinical Electron Microscopy, University of Bergen.)

nent. Plasmids are present (Pfeifer et al., 1981; Gutiérrez et al., 1986).

The mol% G + C of the major DNA component is 63.4 (T_m) and 66.5 (Bd), and that of the minor component, 55.3 (Bd).

Type strain: NCMB 2012 (strain DS2).

2. **Haloferax mediterranei** (Rodriguez-Valera, Juez and Kushner 1983) Torreblanca, Rodriguez-Valera, Juez, Ventosa, Kamekura and Kates 1987, 179.[VP] (Effective publication: Torreblanca, Rodriguez-Valera, Juez, Ventosa, Kamekura and Kates, 1986a, 97.) (*Halobacterium mediterranei* Rodriguez-Valera, Juez and Kushner 1983, 379).

me.di.ter.ra′ne.i. L. gen. n. *mediterranei* of the Mediterranean Sea.

See Table 25.13 and the generic description for many features.

Colonies are pink and highly mucoid after 5–7 days at 37°C. Cells are pleomorphic rods (0.5 × 2 μm). During the late exponential phase and during stationary phase, gas vacuoles are produced. Motile by a tuft of polar flagella.

Growth occurs in media containing 1–5.2 M NaCl. Minimal Mg^{2+} concentration: 0.02 M (Torreblanca et al., 1986a). Temperature range for growth: 25–45°C; optimum temperature: 35–37°C.

Chemoorganotrophic, able to use a wide variety of compounds as carbon and energy sources (glucose, sucrose, fructose, lactose, glycerol, maltose, mannitol, sorbitol, xylose, arabinose, succinate, malate, lactate, pyruvate, citrate, acetate, glutamate, lysine and arginine). Utilization of sugars produces acidification of the medium. Nitrate is reduced. Indole-positive. H$_2$S is not produced. Starch and gelatin are hydrolyzed.

Produces bacteriocins (halocins) active against a range of other halobacteria (Rodriguez-Valera et al., 1982). Resistant to relatively high levels of bacitracin (40 μg ml^{-1}).

Isolated from marine salterns in Spain.

The mol% G + C of the DNA is 60.0 (T_m) and 62.2 (Bd). A minor DNA component has not been detected, but large plasmids are present (Gutiérrez et al., 1986).

Type strain: CCM 3361 (ATCC 33500; NCMB 2177) (strain R-4).

3. **Haloferax gibbonsii** Juez, Rodriguez-Valera, Ventosa and Kushner 1986b, 575.[VP] (Effective publication: Juez, Rodriguez-Valera, Ventosa and Kushner 1986a, 75.)

gib.bon.si′i. M.L. gen. n. *gibbonsii* of Gibbons; named for the Canadian microbiologist, N. E. Gibbons, one of the pioneers in the study of halobacteria.

See Table 23.13 and generic description for many features.

Cells are short pleomorphic rods (0.4 × 0.5–2.5 μm). Motile by tufts of polar flagella.

Growth occurs in media containing 1.5–5.2 M NaCl; optimum concentration: 3–4 M NaCl at 40°C and 2–3 M NaCl at 30°C. Temperature range for growth: 25–55°C, optimum temperature: ∼37°C. Mg^{2+} requirement for growth: 0.2 M.

Chemoorganotrophic, acid is produced from a wide range of sugars (arabinose, fructose, galactose, glucose, maltose, mannose, sucrose and xylose). Indole-positive. H$_2$S is produced from thiosulfate. Starch is not hydrolyzed. Tween 20, 40, 60 and 80 are hydrolyzed. A few strains hydrolyze gelatin and reduce nitrate.

Isolated from marine salterns in Spain.

The mol% G + C of the DNA is 61.8 (T_m).

Type strain: ATCC 33959 (strain MA 2.38).

Genus IV. **Halococcus** *Schoop 1935, 817*[AL]

HELGE LARSEN

Hal.o.coc′cus. Gr. n. *halo, halos* the sea, salt; Gr. n. *coccus* a berry; M.L. masc. n. *Halococcus* salt-coccus.

Cocci, 0.8–1.5 μm in diameter, occurring in pairs, tetrads, sarcina packets, or irregular clusters (Fig. 25.32). **Divide by septation.** Nonsporeforming. **Stains mainly Gram-negative with at least some cells Gram-positive. Nonmotile. Strictly aerobic.** Colonies are red to orange due to carotenoids in the cells. Oxidase- and catalase-positive. Chemoorganotrophic. **Require at least 2.5 M NaCl for growth and 3.5–4.5 M NaCl for best growth.** Optimum temperature: 30–37°C. No lysis occurs in hypotonic solutions.

The mol% G + C of the DNA is 61–66 (T_m).

Type species: *Halococcus morrhuae* (Klebahn 1919) Kocur and Hodgkiss 1973, 154.

Further Descriptive Information

Red, extremely halophilic cocci have a thick (30–60 nm), rigid cell wall and form septa, not constrictions, during division (Steensland and Larsen, 1971; Kocur et al., 1972) (Fig. 25.33). The wall material contains, in addition to simple sugars, amino sugars, uronic acids and glycine and forms a complex heteroglycan which is highly sulfated, in some cases sulfonated, and apparently responsible for the rigid structure of the wall and the resistance against lysis in hypotonic solutions (Reistad, 1970, 1975; Steber and Schleifer, 1975).

The main lipids are both C$_{20}$,C$_{20}$ and C$_{20}$,C$_{25}$ derivatives of PG, PGP, TGD-2 and a sulfated diglycosyl glycolipid, probably S-DGD-1. (Kates, 1978; Hunter et al., 1981; Ross and Grant, 1985) The cells contain carotenoids which are of the C$_{50}$ bacterioruberin type, menaquinones, not ubiquinones, and retinal, as also reported for other halobacteria (Kushwaha et al., 1974; Collins et al., 1981).

As in the case of other halobacteria, the proteins are acidic (Reistad, 1970), enzymes are activated by salt (Larsen, 1967), and structural proteinaceous units such as the cell membrane disintegrate in hypotonic solutions (Reistad, 1970).

The mol% G + C of the DNA was determined for nine strains and found to vary from 60.5 to 65.8 (Kocur and Boháček, 1972). Some strains have been reported to contain satellite DNA (31% of total DNA); the mol% G + C of the major DNA component was 67, and that of the minor component, 59 (Moore and McCarthy, 1969). Grant and Ross (1985) reported that the DNA of the type strain contained a major and a minor component.

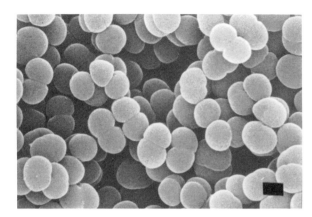

Figure 25.32. *Halococcus morrhuae* strain 24 (DSM 1309; CCM 2226), grown at 30°C in the same medium as listed in the legend to Figure 25.25. *Bar*, 1 μm. (Prepared by A. L. Ustad; photographed by Department of Biophysics, Norwegian Institute of Technology, Trondheim).

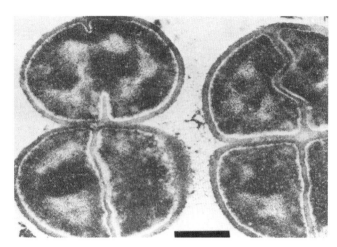

Figure 25.33. *Halococcus morrhuae* strain 24 (DSM 1309; CCM 2226). Thin section of cells at the end of the exponential growth phase. *Bar*, 1 μm. (Reproduced with permission from H. Steensland and H. Larsen, Kgl. Norske Vidensk. Selsk. Skrifter No. 8, Universitetsforlaget, pp. 1–5, 1971,©The Norwegian Research Council for Science and the Humanities, Oslo.)

A yeast extract-salt medium similar to that described for other halobacteria (see under Footnote * under "Genus I. *Halobacterium*") is a suitable growth medium. Good aeration must be provided. Growth is slow even under optimum conditions, and a generation time of ~14 h is the best that has been reported. The strains so far examined have a complex nutrition. A number of amino acids, purines and pyrimidines are required for growth (Onishi et al., 1965), as reported also for some other strains of halobacteria.

The slow growth on laboratory media may be a reason why these halobacteria seem to be less frequently encountered in natural samples. They are, however, found in the same places as other halobacteria, in strongly saline natural lakes and marine salterns, and have been shown to cause spoilage of salted fish and hides. They have also been isolated from seawater (Rodriguez-Valera et al., 1979b) and hypersaline soils (Quesada et al., 1982).

Like other halobacteria, they are insensitive to antibiotics such as penicillin, chloramphenicol, streptomycin and tetracycline, but they are sensitive to bacitracin, anisomycin and novobiocin (H. N. M. Ross and W. D. Grant, unpublished results; Hilpert et al., 1981; Bonelo et al., 1984).

Enrichment and Isolation Procedures

The methods are the same as those given for the genus *Halobacterium*.

Maintenance Procedures

See under *"Halobacterium."*

Differentiation of the genus **Halococcus** *from other genera*

The key to the family *Halobacteriaceae* indicates those characteristics useful for distinguishing *Halococcus* from other genera.

Taxonomic Comments

These organisms are commonly said to have been described first by Farlow (1880), who proposed the name *Sarcina morrhuae* for some colony-forming matter on salt fish, appearing microscopically as tetrad-forming cocci. A reevaluation of the view that Farlow dealt with the red, extremely halophilic cocci is in order, however. Farlow explicitly referred to his coccoid material as "always colorless"; moreover, the cocci measured 5–8 μm in diameter, the tetrads were "surrounded by a thin hyaline envelope," and Farlow never had this cryptically described material in culture. Farlow's description makes it very difficult, if not impossible, to accept him as the discoverer of the red, extremely halophilic cocci. Farlow (1886) later changed the name to *Sarcina litoralis* Poulsen 1879, allegedly for reasons of priority, but Poulsen's description shows rather convincingly that the material he studied was also not the red, extremely halophilic cocci. The name *S. litoralis* was occasionally used in the later literature for these organisms, however.

After Farlow's work, several authors described the occurrence of red-colored cocci from salty material, mostly salted fish. These might well have been of the kind included in this text under the genus *Halococcus*, but they could also have been other kinds of cocci or even involution forms of representatives of the genus *Halobacterium*.

The first to describe the red, extremely halophilic cocci in a satisfactory manner was Klebahn (1919). He isolated and studied several strains from salted fish and proposed two species, *Sarcina morrhuae* Farlow and *Micrococcus (Diplococcus) morrhuae* sp. nov.

Petter (1932) argued that the red, extremely halophilic cocci are variable in that they tend to form packets or pairs and, depending on the growth conditions, vary in size. She therefore proposed that only one species should be retained, *S. morrhuae* Klebahn, giving recognition to Klebahn as being the proper discoverer of these organisms. In 1957, however, in the seventh edition of the *Manual,* two species, *S. litoralis* Poulsen and *M. morrhuae* Klebahn, were listed, and both were described as red, extremely halophilic cocci.

The proposal by Schoop (1935) to accord the red, extremely halophilic cocci generic rank was implemented by Kocur and Hodgkiss (1973). They investigated 22 strains of these organisms and found reasons to propose only one species, *Halococcus morrhuae* (Farlow 1880) comb. nov. This was adopted in the eighth edition of the *Manual* (Gibbons, 1974), and the genus and species were included on the Approved Lists of Bacterial Names in 1980. However, in view of the above discussion, it seems right that Klebahn's name should replace Farlow's to give the more proper designation *Halococcus morrhuae* (Klebahn 1919) Kocur and Hodgkiss 1973, 154.

In a numerical taxonomic analysis of a number of strains of red extremely halophilic cocci, Colwell et al. (1979) found that the strains were less uniform in their characteristics than the strains of *Halobacterium* studied, yet there was no particular reason to distinguish between the strains at a species level. A nucleic acid hybridization study of a more limited number of isolates by Ross and Grant (1985) supports this view. On the basis of present knowledge, it therefore seems best to recognize only a single species in the genus *Halococcus*.

Further Reading

See references provided under "Further Reading" for the family *Halobacteriaceae*.

List of species of the genus **Halococcus**

1. **Halococcus morrhuae** (Klebahn 1919) Kocur and Hodgkiss 1973, 154.[AL] (Not *Sarcina litoralis* Poulsen 1879, 254; not *Sarcina morrhuae* Farlow 1880, 974.) (*Sarcina morrhuae* Klebahn 1919, 38; *Micrococcus (Diplococcus) morrhuae* Klebahn 1919, 42; *Halococcus litoralis* Schoop 1935, 817.)

morr.hu'ae. M.L. n. *morrhuae* from the specific epithet of the codfish, *Gadus morhua* L. (often misspelled *morrhua*); M.L. gen. n. *morrhuae* of the codfish.

The morphology is the same as that described for the genus.

Strictly aerobic. Amino acids are needed for growth and are also used as a source of energy. Glucose is not used as a main source of carbon for growth, and acid and gas are not produced from glucose when tested for by the usual methods. Nitrate is reduced to nitrite without production of gas. Catalase- and oxidase-positive. H_2S is usually produced from thiosulfate and frequently from cysteine. Urease-negative. Some strains produce indole and hydrolyze gelatin, starch and esters.

Optimum pH: 7.2 Some growth occurs at pH 5.5; no growth occurs at pH 8.

Other characteristics are the same as those described for the genus.

The mol% G + C of the DNA is 61–66 (T_m). Appreciable amounts of satellite DNA may occur (mol% G + C of the DNA is 57–59 (Bd)).

Type strain: ATCC 17082 (NCMB 787; DSM 1307).

Genus V. **Natronobacterium** *Tindall, Ross and Grant 1984b, 355* [VP]
(Effective publication: Tindall, Ross and Grant 1984a, 41)

WILLIAM D. GRANT

Na.tro.no.bac.te'ri.um. Gr. n. *natrun* soda, salt; Gr. n. *bakterion* a small rod; M.L. neut. n. *Natronobacterium* soda rod.

Rods in liquid culture in the exponential phase of growth, usually $0.5–1.0 \times 2–15$ μm. Resting stages are not known. Gram-negative. Some strains motile by a tuft of polar flagella. **Strictly aerobic.** Oxidase- and catalase-positive. **Extremely halophilic with growth occurring in media containing 2–5.2 M (saturation) NaCl;** optimum concentration: 3.5 M. Optimum temperature: 35–40°C; maximum: ~50°C; minimum: 20–25°C. **Alkaliphilic with growth occurring at pH 8.5–11.0;** optimum growth occurs at about pH 9.5 at 37°C in media containing 3.5 M NaCl. Chemoorganotrophic. **Glycolipids are absent.**

The DNA is sometimes composed of a major component and a minor component. The latter makes up 10–30% of the total DNA (Bd). Strains that have a minor component usually harbor a large plasmid (~144 kb). The mol% G + C of the major component is 61.2–64.6 (Bd), and that of the minor component, 49.7–51.9 (Bd).

Type species: *Natronobacterium gregoryi* Tindall, Ross and Grant 1984b, 355.[VP]

Further Descriptive Information

Rod-shaped cells are only produced in liquid media under conditions optimal for growth. Even under optimal conditions it is not unusual to see rods of different length and diameters. Cells grown on agar media are spherical; usually 1–1.5 mm in diameter. A large antigenically distinct glycoprotein can be extracted from cell envelopes (A. F. Dixon and W. D. Grant, unpublished results).

Cells contain bacterioruberins and retinal pigments but do not contain bacteriorhodopsin (Bivin and Stoeckenius, 1986). Glycolipids are absent. The polar lipids are based on 2,3-di-*O*-phytanyl-sn-glycerol (C_{20}, C_{20}) and 2-*O*-sesterterpanyl-3-*O*-phytanyl glycerol (C_{25}, C_{20}) diethers (Tindall et al., 1984a). Small amounts of 2,3-di-*O*-sesterterpanyl glycerol (C_{25}, C_{25}) diethers may be present in some strains (Tindall, 1985). Glycolipids are absent. All species have very similar polar lipid patterns, differing only in the presence or absence of a few minor phospholipids (Morth and Tindall, 1985). The main polar lipids are C_{20}, C_{20} and C_{25}, C_{20} derivatives of PG and PGP, with small amounts of one or two uncharacterized phospholipids (Morth and Tindall, 1985).

All species are iinsensitive to penicillin, chloramphenicol, streptomycin and tetracycline and sensitive to anisomycin, bacitracin, novobiocin and vibriostat reagent (0/129).

Organisms like these make up a significant fraction of the microbial population of the Wadi Natrun, Egypt; Lake Magadi, Kenya; and Owens Lake, California. In Lake Magadi, the red of the brine is almost entirely due to a bloom of these organisms. Numbers may reach $10^7–10^8$ cells ml^{-1}. It is to be assumed that very saline soda lakes elsewhere in the world harbor these organisms.

Enrichment and Isolation Procedures

Natronobacterium species may be readily isolated by directly spreading red-pigmented brines from soda lakes or soda salterns on the agar medium (Tindall et al., 1980), which is an alkaline low Mg^{2+} modification of the medium of Payne et al. (1960),* incubating plates in sealed plastic bags to prevent desiccation. Colonies appear after 3–14 days at 37°C. Enrichment is also possible in liquid media of the same composition in shake culture. *N. pharaonis* was originally isolated from the Wadi Natrun by enrichment in a medium containing casamino acids, trisodiuim citrate and glutamic acid, adjusted to pH 10.0 (Soliman and Trüper, 1982). The yeast extract and casein hydrolysate medium of Morth and Tindall (1985) also gives good results.

There are no known selective conditions that will discriminate between *N. pharaonis*, *N. gregoryi* and *N. magadii*.

Maintenance Procedures

See under "*Halobacterium*."

---

*Composition is (in g/l tap water): NaCl, 250.0; Na$_2$CO$_3$·10H$_2$O, 50.0; trisodium citrate, 3.0; KCl, 2.0; MgSO$_4$·7H$_2$O, 1.0; yeast extract, 10.0; and casamino acids, 7.5. Fe^{2+} and Mn^{2+} are added as trace elements at 10 and 0.1 ppm, respectively. The medium has a pH of 10.5 initially but equilibrates to 9.5. The NaCl and Na$_2$CO$_3$·10H$_2$O are autoclaved separately from the other components. Agar media should contain 2% (w/v) agar.

Differentiation of the genus **Natronobacterium** from other genera

The genus *Natronobacterium* is separated from all other rod-shaped halobacteria by its alkaliphily and very low Mg^{2+} requirements. It is readily distinguished from *Natronococcus* by the rod-shaped morphology of the cells in young liquid cultures, the presence of glycoprotein in the cell wall, and the lysis of cells in distilled water.

Taxonomic Comments

The three species of *Natronobacterium* were originally described as having identical polar lipid patterns (Tindall et al., 1984a; Ross and Grant, 1985), but slight differences in minor phospholipid components between the species have now been established (Morth and Tindall, 1985).

N. pharaonis has a DNA/DNA homology of 45% with *N. magadii* and 32% with *N. gregoryi*. The type strain of *N. pharaonis* was originally iso-lated from the Wadi Natrun by Soliman and Trüper (1982). The *N. pharaonis* (SP1) isolate from Lake Magadi (Tindall et al., 1980) has 96% DNA/DNA homology with the Wadi Natrun isolate (Tindall et al., 1984a).

A complete 16S rRNA sequence for *N. magadii* (H. N. M. Ross and W. D. Grant, unpublished results), together with oligonucleotide catalog studies of *N. pharaonis* (SP1) (E. Stackebrandt, personal communication) and 16S rRNA/DNA hybridization studies (Fig. 25.23), has established *Natronobacterium* as a distinct halobacterial group.

Further Reading

See references provided under "Further Reading" for the order *Halobacteriales.*

Differentiation of the species of the genus **Natronobacterium**

Some differential features of the species *N. gregoryi, N. magadii* and *N. pharaonis* are given in Table 25.14.

List of species of the genus **Natronobacterium**

1. **Natronobacterium gregoryi** Tindall, Ross and Grant 1984b, 355.[VP] (Effective publication: Tindall, Ross and Grant 1984a, 41.)

gre.go′ry.i. M.L. gen. n. *gregoryi* of Gregory; named for J. W. Gregory, Scottish geologist who first described the geology of the rift valley.

See Table 25.14 and the generic description for many features.

Colonies are 2–4 mm in diameter after 5–7 days at 37°C, circular, flat, friable and red. In liquid culture, cells are exceptionally long, thin non-motile rods (0.7 × 10–15 μm) (Fig. 25.34). Bending of the cells to give a "hockey stick" appearance is common. Motility has not been convincingly demonstrated, but cells migrate in soft agar media and exhibit twitching in liquid media.

Growth occurs in media containing 2–5.2 M NaCl with an optimum at 3 M. Alkaliphilic with optimum at pH 9.5. Growth occurs at 20–50°C; optimum temperature: 37–40°C.

No definitive studies have been made of the nutrition, but the growth of *N. gregoryi* is stimulated by ribose, fructose, glucose, mannitol and sucrose. Casamino acids are utilized as a nitrogen source. Gelatin is liquefied. H$_2$S is produced from thiosulfate. Does not hydrolyze starch.

N. gregoryi does not have a minor DNA component detectable by density gradient centrifugation. Plasmids have not been detected. The mol% G + C of the DNA is 65.0 (Bd).

Type strain: NCMB 2189 (strain SP2).

2. **Natronobacterium magadii** Tindall, Ross and Grant 1984b, 355.[VP] (Effective publication: Tindall, Ross and Grant 1984a, 41.)

ma.ga′di.i M.L. gen. n. *magadii* of Magadi; named for Lake Magadi, a saline soda lake in Kenya.

See Table 25.14 and the generic description for many features.

Table 25.14.
Characteristics differentiating **Natronobacterium gregoryi, N. magadii** *and* **N. pharaonis**[a]

Characteristic	1. *N. gregoryi*	2. *N. magadii*	3. *N. pharaonis*
Motility	−	+	+
Growth stimulated by sugars	+	−	−
Growth stimulated by acetate	+	−	+[b]
Nitrate reduction	−	−	+[b]
Gelatin liquefaction	−	−	+[c]

Sensitivity to
  Erythromycin
  Flavomycin
  Betoconazole
  Miconazole
  Sulfafurazole
	+	+	−

[a]Symbols: −, 90% or more of strains are negative; +, 90% or more of strains are positive.
[b]There are conflicting reports.
[c]Most strains.

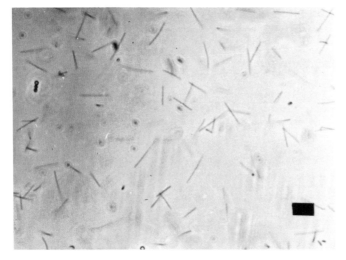

Figure 25.34. Phase-contrast micrograph of *Natronobacterium gregoryi* (NCMB 2189) grown at 37°C in the liquid medium described under *"Natronobacterium."* Note the presence of a few coccoid forms. *Bar,* 10 μm.

Colonies are 2–3 mm in diameter after 5–7 days at 37°C, wrinkled, friable and red. In liquid culture, cells are short rods 0.7–0.9 × 2–4 µm. Motile by a tuft of polar flagella.

Growth occurs in media containing 2–5.2 M NaCl with an optimum at 3.5 M. Growth occurs at 20–50°C; optimum temperature: 37–40°C. Alkaliphilic with optimum pH of 9.5.

Sugars are not utilized, although acetate stimulates growth. Casamino acids are used as nitrogen source. Gelatin is liquefied; sulfide is produced from thiosulfate; does not hydrolyze starch.

The DNA is comprised of a major component and a minor component. A large plasmid (~144 kb) is present. The mol% G + C of the major DNA component is 63.0, and that of the minor component, 49.5 (Bd).

Type strain: NCMB 2190 (strain MS3).

3. **Natronobacterium pharaonis** (Soliman and Trüper 1982) Tindall, Ross and Grant 1984b, 355.[VP] (Effective publication: Tindall, Ross and Grant 1984a, 41). (*Halobacterium pharaonis* Soliman and Trüper, 1982, 327.)

pha.ra.o′nis. L. gen. n. *pharaonis* of Pharaoh, title of the kings of ancient Egypt.

See Table 25.14 and generic description for many features.

Colonies are 1–2 mm in diameter after 5–7 days at 37°C, translucent and red. In liquid culture, cells are short rods (0.8 × 1–3 µm), motile by a tuft of polar flagella.

Growth occurs in media containing 2–5.2 M NaCl; optimum concentration: 3.5 M. Alkaliphilic with optimum pH of 8.5–9.5. Growth occurs at 25–50°C; optimum temperature: 45°C.

Sugars are not utilized. Casamino acids and glutamate are used as nitrogen sources. Gelatin is liquefied by most strains. Sulfide is formed from thiosulfate. Indole is formed from tryptophan. Starch and casein are not hydrolyzed. Nitrate is reduced to nitrite.

The DNA is composed of a major component and a minor component. A large plasmid (~144 kb) is present. The mol% G + C of the major DNA component is 64.3 (T_m) and 61.2 (Bd), and that of the minor component, 51.9 (Bd).

Type strain: DSM 2160 (strain Gabara).

Other Organisms

1. **Strain SP8** (De Rosa et al. 1983). Isolated from Lake Magadi and undoubtedly a *Natronobacterium* species. The lipids of this organism are characterized by a significant proportion of 2,3-di-*O*-sesterterpanyl (C_{25},C_{25}) glycerol diethers. Otherwise, the polar lipid composition is typical. Other details are not available.

Genus VI. **Natronococcus** *Tindall, Ross and Grant 1984b, 355*[VP]
(Effective publication: Tindall, Ross and Grant 1984a, 41)

WILLIAM D. GRANT

Na.tro.no.coc′cus. Gr. n. *natrun* soda, salt; Gr. n. *coccus* a berry; M.L. gen. n. *Natronococcus* soda berry.

Cells coccoid, usually 1–2 µm in diameter, occurring in refractile irregular clusters (Fig. 25.35), also in pairs and as single cells. Resting stages are not known. **Gram reaction is mixed** with some cells staining Gram-positive, others Gram-negative. **Nonmotile, strictly aerobic.** Oxidase- and catalase-positive. **Extremely halophilic with growth occurring in media containing 1.5–5.2 M (saturation) NaCl;** optimum concentration: 3.5 M. Optimum temperature: 35–40°C; maximum: ~45°C; minimum: 20–25°C. **Alkaliphilic with growth occurring at pH 8.5–11.0** and 37°C in media containing 3.5 M MaCl; optimum pH: ~9.5. Chemoorganotrophic. **Glycolipids are absent.**

The DNA is comprised of a major component and a minor component. The mol% G + C of the major component is 64.0 (Bd), and that of the minor component, 55.7.

Type species: *Natronococcus occultus* Tindall, Ross and Grant 1984b, 355.

Further Descriptive Information

Only one isolate has been extensively characterized. In liquid cultures, the arrangement of the cells may be almost exclusively large, refractile, irregular clusters like *Halococcus morrhuae* or may be small, less refractile, irregular groups, pairs and single cells. High NaCl concentrations (>4 M) appear to favor the latter arrangements. Division appears to be by cross-wall formation (Fig. 25.36). A cell wall glycoprotein has not been detected (A. F. Dixon and W. D. Grant, unpublished observation).

Colonies on agar are circular, matt, 2–3 mm in diameter after 5–7 days at 37°C and, unusual for halobacteria, pale brown in color. Occasionally, rough colony variants are produced. It is not known whether bacterioruberins are present. Cells contain retinal pigments but no bacteriorhodopsin (Bivin and Stoeckenius, 1986).

The polar lipids are based on 2,3-di-*O*-phytanyl-*sn*-glycerol (C_{20},C_{20}) and 2-*O*-sesterterpanyl-3-*O*-phytanyl-*sn*-glycerol (C_{25},C_{20}) diethers. Glycolipids are absent (Tindall et al., 1984a; Morth and Tindall, 1985).

The organism has been found only in the soda lake, Lake Magadi, Kenya, and on the basis of direct microscopic observation makes up a numerically insignificant fraction of the population. A number of other uncharacterized isolates exist, originally detected by slightly different colony morphologies (Bivin and Stoeckenius, 1986).

Enrichment and Isolation Procedures

N. occultus was originally isolated by incubating Lake Magadi saltern liquors supplemented with 1.0% (w/v) yeast extract and 0.1% (w/v) KNO$_3$ at 37°C without shaking. However, no comparative studies on the efficacy of this enrichment procedure have been carried out, although at the time several parallel enrichments but with different nutrient sources (tryptone, casamino acids and peptone) also yielded coccoid isolates. The organism grows well in the haloalkaliphile medium[†] (Tindall et al.,

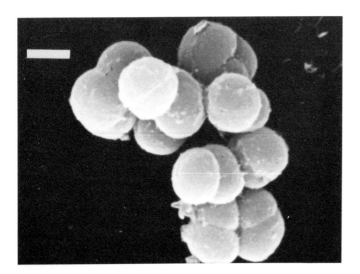

Figure 25.35. *Natronococcus occultus* (NCMB 2192) grown at 37°C in the liquid medium described under *"Natronobacterium."* Bar, 1 µm. (Prepared and photographed by C. F. Norton.)

[†]See under *"Natronobacterium."*

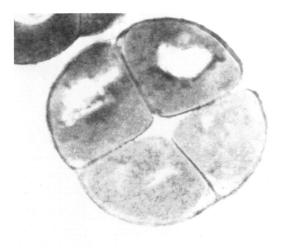

Figure 25.36. *N. occultus* (NCMB 2192) grown at 37°C in the medium described under *"Natronobacterium."* Thin section. *Bar,* 0.25 μm. (Prepared and photographed by A. F. Dixon.)

1980) which is an alkaline low Mg²⁺ modification of the medium of Payne et al. (1960). Agar media are incubated in sealed plastic bags to prevent desiccation. Plates should be perfectly dry before inoculation. The alternative media of Soliman and Trüper (1982) and Morth and Tindall (1985) also give good results.

Natronobacterium species are much more numerous in saline soda lakes, and these also grow well on these media. It is possible that a selective medium for *Natronococcus* species could be devised, based on the relatively low NaCl requirement for growth (1–1.5 M) compared with that for *Natronobacterium* species.

Maintenance Procedures

See under *"Halobacterium."*

Differentiation of the genus **Natronococcus** from other genera

The genus *Natronococcus* is separated from *Halococcus,* the only other halobacterial genus that contains coccoid isolates, by its alkaliphily, low Mg²⁺ requirement and lack of glycolipids. It is also readily distinguished from *Natronobacterium,* the only other genus that contains haloalkaliphiles, since these organisms produce rod-shaped forms in liquid culture.

Grant, 1985) (Fig. 25.23). Oligonucleotide catalogs of 16S rRNA (E. Stackebrandt, personal communication) and 5S rRNA (G. E. Fox, personal communication) are in agreement in this view. Precise knowledge of phylogenetic relationships will depend on future studies of other coccoid haloalkaliphiles.

Taxonomic Comments

DNA/16S rRNA hybridization studies indicate that *Natronococcus occultus* represents a separate and distinct halobacterial line (Ross and

Further Reading

See references provided under "Further Reading" for the order *Halobacteriales.*

List of species of the genus **Natronococcus**

1. **Natronococcus occultus** Tindall, Ross and Grant 1984b, 355.[VP] (Effective publication: Tindall, Ross and Grant 1984a, 41.)

oc.cul′tus. L. m. adj. *occultus* hidden, the hidden *Natronococcus.*

See the generic description for many features.

The morphology is the same as that described for the genus.

Stimulation of growth occurs in the presence of glucose, ribose, sucrose and xylose. Indole is produced from tryptophan. Starch is not hydrolyzed, but gelatin is liquefied. Nitrate is reduced to nitrite.

Sensitive to anisomycin, bacitracin, erythromycin, novobiocin and vibriostat reagent (0/129). Insensitive to penicillin, chloramphenicol, flavomycin, streptomycin and tetracycline.

The polar lipid composition is characterized by C₂₀,C₂₀ and C₂₅,C₂₀ versions of phosphatidylglycerol (PG), phosphatidylglycerol phosphate (PGP) and two unknown phospholipids.

The DNA is composed of a major component and a minor component. A large plasmid (~144 kb) is present. The mol% G + C of the DNA is 64.0 (Bd) for the major component and 55.7 (Bd) for the minor component. (Bd).

Type strain: NCMB 2192 (strain SP4).

GROUP IV. **CELL WALL-LESS ARCHAEOBACTERIA**

THOMAS A. LANGWORTHY AND PAUL F. SMITH

Genus **Thermoplasma** Darland, Brock, Samsonoff and Conti 1970, 1418[AL]

Ther.mo.plas′ma. Gr. n. *thermus* heat; Gr. neut. n. *plasma* something formed or molded, a form; M.L. neut. n. *Thermoplasma* heat (-loving) mycoplasma.

Pleomorphic, varying in shape from spherical (0.3–2.0 μm) to filamentous structures. **Cells lack a true cell wall** and are surrounded by a single triple layer membrane, ~5–10 nm thick. Membrane contains ether lipids based on 40-carbon, isopranoid-branched **diglycerol tetraethers**. Resting stages not known. **Gram-negative.** Generally immotile. Facultatively aerobic. **Obligate thermo-acidophile.** Optimum

growth occurs at 55–59°C and pH 1–2. **Cells undergo lysis near neutrality.** On agar at pH 2, colonies attain a diameter of about 0.3 mm and are dark brown in color, flat and coarsely granular, and some exhibit a typical "fried egg" appearance with a translucent peripheral zone. Biochemical and nutritional characteristics relatively poorly defined. Do not require cholesterol. Apparently chemoorganotrophic but have an **ab-**

solute requirement for yeast extract for growth and reproduction. Occur free-living in self-heating coal refuse piles.

The mol% G + C of the DNA is 46 (Bd, T_m).

Type species: *Thermoplasma acidophilum* Darland, Brock, Samsonoff and Conti 1970, 1418.

Further Descriptive Information

When grown in a liquid medium* consisting of Allan's basal salts solution (Allan, 1959) adjusted to pH 2 and supplemented with 0.1% yeast extract and 1.0% glucose, *T. acidophilum* exhibits a typical mycoplasmal morphology by light and phase microscopy. Cells appear as pleomorphic spheres varying in size from 0.3 to 2.0 μm and, in occasional large cells, up to 5 μm in diameter. Filamentous structures exhibiting budding characteristics are also common, particularly in young cultures.

A cell wall is absent, evidenced by electron micrographs of thin-sectioned cells (Darland et al., 1970; Belly et al., 1973; Langworthy, 1979a) (Fig. 25.37). The surrounding cytoplasmic membrane averages about 7 nm in thickness. Membrane lipids lack fatty acid ester residues. The lipids are ether-linked C_{40} biphytanyl diglycerol tetraethers along with small amounts of C_{20} phytanyl glycerol diethers (Langworthy, 1977; Langworthy et al., 1982). Similar ether lipids occur in *Sulfolobus, Halobacteriaceae, Methanobacteriaceae* and *Thermoproteales* (Kates, 1978; Langworthy, 1979a; Tornabene and Langworthy, 1979; Langworthy et al., 1982). No internal membranes or organelles are present.

Cells are generally nonmotile, although flagellalike structures have been observed in negatively stained preparations of one isolate (Black et al., 1979).

Growth on an agar surface is unreliable and difficult to achieve due to drying out at high temperature and hydrolysis of the agar in the presence of acid. These difficulties can sometimes be overcome by combining double-strength liquid medium and agar after cooling to 45–50°C followed by incubation in a humidified atmosphere (see *Thermoplasma* medium*). When growth can be initiated, colonies are small (about 0.3 mm diameter), and some show a fried egg appearance (Belly et al., 1973). Colonies are typically flat, coarsely granular and dark brown. Scanning electron microscopy shows individual cells to have an imbricate surface texture characteristic of cells which lack a cell wall (Mayberry-Carson et al., 1974).

Optimum temperature for growth: 59°C; maximum, 62°C; minimum, about 40°C. Growth is slow to slight at the extremes.

Optimum pH: 2. Growth occurs between the pH limits of 1 and 4, but growth is very slow at the extremes.

Hydrogen ions are specifically required for maintenance of cellular stability. Cells undergo lysis at neutral pH (Belly and Brock, 1972; Smith et al., 1973). Other monovalent cations, divalent cations, or osmotic stabilizers do not substitute for the hydrogen ion requirement. The phenomenon is analogous to the sodium ion requirement by certain *Halobacteriaceae* for the maintenance of cellular integrity. The intracellular hydrogen ion concentration of *T. acidophilum*, however, is not in equilibrium with the external environment, but the internal pH is near neutrality (Hsung and Haug, 1975; Searcy, 1976).

T. acidophilum requires oxygen. It appears to possess cytochromes and menaquinone-7, suggesting the presence of a complete respiratory chain (Belly et al., 1973; Hollander, 1978). Growth is stimulated by slight aeration, but excessive aeration inhibits growth (Smith et al., 1973). Because the amount of dissolved oxygen at 59°C is low, *T. acidophilum* can be considered microaerophilic.

Nutritionally, *T. acidophilum* has an absolute requirement for yeast extract for growth, and thus far no other compounds have been found to substitute (Belly et al., 1973; Smith et al., 1975). At yeast extract concentrations below 0.025%, no growth occurs. At concentrations higher than

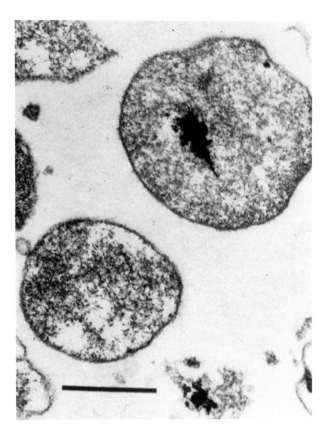

Figure 25.37. Thin section of *Thermoplasma. Bar*, 0.5 μm.

0.25%, growth is inhibited. Between the limiting concentrations, growth is proportional to the concentration of yeast extract used. Growth rates and yields also vary depending upon the manufacturer and the lot of yeast extract employed. The component or components supplied by yeast extract for growth appear to be basic oligopeptide(s) (Smith et al., 1975). No growth occurs aerobically on elemental sulfur or ferrous iron.

Cell yields are influenced by the inoculum size. Total cell yields decrease with inoculum sizes of <5% (v/v). Under optimal conditions, *T. acidophilum* has a generation time of about 5 h (Belly et al., 1973; Smith et al., 1973). Cell numbers increase with optical density (540 nm) to the stationary phase, reaching about 1×10^9 cells/ml, at which point there is a drastic loss in viability, although there is no great reduction in optical density.

Sucrose, glucose, galactose, mannose and fructose, when added in 0.1% concentration to the basal medium containing the growth-limiting concentration of yeast extract (0.025%), appear to stimulate growth of *T. acidophilum* (Belly et al., 1973).

No lysis occurs when cells are suspended in distilled water, when heated to 100°C for 30 min or when treated with EDTA, primary alcohols, digitonin, lysozyme, trypsin or Pronase. Cells are rapidly lysed by sodium lauryl sulfate and more slowly by cetyl trimethylammonium bromide (Belly and Brock, 1972; Smith et al., 1973).

T. acidophilum is resistant to the cell wall inhibitors vancomycin and ristocetin (in concentrations of at least 5 and 1 mg/ml, respectively). Cells are inhibited by novobiocin at a concentration of 0.1 mg/ml. Sensitivity to penicillin has not been determined because of the acid lability of this antibiotic (Darland et al., 1970; Belly et al., 1973; Brock, 1978).

---

* *Thermoplasma* medium contains the following ingredients (in g/l deionized water): KH_2PO_4, 3.0; $MgSO_4$, 0.5; $CaCl_2·2H_2O$, 0.25; $(NH_4)_2SO_4$, 0.2; and yeast extract (Difco), 1.0. Adjust to pH 2 with 10 N H_2SO_4. After the medium is autoclaved, add 10 g of separately sterilized glucose (25 ml of a 40% glucose solution) to give a final concentration of 1.0%. For agar medium, mix equal volumes of separately sterilized double-strength liquid medium and 5.6% Ionagar no. 2 (Consolidated Laboratories, Inc.), after cooling to 45°C, to give a final agar concentration of 2.8%. Incubate in a sealed and humidified atmosphere.

Molecular characteristics which further distinguish *T. acidophilum* include: a membrane-associated linear lipoglycan containing 24 mannose residues and 1 glucose residue (Smith, 1980); a mannosyl membrane glycoprotein (Yang and Haug, 1979); small genome size of from about 8.4×10^8 to 1×10^9 daltons (Christiansen et al., 1975; Searcy and Doyle, 1975) a histonelike protein associated with the DNA (DeLang et al., 1981); a 7-subunit DNA-dependent RNA polymerase that is resistant to rifampicin, streptolydigine and α-amanitine (Sturm et al., 1980); an unusual modification pattern in tRNAs (Gupta and Woese, 1980; Kuchino et al., 1982); an unusual nucleotide sequence in the 16S rRNA (Woese et al., 1980); a 5S rRNA secondary structure which does not conform to the usual models employed for either procaryotic or eucaryotic 5S rRNAs (Luehrsen et al., 1981); occurrence of dipthamide (Kessel and Klink, 1980); an unusual superoxide dismutase (Searcy and Searcy, 1981); coenzyme F_{420} (Lin and White, 1986); and a cytoplasmic membrane which may exist as a lipid monolayer rather than a lipid bilayer and which may account for the characteristic cross-fracture rather than tangential fracture of freeze-etched cells (Langworthy, 1979a, b; Langworthy et al., 1982).

T. acidophilum occurs in self-heating coal refuse piles in southern Indiana and western Pennsylvania. It is found in regions of the piles where temperatures range from 32 to 80°C and pH ranges from 1.17 to 5.21. As far as is known, this is the only natural habitat. It has not been reported in acidic geothermal regions which harbor the thermoacidophiles, *Sulfolobus* and *Bacillus acidocaldarius* (Belly et al., 1973).

Enrichment and Isolation Procedures

Thermoplasma was originally isolated from a coal refuse pile at the Friar Tuck mine in southwestern Indiana by incubating 20 ml of *Thermoplasma* medium with 1.0 g of coal refuse (Darland et al., 1970). The isolation medium has been modified to include the acid-stable antibiotic vancomycin at a concentration of 1225 µg/ml to inhibit the growth of rod-shaped bacteria such as *Bacillus acidocaldarius* (Belly et al., 1973). *Thermoplasma* has also been isolated from water samples by filtration through a membrane filter (0.45-µm pore size), followed by passage of the filtrate through a second filter (0.22-µm pore size), with subsequent incubation in culture medium (Belly et al., 1973). Isolation samples are incubated at 55°C for 4-6 weeks or until the development of visible turbidity. The presence of *Thermoplasma* is confirmed by microscopic examination. Cultures are purified by dilution in liquid medium, since reproducible growth of colonies on agar has not been obtained. The above procedures are selective for the isolation of *Thermoplasma* with the possible exception of *Sulfolobus*, which can be distinguished by its lobed-shape and physiological characteristics.

Maintenance Procedures

The most reliable procedure is to maintain actively growing cultures by continuous passage after 2 or 3 days of incubation. A 10-20% inoculum should be used, and multiple culture tubes should be incubated, since growth is sometimes spurious. Glassware should be free of any trace of detergent or soap residue which will kill the cells. Cells remain viable at room temperature for 10-15 days but die upon refrigeration. Sometimes cells can be recovered from the frozen state, but sufficient time (1-2 weeks) is required for development of visible turbidity. Cells are killed by lyophilization, and neutralization of cultures prior to preservation is precluded by cell lysis.

Differentiation of the genus **Thermoplasma** from other genera

Thermoplasma is distinguished from other genera of mycoplasmas by its stability, by its requirement for hot acid and by its molecular features. Table 25.15 provides the primary characteristics of *Thermoplasma* that distinguish it from other genera of morphologically or physiologically similar thermoacidophilic bacteria.

Taxonomic Comments

Thermoplasma is, by definition, a mycoplasma by virtue of being a free-living organism which morphologically lacks a cell wall. Biochemical characteristics, however, also indicate that *Thermoplasma* is similar to the extremely halophilic, methanogenic and other thermophilic archaeobacteria. Although lacking a cell wall, *Thermoplasma* shares the basic common archaeobacterial features of isopranoid (phytanyl-based) ether lipids, unusual but similar RNA polymerase structure and certain nucleotide sequences in the 16S rRNA, 5S rRNA and tRNA (Fox et al., 1980; Kandler, 1982; Stetter and Zillig, 1985). The precise extent to which *Thermoplasma* is related to the other currently recognized genera of archaeobacteria requires further studies. The lack of DNA/DNA sequence homology (<0.25%) indicates the absence of a close genetic relationship between *Thermoplasma* and *Sulfolobus*; i.e. *Thermoplasma* is not merely a stable L-form derived from *Sulfolobus* (Christiansen et al., 1981). Thus, on biochemical grounds, *Thermoplasma* is an archaeobacterium but is not closely related to these or any other known organisms.

Further Reading

Belly, R.T., B.B. Bohlool and T.D. Brock. 1973. The genus *Thermoplasma*. Ann. N.Y. Acad. Sci. *225*: 94-107.
Brock, T.D. 1978. Thermophilic Microorganisms and Life at High Temperatures. Springer-Verlag, Berlin.
Fox, G.E., E. Stackebrandt, T.B. Hespell, J. Gibson, J. Maniloff, T.A. Dyer, R.S. Wolfe, W.E. Balch, R.R. Tanner, L.J. Magrum, L.B. Zablen, R. Blakemore, R. Gupta, L. Bonen, B.R. Lewis, D.A. Stahl, K.R. Luehrsen, K.N. Chen and C.R. Woese. 1980. The phylogeny of prokaryotes. Science *209*: 457-463.
Kandler. O. (Editor). 1982. Archaebacteria. Gustav Fischer Verlag, Stuttgart.
Langworthy, T.A. 1979a. Special features of thermoplasmas. *In* Barile and Razin (Editors), The Mycoplasmas I: Cell Biology. Academic Press, New York, pp. 495-513.
Langworthy, T.A. 1979b. Membrane structure of thermoacidophilic bacteria. *In* Shilo (Editor), Strategies of Microbial Life in Extreme Environments, Dahlem Konferenzen, Berlin. Verlag-Chemie, Weinheim, pp. 417-432.
Woese, C.R. and R.S. Wolfe (Editors). 1985. The Bacteria, Vol. VIII. Academic Press, New York.

Table 25.15.

Differential characteristics of the genus **Thermoplasma** *and other genera of thermoacidophilic bacteria*[a]

Characteristic	Thermoplasma	Sulfolobus	Bacillus acidocaldarius
Shape			
Pleomorphic spheres	+	−	−
Lobed spheres	−	+	−
Rods, filaments	−	−	+
Cell wall present	−	+[b]	+
Ether lipids present	+	+	−
Endospores formed	−	−	+
Nutrition			
Requires yeast extract	+	−	−
Facultative autotroph	−	+	−
Lysis at neutral pH	+	−	−
Mol% G + C of DNA	46	38	60-64

[a] Symbols: +, positive for all strains; −, negative for all strains.
[b] *Sulfolobus* has a cell wall that lacks peptidoglycan.

Species diversity among *Thermoplasma* isolates has not been established. *Thermoplasma* isolates do exhibit serological diversity and can be differentiated into five antigenic groups by immunofluorescence and immunodiffusion analysis (Belly et al., 1973; Bohlool and Brock, 1974). Of

the variety of original isolates obtained by Darland et al. (1970) and Belly et al. (1973), the following appear to be extant: 122-1B2, 122-1B3, 3-24 and 124-1.

1. **Thermoplasma acidophilum** Darland, Brock, Samsonoff and Conti 1970, 1418.[AL] (*Thermoplasma acidophila* [sic] Darland et al. 1970, 1418.)

a.ci.do′phil.um. M.L. n. *acidum* an acid; Gr. adj. *philus* loving; M.L. neut. adj. *acidophilum* acid-loving.

The characteristics are the same as those described for the genus and listed in Table 25.15.

Occur free-living in self-heating coal refuse piles.

The mol% G + C of the DNA is 46 (T_m, Bd).

Type strain: ATCC 25905 (AMRC-C 165) (isolate 122-1B2 of Darland et al., 1970).

Reference strains: ATCC 27658 (isolate 122-1B3), ATCC 27657 (isolate 3-24) and ATCC 27656 (isolate 124-1).

GROUP V. **EXTREMELY THERMOPHILIC S⁰-METABOLIZERS**

HELMUT KÖNIG AND KARL O. STETTER

Obligately thermophilic aerobic, facultatively aerobic or strictly anaerobic bacteria. Gram-negative rods, filaments or cocci. Optimum temperature for growth: 70–105°C. Acidophiles and neutrophiles.

Autotrophic or heterotrophic growth. Most species are sulfur metabolizers. RNA polymerase is of the BAC type.

Key to the taxa of **Extremely Thermophilic S⁰-Metabolizers**

I. Strictly anaerobic cocci. Obligately heterotrophic. Sulfur can be reduced to H₂S. Tuft of flagella. Optimum temperature for growth: 88–100°C. Can be separated from the *Thermoproteales* mainly by 16S rRNA sequence comparison and by DNA/RNA hybridization.
Order I. *Thermococcales*, p. 2236

II. Strictly anaerobic cocci, plates, rods and filaments. Heterotrophic growth by sulfur respiration. Some groups are able to grow chemolithoautotrophically by reduction of S⁰ with H₂.
Order II. *Thermoproteales*, p. 2240

III. Extreme thermoacidophiles. Coccoid irregularly lobed cells. Strictly or facultatively aerobic. Optimum pH for growth: around 2. Facultatively or obligately chemolithoautotrophic S⁰-metabolizers.
Order III. *Sulfolobales*, p. 2250

ORDER I. **THERMOCOCCALES** ZILLIG 1988, 136[VP] (EFFECTIVE PUBLICATION: ZILLIG *IN* ZILLIG, HOLZ, KLENK, TRENT, WUNDERL, JANEKOVIC, IMSEL AND HAAS 1987, 69)

W. ZILLIG

Ther.mo.coc.ca′les. Gr. fem. n. *therme* heat; Gr. masc. n. *coccos* berry; M.L. fem. pl. n. *Thermococcales* the order of cocci existing in hot environments.

Cells spherical to elongated, about 1 µm in diameter. **Often occur as diplococci** (cell division by constriction) in growing cultures. Cytoplasm is electron-dense in contrast to *Desulfurococcus*. Envelope S layer is composed of subunits.

Strictly anaerobic. Utilize different carbon sources, e.g. peptides and/or carbohydrates by sulfur respiration (forming H₂S from S⁰) but can also use other electron acceptors. Form a strongly smelling product. Produce glycogen. Lipids consist mainly of one bisphytanyl phospholipid component (De Rosa et al., 1986).

Occur in marine solfataric biotopes of neutral pH and 80–103°C or

higher temperature, or in hot springs, or in water holes containing NaCl.

According to DNA/rRNA hybridization and 16S rRNA sequence analyses (Zillig et al., 1983b, 1987; Woese and Olsen, 1986) this group is phylogenetically as close to the methanogens and extreme halophiles as it is to other extreme thermophiles in the genera *Thermoproteus* and *Sulfolobus*. Also *Thermococcales* has a phylogenetic depth that is similar to that of the established branches of the methanogens plus extreme halophiles or the *Thermoproteales* plus *Sulfolobales*.

A single family exists: *Thermococcaceae*.

FAMILY **THERMOCOCCACEAE** ZILLIG 1988, 136 [VP] (EFFECTIVE PUBLICATION: ZILLIG *IN* ZILLIG, HOLZ, KLENK, TRENT, WUNDERL, JANEKOVIC, IMSEL AND HAAS 1987, 69)

Ther.mo.coc.ca′ce.ae. M.L. masc. n. *Thermococcus* type genus of the family; *-aceae* ending to denote a family; M.L. fem. pl. n. *Thermococcaceae* the *Thermococcus* family.

Cell appearance and metabolism and other features are the same as those described for the order.

Key to the genera of the family **Thermococcaceae**

I. Extremely thermophilic (optimum temperature for growth: about 85–90°C) heterotrophic sulfidogens, occurring in heated sea flows. The mol% G + C of the DNA is about 56.
Genus I. *Thermococcus*

II. Ultrathermophiles (optimum temperature for growth: about 100°C), occurring in heated seawaters. The mol% G + C of the DNA is about 38.
Genus II. *Pyrococcus*

Genus I. **Thermococcus** *Zillig 1983, 673* [VP] *(Effective publication: Zillig in Zillig, Holz, Janekovic, Schäfer and Reiter 1983, 93)*

W. ZILLIG

Ther.mo.coc′cus. Gr. fem. n. *therme* heat; Gr. masc. n. *coccos* berry; M.L. masc. n. *Thermococcus* berry existing in a hot environment.

Cocci occurring singly and in pairs, about 1 µm in diameter. **Monopolar, polytrichous flagella.**

Strictly anaerobic. Chemoorganotropic. Reduce sulfur (S⁰) to

H₂S when oxidizing organic carbon sources for energy in the presence of sulfur.

Type species: *Thermococcus celer* Zillig 1983, 673.

List of species of the genus **Thermococcus**

Only one species exists: *Thermococcus celer.*

1. **Thermococcus celer** Zillig 1983, 673. [VP] (Effective publication: Zillig *in* Zillig, Holz, Janekovic, Schäfer and Reiter 1983, 93.)
ce′ler. L. masc. adj. *celer* fast, due to rapid growth rate.

Same description as for genus (Fig. 25.38).
Lives in solfataric marine water holes of Vulcano, Italy, at about 90°C.
Optimum temperature for growth: ∼88°C.
The mol% G + C of the DNA is 56.6 (Bd, T_m).
Type strain: Vu13 (DSM 2476; ATCC 35543).

Genus II. **Pyrococcus** *Fiala and Stetter 1986, 573* [VP] *(Effective publication: Fiala and Stetter 1986, 60)*

G. FIALA AND K. O. STETTER

Pyr.o.coc′cus. Gr. neut. n. *pyr* fire; Gr. masc. n. *coccos* berry; M.L. masc. n. *Pyrococcus* fireball.

Cells slightly **irregular cocci,** 0.8–2.5 µm in width, **occurring singly or in pairs. Monopolar polytrichous flagellated. Strictly anaerobic. Heterotrophic** growth on peptone, tryptone, yeast extract, meat extract, extracts of eubacteria and archaeobacteria, casein, starch, maltose and casamino acids. Temperature for **growth: 70–103°C; optimum: 100°C.** pH for growth: 5–9; optimum: ∼7. Optimum NaCl concentration: ∼2%; maximum: 5%; minimum: 0.5%. Shortest doubling time about 37 min under optimal conditions. Gram-negative. Isopranyl ether lipids present. ADP-ribosylation of elongation factor 2 by diphtheria toxin.

The mol% G + C of the DNA is 38.

Type species: *Pyrococcus furiosus* Fiala and Stetter 1986, 573.

Further Descriptive Information

Cells are surrounded by an envelope about 50 nm thick (Fig. 25.39) which can be differentiated into an inner part of high contrast, measuring about 16 nm in width, and a weakly contrasted outer region. Cells are

stained by the periodate-Schiff reagent and are therefore most likely glycoproteins.

Enrichment and Isolation Procedures

Enrichment of *P. furiosus* can be achieved by using "SME" medium* (Stetter et al., 1983) supplemented with yeast extract and peptone (Fiala et al., 1986). After 1 day of incubation at 100°C, coccoid organisms become visible, which can be purified by repeated serial dilutions whereby the 10⁻⁸ dilutions usually grow overnight. Purification can be achieved alternatively by streaking onto agar-solidified medium. Round, smooth, white colonies of about 0.5 mm in diameter appear after 1 week of anaerobic incubation at 70°C.

Maintenance Procedures

Cultures of *Pyrococcus furiosus* are routinely grown for 10–15 h at 100°C and then transferred into fresh medium. Stock cultures can be stored anaerobically at 4°C for at least 1 year without transfer.

---

*"SME" medium consists of (per liter): NaCl, 13.85 g; MgSO₄·2H₂O, 3.5 g; MgCl₂·6H₂O, 2.75 g; CaCl₂·2H₂O, 1.0 g; KCl, 0.325 g; NaBr, 0.05g; H₃BO₃, 0.015 g; SrCl₂·6H₂O, 0.0075 g; KH₂PO₄, 0.5 g; KI, 0.025 mg; NiNH₄SO₄, 0.002 g; sulfur, 25 g; resazurine, 0.001 g; and trace minerals (Balch et al., 1979), 10 ml.

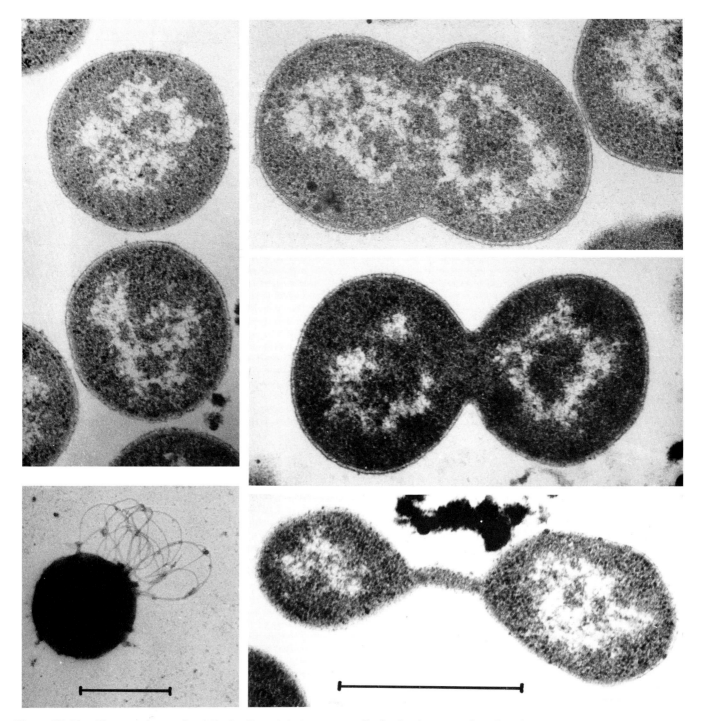

Figure 25.38.   Electron micrographs of *T. celer. Upper left*, thin section of two "normal" cells of *T. celer. Right, top* to *bottom*, thin sections of diplo forms of *T. celer* showing increasing constriction. *Lower left*, cell of *T. celer* showing monopolar polytrichous flagellation. Negatively stained. *Bars*, 1 μm. (Micrographs by D. Janekovic.)

Differentiation of the genus **Pyrococcus** *from other genera*

The genus *Pyrococcus* differs from *Pyrodictium* (Stetter et al., 1983) mainly by its 24 mol% lower G + C content, its flagellation and lack of fiber networks, its growth temperature and its organotrophic mode of nutrition. *Pyrococcus* differs from *Staphylothermus* (Fiala et al., 1986) with respect to its higher temperature optimum and maximum, its much faster growth, its insignificant DNA/DNA hybridization, its morphology and its metabolism. It can be distinguished from *Thermococcus* (Zillig et al., 1983a) in terms of its 18 mol% lower G + C content and its higher optimum and maximum growth temperature.

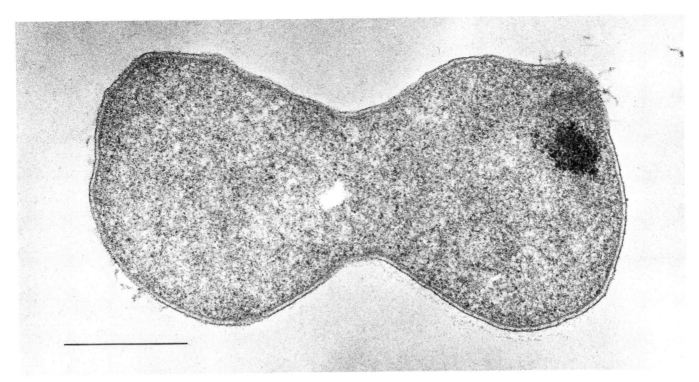

Figure 25.39. Electron micrograph of a thin section of *P. furiosus*. *Bar*, 0.5 μm. (Reproduced with permission from G. Fiala and K. O. Stetter, Archives of Microbiology *145:* 58, 1986, ©Springer-Verlag.)

Taxonomic Comments

16S rRNA total sequencing of *Pyrococcus furiosus* is in progress (C. R. Woese, personal communication).

Further Reading

Fiala, G. and K.O. Stetter. 1986. *Pyrococcus furiosus* sp. nov. represents a novel genus of marine heterotrophic archaebacteria growing optimally at 100°C. Arch. Microbiol. *145:* 56–61.

Zillig, W., I. Holt, H.-P. Klenk, J. Trent, S. Wunderl, D. Janekovic, E. Imsel and B. Haas. 1987. *Pyrococcus Woesei*, sp. nov., an ultra-thermophilic marine archaebacterium, representing a novel order, *Thermococcales*. Syst. Appl. Microbiol. *9:* 62–70.

Differentiation of the species of the genus **Pyrococcus**

Two species have been named, and they are differentiated on the basis of their anaerobic utilization of organic carbon sources.

1. Ferment peptones, yeast extract and polysaccharides.
   1. *P. furiosus*
2. Do not ferment peptones, yeast extract and polysaccharides but do use elemental sulfur as an electron acceptor for these substrates, forming hydrogen sulfide as an end product.
   2. *P. woesei*

List of species of the genus **Pyrococcus**

1. **Pyrococcus furiosus** Fiala and Stetter 1986, 573.[VP] (Effective publication: Fiala and Stetter 1986, 60.)

fur.i.o′sus. L. adj. *furiosus* raging.

Cells are highly motile due to a bundle of about 50 flagella, each about 7 μm long and 7 nm thick. Close to the origin of the flagella an electron-dense granumlike body of up to 1 μm in width can often be seen. H_2 and CO_2 are formed as metabolic products from yeast extract and peptone. In the presence of sulfur, the H_2 concentration is diminished, H_2S is formed, and final cell concentrations are about five times higher than without S^0, indicating a detoxification of H_2 by H_2S formation.

The mol% G + C of the DNA is 38 (T_m).

Type strain: Vc1 (DSM 3638).

2. **Pyrococcus woesei** Zillig 1988, 136.[VP] (Effective publication: Zillig *in* Zillig, Holz, Klenk, Trent, Wunderl, Janekovic, Imsel and Haas 1987, 69.)

woe′se.i. M.L. gen. n. *woesei* of Woese; named for C. R. Woese who recognized archaeobacteria and their testimony for phylogeny.

Roundly spherical to elongated, often constricted cells of 0.5–2 μm in diameter, frequently linked to doublets by short, thin threads. Organism stains Gram-negative with large bundles of smoothly bent filaments (flagella?) attached to one pole when cells grow on solid supports.

Ultrathermophilic anaerobes. Exist in marine solfataras at around 100–103°C in the presence of NaCl, 30 g/l. Upper temperature limit is 104.8°C.

Fermentation not observed. Yeast extract or peptones (e.g., Bacto tryptone) or polysaccharides are used by sulfur respiration. Polysaccharides are used well only in the presence of H_2. Yeast extract may also be used in the absence of elemental sulfur, apparently using an endogenous electron acceptor. Isolated from 102–103°C sediments in vents of marine solfataras of Vulcano Island, Italy.

The mol% G + C of the DNA is 37.5.

Type strain: DSM 3773.

ORDER II. **THERMOPROTEALES** ZILLIG AND STETTER, 1982, 267 ^{VP} (EFFECTIVE PUBLICATION: ZILLIG AND STETTER *IN* ZILLIG, STETTER, SCHÄFER, JANEKOVIC, WUNDERL, HOLZ AND PALM 1981, 224)

W. ZILLIG

Ther.mo.pro.te.a′les. Gr. n. *therme* heat; M.L. masc. n. *proteus* a mythical figure assuming different forms; *-ales* ending to denote an order. M.L. fem. pl. n. *Thermoproteales* the *Thermoproteus* order.

Rod, disc or spherical cells of various sizes; rods are from about 0.1 to 0.5 μm in diameter and from 1 to almost 100 μm long. Spherical forms are from about 0.5 to >5 μm in diameter. **Septa have not been encountered.** Some shape heterogeneity.

Gram-negative. Anaerobic. Extremely thermophilic. Optimal temperature for growth: 85 to more than 100°C.

Grow either chemolithoautotrophically by gaining energy from the reaction of $H_2 + S^0 \rightarrow H_2S$ using CO_2 as sole carbon source, **or by sulfur respiration of various organic substrates** yielding CO_2 and H_2S. Other electron acceptors including disulfides or malate may substitute for S^0. In some genera, heterotrophic growth occurs by unknown fermentations.

Cell envelope S-layer composed of protein or glycoprotein subunits in hexagonal dense packing, devoid of muramic acid.

Lipids contain glycerol ethers of polyisoprenoid C_{40} and, in lesser amounts, C_{20} alcohols.

Transcription is resistant to rifampicin and streptolydigin. RNA polymerases exhibit the complex BAC-component pattern also found in *Sulfolobus* and *Thermoplasma* (Schnabel et al., 1983) and show striking homology to eucaryotic nuclear RNA polymerases (Huet et al., 1983).

Ribosomal 50S rRNA subunits share structural features with *Sulfolobus* and eucaryotes (Henderson et al., 1984).

16S rRNA sequence and rRNA/DNA hybridization data place the *Thermoproteales* close to *Sulfolobus* (Tu et al., 1982; Woese et al., 1984) and distant from the methanogens and extreme halophiles.

Cell division not by septum formation, but by various modes of branching and bud formation.

Occur worldwide in solfataric hot waters and mud holes at high temperatures up to 100°C or higher or in superheated submarine solfataric environments of 103°C or higher.

The order comprises two validly published families, *Thermoproteaceae* and *Desulfurococcaceae*. The genera *Pyrodictium*, *Thermodiscus* and *Staphylothermus* have not yet been taxonomically assigned above the genus level. The phylogenetic position of *Pyrodictium* using 16S rRNA sequencing is already clear (cf. Fig. 25.1). Due to their physiological properties, the three genera are tentatively placed within the *Thermoproteales*.

Key to the families and genera of **Thermoproteales**

I. Cells are rods or filaments (up to 100 μm long). Surface layers composed of sodium dodecyl sulfate-resistant glycoprotein subunits. True branching. Spherical bodies can protrude at the cell ends. The mol% G + C of the DNA is about 56. Optimum temperature: 88°C.

Family I. *Thermoproteaceae*, p. 2241

II. Coccoid cells. Heterotrophic growth by sulfur respiration. Optimum temperature: 85°C. The mol% G + C of the DNA is 51.

Family II. *Desulfurococcaceae*. p. 2244

III. Cells are cocci in aggregates. Heterotrophs. Strictly sulfur-dependent. Cell size about 1 μm. Formation of giant cells (about 15 μm in diameter) on yeast extract. Optimum temperature for growth: 92°C. The mol% G + C of the DNA is 35.

Genus *Staphylothermus*, p. 2247

IV. Cells disk-shaped, forming huge networks of hollow fibers. Optimum temperature for growth: 105°C; maximum, 110°C. Wide salt tolerance (0.2–12% NaCl). Obligate chemolithoautotrophs. The mol% G + C of the DNA is 62.

Genus *Pyrodictium*, p. 2248

V. Disk-shaped cells. Obligate chemoorganotrophs. S^0 not obligately required. Growth occurs between 1 and 4% NaCl. Optimum temperature for growth: 90°C. The mol% G + C of the DNA is 49.

Genus "*Thermodiscus*"*

---

*Editorial note: This genus has not yet been fully characterized and is therefore not included in the *Manual.*

FAMILY I. **THERMOPROTEACEAE** ZILLIG AND STETTER 1982, 267 [VP] (EFFECTIVE PUBLICATION: ZILLIG AND STETTER *IN* ZILLIG, STETTER, SHÄFER, JANEKOVIC, WUNDERL, HOLZ AND PALM 1981, 224)

W. ZILLIG

Ther.mo.pro.te.a′ce.ae. M.L. masc. n. *Thermoproteus* type genus of the family; *-aceae* to denote a family; M.L. fem. pl. n. *Thermoproteaceae* the *Thermoproteus* family.

Rigid rods of variable length without septa, often associated with spherical bodies attached to their ends. **Sometimes with sharp bends, branches and buds.**
Energy production either chemolithoautotrophically by **molecular H_2 and elemental sulfur** (by using CO_2 as sole carbon source and forming H_2S) **or by sulfur respiration by utilizing various organic substrates,** including peptides and organic acids as energy and carbon sources. Store glycogen.

Key to the genera of the family **Thermoproteaceae**

I. Stiff angular rods (0.4 µm in diameter). Facultatively autotrophic. C_{20} and C_{40} isopranyl ethers present.
Genus I. *Thermoproteus*
II. Cells are thin filaments about 0.2 µm in diameter. Obligate chemolithotrophs. C_{20} isopranyl ethers only in trace amounts. Many strains require an unknown polar lipid factor of *Thermoproteus*.
Genus II. *Thermofilum*

Genus I. **Thermoproteus** Zillig and Setter 1982, 267 [VP] (Effective publication: Zillig and Stetter in Zillig, Stetter, Shäfer, Janekovic, Wunderl, Holz and Palm 1981, 225)

W. ZILLIG

Ther.mo.pro′te.us Gr. fem. n. *therme* heat; Gr. masc. n. *proteus* a mythical figure able to assume different forms; M.L. masc. n. *Thermoproteus* the genus of thermophilic bacteria of various forms.

Rigid rods of about 0.4 µm in diameter and from <1 to almost 100 µm in length. No cell septa. Otherwise, the description is the same as that for the family.

Has been found in acidic hot springs and water holes in Iceland, Italy, North America, New Zealand, the Azores and Indonesia at pH values 1.7–6.5 and temperatures up to 100°C.
Type species: *Thermoproteus tenax* Zillig and Stetter 1982, 267.

Key to the species of the genus **Thermoproteus**

I. Grows best at pH 5.
1. *T. tenax*
II. Grows best at pH 6.5.
2. *T. neutrophilus*

List of species of the genus **Thermoproteus**

1. **Thermoproteus tenax** Zillig and Stetter 1982, 267.[VP] (Effective publication: Zillig and Stetter *in* Zillig, Stetter, Shäfer, Janekovic, Wunderl, Holz and Palm 1981, 225.)

te′nax. L. masc. adj. *tenax* tenacious, resistant.

Cell shapes typical of genus (Figs. 25.40 and 25.41). Nonmotile. Pili attached laterally and/or terminally. Grows chemolithoautotrophically with H_2 and S^0 as energy sources and CO_2 as carbon source, or by sulfur respiration of different compounds serving as carbon sources, including glucose, starch, glycogen, fumarate and amino acids, but not lactate, acetate and pyruvate. Malate replaces sulfur as electron acceptor. Growth on organic substrates stimulated by yeast extract, at concentrations of 0.2–0.5 g/l. Forms CO_2. Fermentation pathways are unknown.

Grows best at about pH 5 and 90°C but grows even up to 96°C. The DNA-dependent RNA polymerase is stable at 95°C.

Strain Kra 1 is from Krafla, Iceland, and is host to four different rod-shaped viruses (Fig. 25.42) of a previously unknown type containing double-stranded DNA (Janekovic et al., 1983; Zillig et al., 1986).

The mol% G + C of the DNA is 55.5.

Type strain: Kra 1 (DSM 2076; ATCC 35583).

2. **Thermoproteus neutrophilus** Stetter and Zillig sp. nov.

neu.tro.phi′lus. L. adj. *neutralis* neutral; Gr. adj. *philus* liking, preferring; M.L. adj. *neutrophilus* preferring neutral pH.

Facultative chemolithotroph which can utilize acetate instead of CO_2 as carbon source, gaining energy by the formation of H_2S from H_2 and S^0 (Schäfer et al., 1986). Grow optimally at pH 6.5 but also as high as pH 7.0. In other respects resembles *T. tenax* but not as a host to its viruses.

Type strain: DSM 2338.

Genus II. **Thermofilum** Zillig and Gierl 1983, 673 [VP] (Effective publication: Zillig and Gierl in Zillig, Gierl, Schreiber, Wunderl, Janekovic, Stetter and Klenk 1983, 86)

W. ZILLIG

Ther.mo.fi′lum. Gr. fem. n. *therme* heat; L. neut. n. *filum* thread, filament; M.L. neut. n. *Thermofilum* filament existing in a hot environment.

Thin rods of 0.15–0.35 µm in diameter and 1 to >100 µm in length with terminal pili. In contrast to *Thermoproteus*, **only rarely branched or with sharp bends**; often with terminal spherical protrusions on both ends; sometimes with swollen sections; ghosts become spiral shaped. Stain as Gram-negative.

Anaerobic; thermoacidophilic; utilize peptides by sulfur respiration.

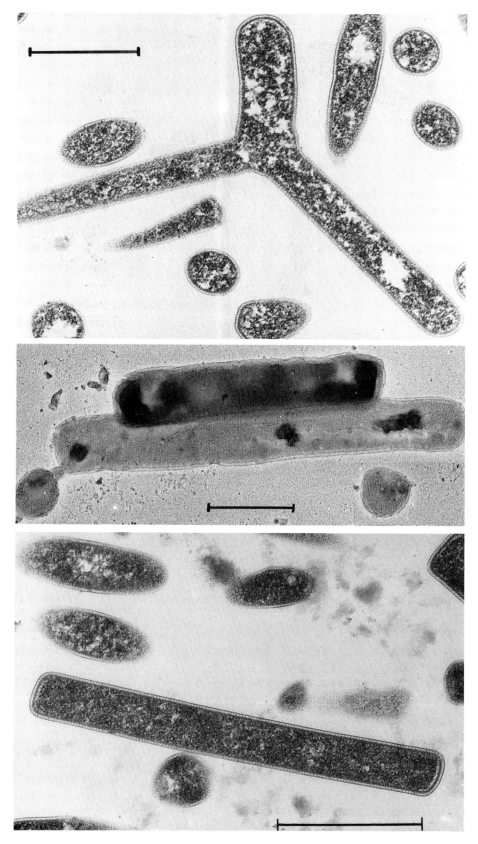

Figure 25.40.   Electron micrographs of *Thermoproteus. Top*, branched form of *T. tenax*, thin section. *Middle*, golf club and released spheroid of *Thermoproteus* species isolate H3, platinum-shadowed. *Bottom*, normal rod of *T. tenax*, thin section. *Bars*, 1 μm. (Micrographs courtesy of D. Janekovic.)

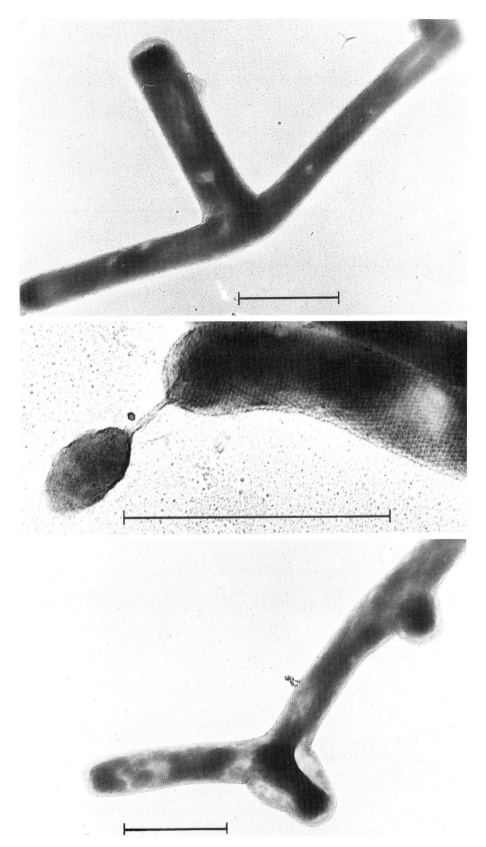

Figure 25.41. *Top,* branched form of *T. tenax. Middle,* golf club of *T. tenax. Bottom,* budding form of *T. tenax.* All platinum-shadowed. *Bars,* 1 μm. (Micrographs by D. Janekovic.)

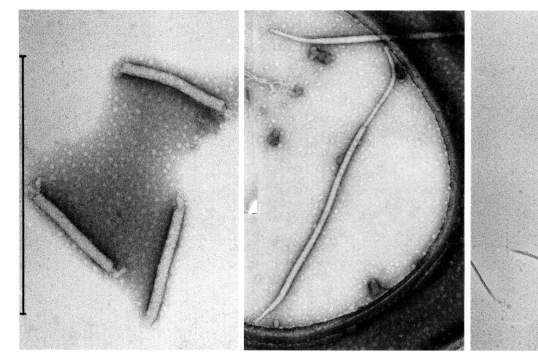

Figure 25.42. Electron micrographs of viruses of *T. tenax. Left to right*, TTV1, TTV2 and TTV3, respectively. *Bar* on the *left*, 1 μm for the left and the middle section of the figure. *Bar* on the *right*, 1 μm for the right section of the figure. Negatively stained. (Micrographs by D. Janekovic.)

Live in solfataric hot springs and water holes at pH 2.8–6.7 and temperatures up to 100°C. Optimum pH for growth: about 5. Optimum temperature: 85–90°C.

Type species: *Thermofilum pendens* Zillig and Gierl 1983, 673.

List of species of the genus **Thermofilum**

Only one species exists.

1. **Thermofilum pendens** Zillig and Gierl 1983, 673.[VP] (Effective publication: Zillig and Gierl *in* Zillig, Stetter, Shäfer, Janekovic, Wunderl, Holz and Palm 1983, 86.)

pen'dens. L. neut. part. adj. *pendens* depending; growth depends on factor from *Thermoproteus* species.

Description is the same as for the genus, except that it requires a polar lipid component of *Thermoproteus tenax* for growth. See Figure 25.43.

The mol% G + C of the DNA is 57.4

Type strain: Hrk 5 (DSM 2475; ATCC 35544).

FAMILY II. **DESULFUROCOCCACEAE** ZILLIG AND STETTER 1983, 438[VP]
(EFFECTIVE PUBLICATION: ZILLIG AND STETTER *IN* ZILLIG, STETTER, PRANGISHVILLI, SCHÄFER, WUNDERL, JANEKOVIC, HOLZ AND PALM 1982, 315)

W. ZILLIG

De.sul.fu.ro.coc.ca′ce.ae. M.L. masc. n. *Desulfurococcus* type genus of family; *-aceae* ending to denote a family; M.L. fem. pl. n. *Desulfurococcaceae* the *Desulfurococcus* family.

Cells cocci. Stains Gram-negative.

Anaerobic; utilize protein, peptides or carbohydrates facultatively by sulfur respiration or fermentation.

Cell envelope flexible, composed of subunits. Lipids, RNA polymerase and resistance to antibiotics are the same as those described for the order.

Only one genus exists.

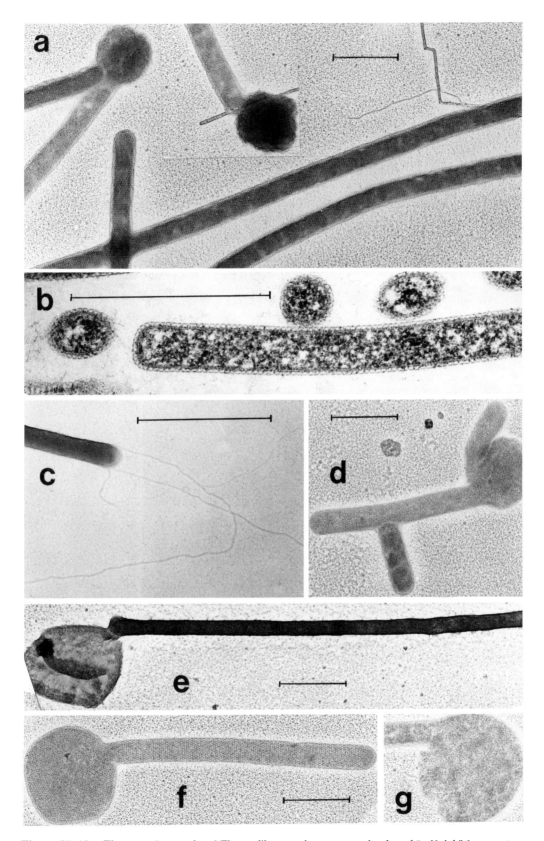

Figure 25.43. Electron micrographs of *Thermofilum pendens*. *a*, normal rods and "golf club" forms, rotary-shadowed with platinum. *b*, normal rods, longitudinal sections and cross-sections, doubly contrasted with lead citrate and uranyl acetate. *c*, end of rod with pili. *d*, branching or budding. *e*, golf club form. *f* and *g*, spiralized forms. *c–g*, rotary shadowed with platinum. *Bars*, 1 μm. (Micrographs by D. Janekovic.)

Genus **Desulfurococcus** Zillig and Stetter 1983, 438 VP (Effective publication: Zillig and Stetter in Zillig, Stetter, Prangishvilli, Schäfer, Wunderl, Janekovic, Holz and Palm 1982, 316)

W. ZILLIG

De.sul.fu.ro.coc'cus. L. pref. de from; L. n. sulfur sulfur; Gr. n. coccos berry; M.L. masc. n. Desulfurococcus sulfur-reducing coccus.

The description for the genus is the same as that for the family. See Figure 25.44 for appearance of cells.

Type species: *Desulfurococcus mucosus* Zillig and Stetter 1983, 438.

List of species of the genus **Desulfurococcus**

1. **Desulfurococcus mucosus** Zillig and Stetter 1983, 438.VP (Effective publication: Zillig and Stetter *in* Zillig, Stetter, Prangishvilli, Schäfer, Wunderl, Janekovic, Holz and Palm 1982, 316.)

mu.co'sus. L. masc. adj. *mucosus* slimy.

The description is the same as that for the family with the addition that it forms a strongly smelling unknown product and produces a slimy polymer attached to its surface. Nonmotile. Optimum pH for growth: 6. Optimum temperature for growth: 85°C.

Lives in solfataric hot springs at pH 2.2–6.5 and up to 97°C.

The mol% G + C of the DNA is 51.3.

Type strain: 07 (DSM 2162; ATCC 35584).

2. **Desulfurococcus mobilis** Zillig and Stetter 1983, 438.VP (Effective publication: Zillig and Stetter *in* Zillig, Stetter, Prangishvilli, Schäfer, Wunderl, Janekovic, Holz and Palm 1982, 316.)

mo'bi.lis. L. masc. adj. *mobilis* motile.

Description is identical with *M. mucosus*, except that cells are motile and do not produce slime. In addition, the 23S rRNA gene contains an intron (Larsen et al., 1986).

Type strain: Hvv3 (DSM 2161; ATCC 35582).

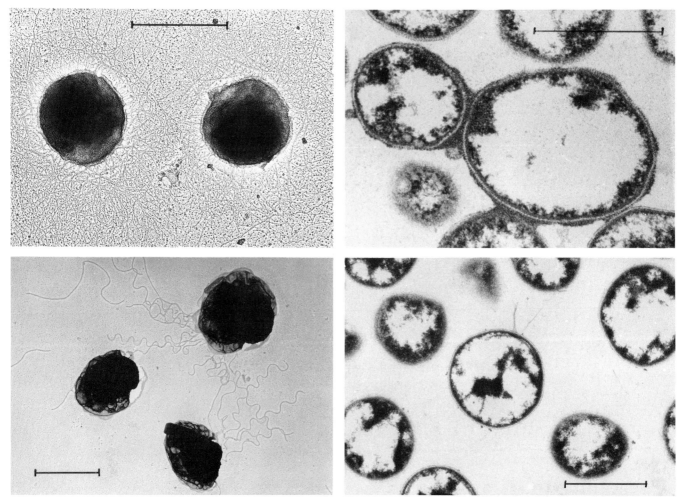

Figure 25.44. Electron micrographs of *Desulfurococcus. Upper left,* two cells of *Desulfurococcus* species with slime filaments on surface. Rotary-shadowed with platinum. *Upper right,* thin section of *D. mucosus* with solid slime layer attached to envelope. *Lower left,* three cells of *D. mobilis,* with one showing monopolar polytrichous flagellation. Rotary-shadowed with platinum. *Lower right,* thin section of *D. mobilis* showing apparatus to which flagella are attached within the cell. *Bars,* 1 μm. (Micrographs courtesy of D. Janekovic.)

OTHER BACTERIA

***Genus* Staphylothermus** *Stetter and Fiala 1986, 573*[VP] *(Effective publication: Stetter and Fiala in Fiala, Stetter, Jannasch, Langworthy and Madon 1986, 112)*

G. FIALA AND K. O. STETTER

Sta.phy.lo.ther´mus. Gr. fem. n. *staphyle* bunch of grapes; Gr. fem. n. *therme* heat; M.L. masc. n. *Staphylothermus* grape (-forming) thermophile.

Cells slightly irregular cocci occurring singly, in pairs, as short chains, and as aggregates of up to 100 cells. Width about 0.5-15 μm, depending on the culture conditions (Fig. 25.45). **Strictly anaerobic. Heterotrophic growth** on peptone, tryptone, yeast extract, meat extract and extracts of eubacteria and archaeobacteria **in the presence of sulfur (S⁰). H₂S, CO₂, acetate and isovalerate are formed as metabolic products. Extreme thermophiles.** With optimal nutrition (0.1% yeast extract + 0.5% peptone), optimum temperature is 92°C, and maximum, 98°C. In minimal medium (0.02% yeast extract + 0.004% *Methanosarcina* extract), optimum temperature is 85°C, and maximum, 92°C. Resistant to vancomycin, kanamycin, streptomycin and chloramphenicol. Gram-negative. Elongation factor 2 is ADP-ribosylable by diphtheria toxin. Phytanyl glycerol diether, dibiphytanyl diglycerol tetraether and a yet unknown ether lipid component are present.

The mol% G + C of the DNA is 35.

Type species: *Staphylothermus marinus* Stetter and Fiala 1986, 573.

Further Descriptive Information

At low substrate concentrations (0.005-0.02% yeast extract), large aggregates are mainly formed; at high substrate concentrations (0.1% yeast extract + 0.5% peptone), single cells, pairs and, very rarely, aggregates of up to 5 cells can be seen. Cells are 0.5-1 μm in diameter. At high yeast extract concentrations (0.2%), giant cells with diameters of up to 15 μm appear, with each containing one to a few highly contrasted dark granules seen by phase-contrast microscopy. Cells consist most likely of glycogen, due to their brownish staining reaction with the Lugol reagent (I − KI solution).

In the presence of oxygen, the titer of viable cells is reduced by 50% within 7 min at 85°C; at 4°C the half-life of survival was about 20 h, thus indicating that the organism is extremely sensitive to oxygen during growth.

S. marinus was isolated both from anaerobic samples taken from the beach of Vulcano, Italy, and from a "black smoker" at the East Pacific Rise.

Enrichment and Isolation Procedures

S. marinus can be enriched anaerobically at 85°C in SME medium (Stetter et al., 1983b) supplemented with yeast extract and peptone. After about 1 week, coccoid cells often appear in aggregates, which can be purified by repeated serial dilutions in fresh medium.

Maintenance Procedures

Cultures of *S. marinus* are grown for 3 days at 85°C. Storage is possible anaerobically at 4°C, conditions at which cells remain viable for at least 2 years.

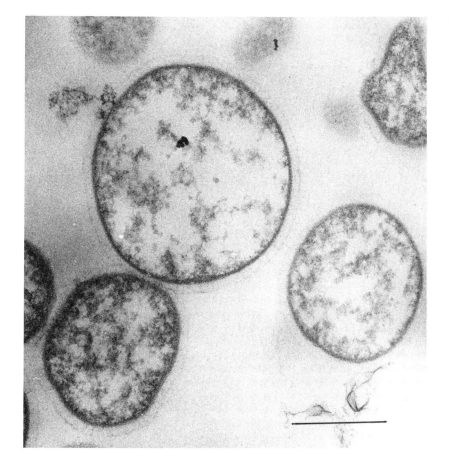

Figure 25.45. Thin section of *S. marinus.* Bar, 0.5 μm.

Differentiation of the genus **Staphylothermus** from other genera

The genus *Staphylothermus* differs from *Pyrodictium* (Stetter et al., 1983b) and *Pyrococcus* (Fiala et al., 1986) by its lower optimum and maximum temperatures, its metabolism and its slower growth. In contrast to *Pyrodictium*, which shows a G + C content 27 mol% higher than that for *Staphylothermus*, the DNAs of *Staphylothermus* and *Pyrococcus* exhibit nearly the same base composition but practically no homology in cross-hybridization experiments. From *Thermococcus* (Zillig et al., 1983a), *Staphylothermus* differs mainly by its 21 mol% lower G + C content and its slower growth. Furthermore, the genus *Staphylothermus* can be distinguished easily by its morphology from the genera mentioned above.

Taxonomic Comments

16S rRNA total sequencing of *S. marinus* is in progress (C. R. Woese, personal communication).

Further Reading

Fiala, G., K.O. Stetter, H.W. Jannasch, T.A. Langworthy and J. Madon. 1986. *Staphylothermus marinus* sp. nov. represents a novel genus of extremely thermophilic submarine heterotrophic archaebacteria growing up to 98°C. Syst. Appl. Microbiol. *8:* 106–113.

Differentiation of the species of the genus **Staphylothermus**

Only one species, *S. marinus*, is currently known.

List of species of the genus **Staphylothermus**

1. **Staphylothermus marinus** Stetter and Fiala 1986.[VP] (Effective publication: Stetter and Fiala *in* Fiala, Stetter, Jannasch, Langworthy and Madon 1986, 112.)

ma.ri′nus. L. masc. adj. *marinus* of the sea.

See the generic description for the features. The mol% G + C of the DNA is 35 (T_m). *Type strain:* F1 (DSM 3639).

Genus **Pyrodictium** Stetter, König and Stackebrandt 1984, 270[VP] (Effective publication: Stetter, König and Stackebrandt 1983, 549)

K. O. STETTER

Pyr.o.dic′ti.um. Gr. neut. n. *pyr* fire; Gr. neut. n. *diktyon* network; M.L. neut. n. *Pyrodictium* fire network.

Cells disk- to dish-shaped, highly variable in diameter, ranging from 0.3 to 2.5 μm, about 0.2 μm thick. **Produce fibers,** 0.04–0.08 μm thick, **which form networks connecting the cells** (Fig. 25.46). Gram-negative. Neither motility nor flagella could be detected. Cell envelope composed of protein subunits (Fig. 25.47) in hexagonal array. Isopranoid ether lipids present (T. Langworthy, personal communication). Elongation factor 2 is ADP-ribosylated by diphtheria toxin (F. Klink, personal communication). **Strictly anaerobic. Optimum temperature: 105°C; maximum: 110°C;** minimum, 82°C. Growth occurs at pH 5–7; optimum pH: around 5.5. Optimal NaCl concentration: around 1.5%; maximum: 12%; minimum: 0.2%. Vigorous shaking prevents cell growth. **Chemolithotrophic, thriving by hydrogen-sulfur autotrophy.** H_2S is formed from molecular sulfur and hydrogen.

The mol% G + C of the DNA is 62.

Type species: *Pyrodictium occultum* Stetter, König and Stackebrandt 1984, 270.

Further Descriptive Information

Cells are fragile and irregular in shape. They occur singly. No septa formation visible. The S-layer consists of subunits 30 nm in diameter. Cells can be disintegrated by sodium dodecyl sulfate (SDS) (1%). The cell envelope of *Pyrodictium* contains a major protein which stains positive with the periodate-Schiff reagent and therefore is most likely a glycoprotein.

The networks composed of fibers and cells can be seen in the light microscope with high-intensity darkfield illumination and in the electron microscope. The fibers often form plectenchymelike bundles. Fibers are hollow cylinders with a diameter of about 23 nm, composed of subunits 5 nm in diameter (Messner and Sleytr, personal communication) in helical array. The thickness of the wall is 2–3 nm. A triple-layered unit membrane was not found. The fibers are up to 40 μm long. They can not be disintegrated by SDS. Granules of sulfur are seen frequently, sticking to the surface of the fibers. Precipitations of zinc and sulfur (B. Sprey, per-

sonal communication), most likely zinc sulfide, can be seen on the fibers, the same as on the cell envelope. In addition to the fibers, pililike appendages up to 5 μm long and 10 nm in diameter, protruding from the disks and the fibers, can be seen.

Antigens against cells of *P. occultum* cross-react with all *Pyrodictium* isolates from 12 different places.

Cell growth is extremely sensitive to oxygen. At 4°C, tolerance to oxygen is variable, depending on unknown factors. Growth is slightly stimulated by yeast extract (0.02%) and citric acid (0.001%). In the fermenter, pyrite is formed during growth (Wauschkuhn, personal communication).

Pyrodictium was isolated from anaerobic samples taken from the hot sea floor and from the beach at Vulcano Island, Italy.

Enrichment and Isolation Procedures

Pyrodictium can be enriched anaerobically in seawater supplemented with sulfur and pressurized with 80% H_2 and 20% CO_2 (300 kPa) and incubated at 100°C without shaking. After 1–3 days, a fluffy layer, strongly reminiscent of the growth of a mold, appears above the sulfur. This layer sticks only very loosely to the sulfur and can be removed easily by gentle shaking. The enrichment cultures can be purified by thrice-repeated serial dilution in SME medium (Stetter et al., 1983b) after vigorous shaking of the enrichment culture. No colonies are formed on medium solidified by agar, polysilicate or starch, due to wetting of the surface during incubation. Packed cells originally grown in liquid medium are white to gray. For growth in fermenters, the steel parts have to be protected, e.g. with halar.

Maintenance Procedures

Stock cultures of *Pyrodictium* can be stored anaerobically at 4°C for at least 2 years without transfer. Storage is also possible at −20°C or under liquid nitrogen (after freezing in the gas phase of the nitrogen vessel). The organisms are transferred routinely into SME medium and incubated at 105°C.

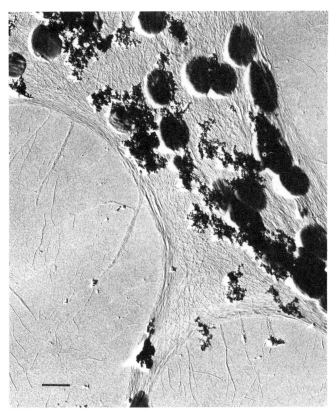

Figure 25.46. Electron micrograph of cells and the large network of fibers of *P. occultum* strain Pl-1. Platinum-shadowed. *Bar*, 2 μm.

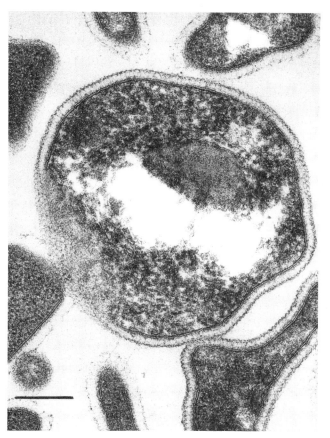

Figure 25.47. Electron micrograph of a thin section of *P. occultum* strain Pl-19. *Bar*, 0.2 μm.

Differentiation of the genus **Pyrodictium** from other genera

The genus *Pyrodictium* belongs to the *Sulfolobus-Thermoproteus* branch within the archaeobacteria, where it is unique because of its growth temperature, morphology and mol% G + C content.

Taxonomic Comments

The phylogenetic relationship of *P. occultum* has been determined by sequence analysis of the 16S rRNA (C. Woese, personal communication). *Pyrodictium* groups with *Thermoproteus* and *Sulfolobus* forming the main branch of extremely thermophilic archaeobacteria (cf. Fig. 25.1).

Further Reading

Stetter, K.O. 1982. Ultrathin mycelia-forming organisms from submarine volcanic areas having an optimum growth temperature of 105°C. Nature *300:* 258–260.

Stetter, K.O., H. König and E. Stackebrandt. 1983. *Pyrodictium* gen. nov., a new genus of submarine disc-shaped sulphur reducing archaebacteria growing optimally at 105°C. Syst. Appl. Microbiol. *4:* 535–551.

Stetter, K.O., H. König and E. Stackebrandt. 1984. Validation of the publication of new names and new combinations previously effectively published outside the IJSB. List no. 14. Int. J. Syst. Bacteriol. *34:* 270–271.

Zillig, W., K.O. Stetter, W. Schäfer, D. Janekovic, S. Wunderl, I. Holz and P. Palm. 1981. *Thermoproteales:* a novel type of extremely thermoacidophilic, anaerobic archaebacteria isolated from Icelandic solfataras. Zentralbl. Bakteriol. Mikrobiol. Hyg. I Abt. Orig. C *2:* 200–227.

Differentiation of the species of the genus **Pyrodictium**

Only two species, *P. occultum* and *P. brockii*, are presently known.

List of species of the genus **Pyrodictium**

1. **Pyrodictium occultum** Stetter, König and Stackebrandt 1984, 270.[VP] (Effective publication: Stetter, König and Stackebrandt 1983, 549.)

oc.cul′tum. L. neut. adj. *occultum* hidden, indicating the invisibility of the network in the phase-contrast microscope.

See the generic description for features. Dominant glycoprotein in the cell envelope with an apparent molecular weight of about 172,000.

Type strain: DSM 2709.

2. **Pyrodictium brockii** Stetter, König and Stackebrandt 1984, 270.[VP] (Effective publication: Stetter, König and Stackebrandt 1983, 549.)

brock′i.i. M.L. gen. n. *brockii* of Brock; named for T. D. Brock for his pioneering work on the extreme thermophiles.

See the generic description for features. Protein components of the envelope are periodate-Schiff-negative or slightly positive.

Type strain: DSM 2708.

ORDER III. **SULFOLOBALES** ORD. NOV.

K. O. Stetter

Sul.fo.lo.ba'les. M.L. fem. n. *Sulfolobaceae* type family of order; *-ales* ending to denote an order; M.L. fem. pl. n. *Sulfolobales* the *Sulfolobaceae* order.

Cells coccoid, irregularly lobed. Extreme thermoacidophiles. Optimum pH for growth: about 2. Strictly or facultatively aerobic.

Facultatively or obligately chemolithoautotrophic S⁰-metabolizers.

FAMILY **SULFOLOBACEAE** FAM. NOV.

Sul.fo.lo.ba'ce.ae. M.L. masc. n. *Sulfolobus* type genus of the family; *-aceae* ending to denote family; M.L. fem. n. the *Sulfolobus* family.

Description of family is the same as for the order.

Key to the genera of the family **Sulfolobaceae**

I. Cells can oxidize H_2S to S^0, and S^0 to sulfuric acid. Some strains oxidize ferrous iron. Most strains are facultative heterotrophs. The mol% G + C of the DNA is about 37.
Genus I. Sulfolobus, p. 2250

II. Cells oxidize H_2S and S^0 aerobically to H_2SO_4 and reduce S^0 to H_2S by H_2 under anaerobic conditions (hydrogen-sulfur autotrophy). Some strains oxidize ferrous iron, and some are facultative heterotrophs. The mol% G + C of the DNA is about 31.
Genus II. Acidianus, p. 2251

Genus I. **Sulfolobus** *Brock, Brock, Belly and Weiss 1972, 66[AL]*

A. Segerer and K. O. Stetter

Sulf.o.lo'bus. L. n. *sulfur* sulfur; L. n. *lobus* lobe; M.L. masc. n. *Sulfolobus* lobed sulfur-oxidizing organism.

Cells coccoid, highly irregular, about 0.8–2 μm in diameter, **usually occurring singly.** Neither motility nor flagella were detected. Cell envelope composed of protein subunits in hexagonal array (Weiss, 1974; Taylor et al., 1982). Isopranyl ether lipids, calditol and caldariella quinone present (Langworthy, 1985). Elongation factor 2 is ADP-ribosylated by diphtheria toxin (Kessel and Klink, 1982). **Aerobic. Lithotrophic growth via oxidation of sulfur, sulfide or tetrathionate** (Brock et al., 1972; Shivvers and Brock, 1973; Wood et al., 1987). No anaerobic growth via S^0 reduction. Organotrophic growth by oxidizing complex organic material (e.g. yeast extract), sugars or amino acids (Brock, 1978). **Thermoacidophilic, growing above 50°C and at pH 1–6.**

The mol% G + C of the DNA is 36–38.

Type species: *Sulfolobus acidocaldarius* Brock, Brock, Belly and Weiss 1972, 66.

Further Descriptive Information

The cells are highly irregular in shape, often lobed, but occasionally spherical. No septum formation visible. The S-layer of *S. acidocaldarius* consists of glycoprotein subunits about 22 nm in width (Michel et al., 1980; Taylor et al., 1982). Piluslike and pseudopodiumlike structures are often found (McClure and Wyckoff, 1982).

Membrane isopranyl glycerol ether lipids consist of 95% tetraethers with cyclopentane rings and 5% diethers (Langworthy, 1985).

Different isolates of the genus *Sulfolobus* are mixotrophic or heterotrophic (Shivvers and Brock, 1973; Wood et al., 1987). Some as yet undescribed strains grow only heterotrophically (Stetter and Zillig, 1985). Sulfur as the electron donor can be replaced by Fe^{2+} ions (Brock et al., 1976). The usual terminal electron acceptor (O_2) can be replaced by Fe^{3+} or MoO_4^{2-} ions, and the cells are therefore able to grow in the absence of air by sulfur oxidation. In contrast to *Acidianus* (Segerer et al., 1986), *Sulfolobus* does not grow anaerobically by S^0 reduction, even in the presence of H_2.

The DNA-dependent RNA polymerase shows incomplete immunochemical cross-reaction between the species of the genus *Sulfolobus* and with the species of the genus *Acidianus*.

Sulfolobus was isolated from acidic continental solfatara fields including Yellowstone National Park (Wyoming), New Mexico, Solfatara Crater and Pisciarelli Solfatara (Naples, Italy), Dominica, El Salvador, New Zealand, Iceland, Japan, The Azores and Sumatra (Stetter, 1986b), indicating worldwide distribution. On the surface of boiling mudholes, oily glimmering films contain large amounts of *Sulfolobus*-shaped cells (up to 10^8/ml).

Thin sections of *Sulfolobus* species strain B6 show hexagonal, densely packed, viruslike particles within the cells (Stetter and Zillig, 1985). A lemon-shaped viruslike particle, SSV1 (previously named SAV1), is known from *Sulfolobus solfataricus* strain B12 (Martin et al., 1984; Zillig et al., 1986). It can be induced by UV light and contains double-stranded DNA of 15-kb length. Infection of *Sulfolobus* cells has not yet been observed.

Enrichment and Isolation Procedures

Sulfolobus can be enriched in modified Allen medium (Allen, 1959; Brock et al., 1972) containing 0.1% yeast extract. Enrichment cultures are incubated by shaking in the presence of air at 80°C. The absence of S^0 prevents growth of *Acidianus infernus*.

Sulfolobus can be isolated by plating under microaerobic conditions onto polysilicate or 10% starch plates containing 0.1% yeast extract.

Maintenance Procedures

Sulfolobus cultures can be stored at 4°C after raising the pH of the medium to 5.5 with $CaCO_3$. They can be used as an inoculum for several weeks. For longer periods of time (at least for 2 years), 50% glycerol is added and the cultures are stored under liquid nitrogen.

Differentiation of the genus **Sulfolobus** from other genera

Sulfolobus differs from the related genus *Acidianus* by its higher mol% G + C content of around 37, its inability to grow anaerobically by means of S⁰ reduction, and the lack of significant DNA homology (Segerer et al., 1986). *Thermoplasma*, the third group of thermoacidophilic archaeobacteria, differs by the lack of a protein cell envelope, its mol% G + C content of 46 and its inability to grow by S⁰ oxidation.

Taxonomic Comments

By 16S rRNA total sequencing, *Sulfolobus* most likely represents a distinct order within the urkingdom of archaeobacteria, the *Sulfolobales* (Woese et al., 1984; Stetter and Zillig, 1985). Due to serological cross-reaction between the RNA polymerases of members of the genera *Sulfolobus* and *Acidianus*, they both belong to the same family, *Sulfolobaceae* (Zillig et al., 1980a; Segerer et al., 1986).

By 16S rRNA cataloging, the two species of *Sulfolobus* (see below) are phylogenetically distant ($S_{AB} = 0.41$; Woese et al., 1984) though phenotypically very similar. Further aerobic *Sulfolobus*-shaped isolates were described, resembling *Sulfolobus* in many physiological and biochemical properties (Huber et al., 1986). They are able to grow lithoautotrophically on sulfidic ores. Due to the incomplete serological cross-reaction of their RNA polymerases with the enzyme of *Sulfolobus* (C. Schiegl, personal communication), they most likely belong to a yet undescribed genus within the *Sulfolobaceae*.

Further Reading

Brock, T.D. 1978. The genus *Sulfolobus. In* Starr (Editor), Thermophilic Microorganisms and Life at High Temperatures. Springer-Verlag, Berlin, pp. 117–179.

Brock, T.D. 1981. The genus *Sulfolobus. In* Starr, Stolp, Trüper, Balows and Schlegel (Editors), The Prokaryotes. A Handbook on Habitats, Isolation, and Identification of Bacteria. Springer-Verlag, Berlin, pp. 981–984.

Stetter, K.O. 1986. Diversity of extremely thermophilic archaebacteria. *In* Brock (Editor), Thermophiles: General, Molecular and Applied Microbiology. John Wiley & Sons, New York, pp. 39–74.

Stetter, K.O. and W. Zillig. 1985. *Thermoplasma* and the thermophilic sulfur-dependent archaebacteria. *In* Woese and Wolfe (Editors), The Bacteria. A Treatise on Structure and Function, Vol. VIII: Archaebacteria. Academic Press, New York, pp. 85–170.

Differentiation of the species of the genus **Sulfolobus**

Only two species, *Sulfolobus acidocaldarius* and *Sulfolobus solfataricus*, are described. A third species, *S. brierleyi*, was found to be a member of the genus *Acidianus* and was renamed *Acidianus brierleyi* (Segerer et al., 1986).

Key to the species of the genus **Sulfolobus**

1. Optimum temperature for growth: 70–75°C. DNA-dependent RNA polymerase stable up to 75°C in vitro.
   1. *S. acidocaldarius*
2. Optimum temperature for growth: 87°C. DNA-dependent RNA polymerase stable up to 85°C in vitro.
   2. *S. solfataricus*

List of species of the genus **Sulfolobus**

1. **Sulfolobus acidocaldarius** Brock, Brock, Belly and Weiss 1972, 66.^AL

a.ci.do.cal.dar′i.us. M.L. neut. n. *acidum* acid; L. masc. adj. *caldarius* pertaining to warm or hot; M.L. masc. adj. *acidocaldarius* organism living in acid-hot environments.

Temperature for growth: 55–85°C; optimum: 70–75°C. pH for growth: 1–6; optimum pH: 2–3. Cells lyse at pH >7.5. DNA-dependent RNA polymerase consists of 10 subunits of different molecular weights. The molecular weights of the subunits are slightly different from the corresponding ones of *Sulfolobus solfataricus* (Zillig et al., 1980a). The enzyme is activated by Mg^{2+} ions (optimum: 20–50 mM Mg^{2+} at 30 mM NH_4^+) and is stable up to 75°C in vitro. No significant DNA homology with *S. solfataricus* (Segerer et al., 1986).

The mol% G + C of the DNA is about 37 (T_m).

See also generic description for features.

Type strain: 98-3 (DSM 639).

2. **Sulfolobus solfataricus** Zillig, Stetter, Wunderl, Schulz, Priess and Scholz 1980, 676.^VP (Effective publication: Zillig, Stetter, Wunderl, Schulz, Priess and Scholz 1980, 268.)

sol.fa.ta′ri.cus. M.L. masc. adj. *solfataricus* living in solfatara biotopes.

Temperature for growth: 50–87°C; optimum: 87°C. pH for growth: 3–5.5; optimum pH: around 4.5. Cells lyse at pH >7.5. DNA-dependent RNA polymerase consists of 11 subunits of different molecular weights. The molecular weights of the subunits are slightly different from the corresponding ones of the above species (Zillig et al., 1980a). The enzyme is activated by Mg^{2+} ions (optimum: 3 mM Mg^{2+} at 30 mM NH_4^+) and is stable up to 85°C in vitro. No significant DNA homology with *S. acidocaldarius* (Segerer et al., 1986).

The mol% G + C of the DNA is around 36 (T_m).

See also generic description for features.

Type strain: DSM 1616.

Genus II. **Acidianus** Segerer, Neuner, Kristjansson and Stetter 1986, 562^VP

A. Segerer and K. O. Stetter

A.cid.i.a′nus. L. masc. adj. *acidus* acid; L. masc. n. *Ianus* a mythical Roman figure with two faces looking in opposite directions; M.L. masc. n. *Acidianus* acidic bifaced (bacterium).

Cells coccoid, highly irregular, about 0.5–2 µm in diameter, **occurring almost exclusively singly.** Neither motility nor flagella were detected. Cell envelope composed of protein subunits in hexagonal array (U. Sleytr, personal communication). Isopranyl ether lipids, calditol and caldariella quinone present (Langworthy, 1985; T. Langworthy and M. Collins, personal communication). Elongation factor 2 is ADP-ribosylated by diphtheria toxin (F. Klink, personal communication).

Facultatively anaerobic. Lithotrophic growth aerobically via S⁰ oxidation or anaerobically via S⁰ reduction with H₂. Thermoacidophilic, growing above 45°C and at pH 1–6. Optimum concentration for growth: around 0.2% NaCl; maximum: 4% NaCl.

The mol% G + C of the DNA is about 31.

Type species: *Acidianus infernus* Segerer, Neuner, Kristjansson and Stetter 1986, 562.

Further Descriptive Information

The cells are highly irregular in shape: lobed, disk- to dish-shaped or appearing as polyhedrons; occasionally spherical (Fig. 25.48). No septa formation visible. The S-layer consists of subunits about 25 nm in width.

The organisms are autotrophic and mixotrophic. Some strains are able to grow heterotrophically on yeast extract in the presence of oxygen. Anaerobic growth via S^0 oxidation takes place in the presence of molybdate. No growth at very low redox potentials (around -300 mV) in the absence of either sulfur or hydrogen or both. Anaerobically grown cells are significantly more resistant to storage and disintegration procedures than are aerobically grown cells.

The DNA-dependent RNA polymerase shows incomplete immunochemical cross-reaction with antibodies against the native enzyme of *Sulfolobus acidocaldarius*.

Acidianus was isolated from anaerobic and aerobic samples taken from acidic solfatara springs and mudholes at Solfatara Crater, Naples, Italy, and Yellowstone National Park, Wyoming, U.S.A. It also occurs in geothermally heated acidic marine environments at the beach of Vulcano Island, Italy. Probably closely related strains were found in solfatara fields from Iceland, The Azores and Java (Indonesia).

Enrichment and Isolation Procedures

Acidianus can be enriched anaerobically in a modified Allen medium (Allen, 1959; Segerer et al., 1985) containing S^0 and an 80% H_2 and 20% CO_2 atmosphere (300 kPa), incubated with shaking at the appropriate temperature. After 2–3 days of incubation, mature cultures are transferred into aerobic medium and further incubated.

Acidianus can be isolated by plating under aerobic or anaerobic conditions onto 10% starch plates containing 0.5–1% colloidal sulfur.

Maintenance Procedures

Since anaerobically grown cells are more resistant to storage procedures than are aerobically grown cells, stock cultures of *Acidianus* are routinely stored anaerobically at 4°C after raising the pH of the medium to 5.5 with $CaCO_3$; they are transferred every 8–12 weeks. The viability of such cultures is variable, depending on the isolate (e.g. the type strain of *A. brierleyi* (DSM 1651) is viable for 6–8 months, while the type strain of *A. infernus* (DSM 3191) is viable even at pH 2.5 for at least 2 years).

Storage of anaerobic or aerobic cultures is also possible in medium (pH 5.5) containing 50% (v/v) glycerol at the temperature of liquid nitrogen.

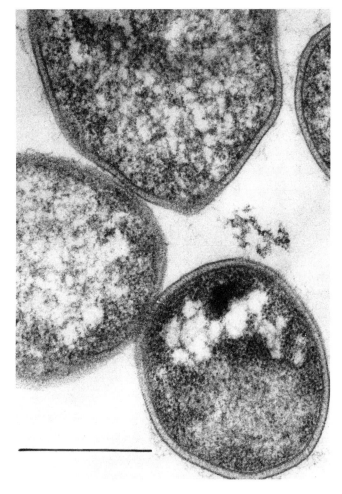

Figure 25.48. Electron micrograph of thin sections of *A. infernus.* *Bar*, 0.5 μm. (Reproduced with permission from A. Segerer, A. Neuer, J. K. Kristjansson and K. O. Stetter, International Journal of Systematic Bacteriology *36*: 559–564, 1986, ©International Union of Microbiological Societies.)

Differentiation of the genus **Acidianus** from other genera

The genus *Acidianus* belongs to the *Sulfolobus* group of S^0-metabolizing archaeobacteria, due to its thermoacidophilic mode of life, morphology, low mol% G + C of the DNA, mode of aerobic energy conservation by means of S^0 oxidation, the presence of caldariella quinone and calditol in the cells and the immunochemical cross-reaction of the DNA-dependent RNA polymerase with antibodies directed against the enzyme of *Sulfolobus*. It differs from *Sulfolobus* by the distinct mol% G + C of the DNA of 31, its ability to grow anaerobically by means of S^0 reduction with H_2, and the lack of significant DNA homology.

Thermoplasma acidophilum, the only other thermoacidophilic archaeobacterium, differs by the lack of a protein cell envelope and a mol% G + C of the DNA of 46. Furthermore, it is unable to grow via S^0 oxidation or S^0/H_2 autotrophy.

Taxonomic Comments

The immunochemical cross-reaction of the DNA-dependent RNA polymerase of *Acidianus* with the enzyme of *Sulfolobus* indicates that

Acidianus belongs to the same family (Stetter et al., 1981), the *Sulfolobaceae*. The exact taxonomic position will have to await 16S rRNA cataloging.

An isolate with physiological properties similar to members of the genus *Acidianus* has been isolated by Zillig et al. (1985) and tentatively named "*Sulfolobus ambivalens*." Recently, it was described as *Desulfurolobus ambivalens*, representing the new genus *Desulfurolobus* (Zillig et al., 1986; Zillig and Böck, 1987). *Desulfurolobus ambivalens* exhibits 60% DNA homology with the type species *Acidianus infernus*, indicating that it is another species of the genus *Acidianus* (Huber et al., 1987).

Further Reading

Segerer, A., K.O. Stetter and F. Klink. 1985. Two contrary modes of chemolithotrophy in the same archaeobacterium. Nature *313:* 787–789.

Segerer, A., A. Neuner, J.K. Kristjansson and K.O. Stetter. 1986. *Acidianus infernus* gen. nov., sp. nov., and *Acidianus brierleyi* comb. nov.: facultatively aerobic, extremely acidophilic thermophilic sulfur-metabolizing archaeobacteria. Int. J. Syst. Bacteriol. *36:* 559–564.

Differentiation of the species of the genus **Acidianus**

Only two species, *A. infernus* and *A. brierleyi*, are currently known.
The latter was previously positioned in the genus *Sulfolobus*.

Key to the species of the genus **Acidianus**

1. Optimum temperature for growth: 85–90°C; maximum: 96°C. Aerobic growth strictly lithotrophically by sulfur oxidation.

   1. *A. infernus*

2. Optimum temperature for growth: 70°C; maximum: 75°C. Aerobic growth lithotrophically by oxidation of S^0 or organotrophically by oxidation of organic material (e.g. yeast extract).

   2. *A. brierleyi*

List of species of the genus **Acidianus**

1. **Acidianus infernus** Segerer, Neuner, Kristjansson and Stetter 1986, 562.[VP]

in.fer′nus. L. masc. adj. *infernus* emerged from Hades, referring to the *locus typicus* at the Solfatara Crater, where Dante placed the gate to hell in his *Divina Commedia*.

Obligately chemolithotrophic. No heterotrophic growth on yeast extract in the presence of O_2. Temperature for growth: 65–96°C; optimum: around 90°C. pH for growth: 1–5.5; optimum: around 2. The cell width depends on the culture conditions, with aerobically grown cells being about 1.5 times larger than anaerobically grown ones of the same growth phase. Cells lyse at pH values >8.5. No significant DNA homology with *A. brierleyi* or with species of the genus *Sulfolobus* (Segerer et al., 1986).

See also the generic description for features.

Type strain: DSM 3191.

2. **Acidianus brierleyi** (Zillig, Stetter, Wunderl, Schulz, Priess and Scholz 1980) Segerer, Neuner, Kristjansson and Stetter 1986, 562.[VP] (*Sulfolobus brierleyi* Zillig, Stetter, Wunderl, Schulz, Priess and Scholz 1980b, 676.)

brier′ley.i. M.L. gen. n. *brierleyi* of Brierley; named for J. A. Brierley who isolated the organism.

Facultatively chemolithotrophic. Heterotrophic growth on yeast extract or lithotrophic growth on sulfur in the presence of O_2. Temperature for growth: 45–75°C; optimum: around 70°C. pH for growth: 1–6; optimum: 1.5–2. Cells lyse at pH values >7. DNA-dependent RNA polymerase requires Mg^{2+} ions and consists of nine subunits of different molecular weight.

See also the generic description for features.

Type strain: DSM 1651.

Bibliography

Aasen, A.J. and S. Liaaen-Jensen. 1966a. The carotenoids of flexibacter. II. A new xanthophyll from *Saprospira grandis*. Acta Chem. Scand. *20:* 811–819.

Aasen, A.J. and S. Liaaen-Jensen. 1966b. Carotenoids of flexibacteria. III. The structures of flexixanthin and deoxy-flexixanthin. Acta Chem. Scand. *20:* 1970–1988.

Aasen, A.J. and S. Liaaen-Jensen. 1966c. Carotenoids of flexibacteria. IV. The carotenoids of two further pigment prototypes. Acta Chem. Scand. *20:* 2322–2324.

Aasen, A.J., S. Liaaen-Jensen and G. Borch. 1972. Carotenoids of flexibacteria. V. The chirality of zeaxanthin from different natural sources. Acta Chem. Scand. *26:* 404–405.

Achenbach, H., A. Böttger, W. Kohl, E. Fautz and H. Reichenbach. 1979c. Untersuchungen zur Biogenese des Flexirubins—Herkunft des Benzolrings A und der aromatischen C-Methylgruppen. Phytochemistry *18:* 961–963.

Achenbach, H., A. Böttger-Vetter, E. Fautz and H. Reichenbach. 1982. On the origin of the branched alkyl substituents on ring B of flexirubin-type pigments. Arch. Microbiol. *132:* 241–244.

Achenbach, H., A. Böttger-Vetter, D. Hunkler, E. Fautz and H. Reichenbach. 1983. Investigations on the biosynthesis of flexirubin—the origin of benzene ring B and its substituents. Tetrahedron *39:* 175–185.

Achenbach, H., W. Kohl, S. Alexanian and H. Reichenbach. 1979a. Neue Pigmente vom Flexirubin-Typ aus *Cytophaga* spec. Stamm Samoa. Chem. Ber. *112:* 196–206.

Achenbach, H., W. Kohl, A. Böttger-Vetter and H. Reichenbach. 1981. Untersuchungen der Pigmente aus *Flavobacterium* spec. Stamm C 1/2. Tetrahedron *37:* 559–563.

Achenbach, H., W. Kohl and H. Reichenbach. 1976. Flexirubin, ein neuartiges Pigment aus *Flexibacter elegans*. Chem. Ber. *109:* 2490–2502.

Achenbach, H., W. Kohl and H. Reichenbach. 1977. 5-Chlorflexirubin, ein Nebenpigment aus *Flexibacter elegans*. Liebigs Ann. Chem. *1977:* 1–7.

Achenbach, H., W. Kohl and H. Reichenbach. 1978a. The flexirubin-type pigments—a novel class of natural pigments from gliding bacteria. Rev. Latinoam. Quim. *9:* 111–124.

Achenbach, H., W. Kohl and H. Reichenbach. 1979b. Die Konstitution der Pigmente vom Flexirubin-Typ aus *Cytophaga johnsonae* Cy j1. Chem. Ber. *112:* 1999–2011.

Achenbach, H., W. Kohl, W. Wachter and H. Reichenbach. 1978b. Investigations of the pigments from *Cytophaga johnsonae* Cy j1. New flexirubin-type pigments. Arch. Microbiol. *117:* 253–257.

Adams, D.G. and N.G. Carr. 1981. The developmental biology of heterocyst and akinete formation in cyanobacteria. CRC Crit. Rev. Microbiol. *9:* 45–100.

Adkins, A.M. and R. Knowles. 1984. Reduction of nitrous oxide by a soil *Cytophaga* in the presence of acetylene and sulfide. FEMS Microbiol. Lett. *23:* 171–174.

Agabian, N. and B. Unger. 1978. *Caulobacter crescentus* cell envelope: effect of growth conditions on murein and outer membrane protein composition. J. Bacteriol. *133:* 987–994.

Agardh, C.A. 1824. Systema Algarum, Litteris Berlingianis. Lund, Sweden, 312 pp.

Agardh, J. 1842. Alg. Mar. Med. Adr.

Agbo, J.A.C. and M.O. Moss. 1979. The isolation and characterization of agarolytic bacteria from a lowland river. J. Gen. Microbiol. *115:* 355–368.

Ahamed, N.M., H. Mayer, H. Biebl and J. Weckesser. 1982. Lipopolysaccharide with 2,3-diamino-2,3-dideoxyglucose containing lipid A in *Rhodopseudomonas sulfoviridis*. FEMS Microbiol. Lett. *14:* 27–30.

Ahlgren, G. 1985. Growth of *Oscillatoria agardhii* in chemostat culture. 3. Simultaneous limitation of nitrogen and phosphorus. Br. Phycol. J. *20:* 249–261.

Ahmadjian, V. 1982. Algal/fungal symbioses. *In* Round and Chapman (Editors), Progress in Phycological Research, Vol. 1. Elsevier, Amsterdam, pp. 179–233.

Ahrens, R. 1968. Taxonomische Untersuchungen an Sternbildenden *Agrobacterium*—Arten aus der westlichen Ostsee. Kiel. Meeresforsch. *24:* 147–173.

Ahrens, R. and G. Moll. 1970. Ein neues knospendes Bakterium aus der Ostsee. Arch. Mikrobiol. *70:* 243–265.

Ahrens, R. and G. Moll. 1971. Über die Fimbriierung sternbildender Bakterien aus Brackwasser. Kiel. Meeresforsch. *27:* 113–116.

Ahrens, R. and G. Rheinheimer. 1967. Über einige sternbildender Bakterien aus der Ostsee. Kiel. Meeresforsch. *23:* 127–136.

Ainsworth, G.C. and P.H.A. Sneath (Editors). 1962. Microbial classification: appendix I. Symp. Soc. Gen. Microbiol. *12:* 456–463.

Akashi, A. 1960. Studies on the cellulose-decomposing bacteria in the rumen. J. Agric. Chem. Soc. Jpn. *34:* 895–900.

Akiba, T., R. Usami and K. Horikoshi. 1983. *Rhodopseudomonas rutila*, a new species of nonsulfur purple bacteria. Int. J. Syst. Bacteriol. *33:* 551–556.

Alam, M. and D. Oesterhelt. 1984. Morphology, function and isolation of halobacterial flagella. J. Mol. Biol. *176:* 459–475.

Albers, H. and G. Gottschalk. 1976. Acetate metabolism in *Rhodopseudomonas gelatinosa* and several other *Rhodospirillaceae*. Arch. Microbiol. *111:* 45–49.

Aleem, M.I.H. 1966. Generation of reducing power in chemosynthesis II. Energy-linked reduction of pyridine nucleotides in the chemoautotroph *Nitrosomonas europaea*. Biochim. Biophys. Acta *113:* 216–224.

Aleem, M.I.H. 1968. Mechanism of oxidative phosphorylation in the chemoautotroph *Nitrobacter agilis*. Biochim. Biophys. Acta *162:* 338–347.

Aleem, M.I.H. and M. Alexander. 1958. Cell-free nitrification by *Nitrobacter*. J. Bacteriol. *76:* 510–514.

Aleem, M.I.H., G.E. Hoch and J.E. Varner. 1965. Water as the source of oxidant and reductant in bacterial chemosynthesis. Proc. Natl. Acad. Sci. *54:* 869–873.

Aleem, M.I.H. and D.L. Sewell. 1981. Mechanism of nitrite oxidation and oxidoreductase systems in *Nitrobacter agilis*. Curr. Microbiol. *5:* 267–272.

Alef, K. and D. Kleiner. 1982. Evidence for an ammonium transport system in the N_2-fixing phototrophic bacterium *Rhodospirillum rubrum*. Arch. Microbiol. *132:* 79–81.

Alexopoulos, C.J. 1962. Introductory Mycology, 2nd Ed. Wiley, New York.

Allen, M.B. 1952. The cultivation of Myxophyceae. Arch. Mikrobiol. *17:* 34–53.

Allen, M.B. 1959. Studies with *Cyanidium caldarium* an anomalously pigmented chlorophyte. Arch. Mikrobiol. *32:* 270–277.

Allen, M.M. 1973. Methods of Cyanophyceae. *In* Stein (Editor), Handbook of Phycological Methods. Cambridge University Press, London, New York, pp. 127–138.

Allen, M.M. 1984. Cyanobacterial cell inclusions. Annu. Rev. Microbiol. *38:* 1–25.

Allsopp, A. 1969. Phylogenetic relationships of the Procaryota and the origin of the eucaryotic cell. New Phytol. *68:* 591–612.

Ambler, R.P. 1976. Amino acid sequences of prokaryotic cytochromes and proteins. *In* Fasman (Editor), Handbook of Biochemistry and Molecular Biology, 3rd Ed., Vol. 3. CRC Press, Cleveland, Ohio, pp. 292–307.

Ambler, R.P., R.G. Bartsch, M. Daniel, M.D. Kamen, L. McLellan, T.E. Meyer and J. van Beeumen. 1981. Amino acid sequences of bacterial cytochromes c_1 and c_{-556}. Proc. Natl. Acad. Sci. U.S.A. *78:* 6854–6857.

Ambler, R.P., M. Daniel, J. Hermoso, T.E. Meyer, T.G. Bartsch and M.D. Kamen. 1979. Cytochrome c_2 sequence variation among the recognized species of purple nonsulphur photosynthetic bacteria. Nature (London) *278:* 659–660.

Ambler, R.P., T.E. Meyer and M.D. Kamen. 1979. Anomalies in amino acid sequences of small cytochromes c and cytochromes c_1 from two species of purple photosynthetic bacteria. Nature (London) *278:* 661–662.

Anacker, R.L. 1956. Studies on the identification, virulence, and distribution of strains of *Chondrococcus columnaris* isolated from fish in the Columbia River system. Ph.D. thesis, University of Washington, Seattle.

Anacker, R.L. and E.J. Ordal. 1955. Study of a bacteriophage infecting the myxobacterium *Chondrococcus columnaris*. J. Bacteriol. *70:* 738–741.

Anacker, R.L. and E.J. Ordal. 1959a. Studies on the myxobacterium *Chondrococcus columnaris*. I. Serological typing. J. Bacteriol. *78:* 25–32.

Anacker, R.L. and E.J. Ordal. 1959b. Studies on the myxobacterium *Chondrococcus columnaris*. II. Bacteriocins. J. Bacteriol. *78:* 33–40.

Anagnostidis, K. 1961. Untersuchungen über die Cyanophyceen einiger Thermen in Griechenland (in Greek, German summary and discussion). Inst. Syst. Bot. Pflanzengeogr., Univ. Thessaloniki *7:* 1–322.

Anagnostidis, K. 1968. Untersuchungen über die Salz- und Süsswasser Thiobiocönosen (Sulfuretum) Griechenlands. Aristotle University, Thessalonika.

Anagnostidis, K. and J. Komárek. 1985. Modern approach to the classification system of cyanophytes. 1. Introduction. Arch. Hydrobiol. Suppl. *71:* 291–302.

Anagnostidis, K. and J. Komárek. 1988. Modern approach to the classification system of cyanophytes. III. Oscillatoriales. Arch. Hydrobiol. Suppl. *80:* 327–472.

Anagnostidis, K. and R. Rathsack-Kuzenbach. 1967. *Isocystis pallida*—Blaualge oder hefeartiger Pilz? Schweiz. Z. Hydrol. *29:* 191–198.

Anderson, J.I.W. and D.A. Conroy. 1969. The pathogenic myxobacteria with special reference to fish diseases. J. Appl. Bacteriol. *32:* 30–39.

Anderson, J.I.W. and W.P. Heffernan. 1965. Isolation and characterization of filterable marine bacteria. J. Bacteriol. *90:* 1713–1718.

Anderson, L. and R.C. Fuller. 1967a. Photosynthesis in *Rhodospirillum rubrum* I. Autotrophic carbon dioxide fixation. Plant Physiol. *42:* 487–490.

Anderson, L. and R.C. Fuller. 1967b. Photosynthesis in *Rhodospirillum rubrum* II. Photoheterotrophic carbon dioxide fixation. Plant Physiol. *42:* 491–496.

Anderson, R.L. and E.J. Ordal. 1961a. *Cytophaga succinicans* sp. n., a facultatively anaerobic, aquatic myxobacterium. J. Bacteriol. *81:* 130–138.

Anderson, R.L. and E.J. Ordal. 1961b. CO₂-dependent fermentation of glucose by *Cytophaga succinicans.* J. Bacteriol. *81:* 139–146.

Andersson, K.K. and A.B. Hooper. 1983. O₂ and H₂O are each the source of one O in NO₂- produced from NH₂ by *Nitrosomonas:* ¹⁵N-NMR evidence. FEBS Lett. *164:* 236–240.

Andersson, K.K., T.A. Kent, J.D. Lipscomb, A.B. Hooper and E. Munck. 1984. Mössbauer, EPR, and optical studies of the P-460 center of hydroxylamine oxidoreductase from *Nitrosomonas.* A ferrous heme with an unusually large quadruple splitting. J. Biol. Chem. *259:* 6833–6840.

Approved Lists of Bacterial Names. 1980. American Society for Microbiology, Washington, D.C. Reprinted from Int. J. Syst. Bacteriol. *30:* 225–420.

Aranki, A. and R. Freter. 1972. Use of anaerobic glove boxes for the cultivation of strictly anaerobic bacteria. Am. J. Clin. Nutr. *25:* 1329–1334.

Archer, D.B. and N.R. King. 1983. A novel ultrastructural feature of a gas-vacuolated *Methanosarcina.* FEMS Microbiol. Lett. *16:* 217–223.

Archer, D.B. and N.R. King. 1984. Isolation of gas vesicles from *Methanosarcina barkeri.* J. Gen. Microbiol. *130:* 167–172.

Aretz, W., H. Kaspari and J.-H. Klemme. 1978. Utilization of purines as nitrogen source by facultative phototrophic bacteria. FEMS Microbiol. Lett. *4:* 249–253.

Arias, J.M., C. Rodriguez and E. Montoya. 1979. Purification and partial characterization of an antibiotic from *Myxococcus coralloides.* J. Antibiot. *32:* 205–211.

Aristovskaya, T.V. 1961. Accumulation of iron in breakdown of organomineral humus complexes by microorganisms (in Russian). Dokl. Akad. Nauk S.S.S.R. *136:* 954–957.

Aristovskaya, T.V. 1963. On the decomposition of organic mineral compounds in podzolic soils. Pochvoved. Akad. Nauk S.S.S.R. *1:* 30–42.

Aristovskaya, T.V. 1964. The taxonomic position of the genus *Seliberia* Aristovskaya et Parinkina. Mikrobiologiya *33:* 929–934.

Aristovskaya, T.V. 1965. Microbiology of podzolic soils. Nauka, Moscow-Leningrad.

Aristovskaya, T.V. 1974. *Seliberia. In* Buchanan and Gibbons (Editors), Bergey's Manual of Determinative Bacteriology, 8th Ed. The Williams and Wilkins Co., Baltimore, p. 160.

Aristovskaya, T.V. and V.V. Parinkina. 1961. New methods of studying soil microorganism associations. Sov. Soil Sci. *1:* 12–20.

Aristovskaya, T.V. and V.V. Parinkina. 1963. New soil microorganism *Seliberia stellata* nov. gen. n. sp. Izv. Akad. Nauk S.S.S.R., Ser. Biol. *28:* 49–56.

Arkesteyn, G.J.M.W. and J.A.M. de Bont. 1980. *Thiobacillus acidophilus:* a study of its presence in *Thiobacillus ferrooxidans* cultures. Can. J. Microbiol. *26:* 1057–1065.

Asenjo, J.A. and P. Dunnill. 1981. The isolation of lytic enzymes from *Cytophaga* and their application to the rupture of yeast cells. Biotechnol. Bioeng. *23:* 1045–1056.

Asselineau, J. and F. Pichinoty. 1983. Lipid composition of strains of *Flavobacterium* and *Sphingobacterium.* FEMS Microbiol. Lett. *20:* 375–378.

Attwood, M.M. and W. Harder. 1972. A rapid and specific enrichment procedure for *Hyphomicrobium* spp. Antonie van Leeuwenhoek J. Microbiol. Serol. *38:* 369–378.

Auran, T.B. and E.L. Schmidt. 1972. Similarities between *Hyphomicrobium* and *Nitrobacter* with respect to fatty acids. J. Bacteriol. *109:* 450–451.

Awramik, S.M. and E.S. Barghoorn. 1977. The Gunflint microbiota. Precambrian Res. *5:* 121–142.

Baalsrud, K. and K.S. Baalsrud. 1954. Studies on *Thiobacillus denitrificans.* Arch. Mikrobiol. *20:* 34–62.

Baas-Becking, L.G.M. 1925. Studies on the sulphur bacteria. Ann. Bot. *39:* 613–650.

Babenzien, H.D. 1965. Über Vorkommen und Kultur von *Nevskia ramosa.* Zentralbl. Bakteriol. Parasitenkd. Infektionskr. Abt. I Suppl. *1:* 111–116.

Babenzien, H.D. 1967. Zur Biologie von *Nevskia ramosa.* Z. Allg. Mikrobiol. *7:* 89–96.

Babenzien, H.D. 1974. Fine structure and systematic position of the caulobacterium *Nevskia ramosa.* XIth conference on the taxonomy of bacteria. Abstracts, Brno, p. 15.

Babenzien, H.D. and P. Hirsch. 1974. Genus *Nevskia. In* Buchanan and Gibbons (Editors), Bergey's Manual of Determinative Bacteriology, 8th Ed. The Williams and Wilkins Co., Baltimore, pp. 161–162.

Babinchak, J.A. and V.F. Gerencser. 1976. Bacteriophage typing of the "*Caulobacter* group." Int. J. Syst. Bacteriol. *26:* 82–84.

Bachmann, B.J. 1955. Studies on *Cytophaga fermentans,* n. sp., a facultatively anaerobic lower myxobacterium. J. Gen. Microbiol. *13:* 541–551.

Bacon, J.S.D., A.H. Gordon, D. Jones, I.F. Taylor and D.M. Webley. 1970. The separation of β-glucanases produced by *Cytophaga johnsonii* and their role in the lysis of yeast cell walls. Biochem. J. *120:* 67–78.

Bacon, K. and E.A. Eiserling. 1968. A unique structure in microcysts of *Myxococcus xanthus.* J. Ultrastruct. Res. *21:* 378–382.

Badian, J. 1930. Z cytologji miksobakteryj (Zur Zytologie der Myxobakterien). Acta Soc. Bot. Pol. *7:* 55–71.

Bahr, H. and U. Schwartz. 1956. Untersuchungen zur Ökologie farblose Schwefelmikroben. Biol. Zeit. *75:* 451–454.

Balashova, V.V. 1967. Structure of the "stalk" fibers in a laboratory culture of *Gallionella filamenta.* Mikrobiologiya *36:* 1050–1053.

Balashova, V.V. 1968. Taxonomy of the genus *Gallionella.* Mikrobiologiya *37:* 715–723.

Balashova, V.V. 1969. The relationship of *Gallionella* to Mycoplasma. Dokl. Akad. Nauk U.S.S.R. Biol. Sci. Sect. *184:* 1429–1432.

Balashova, V.V. 1974. Mycoplasms and Iron Bacteria. Nauka, Moscow, 64 pp. (in Russian).

Balashova, V.V. and N.E. Cherni. 1970. Ultrastructure of *Gallionella filamenta.* Mikrobiologiya *39:* 348–351.

Balashova, V.V., I.Y. Vedenina, G.E. Markosyan and G.A. Zavarzin. 1974. The auxotrophic growth of *Leptospirillum ferrooxidans.* Mikrobiologiya *43:* 581–585 (English translation: *43:* 491–494).

Balashova, V.V. and G.A. Zavarzin. 1972. Oxidation of iron by *Mycoplasma laidlawii.* Mikrobiologiya *42:* 909–911.

Balch, W.E. 1982. Methanogens: their impact on our concept of procaryote diversity. Zentralbl. Bakteriol. Mikrobiol. Hyg. I Abt. Orig. *C3:* 295–303.

Balch, W.E., C.E. Fox, L.J. Magrum, C.R. Woese and R.S. Wolfe. 1979. Methanogens: reevaluation of a unique biological group. Microbiol. Rev. *43:* 260–296.

Balch, W.E. and R.S. Wolfe. 1976. New approach to the cultivation of methanogenic bacteria; 2-mercaptoethane-sulfonic acid (HS-CoM)-dependent growth of *Methanobacterium ruminantium* in a pressurized atmosphere. Appl. Environ. Microbiol. *32:* 781–791.

Balch, W.E. and R.S. Wolfe. 1979a. Specificity and biological distribution of coenzyme M (2-mercaptoethanesulfonic acid). J. Bacteriol. *137:* 256–263.

Balch, W.E. and R.S. Wolfe. 1979b. Transport of coenzyme M (2-mercaptoethanesulfonic acid) in *Methanobacterium ruminantium.* J. Bacteriol. *137:* 264–273.

Balch, W.E. and R.S. Wolfe. 1981. *In* Validation of the publication of new names and new combinations previously effectively published outside the IJSB. List No. 6. Int. J. Syst. Bacteriol. *31:* 215–218.

Balkwill, D.L., D. Maratea and R.P. Blakemore. 1980. Ultrastructure of a magnetotactic spirillum. J. Bacteriol. *141:* 1399–1408.

Balkwill, D.L., S.A. Nierzwicki-Bauer and S.E. Stevens, Jr. 1984. Modes of cell division and branch formation in the morphogenesis of the cyanobacterium *Mastigocladus laminosus.* J. Gen. Microbiol. *130:* 2079–2088.

Bang, S.S., L. Baumann, M.J. Woolkalis and P. Baumann. 1981. Evolutionary relationships in *Vibrio* and *Photobacterium* as determined by immunological studies of superoxide dismutase. Arch. Microbiol. *130:* 111–120.

Barghoorn, E.S. and S.A. Tyler. 1967. Microorganisms from the Gunflint chert. Science *147:* 563–577.

Barker, H.A. 1936. Studies upon the methane-producing bacteria. Arch. Mikrobiol. *7:* 420–438.

Barker, H.A. 1956. Bacterial Fermentations. John Wiley and Sons, New York.

Barksdale, L. 1970. *Corynebacterium diphtheriae* and its relatives. Bacteriol. Rev. *34:* 378–422.

Barrett, J.T., R.H. Croft, D.M. Ferber, C.J. Gerardot, P.V. Schoenlein and B. Ely. 1982a. Genetic mapping with Tn5-derived auxotrophs of *Caulobacter crescentus.* J. Bacteriol. *151:* 888–898.

Barrett, J.T., C.S. Rhodes, D.M. Ferber, B. Jenkins, S.A. Kuhl and B. Ely. 1982b. Construction of a genetic map for *Caulobacter crescentus.* J. Bacteriol. *149:* 889–896.

Barros, M.E.C., D.E. Rawlings and D.R. Woods. 1984. Mixotrophic growth of a *Thiobacillus ferrooxidans* strain. Appl. Environ. Microbiol. *47:* 493–595.

Barton, L.L. and J.M. Shively. 1968. Thiosulfate utilization by *Thiobacillus thiooxidans* ATCC 8085. J. Bacteriol. *95:* 720.

Bartsch, R.G. 1978. Cytochromes. *In* Clayton and Sistrom (Editors), The Photosynthetic Bacteria. Plenum Press, New York and London, pp. 249–279.

Bast, E. 1977. Utilization of nitrogen compounds and ammonia assimilation by *Chromatiaceae.* Arch. Microbiol. *143:* 91–94.

Bauer, C.-A., G.D. Brayer, A.R. Sielecki and M.N.G. James. 1981. Active site of α-lytic protease. Eur. J. Biochem. *129:* 289–294.

Bauer, L. 1962. Untersuchungen an *Sphaeromyxa xanthochlora,* n. sp., einer auf Tropfkörpern vorkommenden Myxobakterienart. Arch. Hyg. Bakteriol. *146:* 392–400.

Bauld, J. 1981. Occurrence of benthic microbial mats in saline lakes. Hydrobiologia *81:* 87–111.

Bauld, J., R. Bigford and J.T. Staley. 1983. *Prosthecomicrobium litoralum,* a new species from marine habitats. Int. J. Syst. Bacteriol. *33:* 613–617.

Bauld, J. and J.T. Staley. 1976. *Planctomyces maris* sp. nov.: a marine isolate of the *Planctomyces-Blastocaulis* group of budding bacteria. J. Gen. Microbiol. *97:* 44–55.

Bauld, J. and J.T. Staley. 1980. *Planctomyces maris* sp. nov., nom. rev. Int. J. Syst. Bacteriol. *30:* 657.

Baumann, L., S.S. Bang and P. Baumann. 1980. Study of relationship among species of *Vibrio, Photobacterium* and terrestrial enterobacteria by an immunological comparison of glutamine synthetase and superoxide dismutase. Curr. Microbiol. *4:* 133–138.

Baur, E. 1905. Myxobakterien Studien. Arch. Protistenkd. *5:* 92–121.

Baur, V.L. 1962. Untersuchungen an *Sphaeromyxa xanthochlora,* n. sp., einer auf tropfkorpern vorkommenden myxobakterienart. Arch. Hyg. Bakteriol. *146:* 392–400.

Bauwens, M. and J. De Ley. 1981. Improvements in the taxonomy of *Flavobacterium* by DNA:rRNA hybridization. *In* Reichenbach and Weeks (Editors),

The *Flavobacterium-Cytophaga* Group. Verlag Chemie, Weinheim, F.R.G., pp. 27-31.

Bavendamm, W. 1924. Die farblosen und roten Schwefelbakterien des Süss- und Salzwassers. *In* Kolkwitz (Editor), Pflanzenforschung. Gustav Fischer Verlag, Jena, pp. 7-156.

Bazylinski, D.A. and R.P. Blakemore. 1983a. Denitrification and assimilatory nitrate reduction in *Aquaspirillum magnetotacticum*. Appl. Environ. Microbiol. *46:* 1118-1124.

Bazylinski, D.A. and R.P. Blakemore. 1983b. Nitrogen fixation (acetylene reduction) in *Aquaspirillum magnetotacticum*. Curr. Microbiol. *9:* 305-308.

Becker, C.D. and M.P. Fujihara. 1978. The Bacterial Pathogen *Flexibacter columnaris* and Its Epizootiology among Columbia River Fish. Monograph No. 2. American Fisheries Society, Washington, D.C., 92 pp.

Beebe, J.M. 1941. The morphology and cytology of *Myxococcus xanthus*, n. sp. J. Bacteriol. *42:* 193-223.

Beebe, J.M. 1943. Studies on the myxobacteria. 3. The utilization of carbohydrates. Iowa State Coll. J. Sci. *17:* 227-240.

Beger, H. 1935. *Leptothrix echinata*, ein neues, vorwiegend Mangan fällendes Eisenbakterium. Zentralbl. Bakteriol. Parasitenkd. Infektionskr. Hyg. Abt. II *92:* 401-406.

Beger, H. 1941. *Naumanniella catenata* und *Sideronema globulifera*, zwei neue Eisenbakterien. Zentralbl. Bakteriol. Parasitenkd. Infektionskr. Hyg. Abt. II *103:* 321-325.

Beger, H. 1949. Beiträge zur Systematik und geographischen Verbreitung der Eisenbakterien. Ber. Dtsch. Bot. Ges. *62:* 7-13.

Beger, H. 1957. Genus *Phragmidiothrix*. *In* Breed, Murray and Smith (Editors), Bergey's Manual of Determinative Bacteriology, 7th Ed. The Williams and Wilkins Co., Baltimore, pp. 273-274.

Beger, H. and G. Bringmann. 1953. Die Scheidenstruktur des Abwasserbakteriums *Sphaerotilus* und des Eisenbakteriums *Leptothrix* im elektronenmikroskopischen Bilde und ihre Bedeutung für die Systematik dieser Gattungen. Zentralbl. Bakteriol. Parasitenkd. Infektionskr. Hyg. Abt. II *107:* 319-334.

Behki, R.M. and S.M. Lesley. 1972. Deoxyribonucleic acid degradation and the lethal effect by myxin in *Escherichia coli*. J. Bacteriol. *109:* 250-261.

Behrens, H. 1978. Charakterisierung der DNA gleitender Bakterien der Ordnung *Cytophagales*. Doctoral thesis, Technical University of Braunschweig, F.R.G., 107 pp.

Behrens, H., J. Flossdorf and H. Reichenbach. 1976. Base composition of deoxyribonucleic acid from *Nannocystis exedens* (*Myxobacterales*). Int. J. Syst. Bacteriol. *26:* 561-562.

Beijerinck, M.W. 1904a. Phénomenes de réduction produits par les microbes. Arch. Neer. Sci. (Sect. 2) *9:* 131-157.

Beijerinck, M.W. 1904b. Über Bakterien welche sich im Dunkeln mit Kohlensäure als Kohlenstoffquelle ernähren können. Zentralbl. Bakteriol. Parasitenkd. Infektionskr. Hyg. Abt. II *11:* 593-599.

Beijerinck, M.W. and A. van Delden. 1903. Ueber eine farblose Bakterie, deren Kohlenstoffnahrung aus der atmosphärischen Luft Herrüht. Zentralbl. Bakteriol. Parasitenkd. Infektionskr Hyg. Abt. II *10:* 33-47.

Belay, N., R. Sparling and L. Daniels. 1984. Dinitrogen fixation by a thermophilic methanogenic bacterium. Nature *312:* 286-288.

Belly, R.T., B.B. Bohlool and T.D. Brock. 1973. The genus *Thermoplasma*. Ann. N.Y. Acad. Sci. *225:* 94-107.

Belly, R.T. and T.D. Brock. 1972. Cellular stability of a thermophilic, acidophilic mycoplasma. J. Gen. Microbiol. *73:* 465-469.

Belly, R.T. and T.D. Brock. 1974. Ecology of iron-oxidizing bacteria in pyritic materials associated with coal. J. Bacteriol. *117:* 726-732.

Belser, L.W. and E.L. Schmidt. 1978a. Nitrification in soils. *In* Schlesinger (Editor), Microbiology 1978. American Society for Microbiology, Washington, D.C., pp. 348-351.

Belser, L.W. and E.L. Schmidt. 1978b. Serological diversity within a terrestrial ammonia-oxidizing population. Appl. Environ. Microbiol. *36:* 589-593.

Belser, L.W. and E.L. Schmidt. 1980. Growth and oxidation kinetics of three genera of ammonia oxidizing nitrifiers. FEMS Microbiol. Lett. *7:* 213-216.

Bensoussan, M. 1977. Contribution à l'étude du genre *Flavobacterium*. Taxonomie numérique et analyse spectrale des pigments de bactéries isolées du milieu marin. Doctoral thesis, Université d'Aix-Marseilles, France, 97 pp.

Bergan, T. 1981. Human- and animal-pathogenic members of the genus *Pseudomonas*. *In* Starr, Stolp, Trüper, Balows and Schlegel (Editors), The Prokaryotes. A Handbook on Habitats, Isolation, and Identification of Bacteria. Springer-Verlag, Berlin, pp. 666-700.

Berger, U. 1963. Reinzüchtung von *Simonsiella* spp. Z. Hyg. *149:* 336-340.

Bergey, D.H., R.S. Breed, B.W. Hammer, F.M. Huntoon, E.G.D. Murray and F.C. Harrison. 1934. Bergey's Manual of Determinative Bacteriology, 4th Ed. The Williams and Wilkins Co., Baltimore, pp. 1-664.

Berkeley, M.J. 1857. Introduction to Cryptogamic Botany. H. Bailliere, London.

Berkeley, M.J. 1874. Notices of North American Fungi. Grevillea *3:* 49-64.

Berkeley, M.J. 1875. Notices of the North American Fungi. Grevillea *3:* 97-112.

Berkeley, M.J. and C.E. Broome. 1873. Enumeration of the fungi of Ceylon. J. Linn. Soc. London Bot. *14:* 29-140.

Berkeley, M.J. and G.H.K. Thwaites. 1849. *In* Engl. Bot., p. 2958.

Bernardi, G. 1969a. Chromatography of nucleic acids on hydroxyapatite. I. Chromatography of native DNA. Biochim. Biophys. Acta *174:* 423-434.

Bernardi, G. 1969b. Chromatography of nucleic acids on hydroxyapatite. II. Chromatography of denatured DNA. Biochim. Biophys. Acta *174:* 435-448.

Bernátová, V., Z. Jor, B. Kopřivik and M. Vychodilová. 1980. Metoda stanovení myxobakterií používaných jako indikátor zemědělského znečištění vody (a method for the determination of myxobacteria used as an indicator of agricultural water pollution). Cesk. Hyg. *25:* 65-70.

Bersa, E. 1920. Über das Vorkommen von kohlensaurem Kalk in einer Gruppe von Schwefelbakterien. Sitzungsber. Saechs Akad. Wiss. Leipzig Math-Naturwiss. Kl. Abt. I *129:* 231-259.

Betti, J.A., R.E. Blankenship, L.V. Natarajan, L.C. Dickinson and R.C. Fuller. 1982. Antenna organization and evidence for the function of a new antenna pigment species in the green photosynthetic bacterium *Chloroflexus aurantiacus*. Biochim. Biophys. Acta *680:* 194-201.

Beudeker, R.F., J.C. Gottschal and J.G. Kuenen. 1982. Reactivity versus flexibility in *Thiobacilli*. Antonie van Leeuwenhoek J. Microbiol. Serol. *48:* 39-51.

Beuscher, N., F. Mayer and G. Gottschalk. 1974. Citrate lyase from *Rhodopseudomonas gelatinosa*, electron microscopy and subunit structure. Arch. Microbiol. *100:* 307-328.

Beveridge, T.J., B.J. Harris, G.B. Patel and G.D. Sprott. 1986a. Cell division and filament splitting in *Methanothrix concilii*. Can. J. Microbiol. *32:* 779-786.

Beveridge, T.J., G.B. Patel, B.J. Harris and G.D. Sprott. 1986b. The ultrastructure of *Methanothrix concilii*, a mesophilic aceticlastic methanogen. Can. J. Microbiol. *32:* 703-710.

Bhandari, B. and D.J.D. Nicholas. 1979a. Ammonia and O_2 uptake in relation to proton translocation in cells of *Nitrosomonas europaea*. Arch. Microbiol. *122:* 249-255.

Bhandari, B. and D.J.D. Nicholas. 1979b. Ammonia, O_2 uptake and proton extrusion by spheroplasts of *Nitrosomonas europaea*. FEMS Microbiol. Lett. *6:* 297-300.

Bicudo, C.E. 1985. *Borzia* Cohn ex Gomont: only a hormogone or a true genus of blue-green algae? Arch. Hydrobiol. Suppl. *71:* 489-493.

Biebl, H. 1973. Die Verbreitung der schwefelfreien Purpurbakterien im Plußsee und anderen Seen Ostholsteins. Ph.D. thesis, University of Freiburg, F.R.G.

Biebl, H. and G. Drews. 1969. Das in-vivo-Spektrum als taxonomisches Merkmal bei Untersuchungen zur Verbreitung von *Athiorhodaceae*. Zentralbl. Bakteriol. Parasitenkd. Infektionskr. Hyg. Abt. II Orig. *123:* 425-452.

Biebl, H. and N. Pfennig. 1978. Growth yields of green sulfur bacteria in mixed cultures with sulfur and sulfate reducing bacteria. Arch. Microbiol. *117:* 9-16.

Biebl, H. and N. Pfennig. 1981. Isolation of members of the family *Rhodospirillaceae*. *In* Starr, Stolp, Trüper, Balows and Schlegel (Editors), The Procaryotes. A Handbook on Habitats, Isolation, and Identification of Bacteria. Springer-Verlag, Berlin, pp. 267-273.

Biedermann, M. and K. Westphal. 1979. Chemical composition and stability of Nb-particles from *Nitrobacter agilis*. Arch. Microbiol. *121:* 187-191.

Biggins, J. and W.E. Dietrich. 1968. Respiratory mechanisms in the *Flexibacteriaceae*. I. Studies on the terminal oxidase system of *Leucothrix mucor*. Arch. Biochem. Biophys. *128:* 40-50.

Bisset, K.A. 1974. The initiation of fruiting body formation in *Myxococcus fulvus*. Differentiation *2:* 47-50.

Bisset, K.A. 1975. The growth and development of fruiting bodies of *Myxococcus fulvus*. Differentiation *4:* 111-113.

Bivin, D.B. and W. Stoeckenius. 1986. Photoactive retinal pigments in haloalkaliphilic bacteria. J. Gen. Microbiol. *132:* 2167-2177.

Björn, L.O. 1979. Photoreversibly photochromic pigments in organisms: properties and role in biological light perception. Q. Rev. Biophys. *12:* 1-23.

Black, F.T., E.A. Freundt, O. Vinther and C. Christiansen. 1979. Flagellation and swimming motility of *Thermoplasma acidophilum*. J. Bacteriol. *137:* 456-460.

Blackmer, A.M., J.M. Bremner and E.L. Schmidt. 1980. Production of nitrous oxide by ammonia-oxidizing chemoautotrophic microorganisms in soil. Appl. Environ. Microbiol. *40:* 1060-1066.

Blakemore, R.P. 1975. Magnetotactic bacteria. Science *190:* 377-379.

Blakemore, R.P. 1982. Magnetotactic bacteria. Annu. Rev. Microbiol. *36:* 217-238.

Blakemore, R.P. and R.B. Frankel. 1981. Magnetic navigation in bacteria. Sci. Am. *245:* 58-65.

Blakemore, R.P., R.B. Frankel and A.J. Kalmijn. 1980. South-seeking magnetotactic bacteria in the Southern hemisphere. Nature *286:* 384-385.

Blakemore, R.P., D. Maratea and R.S. Wolfe. 1979. Isolation and pure culture of a freshwater magnetic spirillum in chemically defined medium. J. Bacteriol. *140:* 720-729.

Blakemore, R.P., K.A. Short, D.A. Bazylinski, C. Rosenblatt and R.B. Frankel. 1984. Microaerobic conditions are required for magnetite formation within *Aquaspirillum magnetotacticum*. Geomicrobiol. J. *4:* 53-71.

Bland, J.A. and T.D. Brock. 1973. The marine bacterium *Leucothrix mucor* as an algal epiphyte. Mar. Biol. *23:* 283-292.

Bland, J.A. and J.T. Staley. 1978. Observations on the biology of *Thiothrix*. Arch. Microbiol. *117:* 79-87.

Blotevogel, K.-H. and U. Fischer. 1985. Isolation and characterization of a new thermophilic and autotrophic methane producing bacterium: *Methanobacterium thermoaggregans* spec. nov. Arch. Microbiol. *142:* 218-222.

Blotevogel, K.-H., U. Fischer and K.H. Lüpkes. 1986. *Methanococcus frisius* sp. nov., a new methylotrophic marine methanogen. Can. J. Microbiol. *32:* 127-131.

Blotevogel, K.-H., U. Fischer, M. Mocha and S. Jannsen. 1985. *Methanobacterium thermoalcaliphilum* spec. nov., a new moderately alkaliphilic and thermophilic autotrophic methanogen. Arch. Microbiol. *142:* 211-217.

Blumer, M., T. Chase and S.W. Watson. 1969. Fatty acids in the lipids of marine and terrestrial nitrifying bacteria. J. Bacteriol. *99:* 366–370.

Böck, A. and O. Kandler. 1985. Antibiotic sensitivity of archaebacteria. *In* Woese and Wolfe (Editors), The Bacteria, Vol. VIII. Academic Press, New York, pp. 525–544.

Bock, E. 1972. Beziehungen zwischen Struktur und Funktion bei reaktivierenden Zellen von *Nitrobacter winogradskyi* Buch. Zentralbl. Bakteriol. Parasitenkd. Infektionskr. Hyg. I Abt. Orig. A *220:* 402–405.

Bock, E. 1976. Growth of *Nitrobacter* in the presence of organic matter. II. Chemoorganotrophic growth of *Nitrobacter agilis*. Arch. Microbiol. *108:* 305–312.

Bock, E. 1980. Nitrifikation—die bakterielle Oxidation von Ammoniak zu Nitrat. Forum Mikrobiologie 1/80: 24–32.

Bock, E. and G. Heinrich. 1969. Morphologische und physiologische Untersuchungen an Zellen von *Nitrobacter winogradskyi* Buch. Arch. Mikrobiol. *69:* 149–159.

Bock, E., H. Sundermeyer-Klinger and E. Stackebrandt. 1983. New facultative lithoautotrophic nitrite-oxidizing bacteria. Arch. Microbiol. *136:* 281–284.

Bohl, M. 1973. Bakterielle Kiemenerkrankungen bei Teichfischen. *In* Liebmann (Editor), Die Furunkulose und neuere Infektionskrankheiten der Süsswasserfische. R. Oldenbourg, München, F.R.G., pp. 89–104.

Bohlool, B.B. and T.D. Brock. 1974. Immunodiffusion analysis of membranes of *Thermoplasma acidophilum*. Infect. Immun. *10:* 280–281.

Bohlool, B.B. and E.L. Schmidt. 1980. The immunofluorescence approach in microbial ecology. Adv. Microb. Ecol. *4:* 203–241.

Bold, H.C. and M.J. Wynne. 1978. Introduction to the Algae. Prentice-Hall, Englewood Cliffs, New Jersey.

Bolotina, I.N. and T.G. Mirchink. 1975. Distribution of manganese-oxidizing organisms in the soil. Pochvovedenie *6:* 64–68.

Bolotina, I.N. and T.G. Mirchink. 1975. Manganese-oxidizing microorganisms inhabiting the phyloplane. Mikrobiologiya *44:* 933–937.

Bolton, R.W. and J.K. Dyer. 1983. Suppression of murine lymphocyte mitogen responses by exopolysaccharide from *Capnocytophaga ochracea*. Infect. Immun. *39:* 476–479.

Bömeke, H. 1951. *Nitrosomonas oligocarbogenes*, eine obligat autotrophes Nitritbakterium. Arch. Mikrobiol. *15:* 414–427.

Bonelo, G., A. Ventosa, M. Megias and F. Ruiz-Berraquero. 1984. The sensitivity of halobacteria to antibiotics. FEMS Microbiol. Lett. *21:* 341–345.

Booker, M.J. and A.E. Walsby. 1979. The relative form resistance of straight and helical blue-green algal filaments. Br. Phycol. J. *14:* 141–150.

Boone, D.R. 1987. Replacement of the type strain of *Methanobacterium formicicum*: request for an opinion and reinstatement of *Methanobacterium bryantii* (ex Balch and Wolfe, 1981) with M.o.H. (= DSM 863) as the type strain. Int. J. Syst. Bacteriol. *37:* 172–173.

Boone, D.R. and M.P. Bryant. 1980. Propionate-degrading bacterium, *Syntrophobacter wolinii* sp. nov. gen. nov., from methanogenic ecosystems. Appl. Environ. Microbiol. *40:* 626–632.

Boone, D.R., J.A.G.F. Menaia, J.E. Boone and R.A. Mah. 1987. Effects of hydrogen pressure during growth and effects of pregrowth with hydrogen on acetate degradation by *Methanosarcina* species. Appl. Environ. Microbiol. *53:* 83–87.

Boone, D.R., S. Worakit, I.M. Mathrani and R.A. Mah. 1986. Alkaliphilic methanogens from high-pH lake sediments. Syst. Appl. Microbiol. *7:* 230–234.

Bootsma, R. and J.P.M. Clerx. 1976. Columnaris disease of cultured carp *Cyprinus carpio* L. Characterization of the causative agent. Aquaculture *7:* 371–384.

Borg, A.F. 1960. Studies on myxobacteria associated with disease in salmonid fishes. Wildl. Dis. *8:* 1–85.

Bornet, E. 1892. Algues de Schousboe. Mem. Soc. Nat. Sci., Cherbourg *28:* 175.

Bornet, E. and C. Flahault. 1886. Revision des Nostocacées hétérocystées. Ann. Sci. Nat. Bot. VII, *4:* 343–373.

Bornet, E. and C. Flahault. 1886. Revision des Nostocacées hétérocystées. Ann. Sci. Nat. Bot. VII, *3:* 323–381.

Bornet, E. and C. Flahault. 1887. Revision des Nostocacées hétérocystées. Am. Sci. Nat. Bot. VII, *5:* 51–129.

Bornet, E. and C. Flahault. 1888. (Reprinted 1959). Revision des Nostocacées hétérocystées. Ann. Sci. Nat. Bot. *7:* 177–262. Reprinted: H.R. Engelmann (J. Cramer), Weinheim.

Borowitzka, L.J. 1986. Osmoregulation in blue-green algae. Prog. Phycol. Res. *4:* 243–256.

Bortels, H. 1956. Die Bedeutung einiger Spurenelemente für *Cellvibrio-* und *Cytophaga*-Arten. Arch. Mikrobiol. *25:* 226–245.

Borzi, A. 1879. Note alla morfologia e biologia delle Alghe ficocromacee. Nuovo G. Bot. Ital. *11:* 347.

Borzi, A. 1882. Note morf. biol. Ficocrom. Nuovo G. Bot. Ital. *14:* 314.

Borzi, A. 1916-1917. Studi sulle Mixficee. Nuovo G. Bot. Ital., Nuova Ser. *21:* 307–360.

Borzi, A. (or Borzoi) 1882. Note alla morfologia e biologia delle Alghe ficocromacee. Nuovo G. Bot. Ital. *12:* 272.

Bounds, H.C. and A.R. Colmer. 1972. Comparison of the kinetics of thiosulfate oxidation by three iron-sulfur oxidizers. Can. J. Microbiol. *18:* 735–740.

Bourrelly, P. 1970. Les Algues d'Eau Douce. III: Les algues bleues et rouges, les Eugleniens, Peridiniens et Cryptomonadines. N. Boubée, Paris.

Bourrelly, P. 1979. Les Cyanophycées, algues ou bacteries? Rev. Algol., N.S. *14:* 5–9.

Bourrelly, P. 1985. Les Algues d'Eau Douce. III. Les algues bleues et rouges, les Eugleniens, Peridiniens et Cryptomonadines. H. Boubée, Paris.

Bousfield, I.J., R.M. Keddie, T.R. Dando and S. Shaw. 1985. Simple rapid methods

of cell wall analysis as an aid in the identification of aerobic coryneform bacteria. *In* Goodfellow and Minnikin (Editors), Chemical Methods in Bacterial Systematics. Academic Press, London, New York, pp. 221–236.

Bovallius, A. 1979. Morphological and chemical characteristics of a *Cytophaga* sp. grown under conditions of magnesium excess and magnesium limitation. J. Gen. Microbiol. *113:* 137–145.

Bøvre, K. 1980. Progress in classification and identification of *Neisseriaceae* based on genetic affinity. *In* Goodfellow and Board (Editors), Microbial Classification and Identification. Academic Press, London, New York, pp. 55–72.

Brand, J.V., S.J. Kirchanski and R. Ramierez-Mitchell. 1979. Chill-induced morphological alterations in *Anacystis nidulans* as a function of growth temperature. Planta *145:* 63–68.

Brandis, A., R.K. Thauer and K.O. Stetter. 1981. Relatedness of strains delta H and Marburg of *Methanobacterium thermoautotrophicum*. Zentralbl. Bakteriol. Parasitenkd. Infektionskr. Hyg. Abt. I Orig. *C2:* 311–317.

Brannan, D.K. and D.E. Caldwell. 1980. *Thermothrix thiopara*: growth and metabolism of a newly isolated thermophile capable of oxidizing sulfur and sulfur compounds. Appl. Environ. Microbiol. *40:* 211–216.

Brannan, D.K. and D.E. Caldwell. 1982. Evaluation of a proposed surface colonization equation using *Thermothrix thiopara* as a model organism. Microb. Ecol. *8:* 15–21.

Brannan, D.K. and D.E. Caldwell. 1983. Growth kinetics and yield coefficients of the extreme thermophile *Thermothrix thiopara* in continuous culture. Appl. Environ. Microbiol. *45:* 169–173.

Brannan, D.K. and D.E. Caldwell. 1986. Ecology and metabolism of *Thermothrix thiopara*. Adv. Appl. Microbiol. *31:* 233–270.

Branson, D. 1972. Methods in Clinical Bacteriology. Charles C Thomas, Springfield, Illinois, p. 36.

Branton, D.W., S. Bullivant, N.G. Giluda, M.J. Karnovsky, H. Moor, K. Muhlentheler, D. Northcote, L. Packer, P. Sater, V. Speth, L.A. Staehelin, R.L. Steere and R.S. Weinstein. 1975. Freeze-etching nomenclature. Science *190:* 54–56.

Braun, A. and A. Grunow. 1865. *In* Rabenhorst's flora Europaea algarum aquae dulcis et submarinae, section II. Eduard Kummer, Leipzig, Germany, pp. 148–149.

Braune, W. 1980. Structural aspects of akinete germination in the cyanobacterium *Anabaena variabilis*. Arch. Microbiol. *126:* 257–261.

Brauss, F.W., W. Heyne and I. Heyne-Katzenberger. 1969. Beschreibung eines neuen lytisch-aktiven Bakterienstammes. Arch. Hyg. Bakteriol. *153:* 457–459.

Brauss, F.W., I. Heyne-Katzenberger and W. Heyne. 1968. Beiträge zur Mikrobiologie von Binnengewässern II. Arch. Hyg. Bakteriol. *152:* 346–349.

Brayer, G.D., L.T.J. Delbaere and M.N.G. James. 1979. Molecular structure of the α-lytic protease from Myxobacter 495 at 2.8 Å resolution. J. Mol. Biol. *131:* 743–775.

Breed, R.S. and J. Smit. 1957. Genus IV. *Sarcina* Goodsir 1842. *In* Breed, Murray and Smith (Editors), Bergey's Manual of Determinative Bacteriology, 7th Ed. The Williams and Wilkins Co., Baltimore, pp. 467–473.

Bremner, J.N. and A.M. Blackmer. 1978. Nitrous oxide: emission from soils during nitrification of fertilizer nitrogen. Science *199:* 295–296.

Brenner, D.J., G.R. Fanning, A.V. Rake and K.E. Johnson. 1969. Batch procedure for thermal elution of DNA from hydroxyapatite. Anal. Biochem. *28:* 447–459.

Bretscher, A.P. and D. Kaiser. 1978. Nutrition of *Myxococcus xanthus*, a fruiting myxobacterium. J. Bacteriol. *133:* 763–768.

Breuil, C. and G.B. Patel. 1980. Composition of *Methanospirillum hungatii* GP1 during growth on different media. Can. J. Microbiol. *26:* 577–582.

Brierley, C.L. and J.A. Brierley. 1982. Anaerobic reduction of molybdenum by *Sulfolobus* species. Zentralbl. Bakteriol. Mikrobiol. Hyg. I Abt. Orig. *C3:* 289–294.

Brierley, J.A. 1978. Thermophilic iron-oxidizing bacteria found in copper leaching dumps. Appl. Environ. Microbiol. *36:* 523–525.

Brimacombe, R., G. Staffer and H.G. Wittmann. 1978. Ribosome structure. Annu. Rev. Biochem. *47:* 217–249.

Broch-Due, M. and J.G. Ormerod. 1978. Isolation of a BChl c mutant from *Chlorobium* with BChl d by cultivation at low light intensity. FEMS Microbiol. Lett. *3:* 305–308.

Brock, T.D. 1964. Knots in *Leucothrix mucor*, a widespread marine microorganism. Science *144:* 870–872 (plus cover).

Brock, T.D. 1966. The habitat of *Leucothrix mucor*, a widespread marine microorganism. Limnol. Oceanogr. *11:* 303–307.

Brock, T.D. 1967. Mode of filament growth of *Leucothrix mucor*. J. Bacteriol. *93:* 985–990.

Brock, T.D. 1969. The neotype of *Leucothrix mucor* Oersted 1844 (emend. mut. char. Harold and Stanier 1955). Int. J. Syst. Bacteriol. *19:* 281–282.

Brock, T.D. 1978. The genus *Thermoplasma*. *In* Starr (Editor), Thermophilic Microorganisms and Life at High Temperatures. Springer-Verlag, Heidelberg, pp. 92–116.

Brock, T.D. 1978. The genus *Sulfolobus*. *In* Starr (Editor), Thermophilic Microorganisms and Life at High Temperatures. Springer-Verlag, Heidelberg, pp. 117–179.

Brock, T.D. 1978. Thermophilic Microorganisms and Life at High Temperatures. Springer-Verlag, Heidelberg, 465 pp.

Brock, T.D. 1981. The genus *Leucothrix*. *In* Starr, Stolp, Trüper, Balows and Schlegel (Editors), The Prokaryotes. A Handbook on Habitats, Isolation, and Identification of Bacteria. Springer-Verlag, Berlin, pp. 400–408.

Brock, T.D., K.M. Brock, R.T. Belly and R.L. Weiss. 1972. *Sulfolobus:* a new genus of sulfur-oxidizing bacteria living at low pH and high temperature. Arch. Microbiol. *84:* 54–68.

Brock, T.D. and S.F. Conti. 1969. Electron microscope studies on *Leucothrix mucor.* Arch. Mikrobiol. *66:* 79–90.

Brock, T.D., S. Cook, S. Peterson and J.L. Mosser. 1976. Biochemistry and bacteriology of ferrous iron oxidation in geothermal habitats. Geochim. Cosmochim. Acta *40:* 493–500.

Brock, T.D. and H. Freeze. 1969. *Thermus aquaticus* gen. n. and sp. n., a nonsporulating extreme thermophile. J. Bacteriol. *98:* 289–297.

Brock, T.D. and J. Gustafson. 1976. Ferric iron reduction by sulfur- and iron-oxidizing bacteria. Appl. Environ. Microbiol. *32:* 567–571.

Brock, T.D. and M. Mandel. 1966. DNA base composition of geographically diverse strains of *Leucothrix mucor.* J. Bacteriol. *91:* 1659–1660.

Brock, T.D. and S. Petersen. 1976. Some effects of light on the viability of rhodopsin-containing halobacteria. Arch. Microbiol. *109:* 199–200.

Brockman, E.R. 1973. Isolation of myxobacteria from marine habitats in the U.S. Virgin Islands. *In* Stevenson and Colwell (Editors), Estuarine Microbial Ecology. University of South Carolina Press, Columbia, pp. 45–52.

Brockman, E.R. 1977. Estimation of fruiting myxobacteria in water by a modified MPN procedure. *In* Skinner and Shewan (Editors), Aquatic Microbiology. Soc. Appl. Bact. Symp. Ser. No. 6. Academic Press, London, p. 356.

Brockman, E.R. and R.L. Todd. 1974. Fruiting myxobacters as viewed with a scanning electron microscope. Int. J. Syst. Bacteriol. *24:* 118–124.

Brockman, H., Jr. and G. Knobloch. 1972. Ein neues Bacteriochlorophyll aus *Rhodospirillum rubrum.* Arch. Mikrobiol. *85:* 123–126.

Brockmann, H., Jr. and A. Lipinski. 1983. Bacteriochlorophyll *g.* A new bacteriochlorophyll from *Heliobacterium chlorum.* Arch. Microbiol. *136:* 17–19.

Broda, P. 1979. Plasmids. W.H. Freeman Co., London, San Francisco.

Bromfield, S.M. 1974. Bacterial oxidation of manganous ions as affected by organic substrate concentration and composition. Soil Biol. Biochem. *6:* 383–392.

Bromfield, S.M. 1979. Manganous ion oxidation at pH values below 5.0 by cell free substances from *Streptomyces* sp. cultures. Soil Biol. Biochem. *11:* 115–118.

Bromfield, S.M. and V.B.D. Skerman. 1950. Biological oxidation of manganese in soils. Soil Sci. *69:* 337–348.

Brooks, B.W., R.G.E. Murray, J.L. Johnson, E. Stackebrandt, C.R. Woese and G.E. Fox. 1980. Red-pigmented micrococci: a basis for taxonomy. Int. J. Syst. Bacteriol. *30:* 627–646.

Brown, C.M. and R.A. Herbert. 1977. Ammonia assimilation in members of the *Rhodospirillaceae.* FEMS Microbiol. Lett. *1:* 43–46.

Brown, N.L., R.P. Burchard, D.W. Morris, J.H. Parish, N.D. Stow and C. Tsopanakis. 1976. Phage and defective phage of strains of *Myxococcus.* Arch. Mikrobiol. *108:* 271–279.

Brown, N.L., M. McClelland and P.R. Whitehead. 1980. *Hgi*AI: a restriction endonuclease from *Herpetosiphon giganteus* HP1023. Gene *9:* 49–68.

Brown, N.L. and J.H. Parish. 1976. Extrachromosomal DNA in chloramphenicol resistant *Myxococcus* strains. J. Gen. Microbiol. *93:* 63–68.

Bruce, B.D., R.C. Fuller and R.E. Blankenship. 1982. Primary photochemistry in the facultatively aerobic green photosynthetic bacterium *Chloroflexus aurantiacus.* Proc. Natl. Acad. Sci. U.S.A. *79:* 6532–6536.

Bryant, M.P. 1965. Rumen methanogenic bacteria. *In* Dougherty, Allen, Burroughs, Jacobson and McGilliard (Editors), Physiology of Digestion in the Ruminant. Buttersworth Publishing, Washington, D.C., pp. 411–418.

Bryant, M.P. 1972. Commentary on the Hungate technique for culture of anaerobic bacteria. Am. J. Clin. Nutr. *25:* 1324–1328.

Bryant, M.P. 1973. Nutritional requirements of the predominant rumen cellulolytic bacteria. Fed. Proc. *32:* 1809–1813.

Bryant, M.P. 1974. Methane-producing bacteria. *In* Buchanan and Gibbons (Editors), Bergey's Manual of Determinative Bacteriology, 8th Ed. The Williams and Wilkins Co., Baltimore, pp. 472–477.

Bryant, M.P. and D.R. Boone. 1987a. Emended description of strain MS (DSM 800), the type strain of *Methanosarcina barkeri.* Int. J. Syst. Bacteriol. *37:* 169–170.

Bryant, M.P. and D.R. Boone. 1987b. Isolation and characterization of *Methanobacterium formicicum* MF. Int. J. Syst. Bacteriol. *37:* 171.

Bryant, M.P. and I.M. Robinson. 1961. An improved nonselective culture medium for ruminal bacteria and its use in determining diurnal variation in number of bacteria in the rumen. J. Dairy Sci. *44:* 1446–1456.

Bryant, M.P., S.F. Tzeng, I.M. Robinson and A.E. Joyner. 1971. Nutrient requirements of methanogenic bacteria. *In* Gould (Editor), Anaerobic Biological Treatment Processes. Advances in Chemistry Series 105. American Chemical Society, Washington, D.C., pp. 23–40.

Bryant, M.P., E.A. Wolin, M.J. Wolin and R.S. Wolfe. 1967. *Methanobacterium omelianskii,* a symbiotic association of two species of bacteria. Arch. Mikrobiol. *59:* 20–31.

Bryant, R.D., K.M. McGroarty, J.W. Costerton and E.J. Laishley. 1983. Isolation and characterization of a new acidophilic *Thiobacillus* species (*T. albertis*). Can. J. Microbiol. *29:* 1159–1170.

Bryant, R.D., K.M. McGroarty, J.W. Costerton and E.J. Laishley. 1988. *In* Validation of the publication of new names and new combinations previously effectively published outside the IJSB. List No. 25. Int. J. Syst. Bacteriol. *38:* 220–222.

Brzin, B. 1966a. Morphology of *Vitreoscilla* grown at different incubation temperatures. Zentralbl. Bakteriol. Parasitenkd. Infektionskr. Hyg. Abt. II *120:* 611–615.

Brzin, B. 1966b. Dependence of the cell morphology of *Vitreoscilla* on the temperature of incubation. Experientia *22:* 1–5.

Buchanan, G.E. and D.A. Kuhn. 1978. Patterns of growth and gliding motility in *Simonsiella.* Curr. Microbiol. *1:* 257–262.

Buchanan, R.E. 1917. Studies on the nomenclature and classification of the bacteria. III. The families of the *Eubacteriales.* J. Bacteriol. *2:* 347–350.

Buchanan, R.E. 1925. General Systematic Bacteriology. The Williams and Wilkins Co., Baltimore.

Buchanan, R.E. 1957. Order VII. *Beggiatoales* Buchanan, Ordo Nov. *In* Breed, Murray and Smith (Editors), Bergey's Manual of Determinative Bacteriology, 7th Ed. The Williams and Wilkins Co., Baltimore, pp. 837–851.

Buchanan, R.E. and N.E. Gibbons (Editors). 1974. Bergey's Manual of Determinative Bacteriology, 8th Ed. The Williams and Wilkins Co., Baltimore.

Büdel, B. and E. Rhiel. 1985. A new cell wall structure in a symbiotic and a free-living strain of the blue-green alga genus *Chroococcidiopsis* (*Pleurocapsales*). Arch. Microbiol. *143:* 117–121.

Buder, J. 1914. *Chloronium mirabile.* Ber. Dtsch. Bot. Ges. *31:* 80–97.

Bullerjahn, G.S., H.C.P. Matthijs, L.R. Mur and L.A. Sherman. 1987. Chlorophyll-protein composition of the thylakoid membrane from *Prochlorothrix hollandica,* a prokaryote containing chlorophyll *b.* Eur. J. Biochem. *168:* 295–300.

Bullock, G.L. 1972. Studies on selected myxobacteria pathogenic on fishes and on bacterial gill disease in hatchery-reared salmonids. Technical Papers of the Bureau of Sport Fisheries and Wildlife No. 60. U.S. Dept. Interior, Fish and Wildlife Service, Washington, D.C., 30 pp.

Bullock, G.L. and J.J.A. McLaughlin. 1970. Advances in knowledge concerning bacteria pathogenic to fishes (1954–1968). *In* Snieszko (Editor), A Symposium on Diseases of Fishes and Shellfishes. American Fisheries Society, Washington, D.C., pp. 231–242.

Bump, F. and R. Schweisfurth. 1981. Zusammenfassende Darstellung der Kenntnisse über *Crenothrix polyspora* Cohn und eigene Untersuchungen. Hochschulsammlung Naturwissenschaft. Biol. *15:* 1–146.

Burchard, R.P. 1980. Gliding motility of bacteria. BioScience *30:* 157–162.

Burchard, R.P. 1984. Inhibition of *Cytophaga* U67 gliding motility by inhibitors of polypeptide synthesis. Arch. Microbiol. *139:* 248–254.

Burchard, R.P. and D.T. Brown. 1973. Surface structure of gliding bacteria after freeze-etching. J. Bacteriol. *114:* 1351–1355.

Burchard, R.P., A.C. Burchard and J.H. Parish. 1977. Pigmentation phenotype instability in *Myxococcus xanthus.* Can. J. Microbiol. *23:* 1657–1662.

Burchard, R.P. and M. Dworkin. 1966a. Light-induced lysis and carotenogenesis in *Myxococcus xanthus.* J. Bacteriol. *91:* 535–545.

Burchard, R.P. and M. Dworkin. 1966b. A bacteriophage for *Myxococcus xanthus*: isolation, characterization and relation of infectivity to host morphogenesis. J. Bacteriol. *9:* 1305–1313.

Burchard, R.P. and J.H. Parish. 1975. Chloramphenicol resistance in *Myxococcus xanthus.* Antimicrob. Agents Chemother. *7:* 233–238.

Burdett, I.D.J. and R.G.E. Murray. 1974. Septum formation in *Escherichia coli*: characterization of septal structure and the effects of antibiotics on cell division. J. Bacteriol. *119:* 303–324.

Burger-Wiersma, T., L.J. Stal and L.R. Mur. 1988. *Prochlorothrix hollandica* gen. nov.: a filamentous oxygenic photoautotrophic prokaryote containing chlorophylls *a* and *b.* Int. J. Syst. Bacteriol., submitted.

Burger-Wiersma, T., M. Veenhuis, H.J. Korthals, C.C.M. Van den Wiel and L.R. Mur. 1986. A new prokaryote containing chlorophylls *a* and *b.* Nature *320:* 262–264.

Burris, R.H., Y. Okon and S.L. Albrecht. 1977. Physiological studies of *Spirillum lipoferum.* *In* Hollaender (Editor), Genetic Engineering for Nitrogen Fixation. Plenum Press, New York, pp. 445–450.

Burton, S.D. and J.D. Lee. 1978. Improved enrichment and isolation procedures for obtaining pure cultures of *Beggiatoa.* Appl. Environ. Microbiol. *35:* 614–617.

Burton, S.D. and R.Y. Morita. 1964. Effect of catalase and cultural conditions on growth of *Beggiatoa.* J. Bacteriol. *88:* 1755–1761.

Burton, S.D., R.Y. Morita and W. Miller. 1966. Utilization of acetate by *Beggiatoa.* J. Bacteriol. *91:* 1192–1200.

Butler, R.F. and S.K. Banerjee. 1975. Theoretical single-domain grain size range in magnetite and titanomagnetite. J. Geophys. Res. *80:* 4049–4058.

Caldwell, D.E., D.K. Brannan and T.L. Kieft. 1983. *Thermothrix thiopara*: selection and adaptation of a filamentous sulfur-oxidizing bacterium colonizing hot spring rufa at pH 7.0 and 74°C. *In* Hallberg (Editor), Environmental Biogeochemistry. Ecol. Bull. (Stockholm) *35:* 129–134.

Caldwell, D.E. and S.J. Caldwell. 1974. The response of littoral communities of bacteria to variations in sulfide and thiosulfate. Abstr. Annu. Meet. Am. Soc. Microbiol. *74:* 59.

Caldwell, D.E. and S.J. Caldwell. 1980. Fine structure of in situ microbial iron deposits. Geomicrobiol. J. *2:* 39–53.

Caldwell, D.E., S.J. Caldwell and J.P. Laycock. 1976. *Thermothrix thiopara* gen. et sp. nov., a facultatively anaerobic facultative chemolithotroph living at neutral pH and high temperature. Can. J. Microbiol. *22:* 1509–1517.

Caldwell, D.E., S.J. Caldwell and J.P. Laycock. 1981. *In* Validation of the publication of new names and new combinations previously effectively published outside the IJSB. List No. 6. Int. J. Syst. Bacteriol. *31:* 215–218.

Caldwell, D.E., T.L. Kieft and D.K. Brannan. 1984. Colonization of sulfide-oxygen interfaces on hot spring tufa by *Thermothrix thiopara.* Geomicrobiol. J. *3:*

181–200.

Callies, E. 1979. Untersuchungen zur Systematik und Physiologie einiger der Gattung *Flavobacterium* Bergey et al., 1923 zugeschriebener, chemoorganotropher Bakteriengruppen. Doctor's thesis, University of Marburg, F.R.G., 117 pp.

Callies, E. and W. Mannheim. 1978. Classification of the *Flavobacterium-Cytophaga* complex on the basis of respiratory quinones and fumarate respiration. Int. J. Syst. Bacteriol. *28:* 14–19.

Callies, E. and W. Mannheim. 1980. Deoxyribonucleic acid relatedness of some menaquinone-producing *Flavobacterium* and *Cytophaga* strains. Antonie van Leeuwenhoek J. Microbiol. Serol. *46:* 41–49.

Cammarano, P., A. Teichner and P. Londei. 1986. Intralineage heterogeneity of archaebacterial ribosomes, evidence for two physicochemically distinct ribosome classes within the third urkingdom. Syst. Appl. Microbiol. *7:* 137–146.

Campbell, A. 1981. Evolutionary significance of accessory DNA elements in bacteria. Annu. Rev. Microbiol. *35:* 55–83.

Campbell, A.C. and J.A. Buswell. 1982. An investigation into the bacterial aetiology of "black patch necrosis" in Dover sole, *Solea solea* L. J. Fish Dis. *5:* 495–508.

Campbell, A.E., J.A. Hellebust and S.W. Watson. 1966. Reductive pentose phosphate cycle in *Nitrosocystis oceanus*. J. Bacteriol. *91:* 1178–1185.

Campos, J.M., J. Geisselsoder and D.R. Zusman. 1978. Isolation of bacteriophage MX4, a generalized transducing phage for *Myxococcus xanthus*. J. Mol. Biol. *119:* 167–178.

Carlile, M.J., J.F. Collins and B.E.B. Moseley (Editors). 1981. Molecular and Cellular Aspects of Microbial Evolution. Cambridge University Press, Cambridge.

Carlson, R.V. and R.E. Pacha. 1968. Procedure for the isolation and enumeration of myxobacteria from aquatic habitats. Appl. Microbiol. *16:* 795–796.

Carmichael, W.W. and P.R. Gorham. 1974. An improved method for obtaining axenic clones of planktonic blue-green algae. J. Phycol. *10:* 238–240.

Carr, N.G., J. Komárek and B.A. Whitton. 1973. Notes on isolation and laboratory culture. *In* Carr and Whitton (Editors), The Biology of Blue-green Algae. Blackwell, Oxford, and University of California Press, Berkeley, pp. 525–530.

Carr, N.G. and B.A. Whitton (Editors). 1982. The Biology of Cyanobacteria. Blackwell, Oxford, and University of California Press, Berkeley.

Carteni-Farina, M., M. Porcelli, G. Cacciapuoti, M. De Rosa, A. Gambacorta, H.N.M. Ross and W.D. Grant. 1985. Polyamines in halophilic archaebacteria. FEMS Microbiol. Lett. *28:* 323–327.

Carver, M.A. and C.W. Jones. 1985. The detection of cytochrome patterns in bacteria. *In* Goodfellow and Minnikin (Editors), Chemical Methods in Bacterial Systematics. Academic Press, London, New York, pp. 383–399.

Casida, L.E. 1980. Bacterial predators of *Micrococcus luteus* in soil. Appl. Environ. Microbiol. *39:* 1035–1041.

Casida, L.E. 1982. *Ensifer adhaerens* gen. nov., sp. nov.: a bacterial predator of bacteria in soil. Int. J. Syst. Bacteriol. *32:* 339–345.

Castenholz, R.W. 1969. Thermophilic blue-green algae and the thermal environment. Bacteriol. Rev. *33:* 476–504.

Castenholz, R.W. 1972. The occurrence of the thermophilic blue-green alga, *Mastigocladus laminosus*, on Surtsey in 1970. Surtsey Prog. Rep. (Reykjavik) *6:* 1–6.

Castenholz, R.W. 1973. The possible photosynthetic use of sulfide by the filamentous phototrophic bacteria of hot springs. Limnol. Oceanogr. *18:* 863–876.

Castenholz, R.W. 1977. The effect of sulfide on the blue-green algae of hot springs. II. Yellowstone National Park. Microb. Ecol. *3:* 79–105.

Castenholz, R.W. 1978. The biogeography of hot spring algae through enrichment cultures. Mitt. Int. Ver. Theor. Angew. Limnol. *21:* 296–315.

Castenholz, R.W. 1981. Isolation and cultivation of thermophilic cyanobacteria. *In* Starr, Stolp, Trüper, Balows and Schlegel (Editors), The Prokaryotes. A Handbook on Habitats, Isolation, and Identification of Bacteria. Springer-Verlag, Berlin, pp. 236–246.

Castenholz, R.W. 1982. Motility and taxes. *In* Carr and Whitton (Editors), The Biology of Cyanobacteria. Blackwell, Oxford, and University of California Press, Berkeley, pp. 413–439.

Castenholz, R.W. 1984a. Composition of hot spring microbial mats: a summary. *In* Cohen, Castenholz and Halvorson (Editors), Microbial Mats: Stromatolites. Alan R. Liss, New York, pp. 101–119.

Castenholz, R.W. 1984b. Habitats of *Chloroflexus* and related organisms. *In* Klug and Reddy (Editors), Current Perspectives in Microbial Ecology. ASM Publications, Washington, D.C., pp. 196–200.

Castenholz, R.W. 1988. Culturing methods for cyanobacteria. Methods Enzymol. *167:* 68–93.

Castenholz, R.W. and B.K. Pierson. 1981. Isolation of members of the family *Chloroflexaceae*. *In* Starr, Stolp, Trüper, Balows and Schlegel (Editors), The Prokaryotes. A Handbook on the Habitats, Isolation, and Identification of Bacteria. Springer-Verlag, Berlin, pp. 290–298.

Cataldi, M.S. 1939. Estudio fisiológico y sistemático de algunas *Chlamydobacteriales*. Thesis, University of Buenos Aires, pp. 1–96.

Cataldi, M.S. 1940. Aislamiento de *Beggiatoa alba* en cultivo puro. Rev. Inst. Bacteriol. Dep. Nacion. Hig. *9:* 393–423.

Cato, E.P., D.E. Hash, L.V. Holdeman and W.E.C. Moore. 1982. Electrophoretic study of *Clostridium* species. J. Clin. Microbiol. *15:* 688–702.

Chang, L.Y.E., J. Pate and R.J. Betzig. 1984. Isolation and characterization of non-spreading mutants of the gliding bacterium *Cytophaga johnsonae*. J. Bacteriol. *159:* 26–35.

Chang, T.P. 1977. Sheath formation in *Oscillatoria agardhii* Gomont. Schweiz. Z. Hydrol. *39:* 178–181.

Chang, W.T.H. and D.W. Thayer. 1975. The growth of *Cytophaga* on mesquite. Dev. Ind. Microbiol. *16:* 456–464.

Chang, W.T.H. and D.W. Thayer. 1977. The cellulase system of a *Cytophaga* species. Can. J. Microbiol. *23:* 1285–1292.

Chang, Y., J.T. Pfeffer and E.S.K. Chian. 1979. Comparative study of different iron compounds in inhibition of *Sphaerotilus* growth. Appl. Environ. Microbiol. *38:* 385–389.

Chang, Y., J.T. Pfeffer and E.S.K. Chian. 1980. Distribution of iron in *Sphaerotilus* and the associated inhibition. Appl. Environ. Microbiol. *40:* 1049–1052.

Charlet, E. and W. Schwartz. 1954. Beiträge zur Biologie der Eisenmikroben. I. Untersuchungen über die Lebensweise von *Leptothrix ochracea* und einigen begleitenden Eisenmikroben. Schweiz. Z. Hydrol. *16:* 318–341.

Cheeseman, P., A. Toms-Wood and R.S. Wolfe. 1972. Isolation and properties of a fluorescent compound, factor $_{420}$, from *Methanobacterium* strain M.o.H. J. Bacteriol. *112:* 527–531.

Chen, C.R.L., H.Y. Chung and G.H. Kuo. 1982. Studies on the pathogenicity of *Flexibacter columnaris*. I. Effects of dissolved oxygen and ammonia on the pathogenicity of *Flexibacter columnaris* to eel (*Anguilla japonica*). CAPD Fisheries Series No. 8. Fish Disease Research (IV), pp. 57–61 (in Chinese with English summary).

Chen, M. and M.J. Wolin. 1979. Effect of monensin and lasalocid on the growth of methanogenic and rumen saccharolytic bacteria. Appl. Environ. Microbiol. *38:* 72–77.

Cheng, L. and R.A. Lewin. 1984. *Prochloron* on *Synaptula*. Bull. Mar. Sci. *35:* 95–98.

Cherni, N.E., J.V. Solovjeva, V.D. Fedorov and E.N. Kondratieva. 1969. Ultrastructure of two species of purple sulfur bacteria. Mikrobiologiya *38:* 479–484.

Cholodny, N. 1924. Über neue Eisenbakterienarten aus der Gattung *Leptothrix* Kütz. Zentralbl. Bakteriol. Parasitenkd. Infektionskr. Hyg. Abt. II *61:* 292–298.

Cholodny, N. 1924. Zur Morphologie der Eisenbakterien *Gallionella* und *Spirophyllum*. Ber. Dtsch. Bot. Gesellsch. *42:* 35–44.

Cholodny, N. 1926. *In* Kolkwitz (Editor), Die Eisenbakterien. Beiträge zur einer Monographie. Pflanzenforsch. Heft 4., G. Fischer, Jena, pp. 1–162.

Cholodny, N. 1953. Iron Bacteria, 2nd Ed. Akad. Nauk S.S.S.R., Moscow.

Christensen, P. 1973. Studies on soil and freshwater cytophagas. Ph.D. thesis, University of Alberta, Edmonton, Canada, 471 pp.

Christensen, P.J. 1977a. The history, biology, and taxonomy of the *Cytophaga* group. Can. J. Microbiol. *23:* 1599–1653.

Christensen, P.J. 1977b. Synonymy of *Flavobacterium pectinovorum* Dorey with *Cytophaga johnsonae* Stanier. Int. J. Syst. Bacteriol. *27:* 122–132.

Christensen, P. 1980. *Flexibacter canadensis* sp. nov. Int. J. Syst. Bacteriol. *30:* 429–432.

Christensen, P. 1980. Description and taxonomic status of *Cytophaga heparina* (Payza and Korn) comb. nov. (Basionym: *Flavobacterium heparinum* Payza and Korn 1956). Int. J. Syst. Bacteriol. *30:* 473–475.

Christensen, P.J. and F.D. Cook. 1972. The isolation and enumeration of cytophagas. Can. J. Microbiol. *18:* 1933–1940.

Christensen, P. and F.D. Cook. 1978. *Lysobacter*, a new genus of nonfruiting, gliding bacteria with a high base ratio. Int. J. Syst. Bacteriol. *28:* 367–393.

Christiansen, C., E.A. Freundt and F.T. Black. 1975. Genome size and deoxyribonucleic acid base composition of *Thermoplasma acidophilum*. Int. J. Syst. Bacteriol. *25:* 99–101.

Christiansen, C., E.A. Freundt and O. Vinther. 1981. Lack of deoxyribonucleic acid-deoxyribonucleic acid homology between *Thermoplasma acidophilum* and *Sulfolobus acidocaldarius*. Int. J. Syst. Bacteriol. *31:* 346–347.

Christison, J. and S.M. Martin. 1971. Isolation and preliminary characterization of an extracellular protease of *Cytophaga* sp. Can. J. Microbiol. *17:* 1207–1216.

Ciferri, O. 1983. *Spirulina*, the edible microorganism. Microbiol. Rev. *47:* 551–578.

Ciferri, O. and O. Tiboni. 1985. The biochemistry and industrial potential of *Spirulina*. Annu. Rev. Microbiol. *39:* 503–526.

Clark, C. and E.L. Schmidt. 1966. Effect of mixed culture on *Nitrosomonas europaea* simulated by uptake and utilization of pyruvate. J. Bacteriol. *91:* 367–373.

Claus, G. 1962. Beiträge zur Kenntnis der Algenflora der abaligeter Höhle. Hydrobiologia *19:* 192–222.

Clausen, V., J.G. Jones and E. Stackebrandt. 1985. 16S ribosomal RNA analysis of *Filibacter limicola* indicates a close relationship to the genus *Bacillus*. J. Gen. Microbiol. *131:* 2659–2663.

Clayton, R.K. and W.R. Sistrom (Editors). 1978. The Photosynthetic Bacteria. Plenum Press, New York and London.

Clements, F.E. 1909. The Genera of Fungi. H.W. Wilson Co., Minneapolis, pp. 1–227.

Clewell, D.B. 1981. Plasmids, drug resistance and gene transfer in the genus *Streptococcus*. Microbiol. Rev. *45:* 409–436.

Cmiech, H.A., G.F. Leedale and C.S. Reynolds. 1984. Morphological and ultrastructural variability of planktonic *Cyanophyceae* in relation to seasonal periodicity. I. *Gloeotrichia echinulata*: vegetative cells, polarity, heterocysts, akinetes. Br. Phycol. J. *19:* 259–275.

Cobley, J.G. 1976a. Energy conserving reactions in phosphorylating electron transport particles from *Nitrobacter winogradskyi*. Biochem. J. *156:* 481–491.

Cobley, J.G. 1976b. Reduction of cytochromes by nitrite in electron-transport particles from *Nitrobacter winogradskyi*. Biochem. J. *156:* 493–498.

Codd, G.A. and W.W. Carmichael. 1982. Toxicity of a cloned isolate of the cyanobacterium *Microcystis aeruginosa* from Great Britain. FEMS Microbiol. Lett. *13:* 409–412.

Cohen, Y. 1984. The Solar Lake cyanobacterial mats: strategies of photosynthetic life under sulfide. *In* Cohen, Castenholz and Halvorson (Editors), Microbial Mats: Stromatolites. Alan R. Liss, New York, pp. 133–148.

Cohen, Y., B.B. Jorgensen, N.P. Revsbech and R. Poplawski. 1986. Adaptation to hydrogen sulfide of oxygenic and anoxygenic photosynthesis among cyanobacteria. Appl. Environ. Microbiol. *51:* 398–407.

Cohen-Bazire, G. and D.A. Bryant. 1982. Phycobilisomes: composition and structure. *In* Carr and Whitton (Editors), The Biology of Cyanobacteria. Blackwell, Oxford, and University of California Press, Berkeley, pp. 143–190.

Cohen-Bazire, G. and R. Kunisawa. 1963. The fine structure of *Rhodospirillum rubrum*. J. Cell Biol. *16:* 401–419.

Cohen-Bazire, G., N. Pfennig and R. Kunisawa. 1964. The fine structure of green bacteria. J. Cell. Biol. *22:* 207–225.

Cohen-Bazire, G., W.R. Sistrom and R.Y. Stanier. 1957. Kinetic studies of pigment synthesis by nonsulfur purple bacteria. J. Cell. Comp. Physiol. *49:* 25–68.

Cohn, F. 1862. Über die Algen des Karlsbader Sprudels, mit Rücksicht auf die Bildung des Sprudelsinters. Abh. Schles. Ges. Vaterl. Kultur, Breslau, Heft *2:* 35–55.

Cohn, F. 1870. Über den Brunnenfaden (*Crenothrix polyspora*) mit Bemerkungen über die mikroskopische Analyse des Brunnenwassers. Beitr. Biol. Pflanz. 1875 *1:* 108–131.

Cohn, F. 1872. Grundzüge einer neuen natürlichen Anordnung der Kryptogamischen Pflanzen. Jahrb. Schles. Ges. Vaterl. Kult. *49:* 83–89.

Cohn, F. 1875. Untersuchungen über Bakterien. II. Beitr. Biol. Pflanz. *1:* 141–207.

Cohn, F. 1882. Sechzigster Jahrsber. Schless. ges. Vaterl. Kult.

Coleman, A.W. and R.A. Lewin. 1983. The disposition of DNA in *Prochloron* (*Prochlorophyta*). Phycologia *22:* 209–212.

Coleman, L.C. 1907/1908. Untersuchungen über Nitrifikation. Zentralbl. Bakteriol. Parasitenkd. Infektionskr. Hyg. II Abt. *20:* 401–420, 484–513.

Colgrove, D.J. and J.W. Wood. 1966. Occurrence and control of *Chrondrococcus columnaris* as related to Fraser River sockeye salmon. Int. Pac. Salmon Fish. Comm. Annu. Rep. No. 15, New Westminster, B.C., Canada, 51 pp.

Collins, F.M. 1964. Cell wall composition of a marine cytophaga. J. Exp. Biol. Med. Sci. *42:* 263–265.

Collins, M.D. 1985. Isoprenoid quinone analyses in bacterial classification and identification. *In* Goodfellow and Minnikin (Editors), Chemical Methods in Bacterial Systematics. Academic Press, London, New York, pp. 267–287.

Collins, M.D., M. Goodfellow and D.E. Minnikin. 1982. A survey of the structures of mycolic acids in *Corynebacterium* and related taxa. J. Gen. Microbiol. *128:* 129–149.

Collins, M.D. and D. Jones. 1981. Distribution of isoprenoid quinone structural types in bacteria and their taxonomic implications. Microbiol. Rev. *45:* 316–354.

Collins, M.D., H.N. Shah, A.S. McKee and R.M. Kroppenstedt. 1982. Chemotaxonomy of the genus *Capnocytophaga* (Leadbetter, Holt and Socransky). J. Appl. Bacteriol. *52:* 409–415.

Collins, M.D., B.J. Tindall and W.D. Grant. 1981. Distribution of isoprenoid quinones in halophilic bacteria. J. Appl. Bacteriol. *50:* 559–565.

Collins, R.R. 1969. Numerical taxonomy of the flexibacteria. J. Gen. Microbiol. *58:* 207–215.

Collins, V.G. 1970. Recent studies of bacterial pathogens of freshwater fish. Water Treat. Exam. *19:* 3–31.

Colwell, R.R. 1969. Numerical taxonomy of the flexibacteria. J. Gen. Microbiol. *58:* 207–215.

Colwell, R.R. 1973. Genetic and phenetic classification of bacteria. Adv. Appl. Microbiol. *16:* 137–175.

Colwell, R.R. (Editor). 1976. The Role of Culture Collections in the Era of Molecular Biology. American Society for Microbiology, Washington, D.C.

Colwell, R.R., R.V. Citarella and P.K. Chen. 1966. DNA base composition of *Cytophaga marinoflava* n. sp. determined by buoyant density measurements in cesium chloride. Can. J. Microbiol. *12:* 1099–1103.

Colwell, R.R., C.D. Litchfield, R.H. Vreeland, L.A. Kiefer and N.E. Gibbons. 1979. Taxonomic studies of red halophilic bacteria. Int. J. Syst. Bacteriol. *29:* 379–399.

Connor, D.T., R.C. Greenough and M. von Strandtmann. 1977. W–7783, a unique antifungal antibiotic. J. Org. Chem. *42:* 3664–3669.

Conrad, R. and H.G. Schlegel. 1977a. Different degradation pathways for glucose and fructose in *Rhodopseudomonas capsulata*. Arch. Microbiol. *112:* 39–48.

Conrad, R. and H.G. Schlegel. 1977b. Influence of aerobic and phototrophic growth conditions on the distribution of glucose and fructose carbon into the Entner-Doudoroff and Embden-Meyerhof pathways in *Rhodopseudomonas sphaeroides*. J. Gen. Microbiol. *101:* 277–290.

Conrad, R. and H.G. Schlegel. 1978a. An alternative pathway for the degradation of endogenous fructose during the catabolism of sucrose in *Rhodopseudomonas capsulata*. J. Gen. Microbiol. *105:* 305–313.

Conrad, R. and H.G. Schlegel. 1978b. Regulation of glucose, fructose and sucrose catabolism in *Rhodopseudomonas capsulata*. J. Gen. Microbiol. *105:* 315–322.

Conti, S.F. and P. Hirsch. 1965. Biology of budding bacteria. III. Fine structure of *Rhodomicrobium* and *Hyphomicrobium* spp. J. Bacteriol. *89:* 503–512.

Conway de Macario, E., H. König and A.J.L. Macario. 1986. Immunological distinctness of archaebacteria that grow in high salt. J. Bacteriol. *168:* 425–427.

Conway de Macario, E. and A.J.L. Macario. 1986. Immunology of archaebacteria: identification, antigenic relationships and immunochemistry of surface structures. Syst. Appl. Microbiol. *7:* 320–324.

Conway de Macario, E., A.J.L. Macario and O. Kandler. 1982c. Monoclonal antibodies for immunochemical analysis of methanogenic bacteria. J. Immunol. *129:* 1670–1674.

Conway de Macario, E., A.J.L. Macario and M.J. Wolin. 1982a. Antigenic analysis of *Methanomicrobiales* and *Methanobrevibacter arboriphilus*. J. Bacteriol. *152:* 762–764.

Conway de Macario, E., A.J.L. Macario and M.J. Wolin. 1982d. Specific antisera and immunological procedures for characterization of methanogenic bacteria. J. Bacteriol. *149:* 320–328.

Conway de Macario, E., M.J. Wolin and A.J.L. Macario. 1981. Immunology of archaebacteria that produce methane gas. Science *214:* 74–75.

Conway de Macario, E., M.J. Wolin and A.J.L. Macario. 1982b. Antibody analysis of relationships among methanogenic bacteria. J. Bacteriol. *149:* 316–319.

Cook, F.D., O.E. Edwards, D.C. Gillespie and E.R. Peterson. 1971. 1-hydroxy 6-methoxy phenazines. U.S. Patent 3,609,153. September 28.

Cook, T.M. and W.W. Umbreit. 1963. The occurrence of cytochrome and coenzyme Q in *Thiobacillus thiooxidans*. Biochemistry *2:* 194–196.

Coombs, R.W., J.A. Verpoorte and K.B. Easterbrook. 1976. Protein conformation in bacterial spinae. Biopolymers *15:* 2353–2369.

Coombs, R.W., J.A. Verpoorte and K.B. Easterbrook. 1978. Physicochemical and immunological homogeneity of spinin, the subunit protein of bacterial spinae. Biochim. Biophys. Acta *535:* 370–387.

Cooper, R., K. Bush, P.A. Principe, W.H. Trejo, J.S. Wells and R.B. Sykes. 1983. Two new monobactam antibiotics produced by a *Flexibacter* sp. I. Taxonomy, fermentation, isolation and biological properties. J. Antibiot. *36:* 1252–1257.

Copeland, H.F. 1956. The Classification of Lower Organisms. Pacific Book, Palo Alto, California.

Copeland, J.J. 1936. Yellowstone thermal *Myxophyceae*. Ann. N.Y. Acad. Sci. *36:* 1–232.

Corbett, L.L. and D.L. Parker. 1976. Viability of lyophilized cyanobacteria (blue-green algae). Appl. Environ. Microbiol. *32:* 777–780.

Corda, A.C.J. 1839. Pracht-Flora Europaeischer Schimmelbildungen. Gerhard Fleischer, Leipzig, pp. 1–55.

Corder, R.E., L.A. Hook, J.M. Larkin and J.I. Frea. 1983. Isolation and characterization of two new methane-producing cocci: *Methanogenium olentangyi*, sp. nov., and *Methanococcus deltae*, sp. nov. Arch. Microbiol. *134:* 28–32.

Costenbader, C.J. and R.P. Burchard. 1978. Effect of cell length on gliding motility of *Flexibacter*. J. Bacteriol. *133:* 1517–1519.

Costerton, J.W.F., R.G.E. Murray and C.F. Robinow. 1961. Observations on the motility and the structure of *Vitreoscilla*. Can. J. Microbiol. *7:* 329–339.

Couch, J.A. 1978. Diseases, parasites, and toxic responses of commercial penaeid shrimps of the Gulf of Mexico and South Atlantic coasts of North America. U.S. Natl. Mar. Fish. Serv. Fish. Bull. *76:* 1–44.

Coughlin, M.F. 1980. M.S. thesis, Dalhousie University, Halifax, Nova Scotia, Canada.

Couté, A. 1982. Ultrastructure d'une cyanophycée aérienne calcifiée cavernicole: *Geitleria calcarea* Friedmann. Hydrobiologia *97:* 255–274.

Couté, A. 1985. Essai préliminaire de comparaison de deux Cyanophycées cavernicoles calcifiées: *Geitleria calcarea* Friedmann et *Scytonema julianum* Meneghini. Arch. Hydrobiol. Suppl. *71:* 91–98.

Cowan, S.T. 1968. A Dictionary of Microbial Taxonomic Usage. Oliver and Boyd, Edinburgh.

Cowan, S.T. 1970. Heretical taxonomy for bacteriologists. J. Gen. Microbiol. *61:* 145–154.

Cowan, S.T. 1978. A Dictionary of Microbial Taxonomy. Cambridge University Press, Cambridge, U.K.

Cox, G. and D.M. Dwarte. 1981. Freeze-etch ultrastructure of a *Prochloron* species, the symbiont of *Didemnum molle*. New Phytol. *88:* 427–438.

Cox, J.C., J.T. Beatty and J.L. Favinger. 1983. Increased activity of respiratory enzymes from photosynthetically grown *Rhodopseudomonas capsulata* in response to small amounts of oxygen. Arch. Microbiol. *134:* 324–328.

Crawford, I.P., B.P. Nichols and C. Yanofsky. 1980. Nucleotide sequence of the trpB gene in *Escherichia coli* and *Salmonella typhimurium*. J. Mol. Biol. *142:* 489–502.

Crerar, D.A., A.G. Fischer and C.L. Plaza. 1980. *Metallogenium* and biogenic deposition of manganese from precambrian to recent time. *In* Geology and Geochemistry of Manganese, Vol. 3: Manganese on the Bottom of Recent Basins. E. Schuleizelbart'sche Verlag, Stuttgart, pp. 285–303.

Crombach, W.H.J., W.L. van Veen, A.W. van der Vlies and W.C.P.M. Bots. 1974. DNA base composition of some sheathed bacteria. Antonie van Leeuwenhoek J. Microbiol. Serol. *40:* 217–220.

Crosa, J.H., D.J. Brenner and S. Falkow. 1973. Use of a single-strand specific nuclease for analysis of bacterial and plasmid deoxyribonucleic acid homo- and heteroduplexes. J. Bacteriol. *115:* 904–911.

Crouan, P.L. and H.M. Crouan. 1858. Note sur quelques algues marines nouvelles de la rade de Brest. Ann. Sci. Nat. Bot. Biol. Veg. *9:* 69–75.

Croucher, S.C. and E.M. Barnes. 1983. The occurrence and properties of *Gemmiger formicilis* and related anaerobic budding bacteria in the avium caecum. J. Appl. Bacteriol. *54:* 7–22.

Crow, W.B. 1927. *Crinalium*. A new genus of *Cyanophyceae* and its bearing on the morphology of the group. Ann. Bot. (London) *41:* 161–165.

Cruden, D.L. and A.J. Markovetz. 1981. Relative numbers of selected bacterial forms in different regions of the cockroach hindgut. Arch. Microbiol. *129:* 129–134.

Cullum, J. and H. Saedler. 1981. DNA rearrangements and evolution. *In* Carlile, Collins and Moseley (Editors), Molecular and Cellular Aspects of Microbial Evolution. Symposium No. 32 of the Society for General Microbiology. Cambridge University Press, London, New York, pp. 131–150.

Cummins, C.S. 1962. Immunochemical specificity and the location of antigens in the bacterial cell. *In* Ainsworth and Sneath (Editors), Microbial Classification. 12th Symposium of the Society for General Microbiology. Cambridge University Press, U.K.

Cummins, C.S. and H. Harris. 1956. The chemical composition of the cell wall in some Gram-positive bacteria and its possible value as a taxonomic character. J. Gen. Microbiol. *14:* 583–600.

Curtiss, R. 1969. Bacterial conjugation. Annu. Rev. Microbiol. *23:* 69–136.

Cyrus, Z. and A. Shadka. 1970. Several interesting organisms present in activated sludge. Hydrobiologia *35:* 383.

Czekalla, C., W. Mevius and H. Hanert. 1985. Quantitative removal of iron and manganese in rapid sand filters (in situ investigations). Water Supply (Berlin) *B3:* 111–123.

Czurda, V. 1935. Über eine neue autotrophe und thermophile Schwefelbakteriengesellschaft. Zentralbl. Bakteriol. Parasitenkd. Infektionskr. Hyg. Abt. II *92B:* 407–414.

Czurda, V. 1937. Weiterer Beitrag zur Kenntnis der neuen autotrophen und thermophilen Schwefelbakteriengesellschaft. Zentralbl. Bakteriol. Parasitenkd. Infektionskr. Hyg. Abt. II *96B:* 138–145.

Czurda, V. and E. Maresch. 1937. Beiträge zur Kenntnis der Athio-rhodobakterien Gesellschaften. Arch. Mikrobiol. *8:* 99–124.

Daft, M.J. and W.D.P. Stewart. 1973. Light and electron microscope observations on algal lysis by bacterium CP-1. New Phytol. *72:* 799–808.

Dagasan, L. and R.M. Weiner. 1986. Contribution of the electrophoretic pattern of cell envelope protein to the taxonomy of *Hyphomonas* spp. Int. J. Syst. Bacteriol. *36:* 192–196.

Daniels, L., N. Belay and B.S. Rajagopal. 1986. Assimilatory reduction of sulfate and sulfite by methanogenic bacteria. Appl. Environ. Microbiol. *51:* 703–709.

Daniels, L. and J.G. Zeikus. 1978. One-carbon metabolism in methanogenic bacteria: analysis of short-term fixation products of $^{14}CO_2$ and $^{14}CH_3OH$ incorporated into whole cells. J. Bacteriol. *136:* 75–84.

Daniels, L.G., G. Fuchs, R.K. Thauer and J.G. Zeikus. 1977. Carbon monoxide oxidation by methanogenic bacteria. J. Bacteriol. *132:* 118–126.

Danon, A. and S.R. Kaplan. 1977. CO_2 fixation by *Halobacterium halobium*. FEBS Lett. *74:* 255–258.

Darland, G., T.D. Brock, W. Samsonoff and S.F. Conti. 1970. A thermophilic, acidophilic mycoplasma isolated from a coal refuse pile. Science *170:* 1416–1418.

Dashekvicz, M.P. and R.L. Uffen. 1979. Identification of a carbon monoxide-metabolizing bacterium as a strain of *Rhodopseudomonas gelatinosa* (Molisch) van Niel. Int. J. Syst. Bacteriol. *29:* 145–148.

DasSarma, S., V.L. RajBhandary and A.G. Khorana. 1984. Bacterioopsin mRNA in wild type and bacterioopsin-deficient *Halobacterium halobium* strains. Proc. Natl. Acad. Sci. U.S.A. *81:* 125–129.

Davis, D.H., M. Doudoroff, R.Y. Stanier and M. Mandel. 1969. Proposal to reject the genus *Hydrogenomonas*: taxonomic implications. Int. J. Syst. Bacteriol. *19:* 375–390.

Davis, H.S. 1922. A new bacterial disease of fresh-water fishes. Bull. U.S. Bureau Fish. *38:* 261–280.

Dawid, W. 1974. *Myxococcus virescens*—ein Schleimbakterium mit grüner Fruchtkörpern. Beobachtungen und Untersuchungen zur Kultur und Biologie eines Schleimbakteriums. Mikrokosmos *6:* 1–7.

Dawid, W. 1975. *Chondrococcus coralloides*—ein weitverbreitetes Myxobakterium unserer Böden. Untersuchungen zur Verbreitung, Fruchtkörperbildung und Biologie. Mikrokosmos *64:* 134–143.

Dawid, W. 1976a. Fruchtkörperbildende Myxobakterien. I. Die *Myxococcus*—Arten: *M. fulvus, M. virescens, M. xanthus, M. stipitatus*. Mikrokosmos *65:* 72–79.

Dawid, W. 1976b. Fruchtkörperbildende Myxobakterien. II. Die *Archangium*—Arten: *A. gephyra, A. primigenium, A. serpens, A. flavum*. Mikrokosmos *65:* 225–231.

Dawid, W. 1976c. Fruchtkörperbildende Myxobakterien. III. Die *Cystobacter*-Arten: *C. fuscus, C. ferrugineus*. Mikrokosmos *65:* 292–298.

Dawid, W. 1977. Fruchtkörperbildende Myxobakterien. V. Die *Polyangium*—Arten: *P. cellulosum, P. fumosum, P. sorediatum, P. vitellinum*. Mikrokosmos *66:* 364–373.

Dawson, R.M.C., D.C. Elliott, W.H. Elliott and K.M. Jones (Editors). 1972. Data for Biochemical Research. Clarendon Press, Oxford.

de Boer, W.E., J.W.M. la Rivière and K. Schmidt. 1971. Some properties of *Achromatium oxaliferum*. Antonie van Leeuwenhoek J. Microbiol. Serol. *37:* 553–563.

de Bont, J.A.M., A. Scholten and T.A. Hansen. 1981. DNA-DNA hybridization of *Rhodopseudomonas capsulata, Rhodopseudomonas sphaeroides* and *Rhodopseudomonas sulfidophila* strains. Arch. Microbiol. *128:* 271–274.

de Bont, J.A.M., J.T. Staley and H.S. Pankratz. 1970. Isolation and description of a non-motile, fusiform, stalked bacterium, a representative of a new genus. Antonie van Leeuwenhoek J. Microbiol. Serol. *36:* 397–407.

Dees, S.B., D.E. Karr, D. Hollis and C.W. Moss. 1982. Cellular fatty acids of *Capnocytophaga* species. J. Clin. Microbiol. *16:* 779–783.

Dees, S.B., C.W. Moss, R.E. Weaver and D. Hollis. 1979. Cellular fatty acid composition of *Pseudomonas paucimobilis* and groups IIk-2, Ve-1, and Ve-2. J. Clin. Microbiol. *10:* 206–209.

Deinema, M.H., S. Henstra and E. Werdmüller von Elgg. 1977. Structural and physiological characteristics of some sheathed bacteria. Antonie van Leeuwenhoek J. Microbiol. Serol. *43:* 19–29.

Delang, R.J., G.R. Green and D.G. Searcy. 1981. A histone-like protein (HTa) from *Thermoplasma acidophilum*. I. Purification and properties. J. Biol. Chem. *256:* 900–904.

De Ley, J., H. Cattoir and A. Reynaerts. 1970. The quantitative measurement of DNA hybridization from renaturation rates. Eur. J. Biochem. *12:* 133–142.

De Ley, J., P. Segers and M. Gillis. 1978. Intra- and intergeneric similarities of *Chromobacterium* and *Janthinobacterium* ribosomal ribonucleic acid cistrons. Int. J. Syst. Bacteriol. *28:* 154–168.

Delwiche, C.C. and M.S. Finstein. 1965. Carbon and energy sources for the nitrifying autotroph *Nitrobacter*. J. Bacteriol. *90:* 102–107.

DeMoll, E. and L. Tsai. 1986. Utilization of purines or pyrimidines as the sole nitrogen source by *Methanococcus vannielii*. J. Bacteriol. *167:* 681–684.

Demoulin, V. and M.P. Janssen. 1981. Relationship between diameter of the filament and cell shape in blue-green algae. Br. Phycol. J. *16:* 55–58.

den Dooren de Jong, L.E. 1926. Bijdrage tot de kennis van het mineralisatieproces. Thesis, Technical University of Delft, The Netherlands, 199 pp.

Denhardt, D.T. 1966. A membrane-filter technique for the detection of complementary DNA. Biochem. Biophys. Res. Commun. *23:* 641–646.

De Rosa, M., A. Gambacorta, B. Nicolaus and W.D. Grant. 1983. A $C_{25}C_{25}$ diether core lipid from alkaliphilic halophiles. J. Gen. Microbiol. *129:* 2333–2337.

De Rosa, M., A. Gambacorta, B. Nicolaus, H.N.M. Ross, W.D. Grant and J.D. Bu'lock. 1982. An asymmetric archaebacterial ether lipid for alkaliphilic halophiles. J. Gen. Microbiol. *128:* 343–348.

De Rosa, M., A. Gambacorta, A. Trincone, A. Basso, W. Zillig and I. Holz. 1987. Lipids of *Thermococcus celer*, a sulfur-reducing archaebacterium: structure and biosynthesis. Syst. Appl. Microbiol. *9:* 1–5.

Desikachary, T.V. 1959. Cyanophyta. Indian Council of Agricultural Research, New Delhi, India, pp. 1–686.

De Smedt, J., M. Bauwens, R. Tytgat and J. De Ley. 1980. Intra- and intergeneric similarities of ribosomal ribonucleic acid cistrons of free-living, nitrogen-fixing bacteria. Int. J. Syst. Bacteriol. *30:* 106–122.

DeSmedt, J. and J. De Ley. 1977. Intra- and intergeneric similarities of *Agrobacterium* ribosomal ribonucleic acid cistrons. Int. J. Syst. Bacteriol. *27:* 222–240.

de Toni, J. 1936. Noterelle nomencl. algolog. 8, Brescia.

Dhar, N.M. and W. Altekar. 1986. Distribution of class I and class II fructose biphosphate aldolases in halophilic archaebacteria. FEMS Microbiol. Lett. *35:* 177–181.

Diakoff, S. and J. Scheibe. 1973. Action spectra for chromatic adaptation in *Tolypothrix tenuis*. Plant Physiol. *51:* 382–385.

Dickerson, R.E. 1980. Cytochrome *c* and the evolution of energy metabolism. Sci. Am. *242:* 137–153.

Dickerson, R.E. 1980. Evolution and gene transfer in purple photosynthetic bacteria. Nature *283:* 210–212.

Diekert, G., U. Konheiser, K. Piechulla and R.K. Thauer. 1981. Nickel requirement and factor F_{430} content of methanogenic bacteria. J. Bacteriol. *148:* 459–464.

Dietrich, C.P. 1969. Enzymatic degradation of heparin. Biochem. J. *111:* 91–95.

DiSpirito, A.A., W.H-T. Loh and O.H. Tuovinen. 1983. A novel method for the isolation of bacterial quinones and its application to appraise the ubiquinone composition of *Thiobacillus ferrooxidans*. Arch. Microbiol. *135:* 77–80.

DiSpirito, A.A., M. Silver, L. Voss and O.H. Tuovinen. 1982. Flagella and pili of iron-oxidizing thiobacilli isolated from a uranium mine in Northern Ontario, Canada. Appl. Environ. Microbiol. *43:* 1196–1200.

Dispirito, A.A., L.R. Taaffe and A.B. Hooper. 1985. Localization and concentration of hydroxylamine oxidoreductase and cytochromes c_{552}, c_{554}, c_{m-552} and *a* in *Nitrosomonas europaea*. Biochim. Biophys. Acta *806:* 320–330.

Ditmar, L.P.F. 1813. Die Pilze Deutschlands. *In* Sturm (Editor), Deutschlands Flora in Abbildungen nach der Natur mit Beschreibungen. *3:* 55–56.

Dobell, C.C. 1912. Researches on the spirochaets and related organisms. Arch. Protistenk. *26:* 117–240.

Dobson, W.J., H.D. McCurdy and T.H. MacRae. 1979. The function of fimbriae in cell-cell interactions. Can. J. Microbiol. *25:* 1359–1372.

Doddema, H.J., J.W.M. Derksen and G.D. Vogels. 1979. Fimbriae and flagella of methanogenic bacteria. FEMS Microbiol. Lett. *5:* 135–138.

Dodson, M.S., J. Mangan and S.W. Watson. 1983. Comparison of deoxyribonucleic acid homologies of six strains of ammonia-oxidizing bacteria. Int. J. Syst. Bacteriol. *33:* 521–524.

Doetsch, R.N., T.M. Cook and Z. Vaituzis. 1967. On the uniqueness of the flagellum of *Thiobacillus thiooxidans*. Antonie van Leeuwenhoek J. Microbiol. Serol. *33:* 196–202.

Dondero, N.C. 1975. The *Sphaerotilus-Leptothrix* group. Annu. Rev. Microbiol. *29:* 407–428.

Doolittle, R.F. 1981. Similar amino acid sequences: chance or common ancestry?

Science (Washington) *214:* 149–159.

Doolittle, W.F. 1979. The cyanobacterial genome, its expression, and the control of that expression. Adv. Microbiol. Physiol. *20:* 1–102.

Dorey, M.J. 1959. Some properties of a pectolytic soil flavobacterium. J. Gen. Microbiol. *20:* 91–104.

Dorff, P. 1934. Die Eisenorganismen. Pflanzenforsch. Heft 16. Hrsg. von Kolkwitz, G. Fischer, Jena, pp. 1–62.

Doronina, N.V., N.J. Govorukhina and Y.A. Trotsenko. 1983. *Blastobacter aminooxidans,* a new species of bacteria growing autotrophically on methylated amines. Mikrobiologiya *52:* 709–715 (English translation: 547–553).

Douglas, C., F. Achatz and A. Böck. 1980. Electrophoretic characterization of ribosomal proteins from methanogenic bacteria. Zentralbl. Bakteriol. Parasitenkd. Infektionskr. Hyg. Abt. I Orig. *C1:* 1–11.

Douglas, D., A. Peat, B.A. Whitton and P. Wood. 1986. Influence of iron status on structure of the cyanobacterium (blue-green alga) *Calothrix parietina.* Cytobios *47:* 155–165.

Drawert, H. and I. Metzner-Küster. 1958. Fluorescenz und elektronmikroskopische Untersuchung an *Beggiatoa alba* und *Thiothrix nivea.* VI. Mitteilung der Reihe: Zellmorphologische und zellphysiologische Studien an Cyanophyceen. Arch. Mikrobiol. *31:* 422–434.

Drews, G. 1981. *Rhodospirillum salexigens,* spec. nov., an obligatory halophilic phototrophic bacterium. Arch. Microbiol. *130:* 325–327.

Drews, G. 1982. *In* Validation of the publication of new names and new combinations previously effectively published outside the IJSB. List No. 9. Int. J. Syst. Bacteriol. *32:* 384–385.

Drews, G. and P. Giesbrecht. 1966. *Rhodopseudomonas viridis,* nov. spec., ein neu isoliertes, obligat phototrophes Bakterium. Arch. Mikrobiol. *53:* 255–262.

Drews, G. and J. Weckesser. 1982. Function, structure and composition of cell walls and external layers. *In* Carr and Whitton (Editors), The Biology of Cyanobacteria. Blackwell, Oxford, and University of California Press, Berkeley, pp. 333–357.

Drouet, F. 1968. Revision of the classification of the *Oscillatoriaceae.* Monogr. Acad. Nat. Sci. (Philadelphia) *67:* 1–341.

Drouet, F. 1973. Revision of the *Nostocaceae* with cylindrical trichomes. Hafner Press, New York.

Drouet, F. 1978. Revision of the *Nostocaceae* with constricted trichomes. Beih. Nova Hedwigia *57:* 1–258.

Drouet, F. 1981. Revision of the *Stigonemataceae* with a summary of the classification of the blue-green algae. J. Cramer, Vaduz.

Drouet, F. and W.A. Daily. 1956. Revision of the coccoid *Myxophyceae.* Butler Univ. Bot. Stud. *10:* 1–218.

Drozd, J.W. 1976. Energy coupling and respiration in *Nitrosomonas europaea.* Arch. Microbiol. *110:* 257–262.

Drozd, J.W. 1980. Respiration in the ammonia-oxidizing chemoautotrophic bacteria. *In* Knowles (Editor), Diversity of Bacterial Respiratory Systems, Vol. II. CRC Press, Boca Raton, Florida, pp. 87–111.

Dubinina, G. and A.V. Zhdanov. 1975. Recognition of the iron bacteria "*Siderocapsa*" as arthrobacters and description of *Arthrobacter siderocapsulatus* sp. nov. Int. J. Syst. Bacteriol. *25:* 340–350.

Dubinina, G.A. 1969. On the inclusion of the genus *Metallogenium* in the order *Mycoplasmatales.* Dokl. Akad. Nauk S.S.S.R. *184:* 1433–1436.

Dubinina, G.A. 1978a. Mechanism of the oxidation of divalent iron and manganese by iron bacteria growing at a neutral pH of the medium. Mikrobiologiya *47:* 591–599.

Dubinina, G.A. 1978b. Functional role of bivalent iron and manganese oxidation in *Leptothrix pseudo-ochraceae.* Mikrobiologiya *47:* 783–789.

Dubinina, G.A. 1984. Infection of procaryotic and eucaryotic microorganisms with *Metallogenium.* Curr. Microbiol. *11:* 349–356.

Dubinina, G.A. and V.M. Gorlenko. 1975. New filamentous photosynthetic green bacteria containing gas vacuoles. Mikrobiologiya *44:* 511–517 (English translation: *44:* 452–458).

Dubinina, G.A. and M.Y. Grabovich. 1983. Isolation of pure *Thiospira* cultures and investigation of their sulfur metabolism. Mikrobiologiya *52:* 5–12.

Dubinina, C.A. and M.Y. Grabovich. 1984. Isolation, cultivation and characteristics of *Macromonas bipunctata.* Mikrobiologiya *53:* 748–755.

Dubinina, G.A. and S.I. Kusnetzov. 1976. The ecological and morphological characteristics of microorganisms in Lesnaya Lamba (Karelia). Int. Rev. Gesamten Hydrobiol. *61:* 1–19.

Dubourguier, H.C., G. Prensier, E. Samain and G. Albagnac. 1985. Granular methanogenic sludge: microbial and structural analysis. *In* Palz, Coombs and Hall (Editors), Energy from Biomass. Proc. 3rd E.C. Conference, Venice. Elsevier Applied Science Publishers, Amsterdam, pp. 542–551.

Dubourguier, H.C., E. Samain, G. Prensier and G. Albagnac. 1986. Characterization of two strains of *Pelobacter carbinolicus* isolated from anaerobic digesters. Arch. Microbiol. *145:* 248–253.

Duchow, A. and H.C. Douglas. 1949. *Rhodomicrobium vannielii,* a new photoheterotrophic bacterium. J. Bacteriol. *58:* 409–416.

Duckworth, M. and J.R. Turvey. 1969. The specificity of an agarase from a *Cytophaga* species. Biochem. J. *113:* 693–696.

Dunn, R., J. McCoy, M. Simsek, A. Majumdar, S.H. Chang, V.L. RajBhandary and H.G. Khorana. 1981. The bacteriorhodopsin gene. Proc. Natl. Acad. Sci. U.S.A. *78:* 6744–6748.

Dussault, H.P. 1955. An improved technique for staining red halophilic bacteria. J. Bacteriol. *70:* 484–485.

Dutton, P.L. and W.C. Evans. 1969. The metabolism of aromatic compounds by *Rhodopseudomonas palustris.* Biochem. J. *113:* 525–536.

Dutton, P.L. and W.C. Evans. 1978. The metabolism of aromatic compounds by *Rhodospirillaceae.* *In* Clayton and Sistrom (Editors), The Photosynthetic Bacteria. Plenum Press, New York, pp. 719–726.

Duxbury, T., B.A. Humphrey and K.C. Marshall. 1980. Continuous observations of bacterial gliding motility in a dialysis microchamber: the effects of inhibitors. Arch. Microbiol. *124:* 169–175.

Dworkin, M. 1962. Nutritional requirements for vegetative growth of *Myxococcus xanthus.* J. Bacteriol. *84:* 250–257.

Dworkin, M. 1969. Sensitivity of gliding bacteria to actinomycin D. J. Bacteriol. *98:* 851–852.

Dworkin, M. 1972. The myxobacteria: new directions in studies of prokaryotic development. CRC Crit. Rev. Microbiol. *1:* 435–452.

Dworkin, M. and S.M. Gibson. 1964. A system for studying microbial morphogenesis: rapid formation of microcysts in *Myxococcus xanthus.* Science *146:* 243–244.

Dworkin, M. and N.J. Niederpruem. 1964. Electron transport system in vegetative cells and microcysts of *Myxococcus xanthus.* J. Bacteriol. *87:* 316–322.

Dyer, J.K. and R.W. Bolton. 1985. Purification and chemical characterization of an exopolysaccharide isolated from *Capnocytophaga ochracea.* Can. J. Microbiol. *31:* 1–5.

Easterbrook, K.B. and S.A. Alexander. 1983. The initiation and growth of bacterial spinae. Can. J. Microbiol. *29:* 476–487.

Easterbrook, K.B. and R.W. Coombs. 1976. Spinin: the subunit protein of bacterial spinae. Can. J. Microbiol. *22:* 438–440.

Easterbrook, K.B., J.B. McGregor-Shaw and R.P. McBride. 1973. Ultrastructure of bacterial spinae. Can. J. Microbiol. *19:* 995–997.

Easterbrook, K.B. and S. Sperker. 1983. Physiological controls of bacterial spinae production in complex medium and their value as indicators of spina function. Can. J. Microbiol. *28:* 130–136.

Easterbrook, K.B. and D.V. Subba Rao. 1984. Conical spinae associated with a picoplanktonic procaryote. Can. J. Microbiol. *30:* 716–718.

Eckersley, K. and C.S. Dow. 1980. *Rhodopseudomonas blastica* sp. nov.: a member of the *Rhodospirillaceae.* J. Gen. Microbiol. *119:* 465–473.

Eckersley, K. and C.S. Dow. 1981. *In* Validation of the publication of new names and new combinations previously effectively published outside the IJSB. List No. 6. Int. J. Syst. Bacteriol. *31:* 216.

Eckhardt, F.E.W., P. Roggentin and P. Hirsch. 1979. Fatty acid composition of various hyphal budding bacteria. Arch. Microbiol. *120:* 81–85.

Edelman, M., D. Swinton, J.A. Schiff, H.T. Epstein and B. Zeldin. 1967. Deoxyribonucleic acid of the blue-green algae (Cyanophyta). Bacteriol. Rev. *31:* 315–331.

Edwards, T. and B.C. McBride. 1975. New method for the isolation and identification of methanogenic bacteria. Appl. Microbiol. *29:* 540–545.

Egorova, A.A. and Z.P. Deryugina. 1963. The spore forming thermophilic thiobacterium: *Thiobacillus thermophilica imschenetskii* nov. spec. Mikrobiologiya *32:* 439–446.

Ehrenberg, C.G. 1838. Die Infusionsthierchen als vollkommene Organismen. L. Voss, Leipzig.

Ehrlich, H.L. 1966. Reaction with manganese by bacteria from marine ferromanganese nodules. Dev. Ind. Microbiol. *7:* 279–286.

Ehrlich, H.L. 1978. Condition for bacterial participation in the initiation of manganese deposition around sediment particles. Environ. Biogeochem. Geomicrobiol. *3:* 839–845.

Eichler, B. and N. Pfennig. 1986. Characterization of a new platelet-forming purple sulfur bacterium, *Amoebobacter pedioformis* sp. nov. Arch. Microbiol. *146:* 295–300.

Eigener, U. 1975. Adenine nucleotide pool variations in intact *Nitrobacter winogradskyi* cells. Arch. Microbiol. *102:* 233–240.

Eigener, U. and E. Bock. 1972. Auf- und Abbau der Polyphosphatfraktion in Zellen von *Nitrobacter winogradskyi* Buch. Arch. Mikrobiol. *81:* 367–378.

Eikelboom, D.H. 1975. Filamentous organisms observed in activated sludge. Water Res. *9:* 365–388.

Eikelboom, D.H. and H.J.J. van Buijsen. 1981. Microscopic sludge investigation manual. Instituut voor milieuhygiene en gezondheidstechniek, TNO Research Institute for Environmental Hygiene, Water and Soil Division, Report A 94a. Delft, The Netherlands, 71 pp., 22 plates.

Eimhjellen, K.E. 1970. *Thiocapsa pfennigii* sp. nov., a new species of phototrophic sulfur bacteria. Arch. Mikrobiol. *73:* 193–194.

Eimhjellen, K.E., H. Steensland and J. Traetteberg. 1967. A *Thiococcus* sp. nov. gen., its pigments and internal membrane system. Arch. Mikrobiol. *59:* 82–92.

Eirich, L.D., G.D. Vogels and R.S. Wolfe. 1979. Distribution of coenzyme F_{420} and properties of its hydrolytic fragments. J. Bacteriol. *140:* 20–27.

Ekiel, I., I.C.P. Smith and G.D. Sprott. 1983. Biosynthetic pathways in *Methanospirillum hungatei* as determined by ^{13}C nuclear magnetic resonance. J. Bacteriol. *156:* 316–326.

Ekiel, I., G.D. Sprott and G.B. Patel. 1985. Acetate and CO_2 assimilation by *Methanothrix concilii.* J. Bacteriol. *162:* 905–908.

Elazari-Volcani, B. 1940. Studies on the microflora of the Dead Sea. Doctoral thesis, Hebrew University, Jerusalem, Israel.

Elazari-Volcani, B. 1957. Genus XII. *Halobacterium. In* Breed, Murray and Smith (Editors), Bergey's Manual of Determinative Bacteriology, 7th Ed. The Williams and Wilkins Co., Baltimore, pp. 207–212.

Elenkin, A.A. 1936, 1938, 1949. Sinezelenye vodorosli SSSR, Monographia algarum cyanophycearum aquidulcium et terrestrium in finibus URSS inventarum, pars generalis, pars specialis I et II. Akad. Nauk S.S.S.R., Moscow.

Elhardt, D. and A. Böck. 1982. An in vitro polypeptide synthesizing system from methanogenic bacteria: sensitivity to antibiotics. Mol. Gen. Genet. 188: 128–134.

Ellis, D. 1932. Sulphur Bacteria. Longmans, Green, London.

Ely, B. 1979. Transfer of drug resistance factors to the dimorphic bacterium Caulobacter crescentus. Genetics 91: 371–380.

Ely, B., A.B.C. Amarasinghe and R.A. Bender. 1978. Ammonia assimilation and glutamate formation in Caulobacter crescentus. J. Bacteriol. 133: 225–230.

Emoto, Y. 1928. Über eine neue schwefeloxydierende Bakterien. Bot. Mag. Tokyo 42: 421–426.

Emoto, Y. 1929. Über drei neue Arten der schwefeloxydierende Bakterien. Proc. Jpn. Acad. 5: 148–151.

Emoto, Y. 1933. Die Mikroorganismen der Thermen. Bot. Mag. Tokyo 47: 405–588.

Emoto, Y. 1934. Chondromyces crocatus in Japan. Shokubutsu Oyobi Dobutsu (Plant and Animal) 2: 1212–1214.

Engelhardt, H., W. Baumeister and W.O. Saxton. 1983. Electron microscopy of photosynthetic membranes containing bacteriochlorophyll b. Arch. Microbiol. 135: 169–175.

Engelhardt, H. and J.-H. Klemme. 1978. Characterization of an allosteric, nucleotide-unspecific glutamate dehydrogenase from Rhodopseudomonas sphaeroides. FEMS Microbiol. Lett. 3: 287–290.

Engler, A. 1882. Im Kieler Hafen in dem sogenannten "Todten Grund" vorkommenden Pilzformen. Verh. Bot. Ver. Brandenb. 24: 17–20.

Engler, A. 1883. Über die Pilzvegetation des Weissen oder Todten Grundes in der Kieler Bucht. Vierter Ber. d. Kommission z. wiss. Untersuchg. der Meere, Abt. I, 187–193.

Epikhina, V.V. and G.A. Zavarzin. 1963. Oxidation-reduction potential in the development of Metallogenium. Mikrobiologiya (English translation) 32: 227–230.

Escalente-Semerena, J.C., R.P. Blakemore and R.S. Wolfe. 1980. Nitrate dissimilation under microaerophilic conditions by a magnetic spirillum. Appl. Environ. Microbiol. 40: 429–430.

Esmarch, E. 1887. Über die Reinkultur eines Spirillum. Zentralbl. Bakteriol. Parasitenkd. Infektionskr. Hyg. Abt. I Orig. 1: 225–230.

Evans, E.H., I. Foulds and N.G. Carr. 1976. Environmental conditions and morphological variation in the blue-green alga Chlorogloea fritschii. J. Gen. Microbiol. 92: 147–155.

Evans, M.C.W., B.B. Buchanan and D.I. Arnon. 1966. A new ferredoxin dependent carbon reduction cycle in a photosynthetic bacterium. Proc. Natl. Acad. Sci. U.S.A. 55: 928–934.

Evans, R.W., S.C. Kushwaha and M. Kates. 1980. The lipids of Halobacterium marismortui, an extremely halophilic bacterium in the Dead Sea. Biochim. Biophys. Acta 619: 533–544.

Fager, E.W. 1969. Recurrent group analysis in the classification of flexibacteria. J. Gen. Microbiol. 58: 179–187.

Fähraeus, G. 1947. Studies in the cellulose decomposition by Cytophaga. Symb. Bot. Ups. 9: 1–128.

Falcone, S.B., A.L. Shug and D.J.D. Nicholas. 1963. Some properties of a hydroxylamine oxidase from Nitosomonas europaea. Biochim. Biophys. Acta 77: 199–208.

Famintzin, A. 1892. Eine neue Bacterienform: Nevskia ramosa. Bull. Acad. Sci. St. Petersb. New Ser. 2, 34: 481–486.

Famurewa, O., H.G. Sonntag and P. Hirsch. 1983. Avirulence of 27 bacteria that are budding, prosthecate, or both. Int. J. Syst. Bacteriol. 33: 565–572.

Farabaugh, P.J., V. Schmeissner, M. Hofer and J.H. Miller. 1978. Genetic studies of the lac repressor. VII. On the molecular nature of spontaneous hotspots in the lacI gene of Escherichia coli. J. Mol. Biol. 126: 847–863.

Farina, M., H. Lins de Barros, D.M.S. Esquivel and J. Danon. 1983. Ultrastructure of a magnetotactic microorganism. Biol. Cell 48: 85–88.

Farlow, W.G. 1880. On the nature of the peculiar reddening of salted codfish during the summer season. Report of the Commissioners for 1878. U.S. Commission of Fish and Fisheries, pp. 969–974.

Farlow, W.G. 1886. Vegetable parasites of codfish. Bull. U.S. Fish Comm. 6: 1–4.

Farquhar, G.J. and W.C. Boyle. 1971. Identification of filamentous microorganisms in activated sludge. J. Water Pollut. Control Fed. 43: 604–622.

Farquhar, G.J. and W.C. Boyle. 1972. Control of Thiothrix in activated sludge. J. Water Pollut. Control. Fed. 44: 12–24.

Fathepure, B.Z. 1983. Isolation and characterization of an acetoclastic methanogen from biogas digester. FEMS Microbiol. Lett. 19: 151–156.

Faull, J. 1916. Chondromyces thaxteri, a new myxobacterium. Bot. Gaz. 62: 226–232.

Faust, L. and R.S. Wolfe. 1961. Enrichment and cultivation of Beggiatoa alba. J. Bacteriol. 81: 99–106.

Fautz, E., L. Grotjahn and H. Reichenbach. 1981. Hydroxy fatty acids as valuable chemosystematic markers in gliding bacteria and flavobacteria. In Reichenbach and Weeks (Editors), The Flavobacterium-Cytophaga Group. Verlag Chemie, Weinheim, F.R.G., pp. 127–133.

Fautz, E., G. Rosenfelder and L. Grotjahn. 1979. Iso-branched 2- and 3-hydroxy fatty acids as characteristic lipid constituents of some gliding bacteria. J.

Bacteriol. 140: 852–858.

Fay, P. 1973. The heterocyst. In Carr and Whitton (Editors), The Biology of Blue-green Algae. Blackwell, Oxford, and University of California Press, Berkeley, pp. 238–259.

Fay, P. 1980. Nitrogen fixation in heterocysts. In Subba-Rao (Editor), Recent Advances in Biological Nitrogen Fixation. Edward Arnold, London, pp. 121–165.

Fay, P. 1983. The Blue-greens (Cyanophyta-Cyanobacteria). Inst. of Biology, Stud. in Biol. Nr. 160. Edward Arnold, London.

Feick, R.G., M. Fitzpatrick and R.C. Fuller. 1982. Isolation and characterization of cytoplasmic membranes and chlorosomes from the green bacterium Chloroflexus aurantiacus. J. Bacteriol. 150: 905–915.

Feldmann, J. and G. Feldmann. 1953. Observations sur les genres Dermocarpa et Dermocarpella (Cyanophyceae). Oesterr. Bot. Z. 100: 505–514.

Fell, J.W. 1966. Sterigmatomyces, a new fungal genus from marine areas. Antonie van Leeuwenhoek J. Microbiol. Serol. 32: 99–104.

Feltham, R.K.A., A.K. Power, P.A. Pell and P.H.A. Sneath. 1978. A simple method of storing bacteria at -76°C. J. Appl. Bacteriol. 44: 313–316.

Ferguson, T.J. and R.A. Mah. 1983. Isolation and characterization of an H$_2$-oxidizing thermophilic methanogen. Appl. Environ. Microbiol. 45: 265–274.

Ferry, J.G., R.D. Sherod, H.D. Peck and L.G. Ljungdahl. 1976. Autotrophic fixation of CO$_2$ via tetrahydrofolate intermediates by Methanobacterium thermoautotrophicum. In Schlegel, Gottschalk and Decker (Editors), Microbial Production and Utilization of Gases (H$_2$, CH$_4$, and CO). Akad. Wiss. Göttingen, Goltz, Göttingen, pp. 173–180.

Ferry, J.G., P.H. Smith and R.S. Wolfe. 1974. Methanospirillum, a new genus of methanogenic bacteria, and characterization of Methanospirillum hungatii sp. nov. Int. J. Syst. Bacteriol. 24: 465–469.

Ferry, J.G. and R.S. Wolfe. 1976. Anaerobic degradation of benzoate to methane by a microbial consortium. Arch. Microbiol. 107: 33–40.

Ferry, J.G. and R.S. Wolfe. 1977. Nutritional and biochemical characterization of Methanospirillum hungatii. Appl. Environ. Microbiol. 34: 371–376.

Fiala, G. and K.O. Stetter. 1986a. Pyrococcus furiosus sp. nov. represents a novel genus of marine heterotrophic archaebacteria growing optimally at 100°C. Arch. Microbiol. 145: 56–61.

Fiala, G. and K.O. Stetter. 1986b. In Validation of the publication of new names and new combinations previously effectively published outside the IJSB. List No. 22. Int. J. Syst. Bacteriol. 36: 573–576.

Fiala, G., K.O. Stetter, H.W. Jannasch, T.A. Langworthy and J. Madon. 1986. Staphylothermus marinus sp. nov. represents a novel genus of extremely thermophilic submarine heterotrophic archaebacteria growing up to 98°C. Syst. Appl. Microbiol. 8: 106–113.

Fijan, N.N. 1969. Antibiotic additives for the isolation of Chondrococcus columnaris from fish. Appl. Microbiol. 17: 333–334.

Fijan, N.N. and P.R. Voorhees. 1969. Drug sensitivity of Chondrococcus columnaris. Vet. Arh. 39: 259–267.

Filer, D. and A.V. Furano. 1980. Portions of the gene encoding elongation factor Tu are highly conserved in prokaryotes. J. Biol. Chem. 255: 728–734.

Filer, D. and A.V. Furano. 1981. Duplication of the tuf gene, which encodes peptide chain elongation factor Tu, is widespread in Gram-negative bacteria. J. Bacteriol. 148: 1006–1011.

Firsov, N.N., I.I. Cherniadiev, R.N. Ivanovsky, E.N. Kondratieva, N.V. Vdovina and N.G. Doman. 1974. Pathways of assimilation of carbon dioxide by Ectothiorhodospira shaposhnikovii. Mikrobiologiya 43: 214–219.

Firsov, N.N. and R.N. Ivanovskii. 1974. Propionate metabolism in Ectothiorhodospira shaposhnikovii. Mikrobiologiya 43: 400–405.

Firsov, N.N. and R.N. Ivanovskii. 1975. Photometabolism of acetate in Ectothiorhodospira shaposhnikovii. Mikrobiologiya 44: 197–201.

Fischer, A., T. Roggentin, H. Schlesner and E. Stackebrandt. 1985. 16S ribosomal RNA oligonucleotide cataloguing and the phylogenetic position of Stella humosa. Syst. Appl. Microbiol. 6: 43–47.

Fischer, F., W. Zillig, K.O. Stetter and G. Schreiber. 1983. Chemolithoautotrophic metabolism of anaerobic extremely thermophilic archaebacteria. Nature 301: 511–513.

Fisher, W.S., E.H. Nilson, J.F. Steenbergen and D.V. Lightner. 1978. Microbial diseases of cultured lobsters: a review. Aquaculture 14: 115–140.

Fitzsimons, A.G. and R.V. Smith. 1984. The isolation and growth of axenic cultures of planktonic blue-green algae. Br. Phycol. J. 19: 156–162.

Flaherty, D.K., F.H. Deck, J. Cooper, K. Bishop, P.A. Winzenburger, L.R. Smith, L. Bynum and W.B. Witmer. 1984a. Bacterial endotoxin isolated from a water spray air humidification system as a putative agent of occupation-related lung disease. Infect. Immun. 43: 206–212.

Flaherty, D.K., F.H. Deck, M.A. Hood, C. Liebert, F. Singleton, P. Winzenburger, K. Bishop, L.R. Smith, L.M. Bynum and W.B. Witmer. 1984b. A Cytophaga species endotoxin as a putative agent of occupation-related lung disease. Infect. Immun. 43: 213–216.

Fliermans, C.B., B.B. Bohlool and E.L. Schmidt. 1974. Autecological study of the chemoautotroph Nitrobacter by immunofluorescence. Appl. Microbiol. 27: 124–129.

Fliesser, S.B. and T.E. Jensen. 1982. Observations on the fine structure of isolates of the blue-green bacteria Calothrix, Fremyella and Gloeotrichia. Cytobios 33: 203–222.

Florenzano, G., W. Balloni and R. Materassi. 1986. Nomenclature of Prochloron didemni (Lewin 1977) sp. nov., nom. rev., Prochloron (Lewin 1976) gen. nov., nom. rev., *Prochloraceae* fam. nov., *Prochlorales* ord. nov., nom. rev. in the class *Photobacteria* Gibbons and Murray 1978. Int. J. Syst. Bacteriol. *36:* 352-353.

Florenzano, G., C. Sili, E. Pelosi and M. Vincenzini. 1985. *Cyanospira rippkae* and *Cyanospira capsulata* (gen. nov. and spp. nov.): new filamentous heterocystous cyanobacteria from Magadi lake (Kenya). Arch. Microbiol. *140:* 301-306.

Flossdorf, J. 1983. A rapid method for the determination of the base composition of bacterial DNA. J. Microbiol. Methods *1:* 305-311.

Focht, D.D. and W. Vestraete. 1977. Biochemical ecology of nitrification and denitrification. Adv. Microb. Ecol. *1:* 135-214.

Fogg, G.E., W.D.P. Stewart, P. Fay and A.E. Walsby. 1973. The Blue-green Algae. Academic Press, London, New York.

Follett, E.A.C. and D.M. Webley. 1965. An electron microscope study of the cell surface of *Cytophaga johnsonii* and some observations on related organisms. Antonie van Leeuwenhoek J. Microbiol. Serol. *31:* 361-382.

Forlenza, S.W., M.G. Newman, A.L. Horikoshi and U. Blachman. 1981. Antimicrobial susceptibility of *Capnocytophaga*. Antimicrob. Agents Chemother. *19:* 144-146.

Forlenza, S.W., M.G. Newman, A.L. Lipsey, S.E. Siegel and U.L. Blachman. 1980. *Capnocytophaga* sepsis: a new recognized clinical entity in granulocytopenic patients. Lancet *i:* 567-568.

Fott, B. and J. Komárek. 1960. Das Phytoplankton der Teiche im Teschner Schlesien. Preslia *32:* 113-141.

Foulds, I.J. and N.G. Carr. 1981. Unequal cell division preceding heterocyst development in *Chlorogloeopsis fritschii*. FEMS Microbiol. Lett. *10:* 223-226.

Fowler, V.J., N. Pfennig, W. Schubert and E. Stackebrandt. 1984. Towards a phylogeny of phototrophic purple bacteria—16S rRNA oligonucleotide cataloguing of 11 species of *Chromatiaceae*. Arch. Microbiol. *139:* 382-387.

Fowler, V.J., F. Widdel, N. Pfennig, C.R. Woese and E. Stackebrandt. 1986. Phylogenetic relationships of sulfate- and sulfur-reducing eubacteria. Syst. Appl. Microbiol. *8:* 32-41.

Fox, G.E. 1985. The structure and evolution of archaebacterial ribosomal RNA. *In* Woese and Wolfe (Editors), The Bacteria, Vol. VIII. Academic Press, New York, pp. 413-457.

Fox, G.E., L.J. Magrum, W.E. Balch, R.S. Wolfe and C.R. Woese. 1977. Classification of methanogenic bacteria by 16S ribosomal RNA characterization. Proc. Natl. Acad. Sci. U.S.A. *74:* 4537-4541.

Fox, G.E., E. Stackebrandt, R.B. Hespell, J. Gibson, J. Maniloff, T.A. Dyer, R.S. Wolfe, W.E. Balch, R.S. Tanner, L.J. Magrum, L.B. Zablen, R. Blakemore, R. Gupta, L. Bonen, B.J. Lewis, D.A. Stahl, K.R. Luehrsen, K.N. Chen and C.R. Woese. 1980. The phylogeny of procaryotes. Science *209:* 457-463.

Frankel, R.B. and R.P. Blakemore. 1980. Navigational compass in magnetic bacteria. J. Magn. Matls. *15-18:* 1562-1564.

Frankel, R.B., R.P. Blakemore, F.F. Torres de Araujo, D.M.S. Esquivel and J. Danon. 1981. Magnetotactic bacteria at the geomagnetic equator. Science *212:* 1269-1270.

Frankel, R.B., G.C. Papaefthymiou, R.P. Blakemore and W. O'Brien. 1983. Fe$_3$O$_4$ precipitation in magnetotactic bacteria. Biochim. Biophys. Acta *763:* 147-159.

Franzmann, P.D. 1983. The aerobic, heterotrophic, non-gliding bacteria of the freshwaters of south-east Queensland. Thesis, University of Queensland, Australia.

Franzmann, P.D. and V.B.D. Skerman. 1981. *Agitococcus lubricus* gen. nov. sp. nov., a lipolytic, twitching coccus from freshwater. Int. J. Syst. Bacteriol. *31:* 177-183.

Franzmann, P.D. and V.B.D. Skerman. 1984. *Gemmata obscuriglobus*, a new genus and species of the budding bacteria. Antonie van Leeuwenhoek J. Microbiol. Serol. *50:* 261-268.

Frémy, P. 1929-1933. Cyanophycées des Côtes d'Europe. Mém. Soc. Natn. Sci. Nat. Math., Cherbourg *41:* 1-236.

Frémy, P. 1936. Remarques sur la morphologie et la biologie de l'*Hapalosiphon laminosus* Hanog. Ann. Protistol. *5:* 175-200.

Friedmann, I. 1955. *Geitleria calcarea* n. gen. et n. sp., a new atmophytic lime-incrusting blue-green alga. Bot. Not. *108:* 439-445.

Friedmann, I. 1961. *Chroococcidiopsis kashaii* sp. n. and the genus *Chroococcidiopsis* (Studies on cave algae from Israel III). Oesterr. Bot. Z. *108:* 354-367.

Friedmann, I. and L.V. Borowitzka. 1982. The symposium on taxonomic concepts in blue-green algae: towards a compromise with the bacteriological code? Taxon *31:* 673-683.

Friedrich, C.G. and G. Mitrenga. 1981. Oxidation of thiosulfate by *Paracoccus denitrificans* and other hydrogen bacteria. FEMS Microbiol. Lett. *10:* 209-212.

Fritsch, F.E. 1945. The Structure and Reproduction of Algae, Vol. II. Cambridge University Press, Cambridge.

Fritsch, F.E. and F. Rich. 1929. Fresh-water algae (exclusive of diatoms) from Griqualand West. Trans. R. Soc. S. Afr. *18:* 1-92.

Fritsche, D. 1975. Untersuchungen zur Struktur der Sphingolipoide von *Bacteroides*-Species. Zentralbl. Bakteriol. Parasitenkd. Infektionskr. Hyg. I Abt. Orig. A *233:* 64-71.

Fuchs, G., E. Stupperich and G. Eden. 1980. Autotrophic CO$_2$ fixation in *Chlorobium limicola*. Evidence for the operation of a reductive tricarboxylic acid cycle in growing cells. Arch. Microbiol. *128:* 64-71.

Fuchs, G., E. Stupperich and R.K. Thauer. 1980. Acetate assimilation and the syn-

thesis of alanine, aspartate and glutamate in *Methanobacterium thermoautotrophicum*. J. Bacteriol. *117:* 61-66.

Füglistaller, P., H. Widmer, W. Sidler, G. Frank and H. Zuber. 1981. Isolation and characterization of the phycoerythrocyanin and chromatic adaptation of the thermophilic cyanobacterium, *Mastigocladus laminosus*. Arch. Microbiol. *129:* 268-274.

Fujihara, M.P. and R.E. Nakatani. 1971. Antibody production and immune responses of rainbow trout and Coho salmon to *Chondrococcus columnaris*. J. Fish. Res. Board Can. *28:* 1253-1258.

Fujita, Y. and S. Shimura. 1974. Phycoerythrin of the marine blue-green alga *Trichodesmium thiebautii*. Plant Cell Physiol. *15:* 939-942.

Fuller, W.H. and A.G. Norman. 1942. A cellulose-dextrin medium for identifying cellulose organisms in soil. Proc. Soil Sci. Soc. Am. *7:* 243-246.

Fuller, W.H. and A.G. Norman. 1943. Cellulose decomposition by aerobic mesophilic bacteria from soil. I. Isolation and description of organisms. J. Bacteriol. *46:* 273-280.

Gabai, V.L. 1985. A one-instant mechanism of phototaxis in the cyanobacterium *Phormidium uncinatum*. FEMS Microbiol. Lett. *30:* 125-129.

Galau, G.A., R.J. Britten and E.H. Davidson. 1977. Studies on nucleic acid reassociation kinetics: rate of hybridization on excess RNA with DNA, compared to the rate of DNA renaturation. Proc. Natl. Acad. Sci. U.S.A. *74:* 1020-1023.

Gal'chenko, V.F. and A.I. Nesterov. 1981. Numerical analysis of protein electrophoregrams of obligate methanotropic bacteria. Mikrobiologiya *50:* 973-979.

Gal'chenko, V.F., V.N. Shishkina, N.E. Suzina and Y.A. Trotsenko. 1977. Isolation and properties of new strains of obligate methanotrophs. Microbiologiya *46:* 890-897.

Galinski, E. and H.G. Trüper. 1982. Betaine, a compatible solute in the extremely halophilic phototrophic bacterium *Ectothiorhodospira halochloris*. FEMS Microbiol. Lett. *13:* 357-360.

Gallardo, V.A. 1977. Large benthic microbial communities in sulphide biota under Peru-Chile subsurface countercurrent. Nature *268:* 331-332.

Gallin, J.I. and E.R. Leadbetter. 1966. Morphogenesis of *Sporocytophaga*. Bacteriol. Proc., p. 75.

Gantt, E., K. Ohki and Y. Fujita. 1984. *Trichodesmium thiebautii* structure of a nitrogen-fixing marine blue-green alga (Cyanophyta). Protoplasma *119:* 188-196.

Garlick, S., A. Oren and E. Padan. 1977. Occurrence of facultative anoxygenic photosynthesis among filamentous and unicellular cyanobacteria. J. Bacteriol. *129:* 623-629.

Garnjobst, L. 1945. *Cytophaga columnaris* (Davis) in pure culture: a myxobacterium pathogenic to fish. J. Bacteriol. *49:* 113-128.

Gaudy, E. and R.S. Wolfe. 1961. Factors affecting filamentous growth of *Sphaerotilus natans*. Appl. Microbiol. *9:* 580-584.

Gaudy, E. and R.S. Wolfe. 1962. Composition of an extracellular polysaccharide produced by *Sphaerotilus natans*. Appl. Microbiol. *10:* 200-205.

Gebauer, A. 1985. Nachweis und Quantifizierung des Autotrophie—Stoffwechsels von *Gallionella ferruginea* Ehrenberg. Ph.D. thesis, University of Braunschweig, pp. 1-75.

Gebauer, A., B. Bowien and H.H. Hanert. 1984. Autotrophic enzymes of *Gallionella ferruginea* and comparison of in vivo activity of its RuBP-carboxylase to *Thiobacillus ferrooxidans* and *Alcaligenes eutrophus*. Abstr. Annu. Meet. German Local Branch Am. Soc. Microbiol. Osnabrück, p. 47.

Gebers, R. 1981. Enrichment, isolation, and emended description of *Pedomicrobium ferrugineum* Aristovskaya and *Pedomicrobium manganicum* Aristovskaya. Int. J. Syst. Bacteriol. *31:* 302-316.

Gebers, R. and P. Hirsch. 1978. Isolation and investigation of *Pedomicrobium* spp., heavy metal-depositing bacteria from soil habitats. *In* Krumbein (Editor), Environmental Biogeochemistry and Geomicrobiology, Vol. 3. Ann Arbor Science Publishers, Ann Arbor, pp. 911-922.

Gebers, R., M. Mandel and P. Hirsch. 1981. Deoxyribonucleic acid base composition and nucleotide distribution of *Pedomicrobium* spp. Zentralbl. Bakteriol. Mikrobiol. Hyg. I Abt. Orig. C*2:* 332-338.

Gebers, R., B. Martens, U. Wehmeyer and P. Hirsch. 1986. Deoxyribonucleic acid homologies of *Hyphomicrobium* spp., *Hyphomonas* spp., and other hyphal, budding bacteria. Int. J. Syst. Bacteriol. *36:* 241-245.

Gebers, R., R.L. Moore and P. Hirsch. 1981. DNA-DNA reassociation studies on the genus *Pedomicrobium*. FEMS Microbiol. Lett. *11:* 283-286.

Gebers, R., R.L. Moore and P. Hirsch. 1984. Physiological properties and DNA-DNA homologies of *Hyphomonas polymorpha* and *Hyphomonas neptunium*. Syst. Appl. Microbiol. *5:* 510-517.

Gebers, R., U. Wehmeyer, T. Roggentin, H. Schlesner, J. Kölbel-Boelke and P. Hirsch. 1985. Deoxyribonucleic acid base compositions and nucleotide distributions of 65 strains of budding bacteria. Int. J. Syst. Bacteriol. *35:* 260-269.

Geitler, L. 1921. Kleine Mitteilung über Blaualgen. Oesterr. Bot. Z. *70:* 158-167.

Geitler, L. 1924. Über *Polyangium parasiticum* n. sp., eine submerse, parasitische *Myxobacteriacee*. Arch. Protistenk. *50:* 67-88.

Geitler, L. 1925. Synoptische Darstellung der Cyanophyceen in morphologischer und systematischer Hinsicht. Beih. Bot. Zentralbl. *41:* 163-294.

Geitler, L. 1927. Bemerkungen über *Paulinella chromatophora*. Zool. Anz. *73:* 333-334.

Geitler, L. 1932. (Reprinted 1971). Cyanophyceae. *In* Rabenhorst (Editor), Kryptogamenflora von Deutschland, Österreich und der Schweiz, Vol. XIV.

Akademische Verlags, Leipzig. Reprinted: Johnson Reprint Co., New York, London.

Geitler, L. 1933. Diagnosen neuer Blaualgen von den Sunda-Inseln. Arch. Hydrobiol. Suppl. *12:* 622-634.

Geitler, L. 1942. Schizophyceae. *In* Engler and Prantl (Editors), Die Natürlichen Pflanzenfamilien, 2nd Ed. Duncker and Humbolt, Berlin, pp. 1-232.

Geitler, L. 1955. *Torulopsidosira* n. gen., ein neuer hefeartiger Pilz, und andere Knospende Mikroorganismen. Arch. Mikrobiol. *22:* 324-334.

Geitler, L. 1960. Schizophyzeen. Gebruder Borntraeger, Berlin-Nikolassee.

Geitler, L. 1963. Die angebliche Cyanophycee *Isocystis pallida* ist ein hefeartiger Pilz *(Torulopsidosira)*. Arch. Mikrobiol. *46:* 238-242.

Geitler, L. 1967. Entwicklungsgeschichtliche und systematische Untersuchungen an einigen Cyanophyceen. Nova Hedwigia Z. Kryptogamenkd. *13:* 403-421.

Geitler, L. 1979. Einige Kritische Bemerkungun zu neuen zusammen fassenden Darstellung der Morphologie und Systematik der Cyanophyceen. Plant Syst. Evol. *132:* 153-160.

Genthner, F.J., L.A. Hook and W.R. Strohl. 1985. Determination of the molecular mass of bacterial genomic DNA and plasmid copy number by high-pressure liquid chromatography. Appl. Environ. Microbiol. *50:* 1007-1013.

Gentile, J.H. and T.E. Maloney. 1969. Toxicity and environmental requirements of a strain of *Aphanizomenon flos-aquae* (L.) Ralfs. Can. J. Microbiol. *15:* 165-173.

Germida, J.J. and L.E. Casida, Jr. 1983. *Ensifer adhaerens* predatory activity against other bacteria in soil, as monitored by indirect phage analysis. Appl. Environ. Microbiol. *45:* 1380-1388.

Gerth, K., H. Irschik, H. Reichenbach and W. Trowitzch. 1980. Myxothiazol and antibiotic from *Myxococcus fulvus* (*Myxobacterales*) I. Cultivation, isolation, physicochemical and biological properties. J. Antibiot. (Tokyo) *33:* 1474-1479.

Gerth, K., H. Irschik, H. Reichenbach and W. Trowitzch. 1982. The myxovirescins, a family of antibiotics from *Myxococcus virescens* (*Myxobacterales*). J. Antibiot. (Tokyo) *35:* 1454-1459.

Gerth, K. and H. Reichenbach. 1978. Induction of myxospore formation in *Stigmatella aurantiaca* (*Myxobacterales*) I. General characterization of the system. Arch. Microbiol. *177:* 173-182.

Gest, H., M.W. Dits and J.L. Favinger. 1983. Characterization of *Rhodopseudomonas sphaeroides* strain 'cordata/81-1'. FEMS Microbiol. Lett. *17:* 321-325.

Gest, H. and J.L. Favinger. 1983. *Heliobacterium chlorum*, an anoxygenic brownish-green photosynthetic bacterium containing a "new" form of bacteriochlorophyll. Arch. Microbiol. *136:* 11-16.

Gest, H. and J.L. Favinger. 1985. *In* Validation List No. 17. Int. J. Syst. Bacteriol. *35:* 223-225.

Ghiorse, W.C. 1984. Biology of iron- and manganese-depositing bacteria. Annu. Rev. Microbiol. *38:* 515-550.

Ghiorse, W.C. and S.D. Chapnick. 1983. Metal-depositing bacteria and the distribution of manganese and iron in swamp waters. *In* Hallberg (Editor), Environmental Biochemistry. Ecol. Bull. (Stockholm) *35:* 367-376.

Ghiorse, W.C. and P. Hirsch. 1979. An ultrastructural study of iron and manganese deposition associated with extracellular polymers of *Pedomicrobium*-like budding bacteria. Arch. Microbiol. *123:* 213-226.

Gibbons, N.E. 1974. Family V. *Halobacteriaceae*. *In* Buchanan and Gibbons (Editors), Bergey's Manual of Determinative Bacteriology, 8th Ed. The Williams and Wilkins Co., Baltimore, pp. 269-273.

Gibbons, N.E. 1974. Reference collections of bacteria—the need and requirements for type and neotype strains. *In* Buchanan and Gibbons (Editors), Bergey's Manual of Determinative Bacteriology, 8th Ed. The Williams and Wilkins Co., Baltimore, pp. 14-17.

Gibbons, N.E. and R.G.E. Murray. 1978. Proposals concerning the higher taxa of bacteria. Int. J. Syst. Bacteriol. *28:* 1-6.

Gibson, C.E. and R.V. Smith. 1982. Freshwater plankton. *In* Carr and Whitton (Editors), The Biology of Cyanobacteria. Blackwell, Oxford, and University of California Press, Berkeley, pp. 463-489.

Gibson, J. 1980. Phylogenetic analysis of photosynthetic bacteria based on comparison of 16S ribosomal RNA catalogues. *In* Halvorson and Van Holde (Editors), The Origins of Life and Evolution. Alan R. Liss, New York.

Gibson, J. 1984. Nutrient transport by anoxygenic and oxygenic photosynthetic bacteria. Annu. Rev. Microbiol. *38:* 133-159.

Gibson, J., W. Ludwig, E. Stackebrandt and C.R. Woese. 1985. The phylogeny of the green photosynthetic bacteria: absence of a close relationship between *Chlorobium* and *Chloroflexus*. Syst. Appl. Microbiol. *6:* 152-156.

Gibson, J., N. Pfennig and J.B. Waterbury. 1984. *Chloroherpeton thalassium* gen. nov. et spec. nov., a non-filamentous, flexing and gliding green sulfur bacterium. Arch. Microbiol. *138:* 96-101.

Gibson, J., N. Pfennig and J.B. Waterbury. 1985. *In* Validation List No. 17. Int. J. Syst. Bacteriol. *35:* 223-225.

Gibson, J., E. Stackebrandt, L.B. Zablen, R. Gupta and C.R. Woese. 1979. A phylogenetic analysis of the purple photosynthetic bacteria. Curr. Microbiol. *3:* 59-64.

Gicklhorn, J. 1920. Über neue farblose Schwefelbakterien. Zentralbl. Bakteriol. Parasitenkd. Infektionskr. Hyg. Abt. II *50:* 415-427.

Gicklhorn, J. 1921. Über den Blauglanz zweier neuer Oscillatorien. Österr. Bot. Z. *70:* 1-11.

Giddings, T.H., Jr. and L.A. Staehelin. 1981. Observation of microplasmodesmata in both heterocyst-forming filamentous cyanobacteria by freeze-fracture electron microscopy. Arch. Microbiol. *129:* 295-298.

Giddings, T.H., N.W. Withers and L.A. Staehelin. 1980. Supramolecular structure of stacked and unstacked regions of the photosynthetic membranes of *Prochloron* sp., a prokaryote. Proc. Natl. Acad. Sci. U.S.A. *77:* 352-356.

Giesberger, G. 1947. Some observations on the culture, physiology and morphology of some brown-red-*Rhodospirillum*-species. Antonie van Leeuwenhoek J. Microbiol. Serol. *13:* 135-148.

Giffhorn, F., N. Beuscher and G. Gottschalk. 1972. Regulation of citrate lyase activity in *Rhodopseudomonas gelatinosa*. Biochem. Biophys. Res. Commun. *49:* 467-471.

Giffhorn, F. and A. Kuhn. 1980. Phototrophic growth on citrate and regulation of citrate lyase in three strains of *Rhodopseudomonas palustris*. FEMS Microbiol. Lett. *7:* 225-228.

Gilbert, H.C. and G.W. Martin. 1933. Myxomycetes found in the bark of living trees. Univ. Iowa Stud. Nat. Hist. *15:* 3-8.

Gillespie, D. and S. Spiegelman. 1965. A quantitative assay for DNA-RNA hybrids with DNA immobilized on a membrane filter. J. Mol. Biol. *12:* 829-842.

Gilligan, P.H., L.R. McCarthy and B.K. Bissett. 1981. *Capnocytophaga ochracea* septicaemia. J. Clin. Microbiol. *13:* 643-645.

Gillis, M., J. Dejonghe, A. Smet, G. Onghenae and J. De Ley. 1982. Intra- and intergeneric similarities of the ribosomal ribonucleic acid cistrons in the *Rhodospirillaceae*. Abstract A 16, IV. Intern. Symp. Photosynthetic Procaryotes, Bombannes-Bordeaux.

Gilmore, D.F. and D. White. 1985. Energy-dependent cell cohesion in myxobacteria. J. Bacteriol. *161:* 113-117.

Gimesi, N. 1924. Hydrobiologiai Tanulmányok (Hydrobiologische Studien). I. *Planctomyces békefii* Gim. nov. gen. et sp. (Ein neues Glied des Phytoplanktons.) Budapest: Kiadja a Magyar Ciszterci Rend, pp. 1-8 (in Hungarian; partial German translation).

Ginsburg-Ardré, F. 1966. *Dermocarpa, Xenococcus, Dermocarpella* (Cyanophycées): nouvelles observations. Oesterr. Bot. Z. *113:* 362-367.

Ginzburg, M., L. Sachs and B.Z. Ginzburg. 1970. Ion metabolism in a *Halobacterium*. I. Influence of age of culture on intracellular concentrations. J. Gen. Physiol. *55:* 187-207.

Giovannoni, S.J., E. Schabtach and R.W. Castenholz. 1987. *Isosphaera pallida*, gen. and comb. nov., a gliding, budding eubacterium from hot springs. Arch. Microbiol. *147:* 276-284.

Giovannoni, S.J., S. Turner, G.J. Olsen, S. Barns, D.J. Lane and N.R. Pace. 1988. Evolutionary relationships among cyanobacteria and green chloroplasts. J. Bacteriol. *170:* 3584-3592.

Giovannoni, S.J., S. Turner, G.J. Olsen, D.J. Lane, N.R. Pace and J.B. Waterbury. 1986. Phylogenetic analysis of cyanobacteria using 16S rRNA sequences. Abstr. Annu. Meet. Am. Soc. Microbiol., Washington, D.C., p. 237.

Glaser, J. and J.L. Pate. 1973. Isolation and characterization of gliding motility mutants of *Cytophaga columnaris*. Arch. Mikrobiol. *93:* 295-309.

Glazer, A.N. 1983. Comparative biochemistry of photosynthetic light-harvesting systems. Annu. Rev. Biochem. *52:* 125-157.

Glazer, A.N. 1984. Phycobilisome: a macromolecular complex optimized for light energy transfer. Biochem. Biophys. Acta *768:* 29-51.

Gleason, F.K. and C.A. Baxa. 1986. Activity of the natural algicide, cyanobacterin, on eukaryotic microorganisms. FEMS Microbiol. Lett. *33:* 85-88.

Gleen, H. and J.H. Quastel. 1953. Sulphur metabolism in soil. Appl. Microbiol. *1:* 70-77.

Gliesche, C.G., N.C. Holm, M. Beese, M. Neumann, H. Völker, R. Gebers and P. Hirsch. 1988. New bacteriophages active on strains of *Hyphomicrobium*. J. Gen. Microbiol. *134:* 1339-1353.

Gloe, A., N. Pfennig, H. Brockmann, Jr. and W. Trowitzsch. 1975. A new bacteriochlorophyll from brown-colored *Chlorobiaceae*. Arch. Microbiol. *102:* 103-109.

Gloe, A. and N. Risch. 1978. Bacteriochlorophyll c_s, a new bacteriochlorophyll from *Chloroflexus aurantiacus*. Arch. Microbiol. *118:* 153-156.

Glover, H.E. 1986. The physiology and ecology of marine cyanobacteria, *Synechococcus* spp. Adv. Aquat. Microbiol. *3:* 49-107.

Gochnauer, M.B. and D.J. Kushner. 1969. Growth and nutrition of extremely halophilic bacteria. Can. J. Microbiol. *15:* 1157-1165.

Godchaux, W. and E.R. Leadbetter. 1980. *Capnocytophaga* spp. contain sulfonolipids that are novel in procaryotes. J. Bacteriol. *144:* 592-602.

Godchaux, W. and E.R. Leadbetter. 1983. Unusual sulfonolipids are characteristic of the *Cytophaga-Flexibacter* group. J. Bacteriol. *153:* 1238-1246.

Godchaux, W. and E.R. Leadbetter. 1984. Sulfonolipids of gliding bacteria. Structure of the *N*-acrylaminosulfonates. J. Biol. Chem. *259:* 2982-2990.

Godden, B. and M.J. Penninckx. 1984. Identification and evolution of the cellulolytic microflora present during composting of cattle manure: on the role of actinomycetes sp. Ann. Microbiol. (Inst. Pasteur) *135B:* 69-78.

Godsy, E.M. 1980. Isolation of *Methanobacterium bryantii* from a deep aquifer by using a novel broth-antibiotic disk method. Appl. Environ. Microbiol. *39:* 1074-1075.

Goldfine, H. and P.O. Hagen. 1968. N-methyl groups in bacterial lipids. III. Phospholipids of hyphomicrobia. J. Bacteriol. *95:* 367-375.

Golecki, J.R. and G. Drews. 1980. Cellular organization of the halophilic, phototrophic bacterium strain WS 68. Eur. J. Cell Biol. *22:* 654-660.

Golecki, J.R. and G. Drews. 1982. Supramolecular organization and composition of membranes. *In* Carr and Whitton (Editors), The Biology of Cyanobacteria. Blackwell, Oxford, and University of California Press, Berkeley, pp. 125–141.

Golovacheva, R.S. 1976. Thermophilic nitrifying bacteria from hot springs. Microbiology *45:* 329–331.

Golovacheva, R.S. and G.I. Karavaiko. 1978. *Sulfobacillus*—a new genus of thermophilic spore-forming bacteria. Mikrobiologiya *47:* 815–822.

Golubic, S. 1973. The relationship between blue-green algae and carbonate deposits. *In* Carr and Whitton (Editors), The Biology of Blue-green Algae. Blackwell, Oxford, and University of California Press, Berkeley, pp. 434–472.

Golubic, S. 1976. Taxonomy of extant stromatolite-building cyanophytes. *In* Walter (Editor), Stromatolites. Elsevier, Amsterdam, pp. 127–140.

Golubic, S. 1979. Cyanobacteria (blue-green algae) under the bacteriological code? An ecological objection. Taxon *28:* 187–188.

Gommers, P.J.F. 1987. Microbiological oxidation of sulfide and acetate in a denitrifying fluidized bed reactor, fundamental and microbiological aspects. Ph.D. dissertation, Delft University of Technology, Delft, The Netherlands.

Gommers, P.J. and J.G. Kuenen. 1987. *Thiobacillus* Q, a chemolithoheterotrophic sulphur bacterium. Arch. Microbiol. *150:* 117–125.

Gomont, M. 1892. Monographie des Oscillariées. Ann. Sci. Nat. Ser. Bot. *15:* 263–368; *16:* 91–264.

Gomont, M. 1895. Note sur le *Scytonema amibiguum* Kütz. J. Bot. *9:* 49–53.

Gonzalez, C., C. Gutierrez and C. Ramirez. 1978. *Halobacterium vallismortis* sp. nov. An amylolytic and carbohydrate-metabolising extremely halophilic bacterium. Can. J. Microbiol. *24:* 710–715.

Goodfellow, M. and D.E. Minnikin (Editors). 1985. Chemical Methods in Bacterial Systematics. Society for Applied Bacteriology, Technical Series 20. Academic Press, London, New York.

Goodwin, T.W. 1980. The Biochemistry of the Carotenoids, Vol. I: Plants. Chapman and Hall, New York.

Gordon, R.E. 1967. The taxonomy of soil bacteria. *In* Gray and Parkinson (Editors), The Ecology of Soil Bacteria. An International Symposium. University of Toronto Press, Toronto, pp. 293–321.

Goreau, T.J., W.A. Kaplan, S.C. Wofsy, M.B. McElroy, F.W. Valois and S.W. Watson. 1980. Production of NO_2^- and N_2O by nitrifying bacteria at reduced concentrations of oxygen. Appl. Environ. Microbiol. *40:* 526–532.

Gorham, P.R., J.S. McLachlan, U.T. Hammer and W.K. Kim. 1964. Isolation and culture of toxic strains of *Anabaena flos-aquae* (Lynb.) de Bréb. Verh. Int. Ver. Theor. Angew. Limnol. *15:* 796–804.

Gorlenko, V.M. 1968. A new species of the green sulphur bacteria. Dokl. Akad. Nauk S.S.S.R. *179:* 1229–1231.

Gorlenko, V.M. 1970. A new phototrophic green sulphur bacterium—*Prosthecochloris aestuarii* nov. gen. nov. sp. Z. Allg. Mikrobiol. *10:* 147–149.

Gorlenko, V.M. 1972. A new species of phototrophic brown sulfur bacteria *Pelodictyon phaeum* nov. spec. Mikrobiologiya *41:* 370–371.

Gorlenko, V.M. 1975. Characteristics of filamentous phototrophic bacteria from the freshwater lakes. Microbiology *44:* 682–684.

Gorlenko, V.M., E.N. Chebotarev and V.I. Kachalkin. 1974. Participation of microorganisms in sulphur turnover in Pomiaretzkoe Lake. Mikrobiologiya *43:* 908–914.

Gorlenko, V.M., G.A. Dubinina and S.I. Kuznetsov. 1983. The Ecology of Aquatic Micro-organisms. E. Schweizerbart'sche Verlag, Stuttgart.

Gorlenko, V.M. and S.A. Korotkov. 1979. Morphological and physiological features of the new filamentous gliding green bacteria *Oscillochloris trichoides* nov. comb. Izv. Akad. Nauk S.S.S.R. Ser. Biol. *5:* 848–857.

Gorlenko, V.M., E.N. Krasil'nikova, O.G. Kikina and N.Y. Tatarinova. 1979. The new motile purple sulfur bacterium *Lamprobacter modestohalophilus* nov. gen., nov. sp. with gas vacuoles. Izv. Akad. Nauk S.S.S.R. Ser. Biol. *5:* 755–767 (in Russian).

Gorlenko, V.M., E.N. Krasil'nikova, O.G. Kikina and N.Y. Tatarinova. 1988. *In* Validation of the publication of new names and new combinations previously effectively published outside the IJSB. Int. J. Syst. Bacteriol. *38:* 220–222.

Gorlenko, V.M. and S.I. Kusnezov. 1972. Über die photosynthetisierenden Bakterien des Kononjer Sees. Arch. Hydrobiol. *70:* 1–13.

Gorlenko, V.M. and E.V. Lebedeva. 1971. New green bacteria with outgrowths. Mikrobiologiya *40:* 1035–1039.

Gorlenko, V.M. and S.I. Lokk. 1979. Vertical distribution and special composition of microorganisms from some stratified estonian lakes. Mikrobiologiya *48:* 351–359.

Gorlenko, V.M. and T.A. Pivovarova. 1977. On the assignment of the blue-green alga *Oscillatoria coerulescens* Gicklhorn, 1921, to the new genus of chlorobacteria *Oscillochloris* nov. gen. Izv. Akad. Nauk S.S.S.R. Ser. Biol. *3:* 396–409.

Gorlenko, V.M., M.B. Vainshtein and V.I. Kachalkin. 1976. Microbiological characteristic of Lake Mogil'noe. Arch. Hydrobiol. *81:* 475–492.

Gorlenko, V.M. and T.N. Zhilina. 1968. A study on a fine structure of green sulfur bacteria, strain SK-413. Mikrobiologiya *37:* 1052–1056.

Gorrell, T.E. and R.L. Uffen. 1977. Fermentative metabolism of pyruvate by *Rhodospirillum rubrum* after anaerobic growth in darkness. J. Bacteriol. *131:* 533–543.

Gorris, L.G.M. and C. van der Drift. 1986. Methanogenic cofactors in pure cultures of methanogens in relation to substrate utilization. *In* Dubourguier, Albagnac, Montreuil, Romond, Santière and Guillaume (Editors), Biology of Anaerobic Bacteria. Elsevier Science Publishers, Amsterdam, pp. 144–150.

Gossling, J. and W.E.C. Moore. 1975. *Gemmiger formicilis*, n. gen., n. sp., an anaer-

obic budding bacterium from intestines. Int. J. Syst. Bacteriol. *25:* 202–207.

Gottschal, J.C. and J.G. Kuenen. 1980. Selective enrichment of facultatively chemolithotrophic thiobacilli and related organisms in continuous culture. FEMS Microbiol. Lett. *7:* 241–247.

Gräf, W. 1961. Anaerobe Myxobakterien, neue Mikroben in der menschlichen Mundhöhle. Arch. Hyg. Bakteriol. *145:* 405–449.

Gräf, W. 1962. Über Wassermyxobakterien. Arch. Hyg. Bakteriol. *146:* 114–125.

Gräf, W. 1975. Myxobakterien der Gattung *Myxococcus* als indirekte Fäkalstoffindikatoren in Oberflächengewässern. Zentralbl. Bakteriol. Parasitenkd. Infektionskr. Hyg. Abt. I Orig. B *160:* 28–39.

Gräf, W. and G. Pelka. 1979. Die Indikatorfunktion der Wassermyxobakterien bei der bakteriologischen Trinkwasseruntersuchung. Zentralbl. Bakteriol. Parasitenkd. Infektionskr. Hyg. Abt. I Orig. B *169:* 225–239.

Gräf, W. and G. Perschmann. 1970. Über eine neue Spezies von *Vitreoscilla (Vitreoscilla proteolytica)* im Bodensee. Arch. Hyg. Bakteriol. *154:* 128–137.

Gräf, W. and E. Pfeiffer. 1967. Serologische Studien an Myxobakterien aus Seen. Arch. Hyg. Bakteriol. *150:* 724–736.

Gräf, W. and P. Stürzenhofecker. 1964. Biologie und Vorkommen von aeroben Wassermyxobakterien *(Sporocytophaga cauliformis)* im Bodensee. Arch. Hyg. Bakteriol. *148:* 79–96.

Gräf, W. and P. Stürzenhofecker. 1965. Myxobakterienquotient als Eutrophierungsindikator bei Oberflächengewässern. Arch. Hyg. Bakteriol. *149:* 265–273.

Grant, W.D., G. Pinch, J.E. Harris, M. De Rosa and A. Gambacorta. 1985. Polar lipids in methanogen taxonomy. J. Gen. Microbiol. *131:* 3277–3286.

Grant, W.D. and H.N.M. Ross. 1986. The ecology and taxonomy of halobacteria. FEMS Microbiol. Rev. *39:* 9–15.

Gray, M.W. and W.F. Doolittle. 1982. Has the endosymbiont hypothesis been proven? Microbiol. Rev. *46:* 1–42.

Greaves, M.P., D. Vaughan and D.M. Webley. 1970. The degradation of nucleic acids by *Cytophaga johnsonii*. J. Appl. Bacteriol. *33:* 380–389.

Greaves, R.I.N. 1956. The preservation of bacteria. Can. J. Microbiol. *2:* 365–371.

Grecz, N. and G.M. Dack. 1961. Taxonomically significant color reactions of *Brevibacterium linens*. J. Bacteriol. *82:* 241–246.

Gregory, E., R.S. Perry and J.T. Staley. 1980. Characterization, distribution, and significance of *Metallogenium* in Lake Washington. Microb. Ecol. *6:* 125–140.

Gregory, E. and J.T. Staley. 1982. Widespread distribution of ability to oxidize manganese among freshwater bacteria. Appl. Environ. Microbiol. *44:* 509–511.

Griffiths, A.J. 1984. A descriptive numericlature for isolates of cyanobacteria. Br. Phycol. J. *19:* 233–238.

Griffiths, D.J., L-V. Thinh and H. Winsor. 1984. Crystals and paracrystalline inclusions of *Prochloron* (Prochlorophyta) symbiotic with the ascidian *Trididemnum cyclops* (Didemnidae). Bot. Mar. *XXVII:* 117–128.

Grilione, P.L. and J. Pangborn. 1975. Scanning electron microscopy of fruiting body formation by myxobacteria. J. Bacteriol. *124:* 1558–1565.

Grimm, K. 1978. Comparison of spontaneous, u.v. induced and nitrosoguanidine-induced mutability to drug resistance in myxobacteria. J. Bacteriol. *135:* 748–753.

Grimm, K. and H. Kühlwein. 1973a. Untersuchungen an spontanen Mutanten von *Archangium violaceum* (*Myxobacterales*) I. Bewegliche und unbewegliche Zellen von *A. violaceum*. Arch. Mikrobiol. *89:* 105–119.

Grimm, K. and H. Kühlwein. 1973b. Untersuchungen an spontanen Mutanten von *Archangium violaceum* (*Myxobacterales*) II. Über den Einfluss des Schleims auf die Bewegung der Zellen und die Entstehung stabiler Suspensionskulturen. Arch. Mikrobiol. *89:* 121–132.

Grobbelaar, N., T.C. Huang, H.Y. Lin and T.J. Chow. 1986. Dinitrogen-fixing endogenous rhythm in *Synechococcus* RF-1. FEMS Microbiol. Lett. *37:* 173–177.

Gromov, B.V., O.G. Ivanov, K.A. Mamkaeva and I.A. Avilov. 1972. The flexibacterium lyzing blue-green algae. Mikrobiologiya *41:* 1074–1079 (in Russian with English summary).

Gross, J. 1911. Über freilebende Spironemaceen. Mitt. Zool. Stat. Neapel *20:* 188–203.

Grunow, A. 1867. Reise Freg. Novara, S. 31.

Guay, R. and M. Silver. 1975. *Thiobacillus acidophilus* sp. nov.; isolation and some physiological characteristics. Can. J. Microbiol. *21:* 281–288.

Güde, H. 1973. Untersuchungen über aerobe pektinzersetzende Bakterien in einem eutrophen See. Arch. Hydrobiol. Suppl. *42:* 483–496.

Güde, H. 1978a. Polysaccharide degradation by aquatic *Cytophaga* populations in a eutrophic lake and in mixed cultures. Verh. Int. Ver. Limnol. *20:* 2233–2237.

Güde, H. 1978b. Model experiments on regulation of bacterial polysaccharide degradation in lakes. Arch. Hydrobiol. Suppl. *55:* 157–185.

Güde, H. 1980. Occurrence of cytophagas in sewage plants. Appl. Environ. Microbiol. *39:* 756–763.

Güde, H., W.R. Strohl and J.M. Larkin. 1981. Mixotrophic and heterotrophic growth of *Beggiatoa alba* in continuous culture. Arch. Microbiol. *129:* 357–360.

Guglielmi, G. 1975. Etude de quelques espèces marines de Rivulariacées en microscopie électronique. Vie Milieu Ser. A *25:* 189–213.

Guglielmi, G. and G. Cohen-Bazire. 1982a. Etude comparée de la structure et de la distribution des filament extracellulaires ou fimbriae chez quelques cyanobactéries. Protistologica *18:* 167–177.

Guglielmi, G. and G. Cohen-Bazire. 1982b. Structure et distribution des pores et des perforations de l'enveloppe de peptidoglycane chez quelques cyanobactéries. Protistologica *18:* 151–165.

Guglielmi, G. and G. Cohen-Bazire. 1984a. Étude taxonomique d'un genre de cyanobactérie Oscillatoriacée: Le genre *Pseudanabaena* Lauterborn. I. Étude ultrastructurali. Protistologica *20:* 377–391.

Guglielmi, G. and G. Cohen-Bazire. 1984b. Étude taxonomique d'un genre de cyanobactérie Oscillatoriacée: Le genre *Pseudanabaena* Lauterborn. II. Analyse de la composition moléculaire et de la structure des phycobilisomes. Protistologica *20:* 393–413.

Guglielmi, G., G. Cohen-Bazire and D.A. Bryant. 1981. The structure of *Gloeobacter violaceus* and its phycobilisomes. Arch. Microbiol. *129:* 181–189.

Gunja-Smith, Z., J.J. Marshall, E.E. Smith and W.J. Whelan. 1970. A glycogen-debranching enzyme from *Cytophaga*. FEBS Lett. *12:* 96–100.

Gunsalus, R.P. and R.S. Wolfe. 1978a. ATP activation and properties of the methyl-coenzyme M reductase system in *Methanobacterium thermoautotrophicum*. J. Bacteriol. *135:* 851–857.

Gunsalus, R.P. and R.S. Wolfe. 1978b. Chromophoric factors F_{342} and F_{430} of *Methanobacterium thermoautotrophicum*. FEMS Microbiol. Lett. *3:* 191–193.

Gupta, R., J.M. Lanter and C.R. Woese. 1983. Sequence of the 16S rRNA from *Halobacterium volcanii*, an archaebacterium. Science *221:* 656–659.

Gupta, R. and C.R. Woese. 1980. Unusual modification patterns in the transfer ribonucleic acids of archaebacteria. Curr. Microbiol. *4:* 245–249.

Gürgün, V., G. Kirchner and N. Pfennig. 1976. Vergärung von Pyruvat durch sieben Arten phototropher Purpurbakterien. Z. Allg. Mikrobiol. *16:* 573–586.

Gutiérrez, M.C., M.T. Garcia, A. Ventosa, J.J. Nieto and F. Ruiz-Berraquero. 1986. Occurrence of megaplasmids in halobacteria. J. Appl. Bacteriol. *61:* 67–71.

Haars, E.G. and J.M. Schmidt. 1974. Stalk formation and its inhibition in *Caulobacter crescentus*. J. Bacteriol. *120:* 1409–1416.

Habib Ali, S. and J.L. Stokes. 1971. Stimulation of heterotrophic and autotrophic growth of *Sphaerotilus discophorus* by manganous ions. Antonie van Leeuwenhoek J. Microbiol. Serol. *37:* 519–528.

Häder, D.P. 1979. Control of locomotion: photomovement. *In* Haupt and Feinleib (Editors), Physiology of Movements. Encycl. Plant Physiol. N.S. Vol. 7. Springer-Verlag, Berlin, pp. 268–309.

Häder, D.P. 1987. Photosensory behavior in procaryotes. Microbiol. Rev. *51:* 1–21.

Halfen, L.N. 1979. Gliding movements. *In* Haupt and Feinleib (Editors), Physiology of Movements Encycl. Plant Physiol. N.S. Vol. 7. Springer-Verlag, Berlin, pp. 250–267.

Halfen, L.N. and R.W. Castenholz. 1971. Gliding motility in the blue-green alga, *Oscillatoria princeps*. J. Phycol. *7:* 133–145.

Halfen, L.N., B.K. Pierson and G.W. Francis. 1972. Carotenoids of a gliding organism containing bacteriochlorophylls. Arch. Mikrobiol. *82:* 240–246.

Hanert, H.H. 1968. Untersuchungen zur Isolierung, Stoffwechselphysiologie und Morphologie von *Gallionella ferruginea* Ehrenberg. Arch. Microbiol. *60:* 348–376.

Hanert, H.H. 1970. Struktur und Wachstum von *Gallionella ferruginea* Ehrenberg am natürlichen Standort in den ersten 6 Stunden der Entwicklung. Arch. Microbiol. *75:* 10–24.

Hanert, H.H. 1974. Untersuchungen zur individuellen Entwicklungskinetik von *Gallionella ferruginea* in statischer Mikrokultur. Arch. Microbiol. *96:* 59–74.

Hanert, H.H. 1975. Entwicklung, Physiologie und Ökologie des Eisenbacteriums *Gallionella ferruginea* Ehrenberg—Beiträge zu einer Monographie. Habilitationsschrift, Faculty of Sciences, University of Braunschweig, pp. 1–104.

Hanert, H.H. 1981. The genus *Gallionella*. *In* Starr, Stolp, Trüper, Balows and Schlegel (Editors), The Prokaryotes. A Handbook on Habitats, Isolation, and Identification of Bacteria. Springer-Verlag, Berlin, pp. 509–515.

Hanert, H.H. 1981. The genus *Siderocapsa* (and other iron- or manganese-oxidizing eubacteria). *In* Starr, Stolp, Trüper, Balows and Schlegel (Editors), The Prokaryotes. A Handbook on the Habitats, Isolation, and Identification of Bacteria. Springer-Verlag, Berlin, pp. 1049–1066.

Hansen, T.A. 1974. Sulfide als electonendonor voor *Rhodospirillaceae*. Ph.D. thesis, University of Groningen, The Netherlands.

Hansen, T.A. and J.F. Imhoff. 1985. *Rhodobacter veldkampii* sp. nov., a new species of the phototrophic purple nonsulfur bacteria. Int. J. Syst. Bacteriol. *35:* 115–116.

Hansen, T.A., A.B.J. Sepers and H. van Gemerden. 1975. A new purple bacterium that oxidizes sulfide to extracellular sulfur and sulfate. Plant Soil *43:* 17–27.

Hansen, T.A. and H. van Gemerden. 1972. Sulfide utilization by purple nonsulfur bacteria. Arch. Mikrobiol. *86:* 49–56.

Hansen, T.A. and H. Veldkamp. 1973. *Rhodopseudomonas sulfidophila*, nov. spec., a new species of the purple nonsulfur bacteria. Arch. Mikrobiol. *92:* 45–58.

Hansgirg, A. 1891. Ueber die Bacteriaceen-gattung *Phragmidiothrix* Engler und einige *Leptothrix* Kutzing-Arten. Bot. Zentralbl. *49:* 314–315.

Happold, F.C., K.I. Johnstone, H.J. Rogers and J.B. Youatt. 1954. The isolation and characteristics of an organism oxidizing thiocyanate. J. Gen. Microbiol. *10:* 261–266.

Happold, F.C. and A. Key. 1937. The bacterial purification of gas works liquor. II. The biological oxidation of ammonium thiocyanate. Biochem. J. *31:* 1323–1329.

Harashima, K., J. Hayasaki, T. Ikari and T. Shiba. 1980. O_2-stimulated synthesis of bacteriochlorophyll and carotenoids in marine bacteria. Plant Cell Physiol. *21:* 1283–1294.

Harashima, K., M. Nakagawa and N. Murata. 1982. Photochemical activities of bacteriochlorophyll in aerobically grown cells of aerobic heterotrophs, *Erythrobacter* species (OCh 114) and *Erythrobacter longus* (OCh 101). Plant Cell Physiol. *23:* 185–193.

Harashima, K., T. Shiba, T. Totsuka, U. Simidu and N. Taga. 1978. Occurrence of bacteriochlorophyll *a* in a strain of an aerobic heterotrophic bacterium. Agric. Biol. Chem. *42:* 1627–1628.

Hardy, K. 1981. Bacterial plasmids. *In* Cole and Knowles (Editors), Aspects of Microbiology Series No. 4. Thomas Nelson and Sons, Walton-on-Thames, U.K.

Harms, H., H.-P. Koops, H. Martiny and M. Wullenweber. 1981. D-Ribulose 1,5-bisphosphate carboxylase and polyhedral inclusion bodies in *Nitrosomonas* spec. Arch. Microbiol. *128:* 280–281.

Harms, H., H.-P. Koops and H. Wehrmann. 1976. An ammonia-oxidizing bacterium, *Nitrosovibrio tenuis* nov. gen. nov. sp. Arch. Microbiol. *108:* 105–111.

Harold, R. and R.Y. Stanier. 1955. The genera *Leucothrix* and *Thiothrix*. Bacteriol. Rev. *19:* 49–58.

Harrison, A.P., Jr. 1981. *Acidiphilium cryptum* gen. nov., sp. nov., heterotrophic bacterium from acidic mineral environments. Int. J. Syst. Bacteriol. *31:* 327–332.

Harrison, A.P. 1982. Genomic and physiological diversity amongst strains of *Thiobacillus ferrooxidans* and genomic comparison with *Thiobacillus thiooxidans*. Arch. Microbiol. *131:* 68–76.

Harrison, A.P. 1983. Genomic and physiological comparisons between heterotrophic thiobacilli and *Acidiphilium cryptum, Thiobacillus versutus*, sp. nov., and *Thiobacillus acidophilus* nom. rev. Int. J. Syst. Bacteriol. *33:* 211–217.

Harrison, A.P. 1984. The acidophilic thiobacilli and other acidophilic bacteria that share their habitat. Annu. Rev. Microbiol. *38:* 265–292.

Harrison, A.P., B.W. Jarvis and J.L. Johnson. 1980. Heterotrophic bacteria from cultures of autotrophic *Thiobacillus ferrooxidans*: relationships as studied by means of deoxyribonucleic acid homology. J. Bacteriol. *143:* 448–454.

Harrison, A.P. and P.R. Norris. 1985. *Leptospirillum ferrooxidans* and similar bacteria: some characteristics and genomic diversity. FEMS Microbiol. Lett. *30:* 99–102.

Harrison, F.C. and M.E. Kennedy. 1922. The red discolouration of cured codfish. Trans. R. Soc. Can. Sect. V *16:* 101–152.

Hartmann, R., H.-D. Sickinger and D. Oesterhelt. 1980. Anaerobic growth of halobacteria. Proc. Natl. Acad. Sci. U.S.A. *77:* 3821–3825.

Harvey, S. and M.J. Pickett. 1980. Comparison of adansonian analysis and deoxyribonucleic acid hybridization results in the taxonomy of *Yersinia enterocolitica*. Int. J. Syst. Bacteriol. *30:* 86–102.

Harwood, C.R. 1980. Plasmids. *In* Goodfellow and Board (Editors), Microbiological Classification and Identification. Academic Press, London, New York, pp. 27–53.

Haselkorn, R. 1986. Organization of the genes for nitrogen fixation in photosynthetic bacteria and cyanobacteria. Annu. Rev. Microbiol. *40:* 525–547.

Hässelbarth, U. and D. Lüdemann. 1967. Die biologische Verockerung von Brunnen durch Massenentwicklung von Eisen- und Manganbakterien. Bohrtechnik-Brunnenbau-Rohr-leitungsbau 10/11 (Ber. DVGW Fachausschuss "Wasserfassung und Wasseranreicherung").

Haubold, R. 1978. Two different types of surface structures of methane utilizing bacteria. Z. Allg. Mikrobiol. *18:* 511–515.

Havenner, J.A., B.A. McCardell and R.M. Weiner. 1979. Development of defined minimal and complete media for the growth of *Hyphomicrobium neptunium*. Appl. Environ. Microbiol. *38:* 18–23.

Hayes, P.R. 1977. A taxonomic study of flavobacteria and related Gram-negative yellow pigmented rods. J. Appl. Bacteriol. *43:* 345–367.

Heaney, S.I. and G.H.M. Jaworski. 1977. A simple separation technique for purifying micro-algae. Br. Phycol. J. *12:* 171–174.

Hedenskog, G. and A.W. Hofsten. 1970. The ultrastructure of *Spirulina platensis*—a new source of microbial protein. Physiol. Plant *23:* 209–216.

Hedges, A. and R.S. Wolfe. 1974. Extracellular enzyme from myxobacter AL-1 that exhibits both β-1,4 glucanase and chitosanase activities. J. Bacteriol. *120:* 844–853.

Hegemann, P., A. Blanck, H. Vogelsang-Wenke, F. Lottspeich and D. Oesterheldt. 1987. The halo-opsin gene 1. Identification and isolation. EMBO J. *6:* 259–264.

Heldal, M. and O. Tumyr. 1981. *Gallionella* from metalimnion in an eutrophic lake: morphology and x-ray energy-dispersive microanalysis of apical cells and stalks. Can. J. Microbiol. *29:* 303–308.

Hemphill, H.E. and S.A. Zahler. 1968. Nutrition of *Myxococcus xanthus* FBa and some of its auxotrophic mutants. J. Bacteriol. *95:* 1011–1017.

Henderson, E., M. Oakes, M.W. Clark, J.A. Lake, A.T. Matheson and W. Zillig. 1984. A new ribosome structure. Science *225:* 510–512.

Henderson, E., B.K. Pierson and J.A. Lake. 1983. *Chloroflexus aurantiacus* has 30s ribosomal subunits of the eubacterial type. J. Bacteriol. *155:* 900–902.

Henis, Y. and B. Kletter. 1963. The effect of some antimicrobial agents on *Myxococcus* species. Can. J. Microbiol. *9:* 646–648.

Henrichs, S.M. 1980. Biogeochemistry of dissolved free amino acids in marine sediments. Ph.D. dissertation, Massachusetts Institute of Technology and Woods Hole Oceanographic Institute.

Henrichsen, J. 1975. On twitching motility and its mechanism. Acta Pathol. Microbiol. Scand. Sect. B *83:* 187–190.

Henrici, A.T. and D.E. Johnson. 1935. Studies on freshwater bacteria. II. Stalked bacteria, a new order of schizomycetes. J. Bacteriol. *30:* 61–93.

Hensel, G. and H.G. Trüper. 1976. Cysteine and *S*-sulfocysteine biosynthesis in phototrophic bacteria. Arch. Microbiol. *109:* 101–103.

Hensel, G. and H.G. Trüper. 1983. *O*-acetylserine sulfhydrylase and *S*-sulfocysteine synthase activities of *Rhodospirillum tenue*. Arch. Microbiol. *134:* 227–232.

Herbert, R.A., E. Siefert and N. Pfennig. 1978. Nitrogen assimilation in *Rhodopseudomonas acidophila*. Arch. Microbiol. *119:* 1–5.

Herdman, M. 1982. Evolution and genetic properties of cyanobacterial genomes. *In* Carr and Whitton (Editors), The Biology of Cyanobacteria. Blackwell, Oxford, and University of California Press, Berkeley, pp. 263–305.

Herdman, M., M. Janvier, R. Rippka and R.Y. Stanier. 1979b. Genome size of cyanobacteria. J. Gen. Microbiol. *111:* 73–85.

Herdman, M., M. Janvier, J.B. Waterbury, R. Rippka and R.Y. Stanier. 1979a. Deoxyribonucleic acid base composition of cyanobacteria. J. Gen. Microbiol. *111:* 63–71.

Herdman, M. and R.Y. Stanier. 1977. The cyanelle: chloroplast or endosymbiotic prokaryote. FEMS Microbiol. Lett. *1:* 7–12.

Herman, L.G. 1978. The slow-growing pigmented water bacteria: problems and sources. Adv. Appl. Microbiol. *23:* 155–171.

Herman, L.G. 1981. The slow growing Gram-negative pigmented water bacteria. *In* Reichenbach and Weeks (Editors), The *Flavobacterium-Cytophaga* Group. Verlag Chemie, Weinheim, F.R.G., pp. 169–178.

Hernández-Muñiz, W. and E. Stevens, Jr. 1987. Characterization of the motile hormogonia of *Mastigocladus laminosus*. J. Bacteriol. *169:* 218–223.

Heynig, H. 1961. Zur Kenntnis des Planktons mitteldeutscher Gewässer. Arch. Protistenk. *105:* 407–416.

Hikida, M., H. Wakabayashi, S. Egusa and K. Masumura. 1979. *Flexibacter* sp., a gliding bacterium pathogenic to some marine fishes in Japan. Bull. Jpn. Soc. Sci. Fish. *45:* 421–428.

Hilpert, R., J. Winter, W. Hammes and O. Kandler. 1981. The sensitivity of archaebacteria to antibiotics. Zentralbl. Bakteriol. Mikrobiol. Hyg. I Abt. Orig. *C2:* 11–20.

Hindák, F. 1985. Morphology of trichomes in *Spirulina fusiformis* Voronichin from Lake Bogoria, Kenya. Arch. Hydrobiol. Suppl. *71:* 201–218.

Hinze, G. 1903. *Thiophysa volutans*, ein neues Schwefelbakterium. Ber. Btsch. Bot. Ges. *21:* 309–316.

Hinze, G. 1913. Beiträge zur Kenntnis der farblosen Schwefelbakterien. Ber. Dtsch. Bot. Ges. *31:* 189–202.

Hinze, H. 1901. Ueber den Bau der Zellen von *Beggiatoa mirabilis* Cohn. Ber. Dtsch. Bot. Ges. *19:* 369–374.

Hippe, H. 1984. Maintenance of methanogenic bacteria. *In* Kirsop and Snell (Editors), Maintenance of Microorganisms. Academic Press, New York, pp. 69–81.

Hippe, H., D. Caspari, K. Fiebig and G. Gottschalk. 1979. Utilization of trimethylamine and other *N*-methyl compounds for growth and methane formation by *Methanosarcina barkeri*. Proc. Natl. Acad. Sci. U.S.A. *76:* 494–498.

Hirosawa, T. and C.P. Wolk. 1979a. Factors controlling the formation of akinetes adjacent to heterocysts in the cyanobacterium *Cylindrospermum licheniforme* Kütz. J. Gen. Microbiol. *114:* 423–432.

Hirosawa, T. and C.P. Wolk. 1979b. Isolation and characterization of a substance which stimulates the formation of akinetes in the cyanobacterium *Cylindrospermum licheniforme* Kütz. J. Gen. Microbiol. *114:* 433–441.

Hirsch, H.-J. 1977. Bacteriocins from *Myxococcus fulvus* (*Myxobacterales*). Arch. Microbiol. *115:* 45–49.

Hirsch, I. 1980. Beiträge zur Taxonomie der *Cytophagales* auf Grund morphologischer und stoffwechselphysiologischer Eigenschaften. Doctor's thesis, Technical University of Braunschweig, F.R.G., 142 pp.

Hirsch, I. and H. Reichenbach. 1981. The *Cytophaga*-like bacteria: a search for key characters. *In* Reichenbach and Weeks (Editors), The *Flavobacterium-Cytophaga* Group. Verlag Chemie, Weinheim, F.R.G., pp. 145–151.

Hirsch, P. 1968. Biology of budding bacteria. IV. Epicellular deposition of iron by aquatic budding bacteria. Arch. Mikrobiol. *60:* 201–216.

Hirsch, P. 1970. Budding, nitrifying bacteria: the nomenclatural status of *Nitromicrobium germinans* Stutzer and Hartleb 1899 and *Nitrobacter*. Int. J. Syst. Bacteriol. *20:* 317–320.

Hirsch, P. 1972. Two identical genera of budding and stalked bacteria: *Planctomyces* Gimesi 1924 and *Blastocaulis* Henrici and Johnson 1935. Int. J. Syst. Bacteriol. *22:* 107–111.

Hirsch, P. 1973. Fine structure of *Thiopedia* spp. *In* Drews (Editor), Abstracts of symposium on prokaryotic photosynthetic organisms, Freiburg, pp. 184–185.

Hirsch, P. 1974a. Budding bacteria. Annu. Rev. Microbiol. *28:* 391–444.

Hirsch, P. 1974b. Genus *Hyphomicrobium* Stutzer and Hartleb 1898, 76. *In* Buchanan and Gibbons (Editors), Bergey's Manual of Determinative Bacteriology, 8th Ed. The Williams and Wilkins Co., Baltimore, pp. 148–150.

Hirsch, P. 1980. Distribution and pure culture studies of morphologically distinct Solar Lake microorganisms. *In* Nissenbaum (Editor), Hypersaline Brines and Evaporitic Environments. Elsevier Science Publishers, Amsterdam, pp. 41–60.

Hirsch, P. 1981a. The genus *Blastobacter*. *In* Starr, Stolp, Trüper, Balows and Schlegel (Editors), The Prokaryotes. A Handbook on Habitats, Isolation, and

Identification of Bacteria. Springer-Verlag, Berlin, pp. 493–495.

Hirsch, P. 1981a. The genus *Toxothrix*. *In* Starr, Stolp, Trüper, Balows and Schlegel (Editors), The Prokaryotes. A Handbook on Habitats, Isolation, and Identification of Bacteria. Springer-Verlag, Berlin, pp. 409–411.

Hirsch, P. 1981b. The genus *Nevskia*. *In* Starr, Stolp, Trüper, Balows and Schlegel (Editors), The Prokaryotes. A Handbook on Habitats, Isolation, and Identification of Bacteria. Springer-Verlag, Berlin, pp. 520–523.

Hirsch, P. 1981c. The family *Pelonemataceae*. *In* Starr, Stolp, Trüper, Balows and Schlegel (Editors), The Prokaryotes. A Handbook on Habitats, Isolation, and Identification of Bacteria. Springer-Verlag, Berlin, pp. 412–421.

Hirsch, P. 1984. Microcolony formation and consortia. *In* Marshall (Editor), Microbial Adhesion and Aggregation. Dahlem Konferenzen. Springer-Verlag, Berlin, pp. 373–393.

Hirsch, P. and S.F. Conti. 1964a. Biology of budding bacteria. I. Enrichment, isolation and morphology of *Hyphomicrobium* spp. Arch. Mikrobiol. *48:* 339–357.

Hirsch, P. and S.F. Conti. 1964b. Biology of budding bacteria. II. Growth and nutrition of *Hyphomicrobium* spp. Arch. Mikrobiol. *48:* 358–367.

Hirsch, P. and S.F. Conti. 1965. Enrichment and isolation of stalked and budding bacteria (*Hyphomicrobium, Rhodomicrobium, Caulobacter*). Sympos. Anreicherungskultur und Mutantenauslese, Göttingen. Zentralbl. Bakteriol. Parasitenkd. Infektionskr. Hyg. I Suppl. *1:* 253–255.

Hirsch, P. and M. Müller. 1985. *Planctomyces limnophilus* sp. nov., a stalked and budding bacterium from freshwater. Syst. Appl. Microbiol. *6:* 276–280.

Hirsch, P. and M. Müller. 1985. *Blastobacter aggregatus* sp. nov., *Blastobacter capsulatus* sp. nov., and *Blastobacter denitrificans* sp. nov., new budding bacteria from freshwater habitats. Syst. Appl. Microbiol. *6:* 281–286.

Hirsch, P. and M. Müller. 1986. *In* Validation of the publication of new names and new combinations previously effectively published outside the IJSB. List No. 20. Int. J. Syst. Bacteriol. *36:* 354–356.

Hirsch, P. and M. Müller. 1986. Methods and sources for the enrichment and isolation of budding, non-prosthecate bacteria from freshwater. Microb. Ecol. *12:* 331–341.

Hirsch, P., M. Müller and H. Schlesner. 1977. New aquatic budding and prosthecate bacteria and their taxonomic position. *In* Skinner and Shewan (Editors), Aquatic Microbiology. Academic Press, London, pp. 107–133.

Hirsch, P. and S.H. Pankratz. 1970. Study of bacterial populations in natural environments by use of submerged electron microscope grids. Z. Allg. Mikrobiol. *10:* 589–605.

Hirsch, P. and G. Rheinheimer. 1968. Biology of budding bacteria. V. Budding bacteria in aquatic habitats: occurrence, enrichment and isolation. Arch. Mikrobiol. *62:* 289–306.

Hirsch, P. and H. Schlesner. 1981. The genus *Stella*. *In* Starr, Stolp, Trüper, Balows and Schlegel (Editors), The Prokaryotes. A Handbook on Habitats, Isolation, and Identification of Bacteria. Springer-Verlag, Berlin, pp. 461–465.

Hodgkin, J. and D. Kaiser. 1977. Cell-to-cell stimulation of movement in nonmotile mutants of *Myxococcus*. Proc. Natl. Acad. Sci. U.S.A. *74:* 2938–2942.

Hoeniger, J.F.M., H.D. Tauschel and J.L. Stokes. 1973. The fine structure of *Sphaerotilus natans*. Can. J. Microbiol. *19:* 309–313.

Höhnl, G. 1955. Ein Beitrag zur Physiologie der Eisenbakterien. Vom Wasser *22:* 176–193.

Holdeman, L.V., E.P. Cato and W.E.C. Moore (Editors). 1977. Anaerobe Laboratory Manual, 4th Ed. Virginia Polytechnic Institute and State University, Blacksburg.

Holdeman, L.V., I.J. Good and W.E.C. Moore. 1976. Human fecal flora: variation in bacterial composition within individuals and a possible effect of emotional stress. Appl. Environ. Microbiol. *31:* 359–375.

Holdeman, L.V., W.E.C. Moore, P.J. Churn and J.L. Johnson. 1982. *Bacteroides oris* and *Bacteroides buccae*, new species from human periodontitis and other human infections. Int. J. Syst. Bacteriol. *32:* 125–131.

Höllander, R. 1978. The cytochromes of *Thermoplasma acidophilum*. J. Gen. Microbiol. *108:* 165–167.

Hollerbach, M.M., K.K. Kossinskaja and G. Poljansky. 1953. Sinezelenye vodorosli (blue-green algae). *In* Opred. presnov. vodoroslei S.S.S.R., 2, Akad. Nauk, Moscow, pp. 1–652.

Hollocher, T.C. 1984. Source of the oxygen atoms of nitrate in the oxidation by nitrite by *Nitrobacter agilis* and evidence against a P-O-N anhydride mechanism in oxidative phosphorylation. Arch. Biochem. Biophys. *233:* 721–727.

Hollocher, T.C., S. Kumar and D.J.D. Nicholas. 1982. Respiration dependent proton translocation in *Nitrosomonas europaea* and its apparent absence in *Nitrobacter agilis* during inorganic oxidations. J. Bacteriol. *149:* 1013–1020.

Hollocher, T.C., M.E. Tate and D.J.D. Nicholas. 1981. Oxidation of ammonia by *Nitrosomonas europaea*. Definitive ^{18}O-tracer evidence that hydroxylamine formation involves a monoxygenase. J. Biol. Chem. *256:* 10834–10836.

Holmes, B. and R.J. Owen. 1979. Proposal that *Flavobacterium breve* be substituted as the type species of the genus in place of *Flavobacterium aquatile* and emended description of the genus *Flavobacterium*: status of the named species of *Flavobacterium*. Int. J. Syst. Bacteriol. *29:* 416–426.

Holmes, N.T.H. and B.A. Whitton. 1981. Phytobenthos of the River Tees and its tributaries. Freshwater Biol. *11:* 139–168.

Holmgren, P.R., H.P. Hostetter and V.E. Scholes. 1971. Ultrastructural observation on the crosswalls in the blue-green alga *Spirulina major*. J. Phycol. *7:* 309–311.

Holst, O., U. Hunger, E. Gerstner and J. Weckesser. 1981. Lipophilic lipopoly-saccharide (O-antigen) in *Rhodomicrobium vannielii* ATCC 17100. FEMS Microbiol. Lett. *10:* 165–168.

Holt, J.G. and R.A. Lewin. 1968. *Herpetosiphon aurantiacus* gen. et sp. n., a new filamentous gliding organism. J. Bacteriol. *95:* 2407–2408.

Holt, S.C., J. Doundowlakis and B.J. Takacs. 1979a. Phospholipid composition of gliding bacteria: oral isolates of *Capnocytophaga* compared with *Sporocytophaga*. Infect. Immun. *26:* 305–310.

Holt, S.C. and M.R. Edwards. 1972. Fine structure of the thermophilic blue-green alga *Synechococcus lividus* Copeland. A study of frozen-fractured-etched cells. Can. J. Microbiol. *18:* 175–181.

Holt, S.C., G. Forcier and B.J. Takacs. 1979b. Fatty acid composition of gliding bacteria: Oral isolates of *Capnocytophaga* compared with *Sporocytophaga*. Infect. Immun. *26:* 298–304.

Holt, S.C., E.R. Leadbetter and S.S. Socransky. 1979c. *Capnocytophaga*: new genus of gram-negative gliding bacteria. II. Morphology and ultrastructure. Arch. Microbiol. *122:* 17–27.

Hook, L.A. 1977. Distribution of myxobacters in aquatic habitats of an alkaline bog. Appl. Environ. Microbiol. *34:* 333–335.

Hook, L.A., J.M. Larkin and E.R. Brockman. 1980. Isolation, characterization, and emendation of description of *Angiococcus disciformis* (Thaxter 1904) Jahn 1924 and proposal of a neotype strain. Int. J. Syst. Bacteriol. *30:* 135–142.

Hooper, A.B. 1968. A nitrite-reducing enzyme from *Nitrosomonas europaea*. Preliminary characterization with hydroxylamine as electron donor. Biochim. Biophys. Acta *162:* 49–65.

Hooper, A.B. 1969. Biochemical basis of obligate autotrophy in *Nitrosomonas europaea*. J. Bacteriol. *97:* 776–779.

Hooper, A.B. 1984. Ammonia oxidation and energy transduction in the nitrifying bacteria. *In* Strohl and Tuovinen (Editors), Microbial Chemoautotrophy. Ohio State University Press, Columbus, pp. 133–167.

Hooper, A.B. and A.A. Dispirito. 1985. In bacteria which grow on simple reductants generation of a proton gradient involves extracytoplasmic oxidation of substrate. Microbiol. Rev. *49:* 140–157.

Hooper, A.B., R.H. Erickson and K.R. Terry. 1972. Electron transport systems in *Nitrosomonas*: isolation of a membrane-envelope fraction. J. Bacteriol. *110:* 430–438.

Hooper, A.B., J. Hansen and R. Bell. 1967. Characterization of glutamate dehydrogenase from the ammonia-oxidizing chemoautotroph *Nitrosomonas europaea*. J. Biol. Chem. *242:* 288–296.

Hooper, A.B., P.C. Maxwell and K.R. Terry. 1978. Hydroxylamine oxidoreductase from *Nitrosomonas*: absorption spectra and content of heme and metal. Biochemistry *17:* 2984–2989.

Hooper, A.B. and K.R. Terry. 1973. Specific inhibitors of ammonia oxidation in *Nitrosomonas*. J. Bacteriol. *115:* 480–485.

Hooper, A.B. and K.R. Terry. 1974. Photoinactivation of ammonia oxidation in *Nitrosomonas*. J. Bacteriol. *119:* 899–906.

Hooper, A.B. and K.R. Terry. 1977. Hydroxylamine oxidoreductase from *Nitrosomonas*: inactivation by hydrogen-peroxide. Biochemistry *16:* 455–459.

Hooper, A.B. and K.R. Terry. 1979. Hydroxylamine oxidoreductase of *Nitrosomonas* production of nitric oxide from hydroxylamine. Biochim. Biophys. Acta *571:* 12–20.

Hooper, A.B., V.M. Tran and C. Balny. 1984. Kinetics of reduction by substrate or dithionite and heme-heme electron transfer in the multiheme hydroxylamine oxidoreductase. Eur. J. Biochem. *141:* 565–571.

Hori, H. and S. Osawa. 1979. Evolutionary change in 5S rRNA secondary structure and a phylogenetic tree of 54 5S RNA species. Proc. Natl. Acad. Sci. U.S.A. *76:* 381–385.

Hortobágyi, T. 1965. Uj Planctomyces fajok. (Neue Planctomyces-Arten.) (Hungarian, with German resume.) Bot. Közl. *52:* 111–115.

Hortobágyi, T. 1968. Planctomyces from Vietnam. Acta Phytopathol. Acad. Sci. Hung. *3:* 271–273.

Hortobágyi, T. 1980. Aquatic bacteria and fungi in Danube River and in the water producing systems of the Budapest waterworks. Acta Microbiol. Acad. Sci. Hung. *27:* 259–268.

Hortobágyi, T. and L. Hajdú. 1984. A critical survey of *Planctomyces* research. Acta Bot. Hung. *30:* 3–9.

Houwink, A.L. 1955. *Caulobacter*. Its morphogenesis, taxonomy and parasitism. Antonie van Leeuwenhoek J. Microbiol. Serol. *21:* 49–64.

Howard, K.S., B.J. Hales and M.D. Socolofsky. 1983. Nitrogen fixation and ammonia switch-off in the photosynthetic bacterium *Rhodopseudomonas viridis*. J. Bacteriol. *155:* 107–112.

Hoyer, B.H., B.J. McCarthy and E.T. Bolton. 1964. A molecular approach in the systematics of higher organisms. Science (Washington) *144:* 959–967.

Hsu, S.C. and J.L. Lockwood. 1975. Powdered chitin agar as a selective medium for enumeration of actinomycetes in water and soil. Appl. Microbiol. *29:* 422–426.

Hsung, J.C. and A. Haug. 1975. Intracellular pH of *Thermoplasma acidophila*. Biochim. Biophys. Acta *389:* 477–482.

Hu, H.-L., J.E. Peterson and E.R. Brockman. 1985. Stalked sporangia of *Polyangium rugiseptum*. Int. J. Syst. Bacteriol. *35:* 362–363.

Huang, T.C. and T.J. Chow. 1986. New type of N₂-fixing cyanobacterium (blue-green alga). FEMS Microbiol. Lett. *36:* 109–110.

Huber, G., H. Huber and K.O. Stetter. 1986. Isolation and characterization of new metal-mobilizing bacteria. Biotechnol. Bioeng. Symp. No. *16:* 239–251.

Huber, H., M. Thomm, H. König, G. Thies and K.O. Stetter. 1982. *Methanococcus thermolithotrophicus*, a novel thermophilic lithotrophic methanogen. Arch. Microbiol. *132:* 47–50.

Huber, R., G. Huber, A. Segerer, J. Seger and K.O. Stetter. 1987. Aerobic and anaerobic extremely thermophilic autotrophs. *In* Van Verseveld and Duine (Editors), Microbial Growth on C₁ Compounds. Martinus Nijhoff Publisher, Dordrecht, pp. 44–51.

Huber-Pestalozzi, G. 1938. Das Phytoplankton des Süsswassers. *In* Thienemann (Editor), Binnengewässer. Vol. 16, Part 1, pp. 1–342.

Huet, J., R. Schnabel, A. Sentenac and W. Zillig. 1983. Archaebacteria and eukaryotes possess DNA-dependent RNA polymerases of a common type. EMBO J. *2:* 1291–1294.

Hugh, R. and E. Leifson. 1953. The taxonomic significance of fermentative versus oxidative metabolism of carbohydrates by various gram-negative bacteria. J. Bacteriol. *66:* 24–26.

Hughes, E.O., P.R. Gorham and A. Zehnder. 1958. Toxicity of a unialgal culture of *Microcystis aeruginosa*. Can. J. Microbiol. *4:* 225–236.

Hui, I. and P.P. Dennis. 1985. Characterisation of rRNA gene clusters in *Halobacterium cutirubrum*. J. Biol. Chem. *260:* 899–906.

Hulshoff Pol, L.W., W.J. de Zeeuw, C.T.M. Velzeboer and G. Lettinga. 1983. Granulation in UASB-reactors. Water Sci. Technol. *15:* 291–304.

Humm, H.J. 1946. Marine agar-digesting bacteria of the south Atlantic coast. Duke Univ. Mar. Stat. Bull. *3:* 44–75.

Humphrey, B.A., M.R. Dickson and K.C. Marshall. 1979. Physicochemical and in situ observations on the adhesion of gliding bacteria to surfaces. Arch. Microbiol. *120:* 231–238.

Humphrey, B.A. and K.C. Marshall. 1980. Fragmentation of some gliding bacteria during the growth cycle. J. Appl. Bacteriol. *49:* 281–289.

Hungate, R.E. 1950. The anaerobic mesophilic cellulolytic bacteria. Bacteriol. Rev. *14:* 1–49.

Hungate, R.E. 1969. A roll tube method for cultivation of strict anaerobes. Methods Microbiol. *3B:* 117–132.

Hunter, M.I.S., T.L. Olawaye and D.A. Saynor. 1981. The effect of temperature on the growth and lipid composition of the extremely halophilic coccus *Sarcina marina*. Antonie van Leeuwenhoek J. Microbiol. Serol. *47:* 25–40.

Huser, B.A., K. Wuhrmann and A.J.B. Zehnder. 1982. *Methanothrix soehngenii* gen. nov. sp. nov., a new acetotrophic nonhydrogen-oxidizing methane bacterium. Arch. Microbiol. *132:* 1–9.

Huser, B.A., K. Wuhrmann and A.J.B. Zehnder. 1983. *In* Validation of the publication of new names and new combinations previously effectively published outside the IJSB. List No. 10. Int. J. Syst. Bacteriol. *33:* 438–440.

Hutchinson, H.B. and J. Clayton. 1919. On the decomposition of cellulose by an aerobic organism (*Spirochaeta cytophaga*, n. sp.). J. Agric. Sci. *9:* 143–173.

Hutchinson, M., K.I. Johnstone and D. White. 1969. Taxonomy of the genus *Thiobacillus*: the outcome of numerical taxonomy applied to the group as a whole. J. Gen. Microbiol. *57:* 397–410.

Hyman, M.R. and P.M. Wood. 1983. Methane oxidation by *Nitrosomonas europaea*. Biochem. J. *212:* 31–37.

Hyman, M.R. and P.M. Wood. 1984a. Ethylene oxidation by *Nitrosomonas europaea*. Arch. Microbiol. *137:* 155–158.

Hyman, M.R. and P.M. Wood. 1984b. Bromocarbon oxidation by *Nitrosomonas europaea*. *In* Crawford and Hanson (Editors), Microbial Growth on C₁ Compounds. American Society for Microbiology, Washington, D.C., pp. 49–52.

Hynes, R.K. and R. Knowles. 1978. Inhibition by acetylene of ammonia oxidation in *Nitrosomonas europaea*. FEMS Microbiol. Lett. *4:* 319–321.

Hynes, R.K. and R. Knowles. 1982. Effect of ethylene on autotrophic and heterotrophic nitrification. Can. J. Microbiol. *28:* 334–340.

Ida, S. and M. Alexander. 1965. Permeability of *Nitrobacter agilis* to organic compounds. J. Bacteriol. *90:* 151–156.

Iizuka, H. and H. Ito. 1971. Taxonomic studies on a radio-resistant *Pseudomonas*. Part XII. Studies on the microorganisms of cereal grain. Agric. Biol. Chem. *35:* 1566–1571.

Imhoff, J.F. 1976. Phototrophe Bakterien salzhaltiger Standorte: Ökologische und taxonomische Aspekte. Diploma thesis, University of Bonn, F.R.G.

Imhoff, J.F. 1981. Response of photosynthetic bacteria to mineral nutrients. *In* Mitsui and Black (Editors), CRC Handbook of Biosolar Resources. CRC Press, Boca Raton, Florida, pp. 135–146.

Imhoff, J.F. 1982. Taxonomic and phylogenetic implications of lipid and quinone compositions in photosynthetic microorganisms. *In* Wintermans and Kuiper (Editors), Biochemistry and Metabolism of Plant Lipids. Elsevier Biomedical Press, Amsterdam and New York, pp. 541–544.

Imhoff, J.F. 1982. Occurrence and evolutionary significance of two sulfate assimilation pathways in the *Rhodospirillaceae*. Arch. Microbiol. *132:* 197–203.

Imhoff, J.F. 1983. *Rhodopseudomonas marina* sp. nov., a new marine phototrophic purple bacterium. Syst. Appl. Microbiol. *4:* 512–521.

Imhoff, J.F. 1984a. Reassignment of the genus *Ectothiorhodospira* Pelsh 1936 to a new family, *Ectothiorhodospiraceae* fam. nov., and emended description of the *Chromatiaceae* Bavendamm 1924. Int. J. Syst. Bacteriol. *34:* 338–339.

Imhoff, J.F. 1984b. Quinones of phototrophic purple bacteria. FEMS Microbiol. Lett. *25:* 85–89.

Imhoff, J.F. 1984c. *In* Validation of the publication of new names and new combinations previously effectively published outside the IJSB. List No. 14. Int. J. Syst. Bacteriol. *34:* 270.

Imhoff, J.F., D.J. Kushner, S.C. Kushwaha and M. Kates. 1982a. Polar lipids in phototrophic bacteria of the *Rhodospirillaceae* and *Chromatiaceae* families. J.

Bacteriol. *150:* 1192–1201.

Imhoff, J.F., H.G. Sahl, G.S.H. Soliman and H.G. Trüper. 1979. The Wadi Natrun: chemical composition and microbial mass developments in alkaline brines of eutrophic desert lakes. Geomicrobiol. J. *1:* 219–234.

Imhoff, J.F., J. Then, F. Hashwa and H.G. Trüper. 1981. Sulfate assimilation in *Rhodopseudomonas globiformis.* Arch. Microbiol. *130:* 234–237.

Imhoff, J.F., B.J. Tindall, W.D. Grant and H.G. Trüper. 1981. *Ectothiorhodospira vacuolata* sp. nov., a new phototrophic bacterium from soda lakes. Arch. Microbiol. *130:* 238–242.

Imhoff, J.F., B.J. Tindall, W.D. Grant and H.G. Trüper. 1982b. *In* Validation of the publication of new names and new combinations previously effectively published outside the IJSB. List No. 8. Int. J. Syst. Bacteriol. *32:* 266.

Imhoff, J.F. and H.G. Trüper. 1977. *Ectothiorhodospira halochloris* sp. nov., a new extremely halophilic phototrophic bacterium containing bacteriochlorophyll *b.* Arch. Microbiol. *114:* 115–121.

Imhoff, J. and H.G. Trüper. 1980a. *Chromatium purpuratum,* sp. nov., a new species of the *Chromatiaceae.* Zentralbl. Bakteriol. Parasitenkd. Infektionskr. Hyg. Abt. I Orig. Reihe C *1:* 61–69.

Imhoff, J. and H.G. Trüper. 1980b. *In* Validation of the publication of new names and new combinations previously effectively published outside the IJSB. List No. 4. Int. J. Syst. Bacteriol. *30:* 601.

Imhoff, J.F. and H.G. Trüper. 1981. *Ectothiorhodospira abdelmalekii* sp. nov., a new halophilic and alkaliphilic phototrophic bacterium. Zentralbl. Bakteriol. Mikrobiol. Hyg. I. Abt. Orig. *C2:* 228–234.

Imhoff, J.F., H.G. Trüper and N. Pfennig. 1984. Rearrangement of the species and genera of the phototrophic "purple nonsulfur bacteria." Int. J. Syst. Bacteriol. *34:* 340–343.

Imhoff, J.F. and H.G. Trüper. 1982. *In* Validation of the publication of new names and new combinations previously effectively published outside the IJSB. List No. 8. Int. J. Syst. Bacteriol. *32:* 266.

Imshenetski, A.A. (spelled Imschenezki). 1959. Mikrobiologie der Cellulose. Akademie-Verlag, Berlin, D.D.R., 466 pp.

Imshenetski, A.A. and L. Solntseva. 1936. On aerobic cellulose-decomposing bacteria. Izv. Akad. Nauk S.S.S.R. Ser. Biol. *6:* 1115–1172 (in Russian with English summary).

Imshenetski, A. and L. Solntseva. 1937. On cellulose decomposing myxobacteria. Mikrobiologiya *6:* 3–15.

Imshenetski, A.A. and L. Solntseva. 1945. On the imperfect forms of myxobacteria. Mikrobiologiya *14:* 220–229 (in Russian with English summary).

Inoue, K. and K. Komagata. 1976. Taxonomic study on obligately psychrophilic bacteria isolated from Antarctica. J. Gen. Appl. Microbiol. *22:* 165–176.

Inouye, S., D. White and M. Inouye. 1980. Development of *Stigmatella aurantiaca:* Effects of light and gene expression. J. Bacteriol. *141:* 1360–1365.

International Code of Nomenclature of Bacteria. 1975. American Society for Microbiology, Washington, D.C.

International Committee on Systematic Bacteriology Subcommittee on the Taxonomy of *Mollicutes.* 1979. Proposal of minimal standards for descriptions of new species of the class *Mollicutes.* Int. J. Syst. Bacteriol. *29:* 172–180.

Irgens, R.L. 1977. *Meniscus,* a new genus of aerotolerant, gas vacuolated bacteria. Int. J. Syst. Bacteriol. *27:* 38–43.

Irschik, H., K. Gerth, T. Kemmer, H. Steinmite and H. Reichenbach. 1983. The myxovalargins, new peptide antibiotic from *Myxococcus fulvus (Myxobacterales).* J. Antibiot. (Tokyo) *36:* 6–12.

Irschik, H. and H. Reichenbach. 1985. Intracellular location of flexirubins in *Flexibacter elegans (Cytophagales).* Biochim. Biophys. Acta *510:* 1–10.

Ishiguro, E.E. and R.S. Wolfe. 1970. Control of morphogenesis in *Geodermatophilus:* ultrastructural studies. J. Bacteriol. *104:* 566–580.

Ivanov, M.V. and J.R. Freney (Editors). 1983. The global biogeochemical sulphur cycle. SCOPE Report No. 19. John Wiley and Sons, New York.

Izumi, Y., M. Takizawa, Y. Tani and H. Yamada. 1982. An obligate methylotrophic *Hyphomicrobium* strain. Identification, growth characteristics and cell composition. Jpn. J. Ferment. Technol. *60:* 371–375.

Izumi, Y., M. Takizawa, Y. Tani and H. Yamada. 1983. *In* Validation of the publication of new names and new combinations previously effectively pubished outside the IJSB. Int. J. Syst. Bacteriol. *33:* 438–440.

Jackman, P.J.H. 1985. Bacterial taxonomy based on electrophoretic whole-cell protein patterns. *In* Goodfellow and Minnikin (Editors), Chemical Methods in Bacterial Systematics. Academic Press, London, New York, pp. 115–129.

Jackson, J.F., D.J.W. Moriarty and D.J.D. Nicholas. 1968. Deoxyribonucleic acid base composition and taxonomy of thiobacilli and some nitrifying bacteria. J. Gen. Microbiol. *53:* 53–60.

Jackson, R.L. and G.R. Matsueda. 1970. Myxobacter AL-1 protease. Methods Enzymol. *19:* 591–599.

Jackson, R.L. and R.S. Wolfe. 1968. Composition, properties and substrate specificities of Myxobacter AL-1 protease. J. Biol. Chem. *243:* 879–888.

Jahn, E. 1911. *Myxobacteriales.* Kryptogamenflora der Mark Brandenburg *5:* 187–206.

Jahn, E. 1924. Beiträge zur botanischen Protistologie. I. Die Polyangiden. Verlag Gebruder Borntraeger, Leipzig, pp. 1–107.

Jahnke, L.S., C. Lyman and A.B. Hooper. 1984. Carbonic anhydrase carbon dioxide levels and growth of *Nitrosomonas.* Arch. Microbiol. *140:* 291–293.

Janekovic, D., S. Wunderl, I. Holz, W. Zillig, A. Gierl and H. Neumann. 1983. TTV1, TTV2 and TTV3, a family of viruses of the extremely thermophilic, anaerobic, sulfur reducing archaebacterium *Thermoproteus tenax.* Mol. Gen.

Genet. *192:* 39–45.

Janke, A. 1924. Allgemeine Technische Mikrobiologie. I. Teil: Die Mikroorganismen. T. Steinkopf, Dresden und Leipzig.

Jannasch, H.W. 1957. Die bakterielle Rotfärbung der Salzseen des Wadi Natrun (Ägypten). Arch. Hydrobiol. *53:* 425–433.

Jannasch, H.W. 1984. Microbial Processes at Deep Sea Hydrothermal Vents. *In* Rona, Bostrom, Laubier and Smith (Editors), Hydrothermal Processes at Seafloor Spreading Centers. Plenum Publishing, New York, pp. 677–709.

Jannasch, H.W. and C.O. Wirsen. 1981. Morphological survey of microbial mats near deep-sea thermal vents. Appl. Environ. Microbiol. *41:* 528–538.

Jannasch, H.W., C.O. Wirsen, D.C. Nelson and L.A. Robertson. 1985. *Thiomicrospira crunogena* sp. nov., a colorless sulfur bacterium from a deep-sea hydrothermal vent. Int. J. Syst. Bacteriol. *35:* 422–424.

Jansen, K., E. Stupperich and G. Fuchs. 1982. Carbohydrate synthesis from acetyl-CoA in the autotroph *Methanobacterium thermoautotrophicum.* Arch. Microbiol. *132:* 355–364.

Janssen, G.R., J.W. Wireman and M. Dworkin. 1977. Effect of temperature on the growth of *Myxococcus xanthus.* J. Bacteriol. *130:* 561–562.

Jarsch, M. and A. Böck. 1985. Sequence of the 16s ribosomal RNA gene of *Methanococcus vannielii:* evolutionary implications. Syst. Appl. Microbiol. *6:* 54–59.

Javor, B. 1984. Growth potential of halophilic bacteria isolated from solar salt environments: carbon sources and salt requirements. Appl. Environ. Microbiol. *48:* 352–360.

Javor, B.J. and R.W. Castenholz. 1981. Laminated microbial mats, Laguna Guerrero Negro, Mexico. Geomicrobiol. J. *2:* 237–273.

Javor, B., C. Requadt and W. Stoeckenius. 1982. Box-shaped halophilic bacteria. J. Bacteriol. *151:* 1532–1542.

Jeeji-Bai, N. 1976. Morphological variation of certain blue-green algae in culture: *Scytonema stuposum* (Kütz.) Born. Schweiz. Z. Hydrol. *38:* 55–62.

Jeeji-Bai, N. 1985. Competitive exclusion or morphological transformation? A case study with *Spirulina fusiformis.* Arch. Hydrobiol. Suppl. *71:* 191–199.

Jeeji-Bai, N., E. Hegewald and C.J. Soeder. 1977. Revision and taxonomic analysis of the genus *Anabaenopsis.* Arch. Hydrobiol. Suppl. *51:* 3–24.

Jeeji-Bai, N. and C.V. Seshadri. 1980. On coiling and uncoiling of trichomes in the genus *Spirulina.* Arch. Hydrobiol. Suppl. *60:* 32–47.

Jeffers, E.E. 1964. Myxobacters of a freshwater lake and its environs. I. New and modified culture media found useful in isolation and characterization of freshwater myxobacters. Int. Bull. Bacteriol. Nomencl. Taxon. *14:* 115–136.

Jeffrey, C. 1977. Biological Nomenclature, 2nd Ed. Edward Arnold, London.

Jeffries, L., M.A. Cawthorne, M. Harris, B. Cook and A.T. Diplock. 1969. Menaquinone determination in the taxonomy of *Micrococcaceae.* J. Gen. Microbiol. *54:* 365–380.

Jenkins, C.L., D.A. Kuhn and K.R. Daly. 1977. Fatty acid composition of *Simonsiella* strains. Arch. Microbiol. *113:* 209–213.

Jensen, A., O. Aasmundrud and K.E. Eimhjellen. 1964. Chlorophylls of photosynthetic bacteria. Biochim. Biophys. Acta *88:* 466–479.

Jensen, H.L. 1940. Nitrogen fixation and cellulose decomposition by soil microorganisms. I. Aerobic cellulose-decomposers in association with *Azotobacter.* Proc. Linn. Soc. N.S.W. *65:* 543–556.

Jensen, T.E. 1985. Cell inclusions in the cyanobacteria. Arch. Hydrobiol. Suppl. *71:* 33–73.

Johannson, B.C. and H. Gest. 1976. Inorganic nitrogen assimilation by the photosynthetic bacterium *Rhodopseudomonas capsulata.* J. Bacteriol. *128:* 683–688.

Johnson, A.H. and J.L. Stokes. 1965. Effect of amino acids on growth of *Sphaerotilus discophorus.* Antonie van Leeuwenhoek J. Microbiol. Serol. *31:* 165–174.

Johnson, D.B. 1983. VI Int. Symp. Environ. Biogeochem. Abstract 5.12, p. 50.

Johnson, D.B. and W.I. Kelso. 1983. Detection of heterotrophic contaminants in cultures of *Thiobacillus ferrooxidans* and their elimination by subculturing in media containing copper sulfate. J. Gen. Microbiol. *129:* 2969–2972.

Johnson, D.E. 1932. Some observations on chitin-destroying bacteria. J. Bacteriol. *24:* 335–340.

Johnson, J.L. 1973. Use of nucleic acid homologies in the taxonomy of anaerobic bacteria. Int. J. Syst. Bacteriol. *23:* 308–315.

Johnson, J.L. 1980. Classification of anaerobic bacteria. *In* Proceedings of International Symposium on Anaerobes (Tokyo, Japan, June 22, 1980). Nippon Merck-Banyu Co., Tokyo, p. 19.

Johnson, J.L. 1981. Genetic characterization. *In* Gerhardt et al. (Editors), Manual of Methods for General Bacteriology. American Society for Microbiology, Washington, D.C., pp. 450–472.

Johnson, J.L. and D.A. Ault. 1978. Taxonomy of the *Bacteroides.* II. Correlation of phenotypic characteristics with deoxyribonucleic acid homology groupings for *Bacteroides fragilis* and other saccharolytic *Bacteroides* species. Int. J. Syst. Bacteriol. *28:* 257–265.

Johnson, J.L. and W.S. Chilton. 1966. Galactosamine glycan of *Chondrococcus columnaris.* Science *152:* 1247–1248.

Johnson, J.L. and E.J. Ordal. 1968. Deoxyribonucleic acid homology in bacterial taxonomy: effect of incubation temperature on reaction specificity. J. Bacteriol. *95:* 893–900.

Johnson, P.W., J.M. Sieburth, C.R. Arnold and M.S. Doty. 1971. *Leucothrix mucor* infestation of benthic crustacea, fish eggs, and tropical algae. Limnol. Oceanogr. *16:* 962–969.

Jones, C.A. and D.P. Kelly. 1983. Growth of *Thiobacillus ferrooxidans* on ferrous iron in chemostat culture: influence of product and substrate inhibition. J.

Chem. Technol. Biotechnol. *33B:* 241–261.

Jones, C.W. 1980. Cytochrome patterns in classification and identification including their relevance to the oxidase test. *In* Goodfellow and Board (Editors), Microbiological Classification and Identification. Academic Press, London, New York, pp. 127–138.

Jones, D. 1978. Composition and differentiation of the genus *Streptococcus*. *In* Skinner and Quesnel (Editors), Streptococci. Academic Press, London, New York, pp. 1–49.

Jones, D. and N.R. Krieg. 1984. Bacterial Classification V. Serology and Chemotaxonomy. *In* Krieg and Holt (Editors), Bergey's Manual of Systematic Bacteriology, Vol. 1. The Williams and Wilkins Co., Baltimore, pp. 15–18.

Jones, D. and P.H.A. Sneath. 1970. Genetic transfer and bacterial taxonomy. Bacteriol. Rev. *34:* 40–81.

Jones, D., J. Watkins and S.K. Erickson. 1973. Taxonomically significant colour changes in *Brevibacterium linens* probably associated with a carotenoid-like pigment. J. Gen. Microbiol. *77:* 145–150.

Jones, H.C. and J.M. Schmidt. 1973. Ultrastructural study of crossbands occurring in the stalks of *Caulobacter crescentus*. J. Bacteriol. *116:* 466–470.

Jones, H.E. and P. Hirsch. 1968. Cell wall composition of *Hyphomicrobium* spp. J. Bacteriol. *96:* 1037–1041.

Jones, J.B., B. Bowers and T.C. Stadtman. 1977. *Methanococcus vannielii:* ultrastructure and sensitivity to detergents and antibiotics. J. Bacteriol. *130:* 1357–1363.

Jones, J.B., G.L. Dilworth and T.C. Stadtman. 1979. Occurrence of selenocysteine in the selenium-dependent formate dehydrogenase of *Methanococcus vannielii*. Arch. Biochem. Biophys. *195:* 255–260.

Jones, J.B. and T.C. Stadtman. 1977. *Methanococcus vannielii:* culture and effects of selenium and tungsten on growth. J. Bacteriol. *130:* 1404–1406.

Jones, J.B. and T.C. Stadtman. 1980. Reconstitution of a formate-NADP⁺ oxidoreductase from formate dehydrogenase and a 5-deazaflavin-linked NADP⁺ reductase isolated from *Methanococcus vannielii*. J. Biol. Chem. *255:* 1049–1053.

Jones, J.B. and T.C. Stadtman. 1981. Selenium-dependent and selenium-independent formate dehydrogenases of *Methanococcus vannielii*. J. Biol. Chem. *256:* 656–663.

Jones, J.G. 1981. The population ecology of iron bacteria (genus *Ochrobium*) in a stratified eutrophic lake. J. Gen. Microbiol. *125:* 85–93.

Jones, R.D. and R.Y. Morita. 1983. Methane oxidation by *Nitrosococcus oceanus* and *Nitrosomonas europaea*. Appl. Environ. Microbiol. *45:* 401–410.

Jones, W.J., J.A. Leigh, F. Mayer, C.R. Woese and R.S. Wolfe. 1983c. *Methanococcus jannaschii* sp. nov., an extremely thermophilic methanogen from a submarine hydrothermal vent. Arch. Microbiol. *136:* 254–261.

Jones, W.J., M.J.B. Paynter and R. Gupta. 1983a. Characterization of *Methanococcus maripaludis* sp. nov., a new methanogen isolated from salt marsh sediment. Arch. Microbiol. *135:* 91–97.

Jones, W.J., W.B. Whitman, R.D. Fields and R.S. Wolfe. 1983b. Growth and plating efficiency of methanococci on agar media. Appl. Environ. Microbiol. *46:* 220–226.

Jooste, P.J. 1985. The taxonomy and significance of *Flavobacterium-Cytophaga* strains from dairy sources. Ph.D. thesis, University of the Orange Free State, Bloemfontein, Republic of South Africa, 169 pp.

Jørgensen, B.B. 1978. Distribution of colorless sulfur bacteria (*Beggiatoa* spp.) in a coastal marine sediment. Mar. Biol. *41:* 19–28.

Jørgensen, B.B. 1982. Ecology of the bacteria of the sulphur cycle with special reference to anoxic-oxic interface environments. Philos. Trans. R. Soc. Lond. B *298:* 543–561.

Jørgensen, B.B. and T. Fenchel. 1974. The sulfur cycle of a marine sediment model system. Mar. Biol. *24:* 189–201.

Jørgensen, B.B. and N.P. Revsbech. 1983. Colorless sulfur bacteria, *Beggiatoa* spp. and *Thiovulum* spp., in O_2 and H_2S microgradients. Appl. Environ. Microbiol. *45:* 1261–1270.

Joshi, M.M. and J.P. Hollis. 1976. Rapid enrichment of *Beggiatoa* from soil. J. Appl. Bacteriol. *40:* 223–224.

Judicial Commission. 1986a. Opinion 62. Transfer of the type species of the genus *Methanococcus* to the genus *Methanosarcina* as *Methanosarcina mazei* (Barker 1936) comb. nov. et emend. Mah and Kuhn 1984 and conservation of the genus *Methanococcus* (Approved Lists, 1980) emend. Mah and Kuhn 1984 with *Methanococcus vannielii* (Approved Lists, 1980) as the type species. Int. J. Syst. Bacteriol. *36:* 491.

Judicial Commission. 1986b. Opinion 63. Rejection of the type species *Methanosarcina methanica* (Approved Lists, 1980) and conservation of the genus *Methanosarcina* (Approved Lists, 1980) emend. Mah and Kuhn 1984 with *Methanosarcina barkeri* (Approved Lists, 1980) as the type species. Int. J. Syst. Bacteriol. *36:* 492.

Juez, G., F. Rodriguez-Valera, A. Ventosa and D.J. Kushner. 1986a. *Haloarcula hispanica* sp. nov. and *Haloferax gibbonsii* sp. nov., two new species of extremely halophilic archaebacteria. Syst. Appl. Microbiol. *8:* 75–79.

Juez, G., F. Rodriguez-Valera, A. Ventosa and D.J. Kushner. 1986b. *In* Validation of the publication of new names and combinations previously effectively published outside the IJSB. List No. 22. Int. J. Syst. Bacteriol. *36:* 573–576.

Jungermann, K. and G. Schön. 1974. Pyruvate formate lyase in *Rhodospirillum rubrum* Ha adapted to anaerobic dark conditions. Arch. Microbiol. *99:* 109–116.

Jurgens, U.J. and T. Burger-Wiersma. 1989. Peptidoglycan-polysaccharide complex in the cell wall of the filamentous *Prochlorothrix hollandica* (*Prochlorophyta*). J. Bacteriol., in press.

Justin, P. and D.P. Kelly. 1978. Growth kinetics of *Thiobacillus denitrificans* in anaerobic and aerobic chemostat culture. J. Gen. Microbiol. *107:* 123–130.

Jüttner, F. 1984. Characterization of *Microcystis* strains by alkyl sulfides and β-cyclocitral. Z. Naturforsch. *39:* 867–871.

Kaars Sijpesteijn, A. and G. Fähraeus. 1949. Adaptation of *Sporocytophaga myxococcoides* to sugars. J. Gen. Microbiol. *3:* 224–234.

Kadota, H. 1956. A study on the marine aerobic cellulose-decomposing bacteria. Mem. Coll. Agric. Kyoto Univ. No. *74:* 1–128.

Kaiser, D., C. Manoil and M. Dworkin. 1979. Myxobacteria: cell interactions, genetics and development. Ann. Rev. Microbiol. *33:* 595–639.

Kaiser, G.E. and M.J. Starzyk. 1973. Ultrastructure and cell division of an oral bacterium resembling *Alysiella filiformis*. Can. J. Microbiol. *19:* 325–327.

Kalbe, L., R. Keil and M. Thiele. 1965. Licht- und elektronenmikroskopische Studien an Arten von *Leptothrix*, *Siderocapsa* und *Planctomyces*. Arch. Protistenkd. *108:* 29–40.

Kalchbrenner, C. and M.C. Cooke. 1880. South African fungi. Grevillia *9:* 17–34.

Kallas, T., M. Rebière, R. Rippka and N. Tandeau de Marsac. 1983. The structural *nif* genes of the cyanobacteria *Gloeothece* sp. and *Calothrix* sp. share homology with those of *Anabaena* sp., but the *Gloeothece* genes have different arrangement. J. Bacteriol. *155:* 427–431.

Kamat, N.K. and J.V. Bhat. 1967. Pectin trans-eliminase activity in *Cytophaga*. Curr. Sci. *36:* 486.

Kämpf, C. and N. Pfennig. 1980. Capacity of *Chromatiaceae* for chemotrophic growth. Specific respiration rates of *Thiocystis violacea* and *Chromatium vinosum*. Arch. Microbiol. *127:* 125–135.

Kandler, O. 1981. Archaebakterien und Phylogenie der Organismen. Naturwissenschaften *68:* 183–192.

Kandler, O. 1982. Cell wall structures and their phylogenetic implications. Zentralbl. Bakteriol. Mikrobiol. Hyg. I Abt. Orig. C3: 149–160.

Kandler, O. (Editor). 1982. Archaebacteria. Gustav Fischer Verlag, Stuttgart.

Kandler, O. and H. Hippe. 1977. Lack of peptidoglycan in the cell walls of *Methanosarcina barkeri*. Arch. Microbiol. *113:* 57–60.

Kandler, O. and H. König. 1978. Chemical composition of the peptidoglycan-free cell walls of methanogenic bacteria. Arch. Microbiol. *118:* 141–152.

Kandler, O. and H. König. 1985. Cell envelopes of archaebacteria. *In* Woese and Wolfe (Editors), The Bacteria, Vol. VIII. Academic Press, New York, pp. 413–457.

Kandler, O., H. König, J. Wiegel and D. Claus. 1983. Occurrence of poly-γ-D-glutamic acid and poly-α-L-glutamine in the genera *Xanthobacter*, *Flexithrix*, *Sporosarcina* and *Planococcus*. Syst. Appl. Microbiol. *4:* 34–41.

Kandler, O. and K.-H. Schleifer. 1980. Taxonomy I: Systematics of bacteria. Prog. Bot. *42:* 234–252.

Kandler, O. and W. Zillig (Editors). 1986. Archaebacteria '85. Gustav Fischer Verlag, Stuttgart and New York.

Kann, E. 1972. Zur Systematik und Okologie der Gattung *Chamaesiphon* (*Cyanophyceae*). I. Systematik. Arch. Hydrobiol. Suppl. 41, Algological Studies 7: 117–171.

Kapke, P.A., A.T. Brown and T.T. Lillich. 1980. Carbon dioxide metabolism by *Capnocytophaga ochracea*: identification, characterization, and regulation of a phosphoenolpyruvate carboxykinase. Infect. Immun. *27:* 756–766.

Kaspari, H. 1979. Reductive pyrimidine catabolism in *Rhodopseudomonas capsulata*. Microbiologica *2:* 231–241.

Katayama, Y. and H. Kuraishi. 1978. Characteristics of *Thiobacillus thioparus* and its thiocyanate assimilation. Can. J. Microbiol. *24:* 804–810.

Katayama-Fujimura, Y., Y. Enokizono, T. Kaneko and H. Kuraishi. 1983a. Deoxyribonucleic acid homologies among species of the genus *Thiobacillus*. J. Gen. Appl. Microbiol. *29:* 287–295.

Katayama-Fujimura, Y., I. Kawashima, N. Tsuzaki and H. Kuraishi. 1983b. Reidentification of *Thiobacillus perometabolis* ATCC 27793 and *Thiobacillus* sp. strain A2 with reference to a new species, *Thiobacillus rapidicrescens* sp. nov. Int. J. Syst. Bacteriol. *33:* 532–538.

Katayama-Fujimura, Y., I. Kawashima, N. Tsuzaki and H. Kuraishi. 1984. Physiological characteristics of the facultatively chemolithotrophic *Thiobacillus* species *Thiobacillus delicatus* nom. rev., emend., *Thiobacillus perometabolis*, and *Thiobacillus intermedius*. Int. J. Syst. Bacteriol. *34:* 139–144.

Katayama-Fujimura, Y. and H. Kuraishi. 1980. Characterization of *Thiobacillus novellus* and its thiosulfate oxidation. J. Gen. Appl. Microbiol. *26:* 357–367.

Katayama-Fujimura, Y. and H. Kuraishi. 1983. Emendation of *Thiobacillus perometabolis* London and Rittenberg 1967. Int. J. Syst. Bacteriol. *33:* 650–651.

Katayama-Fujimura, Y., N. Tsuzaki and H. Kuraishi. 1982. Ubiquinone, fatty acid and DNA base composition determination as a guide to the taxonomy of the genus *Thiobacillus*. J. Gen. Microbiol. *128:* 1599–1611.

Kates, M. 1978. The phytanyl ether-linked polar lipids and isoprenoid neutral lipids of extremely halophilic bacteria. Prog. Chem. Fats Other Lipids *15:* 301–342.

Kates, M. 1986. Influence of salt concentration on membrane lipids of halophilic bacteria. FEMS Microbiol. Rev. *39:* 95–101.

Katoh, T. 1963. Nitrate reductase in photosynthetic bacterium, *Rhodospirillum rubrum*. Purification and properties of nitrate reductase in nitrate-adapted cells. Plant Cell Physiol. *4:* 13–28.

Katz, W. and J.L. Strominger. 1967. Structure of the cell wall of *Micrococcus lysodeikticus*. II. Study of the structure of the peptides produced after lysis with the myxobacterium enzyme. Biochemistry 6: 930–937.

Katzenberger, I. and G.A. Kausche. 1957. Über die Einwirkung von Substanzen aus Myxobacterien auf Viren. Naturwissenschaften 44: 44.

Kauffmann, F. 1966. The Bacteriology of the *Enterobacteriaceae*. Munkssgaard, Copenhagen.

Kawasumi, T., Y. Igarashi, T. Kodama and Y. Minoda. 1980. Isolation of strictly thermophilic and obligately autotrophic hydrogen bacteria. Agric. Biol. Chem. 44: 1985–1986.

Kawasumi, T., Y. Igarashi, T. Kodama and Y. Minoda. 1984. *Hydrogenobacter thermophilus* gen. nov., sp. nov., an extremely thermophilic, aerobic, hydrogen-oxidizing bacterium. Int. J. Syst. Bacteriol. 34: 5–10.

Kawata, S., T. Takemura, K. Yokogawa and S. Kotani. 1984. Isolation of bacteriolytic endopeptidase from a strain of *Cytophaga* and its application to preparation of hydrosoluble polysaccharide peptide from *Staphylococcus epidermidis* peptidoglycan. Agric. Biol. Chem. 48: 2253–2263.

Keddie, R.M. and I.J. Bousfield. 1980. Cell wall composition in the classification and identification of coryneform bacteria. *In* Goodfellow and Board (Editors), Microbiological Classification and Identification. Academic Press, London, New York, pp. 167–188.

Keil, F. 1912. Beiträge zur Physiologie der farblosen Schwefelbakterien. Beitr. Biol. Pflanz. 11: 335–372.

Kellenberger, E., A. Ryter and J. Sechaud. 1958. Electron microscope study of DNA-containing plasmids. II. Vegetative and mature phage DNA as compared with normal bacterial nucleoids in different physiological states. J. Biophys. Biochem. Cytol. 4: 671–678.

Kelley, B.C., R.H. Dunstan and D.J.D. Nicholas. 1982. Respiration-dependent nitrogenase activity in the dark in a denitrifying bacterium *Rhodopseudomonas sphaeroides* forma sp. *denitrificans*. FEMS Microbiol. Lett. 13: 253–258.

Kelly, D.P. 1969. Regulation of chemoautotrophic metabolism. Arch. Mikrobiol. 69: 330–342.

Kelly, D.P. 1971. Autotrophy: concepts of lithotrophic bacteria and their organic metabolism. Annu. Rev. Microbiol. 25: 177–210.

Kelly, D.P. and C.A. Jones. 1978. Factors affecting metabolism and ferrous iron oxidation in suspensions and batch cultures of *Thiobacillus ferrooxidans*: relevance to ferric iron leach solution regeneration. *In* Murr, Torma and Brierley (Editors), Metallurgical Applications of Bacterial Leaching and Related Microbiological Phenomena. Academic Press, New York, pp. 19–44.

Kelly, D.P. and J.G. Kuenen. 1984. Ecology of the colourless sulphur bacteria. *In* Codd (Editor), Aspects of Microbial Metabolism and Ecology. Academic Press, New York, pp. 211–240.

Kelly, D.P. and O.H. Tuovinen. 1972. Recommendation that the names *Ferrobacillus ferrooxidans* Leathen and Braley and *Ferrobacillus sulfooxidans* Kinsel be recognized as synonyms of *Thiobacillus ferrooxidans* Temple and Colmer. Int. J. Syst. Bacteriol. 22: 170–172.

Kelly, M.T. and T.D. Brock. 1969a. Molecular heterogeneity of isolates of the marine bacterium *Leucothrix mucor*. J. Bacteriol. 100: 14–21.

Kelly, M.T. and T.D. Brock. 1969b. Physiological ecology of *Leucothrix mucor*. J. Gen. Microbiol. 59: 153–162.

Kenyon, C.N. 1978. Complex lipids and fatty acids of photosynthetic bacteria. *In* Clayton and Sistrom (Editors), The Photosynthetic Bacteria. Plenum Publishing, New York and London, pp. 281–313.

Kenyon, C.N. and A.M. Gray. 1974. Preliminary analysis of lipids and fatty acids of green bacteria and *Chloroflexus aurantiacus*. J. Bacteriol. 120: 131–138.

Kenyon, C.N., R. Rippka and R.Y. Stanier. 1972. Fatty acid composition and physiological properties of some filamentous blue-green algae. Arch. Mikrobiol. 83: 216–236.

Keppen, O.I. and V.M. Gorlenko. 1975. A new species of purple budding bacteria containing bacteriochlorophyll *b*. Mikrobiologiya 44: 258–264.

Keppen, O.I., A.N. Nozhevnikova and V.M. Gorlenko. 1976. Dark metabolism of *Rhodopseudomonas sulfidophila*. Mikrobiologiya 45: 15–19.

Kersters, K. 1985. Numerical methods in the classification of bacteria by protein electrophoresis. *In* Goodfellow, Jones and Priest (Editors), Computer Assisted Bacterial Systematics. Special Publications of the Society for General Microbiology 15. Academic Press, London, New York, pp. 337–368.

Kersters, K. and J. De Ley. 1975. Identification and grouping of bacteria by numerical analysis of their electrophoretic protein patterns. J. Gen. Microbiol. 87: 333–342.

Kersters, K. and J. De Ley. 1980. Classification and identification of bacteria by electrophoresis of their proteins. *In* Goodfellow and Board (Editors), Microbiological Classification and Identification. Society for Applied Bacteriology Symposium Series 8. Academic Press, London, New York, pp. 273–297.

Kessel, M. and Y. Cohen. 1982. Ultrastructure of square bacteria from a brine pool in Southern Sinai. J. Bacteriol. 150: 851–860.

Kessel, M., Y. Cohen and A.E. Walsby. 1985. Structure and physiology of square-shaped and other halophilic bacteria from the Gavish Sabkha. *In* Friedman and Krumbein (Editors), Ecological Studies, Volume 53: Hypersaline Ecosystems. Springer-Verlag, Berlin, pp. 268–287.

Kessel, M. and F. Klink. 1980. Archaebacterial elongation factor is ADP-ribosylated by diphtheria toxin. Nature (London) 287: 250–251.

Kessel, M. and F. Klink. 1982. Identification and comparison of eighteen archaebacteria by means of the diphtheria toxin reaction. Zentralbl. Bakteriol. Mikrobiol. Hyg. I Abt. Orig. C3: 140–148.

Kessler, C., B.J. Bolton and M.J. Comer. 1986. Screening for novel type II restriction endonucleases. Symposium on Transcriptional Control Mechanisms. 15th Annual Meeting of UCLA Symposia on Molecular and Cellular Biology. J. Cell. Biochem. Suppl. 1986: 101.

Ketchum, P.A. and C.L. Sevilla. 1973. In vitro formation of nitrate reductase using extracts of the nitrate reductase mutant of *Neurospora crassa*, nit-1, and *Rhodospirillum rubrum*. J. Bacteriol. 116: 600–609.

Khakmun, T. 1967. Iron- and manganese-oxidizing microorganisms in soils of South Sakhalin (in Russian). Mikrobiologiya 36: 337–344.

Kieft, T.L. and D.E. Caldwell. 1984a. Weathering of calcite, pyrite, and sulfur by *Thermothrix thiopara* in a thermal spring. Geomicrobiol. J. 3: 201–216.

Kieft, T.L. and D.E. Caldwell. 1984b. Chemostat and in situ colonization kinetics of *Thermothrix thiopara* on calcite and pyrite surfaces. Geomicrobiol. J. 3: 217–229.

Kiene, R.P., R.S. Oremland, A. Catena, L.G. Miller and D.G. Capone. 1986. Metabolism of reduced methylated sulfur compounds in anaerobic sediments and by a pure culture of an estuarine methanogen. Appl. Environ. Microbiol. 52: 1037–1045.

Kiesow, G.A., B.F. Lindsley and J.W. Bless. 1977. Phosphoribulokinase from *Nitrobacter winogradskyi*: activation by reduced nicotinamide adenine dinucleotide and inhibition by pyridoxal phosphate. J. Bacteriol. 130: 20–25.

Kingma-Boltjes, T.Y. 1936. Über *Hyphomicrobium vulgare* Stutzer and Hartleb. Arch. Mikrobiol. 7: 188–205.

Kingsbury, D.T. and E.J. Ordal. 1966. Bacteriophage infecting the myxobacterium *Chondrococcus columnaris*. J. Bacteriol. 91: 1327–1332.

Kinsel, N.A. 1960. New sulfur oxidizing iron bacterium: *Ferrobacillus sulfooxidans* sp. n. J. Bacteriol. 80: 628–632.

Kirchner, O. 1878. Algen. *In* Cohn, Kryptog. Schlesien. 2: 1–284.

Kirchner, O. 1896. Katalog der im Bodensee aufgefundenen Algen und Pilze. *In* Schröter and Kirchner (Editors), Die Vegetation des Bodensees. I. Schrift. der Geschichte des Bodensees. Suppl. 25: 53–122.

Kirchner, O. 1898. *Schizophyceae*. *In* Engler and Prantl (Editors), Die natürlichen Pflanzen familien. W. Engelmann, Leipzig, pp. 45–92.

Kirschvink, J.L. 1983. Biogenic ferrimagnetism: a new biomagnetism. *In* Williamson, Romani, Kaufman and Modena (Editors), Biomagnetism. Plenum Publishing, New York.

Kirsop, B. 1985. The current status of culture collections and their contribution to biotechnology. CRC Crit. Rev. Biotechnol. 2: 287–314.

Kirstein, K.O., E. Bock, D.J. Miller and D.J.D. Nicholas. 1986. Membrane-bound b-type cytochromes in *Nitrobacter*. FEMS Microbiol. Lett. 36: 63–67.

Kisselewa, J.A. 1930. J. Soc. Bot. Russe 15.

Kjems, J., R.A. Garrett and W. Ansorge. 1987. The sequence of the 16s RNA gene and its flanking region from the archaebacterium *Desulfurococcus mobilis*. Syst. Appl. Microbiol. 9: 22–28.

Klas, Z. 1936. Über den Formenkreis von *Beggiatoa mirabilis*. Arch. Mikrobiol. 8: 312–320.

Klaveness, D. 1977. Morphology, distribution and significance of the manganese accumulating microorganisms *Metallogenium* in lakes. Hydrobiology 56: 25–33.

Klaveness, D. 1982. The *Cryptomonas-Caulobacter* consortium: facultative ectocommensalism with possible taxonomic consequences? Nord. J. Bot. 2: 183–188.

Klebahn, H. 1919. Die Schadlinge des Klippfisches. Ein Beitrag zur Kenntnis des salzliebenden organismen. Mitt. Inst. Allg. Bot. Hamb. 4: 11–69.

Kleinig, H. and H. Reichenbach. 1969. Carotenoid pigments of *Stigmatella aurantiaca* (*Myxobacterales*). I. The minor carotenoids. Arch. Mikrobiol. 68: 210–217.

Kleinig, H. and H. Reichenbach. 1970. Carotenoid pigments of *Stigmatella aurantiaca* (*Myxobacterales*). Arch. Mikrobiol. 74: 223–234.

Kleinig, H. and H. Reichenbach. 1977. Carotenoid glucosides and menaquinones from the gliding bacterium *Herpetosiphon giganteus* Hpa2. Arch. Microbiol. 112: 307–310.

Kleinig, H., H. Reichenbach and H. Achenbach. 1970. Carotenoid pigments of *Stigmatella aurantiaca* (*Myxobacterales*) II. Acylated carotenoid glycosides. Arch. Mikrobiol. 7: 223–234.

Kleinig, H., H. Reichenbach, H. Achenbach and J. Stadler. 1971. Carotenoid pigments of *Sorangium compositum* (*Myxobacterales*) including two new carotenoid glucoside esters and two new carotenoid rhamnosides. Arch. Mikrobiol. 78: 224–233.

Kleinig, H., H. Reichenbach, N. Theobald and H. Achenbach. 1974. *Flexibacter elegans* and *Myxococcus fulvus*: aerobic Gram-negative bacteria containing menaquinones as the only isoprenoid quinones. Arch. Microbiol. 101: 91–93.

Klemme, J.-H. 1968. Untersuchungen zur Photoautotrophie mit molekularem Wasserstoff bei neuisolierten schwefelfreien Purpurbakterien. Arch. Mikrobiol. 64: 29–42.

Klemme, J.-H. 1976. Unidirectional inhibition of phosphoenolpyruvate carboxykinase from *Rhodospirillum rubrum* by ATP. Arch. Microbiol. 107: 189–192.

Klemme, J.-H. 1979. Occurrence of assimilatory nitrate reduction in phototrophic bacteria of the genera *Rhodospirillum* and *Rhodopseudomonas*. Microbiologica 2: 415–420.

Klemme, J.-H., I. Chyla and M. Preuss. 1980. Dissimilatory nitrate reduction by strains of the facultative phototrophic bacterium *Rhodopseudomonas palustris*. FEMS Microbiol. Lett. 9: 137–140.

Klemme, J.-H. and C. Pfleiderer. 1977. Production of extracellular proteolytic enzymes by phototrophic bacteria. FEMS Lett. 1: 297–299.

Klenk, H.-P., B. Haas, V. Schwass and W. Zillig. 1986. Hybridization homology: a new parameter for the analysis of phylogenetic relations, demonstrated with the urkingdom of the archaebacteria. J. Mol. Evol. 24: 167–173.

Kluyver, A.J. and C.G.T.P. Schnellen. 1947. On the fermentation of carbon monoxide by pure cultures of methane bacteria. Arch. Biochem. 14: 57–70.

Kluyver, A.J. and C.B. van Niel. 1936. Prospects for a natural system of classification of bacteria. Zentralbl. Bakteriol. Parasitenkd. Infektionskr. Hyg. Abt. II 94: 369–403.

Knoll, A.H. 1985. The distribution and evolution of microbial life in the late Proterozoic era. Annu. Rev. Microbiol. 39: 391–417.

Knudsen, E., E. Jantzen, K. Bryn, J.G. Ormerod and R. Sirevåg. 1982. Quantitative and structural characteristics of lipids in *Chlorobium* and *Chloroflexus*. Arch. Microbiol. 132: 149–154.

Ko, C.Y., J.L. Johnson, L.B. Barnett, H.M. McNair and J.R. Vencellotti. 1977. A sensitive estimation of the percentage of guanine plus cytosine in deoxyribonucleic acid by high performance liquid chromatography. Anal. Biochem. 80: 183–192.

Koch, A.L. 1981. Evolution of antibiotic resistance gene function. Microbiol. Rev. 45: 335–378.

Koch, W. 1964. Verzeichnis der Sammlung von Algenkulturen am Pflanzenphysiologischen Institut der Universität Göttingen. Arch. Mikrobiol. 47: 402–432.

Kocur, M. and J. Boháček. 1972. DNA base composition of extremely halophilic cocci. Arch. Mikrobiol. 82: 280–282.

Kocur, M. and W. Hodgkiss. 1973. Taxonomic status of the genus *Halococcus* Schoop. Int. J. Syst. Bacteriol. 23: 151–156.

Kocur, M., B. Smid and T. Martinec. 1972. The fine structure of extreme halophilic cocci. Microbios 5: 101–107.

Kodaka, H., A.Y. Armfield, G.L. Lombard and V.R. Dowell, Jr. 1982. Practical procedure for demonstrating bacterial flagella. J. Clin. Microbiol. 16: 948–952.

Kofler, L. 1913. Die Myxobakterien der Umgebung von Wien. Sitzungsber. Akad. Wiss. Math. Naturwiss. Kl. Abt. I 122: 845–876.

Kohl, W., H. Achenbach and H. Reichenbach. 1983. The pigments of *Brevibacterium linens*: aromatic carotenoids. Phytochemistry 22: 207–210.

Kohl, W., A. Gloe and H. Reichenbach. 1983. Steroids from the myxobacterium *Nannocystis exedens*. J. Gen. Microbiol. 129: 1629–1635.

Kohler, H.-P.E. 1986. Acetatkatabolismus in *Methanothrix soehngenii*. Thesis No. 8033, Eidgenössische Technische Hochschule, Zürich, 118 pp.

Kohler, H.-P.E. and A.J.B. Zehnder. 1984. Carbon monoxide dehydrogenase and acetate thiokinase in *Methanothrix soehngenii*. FEMS Microbiol. Lett. 21: 287–292.

Köhler, J. and A.C. Schwartz. 1981. Respiratory ubiquinone-9 from *Hyphomicrobium* sp. strain ZV-580. Z. Allg. Mikrobiol. 21: 117–123.

Kohlmiller, E.F., Jr. and H. Gest. 1951. A comparative study of the light and dark fermentations of organic acids by *Rhodospirillum rubrum*. J. Bacteriol. 61: 269–282.

Kölbel-Boelke, J., R. Gebers and P. Hirsch. 1985. Genome size determinations for 33 strains of budding bacteria. Int. J. Syst. Bacteriol. 35: 270–273.

Kolkwitz, R. 1909. Schizomycetes. Spaltpilze (Bacteria). In Botanischer Verein der Provinz Brandenburg, Kryptogamenflora der Mark Brandenburg, Vol. 5. Gebruder Borntraeger, Leipzig, pp. 2–186.

Kolkwitz, R. 1912. Über die Schwefelbakterie *Thioploca ingrica* Wislouch. Ber. Dtsch. Bot. Ges. 30: 662–666.

Kolkwitz, R. 1918. Über die Schwefelbakterien des Solgrabens von Artern. Ber. Dtsch. Bot. Ges. 36: 218–224.

Kolkwitz, R. 1955. Über die Schwefelbakterie *Thioploca ingrica* Wislouch. Ber. Dtsch. Bot. Ges. 68: 374–380.

Komárek, J. 1958. Die taxonomische Revision der planktischen Blaualgen der Tschechoslowakei. In Komárek and Ettl (Editors), Algologischen Studien. Czeck. Akad. Wiss., Prague, pp. 1–206.

Komárek, J. 1972. Reproduction process and taxonomy of unicellular endosporine blue-green algae. In Desikachary (Editor), Proceedings of the Symposium on Taxonomy and Biology of Blue-green Algae. University of Madras, Madras, pp. 41–47.

Komárek, J. 1973. Culture collections. In Carr and Whitton (Editors), The Biology of Blue-green Algae. Blackwell, Oxford, and University of California Press, Berkeley, pp. 519–524.

Komárek, J. 1976. Taxonomic reviews of the genera *Synechocystis* Sauv. 1892; *Synechococcus* Näg, 1849, and *Cyanothece* gen. nov. (*Cyanophyceae*). Arch. Protistenk. 118: 119–179.

Komárek, J. 1983. [Review of Drouet, F. 1981. Summary of the classification of blue-green algae.] Arch. Hydrobiol. Suppl. 67: 113–114.

Komárek, J. and K. Anagnostidis. 1986. Modern approach to the classification system of cyanophytes. 2. *Chroococcales*. Arch. Hydrobiol. Suppl. 73: 157–226.

Komárek, J. and F. Hindak. 1975. Taxonomy of the new isolated strains of *Chroococcidiopsis* (Cyanophyceae). Arch. Hydrobiol. Suppl. 46: 311–329.

Komárek, J., F. Hindak and J. Ludvik. 1985. The cell structure of two *Chamaesiphonaceae*, *Cyanophanon minus* and *Stichosiphon sansibaricus*. Arch. Hydrobiol., Suppl. 71: 75–90.

Komárek, J. and E. Kann. 1973. Zur Taxonomie und Ökologie der Gattung *Homoeothrix*. Arch. Protistenkd. 115: 173–283.

Kompantseva, E.I. 1981. Utilization of sulfide by nonsulfur purple bacteria

Rhodopseudomonas capsulata. Microbiologiya 50: 429–436.

Kompantseva, E.I. 1985. *Rhodobacter euryhalinus* sp. nov., a new halophilic purple bacterial species. Mikrobiologiya 54: 974–982.

Kompantseva, E.I. and V.M. Gorlenko. 1984. A new species of moderately halophilic purple bacterium, *Rhodospirillum mediosalinum*. Mikrobiologiya 53: 954–961.

Kondrat'eva, E.N., R.N. Ivanovsky and E.N. Krasil'nikova. 1981. Light and dark metabolism in purple sulfur bacteria. Sov. Sci. Rev. Amsterdam, pp. 325–364.

Kondratieva, E.N., V.G. Zhukov, R.N. Ivanosky, Y.P. Petrushkova and E.Z. Monosov. 1976. The capacity of the phototrophic sulfur bacterium *Thiocapsa roseopersicina* for chemosynthesis. Arch. Microbiol. 108: 287–292.

Konetzka, W.A. 1977. Microbiology of metal transformations. In Weinberg (Editor), Microorganisms and Minerals. Marcel Dekker, New York, pp. 317–342.

König, E., H. Schlesner and P. Hirsch. 1984. Cell wall studies on budding bacteria of the *Planctomyces/Pasteuria* group and on a *Prosthecomicrobium* sp. Arch. Microbiol. 138: 200–205.

König, H. 1984. Isolation and characterization of *Methanobacterium uliginosum* sp. nov. from a marshy soil. Can. J. Microbiol. 30: 1477–1481.

König, H. 1985. In Validation of the publication of new names and new combinations previously effectively published outside the IJSB. List No. 17. Int. J. Syst. Bacteriol. 35: 375–376.

König, H. 1986. Chemical composition of cell envelopes of methanogenic bacteria isolated from human and animal feces. Syst. Appl. Microbiol. 8: 159–162.

König, H., R. Kralik and O. Kandler. 1982. Structure and modifications of pseudomurein in *Methanobacteriales*. Zentralbl. Bakteriol. Mikrobiol. Hyg. I Abt. Orig. C3: 179–191.

König, H., E. Nusser and K.O. Stetter. 1985. Glycogen in *Methanolobus* and *Methanococcus*. FEMS Microbiol. Lett. 28: 265–269.

König, H. and K.O. Stetter. 1982. Isolation and characterization of *Methanolobus tindarius*, sp. nov., a coccoid methanogen growing only on methanol and methylamines. Zentralbl. Bakteriol. Mikrobiol. Hyg. 1 Abt. Orig. C3: 478–490.

König, H. and K.O. Stetter. 1983. In Validation of the publication of new names and new combinations previously effectively published outside the IJSB. List No. 10. Int. J. Syst. Bacteriol. 33: 438–440.

Koops, H.-P. 1969. Der Nutzeffekt der NH_4^+-Oxydation durch *Nitrosocystis oceanus* Watson. Arch. Mikrobiol. 65: 115–135.

Koops, H.-P. and H. Harms. 1985. Desoxyribonucleic acid homologies among 96 strains of ammonia-oxidizing bacteria. Arch. Microbiol. 141: 214–218.

Koops, H.-P., H. Harms and H. Wehrmann. 1976. Isolation of a moderate halophilic ammonia-oxidizing bacterium, *Nitrosococcus mobilis* nov. sp. Arch. Microbiol. 107: 277–282.

Koppe, F. 1924. Die Schlammflora der ostholsteinischen Seen und des Bodensees. Arch. Hydrobiol. 14: 619–672.

Kott, P. 1980. Algal-bearing didemnid ascidians in the Indo-west Pacific. Mem. Queensl. Mus. 20: 1–47.

Kott, P. 1982. Didemnid-algal symbioses: host species in the western Pacific with notes on the symbiosis. Micronesica 18: 95–127.

Kott, P., D.L. Parry and G.C. Cox. 1984. Prokaryotic symbionts with a range of ascidian hosts. Bull. Mar. Sci. 34: 308–312.

Kowallik, U. and E.G. Pringsheim. 1966. The oxidation of hydrogen sulfide by *Beggiatoa*. Am. J. Bot. 53: 801–806.

Koyasu, S., M. Asada, A. Fukuda and Y. Okada. 1981. Sequential polymerization of flagellin A and flagellin B into *Caulobacter* flagella. J. Mol. Biol. 153: 471–475.

Kran, G., W. Schlote and H.G. Schlegel. 1963. Cytologische Untersuchungen an *Chromatium okenii* Petry. Naturwissenschaften 50: 728–730.

Krasil'nikov, N.A. 1949. Guide to the Bacteria and Actinomycetes. Akad. Nauk S.S.S.R., Moscow, pp. 1–830.

Krasil'nikov, N.A. and S.S. Belyaev. 1970. Morphology and development of *Caulobacter*. Mikrobiologiya 39: 352–356 (English translation: pp. 303–308).

Krasil'nikov, N.A. and S.S. Belyaev. 1973. Taxonomy and classification of the genus *Caulobacter*. Izv. Akad. Nauk S.S.S.R. Ser. Biol. 3: 313–323.

Krasil'nikova, E.N. 1975. Enzymes of carbohydrate metabolism in phototrophic bacteria. Mikrobiologiya 44: 5–10.

Krasil'nikova, E.N. 1981. Assimilation of sulfates by purple sulfur bacteria. Mikrobiologiya 50: 338–344 (in Russian).

Krasil'nikova, E.N. 1985. Enzymes involved in carbon metabolism in a purple sulfur bacterium *Lamprobacter modestohalophilus*. Mikrobiologiya 53: 592–594 (in Russian).

Krasil'nikova, E.N. and E.N. Kondrat'eva. 1979. Possible pathways of acetyl-CoA formation by purple bacteria. Mikrobiologiya 48: 779–784 (in Russian).

Krasil'nikova, E.N., V.G. Zhukov and E.N. Kondrat'eva. 1979. Glycerol metabolism in purple sulfur bacteria. Mikrobiologiya 48: 586–591 (in Russian).

Kratz, W.A. and J. Myers. 1955. Nutrition and growth of several blue-green algae. Am. J. Bot. 42: 282–287.

Krichevsky, M.I. and L.M. Norton. 1974. Sortage and manipulation of data by computers for determinative bacteriology. Int. J. Syst. Bacteriol. 24: 525–531.

Krieg, N.R. 1984. Aerobic/microaerophilic, motile, helical/vibrioid Gram-negative bacteria. In Krieg and Holt (Editors), Bergey's Manual of Systematic Bacteriology, Vol. 1. The Williams and Wilkins Co., Baltimore, p. 71–124.

Krieg, N.R. and P. Gerhardt. 1981. Solid culture. In Gerhardt (Editor), Manual of Methods for General Bacteriology. American Society for Microbiology, Washington, D.C., pp. 143–150.

Kristiansen, J. 1971. On *Planctomyces bekefii* and its occurrence in Danish lakes and ponds. Bot. Tidsskr. *66:* 293–302.

Kristiansen, J.E., A. Bremmelgaard, H.E. Busk, O. Heltberg, W. Fredericksen and T. Justesen. 1984. Rapid identification of *Capnocytophaga* isolated from septicemic patients. Eur. J. Microbiol. *3:* 236–240.

Krul, J.M. 1977. Experiments with *Haliscomenobacter hydrossis* in continuous culture without and with *Zoogloea ramigera*. Water Res. *11:* 197–204.

Krul, J.M. 1978. Denitrification, activity of bacterial flocs, and growth of a filamentous bacterium in relation with the bulking of activated sludge. Ph.D. thesis, University of Wageningen.

Krul, J.M., P. Hirsch and J.T. Staley. 1970. *Toxothrix trichogenes* (Chol.) Beger and Bringmann: the organism and its biology. Antonie van Leeuwenhoek J. Microbiol. Serol. *36:* 409–420.

Krumbein, W.E. and H.J. Altmann. 1973. A new method for the detection and enumeration of manganese oxidizing and reducing microorganisms. Helgol. Wiss. Meeresunters. *25:* 347–356.

Krümmel, A. and H. Harms. 1980. Der Einfluss anorganischer Ionen auf das Wachstum von zwei *Nitrosomonasa*-Stämmen aus verschiedenen Biotopen. Mitt. Inst. Allg. Bot. Hamb. *17:* 89–100.

Krümmel, A. and H. Harms. 1982. Effect of organic matter on growth and cell yield of ammonia-oxidizing bacteria. Arch. Microbiol. *133:* 50–54.

Krych, V.A., J.L. Johnson and A.A. Yousten. 1980. Deoxyribonucleic acid homologies among strains of *Bacillus sphaericus*. Int. J. Syst. Bacteriol. *30:* 476–484.

Kryukov, V.R., N.D. Savelyeva and M.A. Pusheva. 1983. *Calderobacterium hydrogenophilum* nov. gen. nov. sp., an extreme thermophilic hydrogen bacterium, and its hydrogenase activity. Mikrobiologiya *52:* 781–788.

Krzemieniewska, H. 1933. Contribution à l'étude du genre *Cytophaga* (Winogradsky). Arch. Mikrobiol. *4:* 394–408.

Krzemieniewska, H. and S. Krzemieniewski. 1926. Miksobakterje Polski. (Die Myxobakterien von Polen). Acta Soc. Bot. Pol. *4:* 1–54.

Krzemieniewska, H. and S. Krzemieniewski. 1927. Miksobakterje Polski Uzupelnienie. (Die Myxobakterien Von Polen. Anhang.) Acta Soc. Bot. Pol. *5:* 79–98.

Krzemieniewska, H. and S. Krzemieniewski. 1928. Morfologja Komórki miksobakteryj (Zur Morphologie der Myxobakterienzelle). Acta Soc. Bot. Pol. *5:* 46–90.

Krzemieniewska, H. and S. Krzemieniewski. 1930. Miksobakterje Polski Czesc trzecia. (Die Myxobakterien von Polen. III Teil) Acta Soc. Bot. Pol. *7:* 250–273.

Krzemieniewska, H. and S. Krzemieniewski. 1937a. Die zellulosezersetzenden Myxobakterien. Bull. Int. Acad. Cracovie (Acad. Pol. Sci.) Ser. B. Sci. Nat. I, pp. 11–31.

Krzemieniewska, H. and S. Krzemieniewski. 1937b. Über die Zersetzung der Zellulose durch Myxobakterien. Bull. Int. Acad. Cracovie (Acad. Pol. Sci.) Ser. B Sci. Nat. I, pp. 33–59.

Krzemieniewska, H. and S. Krzemieniewski. 1946. Myxobacteria of the species *Chondromyces* Berkeley and Curtis. Bull. Int. Acad. Cracovie. (Acad. Pol. Sci.) Ser. B Sci. Nat. I, pp. 31–48.

Krzycki, J. and J.G. Zeikus. 1980. Quantification of corrinoids in methanogenic bacteria. Curr. Microbiol. *3:* 243–245.

Kucera, S. and R.S. Wolfe. 1957. A selective enrichment method for *Gallionella ferruginea*. J. Bacteriol. *74:* 344–349.

Kuchino, Y., M. Ihara, Y. Yabusaki and S. Nishimura. 1982. Initiator tRNAs from archaebacteria show common unique sequence characteristics. Nature (London) *298:* 684–685.

Kuenen, J.G. 1975. The colourless sulphur bacteria and their role in the sulphur cycle. Plant Soil *43:* 49–76.

Kuenen, J.G. and R.F. Beudeker. 1982. Microbiology of thiobacilli and other sulphur-oxidizing autotrophs, micotrophs and heterotrophs. Philos. Trans. R. Soc. Lond. B *298:* 473–497.

Kuenen, J.G. and O.H. Tuovinen. 1982. The genera *Thiobacillus* and *Thiomicrospira. In* Starr, Stolp, Trüper, Balows and Schlegel (Editors), The Prokaryotes. A Handbook on Habitats, Isolation, and Identification of Bacteria. Springer-Verlag, Berlin, pp. 1023–1036.

Kuenen, J.G. and H. Veldkamp. 1972. *Thiomicrospira pelophila*, gen. n., sp. n., a new obligately chemolithotrophic colourless sulfur bacterium. Antonie van Leeuwenhoek J. Microbiol. Serol. *38:* 241–256.

Kuhl, S.A., D.W. Nix and D.C. Yoch. 1983. Characterization of a *Rhodospirillum rubrum* plasmid: loss of photosynthetic growth in plasmidless strains. J. Bacteriol. *156:* 737–742.

Kühlwein, H. 1950. Beiträge zur Biologie und Entwicklungsgeschichte der Myxobakterien. Arch. Mikrobiol. *14:* 678–704.

Kühlwein, H. 1952. Untersuchungen über *Chondromyces apiculatus* Thaxter. Arch. Mikrobiol. *17:* 403–408.

Kühlwein, H. 1969. Some aspects of morphogenesis and fruiting body formation in myxobacteria. J. Appl. Bacteriol. *32:* 19–21.

Kühlwein, H. and E. Gallwitz. 1958. *Polyangium violaceum* nov. spec. Ein Beitrag zur Kenntnis der Myxobakterien. Arch. Mikrobiol. *31:* 139–145.

Kühlwein, H. and H. Reichenbach. 1964. Ein neuer Vertreter der Myxobakteriengattung *Archangium* Jahn. Arch. Mikrobiol. *48:* 179–184.

Kühlwein, H. and H. Reichenbach. 1965. Anreicherung und Isolierung von Myxobakterien. Zentralbl. Bakteriol. Parasitenkd. Infektionskr. Hyg. Abt. I Orig. Suppl. *1:* 57–80.

Kühlwein, H. and B. Schlicke. 1971. *Polyangium luteum* Krzemieniewski in pure culture. J. Appl. Bacteriol. *34:* 515–519.

Kuhn, D.A. 1981. The genus *Cristispira. In* Starr, Stolp, Trüper, Balows and Schlegel (Editors), The Prokaryotes. A Handbook on Habitats, Isolation, and Identification of Bacteria. Springer-Verlag, Berlin, pp. 555–563.

Kuhn, D.A. and D.A. Gregory. 1978. Emendation of *Simonsiella muelleri* Schmid and description of *Simonsiella steedae* sp. nov., with designations of the respective proposed neotype and holotype strains. Curr. Microbiol. *1:* 11–14.

Kuhn, D.A., D.A. Gregory, G.E. Buchanan, Jr., M.D. Nyby and K.R. Daly. 1978. Isolation, characterization, and numerical taxonomy of *Simonsiella* strains from the oral cavities of cats, dogs, sheep, and humans. Arch. Microbiol. *118:* 235–241.

Kuhn, D.A., D.A. Gregory, M.D. Nyby and M. Mandel. 1977. Deoxyribonucleic acid base composition of *Simonsiellaceae*. Arch. Microbiol. *113:* 205–207.

Kühn, W., K. Fiebig, R. Walther and G. Gottschalk. 1979. Presence of cytochrome b$_{559}$ in *Methanosarcina barkeri*. FEBS Lett. *105:* 271–274.

Kuhrt, M. and J.L. Pate. 1973. Isolation and characterization of tubules and plasma membranes from *Cytophaga columnaris*. J. Bacteriol. *114:* 1309–1318.

Kumar, S. and D.J.D. Nicholas. 1982a. A protonmotive force-dependent adenosine-5′ triphosphate synthesis in spheroplasts of *Nitrosomonas europaea*. FEMS Microbiol. Lett. *14:* 21–25.

Kumar, S. and D.J.D. Nicholas. 1982b. Assimilation of inorganic nitrogen compounds by *Nitrobacter agilis*. J. Gen. Microbiol. *128:* 1795–1801.

Kumar, S. and D.J.D. Nicholas. 1983. Proton electrochemical gradients in washed cells of *Nitrosomonas europaea* and *Nitrobacter agilis*. J. Bacteriol. *154:* 65–71.

Kumar, S., D.J.D. Nicholas and E.H. Williams. 1983. Definitive ^{15}N NMR evidence that water serves as a source of 'O' during nitrite oxidation by *Nitrobacter agilis*. FEBS Lett. *152:* 71–74.

Kuner, J.M. and D. Kaiser. 1981. Introduction of transposon Tn5 in *Myxococcus* for analysis of developmental and other nonselectable mutants. Proc. Natl. Acad. Sci. U.S.A. *78:* 425–429.

Kunkel, D.D. 1982. Thylakoid centers: structures associated with the cyanobacterial photosynthetic membrane system. Arch. Microbiol. *133:* 97–99.

Kunze, B., H. Reichenbach, H. Augustiniak and G. Höfle. 1982. Isolation and identification of althiomycin from *Cystobacter fuscus* (*Myxobacterales*). J. Antibiot. *35:* 635–636.

Künzler, A. and N. Pfennig. 1973. Das Vorkommen von Bacteriochlorophyll a_p and a_{Gg} in Stämmen aller Arten der *Rhodospirillaceae*. Arch. Mikrobiol. *91:* 83–86.

Kuo, S.C., H.Y. Chung and G.H. Kou. 1981. Studies on artificial infection of the gliding bacteria in cultured fishes. Fish Pathol. *15:* 309–314.

Kurowski, W.M. and J.A. Dunleavy. 1976. Pectinase production by bacteria associated with improved preservative permeability in Sitka spruce: synthesis and secretion of polygalacturonate lyase by *Cytophaga johnsonii*. J. Appl. Bacteriol. *41:* 119–128.

Kurtzman, C.P., M.J. Smiley, C.J. Johnson, L.B. Wickerham and G.B. Fuson. 1980. Two new and closely related heterothallic species, *Pichia amylophila* and *Pichia mississippiensis*: characterization by hybridization and deoxyribonucleic acid reassociation. Int. J. Syst. Bacteriol. *30:* 208–216.

Kushner, D.J. 1985. The *Halobacteriaceae. In* Woese and Wolfe (Editors), The Bacteria. A Treatise on Structure and Function, Vol. VIII: Archaebacteria. Academic Press, New York, pp. 171–214.

Kushwaha, S.C., M.B. Gochnauer, D.J. Kushner and M. Kates. 1974. Pigments and isoprenoid compounds in extremely and moderately halophilic bacteria. Can. J. Microbiol. *20:* 241–245.

Kushwaha, S.C., M. Kates, G.D. Sprott and I.C.P. Smith. 1981. Novel complex polar lipids from the methanogenic archaebacterium *Methanospirillum hungatei*. Science *211:* 1163–1164.

Kusuda, R. and H. Kimura. 1982. Characteristics of gliding bacterium isolated from cultured yellowtail *Seriola quinqueradiata*. Bull. Jpn. Soc. Sci. Fish. *48:* 1107–1112 (in Japanese with English summary).

Kutuzova, R.S. 1972. Electron microscope studies of ooze-dwelling microorganisms (in Russian). Mikrobiologiya *41:* 859–861.

Kutuzova, R.S. 1974. Electron microscopic study of ooze overgrowths of an iron-oxidizing coccus related to *Siderococcus limoniticus* Dorff. Mikrobiologiya *43:* 285–288.

Kutuzova, R.S., D.R. Gabe and I.M. Kravkina. 1972. Electron microscope study of overgrowths of iron-manganese microorganisms from ooze. Mikrobiologiya *41:* 1099–1102.

Kützing, F.T. 1833. Beitrag zur Kenntnis über die Entstehung und Metamorphose der niederen vegetalischen Organismen, nebst einer systematischen Zusammensetzung der hierher gehörigen niederen Algenformen. Linnaea *8:* 335–387.

Kützing, F.T. 1843. Phycologia Generales, Leipzig.

Kützing, F.T. 1845. Phycologia Germanica I–X, Nordhausen, 240 pp.

Kützing, F.T. 1849. Species Algarum, I–IV. Leipzig, 922 pp.

Lackey, J.B. and E.W. Lackey. 1961. The habitat and description of a new genus of sulphur bacterium. J. Gen. Microbiol. *26:* 29–39.

Lackey, J.B., E.W. Lackey and G.B. Morgan. 1965. Taxonomy and ecology of the sulfur bacteria. Eng. Prog. Report, No. 119, University of Florida, Gainesville *19:* 3–23.

Laemmli, U.K. 1970. Cleavage of structural proteins during the assembly of the head of bacteriophage T4. Nature (London) *227:* 680–685.

Lafitskaya, T.N. and L.V. Vasilyeva. 1976. A new triangle bacterium. Microbiologiya *45:* 812–816.

Lafitskaya, T.N., L.V. Vasilyeva, E.N. Krasilnikova and N.I. Alexandruskina. 1976. Physiology of *Prosthecomicrobium polyspheroidum* (in Russian). Izv. Akad. Nauk S.S.S.R. Ser. Biol. *6:* 849–857.

Lagenaur, C. and N. Agabian. 1977. *Caulobacter* flagellins. J. Bacteriol. *132:* 731–733.

Lagerheim, G. 1886. Note sur le *Mastigocoleus*, nouveau genre des algues marines de l'ordre des Phycochromacées. Notarisia *1:* 65–69.

Lamont, H.C. 1969. Sacrificial cell death and trichome breakage in an oscillatoriacean blue-green alga: the role of murein. Arch. Mikrobiol. *69:* 237–259.

Lampky, J.R. 1976. Ultrastructure of *Polyangium cellulosum*. J. Bacteriol. *126:* 1278–1284.

Lampky, J.R. and E.R. Brockman. 1977. Fluorescence of *Myxococcus stipitatus*. Int. J. Syst. Bacteriol. *27:* 161.

Lancefield, R.C. 1933. A serological differentiation of human and other groups of hemolytic streptococci. J. Exp. Med. *57:* 571–595.

Lancefield, R.C. 1934. A serological differentiation of specific types of bovine hemolytic streptococci (group B). J. Exp. Med. *59:* 441–458.

Lang, N.J. 1977. *Starria zimbabweénsis* (*Cyanophyceae*) gen. nov. et sp. nov.: a filament triradiate in transverse section. J. Phycol. *13:* 288–296.

Langenberg, K.J., M.P. Bryant and R.S. Wolfe. 1968. Hydrogen-oxidizing methane bacteria. II. Electron microscopy. J. Bacteriol. *95:* 1124–1129.

Langeron, M. 1923. Les oscillariées parasites du tube digestif de l'homme et des animaux. Ann. Parasitol. Hum. Comp. *1:* 113–123.

Langworthy, T.A. 1977. Long-chain diglycerol tetraethers from *Thermoplasma acidophilum*. Biochim. Biophys. Acta *487:* 37–50.

Langworthy, T.A. 1979a. Special features of thermoplasmas. *In* Barile and Razin (Editors), The Mycoplasmas I: Cell Biology. Academic Press, New York, pp. 495–513.

Langworthy, T.A. 1979b. Membrane structure of thermoacidophilic bacteria. *In* Shilo (Editor), Strategies of Microbial Life in Extreme Environments, Berlin: Dahlem Konferenzen. Verlag-Chemie, Weinheim, pp. 417–432.

Langworthy, T.A. 1982. Lipids of bacteria living in extreme environments. Curr. Top. Membr. Transp. *17:* 45–77.

Langworthy, T.A. 1985. Lipids of archaebacteria. *In* Woese and Wolfe (Editors), The Bacteria, Vol. VIII. Academic Press, New York, pp. 459–498.

Langworthy, T.A. and J.L. Pond. 1986. Archaebacterial ether lipids and chemotaxonomy. Syst. Appl. Microbiol. *7:* 253–257.

Langworthy, T.A., T.G. Tornabene and G. Holzer. 1982. Lipids of archaebacteria. Zentralbl. Bakteriol. Mikrobiol. Hyg. I Abt. Orig. C3: 228–244.

Lanyi, J.K. 1986. Halorhodopsin. A light-driven chloride ion pump. Annu. Rev. Biochem. Biophys. Chem. *15:* 11–28.

Lapage, S.P. 1971. Culture collections of bacteria. Biol. J. Linn. Soc. *3:* 197–210.

Lapage, S.P. 1975. Report of the World Federation for Culture Collections. Int. J. Syst. Bacteriol. *25:* 90–94.

Lapidus, I.R. and H.C. Berg. 1982. Gliding motility of *Cytophaga* sp. strain U67. J. Bacteriol. *151:* 384–398.

la Rivière, J.W.M. and K. Schmidt. 1981. Morphologically conspicuous sulfur-oxidizing eubacteria. *In* Starr, Stolp, Trüper, Balows and Schlegel (Editors), The Prokaryotes. A Handbook on Habitats, Isolation, and Identification of Bacteria. Springer-Verlag, Berlin, pp. 1037–1048.

Larkin, J.M. 1980. Isolation of *Thiothrix* in pure culture and observation of a filamentous epiphyte on *Thiothrix*. Curr. Microbiol. *4:* 155–158.

Larkin, J.M. and D.L. Shinabarger. 1983. Characterization of *Thiothrix nivea*. Int. J. Syst. Bacteriol. *33:* 841–846.

Larkin, J.M. and W.R. Strohl. 1983. *Beggiatoa, Thiothrix,* and *Thioploca*. Annu. Rev. Microbiol. *37:* 341–367.

Larsen, H. 1952. On the culture and general physiology of the green sulfur bacteria. J. Bacteriol. *94:* 889–895.

Larsen, H. 1967. Biochemical aspects of extreme halophilism. Adv. Microb. Physiol. *1:* 97–132.

Larsen, H. 1981. The family *Halobacteriaceae*. *In* Starr, Stolp, Trüper, Balows and Schlegel (Editors), The Prokaryotes. A Handbook on Habitats, Isolation, and Identification of Bacteria. Springer-Verlag, Berlin, pp. 985–994.

Larsen, H. 1984. *Halobacteriaceae*. *In* Krieg and Holt (Editors), Bergey's Manual of Systematic Bacteriology, Volume 1. The Williams and Wilkins Co., Baltimore, pp. 261–267.

Larsen, N., H. Leffers, J. Kjems and R.A. Garrett. 1986. Evolutionary divergence between the ribosomal RNA operons of *Halococcus morrhuae* and *Desulfurococcus mobilis*. Syst. Appl. Microbiol. *7:* 49–57.

Larson, R.J. and J.L. Pate. 1975. Growth and morphology of *Asticcacaulis biprosthecum* in defined media. Arch. Microbiol. *106:* 147–157.

Lauerer, G., J.K. Kristjansson, T.A. Langworthy, H. König and K.O. Stetter. 1986a. *Methanothermus sociabilis* sp. nov., a second species within the *Methanothermaceae* growing at 97°C. Syst. Appl. Microbiol. *8:* 100–105.

Lauerer, G., J.K. Kristjansson, T.A. Langworthy, H. König and K.O. Stetter. 1986b. *In* Validation of the publication of new names and new combinations previously effectively published outside the IJSB. List No. 22. Int. J. Syst. Bacteriol. *36:* 573–576.

Laughon, B.E., S.A. Wyed and W.J. Loesche. 1982. API ZYM system for identification of *Bacteroides* spp., *Capnocytophaga* spp., and spirochetes of oral origin. J. Clin. Microbiol. *15:* 97–102.

Lauterborn, R. 1906. Zur Kenntnis der sapropelischen Flora. Allg. Bot. Z. *12:* 196–197.

Lauterborn, R. 1907. Eine neue Gattung der Schwefelbakterien (*Thioploca schmidlei* nov. gen. nov. spec.). Ber. Dtsch. Bot. Ges. *25:* 238–242.

Lauterborn, R. 1913. Zur Kenntnis einiger sapropelischer Schizomyceten. Allg. Bot. Z. *19:* 97–100.

Lauterborn, R. 1915. Die sapropelische Lebewelt. Verh. Naturh.-Med. Ver. Heidelb. *13:* 437–438.

Lauterborn, R. 1916. Die sapropelische Lebewelt. Ein Beitrag zur Biologie des Faulschlammes natürlicher Gewässer. Verh. Naturkundl. Med. Ver. Heidelb. *13:* 395–481.

Lautrop, H. 1965. Gliding motility in bacteria as a taxonomic criterion. Publications de la Faculté des Sciences de l'Université J.E. Purkyne, Brno. Ser. K35, pp. 322–327.

Lawry, N.H., V. Jani and T.E. Jensen. 1981. Identification of the sulfur inclusion body in *Beggiatoa alba* B18LD by energy-dispersive x-ray microanalysis. Curr. Microbiol. *6:* 71–74.

Lazaroff, N. 1973. Photomorphogenesis and nostocacean development. *In* Carr and Whitton (Editors), The Biology of Blue-green Algae. Blackwell, Oxford, and University of California Press, Berkeley, pp. 279–319.

Lazaroff, N. and W. Vishniac. 1964. The relationship of cellular differentiation to colonial morphogenesis of the blue-green alga, *Nostoc muscorum* A. J. Gen. Microbiol. *35:* 447–457.

Leadbetter, E.R. 1963. Growth and morphogenesis of *Sporocytophaga myxococcoides*. Bacteriol. Proc., p. 42.

Leadbetter, E.R. 1974. Family IV. *Methylomonadaceae* Leadbetter 1974. *In* Buchanan and Gibbons (Editors), Bergey's Manual of Determinative Bacteriology, 8th Ed. The Williams and Wilkins Co., Baltimore, pp. 267–269.

Leadbetter, E.R. 1974a. Order II. *Cytophagales* Nomen novum. *In* Buchanan and Gibbons (Editors), Bergey's Manual of Determinative Bacteriology, 8th Ed. The Williams and Wilkins Co., Baltimore, p. 99.

Leadbetter, E.R. 1974b. Genus II. *Flexibacter*. *In* Buchanan and Gibbons (Editors), Bergey's Manual of Determinative Bacteriology, 8th Ed. The Williams and Wilkins Co., Baltimore, pp. 105–107.

Leadbetter, E.R. 1974c. Family II. *Beggiatoaceae*. *In* Buchanan and Gibbons (Editors), Bergey's Manual of Determinative Bacteriology, 8th Ed. The Williams and Wilkins Co., Baltimore, pp. 112–116.

Leadbetter, E.R. and W. Godchaux. 1981. Sulfonolipids novel in procaryotes are significant cellular components of many gliding bacteria. *In* Reichenbach and Weeks (Editors), The *Flavobacterium-Cytophaga* Group. Verlag Chemie, Weinheim, F.R.G., pp. 135–143.

Leadbetter, E.R., S.C. Holt and S.S. Socransky. 1979. *Capnocytophaga:* new genus of Gram-negative bacteria I. General characteristics, taxonomic considerations and significance. Arch. Microbiol. *122:* 9–16.

Leathen, W.W. and S.A. Braley. 1954. A new iron-oxidizing bacterium: *Ferrobacillus ferrooxidans*. Bacteriol. Proc., p. 44.

Lebedinskii, A.V. 1981. Growth of *Hyphomicrobium* with various electron acceptors. Mikrobiologiya *50:* 665–669 (English translation: 492–495).

Lechevalier, M.P. 1977. Lipids in bacterial taxonomy—a taxonomist's view. Crit. Rev. Microbiol. *5:* 109–210.

Lechner, K., G. Wich and A. Bock. 1985. The nucleotide sequence of the 16S rRNA gene and flanking regions from *Methanobacterium formicicium*. On the phylogenetic relationship between methanogenic and halophilic archaebacteria. Syst. Appl. Microbiol. *6:* 157–163.

Lees, H. 1952. The biochemistry of the nitrifying organisms: 1. The ammonia-oxidizing systems of *Nitrosomonas*. Biochem. J. *52:* 134–139.

Leffers, H. and R.A. Garrett. 1984. The nucleotide sequence of the 16S rRNA of the archaebacterium *Halococcus morrhuae*. EMBO J. *3:* 1613–1619.

Lehmann, R. 1976. Wachstumsphysiologische Untersuchungen an fakultative aeroben und mikroaeroben *Rhodospirillaceae* und Charakterisierung ihrer Elektronentransportsysteme. Ph.D. thesis, University of Göttingen, F.R.G.

Lehmann, K.B. and R. Neumann. 1927. Bakteriologie insbesondere Bakteriologische Diagnostik. II. Allgemeine und spezielle Bakteriologie, 7 Aufl. J.F. Lehmann, München.

Lehmann, K.B. and R.O. Neumann. 1931. Bacteriology. Especially Determinative Bacteriology. G.E. Stechert and Co. (Alfred Hafner), New York, p. 516.

Leifson, E. 1960. Atlas of Bacterial Flagellation. Academic Press, New York, pp. 158–159.

Leifson, E. 1962. *Pseudomonas spinosa* n. sp. Int. Bull. Bacteriol. Nomencl. Taxon. *12:* 89–92.

Leifson, E. 1964. *Hyphomicrobium neptunium* sp. n. Antonie van Leeuwenhoek J. Microbiol. Serol. *30:* 249–256.

Leigh, J.A. 1983. The structure of the carbon dioxide reduction factor, a novel carbon carrier in *Methanobacterium thermoautotrophicum*. Ph.D. thesis, University of Illinois.

Leigh, J.A. and R.S. Wolfe. 1983. Carbon dioxide reduction factor and methanopterin, two coenzymes required for CO_2 reduction to methane by extracts of *Methanobacterium*. J. Biol. Chem. *258:* 7536–7540.

Leinfelder, W., M. Jarsch and A. Bock. 1985. The phylogenetic position of the sulphur-dependent archaebacterium *Thermoproteus tenax*: sequence of the 16S RNA gene. Syst. Appl. Microbiol. *6:* 164–170.

Lemmermann, E. 1907. Die Algenflora der Chatham Islands. Bot. Jahrb. Syst. Pflanzengesch. Pflanzengeogr. *38:* 343–382.

Levin, R.A. 1971. Fatty acids of *Thiobacillus thiooxydans*. J. Bacteriol. *108:* 982–995.

Lewin, R.A. 1962. *Saprospira grandis* Gross; and suggestions for reclassifying helical apochlorotic, gliding organisms. Can. J. Microbiol. 8: 555–563.

Lewin, R.A. 1963. Rod-shaped particles in *Saprospira*. Nature 198: 103–104.

Lewin, R.A. 1965a. Isolation and some physiological features of *Saprospira thermalis*. Can. J. Microbiol. 11: 77–86.

Lewin, R.A. 1965b. Freshwater species of *Saprospira*. Can. J. Microbiol. 111: 135–139.

Lewin, R.A. 1969. A classification of flexibacteria. J. Gen. Microbiol. 58: 189–206.

Lewin, R.A. 1970. *Saprospira toviformis* nov. spec. *(Flexibacterales)* from a New Zealand seashore. Can. J. Microbiol. 16: 507–510.

Lewin, R.A. 1970a. *Flexithrix dorotheae* gen. et sp. nov. *(Flexibacterales)*; and suggestions for reclassifying sheathed bacteria. Can. J. Microbiol. 16: 511–515.

Lewin, R.A. 1970b. New *Herpetosiphon* species *(Flexibacterales)*. Can. J. Microbiol. 16: 517–520.

Lewin, R.A. 1972. Growth and nutrition of *Saprospira grandis* Gross *(Flexibacterales)*. Can. J. Microbiol. 18: 361–365.

Lewin, R.A. 1974. *Flexibacter polymorphus*, a new marine species. J. Gen. Microbiol. 82: 393–403.

Lewin, R.A. 1975. A marine *Synechocystis* (Cyanophyta, *Chroococcales*) epizoic on ascidians. Phycologia 14: 153–160.

Lewin, R.A. 1977. *Prochloron*, a type genus of the Prochlorophyta. Phycologia 16: 216.

Lewin, R.A. 1978. Distribution of symbiotic didemnids associated with Prochlorophytes. Proc. Int. Symp. Mar. Biogeogr. Evol. 365–369.

Lewin, R.A. 1979. Formal taxonomic treatment of cyanophytes. Int. J. Syst. Bacteriol. 29: 411–412.

Lewin, R.A. 1980. Uncoiled variants of *Spirulina platensis* (Cyanophyceae: Oscillatoriaceae). Arch. Hydrobiol. Suppl. 60: 48–52.

Lewin, R.A. 1981. The Prochlorophytes. *In* Starr, Stolp, Trüper, Balows and Schlegel (Editors), The Prokaryotes. A Handbook on Habits, Isolation, and Identification of Bacteria. Springer-Verlag, Berlin, pp. 257–266.

Lewin, R.A. 1983. The problems of *Prochloron*. Ann. Microbiol. (Inst. Pasteur) 134B: 37–41.

Lewin, R.A. 1984. *Prochloron*—a status report. Phycologia 23: 203–208.

Lewin, R.A. 1986. The phylogeny of *Prochloron*. G. Bot. Ital. 120: 1–14.

Lewin, R.A. and L. Cheng. 1975. Association of microscopic algae with didemnid ascidians. Phycologia 14: 149–152.

Lewin, R.A., L. Cheng and R.S. Alberte. 1984. *Prochloron*-ascidian symbioses: photosynthetic potential and productivity. Micronesica 19: 165–170.

Lewin, R.A. and E.R. Leadbetter. 1974. Genus V. *Saprospira* Gross 1911, 190; Lewin 1962, 560 emend. mut. char. *In* Buchanan and Gibbons (Editors), Bergey's Manual of Determinative Bacteriology, 8th Ed. The Williams and Wilkins Co., Baltimore, pp. 109–111.

Lewin, R.A. and E.R. Leadbetter. 1974. Genus *Herpetosiphon* Holt and Lewin. *In* Buchanan and Gibbons (Editors), Bergey's Manual of Determinative Bacteriology, 8th Ed. The Williams and Wilkins Co., Baltimore, pp. 107–109.

Lewin, R.A. and D.M. Lounsbery. 1969. Isolation, cultivation and characterization of flexibacteria. J. Gen. Microbiol. 58: 145–170.

Lewin, R.A. and M. Mandel. 1970. *Saprospira toviformis* nov. spec. *(Flexibacterales)* from a New Zealand seashore. Can. J. Microbiol. 16: 507–510.

Liebert, C.A., M.A. Hood, F.D. Deck, K. Bishop and D.K. Flaherty. 1984. Isolation and characterization of a new *Cytophaga* species implicated in a work-related lung disease. Appl. Environ. Microbiol. 48: 936–943.

Lieske, R. 1912. Untersuchungen über die Physiologie die denitrifizierenden Schwefelbakterien. Ber. Dtsch. Bot. Ges. 30: 12–22.

Lieske, R. 1919. Zur Ernährungsphysiologie der Eisenbakterien. Zentralbl. Bakteriol. Parasitenkd. Infektionskr. Hyg. Abt. II 49: 413–425.

Lighthart, B. 1975. A cluster analysis of some bacteria in the water column of Green Lake, Washington. Can. J. Microbiol. 21: 392–394.

Lillich, T.T. and R. Calmes. 1979. Cytochromes and dehydrogenases in membranes of a new human periodontal bacterial pathogen, *Capnocytophaga ochracea*. Arch. Oral Biol. 24: 699–702.

Lin, X.L. and R.H. White. 1986. Occurrence of coenzyme F420 and its γ-monoglutamyl derivative in nonmethanogenic archaebacteria. J. Bacteriol. 168: 444–448.

Link, H.F. 1809. Observationes in Ordines plantarum naturales. Disseratio Ima complectens. Anandrarum ordines Epiphytas, Mucedines Gastromycos et Fungos. Magaz. Ges. Nat. Freunde Berlin 3: 3–42.

Linnaeus, C. 1753. Species plantarum, exhibentes plantas rite Cognitas, and genera relatas, cum differentüs specificis, nominibus trivialibus, synonymis selectis, locis natalibus, secundum systema sexuale digestas. Tomus II, Stockholm, pp. 561–1200.

Lipscomb, J.D. and A.B. Hooper. 1982. Resolution of multiple heme centers of hydroxylamine oxidoreductase from *Nitrosomonas*. 1. Electron paramagnetic resonance spectroscopy. Biochemistry 21: 3965–3972.

Liston, J., W. Weibe and R.R. Colwell. 1963. Quantitative approach to the study of bacterial species. J. Bacteriol. 85: 1061–1070.

Liu, K.-C. and L.E. Casida, Jr. 1983. Survival of myxobacter strain 8 in natural soil in the presence and absence of host cells. Soil Biol. Biochem. 15: 551–555.

Liu, Y., D.R. Boone, R. Sleat and R.A. Mah. 1985. *Methanosarcina mazei* LYC, a new methanogenic isolate which produces a disaggregating enzyme. Appl. Environ. Microbiol. 49: 608–613.

Livingstone, D., T.M. Khoja and B.A. Whitton. 1983. Influence of phosphorus on physiology of a hair-forming blue-green alga (*Calothrix parietina*) from an upland stream. Phycologia 22: 345–350.

Livingstone, D. and B.A. Whitton. 1983. Influence of phosphorus on morphology of *Calothrix parietina* (Cyanophyta) in culture. Br. Phycol. J. 18: 29–38.

Livingstone, D. and B.A. Whitton. 1984. Water chemistry and phosphatase activity of the blue-green alga *Rivularia* in Upper Teesdale streams. J. Ecol. 72: 405–421.

Lobos, J.H., T.E. Chisolm, L.H. Bopp and D.S. Holmes. 1986. *Acidiphilium organosvorum* sp. nov., an acidophilic heterotroph isolated from a *Thiobacillus ferrooxidans* culture. Int. J. Syst. Bacteriol. 36: 139–144.

Lochhead, A.G. 1934. Bacteriological studies on the red discolouration of salted hides. Can. J. Res. 10: 275–286.

Lockhart, W.R. and J. Liston. 1970. Methods for Numerical Taxonomy. American Society for Microbiology, Washington, D.C.

Lodwick, D., H.N.M. Ross, J.G. Harris, J.W. Almond and W.D. Grant. 1986. *dam* methylation in the archaebacteria. J. Gen. Microbiol. 132: 3055–3059.

Loginova, N.V. and Y.A. Trotsenko. 1979. *Blastobacter viscosus*—a new species of autotrophic bacteria utilizing methanol. Mikrobiologiya 48: 644–651.

Løken, O. and R. Sirevåg. 1982. Evidence for the presence of the glyoxylate cycle in *Chloroflexus*. Arch. Microbiol. 132: 276–279.

London, J. 1963. *Thiobacillus intermedius* nov. sp. A novel type of facultative autotroph. Arch. Mikrobiol. 46: 329–337.

London, J., R. Celesk and P. Kolenbrander. 1982. Physiological and ecological properties of the oral Gram-negative gliding bacteria capable of attaching to hydroxyapatite. *In* Genco and Mergenhagen (Editors), Host-Parasite Interactions in Periodontal Disease. American Society for Microbiology, Washington, D.C., pp. 76–85.

London, J. and K. Kline. 1973. Aldolases of lactic acid bacteria: a case history in the use of an enzyme as an evolutionary marker. Bacteriol. Rev. 37: 453–478.

London, J. and S.C. Rittenberg. 1967. *Thiobacillus perometabolis* nov. sp., a nonautotrophic *Thiobacillus*. Arch. Microbiol. 59: 218–225.

Lovley, D.R., R.C. Greening and J.G. Ferry. 1984. Rapidly growing rumen methanogenic organism that synthesizes coenzyme M and has a high affinity for formate. Appl. Environ. Microbiol. 48: 81–87.

Lu, W.-P. and D.P. Kelly. 1984a. Purification and characterization of two essential cytochromes of the thiosulfate-oxidizing multienzyme system from *Thiobacillus* A2 (*T. versutus*). Biochim. Biophys. Acta 765: 106–117.

Lu, W.-P. and D.P. Kelly. 1984b. Properties and role of sulphite:cytochrome c oxidoreductase purified from *Thiobacillus versutus* (A2). J. Gen. Microbiol. 130: 1683–1692.

Lu, W.-P. and D.P. Kelly. 1984c. Oxidation of inorganic sulfur compounds by thiobacilli. *In* Crawford and Hanson (Editors), Microbial Growth on C₁ Compounds. American Society for Microbiology, Washington, D.C., pp. 34–41.

Lüderitz, R. and J.-H. Klemme. 1977. Isolierung und Charakterisierung eines membrangebundenen Pyruvatdehydrogenase-Komplexes aus dem phototrophen Bakterium *Rhodospirillum rubrum*. Z. Naturforsch. 32C: 351–361.

Ludwig, W., K.H. Schleifer, H. Reichenbach and E. Stackebrandt. 1983. A phylogenetic analysis of the myxobacteria *Myxococcus fulvus*, *Stigmatella aurantiaca*, *Cystobacter fuscus*, *Sorangium cellulosum* and *Nannocystis exedens*. Arch. Microbiol. 135: 58–62.

Luedemann, G.M. 1968. *Geodermatophilus*, a new genus of the *Dermatophilaceae* (*Actinomycetales*). J. Bacteriol. 96: 1848–1858.

Luehrsen, K., G.E. Fox, M.W. Kilpatrick, R.T. Walker, H. Domdey, G. Krupp and H.J. Gross. 1981. The nucleotide sequence of the 5S rRNA from the archaebacterium *Thermoplasma acidophilum*. Nucleic Acids Res. 9: 965–970.

Lueking, D., L. Pike and G. Sojka. 1976. Glycerol utilization by a mutant of *Rhodopseudomonas capsulata*. J. Bacteriol. 125: 750–752.

Lund, B.M. 1969. Properties of some pectolytic, yellow pigmented, Gram negative bacteria isolated from fresh cauliflowers. J. Appl. Bacteriol. 32: 60–67.

Lundin, S.J. 1968. A bacterial factor capable of solubilizing cholinesterase from plaice foot muscle. Acta Chem. Scand. 22: 2519–2528.

Lütters, S. 1985. Ultrastruktur von *Gallionella ferruginea* Ehrenberg und *Thiobacillus ferrooxidans*. Diplomarbeit, University of Braunschweig, pp. 1–104.

Lysenko, A.M., A.M. Semenov and L.V. Vasilyeva. 1984. DNA nucleotide composition of prosthecate bacteria with radial cell symmetry. Mikrobiologiya 53: 859–861.

Lysenko, A.M. and T.N. Zhilina. 1985. Taxonomic position of *Methanosarcina vacuolata* and *Methanococcus halophilus* determined by the technique of DNA-DNA hybridization. Mikrobiologiya 54: 501–502.

Macario, A.J.L. and E. Conway de Macario. 1983. Antigenic fingerprinting of methanogenic bacteria with polyclonal antibody probes. Syst. Appl. Microbiol. 4: 451–458.

Macario, A.J.L. and E. Conway de Macario (Editors). 1985. Monoclonal Antibodies against Bacteria, Vols. 1 and 2. Academic Press, New York.

Macario, A.J.L., C.B. Dugan and E. Conway de Macario. 1987. Antigenic mosaic of *Methanogenium* spp.: analysis with poly and monoclonal antibody probes. J. Bacteriol. 169: 666–669.

MacKay, R.M., L.B. Zablen, C.R. Woese and W.F. Doolittle. 1979. Homologies in processing and sequence between the 23S ribosomal ribonucleic acids of *Paracoccus denitrificans* and *Rhodopseudomonas sphaeroides*. Arch. Microbiol. 123: 165–172.

MacRae, J.H. and H.D. McCurdy. 1975. Ultrastructural studies of *Chondromyces crocatus* vegetative cells. Can. J. Microbiol. *21:* 1815-1926.

MacRae, T.H., W. Dobson and H.D. McCurdy. 1977. Fimbriation in gliding bacteria. Can. J. Microbiol. *23:* 1096-1108.

MacRae, T.H. and H.D. McCurdy. 1976. The isolation and characterization of gliding motility mutants of *Myxococcus xanthus.* Can. J. Microbiol. *22:* 1282-1292.

Madigan, M., S.S. Cox and R.E. Stegeman. 1984. Nitrogen fixation and nitrogenase activities in members of the family *Rhodospirillaceae.* J. Bacteriol. *157:* 73-78.

Madigan, M.T. 1976. Studies on the physiological ecology of *Chloroflexus aurantiacus,* a filamentous photosynthetic bacterium. Ph.D. thesis, University of Wisconsin, Madison, 239 pp.

Madigan, M.T. 1986. *Chromatium tepidum* sp. nov., a thermophilic photosynthetic bacterium of the family *Chromatiaceae.* Int. J. Syst. Bacteriol. *36:* 222-227.

Madigan, M.T. and T.D. Brock. 1975. Photosynthetic sulfide oxidation by *Chloroflexus aurantiacus,* a filamentous, photosynthetic, gliding bacterium. J. Bacteriol. *122:* 782-784.

Madigan, M.T. and T.D. Brock. 1977. CO_2 fixation in photosynthetically grown *Chloroflexus aurantiacus.* FEMS Microbiol. Lett. *1:* 301-304.

Madigan, M.T. and S.S. Cox. 1982. Nitrogen metabolism in *Rhodopseudomonas globiformis.* Arch. Microbiol. *133:* 6-10.

Madigan, M.T., S.S. Cox and R.A. Stegeman. 1984. Nitrogen fixation and nitrogenase activities in members of the family *Rhodospirillaceae.* J. Bacteriol. *157:* 73-78.

Madigan, M.T. and H. Gest. 1978. Growth of a photosynthetic bacterium anaerobically in darkness, supported by "oxidant-dependent" sugar fermentation. Arch. Microbiol. *117:* 119-122.

Madigan, M.T. and H. Gest. 1979. Growth of the photosynthetic bacterium *Rhodopseudomonas capsulata* chemoautotrophically in darkness with H_2 as the energy source. J. Bacteriol. *137:* 524-530.

Madigan, M.T., S.R. Petersen and T.D. Brock. 1974. Nutritional studies on *Chloroflexus,* a filamentous photosynthetic, gliding bacterium. Arch. Microbiol. *100:* 97-103.

Madigan, M.T., J.D. Wall and H. Gest. 1979. Dark anaerobic dinitrogen fixation by a photosynthetic microorganism. Science *204:* 1429-1430.

Maehr, H. and J.M. Smallheer. 1984. Rivularins. Preliminary synthetic studies. J. Org. Chem. *49:* 1549-1553.

Mague, T.H. and R.A. Lewin. 1974. *Leucothrix:* absence of demonstrable fixation of N_2. J. Gen. Microbiol. *85:* 365-367.

Mah, R.A. 1980. Isolation and characterization of *Methanococcus mazei.* Curr. Microbiol. *3:* 321-326.

Mah, R.A. and D.A. Kuhn. 1984a. Transfer of the type species of the genus *Methanococcus* to the genus *Methanosarcina,* naming it *Methanosarcina mazei* (Barker 1936) comb. nov. et emend. and conservation of the genus *Methanococcus* (Approved Lists 1980) with *Methanococcus vannielii* (Approved Lists 1980) as the type species. Int. J. Syst. Bacteriol. *34:* 263-265.

Mah, R.A. and D.A. Kuhn. 1984b. Rejection of the type species *Methanosarcina methanica* (Approved Lists 1980), conservation of the genus *Methanosarcina* with *Methanosarcina barkeri* (Approved Lists 1980) as the type species, and emendation of the genus *Methanosarcina.* Int. J. Syst. Bacteriol. *34:* 266-267.

Mah, R.A. and M.R. Smith. 1981. The methanogenic bacteria. *In* Starr, Stolp, Trüper, Balows and Schlegel (Editors), The Prokaryotes. A Handbook on Habitats, Isolation, and Identification of Bacteria. Springer-Verlag, Berlin, pp. 948-977.

Mah, R.A., M.R. Smith and L. Baresi. 1977. Isolation and characterization of a gas vacuolated methanosarcina. Abst. Annu. Meet. Am. Soc. Microbiol. Q29, p. 195.

Mah, R.A., M.R. Smith and L. Baresi. 1978. Studies on an acetate-fermenting strain of *Methanosarcina.* Appl. Environ. Microbiol. *35:* 1174-1184.

Mah, R.A., M.R. Smith, T. Ferguson and S. Zinder. 1981. Methanogenesis from H_2-CO_2, methanol, and acetate by *Methanosarcina. In* Dalton (Editor), Microbial Growth on C_1 Compounds. Heyden & Sons, Philadelphia, pp. 131-142.

Mahoney, R.P. and M.R. Edwards. 1966. Fine structure of *Thiobacillus thiooxidans.* J. Bacteriol. *92:* 487-495.

Maier, S. 1963. A cytological study of *Thioploca ingrica* Wislouch. Ph.D. dissertation, Ohio State University.

Maier, S. 1974. Genus III. *Thioploca* Lauterborn. *In* Buchanan and Gibbons (Editors), Bergey's Manual of Determinative Bacteriology, 8th Ed. The Williams and Wilkins Co., Baltimore, pp. 115-116.

Maier, S. 1980. Growth of *Thioploca ingrica* in a mixed culture system. Ohio J. Sci. *80:* 30-32.

Maier, S. 1984. Description of *Thioploca ingrica* sp. nov., nom. rev. Int. J. Syst. Bacteriol. *34:* 344-345.

Maier, S. and V.A. Gallardo. 1984a. Nutritional characteristics of two marine thioplocas determined by autoradiography. Arch. Microbiol. *139:* 218-220.

Maier, S. and V.A. Gallardo. 1984b. *Thioploca araucae* sp. nov. and *Thioploca chileae* sp. nov. Int. J. Syst. Bacteriol. *34:* 414-418.

Maier, S. and R.G.E. Murray. 1965. The fine structure of *Thioploca ingrica* and a comparison with *Beggiatoa.* Can. J. Microbiol. *11:* 645-655.

Maier, S. and W.C. Preissner. 1979. Occurrence of *Thioploca* in Lake Constance and Lower Saxony, Germany. Microb. Ecol. *5:* 117-119.

Malik, K.A. 1984. A new method for liquid nitrogen storage of phototrophic bacteria under anaerobic conditions. J. Microbiol. Methods *2:* 41-47.

Malofeeva, I.V., E.N. Kondratieva and A.B. Rubin. 1975. Ferredoxin-linked nitrate reductase from the phototrophic bacterium *Ectothiorhodospira shaposhnikovii.* FEBS Lett. *53:* 188-189.

Malofeeva, I.V. and D. Laush. 1976. Utilization of various nitrogen compounds by phototrophic bacteria. Microbiologiya *45:* 512-514.

Mandel, M., P. Hirsch and S.F. Conti. 1972. Deoxyribonucleic acid base compositions of hyphomicrobia. Arch. Mikrobiol. *81:* 289-294.

Mandel, M. and E.R. Leadbetter. 1965. Deoxyribonucleic acid base composition of myxobacteria. J. Bacteriol. *90:* 1795-1796.

Mandel, M., E.R. Leadbetter, N. Pfennig and H.G. Trüper. 1971. Deoxyribonucleic acid base composition of phototrophic bacteria. Int. J. Syst. Bacteriol. *21:* 222-230.

Mandel, M. and R.A. Lewin. 1969. Deoxyribonucleic acid base composition of flexibacteria. J. Gen. Microbiol. *71:* 171-178.

Mankin, A.S., V.K. Kagramanova, N.L. Teterina, P. Rubtsov, E.N. Belova, A.M. Kopylov, L.A. Baratova and A.A. Bogdanov. 1985. The nucleotide sequence of the gene coding for the 16S rRNA from the archaebacterium *Halobacterium halobium.* Gene *37:* 181-189.

Mann, S., R.B. Frankel and R.P. Blakemore. 1984a. Structure, morphology and crystal growth of bacterial magnetite. Nature *310:* 405-407.

Mann, S., T.T. Moench and R.J.P. Williams. 1984b. A high resolution electron microscopic investigation of bacterial magnetite; implications for crystal growth. Proc. R. Soc. London *221:* 385-393.

Mannheim, W. 1981a. Taxonomically useful test procedures pertaining to bacterial lipoquinones and associated functions, with special reference to *Flavobacterium* and *Cytophaga. In* Reichenbach and Weeks (Editors), The *Flavobacterium-Cytophaga* Group. Verlag Chemie, Weinheim, F.R.G., pp. 115-125.

Mannheim, W. 1981b. Lipoquinones of *Flavobacterium aquatile* strain Taylor F36. *In* Reichenbach and Weeks (Editors), The *Flavobacterium-Cytophaga* Group. Verlag Chemie, Weinheim, F.R.G., p. 125.

Manning, H.L. 1975. New medium for isolating iron-oxidizing and heterotrophic acidophilic bacteria from acid mine drainage. Appl. Microbiol. *30:* 1010-1016.

Maratea, D. and R.P. Blakemore. 1981. *Aquaspirillum magnetotacticum* sp. nov., a magnetic spirillum. Int. J. Syst. Bacteriol. *31:* 452-455.

Margulis, L., D.B.D. Grozovsky, J.F. Stolz, E.J. Gong-Collins, S. Lenk, D. Read and A. Lopes-Cortes. 1983. Distinctive microbial structures and the prephanerozoic fossil record. Precambrian Res. *20:* 443-477.

Markiewicz, Z., B. Glauner and U. Schwarz. 1983. Murein structure and lack of DD- and LD-carboxypeptidase activities in *Caulobacter crescentus.* J. Bacteriol. *156:* 649-655.

Markosyan, G.E. 1973. A new mixotrophic sulfur bacterium developing in acid media, *Thiobacillus organoparus* sp. n. Dokl. Akad. Nauk S.S.S.R. *211:* 1205-1208.

Marks, J.E., D.H. Lewis and G.S. Trevino. 1980. Mixed infection in columnaris disease of fish. J. Am. Vet. Med. Assoc. *177:* 811-814.

Marmur, J. and P. Doty. 1961. Thermal renaturation of deoxyribonucleic acids. J. Mol. Biol. *3:* 585-594.

Marmur, J. and P. Doty. 1962. Determination of the base composition of deoxyribonucleic acid from its thermal denaturation temperature. J. Mol. Biol. *5:* 109-118.

Marquez, M.C., A. Ventosa and F. Ruiz-Baquerro. 1987. A taxonomic study of heterotrophic halophilic and non-halophilic bacteria from a solar saltern. J. Gen. Microbiol. *133:* 45-56.

Marsh, R.M. and P.R. Norris. 1983. The isolation of some thermophilic, autotrophic iron- and sulphur-oxidizing bacteria. FEMS Microbiol. Lett. *17:* 311-315.

Marshall, J.J. 1973. Separation and characterization of the β-D-glucan hydrolases from a species of *Cytophaga.* Carbohydr. Res. *26:* 274-277.

Martin, A., S. Yeats, D. Janekovic, W.D. Reiter, W. Aicher and W. Zillig. 1984. SAV1, a temperate u.v.-inducible DNA virus-like particle from the archaebacterium *Sulfolobus acidocaldarius* isolate B12. EMBO J. *3:* 2165-2168.

Martin, H.H., H.J. Preusser and J.P. Verma. 1968. Über die Oberflächenstruktur von Myxobakterien II. Anionische Heteropolysaccharide als Baustoffe der Schleimhülle von *Cytophaga hutchinsonii* und *Sporocytophaga myxococcoides.* Arch. Mikrobiol. *62:* 72-84.

Martin, S., E. Sodergren, T. Masuda and D. Kaiser. 1978. Systematic isolation of transducing phages for *Myxococcus xanthus.* Virology 88: 44-53.

Martin, S.M. (Editor). 1963. Culture Collections: Perspectives and Problems. Proceedings of the Specialists' Conference on Culture Collections, Ottawa, 1962. University of Toronto Press, Toronto.

Martin, S.M. and V.B.D. Skerman. 1972. World Directory of Collections of Cultures of Microorganisms. Wiley-Interscience, New York.

Martin, S.M. and V. So. 1969. Solubilization of autoclaved feathers and wool by myxobacteria. Can. J. Microbiol. *15:* 1393-1397.

Martin, T.C. and J.T. Wyatt. 1974. Comparative physiology and morphology of six strains of stigonematacean blue-green algae. J. Phycol. *10:* 57-65.

Martiny, H. and H.-P. Koops. 1982. Incorporation of organic compounds into cell protein by lithotrophic, ammonia-oxidizing bacteria. Antonie van Leeuwenhoek J. Microbiol. Serol. *48:* 327-336.

Mashimo, P.A., Y. Yamamoto, M. Nakamura and J. Slots. 1983. Selective recovery of oral *Capnocytophaga* spp. with sheep blood agar containing bacitracin and polymyxin B. J. Clin. Microbiol. *17:* 187-191.

Masters, R.A. and M.T. Madigan. 1983. Nitrogen metabolism in the phototrophic bacteria *Rhodocyclus purpureus* and *Rhodospirillum tenue*. J. Bacteriol. *155:* 222-227.

Matheron, R. and R. Baulaigue. 1972. Bactéries photosynthétiques sulfureases marines. Arch. Mikrobiol. *86:* 291-304.

Mathrani, I.M. and D.R. Boone. 1985. Isolation and characterization of a moderately halophilic methanogen from a solar saltern. Appl. Environ. Microbiol. *50:* 140-143.

Matin, A. 1978. Organic nutrition of chemolithotrophic bacteria. Annu. Rev. Microbiol. *32:* 433-468.

Matin, A., F.J. Kahan and R.H. Leefeldt. 1980. Growth factor requirement of *Thiobacillus novellus*. Arch. Microbiol. *124:* 91-95.

Matsuda, T., J. Endo, N. Osakube, A. Tonomura and T. Arii. 1983. Morphology and structure of biogenic magnetite particles. Nature *302:* 411-412.

Matzen, N. and P. Hirsch. 1982a. Improved growth conditions for *Hyphomicrobium* sp. B-522 and two additional strains. Arch. Microbiol. *131:* 32-35.

Matzen, N. and P. Hirsch. 1982b. Continuous culture and synchronization of *Hyphomicrobium* sp. B-522. Arch. Microbiol. *132:* 96-99.

Maxam, A.M. and W. Gilbert. 1977. A new method for sequencing DNA. Proc. Natl. Acad. Sci. U.S.A. *74:* 560-564.

Mayberry-Carson, K.J., I.L. Roth, J.L. Harris and P.F. Smith. 1974. Scanning electron microscopy of *Thermoplasma acidophilum*. J. Bacteriol. *120:* 1472-1475.

Mayer, D. 1967. Ernahrungsphysiologische Untersuchungen an *Archangium violaceum*. Arch. Mikrobiol. *58:* 186-200.

Mayer, H., E. Bock and J. Weckesser. 1983. 2,3-diamino-2,3-dideoxyglucose containing lipid A in the *Nitrobacter* strain X$_{14}$. FEMS Microbiol. Lett. *17:* 93-96.

Mayer, H. and H. Reichenbach. 1978. Restriction endonucleases: general survey procedures and survey of gliding bacteria. J. Bacteriol. *136:* 708-713.

Mayer, H., P.V. Salimath, O. Holst and J. Weckesser. 1984. Unusual lipid A types in phototrophic bacteria and related species. Rev. Infect. Dis. *6:* 542-545.

Mayfield, D.C. and A.S. Kester. 1972. Some physiological studies on *Vitreoscilla stercoraria*. J. Bacteriol. *112:* 1052-1056.

Mayfield, D.C. and A.S. Kester. 1975. Nutrition of *Vitreoscilla stercoraria*. Can. J. Microbiol. *21:* 1947-1951.

Mays, T.D., L.V. Holdeman, W.E.C. Moore, M. Rogosa and J.L. Johnson. 1982. Taxonomy of the genus *Veillonella* Prévot. Int. J. Syst. Bacteriol. *32:* 28-36.

Mazé, P. 1903. Sur la fermentation formènique et le ferment qui la produit. C.R. Hebd. Sèanc. Acad. Sci. (Paris) *137:* 887-889.

Mazé, P. 1915. Ferment formènique. Fermentation formènique de l'acétone. Procédé de culture simple du ferment formènique. C.R. Hebd. Soc. Biol. (Paris) *78:* 398-405.

McCarthy, B.J. and E.T. Bolton. 1963. An approach to the measurement of genetic relatedness among organisms. Proc. Natl. Acad. Sci. U.S.A. *50:* 156-164.

McClure, M. and W.G. Wyckoff. 1982. Ultrastructural characteristics of *Sulfolobus acidocaldarius*. J. Gen. Microbiol. *128:* 433-437.

McCowan, R.P., K.-J. Cheng and J.W. Costerton. 1979. Colonization of a portion of the bovine tongue by unusual filamentous bacteria. Appl. Environ. Microbiol. *37:* 1224-1229.

McCurdy, H.D. 1963. A method for the isolation of myxobacteria in culture. Can. J. Microbiol. *9:* 282-285.

McCurdy, H.D. 1964. Growth and fruiting body formation of *Chondromyces crocatus* in pure culture. Can. J. Microbiol. *10:* 935-936.

McCurdy, H.D. 1969a. Light and electron microscope studies on the fruiting bodies of *Chondromyces crocatus*. Arch. Mikrobiol. *65:* 380-390.

McCurdy, H.D. 1969b. Studies on the taxonomy of the *Myxobacterales*. I. Record of Canadian isolates and survey of methods. Can. J. Microbiol. *15:* 1453-1461.

McCurdy, H.D. 1970. Studies on the taxonomy of the *Myxobacterales*. II. *Polyangium* and the demise of the *Sorangiaceae*. Int. J. Syst. Bacteriol. *20:* 283-296.

McCurdy, H.D. 1971a. Studies on the taxonomy of the *Myxobacterales*. III. *Chondromyces* and *Stigmatella*. Int. J. Syst. Bacteriol. *21:* 40-49.

McCurdy, H.D. 1971b. Studies on the Taxonomy of the *Myxobacterales*. IV. *Melittangium*. Int. J. Syst. Bacteriol. *21:* 50-54.

McCurdy, H.D. 1974. Order I. *Myxobacterales*. Thaxter emend Stanier 1957, 854. The fruiting myxobacteria. *In* Buchanan and Gibbons (Editors), Bergey's Manual of Determinative Bacteriology, 8th Ed. The Williams and Wilkins Co., Baltimore, pp. 76-98.

McCurdy, H.D., Jr. and W. Hodgson. 1974. The isolation of blue-green bacteria in pure culture. Can. J. Microbiol. *20:* 272-273.

McCurdy, H.D. and B.T. Khouw. 1969. Studies on *Stigmatella brunnea*. Can. J. Microbiol. *15:* 731-738.

McCurdy, H.D. and T.H. MacRae. 1974. Xanthacin. A bacteriocin from *Myxococcus xanthus* fb. Can. J. Microbiol. *20:* 131-135.

McCurdy, H.D. and S. Wolf. 1967. Deoxyribonucleic acid base compositions of fruiting *Myxobacterales*. Can. J. Microbiol. *13:* 1707-1708.

McEwan, A.G., S.J. Ferguson and J.B. Jackson. 1983. Electron flow to dimethylsulphoxide or trimethyl-*N*-oxide generates a membrane potential in *Rhodopseudomonas capsulata*. Arch. Microbiol. *136:* 300-305.

McGowan, V.F. and V.B.D. Skerman (Editors). 1982. World Directory of Collections of Cultures of Microorganisms, 2nd Ed. World Data Centre on

Microorganisms, University of Queensland, Brisbane.

McGregor-Shaw, J.B., K.B. Easterbrook and R.P. McBride. 1973. A bacterium with echinuliform (nonprosthecate) appendages. Int. J. Syst. Bacteriol. *23:* 267-270.

McGuire, R.F. 1984. A numerical taxonomic study of *Nostoc* and *Anabaena*. J. Phycol. *20:* 454-460.

McInerney, M.J., M.P. Bryant, R.B. Hespell and J.W. Costerton. 1981. *Syntrophomonas wolfei* gen. nov. sp. nov., an anaerobic, syntrophic, fatty acid-oxidizing bacterium. Appl. Environ. Microbiol. *41:* 1029-1039.

McLachlan, J. 1973. Growth media—marine. *In* Stein (Editor), Handbook of Phycological Methods: Culture Methods and Growth Measurements. Cambridge University Press, Cambridge, New York, pp. 25-51.

McLachlan, J.L., U.T. Hammer and P.R. Gorham. 1963. Observations on the growth and colony habits of ten strains of *Aphanizomenon flos-aquae*. Phycologia *2:* 157-168.

McNeil, K.E. and V.B.D. Skerman. 1972. Examination of myxobacteria by scanning electron microscopy. Int. J. Syst. Bacteriol. *22:* 243-250.

Mechsner, K. 1957. Physiologische und morphologische Untersuchungen an Chlorobakterien. Arch. Mikrobiol. *26:* 32-51.

Meckel, R.A. and A.S. Kester. 1980. Extractability of carotenoid pigments from non-photosynthetic bacteria with solvents and detergents: implications for the location and binding of pigments. J. Gen. Microbiol. *120:* 111-116.

Meffert, M.E. and T.P. Chang. 1978. The isolation of planktonic blue-green algae (*Oscillatoria* species). Arch. Hydrobiol. *82:* 231-239.

Mehra, I.J., G.M. Warke and S.A. Dhala. 1967. Effect of zinc salts on *Cytophaga* spp. Indian J. Microbiol. *7:* 75-78.

Mendoza, N.S. and A. Amemura. 1983. (1→2)-β-D-glucan-hydrolyzing enzymes in *Cytophaga arvensicola*: partial purification and some properties of endo-(1→2)-β-D-glucanase specific for (1→2)- and (1→3)-linkages. J. Ferment. Technol. *61:* 473-481.

Mertens, K.H. 1822. *In* Jürgens, Algae Aquaticae. Decas XV, No. 4.

Metchnikoff, E. 1888. *Pasteuria ramosa* un representant des bactéries a division longitudinale. Ann. Inst. Pasteur (Paris) *2:* 165-170.

Mevius, W., Jr. 1953. Beiträge zur Kenntnis von *Hyphomicrobium vulgare* Stutzer and Hartleb. Arch. Mikrobiol. *19:* 1-29.

Meyer, D.J. and C.W. Jones. 1973. Distribution of cytochromes in bacteria: relationship to general physiology. Int. J. Syst. Bacteriol. *23:* 459-467.

Meyer, O., J. Lalucat and H.G. Schlegel. 1980. *Pseudomonas carboxydohydrogena* (Sanjieva and Zavarzin) comb. nov., a monotrichous, nonbudding, strictly aerobic, carbon monoxide-utilizing hydrogen bacterium previously assigned to *Seliberia*. Int. J. Syst. Bacteriol. *30:* 189-195.

Meyer, R.C. 1961. Studies on the cellulose-digesting *Cytophaga* of the soil. Ph.D. thesis, Ohio State University, Columbus, 101 pp.

Meyer, T.E. 1982. Electron transport proteins and taxonomic position of the *Ectothiorhodospira* species including *E. halophila*, *E. halochloris*, *E. abdelmalekii* and *E. vacuolata*. Abstract A 46, IV. Int. Symp. Photosynthetic Procaryotes, Bombannes-Bordeaux.

Meyer, T.E., R.G. Bartsch, M.A. Cusanovich and J.H. Mathewson. 1968. The cytochrome of *Chlorobium thiosulfatophilum*. Biochim. Biophys. Acta *153:* 854-861.

Mezzino, M.J., W.R. Strohl and J.M. Larkin. 1984. Characterization of *Beggiatoa alba*. Arch. Microbiol. *137:* 139-144.

Michalski, T.J., J.E. Hunt, M.K. Bowman, U. Smith, K. Bardeen, H. Gest, J.R. Norris and J.J. Katz. 1987. Bacteriopheophytin *g*: properties and some speculations on a possible primary role for bacteriochlorophylls *b* and *g* in the biosynthesis of chlorophylls. Proc. Natl. Acad. Sci. U.S.A. *84:* 2570-2574.

Michel, H., D.-C. Neugebauer and D. Oesterhelt. 1980. The 2-D crystalline cell wall of *Sulfolobus acidocaldarius*: structure, solubilization and reassembly. *In* Baumeister and Vogell (Editors), Electron Microscopy at Molecular Dimension. Springer-Verlag, Heidelberg, pp. 27-35.

Middleton, C.A. and J.L. Pate. 1976. Isolation and partial characterization of some new bacteriophages active against *Asticcacaulis* strains. Int. J. Syst. Bacteriol. *26:* 269-277.

Migula, W. 1894. Ueber ein neues System der Bakterien. Arb. Bakteriol. Inst. Karlsruhe *1:* 235-238.

Migula, W. 1900. System der Bakterien, Vol. 2. Gustav Fischer, Jena.

Milde, K. and E. Bock. 1984. Isolation and partial characterization of inner and outer membrane fractions of *Nitrobacter hamburgensis*. FEMS Microbiol. Lett. *21:* 137-141.

Miller, M.M. and N.J. Lang. 1971. The effect of aging on thylakoid configuration and granular inclusions in *Gloeotrichia*. *In* Parker and Lang (Editors), Contributions in Phycology. Allen Lane Press, Lawrence, Kansas, pp. 53-58.

Miller, T.L. and M.J. Wolin. 1974. A serum bottle modification of the Hungate technique for cultivating obligate anaerobes. Appl. Microbiol. *27:* 985-987.

Miller, T.L. and M.J. Wolin. 1982. Enumeration of *Methanobrevibacter smithii* in human feces. Arch. Microbiol. *131:* 14-18.

Miller, T.L. and M.J. Wolin. 1983. Oxidation of hydrogen and reduction of methanol to methane is the sole energy source for a methanogen isolated from human feces. J. Bacteriol. *153:* 1051-1055.

Miller, T.L. and M.J. Wolin. 1985a. *Methanosphaera stadtmaniae* gen. nov.; sp. nov.; a species that forms methane by reducing methanol with hydrogen. Arch. Microbiol. *141:* 116-122.

Miller, T.L. and M.J. Wolin. 1985b. *In* Validation of the publication of new names and new combinations previously effectively published outside the IJSB. List

19. Int. J. Syst. Bacteriol. *35:* 535.

Miller, T.L. and M.J. Wolin. 1986. Methanogens in human and animal intestinal tracts. Syst. Appl. Microbiol. *7:* 223–229.

Miller, T.L., M.J. Wolin, E. Conway de Macario and A.J.L. Macario. 1982. Isolation of *Methanobrevibacter smithii* from human feces. Appl. Environ. Microbiol. *43:* 227–232.

Miller, T.L., M.J. Wolin, Z. Hongxue and M.P. Bryant. 1986b. Characteristics of methanogens isolated from bovine rumen. Appl. Environ. Microbiol. *51:* 201–202.

Miller, T.L., M.J. Wolin and E.A. Kusel. 1986a. Isolation and characterization of methanogens from animals. Syst. Appl. Microbiol. *8:* 234–238.

Miller, V. 1923. Zum Systematik der Gattung *Anabaena* Bory. Arch. Protistol. *2:* 116–126.

Minges, C.G., J.A. Titus and W.R. Strohl. 1983. Plasmid DNA in colorless filamentous gliding bacteria. Arch. Microbiol. *134:* 38–44.

Mink, R.W. and P.R. Dugan. 1977. Tentative identification of methanogenic bacteria by fluorescence microscopy. Appl. Environ. Microbiol. *33:* 713–717.

Minnikin, D.E. and M. Goodfellow. 1980. Lipid composition in the classification and identification of acid fast bacteria. *In* Goodfellow and Board (Editors), Microbiological Classification and Identification. Academic Press, London, New York, pp. 189–256.

Mishustin, E.N. 1938. Cellulose-decomposing myxobacteria. Mikrobiologiya *7:* 427–444.

Mishustin, E.N. 1942. *Chondrococcus coralloides* (Thaxter) and factors influencing its cycle of development. Mikrobiologiya *11:* 178–194 (in Russian with English summary).

Mitchell, T.G., M.S. Hendrie and J.M. Shewan. 1969. The taxonomy, differentiation and identification of *Cytophaga* species. J. Appl. Bacteriol. *32:* 40–50.

Mitra, A.K. and D.C. Pandey. 1966. On a new genus of the blue-green alga *Chlorogloeopsis* with remarks on the heterocysts in the alga. Phykos *5:* 106–114.

Mitsui, A., S. Kumazawa, T. Takahashi, H. Ikemoto, S. Cao and T. Arai. 1986. Strategy by which nitrogen-fixing unicellular cyanobacteria grow photoautotrophically. Nature *323:* 730–732.

Mitsuoka, T. 1980. A Color Atlas of Anaerobic Bacteria. Gyōbunsha, Tokyo, Japan.

Miyazawa, Y. and C.A. Thomas. 1965. Composition of short segments of DNA molecules. J. Mol. Biol. *11:* 223–237.

Mizoguchi, T., T. Sato and T. Okabe. 1976. New sulfur-oxidizing bacteria capable of growing heterotrophically, *Thiobacillus rubellus* nov. sp. and *Thiobacillus delicatus* nov. sp. J. Ferment. Technol. *54:* 181–191.

Moench, T.T. 1978. Distribution, isolation and characterization of a magnetotactic bacterium. Thesis, Indiana University, pp. 1–109.

Moench, T.T. and W.A. Konetzka. 1978. A novel method for the isolation and study of a magnetotactic bacterium. Arch. Microbiol. *119:* 203–212.

Molisch, H. 1906. Zwei neue Purpurbakterien mit Schwebe körperchen. Bot. Ztg. Abt. I *64:* 223–232.

Molisch, H. 1907. Die Purpurbakterien nach neueren Untersuchungen. Gustav Fischer Verlag, Jena, pp. 1–95.

Molisch, H. 1909. *Siderocapsa treubii* Molisch, eine neue, weit verbreitete Eisenbakterie. Ann. Jard. Bot. Buitenzorg. Ser. 2 Suppl. *3:* 29–34.

Molisch, H. 1910. Die Eisenbakterien. Gustav Fischer Verlag, Jena, pp. 1–83.

Molisch, H. 1910. *Siderocapsa treubii* Molisch, eine neue, weit verbreitete Eisenbakterie. Ann. Jard. Bot. Buitenzorg Suppl. *3:* 29–34.

Molisch, H. 1912. Neue farblose Schwefelbakterien. Zentralbl. Bakteriol. Parasitenkd. Infektionskr. Hyg. Abt. II *33:* 55–62.

Molisch, H. 1925. Botanische Beobachtungen in Japan. VIII. Die Eisenorganismen Japan. Sci. Rep. Tohoku Imp. Univ. Ser. IV Biol. *1:* 135–168.

Moll, G. and R. Ahrens. 1970. Ein neuer Fimbrientyp. Arch. Mikrobiol. *70:* 361–368.

Mollenhauer, D. 1970. Beiträge zm Kenntnis der Gattung *Nostoc*. Waldemar Kramer, Frankfurt a. Main. Abh. Senckenb. Naturforsch. Ges. *524:* 1–80.

Mollenhauer, H.H. 1964. Plastic embedding mixtures for use in electron microscopy. Stain Technol. *39:* 111–141.

Møller, M.M., L.P. Nielsen and B.B. Jørgensen. 1985. Oxygen responses and mat formation by *Beggiatoa* spp. Appl. Environ. Microbiol. *50:* 373–382.

Möller, U. 1983. Serologische Untersuchungen zur Taxonomie nitrifizierender Bakterien. Diplomarbeit, FB Biol., University of Hamburg.

Moore, R.L. 1977. Ribosomal ribonucleic acid cistron homologies among *Hyphomicrobium* and various other bacteria. Can. J. Microbiol. *23:* 478–481.

Moore, R.L. 1981a. The genera *Hyphomicrobium*, *Pedomicrobium*, and *Hyphomonas*. *In* Starr, Stolp, Trüper, Balows and Schlegel (Editors), The Prokaryotes. A Handbook on Habitats, Isolation, and Identification of Bacteria. Springer-Verlag, Berlin, pp. 480–487.

Moore, R.L. 1981b. The biology of *Hyphomicrobium* and other prosthecate, budding bacteria. Annu. Rev. Microbiol. *35:* 567–594.

Moore, R.L. and P. Hirsch. 1972. Deoxyribonucleic acid base sequence homologies of some budding and prosthecate bacteria. J. Bacteriol. *110:* 256–261.

Moore, R.L. and P. Hirsch. 1973. Nuclear apparatus of *Hyphomicrobium*. J. Bacteriol. *116:* 1447–1455.

Moore, R.L. and B.J. McCarthy. 1969. Base sequence homology studies and renaturation studies of the deoxyribonucleic acid of extremely halophilic bacteria. J. Bacteriol. *99:* 255–262.

Moore, R.L., J. Schmidt, J. Poindexter and J.T. Staley. 1978. Deoxyribonucleic acid homology among the caulobacters. Int. J. Syst. Bacteriol. *28:* 349–353.

Moore, R.L. and J.T. Staley. 1976. Deoxyribonucleic acid homology of *Prosthecomicrobium* and *Ancalomicrobium* strains. Int. J. Syst. Bacteriol. *26:* 283–285.

Moore, R.L., R.M. Weiner and R. Gebers. 1984. Genus *Hyphomonas* Pongratz 1957 nom. rev. emend., *Hyphomonas polymorpha* Pongratz 1957 nom. rev. emend., and *Hyphomonas neptunium* (Leifson 1964) comb. nov. emend. (*Hyphomicrobium neptunium*). Int. J. Syst. Bacteriol. *34:* 71–73.

Moore, W.E.C., D.E. Hash, L.V. Holdeman and E.P. Cato. 1980. Polyacrylamide slab gel electrophoresis of soluble proteins for studies of bacterial floras. Appl. Environ. Microbiol. *39:* 900–907.

Moore, W.E.C. and L.V. Holdeman. 1974. Human fecal flora: the normal flora of 20 Japanese-Hawaiians. Appl. Microbiol. *27:* 961–979.

Morel, F.M.M. and J.G. Rueter. 1979. Aquil: a chemically defined phytoplankton culture medium for trace metal studies. J. Phycol. *15:* 135–141.

Morgan, H.W. and M. Daniel. 1982. Isolation of a new species of sulphur reducing extreme thermophile. Proc. XIII Int. Congr. Microbiol. Boston, Massachusetts, U.S.A., August 1982.

Morii, H., M. Nishihara and Y. Koga. 1983. Isolation, characterization and physiology of a new formate-assimilable methanogenic strain (A2) of *Methanobrevibacter arboriphilus*. Agric. Biol. Chem. *47:* 2781–2789.

Morita, R.Y., R. Iturriaga and V.A. Gallardo. 1981. *Thioploca*: methylotroph and significance in the food chain. Kiel. Meeresforsch. *5:* 384–389.

Morita, R.Y. and P.W. Stave. 1963. Electron micrograph of an ultrathin section of *Beggiatoa*. J. Bacteriol. *85:* 940–942.

Morren, C. 1838. Mém. Acad. R. Belg. *11:* 5–20.

Morris, D.W., S.R. Ogden-Swift, V. Virrankoski-Castrodeza, K. Ainley and J.H. Parish. 1978. Transduction of *Myxococcus virescens* by coliphage P1CM: generation of plasmids containing both phage and myxococcus genes. J. Gen. Microbiol. *107:* 73–83.

Morrison, C., J. Cornick, G. Shum and B. Zwicker. 1981. Microbiology and histopathology of "saddleback" disease of underyearling Atlantic salmon, *Salmo salar* L. J. Fish Dis. *4:* 243–258.

Morth, S. and B.J. Tindall. 1985. Variation of polar lipid composition within haloalkaliphilic archaebacteria. Syst. Appl. Microbiol. *6:* 247–250.

Moss, C.W. and S.B. Dees. 1978. Cellular fatty acids of *Flavobacterium meningosepticum* and *Flavobacterium* species group IIb. J. Clin. Microbiol. *8:* 772–774.

Mouches, C., J.C. Vignault, J.G. Tully, R.F. Whitcomb and J.M. Bové. 1979. Characterization of spiroplasmas by one- and two-dimensional protein analysis on polyacrylamide slab gels. Curr. Microbiol. *2:* 69–74.

Mountfort, D.O. and M.P. Bryant. 1982. Isolation and characterization of an anaerobic syntrophic benzoate-degrading bacterium from sewage sludge. Arch. Microbiol. *133:* 249–256.

Muehlstein, L. and R.W. Castenholz. 1983. Sheath pigment formation in blue-green alga, *Lyngbya aestuarii*, as an adaptation to high light. Biol. Bull. *165:* 521–522 (abstract).

Mulder, E.G. 1964. Iron bacteria, particularly those of the *Sphaerotilus-Leptothrix* group, and industrial problems. J. Appl. Bacteriol. *27:* 151–173.

Mulder, E.G. and M.H. Deinema. 1981. The sheathed bacteria. *In* Starr, Stolp, Trüper, Balows, and Schlegel (Editors), The Prokaryotes. A Handbook on Habitats, Isolation, and Identification of Bacteria. Springer-Verlag, Berlin, pp. 425–440.

Mulder, E.G. and W.L. van Veen. 1963. Investigations on the *Sphaerotilus-Leptothrix* group. Antonie van Leeuwenhoek J. Microbiol. Serol. *29:* 121–153.

Mulder, E.G. and W.L. van Veen. 1965. Anreicherung von Organismen der *Sphaerotilus-Leptothrix*-Gruppe. Aus: Anreicherungskultur und Mutantenauslese, Symp. Göttingen, 1964. Zentralbl. Bakteriol. Parasitenkd. Infektionskr. Hyg. Abt. I Suppl. *1:* 28–46.

Mulder, E.G. and W.L. van Veen. 1968. Effect of microorganisms on the transformation of mineral fractions in soil. *In* Ninth International Congress on Soil Science Transactions, Vol. 4. Adelaide, Australia, pp. 651–661.

Mulder, E.G. and W. van Veen. 1974. Genus *Streptothrix*. *In* Buchanan and Gibbons (Editors), Bergey's Manual of Determinative Bacteriology, 8th Ed. The Williams and Wilkins Co., Baltimore, p. 133.

Mullakhanbhai, M.F. and H. Larsen. 1975. *Halobacterium volcanii* sp. nov.: a Dead Sea halobacterium with a moderate salt requirement. Arch. Microbiol. *104:* 207–214.

Müller, O.F. 1773. Vermium Terrestrium et Fluviatilium, seu Animalium Infusoriorum, Helminthicorum et Testaceorum, non Marionorum. Succincta Historia *1:* 1–135.

Müller, R. 1911. Zur Stellung der Krankheitserreger im Natursystem. Muench. Med. Wochenschr. *58:* 2246–2247.

Müller, V., M. Blaut and G. Gottschalk. 1986. Utilization of methanol plus hydrogen by *Methanosarcina barkeri* for methanogenesis and growth. Appl. Environ. Microbiol. *52:* 269–274.

Mullings, R. and J.H. Parish. 1981. Distribution of cellulose degrading Gram-negative bacteria. *In* Reichenbach and Weeks (Editors), The *Flavobacterium-Cytophaga* Group. Verlag Chemie, Weinheim, F.R.G., pp. 179–187.

Mullings, R. and J.H. Parish. 1984. Mesophilic aerobic Gram-negative cellulose degrading bacteria from aquatic habitats and soils. J. Appl. Bacteriol. *57:* 455–468.

Mur, L.R. 1983. Some aspects of the ecophysiology of cyanobacteria. Ann. Microbiol. (Inst. Pasteur) *134B:* 61–72.

Murayama, Y., P.A. Mashimo, L.A. Tabak, M.J. Levine and S.A. Ellison. 1982. Isolation and partial characterization of a genus common antigen and species specific antigen of *Capnocytophaga*. Jpn. J. Med. Sci. Biol. *35:* 153–170.

Murray, P.A. and S.H. Zinder. 1984. Nitrogen fixation by a methanogenic archaebacterium. Nature *312:* 284–285.

Murray, P.A. and S.H. Zinder. 1985. Nutritional requirements of *Methanosarcina* sp. strain TM-1. Appl. Environ. Microbiol. *50:* 49–55.

Murray, R.G.E. 1962. Fine structure and taxonomy of bacteria. *In* Ainsworth and Sneath (Editors), Microbial Classification. Cambridge University Press, Cambridge.

Murray, R.G.E. 1968. Microbial structure as an aid to microbial classification and taxonomy. Spisy (Faculte des Sciences de l'Universite J.E. Purkyne, Brno) *43:* 249–252.

Murray, R.G.E. 1974. A place for bacteria in the living world. *In* Buchanan and Gibbons (Editors), Bergey's Manual of Determinative Bacteriology, 8th Ed. The Williams and Wilkins Co., Baltimore.

Murray, R.G.E. and S.W. Watson. 1965. Structure of *Nitrosocystis oceanus* and comparison with *Nitrosomonas* and *Nitrobacter.* J. Bacteriol. *89:* 1594–1609.

Mylroie, R.L. and R.E. Hungate. 1954. Experiments on the methane bacteria in sludge. Can. J. Microbiol. *1:* 55–64.

Nadson, G.A. 1906. The morphology of inferior algae. III: *Chlorobium limicola* Nads., the green chlorophyll bearing microbe. Bull. Jard. Bot. St. Petersb. *6:* 190.

Nägeli, C. 1847. Die neuern Algensysteme und versuch zur Begrundung eines eigenen Systems der Algen und Florideen. Neue Denckschriften der allgemeinen schweizerischen Gesellschaft für die gesammten Naturwissenschaften, Vol. 9, Zurich.

Nägeli, C. 1849. Galtungen einzelliger Algen physiologisch und systematisch bearbeitet. Neue Denckschriften der allgemeinen schweizerischen Gesellschaft für die gesammten Naturwissenschaften, Vol. 10, Zurich.

Nakamura, M. and J. Slots. 1981. Aminopeptidase activity of *Capnocytophaga.* J. Periodontal Res. *17:* 597–603.

Namsaraev, B.B. and G.A. Zavarzin. 1972. Trophic relationship in a methane-oxidizing culture. Mikrobiologiya *41:* 999–1006 (English translation: 887–892).

Namsaraev, B.B. and G.A. Zavarzin. 1974. Growth of the budding bacterium "*tetrahedron*" on monocarbon compounds. Microbiologiya *43:* 406–409.

Napier, E.J. 1966. Microbiological Process. British Patent No. 1,048,887, Nov. 23 (Glaxo Laboratories).

Nathansohn, A. 1902. Über eine neue Gruppe von Schwefelbakterien und ihren Stoffwechsel. Mitt. Zool. Sta. Neapel. *15:* 655–680.

Naumann, E. 1921. Untersuchungen über die Eisenorganismen Schwedens. I. Die Erscheinungen der Sideroplastie in den Gewässern des Teichgebietes Aneboda. K. Sven. Vetenskapsakad. Handl. *62:* 1–68.

Naumann, E. 1929. Die eisenspeichernden Bakterien. Kritische Übersicht der bisher bekannten Formen. Zentralbl. Bakteriol. Parasitenkd. Infektionskr. Hyg. Abt. II *78:* 512–515.

Nealson, K.H. 1978. The isolation and characterization of marine bacteria which catalyze manganese oxidation. Environ. Biogeochem. Geomicrobiol. *3:* 847–858.

Nealson, K.H. 1983a. The microbial iron cycle. *In* Krumbein (Editor), Microbial Geochemistry. Blackwell Scientific, Oxford, pp. 159–190

Nealson, K.H. 1983b. The microbial manganese cycle. *In* Krumbein (Editor), Microbial Geochemistry. Blackwell Scientific, Oxford, pp. 191–222.

Nealson, K.H. and J. Ford. 1980. Surface enhancement of bacterial manganese oxidation: implications for aquatic environments. Geomicrobiol. J. *2:* 21–37.

Nelson, D.C. 1989. Physiology and biochemistry of filamentous sulfur bacteria. *In* Schlegel and Bowien (Editors), Autotrophic Bacteria. Science Tech Publishers, Madison, Wisconsin, in press.

Nelson, D.C. and R.W. Castenholz. 1981a. Use of reduced sulfur compounds by *Beggiatoa* sp. J. Bacteriol. *147:* 140–154.

Nelson, D.C. and R.W. Castenholz. 1981b. Organic nutrition of *Beggiatoa* sp. J. Bacteriol. *147:* 236–247.

Nelson, D.C. and R.W. Castenholz. 1982. Light responses of *Beggiatoa.* Arch. Microbiol. *131:* 146–155.

Nelson, D.C. and H.W. Jannasch. 1983. Chemoautotrophic growth of a marine *Beggiatoa* in sulfide-gradient cultures. Arch. Microbiol. *136:* 262–269.

Nelson, D.C., B.B. Jørgensen and N.P. Revsbech. 1986b. Growth pattern and yield of chemoautotrophic *Beggiatoa* sp. in oxygen-sulfide microgradients. Appl. Environ. Microbiol. *52:* 225–233.

Nelson, D.C., N.P. Revsbech and B.B. Jørgensen. 1986a. The microoxic/anoxic niche of *Beggiatoa:* a microelectrode survey of marine and freshwater strains. Appl. Environ. Microbiol. *52:* 161–168.

Nelson, D.C., J.B. Waterbury and H.W. Jannasch. 1982. Nitrogen fixation and nitrate utilization by marine and freshwater *Beggiatoa.* Arch. Microbiol. *133:* 172–177.

Nelson, D.C., C.A. Williams, B.A. Farah, and J.M. Shively. 1989. Occurrence and regulation of Calvin cycle enzymes in non-autotrophic *Beggiatoa* strains. Arch. Microbiol., in press.

Neutzling, O., J.F. Imhoff and H.G. Trüper. 1984a. *Rhodopseudomonas adriatica* spec. nov., a new species of the *Rhodospirillaceae,* dependent on reduced sulfur compounds. Arch. Microbiol. *137:* 256–261.

Neutzling, O., J.F. Imhoff and H.G. Trüper. 1984b. *In* Validation of the publication of new names and new combinations previously effectively published outside the IJSB. List No. 16. Int. J. Syst. Bacteriol. *34:* 503–504.

Neutzling, O. and H.G. Trüper. 1982. Assimilatory sulfur metabolism in *Rhodopseudomonas sulfoviridis.* Arch. Microbiol. *133:* 145–148.

Newcomb, E.H. and T.D. Pugh. 1975. Blue-green algae associated with ascidians of the Great Barrier Reef. Nature (London) *253:* 533–534.

Newman, M.G., V.L. Sutter, M.J. Pickett, U. Blachman, J.R. Greenwood, V. Grinenko and D. Citron. 1979. Detection, identification, and comparison of *Capnocytophaga, Bacteroides ochraceus* and DF-1. J. Clin. Microbiol. *10:* 557–562.

Nichols, J.M. and D. G. Adams. 1982. Akinetes. *In* Carr and Whitton (Editors), The Biology of Cyanobacteria. Blackwell, Oxford, and University of California Press, Berkeley, pp. 387–412.

Nichols, P., B.K. Stulp, J.G. Jones and D.C. White. 1986. Comparison of fatty acid content and DNA homology of the filamentous gliding bacteria *Vitreoscilla, Flexibacter, Filibacter.* Arch. Microbiol. *146:* 1–6.

Nicholson, D.E. and G.E. Fox. 1983. Molecular evidence for a close phylogenetic relationship among box-shaped halobacteria. *Halobacterium vallismortis* and *Halobacterium marismortui.* Can. J. Microbiol. *29:* 52–59.

Nicolet, J., P. Paroz and M. Krawinkler. 1980. Polyacrylamide gel electrophoresis of whole-cell proteins of porcine strains of *Haemophilus.* Int. J. Syst. Bacteriol. *30:* 69–76.

Nielsen, A.M., R.J. Rampsch and G.A. Sojka. 1979. Regulation of isocitrate lyase in a mutant of *Rhodopseudomonas capsulata* adapted to growth on acetate. Arch. Microbiol. *120:* 43–46.

Nierzwicki, S.A., D. Maratea, D.L. Balkwill, L.P. Hardie, V.B. Mehta and S.E. Stevens, Jr. 1982b. Ultrastructure of the cyanobacterium, *Mastigocladus laminosus.* Arch. Microbiol. *133:* 11–19.

Nierzwicki-Bauer, S.A., D.L. Balkwill and S.E. Stevens, Jr. 1983. Three-dimensional ultrastructure of a unicellular cyanobacterium. J. Cell Biol. *97:* 713–722.

Nierzwicki-Bauer, S.A., D.L. Balkwill and S.E. Stevens, Jr. 1984. Morphology and ultrastructure of the cyanobacterium *Mastigocladus laminosus* growing under nitrogen-fixing conditions. Arch. Microbiol. *137:* 97–103.

Nies, M. and W. Wehrmeyer. 1981. Biliprotein assembly in the hemisdiscoidal phycobilisomes of the thermophilic cyanobacterium *Mastigocladus laminosus* Cohn. Characterization of dissociation products with special reference to the peripheral phycoerythrocyanin-phycocyanin complexes. Arch. Microbiol. *129:* 374–379.

Nikitin, D.I. and L.V. Vasilyeva. 1968. A new soil microorganism *Agrobacterium polyspheroidum,* n. sp. (in Russian). Izv. Akad. Nauk S.S.S.R. Ser. Biol. *3:* 443–444.

Nikitin, D.I., L.V. Vasilyeva and R.A. Lokhmacheva. 1966. New and Rare Forms of Soil Microorganisms. Nauka, Moscow.

Nishimura, Y., M. Shimadzu and H. Iizuka. 1981. Bacteriochlorophyll formation in radiation-resistant *Pseudomonas radiora.* J. Gen. Microbiol. *27:* 427–430.

Nissen, H. and I.D. Dundas. 1984. *Rhodospirillum salinarum* sp. nov., a halopholic photosynthetic bacterium isolated from a Portugese saltern. Arch. Microbiol. *138:* 251–256.

Nissen, H. and I.D. Dundas. 1985. *In* Validation of the publication of new names and new combinations previously effectively published outside the IJSB. Int. J. Syst. Bacteriol. *35:* 223–225.

Nissenbaum, A. 1975. The microbiology and biogeochemistry of the Dead Sea. Microbiol. Ecol. *2:* 139–161.

Noel, K.D. and W.J. Brill. 1980. Diversity and dynamics of indigenous *Rhizobium japonicum* populations. Appl. Environ. Microbiol. *40:* 931–938.

Nolte, E.M. 1957. Untersuchungen über Ernahrung und Fruchtkörperbildung von Myxobakterien. Arch. Mikrobiol. *28:* 191–218.

Nordin, R.N. and J.R. Stein. 1980. Taxonomic revision of *Nodularia* (*Cyanophyceae*/Cyanobacteria). Can. J. Bot. *58:* 1211–1224.

Norris, P.R. 1984. Iron and mineral oxidation with *Leptospirillum*-like bacteria. *In* Rossi and Torma (Editors), Recent Progress in Biohydrometallurgy. Associazione Mineraria Sardia, Inglesias, pp. 83–96.

Norton, R.S. and R.J. Wells. 1982. A series of chiralpolybrominated biindoles from the marine blue-green alga *Rivularia firma.* Application of ^{13}C NMR spin-lattice relaxation data and $^{13}C–^1H$ coupling constants to structure elucidation. J. Am. Chem. Soc. *1982:* 3628–3635.

Nottingham, P.M. and R.E. Hungate. 1968. Isolation of methanogenic bacteria from feces of man. J. Bacteriol. *96:* 2178–2179.

Novick, R.P. 1969. Extrachromosomal inheritance in bacteria. Bacteriol. Rev. *33:* 210–235.

Novikova, L.M. 1971. Formation and utilization of reserve products by *Ectothiorhodospira shaposhnikovii.* Mikrobiologiya *40:* 28–33.

Nozhevnikova, A.N. and V.I. Chudina. 1984. Morphology of the thermophilic acetate methane bacterium *Methanothrix thermoacetophila* sp. nov. Mikrobiologiya *53:* 756–760.

Nozhevnikova, A.N. and T.G. Yagodina. 1982. A thermophilic acetate methane-producing bacterium. Mikrobiologiya *51:* 642–649.

Nultsch, W. and K. Wenderoth. 1983. Partial irradiation experiments with *Anabaena variabilis* (Kütz). Z. Pflanzenphysiol. *111:* 1–7.

Nunley, J.W. and N.R. Krieg. 1968. Isolation of *Gallionella ferruginea* by use of formalin. Can. J. Microbiol. *14:* 385–389.

Nurmiaho-Lassila, E.-L., K. Haahtela and V. Sundman. 1981. A new spiral structure associated with the flagellum of *Azospirillum lipoferum*. Can. J. Microbiol. *27:* 1267–1271.

Nygaard, A.P. and B.D. Hall. 1963. A method for detection of RNA-DNA complexes. Biochem. Biophys. Res. Commun. *12:* 98–104.

O'Connor, K.A. and D.R. Zusman. 1983. Coliphage Pl-mediated transduction of cloned DNA from *Escherichia coli* to *Myxococcus xanthus*: use for complementation and recombinational analysis. J. Bacteriol. *155:* 317–329.

Oelze, J. and R.C. Fuller. 1983. Temperature dependence of growth and membrane-bound activities of *Chloroflexus aurantiacus* energy metabolism. J. Bacteriol. *155:* 90–96.

Oetker, H. 1953. Untersuchungen über die Ernährung einiger Myxobakterien. Arch. Mikrobiol. *19:* 206–246.

Oettmeier, W., D. Godde, B. Kunze and G. Höfle. 1985. Stigmatellin. A dual type inhibitor of photosynthetic electron transport. Biochim. Biophys. Acta *807:* 216–219.

O'Farrell, P. 1975. High resolution two-dimensional electrophoresis of proteins. J. Biol. Chem. *250:* 4007–4021.

O'Flaherty, L.M. and H.K. Phinney. 1970. Requirements for the maintenance and growth of *Aphanizomenon flos-aquae* in culture. J. Phycol. *6:* 95–97.

Ohki, K. and Y. Fujita. 1982. Laboratory culture of the pelagic blue-green alga *Trichodesmium thiebautii*: conditions for unialgal culture. Mar. Ecol. Prog. Ser. *7:* 185–190.

Ohki, K., J.G. Rueter and Y. Fujita. 1986. Cultures of the pelagic cyanophytes *Trichodesmium erythraeum* and *T. thiebautii* in synthetic medium. Mar. Biol. *91:* 9–13.

O'Kelley, J.C., G.E. Becker and A. Nason. 1970. Characterization of the particulate nitrite oxidase and its component activities from the chemoautotroph *Nitrobacter agilis*. Biochim. Biophys. Acta *205:* 409–425.

Oláh, J. and L. Hajdú. 1973. Electron microscopic morphology of *Planctomyces bekeffi* [sic] Gimesi. Arch. Hydrobiol. *71:* 271–275.

Ollivier, B.M., R.A. Mah, J.L. Garcia and D.R. Boone. 1986. Isolation and characterization of *Methanogenium bourgense* sp. nov. Int. J. Syst. Bacteriol. *36:* 297–301.

Ollivier, B.M., R.A. Mah, J.L. Garcia and R. Robinson. 1985. Isolation and characterization of *Methanogenium aggregans* sp. nov. Int. J. Syst. Bacteriol. *35:* 127–130.

Olsen, G.J., D.J. Lane, S.J. Giovannoni and N.R. Pace. 1986. Microbial ecology and evolution: a ribosomal RNA approach. Annu. Rev. Microbiol. *40:* 337–365.

Olson, M.O.J., N. Nagabhushan, M. Dzwiniel, L.B. Smillie and D.R. Whitaker. 1970. Primary structure of α-lytic protease: a bacterial homologue of the pancreatic serine proteases. Nature (London) *228:* 438–442.

Olson, T.C. and A.B. Hooper. 1983. Energy coupling in the bacterial oxidation of small molecules: an extracytoplasmic dehydrogenase in *Nitrosomonas*. FEMS Microbiol. Lett. *19:* 47–50.

Omar, A.S., H.T. Flammann, D. Borowiak and J. Weckesser. 1983. Lipopolysaccharides of two strains of the phototrophic bacterium *Rhodopseudomonas capsulata*. Arch. Microbiol. *134:* 212–216.

Omata, T. and H. Murata. 1984. Isolation and characterization of three types of membranes from the cyanobacterium (blue-green alga) *Synechocystis* PCC 6714. Arch. Microbiol. *139:* 113–116.

Omelianski, W. 1905. Über eine neue Art farbloser Thiospirillen. Zentralbl. Bakteriol. Parasitenkd. Infektionskr. Hyg. Abt. II *14:* 769–772.

Ong, L.J., A.N. Glazer and J.B. Waterbury. 1984. An unusual phycoerythrin from a marine cyanobacterium. Science *224:* 80–83.

Onishi, H., T. Kobayashi, S. Iwao and M. Kamekura. 1985. Archaebacterial diether lipids in non-pigmented extremely halophilic bacterium. Agric. Biol. Chem. (Tokyo) *49:* 3053–3056.

Onishi, H., M.E. McCance and N.E. Gibbons. 1965. A synthetic medium for extremely halophilic bacteria. Can. J. Microbiol. *11:* 365–373.

Ordal, E.J. and R.R. Rucker. 1944. Pathogenic myxobacteria. Proc. Soc. Exp. Biol. Med. *56:* 15–18.

Oren, A. 1983a. *Halobacterium sodomense* sp. nov., a Dead Sea halobacterium with an extremely high magnesium requirement. Int. J. Syst. Bacteriol. *33:* 381–386.

Oren, A. 1983b. Bacteriorhodopsin-mediated CO_2 photoassimilation in the Dead Sea. Limnol. Oceanogr. *28:* 33–41.

Oren, A. and M. Shilo. 1981. Bacteriorhodopsin in a bloom of halobacteria in the Dead Sea. Arch. Microbiol. *130:* 185–187.

Orla-Jensen, S. 1909. Die Hauptlinien des natürlichen Bakteriensystems. Zentralbl. Bakteriol. Parasitenkd. Infektionskr. Hyg. Abt. II *22:* 305–346.

Osipov, G.A., E.A. Shabanova, O.V. Morozov, G.I. ál'-Registan, A.N. Kozlova and T.N. Zhilina. 1985. Lipids of *Methanosarcina vacuolata* and *Methanococcus halophilus*. Microbiology (English Translation) *54:* 514–519.

Öström, B. 1976. Fertilization of the Baltic by nitrogen fixation in the blue-green alga *Nodularia spumigena*. Remote Sens. Environ. *4:* 305–310.

Owen, R.J. and J.J.S. Snell. 1976. Deoxyribonucleic acid reassociation in the classification of flavobacteria. J. Gen. Microbiol. *93:* 89–102.

Oyaizu, H., B. Debrunner-Vossbrinck, L. Mandelco, J.A. Studier and C.R. Woese. 1987. The green non-sulfur bacteria: a deep branching in the eubacterial line of descent. Syst. Appl. Microbiol. *9:* 47–53.

Oyaizu, H. and K. Komagata. 1981. Chemotaxonomic and phenotypic characterization of the strains of species in the *Flavobacterium-Cytophaga* complex. J. Gen. Appl. Microbiol. *27:* 57–107.

Oyaizu, H., K. Komagata, A. Amemura and T. Harada. 1982. A succinoglycan-decomposing bacterium, *Cytophaga arvensicola* sp. nov. J. Gen. Appl. Microbiol. *28:* 369–388.

Oyaizu, H., K. Komagata, A. Amemura and T. Harada. 1983. *In* Validation of the publication of new names and new combinations previously effectively published outside the IJSB. List No. 10. Int. J. Syst. Bacteriol. *33:* 438–440.

Pacha, R.E. 1968. Characteristics of *Cytophaga psychrophila* (Borg) isolated during outbreaks of bacterial cold-water disease. Appl. Microbiol. *16:* 97–101.

Pacha, R.E. and E.J. Ordal. 1970. Myxobacterial diseases of salmonids. *In* Snieszko (Editor), A Symposium on Diseases of Fishes and Shellfishes. American Fisheries Society, Washington, D.C., pp. 243–257.

Pacha, R.E. and S. Porter. 1968. Characteristics of myxobacteria isolated from the surface of freshwater fish. Appl. Microbiol. *16:* 1901–1906.

Padan, E. and Y. Cohen. 1982. Anoxygenic photosynthesis. *In* Carr and Whitton (Editors), The Biology of Cyanobacteria. Blackwell, Oxford, and University of California Press, Berkeley, pp. 215–235.

Paerl, H.W. 1984. N_2 fixation (nitrogenase activity) attributable to a specific *Prochloron* (*Prochlorophyta*)-ascidian association in Palau, Micronesia. Mar. Biol. *81:* 251–254.

Paerl, H.W., R.A. Lewin and L. Cheng. 1984. Variations in chlorophyll and carotenoid pigmentation among *Prochloron* (*Prochlorophyta*) symbionts in diverse marine ascidians. Bot. Mar. *27:* 257–264.

Palleroni, N.J. 1984. Genus *Pseudomonas*. *In* Krieg and Holt (Editors), Bergey's Manual of Systematic Bacteriology, Vol. 1. The Williams and Wilkins Co., Baltimore, p. 191.

Palmer, F.E., J.T. Staley, R.G.E. Murray, T.Counsell and J.B. Adams. 1985. Identification of manganese-oxidizing bacteria from desert varnish. Geomicrobiol. J. *4:* 343–360.

Pan, P. and W.W. Umbreit. 1972. Growth of obligate autotrophic bacteria on glucose in a continuous flow-through apparatus. J. Bacteriol. *109:* 1149–1155.

Pangborn, J., D.A. Kuhn and J.R. Woods. 1977. Dorsal-ventral differentiation in *Simonsiella* and other aspects of its morphology and ultrastructure. Arch. Microbiol. *13:* 197–204.

Pankratz, H.S. and C.C. Bowen. 1963. Cytology of blue-green algae. I. The cells of *Symploca muscorum*. Am. J. Bot. *50:* 387–399.

Parish, J.H. 1979. Myxobacteria. *In* Parish (Editor), Developmental Biology of Prokaryotes. Blackwell, London.

Park, C.-E. and L.R. Berger. 1967. Fatty acids of extractable and bound lipids of *Rhodomicrobium vannielii*. J. Bacteriol. *93:* 230–236.

Parker, C.D. 1945. The corrosion of concrete. I. The isolation of a species of bacterium associated with the corrosion of concrete exposed to atmosphere containing hydrogen sulphide. Aust. J. Exp. Biol. Med. Sci. *23:* 81–90.

Parker, C.D. 1957. Genus V. *Thiobacillus* Beijerinck 1904. *In* Breed, Murray and Smith (Editors), Bergey's Manual of Determinative Bacteriology, 7th Ed. The Williams and Wilkins Co., Baltimore, pp. 83–88.

Parker, C.D. and J. Prisk. 1953. The oxidation of inorganic compounds of sulphur by various sulphur bacteria. J. Gen. Microbiol. *8:* 344–364.

Parker, D.L. 1982. Improved procedures for the cloning and purification of *Microcystis* cultures (Cyanophyta). J. Phycol. *18:* 471–477.

Parra, O. 1972. Presencia del género *Planctomyces* (Fungi Imperfecti—Moniliales) en Chile. Bol. Soc. Arg. Bot. *14:* 282–284.

Paster, B.J., W. Ludwig, W.G. Weisburg, E. Stackebrandt, R.B. Hespell, C.M. Hahn, H. Reichenbach, K.O. Stetter and C.R. Woese. 1985. A phylogenetic grouping of the bacteroides, cytophagas and certain flavobacteria. Syst. Appl. Microbiol. *6:* 34–42.

Pate, J.L. and L.Y.E. Chang. 1979. Evidence that gliding motility in prokaryotic cells is driven by rotary assemblies in the cell envelope. Curr. Microbiol. *2:* 59–64.

Pate, J.L., J.L. Johnson and E.J. Ordal. 1967. The fine structure of *Chondrococcus columnaris*. II. Structure and formation of rhapidosomes. J. Cell. Biol. *35:* 15–35.

Pate, J.L. and E.J. Ordal. 1965. The fine structure of two unusual stalked bacteria. J. Cell Biol. *27:* 133–150.

Pate, J.L. and E.J. Ordal. 1967a. The fine structure of *Chondrococcus columnaris* I. Structure and formation of mesosomes. J. Cell. Biol. *35:* 1–13.

Pate, J.L. and E.J. Ordal. 1967b. The fine structure of *Chondrococcus columnaris* III. The surface layers of *Chondrococcus columnaris*. J. Cell. Biol. *35:* 37–51.

Pate, J.L., S.J. Petzold and L.Y.E. Chang. 1979. Phages for the gliding bacterium *Cytophaga johnsonae* that infect only motile cells. Curr. Microbiol. *2:* 257–262.

Pate, J.L., S.J. Petzold and T.H. Umbreit. 1979. Two flagellotropic phages and one pilus-specific phage active against *Asticcacaulis biprosthecum*. Virology *94:* 24–37.

Pate, J.L., J.S. Porter and T.L. Jordan. 1973. *Asticcacaulis biprosthecum* sp. nov. Life cycle, morphology and cultural characteristics. Antonie van Leeuwenhoek J. Microbiol. Serol. *39:* 569–583.

Patel, G.B. 1984. Characterization and nutritional properties of *Methanothrix concilii* sp. nov., a mesophilic, aceticlastic methanogen. Can. J. Microbiol. *30:* 1383–1396.

Patel, G.B. 1985. *In* Validation of the publication of new names and new combinations previously effectively published outside the IJSB. List No. 17. Int. J. Syst. Bacteriol. *35:* 223–225.

Patel, G.B., L.A. Roth and G.D. Sprott. 1979. Factors influencing filament length of *Methanospirillum hungatii*. J. Gen. Microbiol. *112:* 411–415.

Patel, G.B., L.A. Roth, L. van den Berg and D.S. Clark. 1976. Characterization of a strain of *Methanospirillum hungatii*. Can. J. Microbiol. *22:* 1404–1410.

Patel, G.B., G.D. Sprott, R.W. Humphrey and T.J. Beveridge. 1986. Comparative analyses of the sheath structures of *Methanothrix concilii* GP6 and *Methanospirillum hungatei* strains GP1 and JF1. Can. J. Microbiol. *32:* 623-631.

Paterek, J.R. and P.H. Smith. 1985. Isolation and characterization of a halophilic methanogen from Great Salt Lake. Appl. Environ. Microbiol. *50:* 877-881.

Patterson, G.M. and N.W. Withers. 1982. Laboratory cultivation of *Prochloron*, a tryptophan auxotroph. Science *217:* 1934-1935.

Payne, J.I., S.N. Sehgal and N.E. Gibbons. 1960. Immersion refractometry of some halophilic bacteria. Can. J. Microbiol. *6:* 9-15.

Paynter, M.J.B. and R.E. Hungate. 1968. Characterization of *Methanobacterium mobilis*, sp. n., isolated from the bovine rumen. J. Bacteriol. *95:* 1943-1951.

Payza, A.N. 1956. Bacterial degradation of heparin. Nature *177:* 88-89.

Payza, A.N. and E.D. Korn. 1956. The degradation of heparin by bacterial enzymes. I. Adaptation and lyophilized cells. J. Biol. Chem. *223:* 853-858.

Pearson, H.W., R. Howsley, C.K. Kjeldsen and A.E. Walsby. 1979. Aerobic nitrogenase activity associated with a non-heterocystous filamentous cyanobacterium. FEMS Microbiol. Lett. *5:* 163-167.

Pearson, H.W., G. Malin and R. Howsley. 1981. Physiological studies on *in vitro* nitrogenase activity by axenic cultures of the blue-green alga *Microcoleus chthonoplastes*. Br. Phycol. Soc. *16:* 139 (abstract).

Pearson, J.E. and J.M. Kingsbury. 1966. Culturally induced variation in four morphologically diverse blue-green algae. Am. J. Bot. *53:* 192-200.

Peattie, D.A. 1979. Direct chemical method for sequencing RNA. Proc. Natl. Acad. Sci. U.S.A. *76:* 1760-1764.

Pecher, T. and A. Böck. 1981. In vivo susceptability of halophilic and methanogenic organisms to protein synthesis inhibitors. FEMS Microbiol. Lett. *10:* 295-297.

Pedersen, M. and E.J. DaSilva. 1973. Simple brominated phenols in the blue-green alga *Calothrix brevissima* West. Planta *115:* 83-86.

Peel, D. and J.R. Quayle. 1961. Microbial growth on C_1 compounds. I. Isolation and characterization of *Pseudomonas* AM 1. Biochem. J. *81:* 465-469.

Pellerin, N.B. and H. Gest. 1983. Diagnostic features of the photosynthetic bacterium *Rhodopseudomonas sphaeroides*. Curr. Microbiol. *9:* 339-344.

Pellerin, P., B. Gruson, G. Prensier, G. Albagnac and P. Debeire. 1987. Glycogen in *Methanothrix*. Arch. Microbiol. *146:* 377-381.

Pelsh, A.D. 1936. Hydrobiology of Karabugaz Bay of the Caspian Sea. Tr. Vses. Nauchno-Issled. Inst. Galurgii Leningrad *5:* 49-126.

Pelsh, A.D. 1937. Photosynthetic sulfur bacteria of the eastern reservoir of Lake Sakskoe. Mikrobiologiya *6:* 1090-1100.

Penso, G. 1947. Il rosso der baaccalari—Etiologia, commestibilite bonificial e prevenzione. Rend. 1st Super Sanita. *10:* 563-605.

Perfil'ev, B.V. 1921. On the knowledge of microorganisms of the Nevsky Bay. Bull. Inst. Hydrol. Leningrad *1:* 84-96.

Perfil'ev, B.V. 1926. New data on the role of microbes in ore formation. Izv. Geol. Komiteta *45:* 795.

Perfil'ev, B.V. 1927. Die Rolle der Mikroben in der Erzbildung. Verhandl. Int. Ver. Limnol. *3:* 330-359.

Perfil'ev, B.V. 1964. The capillary microbial-landscape method in geomicrobiology. *In* Perfil'ev, Gabe, Gal'perina, Rabinovich, Sapotnitskii, Sherman and Troshanov (Editors), Applied Capillary Microscopy. The Role of Microorganisms in the Formation of Iron-manganese Deposits. Izv. Akad. Nauk. S.S.S.R., Savarenskii Laboratory for Hydrogeological Problems, Moscow (in Russian.) (Translation: Consultants Bureau Enterprise Inc., 1965, New York.)

Perfil'ev, B.V. 1969. On a new iron sulfide microorganism *Thiodendron latens* n.g.n.sp. and on methods of its growing in elective culture. Izv. Akad. Nauk S.S.S.R. Ser. Biol. *2:* 181-198.

Perfil'ev, B.V. and D.R. Gabe. 1961. Capillary methods of investigating microorganisms. Izv. Akad. Nauk S.S.S.R. (in Russian). (English translation: J.M. Shewan, University of Toronto Press, Toronto, 1969.)

Perfil'ev, B.V. and D.R. Gabe. 1964. Methods for the study of bacteria accumulating manganese and iron in bottom deposits. *In* Gurevich (Editor), The Role of Microorganisms in the Formation of Iron Manganese Lake Ores. Nauka, Moscow, pp. 16-53.

Perkins, F.O., L.W. Haas, D.E. Phillips and K.L. Webb. 1981. Ultrastructure of a marine *Synechococcus* possessing spinae. Can. J. Microbiol. *27:* 318-329.

Perry, L.B. 1973. Gliding motility in some non-spreading flexibacteria. J. Appl. Bacteriol. *36:* 227-232.

Perski, H.J., P. Schönheit and R.K. Thauer. 1982. Sodium dependence of methane formation in methanogenic bacteria. FEBS Lett. *143:* 323-326.

Perty, M. 1852. Zur Kenntnis kleinster Lebensformen. Jent and Reinert, Bern I-VIII, pp. 1-228.

Peshkoff, M.A. 1948. Order *Caryophanales*. *In* Breed, Murray and Hitchens (Editors), Bergey's Manual of Determinative Bacteriology, 6th Ed. The Williams and Wilkins Co., Baltimore, pp. 1002-1005.

Peterson, J.E. 1959. New species of myxobacteria from the bark of living trees. Mycologia *51:* 163-172.

Peterson, J.E. 1959. A monocystic genus of the *Myxobacterales (Schizomycetes)*. Mycologia *51:* 1-8.

Peterson, J.E. 1969. Isolation, cultivation and maintenance of the myxobacteria. Methods Microbiol. *3B:* 185-210.

Peterson, J.E. 1974. *Polyangium sorediatum*. *In* Buchanan and Gibbons (Editors),

Bergey's Manual of Determinative Bacteriology, 8th Ed. The Williams and Wilkins Co., Baltimore, p. 95.

Petitprez, M., A. Petitprez, H. Leclerc and E. Vivier. 1969. Quelques aspects structuraux de *Sphaerotilus natans*. Ann. Inst. Pasteur Lille *20:* 108-114.

Petter, H.F.M. 1931. On bacteria of salted fish. Proc. Koninkl. Nederl. Akad. Wetensch. Amsterdam *34:* 1417-1423.

Petter, H.F.M. 1932. Over roode en andere bacterien van gezouten visch. Doctoral thesis, Rijks-Universitat de Utrecht, pp. 1-116.

Pfeifer, F. 1987. Genetics of halobacteria. *In* Rodriguez-Valera (Editor), Halophilic Bacteria. CRC Press, Boca Raton, Florida.

Pfeifer, F., G. Weidinger and W. Goebel. 1981. Characterisation of plasmids in halobacteria. J. Bacteriol. *145:* 369-374.

Pfeiffer, E. 1967. Eine koprophile Wassermyxobakterienspezies aus der Gattung *Sporocytophaga*. Arch. Hyg. Bakteriol. *151:* 258-265.

Pfennig, N. 1962. Beobachtungen über das Schwärmen von *Chromatium okenii*. Arch. Mikrobiol. *42:* 90-95.

Pfennig, N. 1965. Anreicherungskulturen für rote und grüne Schwefelbakterien. Zentralbl. Bakteriol. Parasitenkd. Infektionskr. Hyg. Abt. I Suppl. I, 179-189, 503-505.

Pfennig, N. 1968. *Chlorobium phaeobacteroides* nov. spec. und *Chlorobium phaeovibrioides* nov. spec., zwei neue Arten der grünen Schwefelbakterien. Arch. Mikrobiol. *63:* 224-226.

Pfennig, N. 1969a. *Rhodopseudomonas acidophila*, sp. n., a new species of the budding purple nonsulfur bacteria. J. Bacteriol. *99:* 597-602.

Pfennig, N. 1969b. *Rhodospirillum tenue* sp. n., a new species of the purple nonsulfur bacteria. J. Bacteriol. *99:* 619-620.

Pfennig, N. 1973. Culture and ecology of *Thiopedia rosea*. *In* Drews (Editor), Abstracts of Symposium on Prokaryotic Photosynthetic Organisms. Freiburg, pp. 75-76.

Pfennig, N. 1974. *Rhodopseudomonas globiformis*, sp. n., a new species of the *Rhodospirillaceae*. Arch. Microbiol. *100:* 197-206.

Pfennig, N. 1977. Phototrophic green and purple bacteria: a comparative systematic survey. Annu. Rev. Microbiol. *31:* 275-290.

Pfennig, N. 1978. *Rhodocyclus purpureus* gen. nov. and sp. nov., a ring-shaped, vitamin B_{12}-requiring member of the family *Rhodospirillaceae*. Int. J. Syst. Bacteriol. *28:* 283-288.

Pfennig, N. 1980. Syntrophic mixed cultures and symbiotic consortia with phototrophic bacteria: a review. *In* Gottschalk, Pfennig, Werner (Editors), Anaerobes and Anaerobic Infections. Gustav Fischer Verlag, Stuttgart, New York, pp. 127-131.

Pfennig, N. and G. Cohen-Bazire. 1967. Some properties of the green bacterium *Pelodictyon clathratiforme*. Arch. Microbiol. *59:* 226-236.

Pfennig, N., K.E. Eimhjellen and S. Liaaen-Jensen. 1965. A new isolate of the *Rhodospirillum fulvum* group and its photosynthetic pigments. Arch. Mikrobiol. *51:* 258-266.

Pfennig, N. and K.D. Lippert. 1966. Über das Vitamin B_{12}-Bedürfnis phototropher Schwefelbakterien. Arch. Mikrobiol. *55:* 245-256.

Pfennig, N., M.C. Markham and S. Liaaen-Jensen. 1968. Carotenoids of *Thiorhodaceae*. 8. Isolation and characterization of a *Thiothece, Lamprocystis* and *Thiodictyon* strain and their carotenoid pigments. Arch. Mikrobiol. *62:* 178-191.

Pfennig, N. and H.G. Trüper. 1971. New nomenclatural combinations in the phototrophic sulfur bacteria. Int. J. Syst. Bacteriol. *21:* 11-14.

Pfennig, N. and H.G. Trüper. 1971. Higher taxa of the phototrophic bacteria. Int. J. Syst. Bacteriol. *21:* 17-18.

Pfennig, N. and H.G. Trüper. 1974. Family III. *Chlorobiaceae*. *In* Buchanan and Gibbons (Editors). Bergey's Manual of Determinative Bacteriology, 8th Ed. The Williams and Wilkins Co., Baltimore, pp. 51-60.

Pfennig, N. and H.G. Trüper. 1974. The phototrophic bacteria. *In* Buchanan and Gibbons (Editors), Bergey's Manual of Determinative Bacteriology, 8th Ed. The Williams and Wilkins Co., Baltimore, pp. 24-64.

Pfennig, N. and H.G. Trüper. 1974. Family II. *Chromatiaceae*. *In* Buchanan and Gibbons (Editors), Bergey's Manual of Determinative Bacteriology, 8th Ed. The Williams and Wilkins Co., Baltimore, pp. 34-51.

Pfennig, N. and H.G. Trüper. 1981. Isolation of members of the families *Chromatiaceae* and *Chlorobiaceae*. *In* Starr, Stolp, Trüper, Balows and Schlegel (Editors), The Prokaryotes. A Handbook on Habitats, Isolation, and Identification of Bacteria. Springer-Verlag, Berlin, pp. 279-289.

Phaup, J.D. 1968. The biology of *Sphaerotilus* species. Water Res. *2:* 597-614.

Pierson, B.K. 1979. Cytochromes of *Chloroflexus* grown with and without oxygen. Abstracts of III International Symposium on Photosynthetic Prokaryotes, Oxford, published by Department of Biochemistry, University of Liverpool, p. B40.

Pierson, B.K. and R.W. Castenholz. 1971. Bacteriochlorophylls in gliding filamentous prokaryotes from hot springs. Nature (New Biol.) *233:* 25-27.

Pierson, B.K. and R.W. Castenholz. 1974a. A phototrophic gliding filamentous bacterium of hot springs, *Chloroflexus aurantiacus*, gen. and sp. nov. Arch. Microbiol. *100:* 5-24.

Pierson, B.K. and R.W. Castenholz. 1974b. Studies of pigments and growth in *Chloroflexus aurantiacus*, a phototrophic filamentous bacterium. Arch. Microbiol. *100:* 283-305.

Pierson, B.K., S.J. Giovannoni and R.W. Castenholz. 1984a. Physiological ecology of a gliding bacterium containing bacteriochlorophyll *a*. Appl. Environ. Microbiol. *47:* 576-584.

Pierson, B.K., S.J. Giovannoni, D.A. Stahl and R.W. Castenholz. 1985. *Heliothrix oregonensis*, gen. nov., sp. nov., a phototrophic filamentous bacterium containing bactriochlorophyll *a*. Arch. Microbiol. *142*: 164–167.

Pierson, B.K., S.J. Giovannoni, D.A. Stahl and R.W. Castenholz. 1986. *In* Validation of the publication of new names and new combinations previously effectively published outside the IJSB. List No. 20. Int. J. Syst. Bacteriol. *36*: 354–356.

Pierson, B.K., L. Keith and J. Leovy. 1984b. The isolation of pigmentation mutants of the green filamentous photosynthetic bacterium, *Chloroflexus aurantiacus*. J. Bacteriol. *159*: 222–227.

Pierson, B.K. and J.P. Thornber. 1983. Isolation and spectral characterization of photochemical reaction centers from the thermophilic green bacterium *Chloroflexus aurantiacus* strain J-10-fl. Proc. Natl. Acad. Sci. U.S.A. *80*: 80–84.

Pierson, B.K., J.P. Thornber and R.E.B. Seftor. 1983. Partial purification, subunit structure and thermal stability of the photochemical reaction center of the thermophilic green bacterium *Chloroflexus aurantiacus*. Biochim. Biophys. Acta *723*: 322–326.

Pivovarova, T.A. and V.M. Gorlenko. 1977. Fine structure of *Chloroflexus aurantiacus* var. *mesophilus* (Nom. prof.) grown in light under aerobic and anaerobic conditions. Microbiology *46*: 276–282.

Poffe, R., J. Vanderleyden and H. Verachtert. 1979. Characterization of a *Leucothrix*-type bacterium causing sludge bulking during petrochemical waste-water treatment. Eur. J. Appl. Microbiol. *8*: 229–235.

Poindexter, J.S. 1964. Biological properties and classification of the *Caulobacter* group. Bacteriol. Rev. *28*: 231–295.

Poindexter, J.S. 1981. The caulobacters: ubiquitous unusual bacteria. Microbiol. Rev. *45*: 123–179.

Poindexter, J.S. 1984. The role of calcium in stalk development and in phosphate acquisition in *Caulobacter crescentus*. Arch. Microbiol. *138*: 140–152.

Poindexter, J.S. and J.G. Hagenzieker. 1982. Novel peptidoglycans in *Caulobacter* and *Asticcacaulis* spp. J. Bacteriol. *150*: 332–347.

Poindexter, J.S. and R.F. Lewis. 1966. Recommendations for revision of the taxonomic treatment of stalked bacteria. Int. J. Syst. Bacteriol. *16*: 377–382.

Poirier, T.P. and S.C. Holt. 1983a. Acid and alkaline phosphatase of *Capnocytophaga* species. I. Production and cytological localization of the enzymes. Can. J. Microbiol. *28*: 1350–1360.

Poirier, T.P. and S.C. Holt. 1983b. Acid and alkaline phosphatases of *Capnocytophaga* species. II. Isolation, purification, and characterization of the enzymes from *Capnocytophaga ochracea*. Can. J. Microbiol. *29*: 1361–1368.

Poirier, T.P. and S.C. Holt. 1983c. Acid and alkaline phosphatases of *Capnocytophaga* species. III. The relationship of the enzymes to the cell wall. Can. J. Microbiol. *29*: 1369–1381.

Poirier, T.P., R. Mishell, C.L. Trummel and S.C. Holt. 1983. Biological and chemical comparison of butanol- and phenol-water extracted lipopolysaccharide from *Capnocytophaga sputigena*. J. Periodontal Res. *18*: 541–557.

Poirier, T.P., S.J. Tonelli and S.C. Holt. 1979. Ultrastructure of gliding bacteria: scanning electron microscopy of *Capnocytophaga sputigena*, *Capnocytophaga gingivalis*, and *Capnocytophaga ochracea*. Infect. Immun. *26*: 1146–1158.

Politi, I. 1941. Alcune osservazioni sui microrganismi aerobi decomponenti la cellulosa. Tentativi di isolamento in coltura pura. Boll. Soc. Ital. Microbiol. *13*: 143–149.

Polman, J.K., and J.M. Larkin. 1988. Properties of in vivo nitrogenase activity in *Beggiatoa alba*. Arch. Microbiol. *150*: 126–130.

Pongratz, E. 1957. D'une bacterie pediculee isolee d'un pus de sinus. Schweiz. Z. Allg. Pathol. Bakteriol. *20*: 593–608.

Ponomareva, W.W. 1964. Theory of Podzolization. Academy of Science, Moscow, pp. 41–73.

Poos, J.C., F.R. Turner, D. White, G.D. Simon, K. Bacon and C.T. Russell. 1972. Growth, cell division, and fragmentation in a species of *Flexibacter*. J. Bacteriol. *112*: 1387–1395.

Porter, J.R. 1976. The world view of culture collections. *In* Colwell (Editor), The Role of Culture Collections in the Era of Molecular Biology. American Society for Microbiology, Washington, D.C., pp. 62–72.

Porter, J.S. and J.L. Pate. 1975. Prosthecae of *Asticcacaulis biprosthecum*: system for the study of membrane transport. J. Bacteriol. *122*: 976–986.

Post, F.J. 1977. The microbial ecology of the Great Salt Lake. Microb. Ecol. *3*: 143–165.

Potts, M., R. Ocampo-Friedmann, M.A. Bowman and B. Tözün. 1983. *Chroococcus* S24 and *Chroococcus* N41 (cyanobacteria): morphological, biochemical and genetic characterization and effects of water stress on ultrastructure. Arch. Microbiol. *135*: 81–90.

Poulsen, V.A. 1879. Om nogle mikroskopiske Planteorganismes. Vidensk. Medd. Naturhist. Foren. Kjobenhaum *1879–1880*: pp. 231–254.

Powell, D.M., B.S. Roberson and R.M. Weiner. 1980. Serological relationships among budding, prosthecate bacteria. Can. J. Microbiol. *26*: 209–217.

Präve, P. 1957. Untersuchungen über die Stoffwechselphysiologie des Eisenbakteriums *Leptothrix ochracea* Kützing. Arch. Mikrobiol. *27*: 33–62.

Preissner, W.C., S. Maier, H. Völker and P. Hirsch. 1988. Isolation and characterization of a bacteriophage active on *Hyphomicrobium* WI-926. Can. J. Microbiol. *34*: 101–106.

Pribram, E. 1929. A contribution to the classification of microorganisms. J. Bacteriol. *18*: 361–394.

Price, K.W. 1977. A study of the taxonomy of flavobacteria isolated in clinical laboratories. Doctor's thesis, University of California, Los Angeles.

Pridham, T.G. 1974. Micro-organism Culture Collections: Acronyms and Abbreviations. ARS-NC-17. Agricultural Research Service, U.S. Department of Agriculture, North Central Region, Peoria, Illinois.

Prince, R.C., K.E. Stokley, C.E. Haith, and H.W. Jannasch. 1988. The cytochromes of a marine *Beggiatoa*. Arch. Microbiol. *150*: 193–196.

Prince, R.L., C. Larroque and A.B. Hooper. 1983. Resolution of the hemes of hydroxylamine oxidoreductase by redox potentiometry and optical spectroscopy. FEBS Lett. *163*: 25–27.

Pringsheim, E.G. 1949a. Iron bacteria. Biol. Rev. Cambridge Philos. Soc. *24*: 200–245.

Pringsheim, E.G. 1949b. The filamentous bacteria *Sphaerotilus*, *Leptothris*, *Cladothrix*, and their relation to iron and manganese. Philos. Trans. R. Soc. London Ser. B *223*: 453–482.

Pringsheim, E.G. 1949b. The relationship between bacteria and the *Myxophyceae*. Bacteriol. Rev. *13*: 47–91.

Pringsheim, E.G. 1951. The *Vitreoscillaceae*: a family of colourless, gliding, filamentous organisms. J. Gen. Microbiol. *5*: 124–149.

Pringsheim, E.G. 1957. Observations on *Leucothrix mucor* and *Leucothrix cohaerens* nov. sp. Bacteriol. Rev. *21*: 69–76.

Pringsheim, E.G. 1963. Farblose Algen. Gustav Fischer Verlag, Stuttgart.

Pringsheim, E.G. 1964. Heterotrophism and species concepts in *Beggiatoa*. Am. J. Bot. *51*: 893–913.

Pringsheim, E.G. 1967. Die Mixotrophie von *Beggiatoa*. Arch. Mikrobiol. *59*: 247–254.

Pringsheim, E.G. 1967. Bakterien und Cyanophyceen. Oesterr. Bot. Z. *114*: 324–340.

Pringsheim, E.G. 1970. Prefatory chapter: contributions toward the development of general microbiology. Annu. Rev. Microbiol. *24*: 1–16.

Pringsheim, E.G. and W. Wiessner. 1963. Minimum requirements for heterotrophic growth and reserve substance in *Beggiatoa*. Nature *197*: 102.

Printz, H. 1921. Subaerial algae from South Africa. K. Nor. Vidensk. Selsk. Skr. *1*: 35–36.

Pronina, N.I. 1962. Description of new species and varieties of cellulose-decomposing myxobacteria. Microbiology *31*: 384–390.

Provasoli, L. 1963. Growing marine seaweeds. *In* Proceedings of the 4th International Seaweed Symposium, Biarritz, France, September, 1961. Pergamon Press, New York, pp. 9–17.

Puchkova, N.N. 1984. Green sulphur bacteria as a component of the "sulfureta" of shallow saline waters of the Crimea and northern Caucasus. Mikrobiologiya *53*: 324–328.

Puchkova, N.N. and V.M. Gorlenko. 1976. New brown chlorobacteria *Prosthecochloris phaeoasteroidea* nov. sp. Mikrobiologiya *45*: 656–660.

Puchkova, N.N. and V.M. Gorlenko. 1982. *Chlorobium chlorovibrioides* nov. sp., a new green sulfur bacterium. Mikrobiologiya *51*: 118–124.

Pyle, S.W. and E.B. Shotts. 1980. A new approach for differentiating flexibacteria isolated from cold-water and warm-water fish. Can. J. Fish. Aquat. Sci. *37*: 1040–1042.

Pyle, S.W. and E.B. Shotts. 1981. DNA homology studies of selected flexibacteria associated with fish disease. Can. J. Fish. Aquat. Sci. *38*: 146–151.

Qinsheng, L., L. Shanghao and W. Dasi. 1984. Isolation and characterization of *Flexibacter chinenses* sp. nov. Acta Microbiol. Sin. *24*: 7–13 (in Chinese with English summary).

Qualls, G.T., K. Stephens and D. White. 1978. Light stimulated morphogenesis in the fruiting myxobacterium *Stigmatella aurantiaca*. Science *201*: 444–445.

Quayle, J.R. and N. Pfennig. 1975. Utilization of methanol by *Rhodospirillaceae*. Arch. Microbiol. *102*: 193–198.

Quehl, A. 1906. Untersuchungen über die Myxobakterien. Zentralbl. Bakteriol. Parasitenkd. Infektionskr. Hyg. Abt. II *16*: 9–34.

Quesada, E., A. Ventosa, F. Rodriguez-Valera and A. Ramos-Cormenzana. 1982. Types and properties of some bacteria isolated from hypersaline soils. J. Appl. Bacteriol. *53*: 155–161.

Quinn, G.R. and V.B.D. Skerman. 1980. *Herpetosiphon*—nature's scavenger? Curr. Microbiol. *4*: 57–62.

Rabenhorst, L. 1865. Flora Europaea Algarum aguae dulcis et submarinae. Sectio II, Algas physochromaceas complectens, Leipzig, 319 pp.

Raj, H.D. 1977. *Leucothrix*. Crit. Rev. Microbiol. *5*: 270–304.

Rambler, M., L. Margulis and E.S. Barghoorn. 1977. Natural mechanisms of protection of a blue-green alga against ultraviolet light. *In* Ponnamperuma (Editor), Chemical Evolution of the Early Precambrian. Academic Press, London, New York, pp. 133–141.

Raverdy, J. 1973. Sur l'isolement et l'activite bacteriolytique de quelques myxobacteries isolees de l'eau. Water Res. *7*: 687–693.

Ravin, A.W. 1963. Experimental approaches to the study of bacterial phylogeny. Am. Nat. *97*: 307–318.

Raymond, J.C. and W.R. Sistrom. 1969. *Ectothiorhodospira halophila*: A new species of the genus *Ectothiorhodospira*. Arch. Mikrobiol. *69*: 121–126.

Razin, S. and S. Rottem. 1967. Identification of *Mycoplasma* and other microorganisms by polyacrylamide gel electrophoresis of cell proteins. J. Bacteriol. *94*: 1807–1810.

Razumov, A.S. 1949. *Gallionella kljasmiensis* (sp. nov.), a component of the bacterial plankton. Mikrobiologiya *18*: 442–446.

Reanney, D. 1976. Extrachromosomal elements as possible agents of adaptation and development. Bacteriol. Rev. *40:* 552–590.

Redinger, K. 1931. *Siderocapsa coronata* Redinger, eine neue Eisenbakterie aus dem Lunzer Obersee. Arch. Hydrobiol. *22:* 410–414.

Reichardt, W. 1974. Zur Ökophysiologie einiger Gewässerbakterien aus der *Flavobacterium-Cytophaga*-Gruppe. Zentralbl. Bakteriol. Parasitenkd. Infektionskr. Hyg. Abt. I Orig. A *227:* 85–93.

Reichardt, W. 1975. Bacterial decomposition of different polysaccharides in a eutrophic lake. Verh. Int. Ver. Limnol. *19:* 2636–2642.

Reichardt, W. 1981. Some ecological aspects of aquatic cytophagas. *In* Reichenbach and Weeks (Editors), The *Flavobacterium-Cytophaga* Group. Verlag Chemie, Weinheim, F.R.G., pp. 189–199.

Reichardt, W., B. Gunn and R.R. Colwell. 1983. Ecology and taxonomy of chitinoclastic *Cytophaga* and related chitin-degrading bacteria isolated from an estuary. Microb. Ecol. *9:* 273–294.

Reichardt, W. and R.Y. Morita. 1982a. Influence of temperature adaptation on glucose metabolism in a psychrotrophic strain of *Cytophaga johnsonae*. Appl. Environ. Microbiol. *44:* 1282–1288.

Reichardt, W. and R.Y. Morita. 1982b. Survival stages of a psychrotrophic *Cytophaga johnsonae* strain. Can. J. Microbiol. *28:* 841–850.

Reichenbach, H. 1962. Über verschiedene Arten von Cystenmustern bei *Chondrococcus coralloides* (*Myxobacteriales*). Ber. Dtsch. Bot. Ges. *75:* 85–90.

Reichenbach, H. 1966. *Myxococcus* spp. (*Myxobacteriales*). *In* Wolf (Editor), Encyclopedia Cinematographica. Institut für den wissenschaftlichen Film, Göttingen, F.R.G, pp. 557–578.

Reichenbach, H. 1967. Die wahre Natur der Myxobakterien-"Rhapidosomen." Arch. Mikrobiol. *56:* 371–383.

Reichenbach, H. 1970. *Nannocystis exedens* gen. nov., spec. nov., a new myxobacterium of the family *Sorangiaceae*. Arch. Mikrobiol. *70:* 119–138.

Reichenbach, H. 1974a. Die Biologie der Myxobakterien. Biologie in unserer Zeit. *4:* 33–45.

Reichenbach, H. 1974b. *Chondromyces apiculatus* (*Myxobacterales*) Schwarmentwicklung und Morphogenese. *In* Wolf (Editor), Publikat. wissensch. Filmen, Institut für den wissenschaftlichen Film Göttingen, Sektion Biologie *7:* 245–263.

Reichenbach, H. 1980. *Saprospira grandis* (*Leucotrichales*). Growth and movement. Publikat. wissensch. Filmen, Institut für den wissenschaflichen Film Göttingen, Ser. *13:* 1–21.

Reichenbach, H. 1983. A simple method for the purification of myxobacteria. J. Microbiol. Methods *1:* 77–79.

Reichenbach, H., P. Boyer and H. Kleinig. 1978. The pigments of the gliding bacterium *Herpetosiphon giganteus*. FEMS Microbiol. Lett. *3:* 155–156.

Reichenbach, H. and M. Dworkin. 1969. Studies on *Stigmatella aurantiaca* (*Myxobacterales*). J. Gen. Microbiol. *58:* 3–14.

Reichenbach, H. and M. Dworkin. 1970. Induction of myxospore formations in *Stigmatella aurantiaca* (*Myxobacterales*) by monovalent cations. J. Bacteriol. *101:* 325–326.

Reichenbach, H. and M. Dworkin. 1981a. Introduction to the gliding bacteria. *In* Starr, Stolp, Trüper, Balows and Schlegel (Editors), The Prokaryotes. A Handbook on Habitats, Isolation and Identification of Bacteria. Springer-Verlag, Berlin, pp. 315–327.

Reichenbach, H. and M. Dworkin. 1981b. The order *Myxobacterales*. *In* Starr, Stolp, Trüper, Balows and Schlegel (Editors), The Prokaryotes. A Handbook on Habitats, Isolation and Identification of Bacteria. Springer-Verlag, Berlin, pp. 328–355.

Reichenbach, H. and M. Dworkin. 1981c. The order *Cytophagales* (with addenda on the genera *Herpetosiphon*, *Saprospira*, and *Flexithrix*). *In* Starr, Stolp, Trüper, Balows and Schlegel (Editors), The Prokaryotes. A Handbook on Habitats, Isolation, and Identification of Bacteria. Springer-Verlag, Berlin, pp. 356–379.

Reichenbach, H., H.K. Galle and H.H. Heunert. 1975–1976. *Stigmatella aurantiaca* (*Myxobacterales*). Schwarmentwicklung und Fruchtkorperbildung. *In* Encyclopaedia Cinematographica E2421. Institut für den wissenschaftlichen Film, Göttingen, F.R.G.

Reichenbach, H., H.K. Galle and H.H. Heunert. 1975–1976. *Saprospira grandis* (*Leucotrichales*). Wachstum und Bewegung. *In* Encyclopaedia Cinematographica E 2424. Institut für den wissenschaftlichen Film, Göttingen, F.R.G.

Reichenbach, H. and J.R. Golecki. 1975. The fine structure of *Herpetosiphon*, and a note on the taxonomy of the genus. Arch. Microbiol. *102:* 281–291.

Reichenbach, H. and H. Kleinig. 1971. The carotenoids of *Myxococcus fulvus* (*Myxobacterales*). Arch. Mikrobiol. *76:* 364–380.

Reichenbach, H. and H. Kleinig. 1984. Pigments of myxobacteria. *In* Rosenberg (Editor), Myxobacteria, Development and Cell Interactions. Springer-Verlag, New York, pp. 127–137.

Reichenbach, H., H. Kleinig and H. Achenbach. 1974. The pigments of *Flexibacter elegans*: novel and chemosystematically useful compounds. Arch. Microbiol. *101:* 131–144.

Reichenbach, H., W. Kohl and H. Achenbach. 1981. The flexirubin-type pigments, chemosystematically useful compounds. *In* Reichenbach and Weeks (Editors), The *Flavobacterium-Cytophaga* Group. Verlag Chemie, Weinheim, F.R.G., pp. 101–108.

Reichenbach, H., W. Ludwig and E. Stackebrandt. 1986. Lack of relationship between gliding cyanobacteria and filamentous gliding heterotrophic eubacteria: comparison of 16S rRNA catalogues of *Spirulina*, *Saprospira*, *Vitreoscilla*, *Leucothrix*, and *Herpetosiphon*. Arch. Microbiol. *145:* 391–395.

Reichenbach, H., H. Voelz and M. Dworkin. 1969. Structural changes in *Stigmatella aurantiaca* during myxospore induction. J. Bacteriol. *97:* 905–911.

Reistad, R. 1970. On the composition and nature of the bulk protein of extremely halophilic bacteria. Arch. Mikrobiol. *71:* 353–360.

Reistad, R. 1975. Amino sugar and amino acid constituents of the cell wall of the extremely halophilic cocci. Arch. Mikrobiol. *102:* 71–73.

Remsen, C.C. 1978. Comparative subcellular architecture of photosynthetic bacteria. *In* Clayton and Sistrom (Editors), The Photosynthetic Bacteria. Plenum Press, New York and London, pp. 31–60.

Remsen, C.C. and S.W. Watson. 1972. Freeze-etching of bacteria. Int. Rev. Cytol. *33:* 253–296.

Resch, C.M. and J. Gibson. 1983. Isolation of the carotenoid-containing cell wall of three unicellular cyanobacteria. J. Bacteriol. *155:* 345–350.

Revsbech, N.P. and D.M. Ward. 1984. Microprofiles of dissolved substances and photosynthesis in microbial mats measured with microelectrodes. *In* Cohen, Castenholz and Halvorson (Editors), Microbial Mats: Stromatolites. Alan R. Liss, New York, pp. 171–188.

Reynolds, D.M., E.J. Laishley and J.W. Costerton. 1981. Physiological and ultrastructural characterization of a new acidophilic *Thiobacillus* species (*T. kabobis*). Can. J. Microbiol. *27:* 151–161.

Richardson, L.L. and R.W. Castenholz. 1987. Enhanced survival of the cyanobacterium *Oscillatoria terebriformis* in darkness under anaerobic conditions. Appl. Environ. Microbiol. *53:* 2151–2158.

Ridgway, H.F. 1977a. Ultrastructural characterization of globlet-shaped particles from the cell of *Flexibacter polymorphus*. Can. J. Microbiol. *23:* 1201–1213.

Ridgway, H.F. 1977b. Source of energy for gliding motility in *Flexibacter polymorphus*: effects of metabolic and respiratory inhibitors on gliding motility. J. Bacteriol. *131:* 544–556.

Ridgway, H.F. and R.A. Lewin. 1973. Goblet-shaped sub-units from the wall of a marine gliding microbe. J. Gen. Microbiol. *79:* 119–128.

Ridgway, H.F. and R.A. Lewin. 1983. Subunit composition of goblet-shaped particles from the cell wall of *Flexibacter polymorphus*. Can. J. Microbiol. *29:* 1689–1693.

Ridgway, H.F., R.M. Wagner, W.T. Dawsey and R.A. Lewin. 1975. Fine structure of the cell envelope layers of *Flexibacter polymorphus*. Can. J. Microbiol. *21:* 1733–1750.

Ringel, S.M., R.C. Greenough, S. Roemer, D. Connor, A.L. Gutt, B. Blair, G. Kanter and M. Von Strandtmann. 1977. Ambruticin (W7783). A new antifungal antibiotic. J. Antibiot. (Tokyo) *30:* 371–375.

Rippka, R. 1982. Citation. *In* Carr and Whitton (Editors), The Biology of Cyanobacteria. Blackwell, Oxford, and University of California Press, Berkeley, p. 292.

Rippka, R. and G. Cohen-Bazire. 1983. The *Cyanobacteriales*: a legitimate order based on the type strain *Cyanobacterium stanieri*? Ann. Microbiol. (Inst. Pasteur) *134B:* 21–36.

Rippka, R., J. Deruelles, J.B. Waterbury, M. Herdman and R.Y. Stanier. 1979. Generic assignments, strain histories and properties of pure cultures of cyanobacteria. J. Gen. Microbiol. *111:* 1–61.

Rippka, R., J. Waterbury and G. Cohen-Bazire. 1974. A cyanobacterium which lacks thylakoids. Arch. Microbiol. *100:* 419–436.

Rippka, R., J.B. Waterbury and R.Y. Stanier. 1981a. Isolation and purification of cyanobacteria: some general principles. *In* Starr, Stolp, Trüper, Balows and Schlegel (Editors), The Prokaryotes. A Handbook on Habitats, Isolation, and Identification of Bacteria. Springer-Verlag, Berlin, pp. 212–220.

Rippka, R., J.B. Waterbury and R.Y. Stanier. 1981b. Provisional generic assignments for cyanobacteria in pure culture. *In* Starr, Stolp, Trüper, Balows and Schlegel (Editors), The Prokaryotes. A Handbook on Habitats, Isolation, and Identification of Bacteria. Springer-Verlag, Berlin, pp. 247–256.

Ritchie, G.A.F. and D.J.D. Nicholas. 1972. Identification of the sources of nitrous oxide produced by oxidative and reductive processes in *Nitrosomonas europaea*. Biochem. J. *126:* 1181–1191.

Ritchie, G.A.F. and D.J.D. Nicholas. 1974. The partial characterization of purified nitrite reductase and hydroxylamine oxidase from *Nitrosomonas europaea*. Biochem. J. *138:* 471–480.

Rittenberg, S.C. 1972. The obligate autotroph—the demise of a concept. Antonie van Leeuwenhoek J. Microbiol. Serol. *38:* 457–478.

Rivard, C.J., J.M. Henson, M.V. Thomas and P.H. Smith. 1983. Isolation and characterization of *Methanomicrobium paynteri* sp. nov., a mesophilic methanogen isolated from marine sediments. Appl. Environ. Microbiol. *46:* 484–490.

Rivard, C.J., J.M. Henson, M.V. Thomas and P.H. Smith. 1984. *In* Validation of the publication of new names and new combinations previously effectively published outside the IJSB. List No. 13. Int. J. Syst. Bacteriol. *34:* 91–92.

Rivard, C.J. and P.H. Smith. 1982. Isolation and characterization of a thermophilic marine methanogenic bacterium, *Methanogenium thermophilicum* sp. nov. Int. J. Syst. Bacteriol. *32:* 430–436.

Roberts, G.P., W.T. Leps, L.E. Silver and W.J. Brill. 1980. Use of two-dimensional gel electrophoresis to identify and classify *Rhizobium* strains. Appl. Environ. Microbiol. *39:* 414–422.

Robertson, L.A. and J.G. Kuenen. 1983. *Thiosphaera pantotropha* gen. nov. sp. nov., a facultatively anaerobic, facultatively autotrophic sulphur bacterium. J. Gen. Microbiol. *129:* 2847–2855.

Robertson, L.A. and J.G. Kuenen. 1984a. *In* Validation of the publication of new names and new combinations previously effectively published outside the IJSB. List No. 13. Int. J. Syst. Bacteriol. *34:* 91.

Robertson, L.A. and J.G. Kuenen. 1984b. Aerobic denitrification, a controversy revived. Arch. Microbiol. *137:* 351–354.

Robertson, L.A. and J.G. Kuenen. 1984c. Aerobic denitrification—old wine in new bottles? Antonie van Leeuwenhoek J. Microbiol. Serol. *50:* 525–544.

Robinson, I. and M.J. Allison. 1969. Isoleucine biosynthesis from 2-methylbutyric acid by anaerobic bacteria from the rumen. J. Bacteriol. *97:* 1220–1226.

Robinson, R.W. 1986. Life cycles in the methanogenic archaebacterium *Methanosarcina mazei.* Appl. Environ. Microbiol. *52:* 17–27.

Robinson, R.W., H.C. Aldrich, S.F. Hurst and A.S. Bleiweis. 1985. Role of the cell surface of *Methanosarcina mazei* in cell aggregation. Appl. Environ. Microbiol. *49:* 321–327.

Rodriguez-Valera, F., G. Juez and D.J. Kushner. 1982. Halocins: salt-dependent bacteriocins produced by extremely halophilic bacteria. Can. J. Microbiol. *28:* 151–154.

Rodriguez-Valera, F., G. Juez and D.J. Kushner. 1983. *Halobacterium mediterranei,* sp. nov., a new carbohydrate-utilizing extreme halophile. Syst. Appl. Microbiol. *4:* 369–381.

Rodriguez-Valera, F., G. Juez and D.J. Kushner. 1983. *In* Validation of the publication of new names and new combinations previously effectively published outside the IJSB. List No. 12. Int. J. Syst. Bacteriol. *33:* 896–897.

Rodriguez-Valera, F., J.J. Nieto and F. Ruiz-Berraquero. 1983. Light as an energy source in continuous cultures of bacteriorhodopsin-containing halobacteria. Appl. Env. Microbiol. *45:* 868–871.

Rodriguez-Valera, F., F. Ruiz-Berraquero and A. Ramos-Cormenzana. 1979. Isolation of extreme halophiles from seawater. Appl. Environ. Microbiol. *38:* 164–165.

Rodriguez-Valera, F., F. Ruiz-Berraquero and A. Ramos-Cormenzana. 1980. Isolation of extremely halophilic bacteria able to grow in defined organic media with single carbon sources. J. Gen. Microbiol. *119:* 535–538.

Roelofsen, P.A. 1934. On the metabolism of the purple sulfur bacteria. Proc. K. Ned. Akad. Wet. *37:* 660–669.

Rogers, S.R. and J.J. Anderson. 1976a. Measurement of growth and iron deposition in *Sphaerotilus discophorus.* J. Bacteriol. *126:* 257–263.

Rogers, S.R. and J.J. Anderson. 1976b. Role of iron deposition in *Sphaerotilus discophorus.* J. Bacteriol. *126:* 264–271.

Rohmer, M., P. Bouvier-Nave and G. Ourisson. 1984. Distribution of hopanoid triterpens in prokaryotes. J. Gen. Microbiol. *130:* 1137–1150.

Rolls, J.P. and E.S. Lindstrom. 1967. Effect of thiosulfate on the photosynthetic growth of *Rhodopseudomonas palustris.* J. Bacteriol. *94:* 860–866.

Romano, A.H. and J.P. Peloquin. 1963. Composition of the sheath of *Sphaerotilus natans.* J. Bacteriol. *86:* 252–258.

Romesser, J.A. and R.S. Wolfe. 1982. Coupling of Coenzyme M reduction with carbon dioxide activation in extracts of *Methanobacterium thermoautotrophicum.* J. Bacteriol. *152:* 840–847.

Romesser, J.A., R.S. Wolfe, F. Mayer, E. Spiess and A. Walther-Mauruschat. 1979. *Methanogenium,* a new genus of marine methanogenic bacteria, and characterization of *Methanogenium cariaci* sp. nov. and *Methanogenium marisnigri* sp. nov. Arch. Microbiol. *121:* 147–153.

Romesser, J.A., R.S. Wolfe, F. Mayer, E. Spiess and A. Walther-Mauruschat. 1981. *In* Validation of the publication of new names and new combinations previously effectively published outside the IJSB. List No. 6. Int. J. Syst. Bacteriol. *31:* 215–218.

Roper, M.M. and K.C. Marshall. 1977. Lysis of *Escherichia coli* by a marine myxobacter. Microb. Ecol. *3:* 167–171.

Rosenberg, E. (Editor). 1984. Myxobacteria: Development and Cell Interactions. Springer-Verlag, New York.

Rosenberg, E., B. Vaks and A. Zuckerberg. 1973. Bacteriocidal action of an antibiotic produced by *Myxococcus xanthus.* Antimicrob. Agents Chemother. *4:* 507–513.

Rosenberg, R., W.E. Arntz, E.C. de Flores, L.A. Flores, G. Carbajal, I. Finger and J. Tarazona. 1983. Benthos biomass and oxygen deficiency in the upwelling system off Peru. J. Mar. Res. *41:* 263–279.

Rosenfelder, G., O. Lüderitz and O. Westphal. 1974. Composition of lipopolysaccharides from *Myxococcus fulvus* and other fruiting and nonfruiting myxobacteria. Eur. J. Biochem. *44:* 411–420.

Ross, H.N.M. and W.D. Grant. 1985. Nucleic acid studies on halophilic archaebacteria. J. Gen. Microbiol. *131:* 165–173.

Ross, H.N.M., W.D. Grant and J.E. Harris. 1985. Lipids in archaebacterial taxonomy. *In* Goodfellow and Minnikin (Editors), Chemical Methods in Bacterial Systematics. Academic Press, New York, pp. 289–299.

Roth, A.W. 1797. Catalecta botanica quibus plantae novae et minus cognitae describuntur atque illustrantur. Lipsiae in Biblioplio I.G. Mulleriano, fasc. 1.

Rouf, M.A. and J.L. Stokes. 1964. Morphology, nutrition and physiology of *Sphaerotilus discophorus.* Arch. Mikrobiol. *49:* 132–149.

Roustan, J.L., J.P. Touzel, G. Prensier, H.C. Dubourguier and G. Albagnac. 1986. Evidence for a lytic bacteriophage for *Methanothrix* sp. *In* Dubourguier, Albagnac, Montreuil, Romond, Sautière and Guillaume (Editors), Biology of Anaerobic Bacteria. Elsevier Science Publishers, Amsterdam, pp. 200–250.

Roze, E. 1896. Le *Clonothrix,* un nouveau type générique de Cyanophycées. J. Bot. (Paris) *10:* 325–330.

Ruby, E.G. and H.W. Jannasch. 1982. Physiological characteristics of *Thiomicrospira* sp. strain L-12 isolated from deep-sea hydrothermal vents. J. Bacteriol. *149:* 161–165.

Ruby, E.G., C.O. Wirsen and H.W. Jannasch. 1981. Chemolithotrophic sulfur-oxidizing bacteria from the Galapagos rift hydrothermal vents. Appl. Environ. Microbiol. *42:* 317–324.

Rucker, R.R., B.J. Earp and E.J. Ordal. 1953. Infectious diseases of Pacific salmon. Trans. Am. Fish. Soc. *83:* 297–312.

Rückert, G. 1972. Bodenbakterien in Island. Fridericiana. Z. Univ. Karlsruhe *11:* 22–32.

Rückert, G. 1972. Vergleichende Untersuchungen über die Verbreitung einiger Fruchtkörper-bildender Myxobakterien-Arten. Z. Allg. Mikrobiol. *12:* 655–665.

Rückert, G. 1975. Zur Verbreitung bakteriotropher Myxobakterien Waldböden. Mitt. Ver. Forstl. Standortskart Forstpfl. *24:* 43–47.

Ruschke, R. 1968. Die Bedeutung von Wassermyxobakterien für den Abbau organischen Materials. Mitt. Int. Ver. Limnol. *14:* 164–167.

Ruschke, R. and K. Köhn. 1970. Untersuchungen zum Abbau kondensierter Phosphate aus Waschmitteln durch *Sporocytophaga cauliformis* und *Pseudomonas fluorescens.* Zentralbl. Bakteriol. Parasitenkd. Infektionskr. Hyg. Abt. II *124:* 81–90.

Ruschke, R. and M. Rath. 1966. *Sporocytophaga cauliformis* Knorr and Gräf, eine Myxobakterienart mit grosser Bedeutung für den Abbau organischen Materials. Arch. Hydrobiol. Suppl. XXVIII *4:* 377–402.

Sahl, H.G. and H.G. Trüper. 1977. Enzymes of CO_2 fixation in *Chromatiaceae.* FEMS Microbiol. Lett. *2:* 129–132.

Sahm, H., R.B. Cox and J.R. Quayle. 1976. Metabolism of methanol by *Rhodopseudomonas acidophila.* J. Gen. Microbiol. *94:* 313–322.

Saier, M.H., Jr. 1977. Bacterial phosphoenolpyruvate:sugar phosphotransferase systems: structural, functional, and evolutionary interrelationships. Bacteriol. Rev. *41:* 856–871.

Saier, M.H. and J.T. Staley. 1977. Phosphoenolpyruvate: sugar phosphotransferase system in *Ancalomicrobium adetum.* J. Bacteriol. *131:* 716–718.

Salanitro, J.P., P.A. Muirhead and J.R. Goodman. 1976. Morphological and physiological characteristics of *Gemmiger formicilis* isolated from chicken ceca. Appl. Environ. Microbiol. *32:* 623–632.

Samsonoff, W.A., T. Hashimoto and S.F. Conti. 1970. Ultrastructural changes associated with germination and outgrowth of an appendage-bearing clostridial spore. J. Bacteriol. *101:* 1038–1045.

Sanfilippo, A. and R.A. Lewin. 1970. Preservation of viable flexibacteria at low temperatures. Can. J. Microbiol. *16:* 441–444.

Sanger, F., G.G. Brownlee and B.G. Barrell. 1965. A two-dimensional fractionation procedure for radioactive nucleotides. J. Mol. Biol. *13:* 373–398.

Sanger, F., S. Nicklen and A.R. Coulson. 1977. DNA sequencing with chain-terminating inhibitors. Proc. Natl. Acad. Sci. U.S.A. *74:* 5463–5467.

Sangkhobol, V. and V.B.D. Skerman. 1981. *Chitinophaga,* a new genus of chitinolytic myxobacteria. Int. J. Syst. Bacteriol. *31:* 285–293.

Sanzhieva, E.U. and G.A. Zavarzin. 1971. A bacterium which oxidizes carbon monoxide. Dokl. Akad. Nauk S.S.S.R. *196:* 956–958.

Sarao, R., H.D. McCurdy and L. Passador. 1985. Enzymes of the intermediary carbohydrate metabolism of *Polyangium cellulosum.* Can. J. Microbiol. *31:* 1142–1146.

Sarkar, P.K. and A.K. Banerjee. 1980. Nicotinic acid as an essential growth factor of *Rhodospirillum photometricum* and a new *Rhodospirillum* isolate. Naturwissenschaften *67:* 41–42.

Sarles, L.S. and F.R. Tabita. 1983. Derepression of the synthesis of D-ribulose 1,5-bisphosphate carboxylase/oxygenase from *Rhodospirillum rubrum.* J. Bacteriol. *153:* 458–464.

Sarokin, D.J. and E.J. Carpenter. 1981. Cyanobacterial spinae. Bot. Mar. *24:* 389–392.

Sato, K. 1978. Bacteriochlorophyll formation by facultative methylotrophs, *Protaminobacter ruber* and *Pseudomonas* AM 1. FEBS Lett. *85:* 207–210.

Sato, K., K. Ishida, T. Kuno, A. Mizuno and S. Shimizu. 1981. Regulation of vitamin B_{12} and bacteriochlorophyll biosynthesis in a facultative methylotroph, *Protaminobacter ruber.* J. Nutr. Sci. Vitaminol. *27:* 439–441.

Sato, K. and S. Shimizu. 1979. The conditions for bacteriochlorophyll formation and the ultrastructure of a methanol-utilizing bacterium, *Protaminobacter ruber,* classified as non-photosynthetic bacteria. Agric. Biol. Chem. *43:* 1669–1675.

Satoh, T., Y. Hoshina and H. Kitamura. 1974. Isolation of denitrifying photosynthetic bacteria. Agric. Biol. Chem. *38:* 1749–1751.

Satoh, T., Y. Hoshino and H. Kitamura. 1976. *Rhodopseudomonas sphaeroides* forma sp. *denitrificans,* a denitrifying strain as a subspecies of *Rhodopseudomonas sphaeroides.* Arch. Microbiol. *108:* 265–269.

Saunders, V.A. 1978. Genetics of *Rhodospirillaceae.* Microbiol. Rev. *42:* 357–384.

Sayre, R.M. and M.P. Starr. 1985. *Pasteuria penetrans* (ex Thorne 1940) nom. rev., comb. nov., sp. nov., a mycelial and endospore-forming bacterium parasitic in plant-parasitic nematodes. Proc. Helminthol. Soc. Wash. *52:* 149–165.

Schaab, C., F. Giffhorn, S. Schobert, N. Pfennig and G. Gottschalk. 1972. Phototrophic growth of *Rhodopseudomonas gelatinosa* on citrate: accumulation and subsequent utilization of cleavage products. Z. Naturforsch. *27b:* 962–967.

Schachte, J.H. and E.C. Mora. 1973. Production of agglutinating antibodies in the channel catfish *(Ictalurus punctatus)* against *Chondrococcus columnaris.* J. Fish. Res. Board Can. *30:* 116–118.

Schäfer, S., C. Barkowski and G. Fuchs. 1986. Carbon assimilation by the autotrophic thermophilic archaebacterium *Thermoproteus neutrophilus.* Arch.

Microbiol. *146:* 301–308.

Schauer, N.L., D.P. Brown and J.G. Ferry. 1982. Kinetics of a formate metabolism in *Methanobacterium formicicum* and *Methanospirillum hungatei.* Appl. Environ. Microbiol. *44:* 549–554.

Schauer, N.L. and J.G. Ferry. 1980. Metabolism of formate in *Methanobacterium formicicum.* J. Bacteriol. *142:* 800–807.

Scheminzky, F., Z. Klas and C. Job. 1972. Über das Vorkommen von *Thiobacterium bovista* in Thermalwässern. Int. Rev. Gesamten Hydrobiol. *57:* 801–813.

Scherer, P. and H. Kneifel. 1983. Distribution of polyamines in methanogenic bacteria. J. Bacteriol. *154:* 1315–1322.

Schewiakoff, W. 1893. Über einen neuen bacterienähnlichen Organismus des Süsswassers., Habilitationsschrift, Universität Heidelberg, C. Winter, pp. 1–36.

Schildkraut, C.L., J. Marmur and P. Doty. 1962. Determination of the base composition of deoxyribonucleic acid from its buoyant density in CsCl. J. Mol. Biol. *4:* 430–443.

Schlegel, H.G. and N. Pfennig. 1961. Die Anreicherungskultur einiger Schwefelpurpurbakterien. Arch. Mikrobiol. *38:* 1–39.

Schleifer, K.H. and O. Kandler. 1967. Zur chemischen zusammensetzung der zellwand der Streptokokken. I. Die aminosäuresequenz des mureins von *Str. thermophilus* und *Str. faecalis.* Arch. Mikrobiol. *57:* 335–364.

Schleifer, K.H. and O. Kandler. 1972. Peptidoglycan types of bacterial cell walls and their taxonomic implications. Bacteriol. Rev. *36:* 407–477.

Schleifer, K.H. and P.H. Seidl. 1985. Chemical composition and structure of murein. *In* Goodfellow and Minnikin (Editors), Chemical Methods in Bacterial Systematics. Academic Press, London, New York, pp. 201–219.

Schleifer, K.H. and E. Stackebrandt. 1983. Molecular systematics of prokaryotes. Annu. Rev. Microbiol. *37:* 143–187.

Schlesner, H. 1983. Isolierung und Beschreibung knospender und prosthekater Bakterien aus der Kieler Förde. Ph.D. thesis, Christian-Albrechts-Universität, Kiel, F.R.G

Schlesner, H. and P. Hirsch. 1984. Assignment of ATCC 27377 to *Pirella* gen. nov. as *Pirella staleyi* comb. nov. Int. J. Syst. Bacteriol. *34:* 492–495.

Schlesner, H. and E. Stackebrandt. 1986. Assignment of the genera *Planctomyces* and *Pirella* to a new family *Planctomycetaceae* fam. nov. and description of the order *Planctomycetales* ord. nov. Syst. Appl. Microbiol. *8:* 174–176.

Schmid, K., M. Thomm, A. Laminet, F.G. Laue, C. Kessler, K.O. Stetter and R. Schmitt. 1984. Three new restriction endonucleases *Mae*I, *Mae*II and *Mae*III from *Methanococcus aeolicus.* Nucleic Acids Res. *12:* 2619–2628.

Schmidle, W. 1901. Neue Algen aus dem Gibiete des Oberrheins. Beih. Bot. Zentralbl. *10:* 179–180.

Schmidt, J. 1901. Plankt. Röde Hav og Adenb., Vidensk. Med. Nat. Foren. Kjöbenh., p. 147.

Schmidt, J.M. 1978. Isolation and ultrastructure of freshwater strains of *Planctomyces.* Curr. Microbiol. *1:* 65–70.

Schmidt, J.M. 1981a. The genera *Caulobacter* and *Asticcacaulis. In* Starr, Stolp, Trüper, Balows and Schlegel (Editors), The Prokaryotes. A Handbook on Habitats, Isolation, and Identification of Bacteria. Springer-Verlag, Berlin, pp. 466–476.

Schmidt, J.M. 1981b. The genus *Thiodendron. In* Starr, Stolp, Trüper, Balows and Schlegel (Editors), The Prokaryotes. A Handbook on Habitats, Isolation, and Identification of Bacteria. Springer-Verlag, Berlin, pp. 488–489.

Schmidt, J.M., P.R. Dong and M.P. Starr. 1980. Cell envelope features, antibiotic resistance, and related properties of isolates of the *Blastocaulis-Planctomyces* group. Abst. Annu. Meet., Am. Soc. Microbiol. *1980:* 102.

Schmidt, J.M., W.P. Sharp and M.P. Starr. 1981. Manganese and iron encrustations and other features of *Planctomyces crassus* Hortobágyi 1965, morphotype Ib of the *Blastocaulis-Planctomyces* group of budding and appendaged bacteria, examined by electron microscopy and x-ray micro-analysis. Curr. Microbiol. *5:* 241–246.

Schmidt, J.M., W.P. Sharp and M.P. Starr. 1982. Metallic-oxide encrustations of the nonprosthecate stalks of naturally occurring populations of *Planctomyces bekefii.* Curr. Microbiol. *7:* 389–394.

Schmidt, J.M. and R.Y. Stanier. 1965. Isolation and characterization of bacteriophages active against stalked bacteria. J. Gen. Microbiol. *39:* 95–107.

Schmidt, J.M. and R.Y. Stanier. 1966. The development of cellular stalks in bacteria. J. Cell Biol. *28:* 423–436.

Schmidt, J.M. and M.P. Starr. 1978. Morphological diversity of freshwater bacteria belonging to the *Blastocaulis-Planctomyces* group as observed in natural populations and enrichments. Curr. Microbiol. *1:* 325–330.

Schmidt, J.M. and M.P. Starr. 1979a. Morphotype V of the *Blastocaulis-Planctomyces* group of budding and appendaged bacteria: *Planctomyces guttaeformis* Hortobágyi (sensu Hajdú). Curr. Microbiol. *2:* 195–200.

Schmidt, J.M. and M.P. Starr. 1979b. Corniculate cell surface protrusions in morphotype II of the *Blastocaulis-Planctomyces* group of budding and appendaged bacteria. Curr. Microbiol. *3:* 187–190.

Schmidt, J.M. and M.P. Starr. 1980a. Current sightings, at the respective type localities and elsewhere, of *Planctomyces bekefii* Gimesi 1924 and *Blastocaulis sphaerica* Henrici and Johnson 1935. Curr. Microbiol. *4:* 183–188.

Schmidt, J.M. and M.P. Starr. 1980b. Some ultrastructural features of *Planctomyces bekefii,* morphotype I of the *Blastocaulis-Planctomyces* group of budding and appendaged bacteria. Curr. Microbiol. *4:* 189–194.

Schmidt, J.M. and M.P. Starr. 1981. The *Blastocaulis-Planctomyces* group of budding and appendaged bacteria. *In* Starr, Stolp, Trüper, Balows and Schlegel

(Editors), The Prokaryotes. A Handbook on Habitats, Isolation, and Identification of Bacteria. Springer-Verlag. Berlin, pp. 496–504.

Schmidt, J.M. and M.P. Starr. 1982. Ultrastructural features of budding cells in a prokaryote belonging to morphotype IV of the *Blastocaulis-Planctomyces* group. Curr. Microbiol. *7:* 7–11.

Schmidt, J.M. and M.P. Starr. 1984. Unidirectional polar growth of cells of *Seliberia stellata* and aquatic *Seliberia*-like bacteria revealed by immunoferritin labeling. Arch. Microbiol. *138:* 89–95.

Schmidt, J.M. and J.R. Swafford. 1975. Ultrastructure of crossbands in prosthecae of *Asticcacaulis* species. J. Bacteriol. *124:* 1601–1603.

Schmidt, J.M. and J.R. Swafford. 1979. Isolation and morphology of helically sculptured, rosette-forming, freshwater bacteria resembling *Seliberia.* Curr. Microbiol. *3:* 65–70.

Schmidt, J.M. and J.R. Swafford. 1981. The genus *Seliberia. In* Starr, Stolp, Trüper, Balows and Schlegel (Editors), The Prokaryotes. A Handbook on Habitats, Isolation, and Identification of Bacteria. Springer-Verlag, Berlin, pp. 516–519.

Schmidt, K. 1978. Biosynthesis of carotenoids. *In* Clayton and Sistrom (Editors), The Photosynthetic Bacteria. Plenum Press, New York, London, pp. 729–750.

Schmidt, K. 1980. A comparative study on the composition of chlorosomes (chlorobium vesicles) and cytoplasmic membranes from *Chloroflexus aurantiacus* strain OK-70-fl and *Chlorobium limicola* f. *thiosulfatophilum* strain 6230. Arch. Microbiol. *124:* 21–31.

Schmidt, K. and B. Bowien. 1983. Notes on the description of *Rhodopseudomonas blastica.* Arch. Microbiol. *136:* 242.

Schmidt, K. and S. Liaaen-Jensen. 1973. Bacterial carotenoids. XLII. New ketocarotenoids from *Rhodopseudomonas globiformis.* Acta Chem. Scand. *27:* 3040–3052.

Schmidt, K., M. Maarzahl and F. Mayer. 1980. Development and pigmentation of chlorosomes in *Chloroflexus aurantiacus* strain OK-70-fl. Arch. Microbiol. *123:* 87–97.

Schmidt, K., N. Pfennig and S. Liaaen-Jensen. 1965. Carotenoids of *Thiorhodaceae.* IV. The carotenoid composition of 25 pure isolates. Arch. Mikrobiol. *52:* 132–146.

Schmidt, K. and R. Schiburr. 1970. Die Carotinoide der grünen Schwefel bakterien: Carotinoidzusammensetzung in 18 Stämmen. Arch. Mikrobiol. *74:* 350–355.

Schmidt, K. and H.G. Trüper. 1971. Carotenoid composition in the genus *Ectothiorhodospira* Pelsh. Arch. Mikrobiol. *80:* 38–42.

Schmidt, T.M. 1985. Anaerobic reduction of elemental sulfur by *Chromatium vinosum* and *Beggiatoa alba. In* Sagan (Editor), The Global Sulfur Cycle. NASA Office of Space Science Applications, Washington, D.C., pp. 108–113.

Schmidt, T.M., B. Arieli, Y. Cohen, E. Padan, and W.R. Strohl. 1987. Sulfur metabolism in *Beggiatoa alba.* J. Bacteriol. *169:* 5466–5472.

Schmidt, T.M., V.A. Vinci and W.R. Strohl. 1986. Protein synthesis by *Beggiatoa alba* B18LD in the presence and absence of sulfide. Arch. Microbiol. *144:* 158–162.

Schmidt, W., G. Drews, J. Weckesser, I. Fromme and D. Borowiak. 1980. Characterization of the lipopolysaccharides from eight strains of the cyanobacterium *Synechococcus.* Arch. Microbiol. *127:* 209–215.

Schmidt, W.D. 1984. Die Eisenbakterien des Plussees. II. Morphologie und Feinstruktur von *Siderocapsa geminata* (Skuja 1954/57). Z. Allg. Mikrobiol. *24:* 391–396.

Schnabel, R., M. Thomm, R. Gerardy-Schahn, W. Zillig, K.O. Stetter and J. Huet. 1983. Structural homology between different archaebacterial DNA-dependent RNA polymerases analyzed by immunological comparison of their components. EMBO J. *2:* 751–755.

Schnellen, C.G.T.P. 1947. Onderzoekingen over de methaanginsting. Thesis, Technisches Hoogeschool Delft, Druckkerij "De Maasstad," Rotterdam, The Netherlands, pp. 1–137.

Schoenichen, W. 1925. Einfachsten Lebensformen des Tier- und Pflanzenteiches, 5th Ed. Spaltpflanzen, Geissellinge, Algen. Behrmuhler, Berlin *1:* 1–519.

Schoenlein, P.V. and B. Ely. 1983. Plasmids and bacteriocins in *Caulobacter* species. J. Bacteriol. *153:* 1092–1094.

Schönichen, W. and A. Kalberlah. 1900. IV Fam. *Chlamydobacteriaceae. In* Eyferth's Lebensformen des Tier- und Pflanzenreiches. Benno Goeritz, Braunschweig, pp. 43–47.

Schook, L.B. and R.S. Berk. 1978. Nutritional studies with *Pseudomonas aeruginosa* grown on inorganic sulfur sources. J. Bacteriol. *133:* 1377–1382.

Schoop, G. 1935. *Halococcus litoralis,* ein obligat halophiles Farbstoffbildner. Dtsch. Tierarzl. Wochenschr. *43:* 817–820.

Schopf, J.W. and M.R. Walter. 1982. Origin and evolution of cyanobacteria: the geological evidence. *In* Carr and Whitton (Editors), The Biology of Cyanobacteria. Blackwell, Oxford, and University of California Press, Berkeley, pp. 543–564.

Schorler, B. 1904. Beiträge zur Kenntnis der Eisenbakterien. Zentralbl. Bakteriol. Parasitenkd. Infektionskr. Hyg. Abt. II *12:* 681–695.

Schrader, M., G. Drews, J.R. Golecki and J. Weckesser. 1982. Isolation and characterization of the sheath from the cyanobacterium, *Chlorogloeopsis* PCC 6912. J. Gen. Microbiol. *128:* 267–272.

Schröder, J. and H. Reichenbach. 1970. The fatty acid composition of vegetative cells and myxospores of *Stigmatella aurantiaca* (*Myxobacterales*). Arch. Mikrobiol. *71:* 384–390.

Schroeter, J. 1885–1889. *In* Cohn (Editor), Kryptogamenflora von Schlesien Bd. 3,

Heft 3, Pilze. J.U. Kern's Verlag, Breslau, pp. 1-814.

Schultz, J.E. and P.F. Weaver. 1982. Fermentation and anaerobic respiration by *Rhodospirillum rubrum* and *Rhodopseudomonas capsulata*. J. Bacteriol. *149:* 181-190.

Schulz, E. and P. Hirsch. 1973. Morphologically unusual bacteria in acid bog water habitats. Abstr. Annu. Meet. Am. Soc. Microbiol. *73:* 60.

Schulz-Baldes, M. and R.A. Lewin. 1976. Fine structure of *Synechocystis didemni* (Cyanophyta: Chroococcales). Phycologia *15:* 1-6.

Schürmann, C. 1967. Growth of myxococci in suspension in liquid media. Appl. Microbiol. *15:* 971-974.

Schwabe, G.H. 1960. Über den thermobionten Kosmopoliten *Mastigocladus laminosus* Cohn. Schweiz. Z. Hydrol. *22:* 759-792.

Schwabe, H. 1827. *In* Sprengel, Syst. Veg. 4, Part 1, p. 314.

Schwartz, R.M. and M.O. Dayhoff. 1978. Origins of prokaryotes, eukaryotes, mitochondria, and chloroplasts. Science (Washington) *199:* 395-403.

Schwers, E. 1912. *Megalothrix discophora*, eine neue Eisenbakterie. Zentralbl. Bakteriol. Parasitenkd. Infektionskr. Hyg. Abt. II *33:* 273-276.

Scott, O.T., R.W. Castenholz and H.T. Bonnett. 1984. Evidence for a peptidoglycan envelope in the cyanelles of *Glaucocystis nostochinearum* Itzigsohn. Arch. Microbiol. *139:* 130-138.

Scotten, H.L. and J.L. Stokes. 1962. Isolation and properties of *Beggiatoa*. Arch. Mikrobiol. *42:* 353-368.

Searcy, D.G. 1976. *Thermoplasma acidophilum:* intracellular pH and potassium concentration. Biochim. Biophys. Acta *451:* 278-286.

Searcy, D.G. and E.K. Doyle. 1975. Characterization of *Thermoplasma acidophilum* deoxyribonucleic acid. Int. J. Syst. Bacteriol. *25:* 286-289.

Searcy, K.B. and D.G. Searcy. 1981. Superoxide dismutase from the archaebacterium *Thermoplasma acidophilum*. Biochim. Biophys. Acta *670:* 39-46.

Seewaldt, E., K.-H. Schleifer, E. Bock and E. Stackebrandt. 1982. The close phylogenetic relationship of *Nitrobacter* and *Rhodopseudomonas palustris*. Arch. Microbiol. *131:* 287-290.

Seewaldt, E. and E. Stackebrandt. 1982. Partial sequence of 16S ribosomal RNA and the phylogeny of *Prochloron*. Nature (London) *295:* 618-620.

Segerer, A., A. Neuner, J.K. Kristjansson and K.O. Stetter. 1986. *Acidianus infernus* gen. nov., sp. nov., and *Acidianus brierleyi* comb. nov.: facultatively aerobic, extremely acidophilic thermophilic sulfur-metabolizing archaebacteria. Int. J. Syst. Bacteriol. *36:* 559-564.

Segerer, A., K.O. Stetter and F. Klink. 1985. Two contrary modes of chemolithotrophy in the same archaebacterium. Nature *313:* 787-789.

Sewell, D.L. and M.I.H. Aleem. 1979. NADH-linked oxidative phosphorylation in *Nitrobacter agilis*. Curr. Microbiol. *2:* 35-37.

Sgorbati, B. 1979. Preliminary quantification of immunological relationships among the transaldolases of the genus *Bifidobacterium*. Antonie van Leeuwenhoek J. Microbiol. Serol. *45:* 557-564.

Sgorbati, B. and V. Scardovi. 1979. Immunological relationships among transaldolases in the genus *Bifidobacterium*. Antonie van Leeuwenhoek J. Microbiol. Serol. *49:* 129-140.

Shafia, F., K.R. Brinson, M.W. Heinzman and J.M. Brady. 1972. Transition of chemolithotroph *Ferrobacillus ferrooxidans* to obligate organotrophy and metabolic capabilities of glucose grown cells. J. Bacteriol. *111:* 56-65.

Shah, H.N., R.A. Nash, J.M. Hardie, D.A. Weetman, D.A. Geddes and T.W. MacFarlane. 1985. Detection of acidic end-products of metabolism of anaerobic Gram-negative bacteria. *In* Goodfellow and Minnikin (Editors), Chemical Methods in Bacterial Systematics. Academic Press, London, New York, pp. 317-340.

Sharak Genthner, B.R., C.L. Davis and M.P. Bryant. 1981. Features of rumen and sewage sludge strains of *Eubacterium limosum*, a methanol and H_2-CO_2-utilizing species. Appl. Environ. Microbiol. *42:* 12-19.

Shaw, N. 1975. Bacterial glycolipids and glycophospholipids. Adv. Microb. Physiol. *12:* 141-167.

Shelton, R.G.J., P.M.J. Shelton and A.S. Edwards. 1975. Observations with the scanning electron microscope on a filamentous bacterium present on the aesthetic setae of the brown shrimp *Crangon crangon* (L.). J. Mar. Biol. Assoc. U.K. *55:* 795-800.

Shewan, J.M. 1971. The microbiology of fish and fishery products—a progress report. J. Appl. Bacteriol. *34:* 299-315.

Shewan, J.M. and T.A. McMeekin. 1983. Taxonomy (and ecology) of *Flavobacterium* and related genera. Annu. Rev. Microbiol. *37:* 233-252.

Shiba, H., T. Kawasumi, Y. Igarashi, T. Kodama and Y. Minoda. 1982. The deficient carbohydrate metabolic pathways and the incomplete tricarboxylic acid cycle in an obligately autotrophic hydrogen-oxidizing bacterium. Agric. Biol. Chem. *46:* 2341-2345.

Shiba, T. 1984. Utilization of light energy by the strictly aerobic bacterium *Erythrobacter* sp. OCH 114. J. Gen. Appl. Microbiol. *30:* 239-244.

Shiba, T. and U. Simidu. 1982. *Erythrobacter longus* gen. nov., sp. nov., an aerobic bacterium which contains bacteriochlorophyll *a*. Int. J. Syst. Bacteriol. *32:* 211-217.

Shiba, T., U. Simidu and N. Taga. 1979. Distribution of aerobic bacteria which contain bacteriochlorophyll *a*. Appl. Environ. Microbiol. *38:* 43-45.

Shiba, T. and N. Taga. 1980. Heterotrophic bacteria attached to seaweeds. J. Exp. Mar. Biol. Ecol. *47:* 251-258.

Shilo, M. 1970. Lysis of blue-green algae by myxobacter. J. Bacteriol. *104:* 453-461.

Shimkets, L. and T.W. Seale. 1975. Fruiting-body formation and myxospore differentiation and germination in *Myxococcus xanthus* viewed by scanning

electron microscopy. J. Bacteriol. *121:* 711-720.

Shishkina, V.M. and Yu. A. Trotsenko. 1974. Characteristics of a new *Hyphomicrobium* strain utilizing one-carbon compounds. Mikrobiologiya *43:* 765-770 (English translation: 653-657).

Shively, J.M. 1974. Inclusion bodies of prokaryotes. Annu. Rev. Microbiol. *28:* 167-187.

Shively, J.M., E. Bock, K. Westphal and G.C. Cannon. 1977. Isohedral inclusions (carboxysomes) of *Nitrobacter agilis*. J. Bacteriol. *132:* 673-675.

Shively, J.M., G.L. Decker and J.W. Greenawalt. 1970. Comparative ultrastructure of the thiobacilli. J. Bacteriol. *101:* 618-627.

Shivvers, D.W. and T.D. Brock. 1973. Oxidation of elemental sulfur by *Sulfolobus acidocaldarius*. J. Bacteriol. *114:* 706-710.

Shotts, E.B. and G.L. Bullock. 1975. Bacterial diseases of fishes: diagnostic procedures for Gram-negative pathogens. J. Fish. Res. Board Can. *32:* 1243-1247.

Shporer, M. and M.M. Civan. 1977. Pulsed nuclear magnetic resonance study of ^{39}K within halobacteria. J. Membr. Biol. *33:* 385-400.

Shuttleworth, K.L., R.F. Unz and P.L. Wichlacz. 1985. Glucose catabolism in strains of acidophilic, heterotrophic bacteria. Appl. Environ. Microbiol. *50:* 573-579.

Siefert, E. 1976. Die Fixierung von molekularem Stickstoff bei phototrophen Bakterien am Beispiel von *Rhodopseudomonas acidophila*. Ph.D. thesis, University of Göttingen, F.R.G.

Siefert, E., R.L. Irgens and N. Pfennig. 1978. Phototrophic purple and green bacteria in a sewage treatment plant. Appl. Environ. Microbiol. *35:* 38-44.

Siefert, E. and V.B. Koppenhagen. 1982. Studies on the vitamin B_{12} auxotrophy of *Rhodocyclus purpureus* and two other vitamin B_{12}-requiring purple nonsulfur bacteria. Arch. Microbiol. *132:* 173-178.

Siefert, E. and N. Pfennig. 1979. Chemoautotrophic growth of *Rhodopseudomonas* species with hydrogen and chemotrophic utilization of methanol and formate. Arch. Microbiol. *122:* 177-182.

Siefert, E. and N. Pfennig. 1980. Diazotrophic growth of *Rhodopseudomonas acidophila* and *Rhodopseudomonas capsulata* under microaerobic conditions in the dark. Arch. Microbiol. *125:* 73-77.

Siefert, E. and N. Pfennig. 1984. Convenient method to prepare neutral sulfide solution for cultivation of phototrophic sulfur bacteria. Arch. Microbiol. *139:* 100-101.

Sijderius, R. 1946. Heterotrophe bacterien, die thiosulfaat oxydeeren. Ph.D. thesis, University of Amsterdam.

Silver, M., S. Friedman, R. Guay, J. Couture and R. Tanguay. 1971. Base composition of deoxyribonucleic acid isolated from *Athiorhodaceae*. J. Bacteriol. *107:* 368-370.

Silverman, M.P. and D.G. Lundgren. 1959. Studies on the chemoautotrophic iron bacterium *Ferrobacillus ferrooxidans*. I. An improved medium and harvesting procedure for obtaining high cell yields. J. Bacteriol. *77:* 642-647.

Silvestri, L., M. Turri, L.R. Hill and E. Gilardi. 1962. A quantitative approach to the systematics of actinomycetes based on overall similarity. Symp. Soc. Gen. Microbiol. *12:* 333-360.

Simon, G.D. and D. White. 1971. Growth and morphological characteristics of a species of *Flexibacter*. Arch. Mikrobiol. *78:* 1-16.

Simons, H. 1922. Saprophytische oscillarien des menschen und der tiere. Zentralbl. Bakteriol. Parasitenkd. Infektionskr. Hyg. Abt. I Orig. *88:* 501-510.

Sinclair, C. and B.A. Whitton. 1977a. Influence of nutrient deficiency on hair formation in the *Rivulariaceae*. Br. Phycol. J. *12:* 297-313.

Sinclair, C. and B.A. Whitton. 1977b. Influence of nitrogen source on morphology of *Rivulariaceae* (Cyanophyta). J. Phycol. *13:* 335-340.

Singh, B.N. 1947. Myxobacteria in soils and composts; their distribution, number and lytic action on bacteria. J. Gen. Microbiol. *1:* 1-10.

Singh, B.N. and N.B. Singh. 1971. Distribution of fruiting myxobacteria in Indian soils, bark of trees and dung of herbivorous animals. Indian J. Microbiol. *11:* 47-92.

Sirevåg, R. and R.W. Castenholz. 1979. Aspects of carbon metabolism in *Chloroflexus*. Arch. Microbiol. *120:* 151-153.

Sirevåg, R. and J.G. Ormerod. 1977. Synthesis, storage and degradation of polyglucose in *Chlorobium thiosulfatophilum*. Arch. Microbiol. *111:* 239-244.

Skerman, V.B.D. 1967. A Guide to the Identification of the Genera of Bacteria, 2nd Ed. The Williams and Wilkins Co., Baltimore.

Skerman, V.B.D. 1968. A new type of micromanipulator and microforge. J. Gen. Microbiol. *54:* 287-297.

Skerman, V.B.D., G. Dementjeva and B.J. Carey. 1957. Intracellular deposition of sulfur by *Sphaerotilus natans*. J. Bacteriol. *73:* 504-512.

Skerman, V.B.D., V. McGowan and P.H.A. Sneath (Editors). 1980. Approved Lists of Bacterial Names. American Society for Microbiology, Washington, D.C. Reprinted from Int. J. Syst. Bacteriol. *30:* 225-420, 1980.

Skerman, V.B.D., G.R. Quinn, L.I. Sly and J.V. Hardy. 1977. Sheath formation by strains of *Herpetosiphon* species. Int. J. Syst. Bacteriol. *27:* 274-278.

Skuja, H. 1948. Taxonomie des Phytoplanktons einiger Seen in Uppland, Schweden. Symb. Bot. Ups. *9:* 1-399.

Skuja, H. 1956. Taxonomische und biologische Studien über das Phytoplankton schwedischer Binnengewässer. Nova Acta Reg. Soc. Sci. Ups. Ser. IV *16:* 1-404.

Skuja, H. 1958. Die Pelonemataceen *Desmanthos thiokrenophilum*, ein Vertreter der apochromatischen Blaualgen aus Schwefelquellen. Sven. Bot. Tidskr. *52:*

437–444.

Skuja, H. 1964. Grundzüge der Algenflore und Algenvegetation der Fjeldgegenden um Abisko in Schwedish-Lappland. Nova Acta Reg. Soc. Sci. Ups. Ser. IV *18:* 1–465.

Skuja, H. 1974. Genus *Siderocapsa* Molisch 1910. *In* Buchanan and Gibbons (Editors), Bergey's Manual of Determinative Bacteriology, 8th Ed. The Williams and Wilkins Co., Baltimore, pp. 465–466.

Skuja, H. 1974. Family *Pelonemataceae* Skuja 1956, 81. *In* Buchanan and Gibbons (Editors), Bergey's Manual of Determinative Bacteriology, 8th Ed. The Williams and Wilkins Co., Baltimore, pp. 122–127.

Skulberg, O.M., G.A. Codd and W.W. Carmichael. 1984. Toxic blue-green algal blooms in Europe: a growing problem. Ambio *13:* 244–247.

Sleytr, U.B. and P. Messner. 1983. Crystalline surface layers on bacteria. Annu. Rev. Microbiol. *37:* 311–339.

Slots, J. 1981. Enzymatic characterization of some oral and nonoral Gram-negative bacteria with the API ZYM system. J. Clin. Microbiol. *14:* 288–294.

Sly, L.I. 1985. Emendation of the genus *Blastobacter* Zavarzin 1961 and description of *Blastobacter natatorius* sp. nov. Int. J. Syst. Bacteriol. *35:* 40–45.

Šmarda, J. 1985. A new epiphytic bacterium of a cyanophyte. Syst. Appl. Microbiol. *6:* 298–301.

Smit, M. and A.G. Clark. 1971. The observation of myxobacterial fruiting bodies. J. Appl. Bacteriol. *34:* 399–401.

Smith, A.J. 1982. Modes of cyanobacterial carbon metabolism. *In* Carr and Whitton (Editors), The Biology of Cyanobacteria. Blackwell, Oxford, and University of California Press, Berkeley, pp. 47–85.

Smith, A.J. and D.S. Hoare. 1968. Acetate assimilation by *Nitrobacter agilis* in relation to its "obligate autotrophy". J. Bacteriol. *95:* 844–855.

Smith, A.J. and D.S. Hoare. 1977. Specialist phototrophs, lithotrophs, and methylotrophs: a unity among a diversity of procaryotes. Bacteriol. Rev. *41:* 419–448.

Smith, P.F. 1980. Sequence and glycosidic bond arrangement of sugars in lipopolysaccharide from *Thermoplasma acidophilum*. Biochim. Biophys. Acta *619:* 367–373.

Smith, P.F., T.A. Langworthy, W.R. Mayberry and A.E. Hougland. 1973. Characterization of the membranes of *Thermoplasma acidophilum*. J. Bacteriol. *116:* 1019–1028.

Smith, P.F., T.A. Langworthy and M.R. Smith. 1975. Polypeptide nature of growth requirement in yeast extract for *Thermoplasma acidophilum*. J. Bacteriol. *124:* 884–892.

Smith, P.H. 1966. The microbial ecology of sludge methanogenesis. Dev. Ind. Microbiol. *7:* 156–160.

Smith, P.H. and R.E. Hungate. 1958. Isolation and characterization of *Methanobacterium ruminantium* n. sp. J. Bacteriol. *75:* 713–718.

Sneath, P.H.A. 1972. Computer taxonomy. Methods Microbiol. *7A:* 29–98.

Sneath, P.H.A. 1974. Phylogeny of microorganisms. Symp. Soc. Gen. Microbiol. *24:* 1–39.

Sneath, P.H.A. 1977. The maintenance of large numbers of strains of microorganisms, and the implications for culture collections. FEMS Microbiol. Lett. *1:* 333–334.

Sneath, P.H.A. 1977. A method for testing the distinctness of clusters: a test for the disjunction of two clusters in euclidean space as measured by their overlap. J. Int. Assoc. Math. Geol. *9:* 123–143.

Sneath, P.H.A. 1978. Classification of microorganisms. *In* Norris and Richmond (Editors), Essays in Microbiology. John Wiley and Sons, Chichester, U.K., pp. 9/1–9/31.

Sneath, P.H.A. 1979a. BASIC program for a significance test for clusters in UPGMA dendrograms obtained from square euclidean distances. Comput. Geosci. *5:* 127–137.

Sneath, P.H.A. 1979b. BASIC program for a significance test for two clusters in euclidean space as measured by their overlap. Comput. Geosci. *5:* 143–155.

Sneath, P.H.A. and R.R. Sokal. 1973. Numerical Taxonomy. The Principles and Practice of Numerical Classification. W.H. Freeman, San Francisco.

Snellen, J.E. and H.D. Raj. 1970. Morphogenesis and fine structure of *Leucothrix mucor* and effects of calcium deficiency. J. Bacteriol. *101:* 240–249.

Snieszko, S.F. 1974. The effects of environmental stress on outbreaks of infectuous diseases of fishes. J. Fish. Biol. *6:* 197–208.

Socransky, S.S., S.C. Holt, E.R. Leadbetter, A.C. Tanner, E. Savitt and B.F. Hammond. 1979. *Capnocytophaga*: new genus of Gram-negative gliding bacteria. III. Physiological characterization. Arch. Microbiol. *122:* 29–33.

Söhngen, N.L. 1906. Het ontstaan en verdwijnen van waterstof en methaan onder den invloed van het organische leven. Proefschrift. Technische Hoogeschool, Delft, pp. 138.

Söhngen, N.L. 1914. Umwandlungen von Manganverbindungen unter dem Einfluss mikrobiologischer Prozesse. Zentralbl. Bakteriol. Parasitenkd. Infektionskr. Hyg. Abt. II *40:* 545–554.

Solangi, M.A., R.M. Overstreet and A.L. Gannam. 1979. A filamentous bacterium on the brine shrimp and its control. Gulf Res. Rep. *6:* 275–281.

Soliman, G.S.H. and H.G. Trüper. 1982. *Halobacterium pharaonis* sp. nov., a new, extremely haloalkaliphilic archaebacterium with low magnesium requirement. Zentralbl. Bakteriol. Mikrobiol. Hyg. I Abt. Orig. *C3:* 318–329.

Solntseva, L.I. 1939. Methods of cultivation of myxobacteria. Mikrobiologiya *8:* 959–964.

Solntseva, L.I. 1940. Biology of myxobacteria. I. *Myxococcus.* Mikrobiologiya *9:* 217–232 (in Russian with English summary).

Solntseva, L.I. 1941. Biology of the Myxobacteria. II. Genera *Melittangium* and *Chondromyces.* Mikrobiologiya *10:* 505–524.

Sone, N., Y. Yanagita, K. Hon-Nami, Y. Fukomori and T. Yamanaka. 1983. Proton-pump activity of *Nitrobacter agilis* and *Thermus thermophilus* cytochrome *c* oxidase. FEBS Lett. *155:* 150–154.

Sonea, S. 1971. A tentative unifying view of bacteria. Rev. Can. Biol. *30:* 239–244.

Sonea, S. and M. Panisset. 1976. Pour une nouvelle bacteriologie. Rev. Can. Biol. *35:* 103–167.

Sonea, S. and M. Panisset. 1980. Introduction a la nouvelle bacteriologie. Les Presses de l'Université de Montréal et Masson, Montréal and Paris.

Soriano, S. 1945. Un nuevo orden de bacterias: *Flexibacteriales.* Cienc. Invest. B. Aires *1:* 92–93.

Soriano, S. 1947. The *Flexibacteriales* and their systematic position. Antonie van Leeuwenhoek J. Microbiol. Serol. *12:* 215–222.

Soriano, S. 1973. Flexibacteria. Annu. Rev. Microbiol. *27:* 155–170.

Sournia, A. 1968. La cyanophycée *Oscillatoria* (=*Trichodesmium*) dans le plancton marin. Nova Hedwigia *15:* 1–12.

Sowers, K.R., S.F. Baron and J.G. Ferry. 1984. *Methanosarcina acetivorans* sp. nov., an acetotrophic methane-producing bacterium isolated from marine sediments. Appl. Environ. Microbiol. *47:* 971–978.

Sowers, K.R. and J.G. Ferry. 1983. Isolation and characterization of a methylotrophic marine methanogen, *Methanococcoides methylutens* gen. nov., sp. nov. Appl. Environ. Microbiol. *45:* 684–690.

Sowers, K.R. and J.G. Ferry. 1985. Trace metal and vitamin requirements of *Methanococcoides methylutens* grown with trimethylamine. Arch. Microbiol. *142:* 148–151.

Sowers, K.R. and J.G. Ferry. 1985. *In* Validation of the publication of new names and new combinations previously effectively published outside the IJSB. List No. 17. Int. J. Syst. Bacteriol. *35:* 223–225.

Sowers, K.R. and R.P. Gunsalus. 1988. Adaptation for growth at various saline concentrations by the archaebacterium *Methanosarcina thermophila*. J. Bacteriol. *170:* 998–1002.

Sowers, K.R., J.L. Johnson and J.G. Ferry. 1984. Phylogenetic relationships among the methylotrophic methane-producing bacteria and emendation of the family *Methanosarcineae*. Int. J. Syst. Bacteriol. *34:* 444–450.

Spencer, R. 1960. Indigenous marine bacteriophages. J. Bacteriol. *79:* 614.

Spormann, A.M. and R.S. Wolfe. 1984. Chemotactic, magnetotactic and tactile behavior in a magnetic spirillum. FEMS Microbiol. Lett. *22:* 171–177.

Sprague, S.G., L.A. Staehelin and R.C. Fuller. 1981a. Semiaerobic induction of bacteriochlorophyll synthesis in the green bacterium *Chloroflexus aurantiacus*. J. Bacteriol. *147:* 1032–1039.

Sprague, S.G., L.A. Staehelin, M.J. DiBartolomeis and R.C. Fuller. 1981b. Isolation and development of chlorosomes in the green bacterium *Chloroflexus aurantiacus*. J. Bacteriol. *147:* 1021–1031.

Sprott, G.D., T.J. Beveridge, G.B. Patel and G. Ferrante. 1987. Sheath disassembly in *Methanospirillum hungatei* strain GP1. Can. J. Microbiol. *32:* 847–854.

Sprott, G.D., J.R. Colvin and R.C. McKellar. 1979. Spheroplasts of *Methanospirillum hungatii* formed upon treatment with dithiothreitol. Can. J. Microbiol. *25:* 730–738.

Sprott, G.D. and K.F. Jarrell. 1981. K⁺, Na⁺ and Mg²⁺ content and permeability of *Methanospirillum hungatei* and *Methanobacterium thermoautotrophicum*. Can. J. Microbiol. *27:* 444–451.

Sprott, G.D. and K.F. Jarrell. 1982. Sensitivity of methanogenic bacteria to dicyclohexylcarbodiimide. Can. J. Microbiol. *28:* 982–986.

Sprott, G.D. and R.C. McKellar. 1980. Composition and properties of the cell wall of *Methanospirillum hungatii*. Can. J. Microbiol. *26:* 115–120.

Sprott, G.D., R.C. McKellar, K.M. Shaw, J. Giroux and W.G. Marten. 1979. Properties of malate dehydrogenase isolated from *Methanospirillum hungatii*. Can. J. Microbiol. *25:* 192–200.

Sprott, G.D., K.M. Shaw and K.F. Jarrell. 1983. Isolation and chemical composition of the cytoplasmic membrane of the archaebacterium *Methanospirillum hungatei*. J. Biol. Chem. *258:* 4026–4031.

Spudich, J.L. and W. Stoeckenius. 1979. Photosensory and chemosensory behaviour of *Halobacterium halobium*. Photochem. Photophys. *1:* 43–53.

Stackebrandt, E. 1985. Phylogeny and phylogenetic classification of prokaryotes. *In* Schleifer and Stackebrandt (Editors), The Evolution of Prokaryotes. Academic Press, London, pp. 309–334.

Stackebrandt, E., V.J. Fowler, W. Schubert and J.F. Imhoff. 1984. Towards a phylogeny of phototrophic purple sulfur bacteria—the genus *Ectothiorhodospira*. Arch. Microbiol. *137:* 366–370.

Stackebrandt, E., W. Ludwig, W. Schubert, F. Klink, H. Schlesner, T. Roggentin and P. Hirsch. 1984. Molecular genetic evidence for early evolutionary origin of budding peptidoglycan-less eubacteria. Nature (London) *307:* 735–737.

Stackebrandt, E., E. Seewaldt, V.J. Fowler and K.-H. Schleifer. 1982. The relatedness of *Prochloron* sp. isolated from different didemnid ascidian hosts. Arch. Microbiol. *132:* 216–217.

Stackebrandt, E., E. Seewaldt, W. Ludwig, K.-H. Schleifer and B.A. Huser. 1982. The phylogenetic position of *Methanothrix soehngenii*. Elucidated by a modified technique of sequencing oligonucleotides from 16S rRNA. Zentralbl. Bakteriol. Mikrobiol. Hyg. I Abt. Orig. *C3:* 90–100.

Stackebrandt, E. and C.R. Woese. 1979. A phylogenetic dissection of the family *Micrococcaceae*. Curr. Microbiol. *2:* 317–322.

Stackebrandt, E. and C.R. Woese. 1981. The evolution of procaryotes. *In* Carlile, Collins, and Mosely (Editors), Molecular and Cellular Aspects of Microbial

Evolution. Cambridge University Press, Cambridge, pp. 1–31.

Stackebrandt, E. and C.R. Woese. 1984. The phylogeny of prokaryotes. Microbiol. Sci. *1:* 117–122.

Stadtman, T.C. and H.A. Barker. 1951a. Studies on the methane fermentation. IX. The origin of methane in the acetate and methanol fermentations by *Methanosarcina.* J. Bacteriol. *61:* 81–86.

Stadtman, T.C. and H.A. Barker. 1951b. Studies on the methane fermentation. X. A new formate-decomposing bacterium, *Methanococcus vannielii.* J. Bacteriol. *62:* 269–280.

Staehelin, L.A., J.R. Golecki, R.C. Fuller and G. Drews. 1978. Visualization of the supramolecular architecture of chlorosomes (*Chlorobium*-type vesicles) in freeze-fractured cells of *Chloroflexus aurantiacus.* Arch. Microbiol. *119:* 269–277.

Stahl, D.A., D.J. Lane, G.J. Olsen, D.J. Heller, T.M. Schmidt and N.R. Pace. 1987. A phylogenetic analysis of certain sulfide oxidizing and related morphologically conspicuous bacteria by 5S ribosomal RNA sequences. Int. J. Syst. Bacteriol. *37:* 116–122.

Stahl, D.A., D.J. Lane, G.J. Olsen and N.R. Pace. 1984. Analysis of hydrothermal vent-associated symbionts by ribosomal RNA sequences. Science *224:* 409–411.

Ståhl, S. 1972. Growth variants of *Myxococcus virescens.* Physiol. Plant. *26:* 338–345.

Stal, L.J. 1986. Nitrogen-fixing Cyanobacteria in a Marine Microbial Mat. Littmann-Druck, Oldenburg, F.R.G., 174 pp.

Staley, J.T. 1968. *Prosthecomicrobium* and *Ancalomicrobium*: new freshwater prosthecate bacteria. J. Bacteriol. *95:* 1921–1942.

Staley, J.T. 1971. Incidence of prosthecate bacteria in a polluted stream. Appl. Microbiol. *22:* 496–502.

Staley, J.T. 1973. Budding and prosthecate bacteria. *In* Laskin and Lechevalier (Editors), Handbook of Microbiology, Vol. I. Chemical Rubber Company Press, Cleveland, Ohio, pp. 25–45.

Staley, J.T. 1981a. The genera *Prosthecomicrobium* and *Ancalomicrobium. In* Starr, Stolp, Trüper, Balows and Schlegel (Editors), The Prokaryotes. A Handbook on Habitats, Isolation, and Identification of Bacteria. Springer-Verlag, Berlin, pp. 456–460.

Staley, J.T. 1981b. The genus *Pasteuria. In* Starr, Stolp, Trüper, Balows and Schlegel (Editors), The Prokaryotes. A Handbook on Habitats, Isolation, and Identification of Bacteria. Springer-Verlag, Berlin, pp. 490–492.

Staley, J.T. 1984. *Prosthecomicrobium hirschii,* a new species in a redefined genus. Int. J. Syst. Bacteriol. *34:* 304–308.

Staley, J.T., J.A.M. de Bont and K. de Jonge. 1976. *Prosthecobacter fusiformis* nov. gen. et sp., the fusiform caulobacter. Antonie van Leeuwenhoek J. Microbiol. Serol. *42:* 333–342.

Staley, J.T., J.A.M. de Bont and K. de Jonge. 1980. *Prosthecobacter fusiformis* gen. and sp. nov., nom. rev. Int. J. Syst. Bacteriol. *30:* 595.

Staley, J.T., P. Hirsch and J.M. Schmidt. 1981. Introduction to the budding and/or appendaged bacteria. *In* Starr, Stolp, Trüper, Balows and Schlegel (Editors), The Prokaryotes. A Handbook on Habitats, Isolation, and Identification of Bacteria. Springer-Verlag, Berlin, pp. 451–455.

Staley, J.T. and T.L. Jordan. 1973. Crossbands of *Caulobacter crescentus* stalks serve as indicators of cell age. Nature (London) *246:* 155–156.

Staley, J.T. and M. Mandel. 1973. Deoxyribonucleic acid base composition of *Prosthecomicrobium* and *Ancalomicrobium* strains. Int. J. Syst. Bacteriol. *23:* 271–273.

Staley, J.T., K.C. Marshall and V.B.D. Skerman. 1980. Budding and prosthecate bacteria from freshwater habitats of various trophic states. Microb. Ecol. *5:* 245–251.

Stam, W.T. 1978. A taxonomic study of a number of blue-green algal strains (Cyanophyceae) based on morphology, growth, and deoxyribonucleic acid homologies. Proefschr. Rijksuniv. Groningen, p. 1–116.

Stam, W.T. 1980. Relationships between a number of filamentous blue-green algal strains (Cyanophyceae) revealed by DNA-DNA hybridization. Arch. Hydrobiol. Suppl. *56:* 351–374.

Stam, W.T., S.A. Boele-Bos and B.K. Stulp. 1985. Genotypic relationships between *Prochloron* samples from different localities and hosts as determined by DNA-DNA reassociations. Arch. Microbiol. *142:* 340–341.

Stam, W.T. and H.C. Holleman. 1975. The influence of different salinities on growth and morphological variability of a number of *Phormidium* strains (Cyanophyceae) in culture. Acta Bot. Neerl. *24:* 379–390.

Stam, W.T. and H.C. Holleman. 1979. Cultures of *Phormidium, Plectonema, Lyngbya* and *Synechococcus* (Cyanophyceae) under different conditions: their growth and morphological variability. Acta Bot. Neerl. *28:* 45–66.

Stam, W.T. and G. Venema. 1977. The use of DNA-DNA hybridization for determination of the relationship between some blue-green algae (Cyanophyceae). Acta Bot. Neerl. *26:* 327–342.

Stanier, R.Y. 1940. Studies on the cytophagas. J. Bacteriol. *40:* 619–635.

Stanier, R.Y. 1941. Studies on marine agar-digesting bacteria. J. Bacteriol. *42:* 527–558.

Stanier, R.Y. 1942. The *Cytophaga* group: a contribution to the biology of myxobacteria. Bacteriol. Rev. *6:* 143–196.

Stanier, R.Y. 1947. Studies on nonfruiting myxobacteria. I. *Cytophaga johnsonae* n. sp., a chitin-decomposing myxobacterium. J. Bacteriol. *53:* 297–315.

Stanier, R.Y. 1957. Order VIII. *Myxobacterales* Jahn 1915. *In* Breed, Murray and Smith (Editors), Bergey's Manual of Determinative Bacteriology, 7th Ed. The

Williams and Wilkins Co., Baltimore, pp. 854–891.

Stanier, R.Y. 1961. La place des bactéries dans le monde vivant. Ann. Inst. Pasteur (Paris) *101:* 297–303.

Stanier, R.Y. 1970. Some aspects of the biology of cells and their possible evolutionary significance. *In* Charles and Knight (Editors), Organization and Control in Procaryotic and Eucaryotic Cells. Cambridge University Press, Cambridge.

Stanier, R.Y. 1977. The position of cyanobacteria in the world of phototrophs. Carlsberg Res. Commun. *42:* 77–98.

Stanier, R.Y. and G. Cohen-Bazire. 1977. Phototrophic prokaryotes: the cyanobacteria. Annu. Rev. Microbiol. *31:* 225–274.

Stanier, R.Y., R. Kunisawa, M. Mandel and G. Cohen-Bazire. 1971. Purification and properties of unicellular blue-green algae (order *Chroococcales*). Bacteriol. Rev. *35:* 171–205.

Stanier, R.Y., W.R. Sistrom, T.A. Hansen, B.A. Whitton, R.W. Castenholz, N. Pfennig, V.N. Gorlenko, E.N. Kondratieva, K.E. Eimhjellen, R. Whittenbury, R.L. Gherna and H.G. Trüper. 1978. Proposal to place the nomenclature of the cyanobacteria (blue-green algae) under the rules of the International Code of Nomenclature of Bacteria. Int. J. Syst. Bacteriol. *28:* 335–336.

Stanier, R.Y. and C.B. van Niel. 1962. The concept of a bacterium. Arch. Mikrobiol. *42:* 17–35.

Stanier, R.Y., D. Wachter, D. Gasser and A.C. Wilson. 1970. Comparative immunological studies of two *Pseudomonas* enzymes. J. Bacteriol. *102:* 351–362.

Stanley, P.M. 1976. Isolation and characterization of phages for *Ancalomicrobium adetum.* J. Gen. Virol. *32:* 37–43.

Stanley, P.M., R.L. Moore and J.T. Staley. 1976. Characterization of two new isolates of mushroom-shaped budding bacteria. Int. J. Syst. Bacteriol. *26:* 522–527.

Stanley, P.M., E.J. Ordal and J.T. Staley. 1979. High numbers of prosthecate bacteria in pulp mill waste aeration lagoons. Appl. Environ. Microbiol. *37:* 1007–1011.

Stanley, P.M. and E.L. Schmidt. 1981. Serological diversity of *Nitrobacter* spp. from soil and aquatic habitats. Appl. Environ. Microbiol. *41:* 1069–1071.

Stapp, C. and H. Bortels. 1934. Mikrobiologische Untersuchungen über die Zersetzung von Waldstreu. Zentralbl. Bakteriol. Parasitenkd. Infektionskr. Hyg. Abt. II *90:* 28–66.

Starkey, R.G. 1957. Family I. *Nitrobacteriaceae* Buchanan, 1917. *In* Breed, Murray and Smith (Editors), Bergey's Manual of Determinative Bacteriology, 7th Ed. The Williams and Wilkins Co., Baltimore, pp. 68–73.

Starkey, R.L. 1934. Cultivation of organisms concerned in the oxidation of thiosulfate. J. Bacteriol. *28:* 365–386.

Starkey, R.L. 1934. The production of polythionates from thiosulfate by microorganisms. J. Bacteriol. *28:* 387–400.

Starkey, R.L. 1935. Isolation of some bacteria which oxidize thiosulfate. Soil Sci. *39:* 197–219.

Starkey, R.L. 1948. Family I. *Nitrobacteriaceae* Buchanan 1917. *In* Breed, Murray and Hitchens (Editors), Bergey's Manual of Determinative Bacteriology, 6th Ed. The Williams and Wilkins Co., Baltimore, pp. 69–81.

Starmach, K. 1966. Cyanophyta-Sinice, Glaucophyta-Glaucofity. Flora Slodkowodm. Polski, Pol. Acad. Sci. *2:* 1–807.

Starr, M.P., R.M. Sayre and J.M. Schmidt. 1983. Assignment of ATCC 27377 to *Planctomyces staleyi* sp. nov. and conservation of *Pasteuria ramosa* Metchnikoff 1888 on the basis of type descriptive material. Request for an Opinion. Int. J. Syst. Bacteriol. *33:* 666–671.

Starr, M.P. and J.M. Schmidt. 1981. Prokaryote diversity. *In* Starr, Stolp, Trüper, Balows and Schlegel (Editors), The Prokaryotes. A Handbook on Habitats, Isolation, and Identification of Bacteria. Springer-Verlag, Berlin.

Starr, M.P. and J.M. Schmidt. 1984a. *Planctomyces stranskae* (ex Wawrik 1952) sp. nov. nom. rev. and *Planctomyces guttaeformis* (ex Hortobágyi 1965) sp. nov. nom. rev., distinguishable members of the *Blastocaulis-Planctomyces* group of budding bacteria. Int. J. Syst. Bacteriol. *34:* 470–477.

Starr, M.P., K.A. Short and J.M. Schmidt. 1984. "*Planctomyces gracilis*" (Hortobágyi 1965) nom. dub., an unusual filamentous and rosette-forming bacterium, is not a member of the *Blastocaulis-Planctomyces* group. Int. J. Syst. Bacteriol. *34:* 465–469.

Starr, M.P. and V.B.D. Skerman. 1965. Bacterial diversity: the natural history of selected morphologically unusual bacteria. Annu. Rev. Microbiol. *19:* 420–422.

Starr, R.C. 1978. The culture collection of algae at the University of Texas at Austin. J. Phycol. (Suppl.) *14:* 47–100.

Steber, J. and K.H. Schleifer. 1975. *Halococcus morrhuae:* a sulphated heteropolysaccharide as the structural component of the cell wall. Arch. Microbiol. *105:* 173–177.

Steed, P.D.M. 1962. *Simonsiellaceae* fam. nov. with characterization of *Simonsiella crassa* and *Alysiella filiformis.* J. Gen. Microbiol. *29:* 615–624.

Steensland, H. and H. Larsen. 1969. A study of the cell envelope of the halobacteria. J. Gen. Microbiol. *55:* 325–336.

Steensland, H. and H. Larsen. 1971. The fine structure of the extremely halophilic cocci. Kgl. Norske Vidensk. Selsk. Skrifter No. 8. Universitetsforlaget Oslo, pp. 1–5.

Stefanov, S.B. and D.I. Nikitin. 1965. Submicroscopic bodies in soil suspensions. Mikrobiologiya *34:* 313–317.

Steiner, R., W. Schäfer, I. Blos, H. Wieschoff and H. Scheer. 1981. Δ2,10-phytadienol as esterifying alcohol of bacteriochlorophyll *b* from

Ectothiorhodospira halochloris. Z. Naturforsch. *36C:* 417-420.

Steinmetz, M.A. and U. Fischer. 1982. Cytochromes of green sulfur bacterium *Chlorobium vibrioforme* f. sp. *thiosulfatophilum.* Purification, characterization and sulfur metabolism. Arch. Microbiol. *131:* 19-26.

Steinmüller, W. and E. Bock. 1976. Growth of *Nitrobacter* in the presence of organic matter. I. Mixotrophic growth. Arch. Microbiol. *108:* 299-302.

Stephens, K., G.D. Hegeman and D. White. 1982. Pheromone produced by the myxobacterium *Stigmatella aurantiaca.* J. Bacteriol. *149:* 739-747.

Stetter, K.O. 1982. Ultrathin mycelia-forming organisms from submarine volcanic areas having an optimum growth temperature of 105°C. Nature *300:* 258-260.

Stetter, K.O. 1986a. *In* Validation of the publication of new names and new combinations previously effectively published outside the IJSB. List No. 22. Int. J. Syst. Bacteriol. *36:* 573-576.

Stetter, K.O. 1986b. Diversity of extremely thermophilic archaebacteria. *In* Brock (Editor), Thermophiles: General, Molecular and Applied Microbiology. John Wiley and Sons, New York, pp. 39-74.

Stetter, K.O. 1988a. *Archaeoglobus fulgidus* gen. nov., sp. nov.: a new taxon of extremely thermophilic archaebacteria. Syst. Appl. Microbiol. *10:* 172-173.

Stetter, K.O. 1988b. *In* Validation of the publication of new names and new combinations previously effectively published outside the IJSB. List No. 26. Int. J. Syst. Bacteriol. *38:* 328-329.

Stetter, K.O. and G. Gaag. 1983. Reduction of molecular sulphur by methanogenic bacteria. Nature *305:* 309-311.

Stetter, K.O., H. König and E. Stackebrandt. 1983. *Pyrodictium* gen. nov., a new genus of submarine disc-shaped sulphur reducing archaebacteria growing optimally at 105°C. Syst. Appl. Microbiol. *4:* 535-551.

Stetter, K.O., H. König and E. Stackebrandt. 1984. *In* Validation of the publication of new names and new combinations previously effectively published outside the IJSB. List No. 14. Int. J. Syst. Bacteriol. *34:* 270-271.

Stetter, K.O., G. Lauerer, M. Thomm and A. Neuner. 1987. Isolation of extremely thermophilic sulfate reducers: evidence for a novel branch of archaebacteria. Science *236:* 822-824.

Stetter, K.O., M. Thomm, J. Winter, G. Wildgruber, H. Huber, W. Zillig, D. Janekovic, H. König, P. Palm and S. Wunderl. 1981. *Methanothermus fervidus,* sp. nov., a novel extremely thermophilic methanogen isolated from an Icelandic hot spring. Zentralbl. Bakteriol. Mikrobiol. Hyg. I Abt. Orig. C2: 166-178.

Stetter, K.O., M. Thomm, J. Winter, G. Wildgruber, H. Huber, W. Zillig, D. Janekovic, H. König, P. Palm and S. Wunderl. 1982. *In* Validation of the publication of new names and new combinations previously effectively published outside the IJSB. List No. 8. Int. J. Syst. Bacteriol. *32:* 266-268.

Stetter, K.O., J. Winter and R. Hartlieb. 1980. DNA-dependent RNA polymerase of the archaebacterium *Methanobacterium thermoautotrophicum.* Zentralbl. Bakteriol. Mikrobiol. Hyg. I Abt. Orig. C1: 201-214.

Stetter, K.O. and W. Zillig. 1985. *Thermoplasma* and thermophilic sulfur-dependent archaebacteria. *In* Woese and Wolfe (Editors), The Bacteria. A Treatise on Structure and Function, Vol. VIII: Archaebacteria. Academic Press, New York, pp. 85-170.

Stevens, R.H., B.F. Hammond and C.H. Lai. 1979. Group and type antigens of *Capnocytophaga.* Infect. Immun. *23:* 532-539.

Stevens, S.E., Jr., C.O.P. Patterson and J. Myers. 1973. The production of hydrogen peroxide by blue-green algae: a survey. J. Phycol. *9:* 427-430.

Stewart, J.R. and R.M. Brown, Jr. 1971. Algicidal (sic) nonfruiting myxobacteria with high G + C ratios. Arch. Mikrobiol. *80:* 176-190.

Stewart, W.D.P. 1980. Some aspects of structure and function in N₂-fixing cyanobacteria. Annu. Rev. Microbiol. *34:* 497-536.

Stewart, W.D.P. and M.J. Daft. 1977. Microbial pathogens of cyanophycean blooms. Adv. Aquat. Microbiol. *1:* 177-218.

Stewart, W.D.P., P. Rowell and A.N. Rai. 1983. Cyanobacteria-eukaryotic plant symbioses. Ann. Microbiol. (Inst. Pasteur) *134B:* 205-228.

Stoeckenius, W. 1981. Walsby's square bacterium: fine structure of an orthogonal procaryote. J. Bacteriol. *148:* 352-360.

Stoeckenius, W. and R.A. Bogomolni. 1982. Bacteriorhodopsin and related pigments of halobacteria. Annu. Rev. Biochem. *51:* 587-616.

Stoeckenius, W. and R. Rowen. 1967. A morphological study of *Halobacterium halobium* and its lysis in media of low salt concentration. J. Cell. Biol. *34:* 365-393.

Stokes, J.L. 1954. Studies on the filamentous sheathed iron bacterium *Sphaerotilus natans.* J. Bacteriol. *67:* 278-291.

Stokes, J.L. and A.H. Johnson. 1965. Growth factor requirements of two strains of *Sphaerotilus discophorus.* Antonie van Leeuwenhoek J. Microbiol. Serol. *31:* 175-180.

Stokes, J.L. and M.T. Powers. 1965. Formation of rough and smooth strains of *Sphaerotilus discophorus.* Antonie van Leeuwenhoek J. Microbiol. Serol. *31:* 157-164.

Stolz, J.F. 1984. Fine structure of the stratified microbial community at Laguna Figueroa, Baja California, Mexico: II. Transmission electron microscopy as a diagnostic tool in studying microbial communities *in situ. In* Cohen, Castenholz and Halvorson (Editors), Microbial Mats: Stromatolites. Alan R. Liss, New York, pp. 23-38.

Stouthamer, A.H., W. de Vries and H.G.D. Niekus. 1979. Microaerophily. Antonie van Leeuwenhoek J. Microbiol. Serol. *45:* 5-12.

Strain, H.H. 1951. The pigments of algae. *In* Smith (Editor), Manual of Phycology. Chronica Botanica, Waltham (U.S.A.), pp. 243-262.

Stringfellow, L.A., J. Douglass and T. Blumenthal. 1980. Protein synthesis elongation factors Tu and Tu·Ts from *Caulobacter crescentus:* sensitivity to kirromycin and activity in Qβ replicase. J. Bacteriol. *143:* 389-395.

Strittmatter, W., J. Weckesser, P.V. Salimath and C. Galanos. 1983. Nontoxic lipopolysaccharide from *Rhodopseudomonas sphaeroides* ATCC 17023. J. Bacteriol. *155:* 153-158.

Strohl, W.R. 1979. Ultrastructure of *Cytophaga johnsonae* and *C. aquatilis* by freeze-etching. J. Gen. Microbiol. *112:* 261-268.

Strohl, W.R., G.C. Cannon, J.M. Shively, H. Güde, L.A. Hook, C.M. Lane and J.M. Larkin. 1981b. Heterotrophic carbon metabolism by *Beggiatoa alba.* J. Bacteriol. *148:* 572-583.

Strohl, W.R., I. Geffers and J.M. Larkin. 1981a. Structure of the sulfur inclusion envelopes from four beggiatoas. Curr. Microbiol. *6:* 75-79.

Strohl, W.R., K.S. Howard and J.M. Larkin. 1982. Ultrastructure of *Beggiatoa alba* strain B15LD. J. Gen. Microbiol. *128:* 73-84.

Strohl, W.R. and J.M. Larkin. 1978a. Cell division and trichome breakage in *Beggiatoa.* Curr. Microbiol. *1:* 151-155.

Strohl, W.R. and J.M. Larkin. 1978b. Enumeration, isolation and characterization of *Beggiatoa* from freshwater sediments. Appl. Environ. Microbiol. *36:* 755-770.

Strohl, W.R. and J.M. Larkin. 1980. Sulfide oxidation and metabolism by *Beggiatoa alba.* Abstr. Annu. Meet. Am. Soc. Microbiol. K11, p. 128.

Strohl, W.R., J.M. Larkin, B.H. Good and R.L. Chapman. 1977. Isolation of sporopollenin from four myxobacteria. Can. J. Microbiol. *23:* 1080-1083.

Strohl, W.R. and T.M. Schmidt. 1984. Mixotrophy in *Beggiatoa* and *Thiothrix. In* Strohl and Tuovinen (Editors), Microbial Chemoautotrophy. The Ohio State University Press, Columbus, pp. 79-95.

Strohl, W.R., T.M. Schmidt, N.H. Lawry, M.J. Mezzino and J.M. Larkin. 1986a. Characterization of *Vitreoscilla beggiatoides* and *V. filiformis* sp. nov., nom. rev., and comparison with *V. stercoraria* and *Beggiatoa alba.* Int. J. Syst. Bacteriol. *36:* 302-313.

Strohl, W.R., T.M. Schmidt, V.A. Vinci and J.M. Larkin. 1986b. Electron transport and respiration in *Beggiatoa* and *Vitreoscilla.* Arch. Microbiol. *145:* 71-75.

Strohl, W.R. and L.R. Tait. 1978. *Cytophaga aquatilis* sp. nov., a facultative anaerobe isolated from the gills of freshwater fish. Int. J. Syst. Bacteriol. *28:* 293-303.

Strzeszewski, B. 1914. Beiträge zur Kenntnis der Schwefelflora in der Umgebung von Krakau. Bull. Int. Acad. Sci. Cracovie (Acad. Pol. Sci.) Ser. B Sci. Nat. I, pp. 309-334.

Stulp, B.K. 1982. Morphological variability of *Anabaena* strains under different culture conditions. Arch. Hydrobiol. Suppl. *63:* 165-176.

Stulp, B.K. 1983. Morphological and molecular approaches to the taxonomy of the genus *Anabaena* (Cyanophyceae, Cyanobacteria). Drukkerij van Denderen, Groningen, 115 pp.

Stulp, B.K. and W.T. Stam. 1982. General morphology and akinete germination of *Anabaena* strains (Cyanophyceae) in culture. Arch. Hydrobiol. Suppl. *63:* 35-52.

Stulp, B.K. and W.T. Stam. 1984a. Growth and morphology of *Anabaena* strains (Cyanophyceae, Cyanobacteria) in cultures under different salinities. Br. Phycol. J. *19:* 281-286.

Stulp, B.K. and W.T. Stam. 1984b. Genotypic relationships between strains of *Anabaena* (Cyanophyceae) and their correlation with morphological affinities. Br. Phycol. J. *19:* 287-301.

Stulp, B.K. and W.T. Stam. 1985. Taxonomy of the genus *Anabaena* (Cyanophyceae) based on morphological and genotypic criteria. Arch. Hydrobiol. Suppl. *71:* 257-268.

Stupperich, E. and G. Fuchs. 1981. Products of CO₂ fixation and ¹⁴C labelling pattern of alanine in *Methanobacterium thermoautotrophicum* pulse-labelled with ¹⁴CO₂. Arch. Microbiol. *130:* 294-300.

Sturm, S., U. Schönefeld, W. Zillig, D. Janekovic and K.O. Stetter. 1980. Structure and function of the DNA dependent RNA polymerase of the archaebacterium *Thermoplasma acidophilum.* Zentralbl. Bakteriol. Parasitenkd. Infektionskr. Hyg. Abt. Orig. C1: 12-25.

Stürzenhofecker, P. 1966. Bakteriophagen bei Wassermyxobakterien. Arch. Hyg. Bakteriol. *150:* 153-157.

Stutzer, A. and R. Hartleb. 1898. Untersuchungen über die bei der Bildung von Salpeter beobachteten Mikroorganismen. I. Mitt. Landw. Inst. Königl. Univ. Breslau *1:* 75-100.

Sudo, S.Z. and M. Dworkin. 1969. Resistance of vegetative cells and microcysts of *Myxococcus xanthus.* J. Bacteriol. *98:* 883-887.

Sundarraj, N. and J.V. Bhat. 1971. Endo-polygalacturonate lyase of *Cytophaga johnsonii.* Arch. Mikrobiol. *77:* 155-164.

Sundermeyer, H. and E. Bock. 1981. Energy metabolism of autotrophically and heterotrophically grown cells of *Nitrobacter winogradskyi.* Arch. Microbiol. *130:* 250-254.

Sundermeyer-Klinger, H., W. Meyer, B. Warninghoff and E. Bock. 1984. Membrane-bound nitrite oxidoreductase of *Nitrobacter:* evidence for a nitrate reductase system. Arch. Microbiol. *140:* 153-158.

Sutherland, I.W. and M.L. Smith. 1973. Lipopolysaccharides of fruiting and nonfruiting myxobacteria. J. Gen. Microbiol. *74:* 259-266.

Sutter, V.L., D. Pyeatt and Y.Y. Kwok. 1981. *In vitro* susceptibility of *Capnocytophaga* strains to 18 antimicrobial agents. Antimicrob. Agents Chemother. *20:* 270-271.

Suylen, G.M.H. and J.G. Kuenen. 1986. Chemostat enrichment and isolation of *Hyphomicrobium* EG, a dimethyl sulphide utilizing methylotroph. Antonie van Leeuwenhoek. J. Microbiol. *52:* 281–293.

Suzina, N.E. and B.A. Fikhte. 1977. A new type of surface ultrastructure observed in a methane-oxidizing microorganism. Dokl. Akad. Nauk S.S.S.R. *234:* 470–471.

Suzuki, I., U. Dular and S.-C. Kwok. 1974. Ammonia or ammonium ion as substrate for oxidation by *Nitrosomonas europaea* cells and extracts. J. Bacteriol. *120:* 556–558.

Suzuki, I. and S.-C. Kwok. 1981. A partial resolution and reconstitution of the ammonia-oxidizing system of *Nitrosomonas europaea*: role of cytochrome c_{554}. Can. J. Biochem. *59:* 484–488.

Suzuki, I., S.-C. Kwok and U. Dular. 1976. Competitive inhibition of ammonia oxidation in *Nitrosomonas europaea* by methane, carbon monoxide or methanol. FEBS Lett. *72:* 117–120.

Švorcová, L. 1975. Iron bacteria of the genus *Siderocapsa* in mineral waters. Z. Allg. Mikrobiol. *15:* 553–557.

Švorcová, L. 1979. Diagnostik der Eisenbakterien der Familie *Siderocapsaceae*. Arch. Hydrobiol. *87:* 423–452.

Swafford, J.R. 1980. Stereoscopy of whole mount bacterial cells with a transmission electron microscope. Norelco Rep. *27:* 8–9.

Swarthof, T., H.J.M. Kramer and J. Amesz. 1982. Thin-layer chromatography of pigments of the green photosynthetic bacterium *Prosthecochloris aestuarii*. Biochim. Biophys. Acta *681:* 354–358.

Syed, S. and W. Loesche. 1972. Survival of human dental plaque flora in various transport media. Appl. Microbiol. *24:* 638–644.

Szafer, W. 1911. Zur Kenntnis der Schwefelflora im der Umgebung von Lemberg. Bull. Int. Acad. Sci. Ser. V. Cracovie, pp. 160–167.

Tabita, F.R. and B.A. McFadden. 1972. Regulation of ribulose-1,5-diphosphate carboxylase by 6-phospho-D-gluconate. Biochem. Biophys. Res. Commun. *48:* 1153–1159.

Tabita, F.R. and B.A. McFadden. 1974a. D-Ribulose 1,5-diphosphate carboxylase from *Rhodospirillum rubrum*. I. Levels, purification, and effects of metallic ions. J. Biol. Chem. *249:* 3453–3458.

Tabita, F.R. and B.A. McFadden. 1974b. D-Ribulose 1,5-diphosphate carboxylase from *Rhodospirillum rubrum*. II. Quaternary structure, composition, catalytic, and immunological properties. J. Biol. Chem. *249:* 3459–3464.

Taga, N. 1968. Some ecological aspects of marine bacteria in the Kuroshio current. Bull. Misaki Mar. Biol. Inst. Kyoto Univ. *12:* 56–76.

Takács, B.J. and S.C. Holt. 1971. *Thiocapsa floridana*; a cytological physiological and chemical characterization. I. Cytology of whole cells and isolated chromatophore membranes. Biochim. Biophys. Acta *233:* 258–277.

Takada, N. 1975. A new species of *Hyphomicrobium*. *In* Terui (Editor), Proceedings of the International Symposium on Microbial Growth on C₁ Compounds. The Society of Fermentation Technology, Japan, pp. 29–33.

Takeshita, T., T. Hanioka, H. Tamagawa, C. Hsieh, S. Shizukuishi and Y. Yamamoto. 1983. Neuraminidase activity of some oral anaerobic bacteria. J. Osaka Univ. Dent. Sch. *23:* 87–92.

Tanaka, Y., Y. Fukumori and T. Yamanaka. 1983. Purification of cytochrome a_1c_1 from *Nitrobacter agilis* and characterization of nitrite oxidation system of the bacterium. Arch. Microbiol. *135:* 265–271.

Tandeau de Marsac, N. 1977. Occurrence and nature of chromatic adaptation in cyanobacteria. J. Bacteriol. *130:* 82–91.

Taniguchi, S. and M.D. Kamen. 1963. On the nitrate metabolism of facultative photoheterotrophs. *In* Japanese Society of Plant Physiologists (Editors), Microalgae and Photosynthetic Bacteria. University of Tokyo Press, pp. 465–484.

Tarrand, J.J., N.R. Krieg and J. Döbereiner. 1978. A taxonomic study of the *Spirillum lipoferum* group, with descriptions of a new genus, *Azospirillum* gen. nov. and two species, *Azospirillum lipoferum* (Beijerinck) comb. nov. and *Azospirillum brasilense* sp. nov. Can. J. Microbiol. *24:* 967–980.

Taylor, B.F. and D.S. Hoare. 1969. New facultative *Thiobacillus* and a reevaluation of the heterotrophic potential of *Thiobacillus novellus*. J. Bacteriol. *100:* 487–497.

Taylor, B.F., D.S. Hoare and S.L. Hoare. 1971. *Thiobacillus denitrificans* as an obligate chemolithotroph. Isolation and growth studies. Arch. Mikrobiol. *78:* 193–204.

Taylor, C.D., B.C. McBride, R.S. Wolfe and M.P. Bryant. 1974. Coenzyme M, essential for growth of a rumen strain of *Methanobacterium ruminantium*. J. Bacteriol. *120:* 974–975.

Taylor, G.T., D.P. Kelly and S.J. Pirt. 1976. Intermediary metabolism in methanogenic bacteria *(Methanobacterium)*. *In* Schlegel, Gottschalk and Decker (Editors), Microbial Production and Utilization of Gases (H₂, CH₄, and CO). Akad. Wiss. Göttingen, Goltz, Göttingen, pp. 173–180.

Taylor, K.A., J.F. Deatherage and L.A. Amos. 1982. Structure of the *S*-layer of *Sulfolobus acidocaldarius*. Nature *299:* 840–842.

Tchan, Y.T., J. Pochon and A.R. Prévot. 1948. Études de systématique bactérienne. VIII. Essai de classification des *Cytophaga*. Ann. Inst. Pasteur (Paris) *74:* 394–400.

Tegtmeyer, B., J. Weckesser, H. Mayer and J.F. Imhoff. 1985. Chemical composition of the lipopolysaccharides of *Rhodobacter sulfidophilus*, *Rhodopseudomonas acidophila*, and *Rhodopseudomonas blastica*. Arch. Microbiol. *143:* 32–36.

Teichmann, P. 1935. Vergleichende Untersuchungen über die Kultur und Morphologie einiger Eisenorganismen. Ph.D. thesis, Prague, 134 pp.

Teiling, E. 1942. Schwedische Planktonalgen. 3. Neue oder wenig bekannte Formen. Bot. Not. *1942:* 63–68.

Tekniepe, B.L., J.M. Schmidt and M.P. Starr. 1981. Life cycle of a budding and appendaged bacterium belonging to morphotype IV of the *Blastocaulis-Planctomyces* group. Curr. Microbiol. *5:* 1–6.

Tekniepe, B.L., J.M. Schmidt and M.P. Starr. 1982. Immunoferritin labeling shows de novo synthesis of surface components in buds of a prokaryote belonging to morphotype IV of the *Blastocaulis-Planctomyces* group. Curr. Microbiol. *7:* 1–6.

Tell, G. 1975. Presencia de *Planctomyces bekefii* (Fungi Imperfecti, *Moniliales*) en la Argentina. Physis (B. Aires) *34:* 71.

Temple, K.L. and A.R. Colmer. 1951. The autotrophic oxidation of iron by a new bacterium, *Thiobacillus ferrooxidans*. J. Bacteriol. *62:* 605–611.

Ten, H.M. 1967. Iron- and manganese-oxidizing microorganisms in soils of South Sachalin. Mikrobiologiya *36:* 337–344.

Ten, H.M. 1969. A new manganese-oxidizing soil microorganism. Dokl. Akad. Nauk S.S.S.R. *188:* 697–699.

Teodoresco, E.C. 1901. Verh. Zool. Bot. Gesell. Wien. *51.*

Terekhova, L.P., A.V. Laiko, R.A. Lokhmacheva, T.N. Lafitskaya and L.V. Vasilyeva. 1981. The susceptibility of some genera of prosthecobacteria and budding bacteria to antibiotics. Izv. Akad. Nauk S.S.S.R. Ser. Biol. *1:* 143–147.

Terry, K.R. and A.B. Hooper. 1970. Polyphosphate and orthophosphate content of *Nitrosomonas europaea* as a function of growth. J. Bacteriol. *103:* 199–206.

Terry, K.R. and A.B. Hooper. 1981. Hydroxylamine oxidoreductase: a 20-heme, 200,000 molecular weight cytochrome *c* with unusual denaturation properties which forms a 63,000 molecular weight monomer after heme removal. Biochemistry *20:* 7026–7032.

Thaxter, R. 1892. On the *Myxobacteriaceae*, a new order of Schizomycetes. Bot. Gaz. *17:* 389–406.

Thaxter, R. 1893. A new order of Schizomycetes. Bot. Gaz. *18:* 29–30.

Thaxter, R. 1897. Further observations on the *Myxobacteriaceae*. Bot. Gaz. *23:* 395–411.

Thaxter, R. 1904. Notes on the *Myxobacteriaceae*. Bot. Gaz. *37:* 405–416.

Then, J. and H.G. Trüper. 1981. The role of thiosulfate in sulfur metabolism of *Rhodopseudomonas globiformis*. Arch. Microbiol. *130:* 143–146.

Thiele, H.H. 1968. Die Verwertung einfacher organischer Substrate durch *Thiorhodaceae*. Arch. Mikrobiol. *60:* 124–138.

Thinh, L.-V. 1978. Photosynthetic lamellae of *Prochloron* (*Prochlorophyta*) associated with the ascidian *Diplosoma virens* (Hartmeyer) in the vicinity of Townsville. Aust. J. Bot. *26:* 617–620.

Thinh, L.-V. 1979. *Prochloron* (*Prochlorophyta*) associated with the ascidian *Trididemnum cyclops* Michaelsen. Phycologia *18:* 77–82.

Thinh, L.-V. and D.J. Griffiths. 1977. Studies of the relationship between the ascidian *Diplosoma virens* and its associated microscopic algae. I. Photosynthetic characteristics of the algae. Aust. J. Mar. Freshwater Res. *28:* 673–681.

Thinh, L.-V., D.J. Griffiths and H. Winsor. 1985. Cellular inclusions of *Prochloron* (*Prochlorophyta*) associated with a range of didemnid ascidians. Bot. Mar. *XXVII:* 167–177.

Thomas, I. 1986. Profils Protéiques et Immunochimie des Methanogènes. Thèse No. 77, L'Université des Sciences et Techniques de Lille 1, France.

Thomas, I., D. Verrier, H.D. Dubourguier, N. Hanoune and C. Langrand. 1986. Numerical analysis of whole-cell protein patterns of methanogens. *In* Dubourguier, Albagnac, Montreuil, Romond, Santière and Guillaume (Editors), Biology of Anaerobic Bacteria. Elsevier Science Publishers, Amsterdam, pp. 245–253.

Thomm, M., J. Altenbuchner and K.O. Stetter. 1983. Evidence for a plasmid in a methanogenic bacterium. J. Bacteriol. *153:* 1060–1062.

Thomson, K.S., T.A. McMeekin and C.J. Thomas. 1981. Electron microscopic observations of *Flavobacterium aquatile* NCIB 8694 (= ATCC 11947) and *Flavobacterium meningosepticum* NCTC 10016 (= ATCC 13253). Int. J. Syst. Bacteriol. *31:* 226–231.

Thorne, S.W., E.H. Newcomb and C.B. Osmond. 1977. Identification of chlorophyll *b* in extracts of prokaryotic algae by fluorescence spectroscopy. Proc. Natl. Acad. Sci. U.S.A. *74:* 575–578.

Thuret, G. 1875. Essai de classification des Nostochinées. Ann. Sci. Nat. Bot. VI *1:* 372–382.

Thuret, G. 1880. *Xenococcus schousboei*. *In* Bornet and Thuret (Editors), Notes Algologiques, No. 2. Paris, pp. 73–75.

Thurston, E.L. and L.O. Ingram. 1971. Morphology and fine structure of *Fischerella ambigua*. J. Phycol. *7:* 203–210.

Thwaites, G.H.K. 1848. *In* Engl. Bot., p. 2941.

Tilden, J.E. 1910. Minnesota Algae. I. The *Myxophyceae* of North America. Report Survey, Bot. Ser. 8, Minneapolis.

Timmer ten Hoor, A. 1975. A new type of thiosulphate oxidizing, nitrate reducing microorganism: *Thiomicrospira denitrificans* sp. nov. Neth. J. Sea Res. *9:* 344–350.

Tindall, B.J. 1980. Ph.D. thesis, University of Leicester, Leicester, U.K.

Tindall, B.J. 1985. Qualitative and quantitative distribution of diether lipids in haloalkaliphilic archaebacteria. Syst. Appl. Microbiol. *6:* 243–246.

Tindall, B.J., A.A. Mills and W.D. Grant. 1980. An alkalophilic red halophilic bacterium with a low magnesium requirement from a Kenyan soda lake. J. Gen. Microbiol. *116:* 257–260.

Tindall, B.J., H.N.M. Ross and W.D. Grant. 1984a. *Natronobacterium* gen. nov.

and *Natronococcus* gen. nov., two new genera of haloalkaliphilic archaebacteria. Syst. Appl. Microbiol. *5:* 41-57.

Tindall, B.J., H.N.M. Ross and W.D. Grant. 1984b. *In* Validation of the publication of new names and new combinations previously effectively published outside the IJSB. List No. 15. Int. J. Syst. Bacteriol. *34:* 355-357.

Tindall, B.J., G.A. Tomlinson and L.I. Hochstein. 1987. Polar lipid composition of a new halobacterium. Syst. Appl. Microbiol. *9:* 6-8.

Tindall, B.J. and H.G. Trüper. 1986. Ecophysiology of the aerobic halophilic archaebacteria. Syst. Appl. Microbiol. *7:* 202-212.

Tipper, D.J., J.L. Strominger and J.C. Ensign. 1967. Structure of the cell walls of *Staphylococcus aureus*, strain Copenhagen. VII. Mode of action of the bacteriolytic peptidase from myxobacter and isolation of intact cell wall polysaccharides. Biochemistry *6:* 906-920.

Tolxdorff-Neutzling, R. and J.-H. Klemme. 1982. Metabolic role and regulation of L-alanine dehydrogenase in *Rhodopseudomonas capsulata*. FEMS Microbiol. Lett. *13:* 155-159.

Tomlinson, G.A. and L.I. Hochstein. 1976. *Halobacterium saccharovorum* sp. nov., a carbohydrate-metabolising, extremely halophilic bacterium. Can. J. Microbiol. *22:* 587-591.

Tomlinson, G.A., L.L. Jahnke and L.I. Hochstein. 1986. *Halobacterium denitrificans* sp. nov., an extremely halophilic denitrifying bacterium. Int. J. Syst. Bacteriol. *36:* 66-70.

Tomlinson, G.A., T.K. Koch and L.I. Hochstein. 1974. The metabolism of carbohydrates by extremely halophilic bacteria: glucose metabolism via a modified Entner-Doudoroff pathway. Can. J. Microbiol. *20:* 1085-1091.

Tornabene, T.G. and T.A. Langworthy. 1979. Diphantyl and dibiphantyl glycerol ether lipids of methanogenic archaebacteria. Science *203:* 51-53.

Tornabene, T.G., T.A. Langworthy, G. Holzer and J. Oro. 1979. Squalenes, phytanes and other isoprenoids as major neutral lipids of methanogenic and thermoacidophilic archaebacteria. J. Mol. Evol. *13:* 73-83.

Tornabene, T.G., R.S. Wolfe, W.E. Balch, G. Holzer, G.E. Fox and J. Oró. 1978. Phytanyl-glycerol ethers and squalene in the archaebacterium *Methanobacterium thermoautotrophicum*. J. Mol. Evol. *11:* 259-266.

Torreblanca, M., F. Rodriguez-Valera, G. Juez, A. Ventosa, M. Kamekura and M. Kates. 1986a. Classification of non-alkaliphilic halobacteria based on numerical taxonomy and polar lipid composition, and description of *Haloarcula* gen. nov. and *Haloferax*, gen. nov. Syst. Appl. Microbiol. *8:* 89-99.

Torreblanca, M., F. Rodriguez-Valera, G. Juez, A. Ventosa, M. Kamekura and M. Kates. 1986b. *In* Validation of the publication of new names and new combinations previously effectively published outside the IJSB. List No. 22. Int. J. Syst. Bacteriol. *36:* 573-576.

Torreblanca, M., F. Rodriguez-Valera, G. Juez, A. Ventosa, M. Kamekura and M. Kates. 1987. *In* Validation of the publication of new names and new combinations previously effectively published outside the ISJB. List No. 23. Int. J. Syst. Bacteriol. *37:* 179-180.

Touzel, J.P. and G. Albagnac. 1983. Isolation and characterization of *Methanococcus mazei* strain MC3. FEMS Microbiol. Lett. *16:* 241-245.

Touzel, J.P. and G. Albagnac. 1985. Acetoclastic methanogens in anaerobic digestors. *In* Antonopoulos (Editor), Proceedings, Biotechnological Advances in Processing Municipal Wastes for Fuels and Chemicals. N.T.I.S., U.S. Dept. Comm., Springfield, Virginia, pp. 35-39.

Touzel, J.P., D. Petroff and G. Albagnac. 1985. Isolation and characterization of a new thermophilic *Methanosarcina*, the strain CHTI 55. Syst. Appl. Microbiol. *6:* 66-71.

Towe, K.M. and T.T. Moench. 1981. Electron optical characterization of bacterial magnetite. Earth Plan. Sci. Lett. *52:* 213-220.

Trench, R.K. 1982. Physiology, biochemistry, and ultrastructure of cyanellae. *In* Round and Chapman (Editors), Progress in Phycological Research, Vol. 1. Elsevier Science Publishers, Amsterdam, 257-288.

Trevisan, V. 1842. Prospetto della flora Euganea. Coi Tipi Del Seminario, Padova, pp. 1-68.

Trevisan, V. 1845. Nomenclator algarum. Impr. du seminaire, Padova, pp. 58-59.

Trick, I. and F. Lingens. 1984. Characterization of *Herpetosiphon* spec.—a gliding filamentous bacterium from bulking sludge. Appl. Microbiol. Biotechnol. *19:* 191-198.

Trowitzsch, W., L. Witte and H. Reichenbach. 1981. Geosmin from earthy smelling cultures of *Nannocystis exedens* (*Myxobacterales*). FEMS Microbiol. Lett. *12:* 257-260.

Trüper, H.G. 1968. *Ectothiorhodospira mobilis* Pelsh, a photosynthetic sulfur bacterium depositing sulfur outside the cells. J. Bacteriol. *95:* 1910-1920.

Trüper, H.G. 1976. Higher taxa of the phototrophic bacteria: *Chloroflexaceae* fam. nov., a family for the gliding, filamentous, phototrophic "green" bacteria. Int. J. Syst. Bacteriol. *26:* 74-75.

Trüper, H.G. 1978. Sulfur metabolism. *In* Clayton and Sistrom (Editors), The Photosynthetic Bacteria. Plenum Press, New York, pp. 677-690.

Trüper, H.G. and U. Fischer. 1982. Anaerobic oxidation of sulphur compounds as electron donors for bacterial photosynthesis. Phil. Trans. R. Soc. London *B298:* 529-542.

Trüper, H.G. and S. Genovese. 1968. Characterization of photosynthetic sulfur bacteria causing red water in Lake Faro (Messina, Sicily). Limnol. Oceanogr. *13:* 225-232.

Trüper, H.G. and H. Jannasch. 1968. *Chromatium buderi* nov. spec., eine neue Art der groben *Thiorhodaceae*. Arch. Mikrobiol. *61:* 363-372.

Trüper, H.G. and N. Pfennig. 1971. Family of phototrophic green bacteria: *Chlorobiaceae* Copeland, the correct family name; rejection of *Chlorobacterium* Lauterborn; and the taxonomic situation of the consortium-forming species. Int. J. Syst. Bacteriol. *21:* 8-10.

Tsang, D.C.Y. and I. Suzuki. 1982. Cytochrome c_{554} as a possible electron donor in the hydroxylation of ammonia and carbon monoxide in *Nitrosomonas europaea*. Can. J. Biochem. *60:* 1018-1024.

Tsien, H.C., R. Lambert and H. Laudelout. 1968. Fine structure and the localization of the nitrite oxidizing system in *Nitrobacter winogradskyi*. Antonie van Leeuwenhoek J. Microbiol. Serol. *34:* 483-494.

Tu, J., D. Prangishvilli, H. Huber, G. Wildgruber, W. Zillig and K.O. Stetter. 1982. Taxonomic relations between archaebacteria including 6 novel genera examined by cross hybridization of DNAs and 16s rRNAs. J. Mol. Evol. *18:* 109-114.

Tuovinen, O.H. and D.P. Kelly. 1973. Studies on the growth of *Thiobacillus ferrooxidans*. Arch. Mikrobiol. *88:* 285-298.

Tuovinen, O.H. and D.P. Kelly. 1974. Studies on the growth of *Thiobacillus ferrooxidans* V. Factors affecting growth in liquid culture and development of colonies on solid media containing inorganic sulphur compounds. Arch. Microbiol. *98:* 351-364.

Tuovinen, O.H., D.P. Kelly, C.S. Dow and M. Eccleston. 1978. Metabolic transitions in cultures of acidophilic thiobacilli. *In* Murr, Torma and Brierley (Editors), Metallurgical Applications of Bacterial Leaching and Related Microbiological Phenomena. New York, Academic Press, pp. 83-102.

Tuttle, J.H., P.E. Holmes and H.W. Jannasch. 1974. Growth rate stimulation of marine pseudomonas by thiosulfate. Arch. Microbiol. *99:* 1-14.

Tuttle, J.H. and H.W. Jannasch. 1972. Occurrence and types of *Thiobacillus*-like bacteria in the sea. Limnol. Oceanogr. *17:* 532-543.

Tyler, P.A. and K.C. Marshall. 1967. Pleomorphy in stalked, budding bacteria. J. Bacteriol. *93:* 1132-1136.

Tyulpanova-Mosevich, M.W. 1930. Denitrifikatsya na neorganitcheskoi srede. Arch. Sci. Biol. (U.S.S.R.) *30:* 203-213.

Tzeng, S.F., M.P. Bryant and R.S. Wolfe. 1975a. Factor 420-dependent pyridine nucleotide-linked formate metabolism of *Methanobacterium ruminantium*. J. Bacteriol. *121:* 192-196.

Tzeng, S.F., R.S. Wolfe and M.P. Bryant. 1975b. Factor 420-dependent pyridine nucleotide-linked hydrogenase system of *Methanobacterium ruminantium*. J. Bacteriol. *121:* 184-191.

Uchida, T., L. Bonen, H.W. Schaup, B.J. Lewis, L. Zablen and C.R. Woese. 1974. The use of ribonuclease U_2 in RNA sequence determination: some corrections in the catalog of oligomers produced by ribonuclease T1 digestion of *Escherichia coli* 16s ribosomal RNA. J. Mol. Evol. *3:* 63-77.

Ueda, K., S. Ishikawa, T. Itami and T. Asai. 1952. Studies on the aerobic mesophilic cellulose-decomposing bacteria. Part 5. I. Taxonomic study. J. Agric. Chem. Soc. Jpn. *25:* 543-549.

Uffen, R.L. 1973. Growth properties of *Rhodospirillum rubrum* mutants and fermentation of pyruvate in anaerobic dark conditions. J. Bacteriol. *116:* 874-884.

Uffen, R.L. 1976. Anaerobic growth of a *Rhodopseudomonas* species in the dark with carbon monoxide as sole carbon and energy substrate. Proc. Natl. Acad. Sci. U.S.A. *73:* 3298-3302.

Uffen, R.L. 1983. Metabolism of carbon monoxide by *Rhodopseudomonas gelatinosa*: cell growth and properties of the oxidation system. J. Bacteriol. *155:* 956-965.

Ullman, J.S. and B.J. McCarthy. 1973. The relationship between mismatched base pairs and the thermal stability of DNA duplexes. II. Effects of deamination of cytosine. Biochim. Biophys. Acta *294:* 416-424.

Umbreit, T.H. and J.L. Pate. 1978. Characterization of the holdfast region of wild-type cells and holdfast mutants of *Asticcacaulis biprosthecum*. Arch. Microbiol. *118:* 157-168.

Uphof, J.C.T. 1927. Zur Oekologie der Schwefelbakterien in den Schwefelquellen Mittelfloridas. Arch. Mikrobiol. *18:* 71-84.

Utermöhl, H. 1924. Phaeobakterien. (Bakterien mit braunen Farbstoffen). Biol. Zentralbl. *43:* 605-610.

Utermöhl, H. 1925. Limnologische Phytoplanktonstudien. Arch. Hydrobiol. Suppl. *5:* 251-277.

Vaara, T. 1982. The outermost surface structures in chroococcacean cyanobacteria. Can. J. Microbiol. *28:* 929-942.

Vaccaro, R.F. 1962. The oxidation of ammonia in sea water. J. Cons. Perm. Int. Explor. Mer. *27:* 3-14.

Vaks, B., A. Zuckerberg and E. Rosenberg. 1974. Purification and partial characterization of an antibiotic produced by *Myxococcus xanthus*. Can. J. Microbiol. *20:* 155-161.

Van Baalen, C. and R.M. Brown, Jr. 1969. The ultrastructure of the marine blue-green alga, *Trichodesmium erythraeum*, with special reference to the cell wall, gas vacuoles, and cylindrical bodies. Arch. Mikrobiol. *69:* 79-91.

Van Bruggen, J.J.A., K.B. Zwart, J.G.F. Herman, E.M. van Hove, C.K. Stumm and G.D. Vogels. 1986a. Isolation and characterization of *Methanoplanus endosymbiosus* sp. nov., an endosymbiont of the marine sapropelic ciliate *Metopus contortus* Quennerstedt. Arch. Microbiol. *144:* 367-374.

Van Bruggen, J.J.A., K.B. Zwart, J.G.F. Herman, E.M. van Hove, C.K. Stumm and G.D. Vogels. 1986b. *In* Validation of the publication of new names and new combinations previously effectively published outside the IJSB. List No. 22. Int. J. Syst. Bacteriol. *36:* 573-576.

Van Bruggen, J.J.A., K.B. Zwart, R.M. van Assema, C.K. Stumm and G.D. Vogels.

1984. *Methanobacterium formicicum*, an endosymbiont of the anaerobic ciliate *Metopus striatus* McMurrich. Arch. Microbiol. *139:* 1–7.

van der Meulen, H.J. and W. Harder. 1976. Characterization of the neoagarotetraase and neoagarobiase of *Cytophaga flevensis*. Antonie van Leeuwenhoek J. Microbiol. Serol. *42:* 81–94.

van der Meulen, H.J., W. Harder and H. Veldkamp. 1974. Isolation and characterization of *Cytophaga flevensis* sp. nov., a new agarolytic flexibacterium. Antonie van Leeuwenhoek J. Microbiol. Serol. *40:* 329–346.

Van Ert, M. and J.T. Staley. 1971. Gas-vacuolated strains of *Microcyclus aquaticus*. J. Bacteriol. *108:* 236–240.

van Iterson, G., Jr., L.E. den Dooren de Jong and A.J. Kluyver. 1983. Martinus Willem Beijerinck, his life and his work. Science Tech., Madison, Wisconsin, pp. 146–147.

van Iterson, W. 1958. *Gallionella ferruginea* Ehrenberg in a different light. Verh. K. Ned. Akad. Wet. Afd. Natuurk. Tweede Reeks 2, 52 nr2, pp. 1–185.

Van Liere, L. and L.R. Mur. 1978. Light-limited cultures of the blue-green alga *Oscillatoria agardhii*. Mitt. Int. Ver. Limnol. *21:* 158–167.

Van Liere, L. and A.E. Walsby. 1982. Interactions of cyanobacteria with light. *In* Carr and Whitton (Editors), The Biology of Cyanobacteria. Blackwell, Oxford, and University of California Press, Berkeley, pp. 9–45.

van Neerven, A.R.W. and J.T. Staley. 1988. Mixed acid fermentation by the budding prosthecate, gas vacuolate bacterium *Ancalomicrobium adetum*. Arch. Microbiol. *149:* 335–338.

Van Niel, C.B. 1944. The culture, general physiology, morphology and classification of the nonsulfur purple and brown bacteria. Bacteriol. Rev. *8:* 1–118.

Van Niel, C.B. 1948. Genus I. *Achromatium* Schewiakoff. *In* Breed, Murray and Hitchens (Editors), Bergey's Manual of Determinative Bacteriology, 6th Ed. The Williams and Wilkins Co., Baltimore, pp. 997–1000.

Van Niel, C.B. 1957. The photosynthetic bacteria. Suborder I. *Rhodobacteriineae*. *In* Breed, Murray and Smith (Editors), Bergey's Manual of Determinative Bacteriology, 7th Ed. The Williams and Wilkins Co., Baltimore, pp. 35–67.

van Tieghem, P. 1880. Observations sur des bactériacées vertes, sur des phytochromacées blanches, et sur les affinités de ces deux familles. Bull. Soc. Bot. France (Paris) *27:* 174–179.

van Veen, W.L. 1973. Biological oxidation of manganese in soils. Antonie van Leeuwenhoek J. Microbiol. *39:* 657–662.

van Veen, W.L., J.M. Krul and C.J.E.A. Bulder. 1982. Some growth parameters of *Haliscomenobacter hydrossis* (syn. *Streptothrix hyalina*), a bacterium occurring in bulking activated sludge. Water Res. *16:* 531–534.

van Veen, W.L., E.G. Mulder and M.H. Deinema. 1978. The *Sphaerotilus-Leptothrix* group of bacteria. Microbiol. Rev. *42:* 329–356.

van Veen, W.L., D. van der Kooy, E.C.W.A. Geuze and A.W. van der Vlies. 1973. Investigations on the sheathed bacterium *Haliscomenobacter hydrossis*. J. Microbiol. Serol. *39:* 207–216.

Vanyushin, V., A. Kokurina and A. Belozerskii. 1964. Base composition of *Thiobacillus* DNA. Dokl. Akad. Nauk S.S.S.R. *158:* 722–733.

Vargas, A. and W.R. Strohl. 1985a. Ammonium assimilation and metabolism by *Beggiatoa alba*. Arch. Microbiol. *142:* 275–278.

Vargas, A. and W.R. Strohl. 1985b. Utilization of nitrate by *Beggiatoa alba*. Arch. Microbiol. *142:* 279–284.

Vasilyeva, L.V. 1969. Ultrastructure and cycle of development of *Agrobacterium polyspheroidum*. Izv. Akad. Nauk S.S.S.R. Ser. Biol. *5:* 780–781.

Vasilyeva, L.V. 1970. A star-shaped soil microorganism. Izv. Akad. Nauk S.S.S.R. Ser. Biol. *2:* 308–310.

Vasilyeva, L.V. 1972. On the cycle of development and cytological properties of new soil microorganisms possessing prosthecae (Russian). Izv. Akad. Nauk S.S.S.R. Ser. Biol. *6:* 860–864.

Vasilyeva, L.V. 1972. The peculiarities of ultrastructure and the cycle of development of the bacterium *Stella humosa*. Izv. Akad. Nauk S.S.S.R. Ser. Biol. *5:* 782–788.

Vasilyeva, L.V. 1980. Morphological grouping of prosthecobacteria. Izv. Akad. Nauk S.S.S.R. Ser. Biol. *5:* 719–737.

Vasilyeva, L.V. 1985. *Stella*, gen. nov., a new genus of soil prosthecobacteria, with proposals for *Stella humosa* sp. nov. and *Stella vacuolata* sp. nov. Int. J. Syst. Bacteriol. *35:* 518–521.

Vasilyeva, L.V. and N.T. Lafitskaya. 1976. Assignment of *Agrobacterium polyspheroidum* to the genus *Prosthecomicrobium polyspheroidum* comb. nov. (English translation). Izv. Akad. Nauk S.S.S.R. Ser. Biol. *6:* 768–772.

Vasilyeva, L.V., T.N. Lafitskaya, N.I. Aleksandrushkina and E.N. Krasil'nikova. 1974. Physiologo-biochemical peculiarities of the prosthecobacteria *Stella humosa* and *Prosthecomicrobium* sp. Izv. Akad. Nauk S.S.S.R. Ser. Biol. *5:* 699–714.

Vasilyeva, L.V., T.N. Lafitskaya and B.B. Namsaraev. 1979. A new genus of budding bacteria, *Angulomicrobium tetraedrale*. Mikrobiologiya *46:* 1033–1039.

Vasilyeva, L.V. and A.M. Semenov. 1984. *Labrys monahos*, a new budding prosthecate bacterium with a radial symmetry. Mikrobiologiya *53:* 85–92.

Vasilyeva, L.V. and A.M. Semenov. 1985. *In* Validation of the publication of new names and new combinations previously effectively published outside the IJSB. List No. 18. Int. J. Syst. Bacteriol. *35:* 375–376.

Vásquez, G.M., F. Qualls and D. White. 1985. Morphogenesis of *Stigmatella aurantiaca* fruiting bodies. J. Bacteriol. *163:* 515–521.

Vaucher, J.P. 1803. Histoire des conferves d'eau douce, contenant leurs different modes de reproduction, et la description de leurs principales especes. J.

Paschoud, Geneva, pp. 1–285.

Veldkamp, H. 1955. A study of the aerobic decomposition of chitin by microorganisms. Meded. Landbouwhogesch. Wageningen *55:* 127–174.

Veldkamp, H. 1961. A study of two marine agar-decomposing, facultatively anaerobic myxobacteria. J. Gen. Microbiol. *26:* 331–342.

Veldkamp, H. 1965. Isolation of *Cytophaga* and *Sporocytophaga*. *In* Schlegel (Editor), Anreicherungskultur und Mutantenauslese. Zentralbl. Bakteriol. Parasitenkd. Infektionskr. Hyg. Abt. I Suppl. *1:* 81–90.

Verma, J.P. 1970. The amino acid sequence of mureins of *Cytophaga hutchinsonii* and *Sporocytophaga myxococcoides*. Proc. Indian Natl. Sci. Acad. *36:* 364–368.

Verma, J.P. and H.H. Martin. 1967a. Über die Oberflächenstruktur von Myxobakterien I. Chemie und Morphologie der Zellwände von *Cytophaga hutchinsonii* und *Sporocytophaga myxococcoides*. Arch. Mikrobiol. *59:* 355–380.

Verma, J.P. and H.H. Martin. 1967b. Chemistry and ultrastructure of surface layers in primitive myxobacteria: *Cytophaga hutchinsonii* and *Sporocytophaga myxococcoides*. Folia Microbiol. *12:* 248–254.

Verona, O. 1934. Colture spontanee di cellulositici aerobi: *Cytophaga* Winogradskii n. sp. R. C. Accad. Ital. *19:* 731–734.

Verona, O. and E. Baldacci. 1939. Isolamento di schizomiceti cellulositici (*Cytophaga*), attinomiceti (*Actinomyces*), eumiceti dall'intestino delle termiti, e ricerche sulla attività cellulositica degli attinomiceti. Atti Ist. Bot. Univ. Lab. Crittogam. Pavia (Ser. IV) *11:* 289–301.

Vincent, W.F. and C. Howard-Williams. 1986. Antarctic stream ecosystems: physiological ecology of a blue-green algal epilithon. Freshwater Biol. *16:* 219–233.

Vishniac, W. 1974. Genus *Thiobacillus*. *In* Buchanan and Gibbons (Editors), Bergey's Manual of Determinative Bacteriology, 8th Ed. The Williams and Wilkins Co., Baltimore, pp. 456–461.

Vishniac, W. and M. Santer. 1957. The thiobacilli. Bacteriol. Rev. *21:* 19–21.

Visloukh, S.M. 1911. A new sulfur-microorganism from the Neva, *Thioploca ingrica* Visl. (English translation). Russkii Vrach *10:* 2102–2104.

Visloukh, S.M. 1914. *Spirillum kolkwitzii* nov. sp. (in Russian). Zh. Mikrobiol. *1 (1–2):* 42–51.

Vitolins, M.I. and R.J. Swaby. 1969. Activity of sulphur-oxidizing microorganisms in some Australian soils. Aust. J. Soil Res. *7:* 171–183.

Voelz, H. 1966. The fate of the cell envelopes of *Myxococcus xanthus* during microcyst germination. Arch. Mikrobiol. *55:* 110–115.

Voelz, H. and M. Dworkin. 1962. Fine structure of *Myxococcus xanthus* during morphogenesis. J. Bacteriol. *84:* 943–952.

Voelz, H. and V.F. Gerencser. 1971. A bacteriophage active on *Hyphomicrobium*. Virology *44:* 631–632.

Voelz, H.G. and H. Reichenbach. 1969. Fine structure of fruiting bodies of *Stigmatella aurantiaca* (*Myxobacterales*). J. Bacteriol. *99:* 856–866.

Vogels, G.D., J.T. Keltjens, T.J. Hutten and C. van der Drift. 1982. Coenzymes of methanogenic bacteria. Zentralbl. Bakteriol. Mikrobiol. Hyg. I Abt. Orig. *C3:* 258–264.

Völker, H., R. Schweisfurth and P. Hirsch. 1977. Morphology and ultrastructure of *Crenothrix polyspora*. J. Bacteriol. *131:* 306–313.

von Hofsten, B., B. Berg and S. Beskow. 1971. Observations of bacteria occurring together with *Sporocytophaga myxococcoides* in aerobic enrichment cultures on cellulose. Arch. Mikrobiol. *79:* 69–79.

von Tigerstrom, R.G. 1980. Extracellular nucleases of *Lysobacter enzymogenes*: production of the enzymes and purification and characterization of an endonuclease. Can. J. Microbiol. *26:* 1029–1037.

von Tigerstrom, R.G. 1981. Extracellular nucleases of *Lysobacter enzymogenes*: purification and characterization of a ribonuclease. Can. J. Microbiol. *27:* 1080–1086.

von Tigerstrom, R.G. 1983. The effect of magnesium and manganese ion concentration and medium composition on the production of extracellular enzymes by *Lysobacter enzymogenes*. J. Gen. Microbiol. *129:* 2293–2299.

Voss, E.G. (Editor). 1983. International Code of Botanical Nomenclature. *In* Bohn, Scheltema, and Holkema (Editors), Regnum Vegetabile, Vol. III. Utrecht.

Vozniakovskaya, Y.M. and Z.Z. Rybakova. 1969. Some new data on ecology and properties of bacteria belonging to *Promyxobacterium* genus. Mikrobiologiya *38:* 135–142 (in Russian with English summary).

Wagner, F. 1982. Ursachen, Verhinderung und Bekämpfung der Blähschlammbildung in Belebungsanlagen. Stuttg. Ber. Siedl. Wasserwirt. 76. R. Oldenbourg, München.

Wainwright, M. 1984. Sulfur oxidation in soil. Adv. Agron. *37:* 350–396.

Wakabayashi, H. and S. Egusa. 1974. Characteristics of myxobacteria associated with some freshwater fish diseases in Japan. Bull. Jpn. Soc. Sci. Fish. *40:* 751–757.

Waksman, S.A. 1922. Microorganisms concerned in the oxidation of sulfur in the soil. III. Media used for the isolation of sulfur bacteria from the soil. Soil Sci. *13:* 329–336.

Waksman, S.A. and J.S. Joffe. 1922. Microorganisms concerned in the oxidation of sulfur in the soil. II. The *Thiobacillus thiooxidans*, a new sulfur oxidizing organism isolated from the soil. J. Bacteriol. *7:* 239–256.

Wali, T.M., G.R. Hudson, D.A. Donald and R.M. Weiner. 1980. Timing of swarmer cell cycle morphogenesis and macromolecular synthesis by *Hyphomicrobium neptunium* in synchronous culture. J. Bacteriol. *144:* 406–412.

Walker, E. and F.L. Warren. 1938. Decomposition of cellulose by *Cytophaga*. I. Biochem. J. *32:* 31–43.

Walker, J.D., H.F. Austin and R.R. Colwell. 1975. Utilization of mixed hydrocarbon substrate by petroleum-degrading microorganisms. J. Gen. Appl. Microbiol. 21: 27–39.

Walker, N. and K.N. Wickramasinghe. 1979. Nitrification and autotrophic nitrifying bacteria in acid tea soils. Soil Biol. Biochem. 11: 231–236.

Walker, R.W. 1969. cis-11-Hexadecenoic acid from Cytophaga hutchinsonii lipids. Lipids 4: 15–18.

Walker, R.W., G.L. Howard and W. Litsky. 1968. Lipids of Cytophaga hutchinsonii. Bacteriol. Proc. 1968: 124 (P 77).

Wall, J.D., P.F. Weaver and H. Gest. 1975. Gene transfer agents, bacteriophages, and bacteriocins of Rhodopseudomonas capsulata. Arch. Microbiol. 105: 217–224.

Wallace, W. and D.J.D. Nicholas. 1969. Glutamate dehydrogenase in Nitrosomonas europaea and the effect of hydroxylamine, oximes and related compounds on its activity. Biochim. Biophys. Acta 171: 229–237.

Walsby, A.E. 1977. The gas vacuoles of blue-green algae. Sci. Am. 237: 90–97.

Walsby, A.E. 1980. A square bacterium. Nature (London) 283: 69–71.

Walsby, A.E. 1981. Cyanobacteria: planktonic gas-vacuolate forms. In Starr, Stolp, Trüper, Balows and Schlegel (Editors), The Prokaryotes. A Handbook on Habitats, Isolation, and Identification of Bacteria. Springer-Verlag, Berlin, pp. 224–235.

Walsby, A.E. 1981. Gas-vacuolate bacteria (apart from cyanobacteria). In Starr, Stolp, Trüper, Balows and Schlegel (Editors), The Prokaryotes. A Handbook on Habitats, Isolation, and Identification of Bacteria. Springer-Verlag, Berlin, pp. 441–447.

Walter, M.R. (Editor). 1977. Life in the Precambrian. Precambrian Res. 5(2): 105–219.

Walther-Mauruschat, A., M. Aragno, F. Mayer and H.G. Schlegel. 1977. Micromorphology of Gram-negative hydrogen bacteria. II. Cell envelope, membranes, and cytoplasmic inclusions. Arch. Microbiol. 114: 101–110.

Wang, T.L., P.C. Kao and J.H. Sung. 1964. Numération des bactéries cellulolytiques aérobies sur la couche mince de cellulose précipitée. Acta Microbiol. Sin. 10: 228–235.

Ward, D.M., E. Beck, N.P. Revsbech, K.A. Sandbeck and M.R. Winfrey. 1984. Decomposition of hot spring microbial mats. In Cohen, Castenholz and Halvorson (Editors), Microbial Mats: Stromatolites. Alan R. Liss, New York, pp. 191–214.

Ward, J.M. 1970. The microbial ecology of estuarine methanogenesis. Masters thesis, University of Florida.

Ware, J.C. and M. Dworkin. 1973. Fatty acids of Myxococcus xanthus. J. Bacteriol. 115: 253–261.

Warke, G.M. and S.A. Dhala. 1966. Effect of heat and antimicrobial agents on Cytophaga spp. isolated from various substrates in Bombay. Indian J. Microbiol. 6: 5–8.

Warke, G.M. and S.A. Dhala. 1968. Use of inhibitors for selective isolation and enumeration of cytophagas from natural substrates. J. Gen. Microbiol. 51: 43–48.

Warming, E. 1875. Om nogle ved Danmarks Kyster levende Bakterier. Videnskabelige Meddelelser fra den naturhistoriske Forening i Kjöbenhavn for Aaret 1875: 307–420.

Waterbury, J. 1979. Developmental patterns of pleurocapsalean cyanobacteria. In Parish (Editor), Developmental Biology of Prokaryotes. University of California Press, Berkeley, pp. 203–226.

Waterbury, J.B. and R.Y. Stanier. 1977. Two unicellular cyanobacteria which reproduce by budding. Arch. Microbiol. 115: 249–257.

Waterbury, J.B. and R.Y. Stanier. 1978. Patterns of growth and development in Pleurocapsalean cyanobacteria. Microbiol. Rev. 42: 2–44.

Waterbury, J.B. and R.Y. Stanier. 1981. Isolation and growth of cyanobacteria from marine and hypersaline environments. In Starr, Stolp, Trüper, Balows and Schlegel (Editors), The Prokaryotes. A Handbook on Habitats, Isolation, and Identification of Bacteria. Springer-Verlag, Berlin, pp. 221–223.

Waterbury, J.B., S.W. Watson, F.W. Valois and D.G. Franks. 1986. Biological and ecological characterization of the marine unicellular cyanobacterium Synechococcus. Can. Bull. Fish. Aquat. Sci. 214: 71–120.

Waterbury, J.B., J.M. Willey, D.G. Franks, F.W. Valois and S.W. Watson. 1985. A cyanobacterium capable of swimming motility. Science 230: 74–76.

Watson, S.W. 1965. Characteristics of a marine nitrifying bacterium, Nitrosocystis oceanus sp. n. Limnol. Oceanogr. (Suppl.) 10: R274–289.

Watson, S.W. 1971a. Taxonomic considerations of the family Nitrobacteraceae Buchanan. Requests for opinions. Int. J. Syst. Bacteriol. 21: 254–270.

Watson, S.W. 1971b. Reisolation of Nitrosospira briensis Winogradsky and Winogradsky 1933. Arch. Mikrobiol. 75: 179–188.

Watson, S.W. 1974. Family I. Nitrobacteraceae Buchanan. In Buchanan and Gibbons (Editors), Bergey's Manual of Determinative Bacteriology, 8th Ed. The Williams and Wilkins Co., Baltimore, pp. 450–456.

Watson, S.W., E. Bock, F.W. Valois, J.B. Waterbury and U. Schlosser. 1986a. Nitrospira marina gen. nov., sp. nov.: a chemolithotrophic nitrite-oxidizing bacterium. Arch. Microbiol. 144: 1–7.

Watson, S.W., E. Bock, F.W. Valois, J.B. Waterbury and U. Schlosser. 1986b. In Validation List No. 21. Int. J. Syst. Bacteriol. 36: 489.

Watson, S.W., L.B. Graham, C.C. Remsen and F.W. Valois. 1971. A lobular, ammonia-oxidizing bacterium, Nitrosolobus multiformis nov. gen. nov. sp. Arch. Mikrobiol. 76: 183–203.

Watson, S.W. and M. Mandel. 1971. Comparison of the morphology and deoxyribonucleic acid composition of 27 strains of nitrifying bacteria. J. Bacteriol. 107: 563–569.

Watson, S.W. and C.C. Remsen. 1969. Macromolecular subunits in the walls of marine nitrifying bacteria. Science 163: 685–686.

Watson, S.W. and C.C. Remsen. 1970. Cell envelope of Nitrosocystis oceanus. J. Ultrastruct. Res. 33: 148–160.

Watson, S.W., F.W. Valois and J.B. Waterbury. 1981. The Family Nitrobacteraceae. In Starr, Stolp, Trüper, Balows and Schlegel (Editors), The Prokaryotes. A Handbook on Habitats, Isolation, and Identification of Bacteria. Springer-Verlag, Berlin, pp. 1005–1022.

Watson, S.W. and J.B. Waterbury. 1971. Characteristics of two marine nitrite oxidizing bacteria, Nitrospira gracilis nov. gen. nov. sp. and Nitrococcus mobilis nov. gen. nov. sp. Arch. Microbiol. 77: 203–230.

Wawrik, F. 1952. Planctomyces-Studien. Sydowia 6: 443–452.

Wawrik, F. 1956. Neue Planktonorganismen aus Waldviertler Fishteichen. Österr. Bot. Z. 103: 291–299.

Wawrik, F. 1956. Siderocapsa arlbergensis nova species, eine Eisenbakterie aus den Hochgebirgskleingewässern des Arlberggebietes. Österr. Bot. Z. 103: 19–23.

Weaver, G.A., J.A. Krause, T.L. Miller and M.J. Wolin. 1986. Incidence of methanogenic bacteria in a sigmoidoscopy population: an association of methanogenic bacteria and diverticulosis. Gut 27: 698–704.

Weaver, P.F., J.D. Wall and H. Gest. 1975. Characterization of Rhodopseudomonas capsulata. Arch. Microbiol. 105: 207–216.

Webley, D.M., E.A.C. Follett and I.F. Taylor. 1967. A comparison of the lytic action of Cytophaga johnsonii on a eubacterium and a yeast. Antonie van Leeuwenhoek J. Microbiol. Serol. 33: 159–165.

Webster, J.A. and R. Hugh. 1979. Flavobacterium aquatile and Flavobacterium meningosepticum: glucose nonfermenters with similar flagellar morphologies. Int. J. Syst. Bacteriol. 29: 333–338.

Weckesser, J., G. Drews, R. Indira and H. Mayer. 1977. Lipophilic O-antigens in Rhodospirillum tenue. J. Bacteriol. 130: 629–634.

Weckesser, J., G. Drews and H. Mayer. 1979. Lipopolysaccharides of photosynthetic procaryotes. Annu. Rev. Microbiol. 33: 215–239.

Weckesser, J., G. Drews and H.-D. Tauschel. 1969. Zur Feinstruktur von Rhodopseudomonas gelatinosa. Arch. Mikrobiol. 65: 346–358.

Weckesser, J., H. Mayer, G. Drews and I. Fromme. 1975. Lipophilic O-antigens containing D-glycero-D-mannoheptose as the sole neutral sugar in Rhodopseudomonas gelatinosa. J. Bacteriol. 123: 449–455.

Weckesser, J., H. Mayer, E. Metz and H. Biebl. 1983. Lipopolysaccharide of Rhodocyclus purpureus: taxonomic implication. Int. J. Syst. Bacteriol. 33: 53–56.

Weckesser, J., G. Rosenfelder, H. Mayer and O. Lüderitz. 1971. The identification of 3-O-methyl-D-xylose and 3-O-methyl-L-xylose as constituents of the lipopolysaccharides of Myxococcus fulvus and Rhodopseudomonas viridis respectively. Eur. J. Biochem. 24: 112–115.

Weeks, O.B. 1974. Genus Flavobacterium Bergey et al. 1923, 97. In Buchanan and Gibbons (Editors), Bergey's Manual of Determinative Bacteriology, 8th Ed. The Williams and Wilkins Co., Baltimore, pp. 357–364.

Weeks, O.B. 1981. Preliminary studies of the pigments of Flavobacterium breve NCTC 11099 and Flavobacterium odoratum NCTC 11036. In Reichenbach and Weeks (Editors), The Flavobacterium-Cytophaga Group. Verlag Chemie, Weinheim, F.R.G., pp. 109–114.

Wehrmeyer, W. 1983. Organization and composition of cyanobacterial and Rhodophycean phycobilisomes. In Papageorgiou and Packer (Editors), Photosynthetic Prokaryotes: Cell Differentiation and Function. Elsevier Science Publishers, New York, pp. 1–22.

Weimer, P.J. and J.G. Zeikus. 1978. One carbon metabolism in methanogenic bacteria; cellular characterization and growth of Methanosarcina barkeri. Arch. Mikrobiol. 119: 49–57.

Weiner, R.M., R.A. Devine, D.M. Powell, L. Dagasan and R.L. Moore. 1985. Hyphomonas oceanitis sp. nov., Hyphomonas hirschiana sp. nov., and Hyphomonas jannaschiana sp. nov. Int. J. Syst. Bacteriol. 35: 237–243.

Weisrock, W.P. and R.M. Johnson. 1966. Marine species of Hyphomicrobium. Bacteriol. Proc., p. 22.

Weiss, R.L. 1974. Subunit cell wall of Sulfolobus acidocaldarius. J. Bacteriol. 118: 275–284.

Weissborn, A., H.M. Steinman and L. Shapiro. 1982. Characterization of the proteins of the Caulobacter crescentus flagellar filament: peptide analysis and filament organization. J. Biol. Chem. 257: 2066–2074.

Weitzman, P.D.J. 1980. Citrate synthase and succinate thiokinase in classification and identification. In Goodfellow and Board (Editors), Microbiological Classification and Identification. Academic Press, London, New York, pp. 107–125.

Wellinger, A. and K. Wuhrmann. 1977. Influence of sulfide compounds on the metabolism of Methanobacterium strain AZ. Arch. Microbiol. 115: 13–17.

Went, J.C. and F. De Jong. 1966. Decomposition of cellulose in soils. Antonie van Leeuwenhoek J. Microbiol. Serol. 32: 39–56.

Werber, M.M., J.L. Sussman and H. Eisenberg. 1986. Molecular basis for the special properties of proteins and enzymes from Halobacterium marismortui. FEMS Microbiol. Rev. 39: 129–135.

West, G.S. and B.M. Griffiths. 1913. The lime-sulphur bacteria of the genus Hillhousia. Ann. Bot. 27: 83–91.

West, W. and G.S. West. 1897. J. Bot. London 35.

West, W. and G.S. West. 1898. Notes on fresh water algae. J. Bot. (London) 36: 330–338.

Wetmur, J.G. 1976. Hybridization and renaturation kinetics of nucleic acids. Annu. Rev. Biophys. Bioeng. *5:* 337–361.

Wetmur, J.G. and N. Davidson. 1968. Kinetics of renaturation of DNA. J. Mol. Biol. *31:* 349–370.

Wettstein, F.V. 1924. Handbuch der Systematischen. Botanik Bd. 1, 3rd Ed. Leipzig and Vienna.

Whatley, J. 1977. The fine structure of *Prochloron*. New Phytol. *79:* 309–313.

Whitaker, D.R. 1965. Lytic enzymes of *Sorangium* sp.: isolation and enzymatic properties of the α- and β-lytic proteases. Can. J. Biochem. *43:* 1935–1954.

Whitaker, D.R. 1967. Simplified procedures for production and isolation of the bacteriolytic proteases of *Sorangium* sp. Can. J. Biochem. *45:* 991–993.

Whitaker, D.R. 1970. The α-lytic protease of a myxobacterium. Methods Enzymol. *19:* 599–613.

Whitaker, D.R., F.D. Cook and D.C. Gillespie. 1965a. Lytic enzymes of *Sorangium* sp. Some aspects of enzyme production in submerged culture. Can. J. Biochem. *43:* 1927–1933.

Whitaker, D.R., L. Jurasek and C. Roy. 1966. The nature of the bacteriolytic proteases of *Sorangium* sp. Biochem. Biophys. Res. Commun. *24:* 173–178.

Whitaker, D.R. and C. Roy. 1967. Concerning the nature of the α- and β-lytic proteases of *Sorangium* sp. Can. J. Biochem. *45:* 911–916.

Whitaker, D.R., C. Roy, C.S. Tsai and L. Jurasek. 1965b. Lytic enzymes of *Sorangium* sp. A comparison of the proteolytic properties of the α- and β-lytic proteases. Can. J. Biochem. *43:* 1961–1970.

White, D. 1981. Cell interactions and the control of development in myxobacteria population. Int. Rev. Cytol. *72:* 203–225.

White, D., M. Dworkin and D.J. Tipper. 1968. Peptidoglycan of *Myxococcus xanthus*: structure and relation to morphogenesis. J. Bacteriol. *95:* 2186–2197.

White, D., J.A. Johnson and K. Stephens. 1980b. Effects of specific cations on aggregation and fruiting body morphology in the myxobacterium *Stigmatella aurantiaca*. J. Bacteriol. *144:* 400–405.

White, D., W. Shropshire, Jr. and K. Stephens. 1980a. Photocontrol of development by *Stigmatella aurantiaca*. J. Bacteriol. *142:* 1023–1024.

White, R.H. 1984. Biosynthesis of the sulfonolipid 2-amino-3-hydroxy-15-methylhexadecane-1-sulfonic acid in the gliding bacterium *Cytophaga johnsonae*. J. Bacteriol. *159:* 42–46.

Whitman, W.B. 1985. Methanogenic bacteria. *In* Woese and Wolfe (Editors), The Bacteria. A Treatise on Structure and Function, Vol. VIII: Archaebacteria. Academic Press, New York, pp. 3–84.

Whitman, W.B., E. Ankwanda and R.S. Wolfe. 1982. Nutrition and carbon metabolism of *Methanococcus voltae*. J. Bacteriol. *149:* 852–863.

Whitman, W.B., J. Shieh, S. Sohn, D.S. Caras and U. Premachandran. 1986. Isolation and characterization of 22 mesophilic methanococci. Syst. Appl. Microbiol. *7:* 235–240.

Whittaker, R.H. and L. Margulis. 1978. Protist classification and the kingdoms of organisms. BioSystems *10:* 3–18.

Whittenbury, R., S.L. Davies and J.F. Davey. 1970a. Exospores and cysts formed by methane-utilizing bacteria. J. Gen. Microbiol. *61:* 219–226.

Whittenbury, R. and C.S. Dow. 1977. Morphogenesis and differentiation in *Rhodomicrobium vannielii* and other budding and prosthecate bacteria. Bacteriol. Rev. *41:* 754–808.

Whittenbury, R., K.C. Phillips and J.F. Wilkinson. 1970b. Enrichment, isolation and some properties of methane-utilizing bacteria. J. Gen. Microbiol. *61:* 205–218.

Whittenbury, R.A. and J.M. Nicoll. 1971. A new, mushroom-shaped budding bacterium. J. Gen. Microbiol. *66:* 123–126.

Whitton, B.A. 1968. Effect of light on toxicity of various substances to *Anacystis nidulans*. Plant Cell Physiol. *9:* 23–26.

Whitton, B.A. 1987. The biology of *Rivulariaceae*. *In* Fay and Van Baalen (Editors), The Cyanobacteria. Elsevier Science Publishers, Amsterdam.

Whitton, B.A., B.M. Diaz and N.T.H. Holmes. 1979. A computer orientated numerical coding system for algae. Br. Phycol. J. *14:* 353–360.

Whitton, B.A., S.L.J. Grainger and N. Harris. 1987. Blue heterocysts in the *Rivulariaceae*. Br. Phycol. J. *22:* 338–339.

Wichlacz, P.L. and R.F. Unz. 1981. Acidophilic heterotrophic bacteria of acidic mine waters. Appl. Environ. Microbiol. *41:* 1254–1261.

Wichlacz, P.L. and R.F. Unz. 1982. Taxonomic disposition of acidophilic heterotrophs of acidic mine drainage. Abstract P11.1. XIII Int. Congress Microbiol., Boston, Massachusetts.

Wichlacz, P.L., R.F. Unz and T.A. Langworthy. 1986. *Acidiphilium angustum* sp. nov., *Acidiphilium facilis* sp. nov., *Acidiphilium rubrum* sp. nov. Acidophilic heterotrophic bacteria isolated from acidic coal mine drainage. Int. J. Syst. Bacteriol. *36:* 197–201.

Wickstrom, C.E. and R.W. Castenholz. 1978. Association of *Pleurocapsa* and *Calothrix* (Cyanophyta) in a thermal stream. J. Phycol. *14:* 84–88.

Widdel, F. 1980. Anaerober Abbau von Fettsäuren und Benzoesäure durch neu isolierte Arten Sulfat-reduzierender Bakterien. Doctoral thesis, Universität Göttingen.

Widdel, F. 1981. *In* Validation of the publication of new names and new combinations previously effectively published outside the IJSB. List No. 7. Int. J. Syst. Bacteriol. *31:* 382–383.

Widdel, F. 1983. Methods for enrichment and pure culture isolation of filamentous gliding sulfate-reducing bacteria. Arch. Microbiol. *134:* 282–285.

Widdel, F., G.-W. Kohring and F. Mayer. 1983. Studies on dissimilatory sulfate-reducing bacteria that decompose fatty acids. III. Characterization of the filamentous gliding *Desulfonema limicola* gen. nov. sp. nov., and *Desulfonema magnum* sp. nov. Arch. Microbiol. *134:* 286–294.

Widdel, F. and N. Pfennig. 1981. Studies on dissimilatory sulfate-reducing bacteria that decompose fatty acids. I. Isolation of a new sulfate-reducing bacterium enriched with acetate in saline environments. Description of *Desulfobacter postgatei* gen. nov. sp. nov. Arch. Microbiol. *131:* 395–400.

Widdel, F. and N. Pfennig. 1984. Dissimilatory sulfate- or sulfur-reducing bacteria. *In* Krieg and Holt (Editors), Bergey's Manual of Systematic Bacteriology, Vol. 1. The Williams and Wilkins Co., Baltimore, pp. 663–679.

Wieland, F., J. Lechner and M. Sumper. 1982. The cell wall glycoprotein of halobacteria: structural functional and biosynthetic aspects. Zentralbl. Bakteriol. Mikrobiol. Hyg. I Abt. Orig. *C3:* 161–170.

Wieland, F., G. Paul and M. Sumper. 1985. Halobacterial flagellins are sulphated glycoproteins. J. Biol. Chem. *260:* 15180–15185.

Wiessner, W. 1981. The family *Beggiatoaceae*. *In* Starr, Stolp, Trüper, Balows and Schlegel (Editors), The Prokaryotes. A Handbook on Habitats, Isolation, and Identification of Bacteria. Springer-Verlag, Berlin, pp. 380–389.

Wildgruber, G., M. Thomm, H. König, K. Ober, T. Ricchiuto and K.O. Stetter. 1982. *Methanoplanus limicola*, a plate-shaped methanogen representing a novel family, the *Methanoplanaceae*. Arch. Microbiol. *132:* 31–36.

Wildgruber, G., M. Thomm and K.O. Stetter. 1984. *In* Validation of the publication of new names and new combinations previously effectively published outside the IJSB. List No. 14. Int. J. Syst. Bacteriol. *34:* 270–271.

Williams, B.L. and B.F. Hammond. 1979. *Capnocytophaga*: new genus of Gram-negative gliding bacteria. IV. DNA base composition and sequence homology. Arch. Microbiol. *122:* 35–39.

Williams, B.L., L. Hollis and L.V. Holdeman. 1979. Synonymy of strains of Center for Disease Control group DF-1 with species of *Capnocytophaga*. J. Clin. Microbiol. *10:* 550–560.

Williams, P.J.B. and S.W. Watson. 1968. Autotrophy in *Nitrosocystis oceanus*. J. Bacteriol. *96:* 1640–1648.

Williams, R.A.D. and D.S. Hoare. 1972. Physiology of a new facultatively autotrophic thermophilic *Thiobacillus*. J. Gen. Microbiol. *70:* 555–566.

Williams, T.M. and R.F. Unz. 1985. Filamentous sulfur bacteria of activated sludge: characterization of *Thiothrix*, *Beggiatoa*, and Eikelboom type O21N strains. Appl. Environ. Microbiol. *49:* 887–898.

Willison, J.H.M., K.B. Easterbrook and R.W. Coombs. 1977. The attachment of bacterial spinae. Can. J. Microbiol. *23:* 258–266.

Wilmotte, A.M.R. and W.T. Stam. 1984. Genetic relationships among cyanobacterial strains originally designated as 'Anacystis nidulans' and some other *Synechococcus* strains. J. Gen. Microbiol. *130:* 2737–2740.

Wilson, A.C., S.S. Carlson and T.J. White. 1977. Biochemical evolution. Annu. Rev. Biochem. *46:* 573–639.

Wingard, M., G. Matsueda and R.S. Wolfe. 1972. Myxobacter AL-1 protease II: Specific peptide bond cleavage on the amino side of lysine. J. Bacteriol. *112:* 940–949.

Winkler, M.E., P.V. Schoenlein, C.M. Ross, J.T. Barrett and B. Ely. 1984. Genetic and physical analyses of *Caulobacter crescentus trp* genes. J. Bacteriol. *160:* 279–287.

Winogradsky, H. 1935a. Sur la microflore nitrificatrice des boues activees de Paris. C. R. Acad. Sci. *200:* 1886–1888.

Winogradsky, H. 1935b. On the number and variety of nitrifying organisms. Int. Cong. Soil Sci. *1:* 138–140.

Winogradsky, H. 1937. Contributions a l'étude de la microflore nitrificatrice des boues activees de Paris. Ann. Inst. Pasteur (Paris) *58:* 326–340.

Winogradsky, S. 1887. Über Schwefelbakterien. Bot. Z. *45:* 489–610.

Winogradsky, S. 1888. Über Eisenbakterien. Bot. Z. *46:* 261–270.

Winogradsky, S. 1888. Beiträge zur Morphologie und Physiologie der Bakterien. Heft 1. Zur Morphologie und Physiologie der Schwefelbakterien. Arthur Felix, Leipzig, pp. 1–120.

Winogradsky, S. 1890a. Recherches sur les organismes de la nitrification. Ann. Inst. Pasteur (Paris) *4:* 257–275.

Winogradsky, S. 1890b. Sur les organismes de la nitrification. C. R. Acad. Sci. (Paris) *110:* 1013–1016.

Winogradsky, S. 1891. Recherches sur les organismes de la nitrification. Ann. Inst. Pasteur (Paris) *5:* 577–616.

Winogradsky, S. 1892. Contributions a la morphologie des organismes de la nitrification. Arch. Sci. Biol. (St. Petersb.) *1:* 86–137.

Winogradsky, S. 1904. Die Nitrifikation. *In* Handbuch der technischen Mykologie. Lafar, Jena, pp. 132–181.

Winogradsky, S. 1922. Eisenbakterien als Anorgoxydanten. Zentralbl. Bakteriol. Parasitenkd. Infektionskr. Hyg. Abt. II *57:* 1–21.

Winogradsky, S. 1929. Études sur la microbiologie du sol. Sur la dégradation de la cellulose dans le sol. Ann. Inst. Pasteur (Paris) *43:* 549–633.

Winogradsky, S. 1930. Microbes de la nitrification. Travaux récents. Bull. Inst. Pasteur (Paris) *28:* 683–687.

Winogradsky, S. 1931. Nouvelles recherches sur les microbes de la nitrification. C. R. Acad. Sci. *192:* 1000–1004.

Winogradsky, S. 1935. Travaux récents sur la nitrification. Revue critique. Bull. Inst. Pasteur (Paris) *33:* 1073–1079.

Winogradsky, S. and H. Winogradsky. 1933. Études sur la microbiologie du sol.

VII. Nouvelles recherches sur les organismes de la nitrification. Ann. Inst. Pasteur (Paris) 50: 350–432.

Winslow, C.E.A., J. Broadhurst, R.E. Buchanan, C. Krumwiede, Jr., L.A. Rogers and G.H. Smith. 1917. The families and genera of the bacteria. Preliminary report of the Committee of the Society of American Bacteriologists on characterization and classification of bacterial types. J. Bacteriol. 2: 505–566.

Winslow, C.E.A. and A. Winslow. 1908. The Systematic Relationships of the Coccaceae. John Wiley and Sons, New York, pp. 1–300.

Winter, J. and C. Lerp. 1985. In Validation of the publication of new names and new combinations previously effectively published outside the IJSB. Int. J. Syst. Bacteriol. 35: 223–225.

Winter, J., C. Lerp, H.-P. Zabel, F.X. Wildenauer, H. König and F. Schindler. 1984. Methanobacterium wolfei, sp. nov., a new tungsten-requiring, thermophilic, autotrophic methanogen. Syst. Appl. Microbiol. 5: 457–466.

Wireman, J.W. and M. Dworkin. 1975. Morphogenesis and developmental interactions in myxobacteria. Science 189: 516–523.

Wirsen, C.O. and H.W. Jannasch. 1978. Physiological and morphological observations on Thiovulum sp. J. Bacteriol. 136: 765–774.

Withers, N., W. Vidaver and R.A. Lewin. 1978. Pigment composition, photosynthesis and fine structure of a non-blue-green prokaryotic algal symbiont (Prochloron sp.) in a didemnid ascidian from Hawaiian waters. Phycologia 17: 167–171.

Woese, C.R. 1981. Archaebacteria. Sci. Am. 244: 98–122.

Woese, C.R. 1987. Bacterial evolution. Microbiol. Rev. 51: 221–271.

Woese, C.R. and G.E. Fox. 1977a. Phylogenetic structure of the prokaryote domain: the primary kingdom. Proc. Natl. Acad. Sci. U.S.A. 74: 5088–5090.

Woese, C.R. and G.E. Fox. 1977b. The concept of cellular evolution. J. Mol. Evol. 10: 1–6.

Woese, C.R., G.E. Fox, L. Zablen, T. Uchida, L. Bonen, K. Pechman, B.J. Lewis and D. Stahl. 1975. Conservation of primary structure in 16s ribosomal RNA. Nature (London) 254: 83–86.

Woese, C.R., R. Gupta, C.M. Hahn, W. Zillig and J. Tu. 1984. The phylogenetic relationships of three sulfur-dependent archaebacteria. Syst. Appl. Microbiol. 5: 97–105.

Woese, C.R., L.J. Magrum and G.E. Fox. 1978. Archaebacteria. J. Mol. Evol. 11: 245–252.

Woese, C.R., J. Maniloff and L.B. Zablen. 1980. Phylogenetic analysis of the mycoplasmas. Proc. Natl. Acad. Sci. U.S.A. 77: 494–498.

Woese, C.R. and G.J. Olsen. 1986. Archaebacterial phylogeny: perspectives on the urkingdoms. Syst. Appl. Microbiol. 7: 161–177.

Woese, C.R., E. Stackebrandt, T.J. Macke and G.E. Fox. 1985b. A phylogenetic definition of the major eubacterial taxa. Syst. Appl. Microbiol. 6: 143–151.

Woese, C.R., E. Stackebrandt, W.G. Weisburg, B.J. Paster, M.T. Madigan, V.J. Fowler, C.M. Hahn, P. Blanz, R. Gupta, K.H. Nealson and G.E. Fox. 1984a. The phylogeny of purple bacteria: the alpha subdivision. Syst. Appl. Microbiol. 5: 315–326.

Woese, C.R., W.G. Weisburg, C.M. Hahn, B.J. Paster, L.B. Zablen, B.J. Lewis, T.J. Macke, W. Ludwig and E. Stackebrandt. 1985a. The phylogeny of purple bacteria: the gamma subdivision. Syst. Appl. Microbiol. 6: 25–33.

Woese, C.R., W.G. Weisburg, B.J. Paster, C.M. Hahn, R.S. Tanner, N.R. Krieg, H.-P. Koops, H. Harms and E. Stackebrandt. 1984b. The phylogeny of purple bacteria: the beta subdivision. Syst. Appl. Microbiol. 5: 327–336.

Wolfe, R.S. 1960. Observations and studies of Crenothrix polyspora. J. Am. Water Works Assoc. 52: 915–918.

Wolff, E.K., R.A. Bogolmoni, P.S. Scherrer, B. Hess and W. Stoeckenius. 1986. Color dissemination in halobacteria: spectroscopic characterization of a secondary sensory receptor covering the blue-green region of the spectrum. Proc. Natl. Acad. Sci. U.S.A. 83: 7272–7276.

Wolk, C.P. 1980. Cyanobacteria (blue-green algae). In Tolbert (Editor), The Biochemistry of Plants, Vol. 1: The Plant Cell. Academic Press, New York, pp. 659–686.

Wolk, C.P. 1982. Heterocysts. In Carr and Whitton (Editors), The Biology of Cyanobacteria. Blackwell, Oxford, and University of California Press, Berkeley, pp. 359–386.

Wolkin, R.H. and J.L. Pate. 1984. Translocation of motile cells of the gliding bacterium Cytophaga johnsonae depends on a surface component that may be modified by sugars. J. Gen. Microbiol. 130: 2651–2669.

Wood, A.P. and D.P. Kelly. 1977. Heterotrophic growth of Thiobacillus A2 on sugars and organic acids. Arch. Microbiol. 113: 257–264.

Wood, A.P. and D.P. Kelly. 1978. Comparative radiorespirometric studies of glucose oxidation in three facultatively heterotrophic thiobacilli. FEMS Microbiol. Lett. 4: 283–286.

Wood, A.P. and D.P. Kelly. 1983. Use of carboxylic acids by Thiobacillus A2. Microbios 38: 15–25.

Wood, A.P. and D.P. Kelly. 1984. Growth and sugar metabolism of a thermoacidophilic iron-oxidizing mixotrophic bacterium. J. Gen. Microbiol. 130: 1337–1349.

Wood, A.P. and D.P. Kelly. 1985. Physiological characteristics of a new thermophilic obligately chemolithotrophic Thiobacillus species, Thiobacillus tepidarius. Int. J. Syst. Bacteriol. 35: 434–437.

Wood, A.P., D.P. Kelly and P.R. Norris. 1987. Autotrophic growth of four Sulfolobus strains on tetrathionate and the effect of organic nutrients. Arch. Microbiol. 146: 382–389.

Wood, H.C. 1869. Proc. Am. Philosoph. Soc. Philadelphia II.

Wood, P., A. Peat and B.A. Whitton. 1986. Influence of phosphorus status on fine structure of the cyanobacterium (blue-green alga) Calothrix parietina. Cytobios 47: 89–99.

Worakit, S., D.R. Boone, R.A. Mah, M.-E. Abdel-Samie and M.M. El-Halwagi. 1986. Methanobacterium alcaliphilum sp. nov., an H₂-utilizing methanogen that grows at high pH values. Int. J. Syst. Bacteriol. 36: 380–382.

Woronichin, N.N. 1927. Materiali k agologitscheskoj flore i rastitjelnosti mineralnich istoschnikov gruppi Kaukaskich mineralnich Wod. Trav. Inst. Balneol aux Eaux Miner du Caucase 5: 90–91.

Wullenweber, M., H.-P. Koops and H. Harms. 1977. Polyhedral inclusion bodies in cells of Nitrosomonas spec. Arch. Microbiol. 112: 69–72.

Yabuuchi, E., T. Kaneko, I. Yano, C.W. Moss and N. Miyoshi. 1983. Sphingobacterium, new genus, Sphingobacterium spiritovorum, new combination, Sphingobacterium multivorum, new combination, Sphingobacterium mizutae, new species and Flavobacterium indologenes, new species: glucose non-fermenting Gram-negative rods in CDC groups IIk-2 and IIb. Int. J. Syst. Bacteriol. 33: 580–598.

Yabuuchi, E. and C.W. Moss. 1982. Cellular fatty acid composition of strains of three species of Sphingobacterium gen. nov. and Cytophaga johnsonae. FEMS Microbiol. Lett. 13: 87–91.

Yabuuchi, E., I. Yano, T. Kaneko and A. Ohyama. 1981. Classification of group IIk-2 and related bacteria. In Reichenbach and Weeks (Editors), The Flavobacterium-Cytophaga Group. Verlag Chemie, Weinheim, F.R.G., pp. 79–90.

Yamada, Y., G. Inouye, Y. Tahara and K. Kondo. 1976. The menaquinone system in the classification of coryneform and nocardioform bacteria and related organisms. J. Gen. Appl. Microbiol. 22: 203–214.

Yamanaka, T. and M. Shinra. 1974. Cytochrome C-552 and cytochrome C-554 derived from Nitrosomonas europaea. Purification, properties and their function in hydroxylamine oxidation. J. Biochem. 75: 1265–1273.

Yamazaki, S. 1982. A selenium-containing hydrogenase from Methanococcus vannielii. J. Biol. Chem. 257: 7926–7929.

Yamazaki, S. and L. Tsai. 1980. Purification and properties of 8-hydroxy-5-deazaflavin-dependent NADP⁺ reductase from Methanococcus vannielii. J. Biol. Chem. 255: 6462–6465.

Yamazaki, S., L. Tsai and T.C. Stadtman. 1982. Analogues of 8-hydroxy-5-deazaflavin cofactor: relative activity as substrates for 8-hydroxy-5-deazaflavin-dependent NADP⁺ reductase from Methanococcus vannielii. Biochemistry 21: 934–939.

Yamazaki, S., L. Tsai, T.C. Stadtman, F.S. Jacobson and C. Walsh. 1980. Stereochemical studies of 8-hydroxy-5-deazaflavin-dependent NADP⁺ reductase from Methanococcus vannielii. J. Biol. Chem. 255: 9025–9027.

Yang, D., B.P. Kaine and C.R. Woese. 1985. The phylogeny of archaebacteria. Syst. Appl. Microbiol. 6: 251–256.

Yang, L.L. and A. Haug. 1979. Purification and partial characterization of a procaryotic glycoprotein from the plasma membrane of Thermoplasma acidophilum. Biochim. Biophys. Acta 556: 265–277.

Yano, I., S. Imaizumi, I. Tomiyasu and E. Yabuuchi. 1983. Separation and analysis of free ceramides containing 2-hydroxy fatty acids in Sphingobacterium species. FEMS Microbiol. Lett. 20: 449–453.

Yee, T. and M. Inouye. 1981. Reexamination of the genome size of myxobacteria, including the use of a new method for genome size analysis. J. Bacteriol. 145: 1257–1265.

Yen, H.-C. and B. Marrs. 1977. Growth of Rhodopseudomonas capsulata under anaerobic dark conditions with dimethyl sulfoxide. Arch. Biochem. Biophys. 181: 411–418.

Yoch, D.C. 1978. Nitrogen fixation and hydrogen metabolism by photosynthetic bacteria. In Clayton and Sistrom (Editors), The Photosynthetic Bacteria. Plenum Press, New York and London, pp. 657–676.

Yopp, J.H., D.R. Tindall, D.M. Miller and W.E. Schmid. 1978. Isolation, purification and evidence of the obligate halophilic nature of the blue-green alga Aphanothece halophytica Frémy (Chroococcales). Phycologia 17: 172–177.

Yoshimizu, M. and T. Kimura. 1983. Bacteriological study on lake as ambient water for fish III. Microflora of lake group Onuma (Onuma, Konuma and Junsainuma), 1976–1978. Bull. Fac. Fish. Hokkaido Univ. 34: 361–369 (in Japanese with English summary).

Zabel, H.P., H. König and J. Winter. 1984. Isolation and characterization of a new coccoid methanogen, Methanogenium tatii spec. nov. from a solfataric field on Mount Tatio. Arch. Microbiol. 137: 308–315.

Zabel, H.P., H. König and J. Winter. 1985. Emended description of Methanogenium thermophilicum, Rivard and Smith, and assignment of new isolates to this species. Syst. Appl. Microbiol. 6: 72–78.

Zabel, H.P., H. König and J. Winter. 1986. In Validation of the publication of new names and new combinations previously effectively published outside the IJSB. List No. 20. Int. J. Syst. Bacteriol. 36: 354–356.

Zahler, S.A. and H.D. McCurdy. 1974. Genus Myxococcus. In Buchanan and Gibbons (Editors), Bergey's Manual of Determinative Bacteriology, 8th Ed. The Williams and Wilkins Co., Baltimore, pp. 79–83.

Zanardini, J. 1858. Plantarum in mari rubro hucusque collectarum enumeratio. Memorie del Reale Istituto Veneto 7: 89.

Zanardini, J. 1872. Phycearum indicarum pugillus. Memorie del Reale Istituto Veneto 17: 32–33.

Zavarzin, G.A. 1961. Symbiotic culture of the new manganese-oxidizing microorganism. Mikrobiologiya *30:* 393–395.

Zavarzin, G.A. 1961a. The life cycle and nuclear apparatus in *Hyphomicrobium vulgare* Stutzer and Hartleb. Mikrobiologiya *29:* 38–42 (English translation: 24–27).

Zavarzin, G.A. 1961b. Budding bacteria. Mikrobiologiya *30:* 952–975 (English translation: 774–791).

Zavarzin, G.A. 1962. Symbiotic oxidation of manganese by two species of *Pseudomonas*. Mikrobiologia *31:* 586–588.

Zavarzin, G.A. 1964a. Structure of *Metallogenium*. Mikrobiologiya *32:* 1020–1023.

Zavarzin, G.A. 1964b. *Metallogenium symbioticum*. Z. Allg. Mikrobiol. *4:* 390–395.

Zavarzin, G.A. 1965. Chemoautotrophic Microorganisms. Author's Abstract of Dissertation (in Russian). Inst. Mikrobiol. Akad. Nauk S.S.S.R.

Zavarzin, G.A. 1970. The notion of microflora of dispersion in the carbon cycle. J. Gen. Biol. Akad. Nauk S.S.S.R. *31:* 386–393.

Zavarzin, G.A. 1972. Lithotrophic Microorganisms. Moscow, Nauka.

Zavarzin, G.A. 1972. A heterotrophic satellite of *Thiobacillus ferrooxidans*. Microbiology (English translation) *41:* 323–324.

Zavarzin, G.A. 1974. Genus IV. *Siderococcus* Dorff 1934, 9. *In* Buchanan and Gibbons (Editors), Bergey's Manual of Determinative Bacteriology, 8th Ed. The Williams and Wilkins Co., Baltimore, p. 468.

Zavarzin, G.A. 1981. The genus *Metallogenium*. *In* Starr, Stolp, Trüper, Balows and Schlegel (Editors), The Prokaryotes. A Handbook on Habitats, Isolation, and Identification of Bacteria. Springer-Verlag, Berlin, pp. 524–528.

Zehnder, A. 1985. Isolation and cultivation of large cyanophytes for taxonomic purposes. Arch. Hydrobiol. Suppl. *71:* 281–289.

Zehnder, A.J.B., B.A. Huser, T.D. Brock and K. Wuhrmann. 1980. Characterization of an acetate-decarboxylating, nonhydrogenoxidizing methane bacterium. Arch. Microbiol. *124:* 1–11.

Zehnder, A.J.B. and K. Wuhrmann. 1977. Physiology of a *Methanobacterium* strain AZ. Arch. Microbiol. *111:* 199–205.

Zeikus, J.G., A. Ben-Bassat and P.W. Hegge. 1980. Microbiology of methanogenesis in thermal, volcanic environments. J. Bacteriol. *143:* 432–440.

Zeikus, J.G. and V.G. Bowen. 1975a. Comparative ultrastructure of methanogenic bacteria. Can. J. Microbiol. *21:* 121–129.

Zeikus, J.G. and V.G. Bowen. 1975b. Fine structure of *Methanospirillum hungatii*. J. Bacteriol. *121:* 373–380.

Zeikus, J.G. and D.L. Henning. 1975. *Methanobacterium arboriphilicum* sp. nov., an obligate anaerobe isolated from wetwood of living trees. Antonie van Leeuwenhoek J. Microbiol. Serol. *41:* 543–552.

Zeikus, J.G. and M.R. Winfrey. 1976. Temperature limitation of methanogenesis in aquatic sediments. Appl. Environ. Microbiol. *31:* 99–107.

Zeikus, J.G. and R.S. Wolfe. 1972. *Methanobacterium thermoautotrophicus* sp. n., an anaerobic, autotrophic, extreme thermophile. J. Bacteriol. *109:* 707–713.

Zeikus, J.G. and R.S. Wolfe. 1973. Fine structure of *Methanobacterium thermoautotrophicum*: effect of growth temperature on morphology and ultrastructure. J. Bacteriol. *113:* 461–467.

Zeph, L.R. 1985. Indirect phage analysis studies of the activity of nonobligate predator bacteria in soil. Ph.D. thesis, The Pennsylvania State University, University Park, Pennsylvania.

Zhao, Y., H. Zhang, D.R. Boone and R.A. Mah. 1986. Isolation and characterization of a fast-growing, thermophilic *Methanobacterium* species. Appl. Environ. Microbiol. *52:* 1227–1229.

Zhilina, T.N. 1971. The fine structure of methanosarcina. Microbiology (English translation) *40:* 587–591.

Zhilina, T.N. 1976. Biotypes of *Methanosarcina*. Microbiology (English translation) *45:* 414–421.

Zhilina, T.N. 1978. Growth of a pure *Methanosarcina* culture, biotype 2, on acetate. Microbiology (English translation) *47:* 321–323.

Zhilina, T.N. 1983. New obligate halophilic methane-producing bacterium. Microbiology (English translation) *52:* 290–297.

Zhilina, T.N. 1984. *In* Validation of the publication of new names and new combinations previously effectively published outside the IJSB. List No. 14. Int. J. Syst. Bacteriol. *34:* 270–271.

Zhilina, T.N. 1984. A new obligate halophilic methane-producing bacterium. Mikrobiologiya (English translation) *52:* 375–383.

Zhilina, T.N. 1986. Methanogenic bacteria from hypersaline environments. Syst. Appl. Microbiol. *7:* 216–222.

Zhilina, T.N. and S.A. Ilarionov. 1984. Isolation and comparative characteristics of methanogenic bacteria assimilating formate with the description of *Methanobacterium thermoformicicum* sp. nov. Mikrobiologiya *53:* 785–790.

Zhilina, T.N. and S.A. Ilarionova. 1986. *In* Validation of the publication of new names and new combinations previously effectively published outside the IJSB. List No. 21. Int. J. Syst. Bacteriol. *36:* 489.

Zhilina, T.N. and G.A. Zavarzin. 1979a. Comparative cytology of methanosarcinae and description of *Methanosarcina vacuolata* sp. nov. Microbiology (English translation) *48:* 223–228.

Zhilina, T.N. and G.A. Zavarzin. 1979b. Cyst formation by *Methanosarcina*. Microbiology (English translation) *48:* 349–354.

Zhilina, T.N. and G.A. Zavarzin. 1987. *Methanosarcina vacuolata* sp. nov., a vacuolated methanosarcina. Int. J. Syst. Bacteriol. *37:* 281–283.

Zillig, W. 1983. *In* Validation of the publication of new names and new combinations previously effectively published outside the IJSB. List No. 11. Int. J. Syst. Bacteriol. *33:* 672–674.

Zillig, W. 1988. *In* Validation of the publication of new names and new combinations previously effectively published outside the IJSB. List No. 24. Int. J. Syst. Bacteriol. *38:* 136–137.

Zillig, W. and A. Böck. 1987. *In* Validation of the publication of new names and new combinations previously effectively published outside the IJSB. List No. 23. Int. J. Syst. Bacteriol. *37:* 179–180.

Zillig, W. and A. Gierl. 1983. *In* Validation of the publication of new names and new combinations previously effectively published outside the IJSB. List No. 11. Int. J. Syst. Bacteriol. *33:* 672–674.

Zillig, W., A. Gierl, G. Schreiber, S. Wunderl, D. Janekovic, K.O. Stetter and H.P. Klenk. 1983a. The archaebacterium *Thermofilum pendens* represents a novel genus of the thermophilic, anaerobic sulfur respiring *Thermoproteales*. Syst. Appl. Microbiol. *4:* 79–87.

Zillig, W., F. Gropp, A. Henschen, H. Neumann, P. Palm, W.-D. Reiter, M. Rettenberger, H. Schnabel and S. Yeats. 1986. Archaebacterial virus host systems. Syst. Appl. Microbiol. *7:* 58–66.

Zillig, W., I. Holz, D. Janekovic, W. Schäfer and W.D. Reiter. 1983b. The archaebacterium *Thermococcus celer* represents a novel genus within the thermophilic branch of the archaebacteria. Syst. Appl. Microbiol. *4:* 88–94.

Zillig, W., I. Holz, H.-P. Klenk, J. Trent, S. Wunderl, D. Janekovic, E. Imsel and B. Haas. 1987. *Pyrococcus woesei*, sp. nov., an ultra-thermophilic marine archaebacterium, representing a novel order, *Thermococcales*. Syst. Appl. Microbiol. *9:* 62–70.

Zillig, W., R. Schnabel and K.O. Stetter. 1985. Archaebacteria and the origin of the eukaryotic cytoplasm. Curr. Top. Microbiol. Immunol. *114:* pp. 1–18.

Zillig, W. and K.O. Stetter. 1982. *In* Validation of the publication of new names and new combinations previously effectively published outside the IJSB. List No. 8. Int. J. Syst. Bacteriol. *32:* 266–268.

Zillig, W. and K.O. Stetter. 1983. *In* Validation of the publication of new names and new combinations previously effectively published outside the IJSB. List No. 10. Int. J. Syst. Bacteriol. *33:* 438–440.

Zillig, W., K.O. Stetter, D. Prangishvilli, W. Schäfer, S. Wunderl, D. Janekovic, I. Holz and P. Palm. 1982. *Desulfurococcaceae*, the second family of the extremely thermophilic, anaerobic, sulfur-respiring *Thermoproteales*. Zentralbl. Bakteriol. Mikrobiol. Hyg. I Abt. Orig. *C3:* 304–317.

Zillig, W., K.O. Stetter, W. Schäfer, D. Janekovic, S. Wunderl, I. Holz and P. Palm. 1981. *Thermoproteales*: novel type of extremely thermoacidophilic, anaerobic archaebacteria isolated from Icelandic solfataras. Zentralbl. Bakteriol. Mikrobiol. Hyg. I Abt. Orig. *C2:* 205–227.

Zillig, W., K.O. Stetter, S. Wunderl, W. Schultz, H. Priess and I. Scholz. 1980a. The *Sulfolobus*-"Caldariella" group: taxonomy on the basis of the structure of DNA-dependent RNA-polymerase. Arch. Microbiol. *125:* 259–269.

Zillig, W., K.O. Stetter, S. Wunderl, W. Schultz, H. Priess and I. Scholz. 1980b. *In* Validation of the publication of new names and new combinations previously effectively published outside the IJSB. List No. 5. Int. J. Syst. Bacteriol. *30:* 676–677.

Zillig, W., S. Yeates, I. Holz, A. Böck, F. Gropp, M. Rettenberger and S. Lutz. 1985. Plasmid-related anaerobic autotrophy of the novel archaebacterium *Sulfolobus ambivalens*. Nature *313:* 789–791.

Zillig, W., S. Yeates, I. Holz, A. Böck, M. Rettenberger, F. Gropp and G. Simon. 1986. *Desulfurolobus ambivalens*, sp. nov. gen. nov., an autotrophic archaebacterium facultatively oxidizing or reducing sulfur. Syst. Appl. Microbiol. *8:* 197–203.

Zinder, S.H., S.C. Cardwell and T. Anguish. 1984a. Effects of temperature on methanogenesis in a thermophilic (58°C) anaerobic digestor. Appl. Environ. Microbiol. *47:* 808–813.

Zinder, S.H., S.C. Cardwell, T. Anguish, M. Lee and M. Koch. 1984b. Methanogenesis in a thermophilic (58°C) anaerobic digestor: *Methanothrix* sp. as an important aceticlastic methanogen. Appl. Environ. Microbiol. *47:* 796–807.

Zinder, S.H. and M. Koch. 1984. Non-aceticlastic methanogenesis from acetate: acetate oxidation by a thermophilic syntrophic coculture. Arch. Microbiol. *138:* 263–272.

Zinder, S.H. and R.A. Mah. 1979. Isolation and characterization of a thermophilic strain of *Methanosarcina* unable to use H_2-CO_2 for methanogenesis. Appl. Environ. Microbiol. *38:* 996–1008.

Zinder, S.H., K.R. Sowers and J.G. Ferry. 1985. *Methanosarcina thermophila* sp. nov., a thermophilic, acetotrophic methane-producing bacterium. Int. J. Syst. Bacteriol. *35:* 522–523.

Zobell, C.E. 1941. Studies on marine bacteria. I. The cultural requirements of heterotrophic aerobes. J. Mar. Res. *4:* 42–75.

ZoBell, C.E. and H.C. Upham. 1944. A list of marine bacteria including descriptions of sixty new species. Bull. Scripps Inst. Oceanogr. Univ. Calif. (Techn. Series) *5:* 239–292.

Zuckerkandl, E. and L. Pauling. 1965. Molecules as documents of evolutionary history. J. Theor. Biol. *8:* 357–366.

Zumpft, W.G. and F. Castillo. 1978. Regulatory properties of the nitrogenase from *Rhodopseudomonas palustris*. Arch. Microbiol. *117:* 53–60.

Zusman, D.R., D.M. Krotoski and M. Cumsky. 1978. Chromosome replication in *Myxococcus xanthus*. J. Bacteriol. *133:* 122–129.

Index of Scientific Names of Bacteria

Key to the fonts and symbols used in this index:

Nomenclature
    Lower case, Roman:

Genera, species, and subspecies of bacteria. Every bacterial name mentioned in the *Manual* is listed in the "Index." Specific epithets are listed individually and also under the genus.*

CAPITALS, ROMAN:

Names of taxa higher than genus (tribes, families, orders, classes, divisions, kingdoms).

Pagination
    Roman:

Pages on which taxa are mentioned.

Boldface:

Indicates page on which the description of a taxon is given.†

---

*Infrasubspecific names, such as serovars, biovars, and pathovars, are not listed in the "Index."
†A description may not necessarily be given in the *Manual* for a taxon that is considered as *incertae sedis* or that is listed in an addendum or note added in proof; however, the page on which the complete citation of such a taxon is given is indicated in boldface type.

Index of Scientific Names of Bacteria